Fisher's Contact Dermatitis

Fifth Edition

Fisher's Contact Dermatitis

Fifth Edition

Robert L. Rietschel

Chairman, Department of Dermatology
Oschner Clinic
New Orleans, Louisiana

Clinical Professor of Dermatology
Tulane University Medical Center
and Clinical Associate Professor of Dermatology
Louisiana State University School of Medicine
New Orleans, Louisiana

Joseph F. Fowler, Jr.

Associate Clinical Professor of Dermatology
University of Louisville School of Medicine
Louisville, Kentucky

LIPPINCOTT WILLIAMS & WILKINS
A **Wolters Kluwer** Company

Philadelphia · Baltimore · New York · London
Buenos Aires · Hong Kong · Sydney · Tokyo

Acquisitions Editor: Beth Barry
Developmental Editor: Sarah Fitz-Hugh
Supervising Editor: Mary Ann McLaughlin
Manufacturing Manager: Benjamin Rivera
Production Editor: Janet Domingo, Compset, Inc.
Cover Designer: Mark Lerner
Compositor: Compset, Inc.
Printer: Edwards Brothers

Library of Congress Cataloging-in-Publication Data

Fisher's contact dermatitis.—5th ed. / [edited by] Robert L. Rietschel, Joseph F. Fowler, Jr.
    p. ; cm.
   Includes bibliographical references and index.
   ISBN 0-7817-2252-7 (hardcover)
    1. Contact dermatitis. I. Title: Contact dermatitis. II. Rietschel, Robert L. III. Fowler,
Joseph F. IV. Fisher, Alexander A., 1905– Contact dermatitis.
   [DNLM: 1. Dermatitis, Contact. WR 175 F537 2000]
   RL244.F56 2000
   616.97′3—dc21
                                          00-045339

10 9 8 7 6 5 4 3 2 1

To Alex and his inspiration, Lillian
To Connie, Eric, and Penny
To Lynn

Contents

Preface to the Fifth Edition

In preparing this edition, we continue to stand on a giant's shoulders. Alexander Fisher solo authored the first two editions of this book. For the third edition, he asked a few friends to contribute, but the work was overwhelmingly his. For the fourth edition, we tried to maintain as much of Dr. Fisher's work as possible. We wanted to continue the cohesiveness that comes from a limited number of contributors. We have done much the same for the fifth edition. As much as possible, this is still Dr. Fisher's book. He provided information for the profession that had been shared privately in the **Contact Dermatitis Newsletter.** This source was not available to the dermatological community, but the references he made to this valuable information brought these insights into the open literature. The citations he made to that body of work remain in this edition unless newer information invalidates the findings. At the age of 95, Alexander Fisher continues to critique and compliment us on our efforts to keep his book contemporary.

We recognize that this text is used worldwide. We have endeavored to include information from the world literature that reflects this readership. Contact dermatitis due to grasses in Singapore, poison ivy-like plants in South America, and topical anti-fungals sold in Japan, but not the United States, are included in this volume.

For this edition we have expanded the patient education section. There are more allergens for which we have given sample instructions. These are slanted toward a United States audience and take advantage of our labeling laws. We have also pooled the treatment sections of the fourth edition into a new chapter on treatment. Additional treatment literature has been added to this body of work.

In this Internet age, it is impossible for a text of this nature to capture every reported case of contact dermatitis. A computer search will turn up items that we may have omitted. But this work puts the reports in a context that the Internet cannot. We have attempted to be encyclopedic in our approach. This may make this edition intimidating in size, but we hope it will be found readable, comprehensive, and a credit to Dr. Fisher.

Robert L. Rietschel, MD
Joseph F. Fowler, Jr., MD

CHAPTER 1

The Pathogenesis of Allergic Contact Hypersensitivity

Jadassohn (1), who described contact allergy to mercury in 1895, can be considered the "father" of contact dermatitis. Prior to this time, and indeed for some years thereafter, contact hypersensitivity was essentially unknown except by a few workers in dermatology (2–5). In 1927, Landsteiner (6) published studies regarding antigens containing "simple chemical compounds." Sulzberger (7), in 1929, published one of the earliest American works on the subject.

Another important development was the recognition that a close similarity existed between contact allergy and delayed-type hypersensitivity to microbial antigens, after Landsteiner and Chase published their findings that both contact allergy to small molecular allergens and delayed-type hypersensitivity to microbial antigens could be passively transferred with lymphocytes in guinea pigs (8,9). As a matter of fact, this finding precipitated an era in which many investigators considered contact allergy and microbial allergy to be based on identical mechanisms. Despite many important fundamental similarities, however, certain differences were always evident between these forms of allergy (10,11).

Teleologically, one assumes that cell-mediated hypersensitivity serves the purpose of defending the body against foreign antigens, like those derived from bacteria, fungi, viruses, and foreign tissues, and against autologous tumor antigens and other undesirable autologous antigens. However, although cell-mediated hypersensitivity to these antigens in general helps to preserve the body's integrity, allergic-contact hypersensitivity to small molecular allergens (which, indeed, is hypersensitivity to autologous proteins made "foreign" by complexing with small molecular compounds) is damaging to the skin. In a sense, therefore, contact allergy can be considered a deviant form of cell-mediated hypersensitivity.

OVERVIEW

Contact allergens almost invariably are small-molecule substances of less than 500 daltons (Da) (12). Because of their small size, they penetrate the skin barrier, which is rel-atively impermeable under normal circumstances to large molecules, and reach the living layers of the skin. In order to induce contact allergy, these substances must be presented by antigen-presenting cells, principally epidermal Langerhans cells (LCs), and other dendritic cells, to T lymphocytes in an immunologically effective "processed" form. The effector cells, which mediate allergic contact hypersensitivity, are descendants of these T lymphocytes.

In order to interact with antigen presented by the LCs in the course of both induction of hypersensitivity and elicitation of a reaction, the T lymphocytes must possess surface receptors ("idiotypes") that are complementary to the physicochemical features of that antigen. Furthermore, the antigen-presenting cells must bear immune response–associated antigens for which the T lymphocytes possess receptors. The T lymphocytes must also be activated by interleukin-1 (IL-1), which is released from LCs and keratinocytes.

Under ordinary conditions, exposure to contact allergens sets in motion two competing mechanisms, the one mediated by effector T lymphocytes and leading to a state of hypersensitivity that becomes clinically manifest as an eczematous skin reaction. The other is mediated by suppressor cells and leads to relative or complete tolerance of the allergen. The state of reactivity of the skin at any particular time and site is principally the result of the existing balance between the effector and the suppressor cells present.

CONTACT ALLERGENS

Normally, only small molecular compounds (<500 Da) can penetrate through the horny layer into the living layers of the epidermis. Yet, in order to induce and elicit contact allergy, an antigen with a molecular weight of at least 5,000 Da is required. Antigenicity is accomplished by the conjugation of small molecules with autologous proteins present in the skin. Other requirements for antigenicity are the appropriate number of antigenic determinants and the appropriate tertiary structural features in the resulting molecule. Sensitization is more easily induced when the skin barrier is compromised by dermatitis or ulceration.

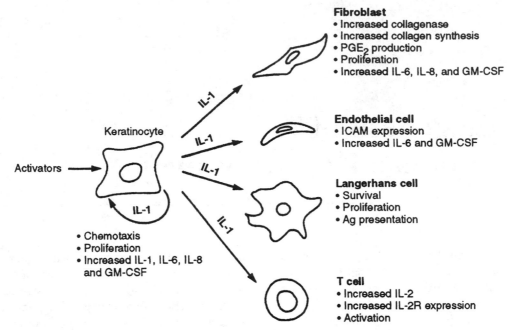

FIG. 1.1 A diagrammatic representation of the mechanism of allergic contact dermatitis.

It was thought originally that such conjugates were formed with the fibrous proteins of prokeratins, keratins, procollagens and collagens, epidermal cell membranes, or soluble tissue, and serum proteins. Although a role for these conjugates cannot be dismissed, it now appears that conjugation takes place mainly with cell membrane proteins in the course of "processing" by the antigen-presenting LCs.

Linkage to the protein moiety is frequently covalent; for example, the epsilon-amino group of lysine and the sulfhydryl groups of cystine and cysteine have been suggested as binding sites for certain allergens. In many instances, however, it is difficult to predict the sensitizing capacity of a substance on the basis of its chemical structure. In the past it has not been adequately emphasized that some of the most common contact allergens, like nickel, chromates, and other metal salts, do not form covalent bonds with proteins; the fact that they can combine in some form with components of LCs provides a reasonable explanation for their allergenicity (13). Current research suggests that a "successful" contact allergen causes an increase in the size of LCs along with an increase of Ia (major histocompatibility complex) molecules on the LC surfaces. In addition, the allergen may induce LC migration to lymph nodes (14).

Genetic Factors

Susceptibility to the development of contact sensitivity is genetically controlled. The mode of inheritance in guinea pigs is autosomal and irregularly dominant (15). Different strains of guinea pigs can make an immune response to dif-

ferent contact allergens. For example, one strain responds to potassium dichromate and beryllium fluoride, but not to mercuric chloride, whereas another strain makes a response to mercuric chloride but responds poorly to potassium dichromate and beryllium fluoride (16). These differences apparently relate to different hapten–amino acid linkages.

Other studies have shown that ultraviolet-B (UVB) exposure inhibits contact sensitivity in certain strains of mice, but not in other genetically distinct strains (17,18). It has been postulated that tumor necrosis factor-α (TNF-α) may be an important mediator of these effects (19).

Studies of the mode of inheritance in humans are still inadequate, but the very limited available data suggest that here also genetic factors control susceptibility to sensitization to particular allergens (20). A number of European studies have compared the frequency of human leucocyte antigens (HLA) antigens in patients with allergic contact dermatitis (ACD), usually to nickel, with local controls (21–23). Several studies have purported to show increased occurrence of one or two HLA types in patients, but for reasons that are obscure, no two studies have found the same HLA antigen to be increased in a statistically significant fashion. Among the antigens reported to be increased to some degree are HLA-B7, -B21, -B12, -Bw22, -B35, -B40, -DR4, and -DRw6. Because the expression of the HLA antigen system is essential for the development of ACD, it is tempting to search for HLA-ACD associations.

Gene products of the TAP-1 and TAP-2 genes (transporter associated with antigen processing) are involved in antigen processing. A Finnish study showed that nickel-allergic persons were much more likely to possess the TAP-

2B gene allele and much less likely to be TAP-2C positive than nonallergic subjects (24). This study further supports the likelihood of inborn genetic factors regulating one's ability to develop contact allergy.

Antigen Presentation

It is not possible for T lymphocytes to interact directly with the contact antigen even when they possess the appropriate surface receptors for that antigen. The antigen must first be "processed" and then be presented in suitable form on the surface of LCs (25) that bear immune response–associated surface antigens (HLA-DR in humans; called Ia in mice) for which the T lymphocytes have the specific receptors. To induce contact allergy, the allergen is displayed in close association with these antigens or perhaps becomes conjugated with them (26,27). Random T lymphocytes circulating through the epidermis, dermis, dermal lymphatics, and regional lymph nodes can become apposed to the LCs, but only T lymphocytes, which have the complementary receptors for the contact antigen that is being presented, can become irreversibly apposed.

Langerhans Cells

Epidermal LCs have properties that make them particularly well suited to serve the function of presenting contact allergens. They have a pronounced capacity to bind small molecular compounds, among them well-recognized contact allergens, to their surface (13). Their capacity to do this binding is greater than that of peripheral blood macrophages (28). Similar antigen-presenting cells are found in the spleen and lymph nodes. These and LCs are all derived from bone marrow precursors.

Antigen-processing capacity of LCs involves, first, plasma membrane changes with endocytosis of the antigen and digestion of proteins to active peptides in acidic organelles (29,30). Birbeck granule expression increases at this time, apparently in relation to antigen processing. As processing continues, LC morphology changes to a more dendritic cell type, which is associated with enhanced antigen-presenting capacity.

Experimental proof of the antigen-presenting functions of LCs derives from studies in inbred guinea pigs and mice and from the demonstration in mice that antigen presentation cannot take place in the absence of adequate numbers of functionally intact LCs at sites of exposure to the allergen (31).

Irradiation with UVB or application of a topical corticosteroid reduces the density of LCs in skin and inhibits induction of contact sensitization (14). In vitro cyclosporine A inhibits the antigen-presenting capability of LCs, apparently without affecting cell surface expression of Ia molecules (32).

INDUCTION OF CONTACT ALLERGY

Shortly after contact with an allergen, various cytokines are released that enhance the development of contact sensitivity (33). Interleukin-1B (IL-1B) increases the level of intercellular adhesive molecule (ICAM-1). Other molecules are then expressed on the LC surface, which facilitates interaction with CD4+ T cells.

Within 24 hours of antigen application, LCs migrate to regional lymph nodes. There they present the antigen to compatible T lymphocytes. The T lymphocytes must bear receptors for complementary major histocompatibility complex protein as well as receptors for the contact allergen. Ultrastructural observations indicate that the contact allergens reside on the surfaces of LCs as well as in the intracyctoplasmic Birbeck granules (34). In the lymph nodes, certain T lymphocytes become physically apposed to the LCs facilitating transfer of antigen. These T cells are CD4+ and CD45RA+ and may be referred to as Th-0 cells (35). Other cytokines are important at this stage of sensitization, including IL-6, TGF-B, and IL-12. Lack of IL-12 can prevent development of Th-1 cells, which cause ACD, and therefore may allow development of tolerance to the particular allergen (36). Through clonal proliferation, a subset of T lymphocytes is produced that will be capable of responding to the particular antigen when future exposure occurs. It will be 7 to 10 days before there are sufficient numbers of these specific T lymphocytes to cause contact dermatitis. After that time, elicitation of contact dermatitis, by patch test or routine exposure, is possible.

Effector and Suppressor Cells

As noted previously, exposure of individuals who are genetically susceptible to sensitization to a specific contact allergen sets in motion two competing mechanisms, namely, allergic sensitization mediated by effector cells and specific immunologic tolerance mediated by suppressor cells. In an unsensitized individual, oral or parenteral administration of an antigen can lead to reduced immune reactivity, whereas the same allergen may cause contact sensitization when applied topically (37). The key role played by lymphocytes as the source and carriers of the hypersensitivity in contact allergy was demonstrated by Landsteiner and Chase (9) 60 years ago in experiments on guinea pigs. Peritoneal exudate cells, predominantly lymphocytes, from contact-allergic donor animals, injected intraperitoneally or intravenously into recipient animals that had not previously been sensitized, passively transferred the hypersensitivity. In humans, however, such passive transfer experiments have yielded contradictory results. Both failure and success have been reported with intracutaneous and intravenous passive transfer of sensitized cells (38–42). The immunologic changes, which ensue during the early days following sensitizing exposure, usually have a lasting impact on the outcome of the competition between effector and suppressor lymphocytes.

The state of specific allergic hypersensitivity may last indefinitely. Once established, it is not possible to deliberately alter it, except for transient hyposensitization. Contact hypersensitivity is thought to often wane spontaneously in elderly people. In some patients, the hypersensitivity wanes spontaneously at a much earlier age (at times within a few years) despite continued exposure to the specific contact allergen. As yet no explanation for this finding has been discovered. Contact allergy can develop from earliest infancy to old age, but it is most common in the intermediate age groups.

Suppressor cells decrease the intensity and duration of the reaction and under appropriate circumstances may abolish the capacity to react and induce a state of specific immunologic tolerance. The spleen plays an important role in generating suppressor cells (43). Tolerance, once established, apparently persists indefinitely in humans. In laboratory animals, tolerance can be broken deliberately with cyclophosphamide (44).

Generalization of Contact Sensitivity

Antigen presentation by LCs to T lymphocytes has been thought to take place primarily in the lymph nodes. Whether antigen presentation occurs in the skin also is uncertain (45). In laboratory animals, enlargement of the regional lymph nodes is observed during this period of proliferation. There they undergo further proliferation, which accounts for the production of large numbers of specifically sensitized effector cells and T memory cells. Their descendants enter the collecting sinus of the lymph node and from there are transferred to the blood, which then circulates them to other parts of the lymphoid system (46). This finding explains why all areas of the body's surface almost invariably become hypersensitive to the contact allergen.

Localized Differences in Sensitivity

Contact sensitivity usually involves the entire integument, but it is not unusual to find differences in degree of sensitivity at different skin sites. For example, a greater degree of sensitivity is often present at the site of originally induced sensitization and at other sites of previous exposure to the particular allergen, such as sites at which patch tests had been done (47). The mechanism for this has not yet been elucidated, but one theory is that clones of sensitized cells have established themselves in the dermis during a previous encounter with the allergen. Reexposure to the allergen may then trigger interaction with and proliferation of the clones of specifically sensitized cells at these particular sites, thus creating the increased capability to react.

ELICITATION OF REACTIONS

After sensitization has taken place, reexposure to the specific allergen leads to a series of events that eventually result in the inflammatory response clinically recognized as an eczematous dermatitis. It is characterized histologically by spongiosis and lymphocytes in the epidermis and by lymphocytes, histiocytes, and varying numbers of eosinophils and basophils in the papillary dermis (see Chapter 4). The spongiosis, at least in part, could be due to the destructive effects of hapten-specific cytotoxic effector cells on keratinocytes and LCs (48). The presence of eosinophils and basophils points to the participation of IgE antibodies and of cutaneous basophil hypersensitivity in the production of contact allergic reactions (49,50). Basophils are sources of transforming growth factor (TGF-β) and therefore may play a role in down-regulating expression of ACD.

Elicitation of ACD in a sensitized individual starts with antigen uptake and presentation by LCs. T lymphocytes specifically reactive to the allergen in question accumulate at the site of exposure. It is uncertain whether this accumulation is due to localized retention or proliferation of the specific T cells once they have arrived at the site, or to preferential migration to the site (51). Kalish (14), however, feels that migration of T lymphocytes is random, and therefore on-site retention or proliferation is likely. Antigen-specific T cells make up only 1% or less of the total T-cell population of the site, but this is still 10 to 100 times more than are present in the circulation.

Both antigen-specific and nonspecific T cells produce a number of inflammatory mediators once they arrive on-site. Tumor necrosis factor β (TNF-β) has direct cytotoxic effects on epidermal cells. In addition, it induces ICAM-1 on keratinocytes, which aids binding of lymphocytes. γ-Interferon also induces ICAM-1 as well as HLA-DR antigen expression on keratinocytes. This, too, facilitates attachment by lymphocytes. Various interleukins stimulate growth and activation of T lymphocytes and attract neutrophils. Granulocyte-monocyte colony-stimulating factor (GM-CSF) activates monocytes and neutrophils (52–54).

MAST CELLS AND BASOPHILS

Mast cells and basophils are routinely found at sites of ACD and are usually confined to the upper dermis. They release histamine, serotonin, and leukotrienes (55). Pruritus and vascular dilation leading to tissue edema may result. Leukotrienes act to attract both neutrophils and lymphocytes. Mast cells and basophils are not essential for the development of ACD, however, as demonstrated by the development of ACD in most cell-deficient mice (56).

KERATINOCYTES

Keratinocytes are not passive bystanders in the process of ACD. Multiple cytokines are produced and/or released by damaged or "activated" keratinocytes. These include interleukin and GM-CSF, with the function noted above. In addition, ICAM-1 is expressed in damaged but not normal keratinocytes and aids T-cell attachment. Furthermore, involved keratinocytes produce HLA-DR antigens in the cell surface, which allows attachment of autoreactive T lymphocytes.

IL-1, which was one of the first cytokines identified from keratinocytes, enhances the activation of accessory dendritic cells, which in turn activates resting T lymphocytes (57). IL-5, also expressed by keratinocytes, further stimulates T-cell proliferation. IL-8 is another keratinocyte product that has a strong chemotactic effect on T cells. Nozaki et al. (58) have prepared an excellent review of currently understood cytokine effects.

NEUROLOGIC FACTORS

Neuropeptides may influence ACD development, because nerve fibers of skin are in direct contact with LCs (59). Substance P may increase ACD by increasing levels of TNF-α and IL-2. Another neuropeptide, calcitonin gene-related peptide, may decrease ACD by stimulating IL-10 production (60, 61). A Substance P antagonist, spantide I, inhibited ACD in mice, whereas Substance P agonists increased it (62).

INHIBITION OF CONTACT SENSITIVITY

Adequate antigen presentation cannot take place when exposure to the contact allergen occurs at a skin site that has an insufficient number of functionally intact LCs. Under such circumstances, the development of specific immunologic tolerance (unresponsiveness) is favored because production of effector T lymphocytes is greatly decreased or absent. Another consequence is that more of the allergen then reaches the central parts of the lymphoid system and induces the production of specific suppressor cells there. However, even when first exposure takes place by contact, a tolerogenic effect is exerted by that fraction of the allergen that bypasses the epidermal LCs and reaches the dermis, the dermal lymphatics, and the regional lymph nodes (63). The ultraviolet radiation–resistant antigen-presenting cell described by Granstein et al. (64) must also be mentioned in this connection.

Under what circumstances can one expect inadequate antigen presentation and consequently suppressor cell predominance to occur? Certain skin sites in laboratory animals have contained a relatively small number of LCs (e.g., the tail skin of mice, which has approximately one-third the number of LCs present in most other areas). Although variations in the number of LCs have been observed in different areas of skin in humans, none has been described to date that is so deprived of these cells that it interferes with adequate antigen presentation (65).

A decrease in the number or functional ability of LCs or a dysfunction of the T-lymphocyte systems can lead to diminished contact sensitivity. Ultraviolet radiation (UVR) decreases the functional capability of LCs and may impair lymphocyte function (14,66). The actual numbers of LCs are not greatly reduced by UVR. Topical corticosteroid usage also results in functional impairment of LCs and suppression of patch test reactions (67). Systemic corticosteroid intake may compromise T-lymphocyte function, as well as LC capability (68). Cyclosporine A impairs LC function in vitro without cytotoxic effects on the LCs or T lymphocytes (69). LC function may be compromised in acquired immunodeficiency syndrome (70). The failure of LCs to stain positively for membrane Ia antigens and adenosine triphosphatase (ATPase) has demonstrated this functional impairment. It should be pointed out that, although the number of LCs, demonstrable by electron microscopy at such sites, is either unchanged or only slightly reduced, many of them are functionally impaired. The number of LCs is temporarily reduced immediately following a contact allergic reaction, but whether this reduction is sufficient to interfere with antigen presentation is not known. Recovery from functional impairment caused by glucocorticosteroids and UVR usually takes 1 to 2 weeks.

Antihistamines, although they inhibit mast cell and basophil function, do not appreciably alter contact hypersensitivity. Likewise, immunosuppressives such as methotrexate do not seem to impair contact sensitivity, as measured by patch testing.

It is safe to assume that other, as yet undiscovered factors and diseases must exist that can also interfere with antigen presentation by LCs.

In Vitro Tests

The interaction between antigen-bearing LCs and sensitized lymphocytes can be demonstrated in vitro. When sensitized T lymphocytes are cultured together with syngeneic Langerhans cell–enriched epidermal cell suspensions in the presence of the specific allergen, they undergo an antigen-specific proliferative response (70,71). Preceding treatment of the epidermal cell suspension with antibodies against Ia antigens abolishes this in vitro response and demonstrates the important role played by the immune response–associated surface antigens in this interaction.

Several in vitro reactions, like the lymphocyte transformation test and the macrophage migration inhibition test, often parallel clinical contact sensitivity. The results of these in vitro procedures, however, do not yet correlate with sufficient regularity with the results of in vivo exposures to justify their regular clinical use. Also, adequate test techniques have been worked out for only a few contact allergens.

Systemic Administration of Contact Allergens

Exposure to contact allergens takes place frequently by the "systemic" route, either by ingestion or by injection and on less frequent occasions by insertion into the body (as in operative procedures and intrauterine devices). As has been discussed earlier, first exposure to contact allergens by the systemic route usually favors the development of partial or complete specific tolerance. In some instances, however, allergic contact sensitization rather than tolerance occurs after such a first exposure. The explanation presumably is that some of the allergen has reached the skin through the blood circulation and has then been taken up by antigen-presenting epidermal or lymph node LCs.

A completely different effect is exerted by contact allergens that are "systemically" administered after specific sensitization has already occurred. Under such circumstances, a clinical reaction may ensue, probably because of take-up of the blood-borne contact allergen by antigen-presenting epidermal cells and subsequent interaction with specifically sensitized lymphocytes.

Hyposensitization

Hyposensitization, a state of decreased sensitivity, occurs in previously sensitized subjects and can sometimes be induced by intravenous administration of the allergen and by prolonged oral administration (72). The allergen then bypasses the epidermal Langerhans cell system and exerts a direct action on effector T lymphocytes. The suppression of hypersensitivity is antigen-specific and is not mediated by suppressor cells, but its exact mechanism is unknown. The possibility of a receptor blockade has been suggested (73). Hyposensitization usually has a short-lived effect, in contrast to specific immunologic tolerance, which is mediated by suppressor cells and tends to be long-lasting.

REFERENCES

1. Jadassohn, J. Zur Kenntnis der medikamentösen Dermatosen. *Verh Dtsch Derm Gesellschaft V Kongress* 1895;103.
2. Low, RC. Skin-sensitiveness to non-bacterial proteins and toxins. *Br J Dermatol* 1924;36:292.
3. Wedroff ES, Dolgoff AP. Über die spezifische Sensibilität der Haut einfachen chemische Stoffen gegenüber. *Arch Dermatol Syphilol* 1935;171:647.
4. Frei W. Über willkürliche Sensibilisierung gegen chemisch definierte Substanzen. I. Untersuchungen mit Neosalvarsan am Menschen. *Klin Wochenschr* 1928;7:539.
5. Mayer RL. Die Überempfindlichkeit gegen Körper von Chinonstruktur. *Arch Dermatol Syphilol* 1928;156:331.
6. Landsteiner K. Über komplexe Antigene. *Klin Wochenschr* 1927;6:103.
7. Sulzberger MB. Hypersensitiveness to arsphenamine in guinea pigs. I. Experiments in prevention and in desensitization. *Arch Dermatol Syphilol* 1929;20:669.
8. Chase MW. The cellular transfer of cutaneous hypersensitivity to tuberculin. *Proc Soc Exp Biol Med* 1945;59:134.
9. Landsteiner K, Chase MW. Experiments on transfer of cutaneous sensitivity to simple compounds. *Proc Soc Exp Biol Med* 1942;49:688.
10. Baer RL. Allergic eczematous sensitization in man 1936 and 1964. *J Invest Dermatol* 1964;43:223.
11. Storck H, Schwarz-Speck M. Different response to experimental sensitization by epicutaneous and intracutaneous application of bacterial antigens. *Monogr Allergy* 1974;8:79.
12. Eisen HN, Orris L, Belman S. Elicitation of delayed skin reactions with haptens: the dependence of elicitation on hapten combination with protein. *J Exp Med* 1952;95:473.
13. Shelley WB, Juhlin L. Langerhans cells form a reticuloepithelial trap for external contact allergens. *Nature* 1976;261:46.
14. Kalish RS. Recent developments in the pathogenesis of allergic contact dermatitis. *Arch Dermatol* 1991;127:1558.
15. Levine B, Ojeda A, Benacerraf B. Studies on artificial antigen. III. The genetic control of the immune response to hapten-poly-L-lysine conjugates in guinea pigs. *J Exp Med* 1963;118:953.
16. Polak L, Barnes JM, Turk JL. The genetic control of contact sensitization to inorganic metal compounds in guinea pigs. *Immunology* 1968;14:707.
17. Satoh T, et al. Effect of the H-2 and Igh complexes on the susceptibility to ultraviolet B–induced immunosuppression in murine contact sensitivity and contact photosensitivity. *Photodermatol Photoimmunol Photomed* 1990;7:73.
18. Streilein JW, Bergstresser PR. Genetic basis of ultraviolet-B effects on contact hypersensitivity. *Immunogenetics* 1988;27:252.
19. Yoshikawa T, Streilein JW. Tumor necrosis factor—alpha and ultraviolet B light have similar effects on contact hypersensitivity in mice. *Regional Immunol* 1990;3:139.
20. Walker FB, et al. Genetic factors in human allergic contact dermatitis. *Int Arch Allergy Appl Immunol* 1967;32:453.
21. Karvonen J, et al. HLA antigens in nickel allergy. *Ann Clin Res* 1984;16:211.
22. Mozzanica N, et al. HLA-A, B, C, and DR antigens in nickel contact sensitivity. *Br J Dermatol* 1990;122:309.
23. Bergstresser PR. Contact dermatitis: old problems and new techniques. *Arch Dermatol* 1989;125:276.
24. Silvennoinen-Kassinen S, Ikaheimo I, Tiilikainen A. TAP1 and TAP2 genes in nickel allergy. *Int Arch Allergy Immunol* 1997;114:94–96.
25. Baer RL, Flotte TJ, Gigli I, Thorbecke GJ. Langerhans cells—the skin-associated antigen-presenting cells. In: Daynes RA, Spikes JD, eds. *Experimental and clinical photoimmunology.* Boca Raton, FL: CRC Press, 1983;1:139.
26. Benacerraf B. Interrelationships between products of the major histocompatibility complex and their relevance to disease. In: Katz DH, Benacerraf B, eds. *The role of products of the histocompatibility gene complex in immune response.* New York: Academic Press, 1976.
27. Nalefski E, Rao A. Nature of the ligand recognized by a hapten- and carrier-specific MHC restricted T-cell receptor. *J Immunol* 1993;150:3806–3816.
28. Braathen LR, Thorsby E. Human epidermal Langerhans cells are more potent than blood monocytes in inducing some antigen-specific T-cell responses. *Br J Dermatol* 1983;108:139.
29. Witmer-Pack MD, et al. Granulocyte-macrophage colony-stimulating factor and interleukin-1 mediate the maturation of murine epidermal Langerhans cells into potent immunostimulatory dendritic cells. *J Exp Med* 1987;167:700.
30. Aiba S, Katz S. Phenotypic and functional characteristics of in vitro activated Langerhans cells. *J Immunol* 1990;145:2791.
31. Toews GB, Bergstresser PR, Streilein JW. Langerhans cells: sentinels of skin-associated lymphoid tissue. *J Invest Dermatol* 1980;75:78.
32. Teunissen MBM, et al. Inhibitory effect of cyclosporin A on antigen and alloantigen presenting capacity of human epidermal Langerhans cells. *Br J Dermatol* 1991;125:309.
33. Enk A, Katz S. Early molecular events in the induction phase of contact sensitivity. *Proc Natl Acad Sci USA* 1992;89:1398–1402.
34. Gawkrodger DJ, et al. The hapten in contact hypersensitivity to dinitrochlorobenzene: immunoelectron microscopic and immunofluorescent studies. *Dermatologica* 1989;178:126.
35. Dearman R, Basketter D, Coleman J, et al. The cellular and molecular basis for divergent allergic responses to chemicals. *Chem Biol Interactions* 1992;84:1–10.
36. Riemann H, Schwarz A, Grabbe S, et al. Neutralization of IL-12 in vivo prevents induction of contact hypersensitivity and induces hapten specific tolerance. *J Immunol* 1996;156:1799–1803.
37. Gautam SC, Battisto JR. Orally induced tolerance generates an efferently acting suppressor T-cell and an acceptor T-cell that together down-regulate contact sensitivity. *J Immunol* 1985;135:2975.
38. Baer RL, Sulzberger MB. Attempts at passive transfer of allergic eczematous sensitivity in man. *J Invest Dermatol* 1952;18:53.
39. Harber LC, Baer RL. Attempts to transfer eczematous contact-type allergy with whole blood transfusions. *J Invest Dermatol* 1961;36:55.
40. Epstein WL, Kligman AM. Transfer of allergic contact–type delayed hypersensitivity in man. *J Invest Dermatol* 1957;28:291.
41. Good RA, Zak SJ, Jensen DR, Pappenheimer AM, Jr. Delayed allergy and agammaglobulinemia. *J Clin Invest* 1957;36:894.

42. Baer RL, Turk JL. Delayed skin reactions. In: Goldsmith LA, ed. *Biochemistry and physiology of the skin.* Oxford: Oxford University Press, 1982.

43. Sommer G, Parker D, Turk JL. Epicutaneous induction of hyporeactivity in contact sensitization: demonstration of suppressor cells induced by contact with 2:4 dinitrothiocyanatebenzene. *Immunology* 1975;29:517.

44. Polak L, Turk JL. Reversal of immunological tolerance by cyclophosphamide through inhibition of suppressor cell activity. *Nature* 1974; 249:654.

45. Silberberg-Sinakin I, Thotbecke G, Baer R, et al. Antigen-bearing Langerhans cells in skin, dermal lymphatics and lymph nodes. *Cell Immunol* 1976;25:137–151.

46. Gowans JL. Life-span, recirculation and transformation of lymphocytes. *Int Rev Exp Pathol* 1966;5:1.

47. Sulzberger MB, Baer RL, Kanof A, Lowenberg C. Skin sensitization to vesicant agents of chemical warfare. *J Invest Dermatol* 1947;8:365.

48. Tamaki K, et al. Hapten-specific TNP reactive cytotoxic effector cells using epidermal cells as targets. *J Invest Dermatol* 1981;77:225.

49. Ray MC, Tharp MD, Sullivan TJ, Tigelaar RE. Contact hypersensitivity reaction to DNFB mediated by monoclonal IgE-DNP antibodies. *J Immunol* 1983;131:1096.

50. Dvorak HF, Mihm MC Jr, Dvorak A. Morphology of delayed-type hypersensitivity in man. *J Invest Dermatol* 1976;67:391.

51. Sterry W, et al. Dominance of memory over naive T cells in contact dermatitis is due to differential tissue immigration. *Br J Dermatol* 1990;123:59.

52. Brasch J, Sterry W. Expression of adhesion molecules in early allergic patch test reactions. *Dermatology* 1992;185:12–17.

53. Lewis R, et al. Intercellular adhesion molecule expression in the evolving human cutaneous delayed hypersensitivity reaction. *J Invest Dermatol* 1989;93:672–677.

54. Heufler C, Koch F, Schuler G. Granulocyte/macrophage colony stimulating factor and interleukin 1 mediate the maturation of murine epidermal Langerhans cells into potent immunostimulatory dendritic cells. *J Exp Med* 1988;167:700–705.

55. Kerdel F, Belsito D, Scotto-Chinnici R, et al. Mast cell participation during the elicitation of murine allergic contact hypersensitivity. *J Invest Dermatol* 1987;88:686–690.

56. Thestrup-Pedersen K, Larsen CG, Ronnevig J. The immunology of contact dermatitis: a review with special references to the pathophysiology of eczema. *Contact Dermatitis* 1989;20:81.

57. Austyn JA, et al. Dendritic cells initiate a two stage mechanism for T lymphocyte proliferation. *J Exp Med* 1983;157:1101.

58. Nozaki S, Feliciani C, Sauder D. Keratinocyte cytokines. In: *Advances in dermatology.* St. Louis: Mosby-Year Book, 1991:7.

59. Hosoi J, et al. Regulation of Langerhans cell function by nerves containing calcitonin gene–related peptide. *Nature* 1993;363:159–163.

60. Calvo C, Chavanel G, Senik A. Substance P enhances IL-2 expression in activated human T-cells. *J Immunol* 1992;148:3498–3504.

61. Fox F, Kubin M, Cassin M, et al. Calcitonin gene–related peptide inhibits proliferation and antigen presentation by human peripheral blood mononuclear cells. *J Invest Dermatol* 1997;108:43–48.

62. Niizeki H, Kurimoto I, Streilein J. A substance P agonist acts as an adjuvant to promote hapten-specific skin immunity. *J Invest Dermatol* 1999;112:437–442.

63. Macher E, Chase MW. Studies on the sensitization of animals with simple chemical compounds. XII. The influence of excision of allergenic depots on onset of delayed hypersensitivity and tolerance. *J Exp Med* 1969;129:103.

64. Granstein RD, Lowy A, Greene MI. Epidermal antigen presenting cells in activation of suppression: identification of a new functional type of ultraviolet radiation–resistant epidermal cell. *J Immunol* 1984;132:563.

65. Bergstresser PR, Toews GB, Gilliam JN, Streilein JW. Unusual numbers and distributions of Langerhans cells in skin with unique immunologic properties. *J Invest Dermatol* 1980;74:312.

66. Aberer W, Schuler G, Stingl G, et al. Ultraviolet light depletes surface markers of Langerhans cells. *J Invest Dermatol* 1981;76:202.

67. Rietschel RL. Irritant and allergic responses as influenced by Triamcinolone in patch test materials. *Arch Dermatol* 1985;121:68.

68. Belsito DV, Flotte TJ, Lim HW, et al. Effect of glucocorticosteroids on epidermal Langerhans cells. *J Exp Med* 1982;155:291.

69. Belsito D, Epstein S, Schulz J, et al. Enhancement by various cytokines or 2-B-mercaptoethanol of Ia antigen expression on Langerhans cells in skin from normal aged and young mice: effect of cyclosporine A. *J Immunol* 1989;143:1530–1536.

70. Belsito DV, Sanchez MR, Baer RL, et al. Reduced Langerhans cell Ia antigen and ATPase activity in patients with acquired immune deficiency syndrome. *N Engl J Med* 1984;310:1279.

71. Stingl G, Katz SI, Shevach EM, et al. Analogous functions of macrophages and Langerhans cells in the initiation of the immune response. *J Invest Dermatol* 1978;71:59.

72. Van Scott E, Kalmanson JD. Complete remissions of mycosis fungoides lymphoma induced by topical nitrogen mustard. *Cancer* 1973;32:18.

73. Polak L, Rinck C. Mechanism of densitization in DNCB-contact sensitivity guinea pigs. *J Invest Dermatol* 1978;20:98.

CHAPTER 2

Practical Aspects of Patch Testing

BASIC ASSUMPTIONS

The patch test is generally required to identify the cause of allergic contact dermatitis. When performed and interpreted properly, it is a scientific method of investigation with definite rules, regulations, and fundamentals. The achievement of valid results from the patch test, which seems simple to apply and read, is in fact a complicated procedure that should not be performed until one has had sufficient experience under the supervision of trained personnel. Modification of the standard methods may lead to confusion and misinterpretation and should not be undertaken lightly.

The patch test is artificial and does not necessarily duplicate clinical exposure, in which sweating, maceration, and multiple applications may play roles in producing dermatitis. The real-life exposure of skin to allergen will have variable contact time for the transfer of allergen to skin, whereas the patch test is applied for a fixed, standardized time. The concentration of allergen in a real-life exposure is seldom known, whereas the patch test exposure is defined and adjusted to minimize the chance for an irritant reaction. Patch testing, however, is a better method of finding an offending contactant than clinical "trial and error." A history of reactions to cheap jewelry, zippers, snaps, or metal buttons might be clinically equated with nickel allergy. This assumption would be incorrect over 53% of the time and would miss true nickel allergy in an additional 35% of those surveyed (1). History simply cannot replace the more complete information obtained by patch testing.

Because the patch test exposes only a small skin area and may be performed on covered parts of the body, even strongly positive reactions need not be disabling or disfiguring. Patch test reactions properly performed and interpreted are acceptable as "scientific proof" of a state of allergic sensitization. If this allergic state can be correlated with known exposures, positive use tests, or improvement by avoidance of substances containing the allergen identified by patch testing, then the validity of the patch test is said to be relevant and may be medicolegally important.

> **Properly applied and correctly interpreted patch tests are, at present, the only scientific "proof" of allergic contact dermatitis.**

Dermatologists who regularly use the patch test realize that the discovery of a specific chemical responsible for dermatitis is fundamentally important to prevent recurrence. That this knowledge is attainable only through intelligent and careful patch testing has been demonstrated time and again, as a review of the medical literature of the past 60 years confirms. Education in the technique of patch testing is as essential to physicians in training as the learning of most surgical procedures.

> **Many otherwise admirable dermatology departments neglect patch testing to the detriment of the patient.**

The four reasons for dermatologists' reluctance to use patch testing are (a) the amount of time required of the physician, (b) the number of visits required of the patient, (c) the unavailability of suitable test materials, and (d) the risk of complications. In general, these beliefs are not supported by the facts: (a) The confirmatory value of patch testing enables the physician to proceed with confidence; (b) patients usually appreciate efforts to investigate their case (the default rate in a dermatology clinic that performs patch tests is lower than that in most other clinics); (c) guidelines have been published on the relative risk of complications and the means to avoid them; and (d) after more than two visits for contact dermatitis, patch testing becomes clearly cost-effective (2). Rajagopalan et al. (3) demonstrated that patch-tested patients have a better outcome than patients who were not patch tested as evidenced by a decrease in disease severity index and percentage of disease activity. They further demonstrated that dermatitis lasting

TABLE 2.1. *Principles of Patch Testing*

1. Test only with known substances in "standard" concentrations. If in doubt, do open or "use" tests with controls. Do not test with industrial substances of unknown concentration.
2. Do not test if the dermatitis is acute. The test site must be *completely* free of dermatitis.
3. Instruct the patient to leave the patches on for 48 hours. If any patch burns and itches severely, the patient should remove that patch carefully without disturbing the others.
4. Instruct the patient not to shower, get the back wet, or engage in sports while the patches are in place. Certain types of heavy work are contraindicated as well, especially if the patient sweats considerably.
5. Patch tests can be read initially at 48 hours after allowing the tape reaction to subside, but an additional reading should be taken between 72 and 120 hours using the interpretation key of the North American Contact Dermatitis Group (see Table 2.5) (14).
6. Irritant and allergic reactions may be difficult to distinguish. As a rule, allergic reactions tend to itch more than irritant reactions. Certain patch test substances commonly produce weak irritant reactions, especially on highly sensitive skin or on skin of subjects who have several strong allergic reactions simultaneously.

from 2 months to 1 year was the most cost-effective group for evaluation by patch tests.

The patch test is not perfect, but as a bioassay it approximates the rigors required in the field of microbiology by the Henle-Koch postulates. These postulates require that a specific microorganism be found in every case in question and account for the pathologic changes and clinical course of the disease, that the organism not occur as a nonpathogen in other clinical disease settings, and that the organism could be grown in pure culture and reintroduced to produce the disease (4). A proper patch test uses a specific substance that produces the disease, contact dermatitis, in miniature; it is the purified etiologic agent reproducing the clinical disease in a susceptible host and causing no disease outside the proper clinical setting (i.e., no reaction in a nonsensitized host). It is a very complete bioassay. To achieve maximum accuracy, the principles in Table 2.1 should be used.

> The patch test is a unique direct in vivo test independent of any laboratory procedure and meets the rigorous requirement of cause and effect contained in the Henle-Koch postulates.

The Provocative Use Test or Open Test

The provocative use test is valuable in confirming positive reactions to nonirritating substances, such as cosmetics, in which at least one of the ingredients was previously found positive by conventional closed testing. The suspected material is rubbed directly onto normal skin in the antecubital fossa, twice daily for 1 week, over an area approximately 3 cm in diameter. If no reaction occurs, the test may be considered negative. False-negative reactions are common with this method of testing. The open "use" or "provocative" test may sometimes distinguish an allergic from an irritant response because open testing is far less likely than closed testing to produce an irritant reaction.

In the detection of contact urticaria, the test may be read 15 to 30 minutes following application, but otherwise the reading is the same as with the open patch test. Cosmetics, such as perfumes, hair sprays, conditioners, aftershave lotions, and plant oleoresins, are tested frequently in this manner. The recommended sites for testing are the retroauricular area, or the outer aspect of the arm immediately above the elbow.

The open or provocative use test is administered (a) before closed patch testing if no safe concentration for closed patch testing is known, (b) to confirm suspected contact urticaria within 15 to 30 minutes by applying the suspect material close to skin that is normally dermatitic and observing for whealing, or (c) to confirm that a substance at its normal "use" concentration in a finished product is capable of inducing contact dermatitis.

> Patch testing for "delayed" eczematous dermatitis is performed only on normal skin, whereas testing for "immediate" urticarial reactions is sometimes done on dermatitic skin (see Chapter 33).

THE CAUSES OF IRRITANT PATCH TEST REACTIONS

Irritant patch test responses are due to either hyperirritability of the skin or the application of an irritating concentration of a test substance. Often a combination of both factors is present. Hyperirritable skin has been attributed to strong allergic responses (the "angry back" or "excited skin state"). However, this is an oversimplification. Memon and Friedmann (5) tried to reproduce a hyperirritable state by patch testing standard allergens adjacent to and various distances from strong allergic and irritant reactions. They could not demonstrate a reproducible effect on the standard substance. Although the ability of positive patch tests in close proximity to influence the responsiveness of each other has been questioned, the ability of distant dermatitis to influence the threshold of reactivity is well established. Patients with active hand eczema are more reactive to irritants applied to the back as compared with similarly tested normal individuals, and patients with healed hand eczema react to such irritants the same as normal subjects (6). The phenomenon of conditioned hyperirritability has been reviewed and an animal model for the production of hyperirritable skin demonstrated (7).

If hyperrritable skin is suspected as the cause of false-positive irritant tests, the test can be repeated in a month or two when the patient's skin may be less irritable. Test only clinically normal skin, and allow the previously active dermatitis to disappear completely. When confronted with a possible irritant test from an industrial or other environmental agent, one must determine the irritancy of the material by patch testing volunteers. This method is not entirely without risk, as one may induce sensitization or produce a severe primary irritant reaction. The concentration that is nonirritating in a few normal test subjects should not be used for patch testing patients. Because patients more frequently have hyperirritable skin than normal volunteers as noted above, one-half or one-third of the concentration that is "safe" in a normal subject will probably prove nonirritating when tested on the patient.

"Open," "use," and "provocative" tests may help distinguish irritants from allergens and may help confirm that the patient is actually allergic to the suspected contactant.

Avoiding Irritant Tests

Because irritant tests can closely mimic allergic patch test responses, it is important to avoid producing irritant tests. Four cardinal rules should be followed:

1. Test only skin that appears completely normal.
2. Avoid concentrations of patch test materials that are irritating.
3. Do not prepare the skin by cleansing it with soaps or solvents.
4. Avoid patch testing with materials other than the standard series to minimize irritant reactions. *Seek consultation for testing with nonstandard substances.*

It is usually stated that one should not patch test patients who are in status eczematicus or who have widespread dermatoses because of the frequent occurrence of irritable skin. Unfortunately, matters are not so simple in practice because patients who have widespread dermatitis may have normally reacting skin, whereas other patients who have only hand dermatitis or other limited processes may have markedly irritable skin. The requirement of normal skin for the patch test site is absolute. Failure to limit patch testing to normal skin may result in false-positive test results, which are worse than useless because they are misleading. Skin to be tested (usually on the back) should be examined with good sidelighting to ensure that not even a minimal trace of dermatitis is present. Unless an area of skin can be cleared completely of dermatitis, reliable patch testing is difficult. Patch testing is best done 2 weeks after a patient is completely clear of dermatitis.

The second requirement, that of not testing with irritant materials, is more difficult. Many allergens, such as forma-lin, chrome, and nickel, are potent irritants. Obtaining a completely nonirritating concentration of these compounds is impossible, as such a concentration would be so diluted it would produce false-negative reactions. It has been the usual practice to determine "safe" or "nonirritating" concentrations by patch testing normal subjects. Even such "safe" concentrations, however, may produce false-positive irritant reactions because the clinician does not test a normal person but a patient whose skin may be more sensitive to irritants than a normal subject.

It should be understood that the term "irritant" as applied to standard commercially available screening allergens is a misnomer or wastebasket term. The test concentration is not one that produces a glazed or scalded patch test reaction typical of what would be generally accepted as an irritant reaction. The false-positive test seen with standard screening allergens more commonly is an erythematous, slightly edematous reaction that would be morphologically a 1+ "allergic" reaction. However, this mild reaction is either unconfirmable on repeated testing or highly suspect because of other circumstances. An example would be an isolated positive patch test to carba mix with a negative reaction to thiuram mix in an individual who was tested while active dermatitis was present elsewhere on the body. Common usage has permitted a broad concept of "irritant" to include these reactions. The patch test is a bioassay that does not by itself distinguish mechanisms. The patch test can result in weak allergic reactions of little or no clinical relevance, mild reactions that do not require specifically sensitized T cells and cannot be morphologically distinguished from reactions that do, or mild reactions that are relevant but may be undervalued by the physician conducting the test. This imprecise terminology has prompted one of us (Robert L. Rietschel) to propose that those nonpapulovesicular patch test reactions consisting of slightly palpable erythema and edema be called Janus reactions. These are reactions that are at or very near the threshold of reactivity. The mythological figure Janus was a symbol found on gates or doorways and looked in both directions simultaneously (double-faced). This would recognize the possibility that this mild reaction may or may not be relevant and only further correlation can establish that (see Table 2.2).

Use testing of mild reactions of this type with cosmetic chemicals showed that 44% of "doubtful" patch test reactions were actually relevant (8). However, weak reactions have also been found to be less likely to have relevance.

TABLE 2.2. *Criteria for a Janus Reaction*

Erythema with or without edema
No vesicles
No necrosis, pustules, or epidermal glazing

The significance of these reactions can only be determined over time based on patient outcomes.
Morphologic criteria alone are insufficient at this level of reaction to be a reliable correlate of allergy.

Fischer and Rystedt (9) found that doubtful reactions to metal salts were relevant 1% to 5% of the time, 1+ reactions were relevant about 20% of the time, 2+ were relevant 80% to 90% of the time, and 3+ reactions were relevant 95% to 100% of the time. Stronger reactions were also associated with greater relevance based on use tests results. Hannuksela and Salo (8) found 1+ and 2+ reactions relevant 80% of the time, in contrast to the 44% relevance of doubtful reactions. The 2+ and 3+ reactions require the presence of papulovesicles. This morphologic criterion more than any other militates against irritation and in favor of an allergic reaction. However, no firm criteria have yet been established that can reliably make this distinction on the basis of one finding. The similarity between irritant and allergic contact dermatitis extends into the immunologic mechanisms that participate in these inflammatory reactions. Virtually all of the events thought to be unique to allergy have also been found in irritant reactions as well (10).

A technique known as the RNase protection assay (RPA), which allows for the measurement of small quantities of RNA obtained from tape stripping of human skin, has been found to be extremely sensitive. In a pilot study, when the RPA was used to analyze tape strippings from patch test reactions, the RPA was able to discriminate between irritant and allergic patch test reactions. Interleukin-4 was found to be increased in allergic but not irritant reactions (11). If this technique is verified in larger trials, then a determination of the true nature of Janus reactions could be readily made.

> **The concentrations of several important allergens with irritant properties have been carefully standardized for use with Finn chamber technology and petrolatum or aqueous vehicles to make irritant reactions a rare event. Potassium dichromate is tested at 0.025% in petrolatum, nickel sulfate at 2.5% to 5% in petrolatum, and formaldehyde at 1% aqueous to minimize false-positive (irritant or Janus) reactions.**

INTERPRETING PATCH TEST REACTIONS

Relevance (Explained or Not Explained)

The clinician's task is not ended once the allergic state of the patient has been established. The fact that certain allergens have been demonstrated reliably by careful patch testing does not prove that such allergens were responsible for the dermatitis. The clinician must determine whether or not the allergy is relevant to the dermatitis, either as a primary cause or as an aggravating factor.

In analyzing the question of relevance, it may be helpful to consider the possibilities as follows:

1. relevance to present dermatitis
   A. primary cause
   B. aggravating factor
2. relevance to a preceding bout of dermatitis
   A. primary cause
   B. aggravating factor
3. not relevant

It is impossible to provide absolute rules for the determining relevance, because it depends on that blend of knowledge and experience known as clinical judgment. Frequently, the clinician must decide among the roles of endogenous factors (atopic eczema, psoriasis) and external factors (irritants, contact allergens). A careful examination of the entire skin and a thorough history are helpful in yielding clues to endogenous dermatitis. The judgment of "not relevant" with regard to a positive patch test often reflects our ignorance about possible exposures rather than a patch test that is actually irrelevant.

Relevance can be considered possible, probable, or certain. If a substance produces an allergic patch test reaction and the patient is exposed to circumstances in which skin contact with materials known to contain the allergen is likely to occur, relevance can be said to be *possible*. For example, when a positive reaction to black rubber mix is found in an auto mechanic who works with black rubber hoses and fan belts, relevance is at least possible. If a chemical component of the black rubber mix can be verified to be present in hoses or fan belts with which the patient comes in contact, relevance is *probable*. If a use test with a black rubber hose rubbed over an area of normal skin produces contact dermatitis, the concentration of allergen in the item is sufficient to elicit dermatitis and relevance is *certain*. The rigor with which relevance evaluation is pursued depends on the clinical circumstances and the impact on lifestyle or job modifications required by the patch test findings.

The absence of positive patch tests does not prove the absence of allergy. "Screening" or battery patch testing is often performed on patients who have eczematous dermatoses of unknown cause as a fishing expedition to help establish etiologic factors. Negative patch tests establish only that the patient is not allergic to the relatively more common and well-established sensitizers included in such patch test batteries. The ability of a screening series to detect contact allergy has been evaluated. In a study of 732 patients referred for possible contact dermatitis, only 15.7% were found to be evaluated adequately by a screening series of 20 allergens (12). In a separate study of 554 patients who were patch tested, a correlation was found between the size of the screening series and the amount of useful information gathered. The 20-allergen screening series detected only 55% of the information obtained by the 50-allergen North American Contact Dermatitis Group (NACDG) series. The 23 allergens of the T.R.U.E. test series identified 65% of the information found by the larger series. The use of additional supplemental series beyond the 50 allergens of the NACDG series found another 103 reactions, of which 59 were relevant (13).

> Larger screening series of allergens yield a more complete evaluation of patients with more relevant allergens identified. Supplemental allergens that are added to screening series based on the patient's history provide additional relevant information.
>
> Unexpected positive patch test reactions that are not relevant to the presenting dermatitis can often be traced to previous exposures. Such reactions may be significant in the future, and the patient should be informed of the test results.

Negative Patch Test Reactions

Just as a positive reaction does not always mean that the cause of the presenting dermatitis has been found, a negative result does not mean that contact dermatitis has been excluded. Standard screening series include only statistically common allergens; we must be constantly alert to the possibility of rare, exotic, or new sensitizers.

Reasons for False-Negative Reactions

False-negative reactions have various causes:

1. Insufficient reproduction by the test of the conditions that produced the dermatitis, such as sweating, friction, pressure, and the presence of damaged, ulcerated, or eczematous skin.
2. A concentration of test substance that is too low. The concentration of test substances is critical and should be "standard" because the threshold of reactivity is a narrow margin and, at even slightly higher concentrations, many substances become irritants.
3. Failure to perform delayed readings (14). When patch tests are read only at 48 hours, some positive reactions are missed. This finding is especially true of substances, such as neomycin, but delayed reactivity may occur with many allergens.
4. Wet or loosened patches.
5. Inappropriate vehicle. For example, testing with nickel suspended in petrolatum as a vehicle may produce negative results, whereas testing with nickel in an aqueous solution may produce positive results.
6. Duration of contact that is too brief. A duration of 24 to 48 hours is probably the minimum for occlusion in the closed patch test; earlier removal may prevent development of some positive reactions.
7. Failure to perform photo patch testing. Testing with a photosensitizing substance may cause a negative result if the test site is completely occluded by opaque material. Sometimes, however, sufficient light penetrates to elicit a definite reaction.
8. Influence of corticosteroids. The application of potent topical steroids to the test site for several days before testing may diminish or even obliterate weak positive results.
9. A fluctuation in the threshold of reactivity that resulted in the level of sensitivity being lower than the patch test concentration at the time chosen for testing. This variable is not under control of the clinician and can result in mild allergens being missed at one time and found on repeated testing.

> Negative patch test reactions are often due to a "missed" allergen, which may be picked up by detailed questioning about the patient's hobbies, home, and work environment or by additional or repeated testing.

Sukanto and associates (15) found that the topical application of corticosteroids had a suppressive effect on both the intensity and the size of epicutaneous reactions; no marked difference in the suppressive effect of the four corticosteroids could be observed. However, intermediate-strength corticosteroids (triamcinolone ointment 0.1%) applied three times per day for a week prior to diagnostic patch testing did not have a significant effect (16). The inclusion of triamcinolone ointment 0.1% directly into a patch test substance such as thimerosal was found to ablate both irritant and allergic reactions (17). Systemic steroids in doses of 20 mg daily or less probably do not inhibit a "significant" patch test.

> Patients on "maintenance" doses of systemic corticosteroids up to 20 mg daily can be patch tested without materially affecting the results of the tests.

What to Tell the Patient about the Results of the Patch Test

When a clinically significant patch test reaction is obtained, the patient should be given the following information, in writing, concerning the sensitizing substance:

1. the various names and guises of the sensitizer
2. immunochemical relatives that might produce cross-reactions with the sensitizer
3. methods of avoiding clinical exposure to the contactant
4. when available, the names of suitable nonsensitizing substitutes

THE SAFETY OF PATCH TESTING

The greatest hazard is *omission* of patch testing procedures in the management of patients who have certain dermatoses. Such omission dooms these patients to repeated

tested may also result in hyperpigmentation. Severe reactions sometimes cause hyperpigmentation or total depigmentation. Irritant reactions in certain patients may result in hyperpigmentation from the inflammation.

Because patch testing is usually performed on the back, which is covered by clothing, these temporary pigmentary changes do not present serious problems. Preparations, such as Covermark corrective makeup, may be used until the pigmentation clears.

Anaphylactoid Reaction from Patch Testing

Rarely, anaphylactoid reactions are seen within 30 minutes after topical testing with certain antibiotics, such as penicillin, neomycin, gentamycin, or bacitracin. Nitrogen mustard may also produce such a reaction (see Chapter 34).

Patch tests with antibiotics may, on rare occasions, produce an anaphylactoid reaction.

In addition to such specific allergic reactions, ammonium persulfate, used as a "booster" of hydrogen peroxide for bleaching "platinum blondes," may rarely produce a nonspecific, idiosyncratic release of histamine that results in an anaphylactoid reaction. Routine patch testing with ammonium persulfate is not advised. If the test is performed under unusual circumstances, such as a medicolegal procedure, readily available injectable epinephrine should be on hand.

Edge Effect

The "edge effect" is an irritant reaction in which the reaction is greatest at the periphery of the patch test, and there is little or no reaction at the center. The effect is probably caused by an increased concentration of an irritant liquid at the margin. The edge effect usually disappears rapidly following removal of the patch. However, the edge effect seen when patch testing corticosteroids is different. This is a sign of allergy and represents the interplay of the pharmacologic and immunologic activities of corticosteroids. Lower concentrations of corticosteroids give a more traditional positive patch test as the pharmacologic effect becomes diluted more than the immunologic effect.

Pustular Patch Test Reactions

These reactions occur occasionally, especially in atopic persons, from application of metallic salts, such as nickel and copper sulfates, arsenic trioxide, and mercuric chloride. Pruritus is often absent or minimal. Pustular reactions usually disappear promptly, although they may persist for some time before they disappear completely. These reactions do not signify allergy.

Pressure Effects

The application of a solid substance to the skin of certain persons produces an edematous area that is almost always most intense at the margins. If the test substance is sufficiently large and heavy, the reaction may cover the entire test area. Persons who have a tendency to dermographism are more likely to develop this reaction. It may even be induced by rubbing the skin while the patches are in place.

Bacterial and Viral Infections

These complications have been described, but fortunately, we have not yet encountered them (26).

Necrosis, Scarring, and Keloids

Foolhardy testing with strong acids, alkalis, or chemicals of unknown composition may produce these adverse effects.

THE ROLE OF THE EXCITED SKIN SYNDROME ("ANGRY BACK") IN PATCH TESTING

There has been a revival of interest in a phenomenon that Dr. Max Jessner of the old New York Skin and Cancer Unit called the "crazy back."

Mitchell (21,27,28) used the term "angry back" to describe a regional phenomenon caused by the presence of a strongly positive reaction, a state of skin hyperreactivity in which other patch test sites become reactive, especially to marginal irritants, such as formalin and potassium dichromate. Mitchell (28) believed that these concomitant "positive" reactions cannot be relied on. He tested 35 patients who showed 90 positive 1+ reactions to 28 substances at 48 hours. He then retested these patients on day 7. On day 9, 42% of the reactions were negative, suggesting that false-positive reactions were common when one strong positive reaction occurred. Mitchell suggested that the true index of sensitivity is falsely exaggerated by concomitant testing. To confirm or deny the significance of individual reactions found on the "angry back," Mitchell recommended sequential testing later with each substance alone.

Strongly positive patch test reactions to nickel sulfate and potassium dichromate (the two "standard" patch test allergens most likely to engender nonspecific reactions in adjacent patch test materials) may be confused with allergic reactions. Whenever the clinical history of a patient suggests strongly that either one of these common allergens may produce a positive reaction, it may be placed on the patient's arm away from the other patches and thus minimize the "crazy back," or what Calnan (26) called the "status eczematicus."

Because patch tests may be performed elsewhere besides the back, Maibach and Mitchell (29,30) have broadened the term "angry back" to the "excited skin syndrome" (ESS).

Some clinical investigators have begun to think seriously about the possibility or indeed the likelihood that some

40% of the positive patch test reactions observed in routine concomitant screening patch testing are in fact false positives. Thus, in order to avoid misinformation, sequential retesting would be mandatory.

Maibach and Mitchell (29,30) have tested patients who have ESS on both arms and have found a similar response; the reproducible or nonreproducible tests could be demonstrated on the arm as well as on the back. In other words, a strong reaction on the right arm can produce a nonspecific response on the left arm. This finding suggests that, whatever the mechanism may be, it is not necessarily localized. This would account for the strong positive and so-called runover effect, for example, the spillover from one site to adjacent sites. But it is not the sole explanation, or one would not see enhanced reactivity over such a wide area as from one arm to the contralateral arm.

> The "angry back" or "excited skin" describes false-positive patch test reactions in a patch test "series" that are nonreproducible when repeated separately, and this nonreproducibility is blamed on the presence of other positive tests.

Since the original description of the angry back syndrome, much has been learned about the reproducibility of patch tests. Gollhausen et al. (31) applied patch tests sequentially to patients and found that 40% were lost (i.e., nonreproducible). These investigators then applied the same patch tests to the left and right side of the back (simultaneously) and again found nonreproducibility of 43.8%. All of these figures are in the range reported for the so-called angry back syndrome and question the explanation of strong reactions influencing other patch test responses. Gollhausen et al. tested allergens from several different manufacturers and found nonreproducibility rates of 17.9% for Pharmacia AB, Uppsala, Sweden; 18.5% for Hermal, Reinback, Germany; and 29.4% for Maser, Herne, Germany. The differences were not statistically significant (32). Discordance of results was found to be in part dependent on the strength of the reaction. With concomitant testing, nonreproducibility of 1+ reactions occurred 36.6% of the time, but with 2+, 3+, or 4+ reactions only 21% of the time. On sequential testing the same trend was found. The 1+ nonreproducibility was 40.4%, and the stronger reactions were nonreproducible 28.4% of the time. This work requires that the explanation for Mitchell's lost reactions be seen as something more than the work of other nearby reactions. Furthermore, entirely too much emphasis was placed on tests that were lost. Retesting leads to new or "found" reactions and does so just as frequently as reactions are "lost." This was demonstrated by Meneghini and Angelini (23), who tested 309 cases of suspected contact dermatitis and found 208 to have one or more positive tests. They used a series of 31 allergens and repeated the patch tests to all 31

from 1 to 36 months after the initial testing. They "lost" 50 cases (25%) but found 55 new cases (26.5%). Likewise, Ayala et al. (33) tested 174 patients with the same 30 allergens 5 years after the original testing. They found one or more patch tests were "lost" in 18% of cases, but 29% had more positive tests on repeat testing and 53% were exactly the same. As noted earlier in this chapter, Memon and Friedmann (5) could not demonstrate an effect on patch test results based on the proximity or distance of patch tests to strong irritants or allergens. Their work does show that reactivity across the back is not uniform to the same patch test, but this lack of uniformity cannot be accounted for by the presence or absence of other test reactions.

We now have patch test reactions that vary with location, vary to a greater degree when they are weaker, and are capable of varying either up or down. It is now known that one factor influencing the reactivity of an area of the back is how recently the area was or was not dermatitic. Nickel-sensitive patients had a controlled nickel dermatitis produced on different quadrants of their backs 8, 4, and 1 months prior to patch testing with a dilution series of nickel over each of these sites and a control site (34). A higher reactivity was found if a previous nickel dermatitis had been present, and, furthermore, a stronger reaction was observed if the antecedent dermatitis was more recent. The findings paint a different picture than envisioned by Mitchell, although his observation was correct. It appears that the closer a patch test exposure is to the patient's threshold of reactivity, the greater the chance that the test will vary over time. Because patch test reactions can vary up or down, the back can be visualized as "twinkling" rather than angry. Because diagnostic patch testing is usually done one time and with only one concentration of an allergen rather than a dilution series, the dynamic aspect of the immunologic variability of the skin will not be noted unless the tests are repeated or placed at varying sites. The proven value of routine testing in patient outcome attests to how well these variables have been overcome with standard screening allergens. This has been achieved by moving away from the threshold of reactivity as much as possible without inducing nonspecific inflammation (Janus-type reactions).

An additional variable that can amplify threshold events is neurogenic inflammation. It has been suggested that "noise" or stochastic resonance may be another factor modifying skin reactivity and that this effect is mediated by cutaneous nerves in contact with Langerhans cells (35). The presence or absence of this neurologic static may modify the threshold response of numerous biological systems.

The concept of spillover was not found by Memon and Friedmann (5), but this author (RLR) has observed this as envisioned originally by Mitchell. A case, which I will describe, illustrates the specificity of spillover that may make the phenomenon very hard to study. At day 2 of diagnostic patch testing a young woman had a 2+ reaction to colophony. No other reactions were present. Patch tests were applied with Scanpor tape to all four quadrants of her back. At the day 4 patch test reading the 2+ colophony reaction was still present, but a tape reaction to Scanpor was now present surrounding the colophony reaction and covering all the area of Scanpor application on the left upper quadrant of her back. There were no reactions at any other sites and no Scanpor reaction at any of the other three quadrants of the back. The Scanpor reaction on the left upper quadrant surrounded all of the standard allergens of the 20-allergen Hermal screening series noted later in this chapter. Not one of those tests turned positive. The enhanced reactivity was confined to an area about 10 cm by 10 cm roughly surrounding the positive colophony test. This enhanced reactivity was specific to colophony interacting with Scanpor. If an attempt had been made to study the influence of a positive colophony reaction on any of the standard allergens, the conclusion would be that no such influence exists and thus spillover does not exist. Spillover appears to be more specific than envisioned by Mitchell (21,28) and not the null event envisioned by the experiments of Memon and Friedmann (5).

> Patch test reactions vary in intensity over time, as the threshold of reactivity is not static. This can cause patch tests to appear positive at times and negative at times and vice versa. This fluctuation occurs equally in both directions: twinkling. All the factors responsible for this fluctuation are not known, but some factors are previous dermatitis at the site of testing, duration of time between prior dermatitis and testing, intensity of reactivity (strength of allergy), patch test concentration vis-à-vis the threshold of reactivity, and possibly the status of the cutaneous nerve endings.

Threshold of Irritancy

In the screening series, the parabens, potassium dichromate, formalin, and wool wax alcohol (lanolin), are notorious for their production of nonreproducible positive responses with greater frequency than other allergens. This finding means that even compounds of extremely low irritancy may produce a false-positive response in some subjects. These rules are relative rather than absolute. Categorization of such reactions requires a determination of relevance as discussed for Janus reactions.

Adhesive Tape Reactions

Adhesive tape produces a localized dermatitis in many subjects for which there are several mechanisms: irritant dermatitis, miliaria, microbial infection, pressure phenomena, allergic contact dermatitis, among others.

Magnusson and Hellgren (36) studied the effect of this dermatitis on patch test reactivity. The thrust of their obser-

vations was on the irritation and adhesive characteristics of different adhesive tapes used in Scandinavia. They recorded diagnostic patch test positivity in men and women, correlating this finding to the degree of adhesive tape reactivity.

With turpentine, potassium dichromate, p-phenylenediamine (PPD), and formalin, they noticed a striking difference in patch test positivity between subjects with and without tape dermatitis. With these four materials, the differences were statistically significant between the groups. For PPD, 17 positive responses (in a group of 26 men) were positive when a tape reaction occurred, and only 4 positive responses occurred with a tape-negative reaction. The investigators observed similar differences with irritants (detergents). Comparable results were obtained for the 26 women in the study only in regard to formalin. (This sex difference in reactivity was not researched further.) Magnusson and Hellgren (36) interpreted the additional responses as a nonspecific increase in skin reactivity secondary to the tape dermatitis.

The Principles of Dealing with Patients Who Have More Than One Positive Patch Test

In verifying the multiple positive responses noted in battery testing, much time and trouble are involved for both patient and physician (refer to Table 2.4). Mitchell and Maibach (30) have developed a strategy that minimizes the task of dealing with the ESS (which is actually a matter of determining relevance and is applicable to any positive patch test result):

1. If more than one positive patch test is noted, the clinical history is retaken. This by itself is often enough to solve the problem.
2. It may not be necessary to retest the positive substances individually. For example, if the material is a chemical that the patient can avoid relatively easily (such as ammoniated mercury, which is rarely used in the United

TABLE 2.4. *Battery Testing: Strategy for Dealing with the Excited Back Syndrome*

When more than one positive is noted, retake the clinical history
May not be necessary to retest positives individually if:
  The material is readily avoided (e.g., ammoniated mercury)
  History strongly negates positive patch test results
Important to retest individually if material is ubiquitous
  Preservatives (paraben mixture)
  Vehicle (wool wax alcohol)
  Medicament (neomycin)
  Fragrance (fragrance mixture)
  Rubber chemical
  Formalin
  Possible job change
  Medicolegal situation
  Regulatory situation

States), the patient can be informed about this and questioned about previous reactions, and testing can be discontinued. If no previous history supports exposure, the impetus for delving into it deeply is diminished.

Equally important, if the subject has a history that strongly negates the relevance of the positive patch test, the patient may not be interested in working through the physician's academic curiosity. It is not as important clinically to repeat that test because it presumably makes little difference to the patient even though it might make significant inroads into the diagnosis.

3. Retesting is unnecessary if the multiple reactions can be reasonably explained by a known chemical similarity or cross-reaction. If formaldehyde, quaternium-15, and imidazolidinyl urea are all positive, the release of formaldehyde by the latter two substances is a sufficient explanation. A positive patch test to benzocaine and paraphenylenediamine need not be reconfirmed because they are known to be potential cross-reactants.

4. It may be helpful to retest the patient if a positive patch test is related to a ubiquitous substance and the physician is uncertain of the validity of the result. The physician can lose credibility when the patient is told that he or she is allergic to something that is known not to cause the difficulty. Attributing the allergy to a chemical such as a preservative (the parabens), a vehicle (wool wax alcohol or lanolin), a medicament (neomycin), a fragrance, rubber chemicals, or formalin has great import. The avoidance of these materials involves considerable effort on the part of the patient, and if it is, in fact, a false-positive response, it is a needless waste of time and causes loss of confidence in the physician.

Maibach et al. (37), in a joint International Contact Dermatitis Research Group (ICDRG) study, attempted to quantify ESS. Fifty-six patients entering the study had two or more positive reactions with the basic ICDRG routine series. At approximately weekly intervals, the patients were retested one at a time with the two most clinically important positive responses. The results of this study revealed that 32 of the 56 subjects were still positive to both substances. In 16 cases, however, the patients reacted to only one of these substances, and in 8 cases, patients reacted to neither substance. This finding suggests that 24 of 56 patients (42%) may have had ESS. However, the study design did not address the number of additional allergens that would be found by retesting the initially negative results. As noted earlier in this chapter, both events occur with similar frequency. Retesting introduces new variables that were not appreciated at the time of the initial studies of excited skin syndrome. Location on the back (5) and prior dermatitis in that region can influence results (33).

TABLE 2.5. *Screening Patch Test Series*

Hermal (based on North American Contact Dermatitis Group recommendations and now of historical interest only)	International Contact Dermatitis Research Group Recommended Series	T.R.U.E Test
Benzocaine 5% in petrolatum, USP	Benzocaine 5% in petrolatum	(Not tested separately; see caine mix)
Mercaptobenzothiazole 1% in petrolatum, USP	Mercaptobenzothiazole 2% in petrolatum	Mercaptobenzothiazole 0.075 mg/cm²
Colophony 20% in petrolatum, USP	Colophony 20% in petrolatum	Colophony 0.85 mg/cm²
p-phenylenediamine 1% in petrolatum, USP	p-phenylenediamine base 1% in petrolatum	p-phenylenediamine 0.09 mg/cm²
Imidazolidinyl urea 2% in water for injection	Not tested	Not tested
Cinnamic aldehyde 1% in petrolatum, USP	Not tested separately; see fragrance mix	Not tested separately; see fragrance mix
Lanolin alcohol (wool wax alcohol) 30% in petrolatum, USP	Wool alcohols 30% in petrolatum	Wool alcohols 1 mg/cm²

Carba mix 3% in petrolatum, USP
  1,3 diphenylguanidine 1%
  zinc diethyldithiocarbamate 1%
  zinc dibutyldithiocarbamate 1%
	Not tested	Carba mix: same 3 as Hermal in equal parts Patch contains 0.25 mg/cm² carba mix

Neomycin sulfate 20% in petrolatum, USP	Neomycin sulfate 20% in petrolatum	Neomycin sulfate 0.23 mg/cm²

Thiuram mix 1% in petrolatum, USP
  Tetramethylthiuram disulfide 0.25%
  Tetramethylthiuram monosulfide (0.25%)
  Tetraethylthiuram disulfide 0.25%
  Dipentamethylenethiuram disulfide 0.25%
	Thiuram mix 1% in petrolatum (same)	Thiuram mix, equal parts: tetramethylthiuram monosulfide, tetramethylthiuram disulfide tetraethylthiuram disulfide, dipentamethylenethiuram disulfide, 0.25 mg/cm² of thiuram mix

continued

TABLE 2.5. *(Continued)*

Hermal (based on North American Contact Dermatitis Group recommendations and now of historical interest only)	International Contact Dermatitis Research Group Recommended Series	T.R.U.E Test
Formaldehyde (contains methanol) 1% in water for injection	Formaldehyde 1% aqueous	N-hydroxymethyl succinimide, which forms formaldehyde in contact with skin 0.18 mg/cm² formaldehyde
Ethylenediamine dihydrochloride 1% in petrolatum, USP	Ethylenediamine dihydrochloride 1% in petrolatum	Ethylenediamine dihydrochloride 0.018 mg/cm²
Epoxy resin 1% in petrolatum, USP	Epoxy resin 1% in petrolatum	Epoxy resin 0.05 mg/cm²
Quaternium-15 [N-(3 chloroallyl)-hexaminium chloride] 2% in petrolatum, USP	Quaternium-15 1% in petrolatum	Quaternium-15 0.081 mg/cm²
p-tert-butylphenol formaldehyde resin 1% in petrolatum, USP	4-tert-butylphenol formaldehyde resin 1% in petrolatum	p-tert-butylphenol formaldehyde resin 0.32 mg/cm²
Mercapto mix 1% in petrolatum, USP N-cyclohexyl-2-benzothiazole-sulfenamide 0.333% 2,2'-benzothiazyl disulfide 0.333% Morpholinyl-2-benzothiazyl disulfide 0.333%	Mercapto mix 2% in petrolatum N-cyclohexylbenzothiazyl sulfenamide 0.5% Mercaptobenzothiazole 0.5% Dibenzothiazyl disulfide 0.5% Morphodinylmercapto-benzothiazole 0.5%	Mercapto mix; equal parts: N-cyclohexylbenzothiazyl-sulphenamide, dibenzothiazyl disulfide, morpholinylmercaptobenzo-thiazole at 0.075 mg/cm²
Black rubber-p-phenylenediamine mix 0.6% in petrolatum, USP N-phenyl-N'-cyclohexyl-p-phenylenediamine 0.25% N-isopropyl-N'-phenyl-p-phenylenediamine 0.10% N,N'-diphenyl-p-phenyl-enediamine 0.25%	Black rubber mix 0.6% in petrolatum (same)	N-isopropyl-N'-phenyl paraphenylenediamine, N-cyclohexyl-N'-phenyl paraphenylenediamine, N,N'-diphenyl paraphenylenediamine in a ratio of 2:5:5 at 0.075 mg mix/cm²
Potassium dichromate, 0.25% in petrolatum, USP	Potassium dichromate 0.5% in petrolatum	Potassium dichromate 0.023 mg/cm²
Balsam of Peru 25% in petrolatum, USP	Balsam of Peru 25% in petrolatum	Balsam of Peru 0.8 mg/cm²
Nickel sulfate (anhydrous) 2.5%	Nickel sulfate (NiSo₄ • 6H₂O) 5% in petrolatum	Nickel sulfate 0.2 mg/cm²
Not tested	Cobalt chloride (CoCl₂ • 6H₂O) 1% in petrolatum	Cobalt chloride 0.02 mg/cm²
Not tested	Quinoline mix 6% in petrolatum and Clioquinol 3% Chlorquinaldol 3%	Quinoline mix, clioquinol, chlorquinaldol in equal parts at 0.19 mg/cm² (omitted from series in 1998)
Not tested	Parabens 15% in petrolatum Methyl-4-hydroxybenzoate 3.0 Ethyl-4-hydroxybenzoate 3.0 Propyl-4-hydroxybenzoate 3.0 Butyl-4-hydroxybenzoate 3.0 Benzyl-4-hydroxybenzoate 3.0	Paraben mix same as European series at 1 mg/cm²
Note tested	Fragrance mix 8% in petrolatum Cinnamic alcohol 1% Cinnamic aldehyde 1% Hydroxycitronellal 1% Amylcinnamaldehyde 1% Geraniol 1% Eugenol 1% Isoeugenol 1% Oak moss absolute 1%	Fragrance mix same 8 ingredients as European series at 0.43 mg/cm²
Not tested	Primin 0.01% in petrolatum	Not tested
Not tested	5-chloro-2-methyl-4-isothiazolin-3-one + 2-methyl-4-isothiazolin-3-one (3:1 in water) 0.01% aqueous	5-chloro-2-methyl-4-isothiazolin-3-one + 2-methyl-4-isothiazolin-3-one (3:1) (Kathon CG) 0.004 mg/cm²

continued

Nickel sulfate (NiSo₄ • 6H₂O)

Cobalt chloride (CoCl₂ • 6H₂O)

TABLE 2.5. *(Continued)*

Hermal (based on North American Contact Dermatitis Group recommendations and now of historical interest only)	International Contact Dermatitis Research Group Recommended Series	T.R.U.E Test
Not tested Tested as benzocaine only	Not tested Tested as benzocaine only	Thimerosal 0.008 mg/cm^2 Caine mix: 　Benzocaine 0.364 mg/patch 　Tetracaine 0.063 mg/patch 　Dibucaine 0.064 mg/patch

In the United States, the Hermal Kit of 20 allergens is no longer distributed by Hermal Pharmaceutical Laboratories, Inc., Oak Hill, NY 12460.

The European series is available in Canada from Pharmascience, Inc., 8400 Ch. Darnley Rd., Montreal, Quebec H4T 1M4 and in Europe from Hermal Kurt Herrmann, P.O. Box 1228, D-2057 Reinbek/Hamburg, Germany, or Chemotechnique Diagnostique AB, Ringugnsgatan 7, S-21616 Malmo, Sweden. Dormer Laboratories has begun distribution of an expanded series of allergens that includes the former 20 allergens of the Hermal series and additional allergens commonly used for screening by the North American Contact Dermatitis Group.

T.R.U.E. Test is distributed by Glaxo Dermatology, Research Triangle Park, NC. The gel vehicles vary among the patches and are listed on the package insert.

Bandmann and Agathos (38) detected a significant number of false-positive reactions by sequential testing, as did Bruynzeel et al. (39).

When more than one positive patch test reaction is obtained, the strongest reaction is probably a true "positive." If weaker tests of uncertain relevance are also present, multiple studies have found that about 30% to 40% of such tests may not be confirmed on retesting, casting serious doubt on their relevance. Correlation with history or known chemical cross-reactivity may be more helpful than retesting.

It is prudent to place notoriously strong sensitizers at a practical distance from similarly strong allergens. Distance will be limited by the size of the patient's back, the number of allergens to be tested, and the application system employed. (Finn chambers are available in single rows of five and double rows of five, all premounted on Scanpor tape.) This provides fixed distances for allergen placement, which may require thoughtful planning when other than "standard" series of allergens are used. (See Table 2.5 for the currently available screening series in the United States and the European counterpart.)

INTERPRETATION OF THE MIXES IN THE SCREENING SERIES

Mixes of closely related chemicals save valuable time and space. By using mixes containing four to five related chemicals from the same family, one can increase considerably the number of test materials.

Occasionally, a sensitive patient shows a negative reaction to a mix but a positive reaction to one of its ingredients tested separately. This finding occurs occasionally with mercapto mix because the concentration of 2-MBT in the mix is lower than in the individual test material. Conversely, testing with tetramethylthiuram disulfide (TMTD) may sometimes be negative, whereas thiuram mix may be positive because the patient is sensitive to the monosulfide but not to the disulfide.

Mixes have assumed a valuable role, but caution must be observed in their preparation so that the concentration of each chemical is sufficient to evoke a reaction. Also, the combination must not react chemically to induce irritation or cause deactivation of one or more of its components, which results in a false-negative reaction.

Patch test "mixes" save time and space. Occasionally, an allergen in the "mix" produces a false-negative reaction because the concentration is too low. The fragrance and paraben mix, however, may rarely produce false-positive (irritant) reactions.

Mitchell (40) states that patch testing with mixes can provide requisite information. Thus, in a patient with clinical findings strongly suggestive of rubber glove dermatitis, a positive reaction to thiuram mix leads to advice on avoidance of rubber, and further testing may be unnecessary. The multitude of allergenic rubber chemicals leads us to test them in groups because it would require too much effort to test each substance individually. The detailed analysis of reactions to rubber chemicals is only necessary in specific cases, for example, for research or legal purposes.

Phenomena of aging, maturity, balance, stability, and quenching have been studied for mixtures of aroma chemicals (fragrances and flavorings). These problems limit the utility of mixes and represent an area for further study.

> **The mercapto mix may miss mercaptobenzothiazole (MBT) sensitivity.**

Naturally Occurring Mixes

In the case of balsam of Peru, a naturally occurring mix of plant origin, patients can show positive patch tests to the balsam but to none of its known allergenic constituents, suggesting that allergens as yet unknown are present in the natural product.

A relatively high patch test concentration is required because most of the material is immunologically indifferent. The allergen(s) may be unstable.

The allergen content of turpentine initially increases and then declines during storage. During the period of increase, patch test sensitization can occur. During the period of decline, false-negative reactions have been noted.

If only a small fraction of a test mixture is allergenic, the very bulk of inert material may preclude an adequate concentration. Lanolin sensitivity is best demonstrated by patch testing with wool alcohols, which contain a concentrate of the allergens.

The Paraben Mix

The name "parabens" is applied to the alkylesters, butyl, ethyl, methyl, and propyl of *p*-hydroxybenzoic acid, which are widely used as preservatives in the pharmaceutical and cosmetic industries, as well as in certain foods. The parabens are the most commonly used preservatives in dermatologic topical medicaments, drugs, dentrifrices, and suppositories.

The high incidence of cross-reactions between the esters and the frequent use of two or more esters in the same preparation makes a paraben mixture desirable for detecting hypersensitivity to any or all of them. The topical application of pharmaceuticals with high concentrations of parabens is not a prerequisite for sensitization. Repeated applications of relatively low concentrations of parabens in medicaments, proprietaries, cosmetics, and dentrifrices appear to be sufficient. Sensitivity reactions to orally ingested parabens, however, have not been reported.

The following facts concerning topical medications should be taken into consideration when treating a paraben-sensitive person:

1. Some corticosteroid ointments are paraben-free.
2. Many corticosteroid creams contain parabens.
3. Many other topical preparations contain parabens.

Some paraben-sensitive patients who develop allergic contact dermatitis when parabens are applied to eczematous skin tolerate their use on normal skin (i.e., cosmetics). It has not been established whether the following medicaments, which contain paraben, are "safe" for paraben-sensitive persons: Lidocaine hydrochloride, prednisone, Solu-Medrol and penicillin, as well as Syrup of Aristocort, Achromycin Pediatric Drops, Maalox, and Terfonyl Suspensions. *Positive weak reactions to the paraben mix should be interpreted with caution because the mixture is near the irritancy threshold for many patients. Testing with the individual paraben components should help clarify these weak responses to the mix or retesting with the mix.*

> **Positive weak reactions with the paraben mix should be interpreted with caution because the mixture is near "irritancy" in many patients.**

A SCREENING PATCH TEST KIT

The Screening Patch Test Kit, which was sold by Hermal in the United States until 1997, contained the 20 clinically common agents known to cause contact dermatitis, as specified by the North American Contact Dermatitis Group (NACDG) (Table 2.5). Many studies were based on this series, and it is included here for historical purposes.

Several allergens grouped together for the purpose of patch testing are referred to as a "test series" or "battery." The series may be general, that is, a "screening" group, or specific, such as a "therapeutic," "metal," or "rubber" series. Such groupings often overlap because the screening series may contain metals, rubber chemicals, and topical therapeutic agents that are common sensitizers. Differences between physician input and regulatory restrictions have led to a slight difference between the two widely used screening series found in Table 2.5 (North American and International Contact Dermatitis Group Series) and the T.R.U.E. test system (Table 2.5).

The Hermal screening allergens were applied on Finn chambers because allergen concentrations have been customized to this system. These shallow aluminum chambers are mounted in units of 10, 5, or single chambers on Scanpor tape. (Available from Allerderm Laboratories, P.O. Box 2070, Petaluma, CA 94953). Petrolatum-based allergens are available today from two North American sources, both in Canada (Omniderm/Pharmascience and Dormer Laboratories). Two strips of 10 patch tests are usually applied to the back of an adult patient. The T.R.U.E. test system is premounted on tape and is applied to the back, as are Finn chambers.

The allergen-petrolatum mixtures are applied directly into the Finn chambers, filling slightly more than half their volume. For the aqueous allergen mixtures, a filter paper disc (Whatman 3 MM) is placed into the chamber and saturated with the mixture. Patient patch test record sheets should be used to record the allergens tested, their position, and the test results.

During application of patch tests to the upper back, the patient should stand erect with shoulders dorsiflexed in a military "attention" posture. This allows the tape to fit tightly against the back when the patient assumes normal standing, sitting, and reclining postures. The lower portion of the test strip is adhered first; the chambers at the lower end of the tape are then fixed by pressing them from below in order to let the air escape from the chambers. Next, the top of the chambers should be pressed gently to obtain an even distribution of the allergen against the skin. The surrounding tape is then pressed against the skin. This process is repeated with each chamber, working up the back to the top of the test strip. A videotape of this process is available from the American Academy of Dermatology, 930 N. Meacham Road, Schaumburg, IL 60173-4965.

After the tests are affixed to the patient's back, the skin around the top and bottom of each strip is outlined by a Pilot Spotlighter pen. This fluoresces a bluish-white under a Wood's light. Upon removal of the Finn chamber, it is helpful to leave the top 0.5 cm of Scanpor tape adherent to the skin as a second marking device for taking delayed readings. The kit comes with a template that aligns with the markings or residual tape to identify patch test sites. The serrated edge of the template can be held against the top of the Finn chambers to keep a small rim of tape in place during removal of the bulk of the patches.

Alternative Marking Systems

Use of a marking paint to delineate the sites of the various tests at the time of test application is an essential step in the technique of testing when several hours or days elapse between the time of test removal and test reading. There is no perfect marking paint. One-half percent gentian violet solution, Castellani's paint, and similar dyestuffs are effective marking paints but permanently smudge overlying clothing. In whites, a concentrated solution of dihydroxyacetone in a mixture of water, alcohol, and acetone provides an effective brown stain that does not discolor clothing. Occasionally this paint fails completely, and it is unsuitable in dark-skinned persons. *Whatever paint is used, it should be reapplied at the time of patch test reading, and also when delayed readings are performed, so that the sites of any delayed positive tests can be identified precisely.*

Aids in Adhesion

In hot weather, extra adhesion can be obtained by spraying a pressure-sensitive silicone adhesive (Hollister Medical Adhesive No. 7730, Hollister Inc., 200 Hollister Drive, Libertyville, IL 60048) to the upper and lower exposed adhesive edges of the tape. This is rarely necessary. An extra strip of 2-in.-wide Scanpor tape is more than adequate. Patch tests should not be applied to the area directly over the vertebrae because false-positive tests from mechanical trauma can result. If one allergen is specifically suspect, it should be applied as a separate test strip so that the patient can remove the patch test if marked itching occurs. The upper arm can be used in this instance to facilitate removal.

SCREENING PATCH TEST SERIES

Some chemicals have proved to be frequent or otherwise important causes of allergic contact dermatitis. These sensitizers may be included in a "screening" patch test series. Such screening series have been variously labeled as "diagnostic," "basic," "standard" or "battery." The term "standard" should be avoided as it implies that other test materials are nonstandard. This is not the case. The proper tests must be selected based on the patient's history. Testing with a screening group of substances has proved of great value when allergic contact dermatitis is suspected and the offending agent cannot be pinpointed by careful history.

Patch test screening only supplements, never supplants, patch testing with suspected environmental agents. *No screening series could ever encompass the many allergens encountered in cosmetics, in industry, and in gardening.*

Screening by a series of patch tests revealed that as many as one-half of all cases of contact dermatitis may be caused or complicated by an allergic contact sensitivity. Hence, patch testing may be a useful procedure for the investigation of any case of dermatitis. The examination is useful as a guide to substances that should be avoided to reduce the risk of a relapse.

New sensitizing chemicals and products are introduced regularly into the environment. Hence, the selection of substances for a screening test series cannot be rigidly defined. Constant revision and additions are needed to adapt the standard series to the sensitivities currently most prevalent in the populations served by any particular clinic.

A positive patch test reaction to one or more substances in the screening series gives the physician and the patient a lead to investigate and may help to determine in retrospect how contact could possibly have been made with the substance that produced the positive patch test reaction. It enables the physician to investigate the possibility that the dermatitis was produced by a chemical that cross-reacts with the substance that produced the reaction. Thus, a positive patch test reaction to paraphenylenediamine not only may incriminate the dye itself but also may alert the physician to the possibility that a group of immunochemically related substances, such as local anesthetics and other chemicals, which have an amino group in the "para" position, may have to be investigated.

PATCH TEST READING AND INTERPRETATION

Reading the Test Results

At each test reading, it is traditional to note the result as negative or positive, and grade the positive results on a quantitative scale. The International Contact Dermatitis

TABLE 2.6. *Interpretation Key*

?	*doubtful* reaction; faint macular erythema only
+	*weak* (nonvesicular) positive reaction; erythema, infiltration, possibly papules
++	*strong* (vesicular) positive reaction; erythema, infiltration, papules, vesicles
+++	*extreme* positive reaction; bullous reaction
−	*negative* reaction
IR	*irritant* reaction of different types
NT	*not tested*

Research Group has recommended a 1+ to 3+ scoring system, with 1+ representing erythema and edema; 2+ representing erythema, edema, and vesicles; and 3+ representing a very severe reaction. Weak and questionable reactions are recorded by a question mark. Irritant reactions are recorded as IR. When the reactions are to be computer codes, the designations are as follows: 1+ = 1; 2+ = 2; 3+ = 3; doubtful = 4; irritant = 5; and negative = 6. This convention is followed by the North American Contact Dermatitis Group and has been adopted by T.R.U.E. test also. The important point in evaluating a positive test response, however, is not how many pluses one should assign to the test response but whether it is a true positive result caused by allergy or a nonspecific irritant reaction. Irritant reactions, also known as false-positive tests, are the bane of patch testing.

Patch test reactions may have features of more than one category. A doubtful reaction is a macular erythema that may not confluently fill the area of the patch test but is sustained beyond a day 2 reading. This level of intensity may represent mild irritancy or weak allergy whether or not the response is confluent. Because the patch test is a bioassay, the point at which irritancy ends or weak allergy begins in any one individual may overlap the contrary reactions in another individual. Only by clinical correlation can the distinction be sorted out; even then, it cannot be done in all cases because there are no *absolute* criteria to morphologically distinguish macular erythema of allergic etiology from that of irritant etiology. If erythema is palpable, accompanied by edema, and covers at least 50% of the patch test site, it is scored 1+. This is considered a morphologic grade in which allergy is probable, although some irritant reactions may still encroach on this level of reactivity. A Janus reaction incorporates both doubtful and 1+ levels of reactivity and gives recognition to the uncertainty associated with this level of response. When papules (microvesicles) occupy up to 50% of the patch test surface, a 2+ reaction is appropriate; however, if greater than 50% of the surface is vesicular or bullous, the reaction is scored 3+. Spreading reactions that are not secondary to overfilling of chambers are by definition scored 3+. Irritant reactions are rare with the standard allergens, but 1+ reactions are commonly encountered and are the most difficult to interpret (Table 2.6).

Distinguishing between Irritant and Allergic Patch Test Responses

Whereas many textbooks indicate that one can reliably decide whether a patch test response is irritant or allergic upon morphologic grounds, in actual practice the morphology of the patch test response is a poor guide to whether the response is allergic or irritant. When the patch test reaction is very strong, it is usually possible to differentiate the sharply demarcated, promptly healing, "burnlike" irritant reaction from the spreading, more slowly disappearing, eczematous reaction to an allergen. Unfortunately, whereas the criteria for distinguishing between irritant and allergic patch test responses are of some value when the patch test is strongly positive, they are of *absolutely no value* when the physician is confronted with a relatively weak reaction. *There is no morphologic way to distinguish a weak irritant patch test from a weak allergic test.*

SUPPLIERS OF PATCH TESTING MATERIALS

1. Screening Series Allergens
   T.R.U.E. Test
   Distributed by Glaxo Dermatology
   Five Moore Drive
   P.O. Box 13438
   Research Triangle Park, NC 27709
   Hermal Kurt Herrmann
   Patch Test Allergens
   P.O. Box 1228
   D-2057 Reinbek bei Hamburg
   Germany
   OmniDerm/Pharmascience (suppliers of Hermal allergens)
   6111 Royalmount Street, Suite 100
   Montreal, Quebec H4P 2T4
   Canada; Tel: (514) 340-1114
   Dormer Laboratories (supplier of Chemotechnique allergens)
   91 Kelfield, Suite 5
   Rexdale, Ontario M9W 5A3
   Canada
   E-mail: www.dormer.com; Tel: (416) 242-6167
   Chemotechnique Diagnostics AB
   Ringugnsgatan 7
   S-216 16 Malmö
   Sweden
2. Patch Testing Devices
   Finn Chambers on Scanpor
   Allerderm Labs
   P.O. Box 2070
   Petaluma, CA 94953
3. Patch Test Adhesive Tapes
   Scanpor Tape
   Allerderm Labs (see above)

Blenderm
3M Company (consult your local surgical supply)
4. Black Light Eastern Division of Spectronics
Westbury, Long Island, New York
Model BLF 6
5. Uni-Solve Adhesive Remover
(Active ingredients 1,1,1, trichloroethane)
United, Division of Howmedica, Inc.
11775 Starkey Road
Largo, FL 33540
6. Hollister Adhesive Remover
No. 7731, 6-oz spray can (contains a fluorocarbon)
Distributed by Hollister, Inc.
211 East Chicago Avenue
Chicago, IL 60611
7. Detachol
Ferndale Laboratories
780 West Eight Mile Road
Ferndale, MI 48220

ADDITIONAL FREQUENTLY USED TEST SUBSTANCES*

1. *Diazolinidyl urea 1% pet and 1% aq.* Both vehicles of this formaldehyde-releasing preservative are used, as cases may be missed by using only one.
2. *DMDM hydrantoin 1% pet and 1% aq.* Both vehicles of this formaldehyde-releasing preservative are tested, as noted in 1 above.
3. *Imidazolidinyl urea 1% pet.* The Hermal screening series includes 1% aq of this formaldehyde-releasing allergen; the additional vehicle detects additional cases.
4. *2-bromo-2-nitropropane-1,3-diol 0.5% pet.* This is another formaldehyde-releasing preservative.
5. *Ethyleneurea nelamine formaldehyde 5% pet.* This textile permanent press finish completes the formaldehyde-related allergens used for screening purposes.
6. *Methyldibromo glutaronitrile 0.4% pet and 2% methyldibromo glutaronitrile/phenoxythanol (Euxyl K400).* This is a preservative, and the ideal concentration is not presently known; both are used to try to determine whether relevant cases are missed by the lower concentrations. Janus reactions were commonly seen at 2.5% Euxyl K400.
7. *Chloroxylenol (PCMX) 1% pet.* A preservative.
8. *Methylchloroisothiazolinone/methylisothiazolinone 100 ppm aq.* A preservative also known as Kathon CG.
9. *Paraben mix 12% pet.* A preservative screening agent.
10. *Iodopropyryl butylcarbamate 0.1% pet.* A preservative.
11. *Thimerosal 0.1% pet.* A perservative also known as merthrolate.
12. *Bacitracin 20% pet.* A topical antibiotic.

*May be obtained from: OmniDerm/Pharmascience or Dormer Laboratories (see above)

13. *Glutaral 1% pet.* An antiseptic better known as glutaraldehyde.
14. *Fragrance mix 8% pet.* Added to balsam of Peru (Myroxylon Perelrae), forms a complete fragrance/perfume screening series.
15. *Mixed dialkyl thioareas 1% pet.* The rubber allergen is associated with neoprene.
16. *Cobalt chloride 1% pet.* Added to detect isolated cobalt allergy–absent nickel allergy.
17. *Gold sodium thiosulfate 0.5% pet.* Considered the best screening substance for gold allergy.
18. *Sesquiterpene/lactone mix 0.1% pet.* Screens for Compositae allergy.
19. *Propylene glycol 30% aq.* An excipient screening agent.
20. *Benzophenone-3 3% pet.* Also known as oxybenzone, this sunscreen is sometimes also used as a preservative.
21. *Ethyl acrylate 0.1% pet.* Screens for acrylate sensitivity, especially artificial fingernails.
22. *Methyl methacrylate 2% pet.* Screens for acrylate sensitivity.
23. *Tosylamide formaldehyde resin 10% pet.* Formerly known as toluene formaldehyde sulfonamide resin, this screens for fingernail polish allergy.
24. *Glyceryl thioglycolate 1% pet.* This was known as glyceryl monothioglycolate and screens for sensitivity to permanent waves of the acid type.
25. *Tixocortol-21-pivalate 1% pet.* This screens for Group A corticosteroid allergy.
26. *Budesonide 0.1% pet.* This screens for corticosteroid allergy in Groups B and D.
27. *Amidoamine 0.1% aq.* This is thought to be the allergenic fraction of cocamidopropyl betaine, a common shampoo and liquid soap ingredient.

REFERENCES

1. Kieffer M. Nickel sensitivity: relationship between history and patch test reaction. *Contact Dermatitis* 1979;5:398.
2. Rietschel RL. Is patch testing cost-effective? *J Am Acad Dermatol* 1989;21:885.
3. Rajagopalan R, Kallal JE, Fowler JF Jr, Sherertz EF. A retrospective evaluation of patch testing in patients diagnosed with allergic contact dermatitis. *Cutis* 1996;57:360.
4. Evans AS. Causation and disease: the Henle-Koch postulates revisited. *Yale J Biol Med* 1976;49:175.
5. Memon AA, Friedmann PS. 'Angry back syndrome': a non-reproducible phenomenon. *Br J Dermatol* 1996;135:924.
6. Bjornberg A. Increased skin reactivity to primary irritants provoked by hand eczema. *Arch Dermatol Forsch* 1974;249:389.
7. Roper SS, Jones HE. An animal model for altering the irritability threshold of normal skin. *Contact Dermatitis* 1985;13:91.
8. Hannuksela M, Salo H. The repeated open application test (ROAT). *Contact Dermatitis* 1986;14:221.
9. Fischer T, Rystedt I. False-positive, follicular and irritant patch test reactions to metal salts. *Contact Dermatitis* 1985;12:93.
10. Rietschel RL. Mechanisms in irritant contact dermatitis. *Clin Dermatol* 1997;15:557.
11. Morhenn VB, Chang E-Y, Rheins LA. A noninvasive method for quantifying and distinguishing inflammatory skin reactions. *J Am Acad Dermatol* 1999;41:687.

12. Cohen DE, Brancaccio R, Andersen D, Belsito DV. Utility of a standard allergen series alone in the evaluation of allergic contact dermatitis: a retrospective study of 732 patients. *J Am Acad Dermatol* 1997;36(6 Pt 1):914.

13. Larkin A, Rietschel RL. The utility of patch tests using larger screening series of allergens. *Am J Contact Dermat* 1998;9:142.

14. Rietschel RL, et al. The case for patch test readings beyond day 2. *J Am Acad Dermatol* 1988;18:42.

15. Sukanto H, et al. Influence of topically applied corticosteroids on patch test reactions. *Contact Dermatitis* 1981;7:180.

16. Clark RA, Rietschel RL. 0.1% triamcinolone acetonide ointment and patch test responses. *Arch Dermatol* 1982;118:163.

17. Rietschel RL. Irritant and allergic responses as influenced by triamcinolone in patch test materials. *Arch Dermatol* 1985;121:68.

18. Bruze M, Hedman H, Bjorkner B, Moller H. The development and course of test reactions to gold sodium thiosulfate. *Contact Dermatitis* 1995;33:386.

19. Agrup G. Sensitization induced by patch testing. *Br J Dermatol* 1968;80:631.

20. Cronin F. Clinical prediction of patch tests. *Trans St. John's Hosp Dermatol Soc* 1972;58:153.

21. Mitchell JC. The angry back syndrome: Eczema creates eczema. *Contact Dermatitis* 1975;1:193.

22. Meneghini CL, et al. A propos de réactions de sensibilisation active après l'execution des tests diagnostiques picutanes: observations sur 281 cas. [Active sensitization reactions after execution of diagnostic epicutaneous tests: 281 cases.] *Annales de Dermatologie et de Syphiliographie* 1972;99:161.

23. Meneghini CL, Angelini G. Behaviour of contact allergy and new sensitivities on subsequent patch tests. *Contact Dermatitis* 1977;3:138.

24. Adams RM. Patch testing—a recapitulation. *J Am Acad Dermatol* 1981;5:637.

25. Malten KE, et al. Patch testing guidelines. Mijnegen, Dekker & van de Begt, 1976.

26. Calnan CD. The use and abuse of patch tests. In: Maibach HI, Gellin GA, eds. *Occupational and Industrial Dermatology.* Chicago: Year Book Medical Publishers, 1982.

27. Mitchell JC. Angry back syndrome [letter]. *Contact Dermatitis* 1981;7:359.

28. Mitchell J. Multiple concomitant positive patch test reactions. *Contact Dermatitis* 1977;3:315.

29. Maibach HI. The ESS-excited skin syndrome (alias the "angry back"). In: Ring J, Burg G, eds. *New Trends in Allergy.* Berlin: Springer-Verlag, 1981.

30. Mitchell JC, Maibach HI. The angry back syndrome—the excited skin syndrome. *Semin Dermatol* 1982;1:9.

31. Gollhausen R, Przybilla B, Ring J. Reproducibility of patch tests. *J Am Acad Dermatol* 1989;21:1196.

32. Gollhausen R, Przybilla B, Ring J. Reproducibility of patch test results: comparison of TRUE Test and Finn Chamber test results. *J Am Acad Dermatol* 1989;21(4 Pt 2):843.

33. Ayala F, Balato N, Lembo G, et al. Statistical evaluation of the persistence of acquired hypersensitivity by standardized patch tests. *Contact Dermatitis* 1996;34:354.

34. Hindsen M, Bruze M, Christensen OB. The significance of previous allergic contact dermatitis for elicitation of delayed hypersensitivity to nickel. *Contact Dermatitis* 1997;37:101.

35. Rietschel RL. Stochastic resonance and angry back syndrome: noisy skin. *Am J Contact Dermat* 1996;7:152.

36. Magnusson B, Hellgren L. Skin irritating and adhesive characteristics of some different tapes. *Acta Derm Venereol* 1962;42:463.

37. Maibach H, et al. Quantification of the excited skin syndrome (the 'angry back'): Retesting one patch at a time. *Contact Dermatitis* 1982;8:78.

38. Bandmann HJ, Agathos M. New results and some remarks to the "angry back syndrome." *Contact Dermatitis* 1981;7:23.

39. Bruynzeel DP, et al. The angry back syndrome—a retrospective study. *Contact Dermatitis* 1981;7:293.

40. Mitchell JC. Patch testing with mixes. *Contact Dermatitis* 1981;7:98.

CHAPTER 3

Predictive Testing for Human Contact Dermatitis

The factors that create the sensitizing potential of a chemical, such as molecular weight, charge, and electrophilic potential, are unique to that chemical. However, a structural analysis of the chemical rarely gives a clue to its sensitizing potential. This is probably because of the complex and poorly understood genetic factors required for sensitization and is related to T-lymphocyte cell surface-receptor expression of the genetic code. It has been estimated that 50% to 70% of the United States population is capable of sensitization to *toxicodendron,* given an adequate sensitizing exposure, but about 30% are genetically incapable of responding regardless of exposure (antigen-specific tolerance) (1). Few compounds rival *toxicodendron* for both sensitizing potential on a chemical basis and abundance of environmental exposures—so much of this potential can be recognized as poison ivy, poison oak, and poison sumac.

Expression of the sensitizing potential of a chemical is restricted by the circumstances of exposure. This has been studied extensively for the preservative methylchloroisothiazolinone/methylisothiazolinone (MCI/MI) (2). The potential of MCI/MI to sensitize at concentrations of 100 to 250 ppm from a single exposure in a closed 48-hour patch test attests to a considerable potential for sensitization. This potential is not always expressed, because this biocide is extremely effective at low concentrations (15 ppm or less); thus, the question arises whether this potential will be recognized in normal use. The answer appears to be dependent on the type of skin exposed to MCI/MI. Application to eczematous skin of products that contain no more than 12.5 ppm appears to be capable of producing sensitizing reactions (3). Similar products applied to normal skin may also produce sensitizing reactions, but products intended for skin application that are subsequently washed off, such as shampoo and liquid soap, were found to pose virtually no problem. This was true even when patients known to be patch test sensitive to MCI/MI bathed in products preserved with 15 ppm MCI/MI (4). This points out the importance of intended skin use, use concentration, duration of skin contact, and type of skin in the assessment of the risk of skin sensitization. These factors, as well as the human genetic variable, make the process of predicting sensitization risk difficult and complex.

> **Expression of cutaneous allergy is dependent on genetic factors, circumstances of exposure (such as concentration and duration of skin contact), and the allergenic potential of the chemical itself.**

THE PATCH TEST CLINIC AS A SOURCE OF EPIDEMIOLOGIC PERSPECTIVE ON SENSITIZATION

Historically, groups of dermatologists have pooled their collective data on the frequency with which positive patch tests occur in patients seeking diagnostic evaluation of persistent or new-onset dermatitis. The frequency of positive tests depends on the knowledge and skill of the clinician, as well as societal or environmental factors, referral patterns, health care systems, and other confounding variables. This type of data can be used to gather clinical insight but cannot be used for epidemiologic purposes. Ability to accurately predict what is occurring in a population requires proper epidemiologic methods (5). When Prystowsky et al. (6) compared the prevalence of ethylenediamine and benzocaine sensitization in a random sample of the population to patch test clinic data, the true prevalence in the population was 10 to 30 times less than expected.

> **The frequency of allergic reactions in patch-tested patients does not predict accurately the frequency with which allergy is occurring in society at large.**

The database for patch test clinic data is historically large, whereas population-based studies are few. Efforts to define the difference between "strong" and "weak" sensitizers have used a 1% threshold from patch test clinic data as a crude guide. That is, if more than 1% of patients test positive in response to a substance, it is deemed a "strong" sensitizer (7). What, then, becomes of materials thought to be sensitizers, which are routinely tested but found positive in less than 1% of patients tested? Are these nonsensitizers or "weak" sensitizers? Or is it the current usage pattern of a product that is increasing or decreasing and thus truly responsible for the number of patients identified in patch test clinics?

For example, in the early 1970s, parabens were found to have sensitized greater than 1% of tested patients, as evaluated by the North American Contact Dermatitis Group (NACDG) (3% of 1,200 patients tested) (8). In the 1980s, the NACDG did not include parabens in its routine screening series of allergens because it had been concluded that most paraben sensitivity occurred in the presence of stasis dermatitis (9). Did the sensitizing potential of parabens change? It is more likely that the sample drawn from clinic-based patch test data rather than from population-based data will always show this type of variation and cannot be used to accurately gauge the sensitizing potential of a substance, even on a scale as simple as "strong" versus "weak."

> **Comparisons of patch test clinic data from different centers is meaningless unless corrected for factors such as age, sex, occupation, climate, and usage patterns of products.**

The same phenomena were recently seen with patch test clinic-based reports of the prevalence of sensitivity to MCI/MI. Patients were reported to have anywhere from 1% to 16% frequency of positive reactions to MCI/MI. A critical analysis of these findings revealed an inverse linear correlation between the "prevalence" and the log size of the population tested (10). The sample sizes used to generate the reports did not provide sufficient reliability, nor were study groups matched for age, sex, occupation, usage, or climate. Because patch test clinic data do not report on the same group of patients tested sequentially, the finding may reflect different percentages of varying occupations or similar factors in the study population. One obvious example of the importance of controlling such variables is the degree to which nickel sensitivity is found in patch test clinics. Sound epidemiologic studies have repeatedly and overwhelmingly found nickel allergy to be a female allergen (10:1) (11). Nickel allergy is found in patch test clinic "epidemiologic" reports of from 4% of 2,897 tested (12) to 16% of 4,500 patients tested (13). Without correcting for the proportion of women (or other important variables) in the two separate trials, comparison of these figures becomes meaningless.

The importance of the use of proper epidemiologic methods is required if we are to assess the potency of a sensitizer. We cannot rely solely on data derived from patients in patch test clinics. This type of information can only be used as a guide to more carefully controlled studies that address relevant variables appropriate to the material in question. Does the population at risk have intact skin or eczematous skin? Is the duration of contact an issue? What concentrations will be encountered in actual use?

LIMITS OF PREDICTIVE TESTING

A great deal of predictive patch testing is performed on populations likely to be exposed to the products under scrutiny. Sample size immediately becomes an issue; as the mathematical calculations of Henderson and Riley (14) have shown, at the 95% confidence interval there may be no reactions detected in a sample size of 200 subjects, but up to 15 of every 1,000 in the general population might still be sensitized. If the confidence limits were increased to 99% without a change in sample size, 22 of every 1,000 could still react. If only one member of a panel of 200 is sensitized, we can state with 95% confidence that between 1 and 275 of every 10,000 subjects would be sensitized. Because panel sizes of 200 humans are commonly used in such tests as the modified Draize test, these limitations must be borne in mind when results are discussed.

ANIMAL TESTING

Although the thrust of this chapter is human testing, it is helpful to know some of the common methods used for screening and preclinical work. The United States Environmental Protection Agency (EPA) recognizes seven methods of animal testing as acceptable for use under the Toxic Substances Control Act (15). These are the Buehler method, the open epicutaneous test, the guinea pig maximization test (GPMT), the split adjuvant technique, Freund's complete adjuvant test, the Maurer optimization test, and the footpad technique (16). The GPMT has been adopted by the OECD Test Guideline 406 along with the local lymph-node assay (LLNA) as a screen for sensitization. This in effect has created a worldwide standard. However, to eliminate laboratory variation, the guideline stipulates that three sensitizers be used and demonstrated as positive to show proficiency in performing the tests. These three chosen standards are hexyl cinnamic aldehyde, mercaptobenzothiazole, and benzocaine. The first two of these perform well in both the GPMT and the LLNA, but widely divergent results are obtained with benzocaine. In the GPMT, 0% to 60% of animals were positive, and in the LLNA 12 tests in two laboratories only occasionally found positive results (17).

The guinea pig maximization test bears comment. The method uses Freund's complete adjuvant to facilitate a heightened immune response to the test substance (18). To further augment the opportunity for sensitization, 10% sodium lauryl sulfate (SLS) is applied in conjunction with the test substance if the substance fails to produce irritation by

TABLE 3.1. *Degree of Sensitization in Different Phases of Animal Testing*

Percentage of animals sensitized	Sensitizer grade	Class
0–8	Weak	I
9–28	Mild	II
29–64	Moderate	III
65–80	Strong	IV
81–100	Extreme	V

TABLE 3.2. *Human Sensitizer Risk Assessment Variables*

- Normal versus dermatitic skin
- Vehicle effects on absorption
- Percutaneous absorption variables such as body site
- Open or occluded use
- Leave-on or rinse-off exposure
- Duration of skin contact
- Frequency of skin exposure
- Use concentration

itself on day 7 of the test. After a rest period, the animals are challenged. Usually 20 to 25 animals are used in each phase of the test, and the degree of sensitization is assessed, as shown in Table 3.1. Efforts have been made to improve on the predictive value of the GPMT by focusing on the minimum induction concentration that induces a positive response and comparing the challenge concentrations that produce a standardized reaction intensity with the highest concentration for induction. This correlated well with allergen levels in causative products in human cases of contact dermatitis (19).

EXTRAPOLATING TO HUMANS

Maurer (20) has equated strong sensitizing capacity with a frequency of 100 individuals sensitized per 100,000 population and weak allergy with a frequency of 10 per 100,000. He believes that adjuvant-enhanced animal models like the GPMT can detect most weak sensitizers, leaving compounds with allergenicity in the 1:10,000 range as those expected to enter the marketplace. It is generally recognized that the incidence of sensitization will never be zero. Animal tests that do not employ adjuvant are less sensitive for allergen screening. These animal tests are useful guides but

still do not address the issues of concentration to be employed in finished products where skin contact is intended or inevitable, contact time, vehicle and solubility, or penetration of human stratum corneum. It is generally acknowledged that hexavalent chromium is a sensitizer and potential hazard, whereas trivalent chromium is less soluble and thus frequently behaves as a nonsensitizer, because it fails to penetrate human stratum corneum (21). These factors are required if an evaluation of the sensitizing potential of a substance is to become a human risk assessment (Table 3.2).

> "Strong" allergens sensitize about 100 of every 100,000 in the general population, whereas "weak" allergens sensitize about 10 per 100,000.

According to Cronin and Agrup (22), human test panels have statistical limitations. In order to ensure with a confidence limit of 99.5% that no more than 0.1% of a population would be sensitized, a human panel of 5,300 subjects would have to be tested. This would still be 10 times more people sensitized than if screening were done with adjuvant

TABLE 3.3. *Modified Draize and Human Maximization Tests*

Substance	Human predictive test sensitized/tested	Percentage sensitized by patch test clinic data (NACDG)[b]
Formaldehyde	4.5%–7.8%/331	4
Parabens	0.3%/397	3
p-paraphenylenediamine	53%/NA	8
Balsam of Peru	28%/25[a]	3.2–4.5
Nickel	48%/25[a]	11
Chromium	48%/23	8
Ammoniated mercury	59%/74[a]	5
Neomycin	28%/25[a]	6
Thiuram	16%/25[a]	4
Benzocaine	6%/99	
	22%/23[a]	5
Ethylenediamine	8%/61	7

[a]Indicates human maximization test. All others are from modified Draize test. Summarized from Marzulli, FN, Maibach HI. Predictive testing in humans for contact allergy. In: Fisher AA, ed. *Contact dermatitis.* 3rd ed. Philadelphia: Lea & Febiger, 1986;30–44.
[b]NACDG, North American Contact Dermatitis Group.

animal testing. The customary human panel consists of about 200 subjects.

The most commonly cited human predictive tests are the modified Draize test and the maximization test. In the modified Draize test, a high concentration of 0.5 mL or 0.5 g of material is suspended in petrolatum applied to the arm with occlusive bandages for 48 hours on 10 occasions. After 2 weeks' rest, a nonirritant concentration is applied to a new site for 72 hours (23). The human maximization test usually uses 25 volunteers instead of the 200 used for the modified Draize test (24). For the maximization test, 1 mL of 5% SLS followed by 1 mL of 25% test substance in petrolatum is applied to the arm on Webril, a type of gauze, and occluded with Blenderm tape. First, the SLS is applied for 24 hours; then the subject undergoes five successive 48-hour challenges of the SLS-treated site followed by a 10-day rest. The challenge for elicitation of sensitization is performed at a different site on the back. The skin is pretreated with 0.4 mL of 10% SLS for 1 hour, followed 24 hours later by 0.4 mL of test material at 10% concentration for 48 hours.

Some sample results of common patch test allergens evaluated by "predictive" methods, such as the modified Draize and human maximization tests, are seen in Table 3.3 (25).

Most substances commonly employed for diagnostic patch test purposes would be labeled as sensitizers by such predictive tests, but the frequency with which these materials are found in patch test clinics indicates the importance of the variables seen in Table 3.1. Sensitizers that affect 10 to 100 persons per 100,000 are generally identifiable with current methodology.

REFERENCES

1. Lampe KF. Cutaneous toxicology. In: Drill VA, Lazar P, eds. New York: Raven Press, 1984.
2. Rietschel RL, et al. Methylchloroisothiazolinone-methylisothiazolinone reactions in patients screened for vehicle and preservative hypersensitivity. *J Am Acad Dermatol* 1990;22:734.
3. de Groot AC, Liem DH, Weyland JW, Kathron CG. Cosmetic allergy and patch test sensitization. *Contact Dermatitis* 1985;12:76.
4. Weaver JE, Cardin CW, Maibach HI. Dose-response assessments of Kathron biocide (I). Diagnostic use and diagnostic threshold patch testing with sensitized humans. *Contact Dermatitis* 1985;12:141.
5. Allen AM. Use and misuse of "epidemiology" [Letter]. *Arch Dermatol* 1974;110:131.
6. Prystowsky SD, et al. Allergic contact hypersensitivity to nickel, neomycin, ethylenediamine and benzocaine: relationships between age, sex, history of exposure, and reactivity to standard patch tests and use tests in a general population. *Arch Dermatol* 1979;115:959.
7. Meneghini CL, Rantuccio F, Lomuto A. Additives, vehicles and active drugs of topical medicaments as causes of delayed type allergic dermatitis. *Dermatologica* 1971;143:137.
8. North American Contact Dermatitis Group. Epidemiology of contact dermatitis in North America: 1972. *Arch Dermatol* 1973;108:537.
9. Nethercott JR, et al. Patch testing with a routine screening tray in North America, 1985 through 1989: frequency of response. *Am J Contact Dermatitis* 1991;2:122.
10. Shuster S. Patch-test sensitivity and reproducibility in individuals and populations. *Am J Contact Dermatitis* 1992;3:74.
11. Menné T, Christopherson J, Green A. Epidemiology of nickel dermatitis. In: Maibach HI, Menné T, eds. *Nickel and the skin: immunology and toxicology.* Boca Raton, FL: CRC Press, 1989.
12. Korossy S. Zur Epidemiologie der allergischen Kontakt Dermatitis in Ungarn. *Dermatosen* 1978;27:119.
13. Husain SL. Contact dermatitis in the west of Scotland. *Contact Dermatitis* 1977;3:327.
14. Henderson CR, Riley EC. Certain statistical considerations in patch testing. *J Invest Dermatol* 1945;6:227.
15. Health Effects Test Guidelines. EPA 560/6–82–001. Washington, DC: Office of Pesticides and Toxic Substances, U.S. Environmental Protection Agency, 1982.
16. Henningsen GM. Dermal hypersensitivity: immunologic principles and current methods of assessment. In: Hubson DW, ed. *Dermal and ocular toxicology fundamentals and methods.* Boca Raton, FL: CRC Press, 1991;153.
17. Basketter DA, Scholes EW, Wahlkvist H, Montelius J. An evaluation of the suitability of benzocaine as a positive control skin sensitizer. *Contact Dermatitis* 1995;33:28.
18. Magnusson B, Kligman AM. The identification of contact allergens by animal assay. The guinea pig maximization test. *J Invest Dermatol* 1969;52:268.
19. Nakamura A, et al. A new protocol and criteria for quantitative determination of sensitization potencies of chemicals by guinea pig maximization test. *Contact Dermatitis* 1994:31:72.
20. Maurer T. *Contact and photocontact allergens: a manual of predictive test methods.* New York: Marcel Dekker, 1983.
21. Burrows D. Adverse chromate reactions on the skin. In: Burrows D, ed. *Chromium metabolism and toxicity.* Boca Raton, FL: CRC Press, 1983:137.
22. Cronin E, Agrup G. Contact dermatitis C. *Br J Dermatol* 1970;82:428.
23. Marzulli FN, Maibach HI. Contact allergy: predictive testing in man. *Contact Dermatitis* 1976;2:1.
24. Kligman AM. The identification of contact allergens by human assay. III. The maximization test: a procedure for screening and rating contact sensitizers. *J Invest Dermatol* 1966;47:393.
25. Marzulli FN, Maibach HI. Predictive testing in humans for contact allergy in contact dermatitis. In: Fisher AA, ed. *Contact dermatitis.* 3rd ed. Philadelphia: Lea & Febiger, 1986;30–45.

CHAPTER 4

Histology of Contact Dermatitis

Contact dermatitis is normally differentiated from other types of dermatitis on the basis of clinical findings, knowledge of exposure to potential allergens or irritants, and diagnostic patch testing. The histopathology of contact dermatitis shows much overlap with that of the other forms of dermatitis and is, therefore, not usually helpful in distinguishing the various forms of dermatitis. Both irritant (ICD) and allergic contact dermatitis (ACD), however, have certain histopathologic features that may at times add weight to the evidence in favor of the diagnosis.

HISTOLOGY OF ACD

Cutaneous changes viewed by light microscopy are dependent on two factors, severity of the response to an allergen and time of biopsy after allergen exposure. Severity of the response in turn is dependent on both the potency of the allergen and the degree of immunologic sensitivity of the affected individual.

Biopsies of experimentally induced ACD (e.g., to 1% dinitrochlorobenzene [DNCB]) show changes as early as 4 to 8 hours after allergen application (1). The earliest change noted is the appearance of a few lymphocytes perivascularly in the dermis. By 6 to 8 hours, some lymphocytes migrate into the epidermis as the dermal infiltrate increases. Also at about 6 to 8 hours, focal spongiosis (intercellular edema) in the malpighian and basal layers occurs. Both of these findings peak at 24 to 48 hours after application. A study comparing punch biopsies from allergic patch tests (quaternium-15 or colophony) with irritant patch tests (benzalkonium chloride) demonstrated follicular spongiosis in six of seven allergic reactions but only one of seven irritant reactions (2). Vesiculation occurs when the focal areas of spongiosis coalesce. With severe reactions, an occasional neutrophil may be seen, but this is rare in comparison to ICD. Eosinophils may be found in both the dermis and the epidermis and, if present, suggest ACD rather than another form of dermatitis. Starting at about 24 hours, and perhaps even earlier, basophils begin to appear. They may comprise up to 15% of the infiltrate by day 3, at which time tissue mast cells begin to increase in number. Whereas basophils enter the site from the blood, mast cells are formed by local replication, accounting for their delayed appearance. Other changes within the 24- to 48-hour time frame may include increased vascular permeability resulting in rare erythrocyte extravasation and dermal papillary edema, as well as fibrin deposition in the reticular dermis. After 48 to 72 hours, the activity of inflammation subsides. Rebuilding and "cleanup" processes occur with infiltration of macrophages needed for removal of keratinocyte debris (3).

In contrast to the above experimentally derived data, biopsy of suspected contact dermatitis in the clinical setting usually occurs days or even months after onset. In this case, a pattern of subacute or chronic dermatitis may be seen, which may be impossible to distinguish from nummular dermatitis or lichen simplex chronicus (4). The inflammatory infiltrate, again primarily lymphocytes and other mononuclear cells, is less prominent and, in fact, may be absent from the epidermis. In the dermis, a perivascular pattern is likely. Mild spongiosis and microvesicle formation may be seen, but these changes may be absent in long-standing dermatitis. Chronically, acanthosis with hyperkeratosis and some parakeratosis may be seen. Apparent intracellular edema may actually be due to glycogen distribution. Upper dermal fibrosis may occur as the result of thickened collagen.

HISTOLOGY OF ICD

Experimentally induced irritant contact dermatitis gives a very different histopathologic picture as compared to ACD when biopsies are taken during the first day or two following exposure. This would be expected because in ICD the epidermal damage is caused directly by the toxic agent, whereas in ACD the damage is due to the host's immune reactions. Although it varies with the strength and type of irritant, ICD generally develops much more quickly than ACD (5). Within a few hours of exposure to a moderately strong irritant such as 10% DNCB, dermo-epidermal separation begins. By 24 hours, epidermal necrosis is observed, often with subepidermal blister formation (1). Lymphocytes are relatively rare in either the dermis or the epidermis. In contrast, the bulk of the inflammatory infiltrate is made up of neutrophils, which first appear within 6 to 8 hours of exposure. In guinea pigs, Anderson (6) has shown that basophils are much more plentiful in early allergic as opposed to irritant reactions. Although presumably all allergens induce a similar immune response, different irritants produce different histologic findings, depending on their mechanism of cell damage. For example, after 48 hours the cytotoxic agent dithranol produced a balloon degeneration of the upper dermis with disruption of mitochondria, whereas the detergent sodium lauryl sulfate induced parakeratosis and intracytoplasmic vesicles and lipid vacuoles.

Unfortunately, these differences between early ACD and ICD are rarely of clinical benefit because biopsies within the first few days of onset are usually unavailable. The histologic findings of a chronic low-grade ICD may be identical to those described above for ACD. Although by no means pathognomonic, the presence of eosinophils might suggest ACD, whereas the absence of exocytosis of lymphocytes might suggest ICD.

DIFFERENTIATING CONTACT DERMATITIS FROM OTHER DERMATOSES

At times, biopsy may shed light on a confusing clinical picture to help determine if the diagnosis is within the broad category of dermatitis as opposed to some other entity. Acute ICD or ACD, for example, may be simulated by bullous impetigo or a viral vesicular eruption such as herpes. The histologic pattern of these conditions would be readily distinguished from contact dermatitis. Contact urticaria or urticarial vasculitis can likewise be suggested by biopsy examination. Persistent or "dermal" contact dermatitis may be differentiated histologically from infiltrative processes such as rosacea, sarcoid, or cutaneous T-cell lymphoma. Generalized ACD, as sometimes seen in formaldehyde allergy, for example, can be histologically separated from erythroderma due to psoriasis, a drug reaction, or Sézary syndrome. The histopathology of these other conditions is beyond the scope of this text and is thoroughly reviewed in texts on that subject.

UNUSUAL HISTOLOGIC PATTERNS OF CONTACT DERMATITIS

Occasional cases of ACD, either systemic or exogenous, may show histologic and clinical patterns simulating other diseases. These include erythema multiforme, vasculitis, and granuloma formation (7). These rare variants are reviewed in the chapters covering the allergens involved.

REFERENCES

1. Medenica M, Rostenberg A. A comparative light and electron microscopic study of primary irritant contact dermatitis and allergic contact dermatitis. *J Invest Dermatol* 1971;56:259–271.
2. Vestergaard L, Clemmensen O, Sorensen F, Andersen K. Histologic distinction between early allergic and irritant patch test reactions: follicular spongiosis may be characteristic of early allergic contact dermatitis. *Contact Dermatitis* 1999;41:207–210.
3. Dvorak H, Mihm M, Dvorak A. Morphology of delayed-type hypersensitivity reactions in man. *J Invest Dermatol* 1976;67:391–401.
4. Lever WF, Schaumburg-Lever G. *Histopathology of the skin.* 7th ed. Philadelphia: WB Saunders, 1990:106–110.
5. Willis C, Stephens C, Wilkinson J. Epidermal damage induced by irritants in man: a light and electron microscopic study. *J Invest Dermatol* 1989;5:695–699.
6. Anderson C. Dermal cell infiltrates: allergic, toxic, irritant, and type I reactions. *Acta Derm Venereol Suppl* (Stockh) 1988;68:24–27.
7. White C. Histopathology of exogenous and systemic contact eczema. *Semin Dermatol* 1990;9:226–229.

CHAPTER 5

The Role of Age, Sex, and Color of Skin in Contact Dermatitis

AGE FACTORS

Contact Dermatitis in Childhood

Both allergic and irritant varieties of contact dermatitis occur during childhood and infancy (1). The skin is less reactive to potent contact sensitizers in early infancy than it is later in life. Irritant dermatitis readily takes place in persons of all ages, including newborns. Allergic dermatitis due to poison ivy oleoresin and to certain topical medications is by no means rare in early life (2). Dermatitis due to wearing apparel, particularly wool, and to sensitizers in shoes is frequent.

> **Irritant or allergic contact dermatitis from topical medications readily occurs in infancy and may resemble prickly heat.**

Certain topical medications that produce sensitization in adults, including mercury, benzocaine, and antihistamines, also produce dermatitis in children. Antibiotic ointments may be prescribed in the same strength as for adults. Children are also susceptible to photosensitizing reactions from tar preparations used for topical medications and to the essential oils of perfumes.

Children may acquire severe irritant dermatitis and burns from accidental contact with a host of potentially harmful household products, including caustics.

Caustic Burns

So many caustic substances are used in the home that it is inevitable that children will suffer caustic burns. Proper treatment depends on whether the burn was caused by an acidic or an alkaline substance. The burn should be touched with the pH portion of a urine dipstick. Alkali burns may be treated with orange juice or vinegar; acid burns should be treated with bicarbonate paste or milk of magnesia.

Other household irritants include polishes, waxes, solvents, detergents, bleaching agents, disinfectants, and insecticides. Widespread dermatitis may be produced by baby oils containing antiseptics, such as 8-hydroxyquinoline sulfate (oxyquinoline sulfate). The eruptions may resemble prickly heat.

Highly perfumed oils, toilet soaps, and dusting powders may also cause infantile dermatitis. These preparations may accumulate in the folds of the skin, particularly in the axillary and inguinal folds, in which staphylococcal infections may become superimposed on the dermatitis. In general, infant skin tolerates lotions better than it does oils.

The use of nonperfumed oils, powders, and soaps free of antiseptics is recommended for infants. When the infant begins to crawl, dermatitis of the legs, knees, and elbows may be produced by floor polish, floor wax, rough fabrics used in rugs and carpets, and oily dust on furniture. The wearing of cotton coveralls prevents such dermatitis.

Dermatitis in children may result from exposure to irritants and sensitizers while participating in activities such as finger painting, shop work, and chemistry experiments. Crayons may also produce dermatitis.

Soap and Detergent Dermatitis

"Detergent hands" may occur in young girls who wash doll clothes. Honigman (3) showed that a subacute primary irritant dermatitis is brought about usually by prolonged bubble baths, bathing too frequently, using excessive amounts of bubble bath concentrate, or a combination of these factors. Children who have atopic eczema and who normally have xerotic skin are often severely affected.

Asteatosis and primary irritations are the inevitable results of overindulgence in bathing. Bubble baths assuredly can contribute to this problem.

Bubble baths are available as powders, liquids, and aerosol foams. They are often packaged in containers shaped appropriately for subsequent use as a toy when empty. The attractive container, the ease of bathing the child, and the child's preference for bubble baths account for their popularity with both parents and children.

Diaper Dermatitis

Diaper dermatitis (napkin dermatitis, erythema of Jacquet), the most common form of contact dermatitis in infancy, is produced by prolonged contact with urine or feces or both; by residual antiseptics, soaps, and detergents in the diapers; and by friction.

The sequence of events leading to diaper dermatitis is thought to be initiated by moisture-induced increases in the coefficient of friction and skin abrasion. The increased wetness is accompanied by enhanced permeability and increased numbers of microorganisms. Ammonia, once thought to be a key factor, was found by Leyden et al. (4) to be present in equivalent amounts in morning diapers for infants with and without diaper dermatitis. Because ammonia is a known irritant, it cannot be dismissed as a cofactor on abraded skin.

The diaper can produce a higher than normal skin pH by relative occlusion, which can increase the enzymatic activity of fecal bacterial urease, fecal proteases, lipases, and bile salts and lead to further irritation (due to increased ammonia production or to the higher pH alone) or to enhanced enzyme irritation (5–7).

The Role of Microorganisms in Diaper Dermatitis

Brown and Wilson (8) stated that the urea-splitting *Bacillus proteus* occurs much more frequently than *B. ammoniagenes* in some cases of diaper dermatitis. Montes et al. (9) isolated *Candida albicans* from lesions of 27 patients who had diaper dermatitis but from the skin of only 5 control subjects. Its frequency decreased following cure of the rash. *Escherichia coli* and *Staphylococcus aureus* were found in many lesions of diaper dermatitis, but they were also frequent in normal skin. A synergistic action between these bacteria and *C. albicans* is possible. In many infants, regardless of the presence of dermatitis, the microbial population of the diaper region was high.

Leyden and Kligman (10) studied the role of microorganisms in diaper dermatitis. This work was inspired by the vast number of studies concerning this problem, with no consensus reached regarding which organisms, if any, play a central role in the pathogenesis of diaper rash. The authors performed a quantitative microbiologic study in the diaper area of 40 normal infants and 100 infants who had diaper dermatitis. They stressed that diaper dermatitis, like hand dermatitis, is a regional diagnosis with many different causes.

It was found that the common but usually mild chafing dermatitis did not show microbiologic differences from normal diaper areas except for low numbers of *S. aureus*. This form of diaper rash is caused by friction and maceration, whereas ammonia has no role at all. *S. aureus* was found in all cases of atopic dermatitis and, as in other locations of atopic dermatitis, was considered a secondary invader. *S. aureus* also occurred in low numbers in psoriasis.

In the infants who had seborrheic dermatitis, *S. aureus* and *C. albicans* were isolated, and a pathogenic role of *C. albicans* could not be ruled out. *C. albicans* occurred in 80% of cases clinically diagnosed as moniliasis but in only 5 of 145 culture sites in 40 normal infants. It was concluded that *C. albicans* has a primary instigating role in certain severe forms of diaper rash.

C. albicans is a primary cause of certain severe forms of diaper rash.

Clinical Picture of Diaper Dermatitis

The dermatitis is present over the external genitalia and buttocks, *usually sparing the creases*. The eruption may spread to include the entire lower half of the abdomen, and even the skin of the feet coming in contact with ammoniacal urine may become involved.

In mild cases, only a slight erythema confined to the diaper area is found. When neglected, the affected skin becomes scalded and edematous. Vesicles and bullae may supervene. Eroded bullae may become eczematous, and pyodermic lesions may appear. Herpetiform ulcers are not uncommon.

In male infants, diaper dermatitis may appear as ulcers of the meatus of the glans; the ulcers may become covered with a diphtheritic type of membrane. Urination is painful, and the infant may become restless.

Disposable Diapers

Disposable diapers were introduced in the United States in the early 1960s and are estimated to be used exclusively on 71% of infants; they are used along with cloth diapers in 22% of infants, and only 7% of infants now use cloth diapers (11). There are two main types of disposable diapers: conventional cellulose-core diapers and extra-absorbent diapers containing absorbent gelling material (AGM). There is usually an inner topsheet in contact with the child's skin to decrease friction and distance the skin from the moisture in the cellulose-core diapers. The AGM is positioned in different locations in various manufacturers' products and is composed of high-molecular-weight polymers that gel on hydration. The outer covering is either polypropylene or polyethylene.

AGM-containing diapers have shown superiority over home-laundered cloth diapers in preventing diaper dermatitis, reducing wetness, and normalizing pH with the buffering capacity of sodium polyacrylate (11).

> **Disposable diapers are superior to cloth in the prevention of diaper dermatitis.**

Psoriasiform Diaper Dermatitis

This syndrome has been variously interpreted as an early manifestation of psoriasis, a seborrheic dermatitis, a candida infection, and a disease sui generis. Fergusson et al. (12) stated that treatment with antimonilial dyes in the diaper area is superior to therapy with steroid creams. The clinical appearance of the diaper eruption and the fact that all infants were hospital born were thought to support a monilial etiology.

Psoriasiform diaper dermatitis can be treated with the use of equal parts of a corticosteroid cream and Lassar's paste. This combination adheres well to the diaper area and is more efficacious than a corticosteroid cream or ointment alone (13).

Perianal Dermatitis

Frequent soft or liquid stools and undigested food particles or their split products in feces may produce perianal dermatitis. Coating the area with zinc oxide ointment is protective and healing in such instances. Mercurial, formaldehyde, or strong detergent disinfectants on a thermometer may produce contact dermatitis in the perianal area.

Toilet seat dermatitis may be produced by strong detergents used to cleanse the seat. In addition, lacquer or paint covering the seat may cause a clearly defined pattern of dermatitis on the posterior aspect of the thighs and buttocks.

Clothing Dermatitis

Irritant contact dermatitis in childhood is not uncommonly due to woolen clothing. Rough cuffs and collars, particularly when wet, readily irritate the skin, especially in children who have atopic dermatitis.

Residues of soap and detergent in laundered clothes can also be irritating. Highly starched garments may initiate dermatitis. Clothing dyes rarely cause dermatitis in infants. New clothing and bed linens should be washed before coming in contact with the inflamed skin of children. Clothing that has been dry cleaned or contaminated with moth preventatives or insecticides should be thoroughly aired before being worn by the child.

Children's flame-retardant night clothing no longer contains TRIS (2,3-dibromopropyl) phosphate, a flame retardant that was once used frequently on acetate, acetate blends, triacetate, triacetate blends, and 100% polyester children's sleepwear.

The principal manner in which children's sleepwear has to comply with the flammability standards, however, is with the use of inherently flame-resistant fibers. Examples are modacrylic (brand names Verel, SEF, Kanecaron), modacrylic blends, matrix (brand name Cordelan), matrix blends, vinyon (brand name Leavil), vinyon blends, and polyester.

Wool is not flammable but cannot be tolerated by atopic persons. Cotton is not used in children's sleepwear at present. It has been replaced by the aforementioned synthetic fibers, which are flame resistant without further treatment (report from U.S. Consumer Products Commission, Washington, DC).

> **Rough-textured and woolen clothing and occlusive footwear frequently cause dermatitis in children. "Flame-proof" chemicals are no longer added to children's sleepwear. Certain flame-resistant synthetic fibers are used.**

Dermatitis of the Feet

Dermatitis Due to Shoes

This type of dermatitis in children may be due to allergic sensitization to ingredients in shoes, particularly rubber. Frequently a nonspecific dermatitis is produced by the friction and irritation of an ill-fitting shoe. The dorsal aspect of the first toe may be involved in both allergic and irritant types of shoe dermatitis. It is not uncommon for friction of tight-fitting shoes to localize atopic dermatitis to this site. It may be necessary to perform patch tests with shoe ingredients in order to differentiate such atopic dermatitis from allergic contact dermatitis due to shoes.

Dermatitis Due to Hyperhidrosis and Occlusive Footwear

Children whose feet perspire excessively and who wear socks containing synthetic fibers or sneakers, rubbers, or rubber-soled shoes for prolonged periods may suffer from sweaty sock dermatitis, an eruption of the toes and interweb areas due to maceration by unabsorbed sweat (14). These areas readily become eczematous and infected. Paronychial infections and dystrophic nail changes in neglected cases are not uncommon.

This syndrome must be distinguished from tinea pedis, contact dermatitis from shoes, and atopic dermatitis. Scrapings and cultures for tinea may be necessary in the differential diagnosis. Allergic contact dermatitis to shoes usually spares the interdigital areas. Patch tests may be necessary to rule out sensitization to chemicals in footwear. Sweaty sock dermatitis is often confused with atopic dermatitis of the feet, particularly if hyperhidrosis also causes dermatitis of the antecubital fossae.

Juvenile plantar dermatosis (JPD) is probably the same condition, and the precise role of atopy in producing JPD is still not understood. A glazed and fissured plantar dermatitis is found as a morphologic marker of JPD. A personal or family history of atopic dermatitis is encountered in nearly half of children with JPD (15,16).

Children with hyperhidrosis of the feet should wear all-cotton hose and, whenever feasible, shoes with perforated uppers or sandals. Prolonged wearing of rubbers, boots, sneakers, or other occlusive footwear should be avoided. Foot baths of potassium permanganate made by dissolving a 5-grain tablet in 2 qt of water should be used nightly for 20 minutes. Each morning Zea-SORB Powder (Stiefel) should be dusted onto the feet and into hose and footwear.

Sweaty sock dermatitis should be combated by use of nonocclusive footwear, permanganate baths, and dusting powder.

Contact Cheilitis and Perioral Dermatitis

In children, the lips and adjacent skin are commonly irritated. Children who have a habit of licking often have inflammation of this area. In addition, saliva trapped between the thumb and the mouth of a thumb-sucking child may produce dermatitis of the lips and cheeks. Similarly, children who salivate when teething may develop facial dermatitis. The constant chewing of bubble gum can produce dermatitis of the face and cheilitis because of the macerating effect of the moist gum and the irritation of essential oils.

Children whose eating habits permit foods such as spinach, carrots, and citrus fruit to remain on the cheeks may have dermatitis from the irritation of food juices. The facial dermatitis produced by saliva or food juices may closely resemble atopic eczema. Regurgitation of food particles may cause contact dermatitis around the mouth and on the neck and chin. Rubber-sensitive children may acquire a perioral dermatitis resembling perleche from chewing rubber pencil erasers or rubber bands.

Plant Dermatitis

Poison ivy, poison sumac, and poison oak are the most common causes of allergic eczematous contact dermatitis in children. Contact with resins of trees may also produce allergic dermatitis. Anemones and buttercups contain a blister-producing lactone that can cause vesiculation in children who crush or chew the plants.

Although allergic rhinitis due to ragweed protein is common throughout childhood, ragweed oil dermatitis is extremely rare during this period.

Vick's Vaporub contains several plant substances, including oil of turpentine, oil of eucalyptus, and oil of cedar, which may irritate or sensitize a child's skin. In addition, this nostrum contains camphor, menthol, oil of nutmeg, and thymol.

Although poison ivy dermatitis is essentially a summer disease, it may occur whenever children come into contact with the dried oleoresin on the twigs of the dormant plant. Not infrequently, pets, particularly long-haired dogs, come into contact with poison ivy plants and transmit the oleoresin to children. Ingestion of *toxicodendron* plants may produce systemic symptoms, such as vomiting, diarrhea, fever, convulsions, and stupor. Acute nephritis may accompany ingestion or marked cutaneous involvement.

There is no difficulty in sensitizing newborn infants to poison ivy oleoresin (17). Although clinically one may see many severe cases of poison ivy dermatitis in children, experimental evidence indicates that poison ivy reactions are more intense in adults and that the reactivity does not reach its zenith for several years.

Cosmetic Dermatitis

Infants and children may acquire cosmetic dermatitis by contact with cosmetics worn by the mother and other attendants or by cosmetics in play.

The cheeks and forehead of an infant may be affected by the mother's perfume, face powder, lipstick, or hair spray. Dermatitis may occur if an attendant handles a child before her nail polish is dry. Berloque dermatitis in children, resulting in patchy pigmentation, may be seen from the photosensitizing effect of perfumes and toilet waters. Occasionally, children use irritating or sensitizing eye makeup.

Atopic Dermatitis Due to Contact with Proteins

Rarely, atopic infants, particularly those allergic to eggs or fish, acquire marked edema of the skin or oral mucosa from contact with the foods to which they are allergic. In addition, contact with egg white in susceptible infants may produce the clinical picture of atopic dermatitis. The eruption from contact with proteins is usually urticarial rather than eczematous.

Protein allergens, such as wool and silk, are said to produce wheals when they come into contact with infantile skin (18). Atopic dermatitis may also be produced. Such eruptions may be due theoretically to transepidermal penetration of protein allergens into the corium.

Contact Urticaria Due to Milk in Childhood

Edwards (19) described contact urticaria that developed in an 18-month-old girl as a reaction to cow's milk. The child did not have a similar reaction after the milk was heated to 80°C for 30 seconds. This child presented with urticaria on the neck, perioral, and chest areas that developed immediately after her diet was changed from an infant formula without iron to commercial, pasteurized cow's milk. A few minutes after first drinking warm cow's milk, the child developed a red eruption on the face that disappeared after 30 minutes. No systemic manifestations of allergy were present.

Lecks (20) reported that a child developed a severe urticarial reaction of the diaper area with an anaphylactoid reaction from the use of Diaparene neonatal ointment, which contains a milk protein (casein). This case report is presented to alert pediatricians, allergists, and other practicing physicians of the hazards of using Diaparene neonatal ointment in infants and young children exquisitely sensitive to cow's milk proteins (see also Chapter 34).

> **Diaparene neonatal ointment containing casein may produce contact urticaria in milk-sensitive infants.**

Patch Tests in Atopic Infants

Cow's milk allergy is a common consideration in children with atopic dermatitis. Double-blind, placebo-controlled oral challenges identified cow's milk allergy in 54 infants age 2 to 24 months. The reactions were immediate in 36 and delayed in 18 of these children (21). Immediate reactions were detected with prick tests, and the delayed reactions were identified with a patch test to powdered cow's milk. Altogether, 26% of cases were identifiable only by patch testing. Immediate reactions were characterized by pruritus, urticaria, and exanthema, whereas delayed cases exhibited eczematous lesions (22). In a second study, prick tests detected 67% of immediate reactions to oral challenge, whereas patch tests detected 89% of delayed onset reactions (22). Similar results can be found in children who react to oral challenges with cereals such as wheat, rye, barley, and oats. Some reactions can only be detected by patch testing, which, unfortunately, is not yet standardized (23).

Patch Testing in Childhood

Veien et al. (24) studied 168 children, 14 years of age or younger, who were patch tested with the Standard Series of the International Contact Dermatitis Research Group (ICDRG) over a 5-year period. Seventy-seven of the children had one or more positive reactions; relevant test results were found in 80% of them.

Eight boys and 24 girls were allergic to nickel, which proved to be the most common allergen. Five boys and 6 girls reacted to chromate, and 5 boys and 4 girls reacted to one or more of the rubber chemicals.

Although it was suggested that patch testing of children may result in nonspecific reactions, these investigators encountered no difficulty in the classification of allergic or toxic patch test results. This finding was in accord with the fact that most of the positive patch tests were relevant to the current dermatitis. Therefore, they prefer the same patch test allergens and concentrations used for adults rather than the lower concentration of allergens for children suggested by Fisher (1).

In an evaluation of the currently available screening allergens sold by Hermal, the North American Contact Dermatitis Group (25) found that irritant reactions were not a problem for children when Finn chambers were used. This proved to be the case even though some allergens were tested at concentrations later deemed to be marginal irritants in adults: 2% cinnamic aldehyde in petrolatum, 2% formaldehyde aqueous, and 0.5% potassium dichromate in petrolatum. These three marginal irritant concentrations were later halved; nonetheless, irritant reactions were always less frequent in children than in adults, and relevant positive patch tests were found in 68% of children. A study from Scotland (26) of children tested with standard diagnostic patch test concentrations found 48% of 125 reactions to be positive and 92% to be relevant.

Five recent studies confirm the value of patch testing children (27–31). The frequency of positive patch tests ranged from 37% to 66%. Relevance ranged from 40% to 54%. The recurring theme of these reports is that nickel is the most commonly encountered allergen along with other metals. Mercury and thimerosal are frequently found, probably due to thimerosal in immunizations. Fragrance and rubber chemical additives are also common. Roul et al. (27) found the peak incidence around 3 years of age, whereas Giordano-Labadie et al. (28) found the peak to occur after the age of 5. The relevance of nickel in children was uncommon enough to be called rare by Roul et al. They believe that atopic dermatitis in children leads to frequent false-positive nickel patch tests. Whereas Roul et al. tested children of all types, Giordano-Labadie et al. focused on children with atopic dermatitis. Among the children with atopic dermatitis, metals were positive in 19.3% (28), whereas in a German study of children (regardless of atopic status), 15.9% were sensitive to nickel (29). The German study found a lower prevalence of atopic dermatitis among children with positive patch tests. Although there may be disagreement about the relevance of positive patch tests to metals in children, particularly atopic children, there is general agreement on the value of patch testing children with suspected contact dermatitis.

Epstein (17) stated that although allergic contact dermatitis in neonates and young infants is unusual, an occasional case may be overlooked because patch testing is rarely performed in this age group. Neonates and young infants can be sensitized. The lack of contact sensitization in this age group is a consequence of the lack of exposure to the more potent allergens in the environment.

Allergic Dermatitis Due to Specific Sensitizers in Children

Table 5.1 lists the most common causes of allergic contact dermatitis in childhood, which are not very different from those of the general population.

TABLE 5.1. *The Most Common Sensitizers in Childhood*

Poison ivy, oak, and sumac
Mercaptobenzothiazole (in shoes)
Potassium dichromate (in shoes)
Nickel (in earrings)
Ethylenediamine hydrochloride
Topical antihistamines
Ethyl aminobenzoate (benzocaine)
Neomycin
Cosmetics
Perfumes
Balsam of Peru
Thimerosal (merthiolate)
Merbromin (mercurochrome)

Nickel Dermatitis

Sensitization to nickel in childhood is caused most frequently by the piercing of ears and insertion of nickel-plated earrings. Such sensitization has been reported in the first few weeks of life. Identification bands with a plastic strap and metal clip, zippers, metal tips of shoelaces, and coins have produced dermatitis in nickel-sensitive children. Once sensitization to nickel occurs, the child is subject to nickel dermatitis indefinitely (32,33).

Neomycin

This antibiotic applied as a powder to circumcisions at certain hospitals has sensitized many infants (34).

Mercaptobenzothiazole

This rubber chemical, present in many shoes and used as a rubber adhesive to cement shoe linings to shoe uppers, is one of the most common causes of allergic contact reactions in childhood, particularly in boys who have hyperhidrosis (35).

Thimerosal (Merthiolate) and Merbromin (Mercurochrome)

These antiseptics, used frequently in infancy and childhood, may cause cases of allergic contact dermatitis (32).

Balsam of Peru

Several topical medications for use in the diaper area containing balsam of Peru (Balmex baby powder, emollient, lotion, and ointment, as well as Diaprox ointment) have produced allergic contact dermatitis (see Chapter 11) (18).

Ethylenediamine Hydrochloride

This stabilizer in original Mycolog Cream used on the diaper area has sensitized many infants. Mycolog II does not contain ethylenediamine, and the original formula is available only from generic suppliers.

> Neonatal infants have acquired allergic contact dermatitis from vinyl identification bands, nickel, neomycin, ethylenediamine, thimerosal (merthiolate), merbromin (mercurochrome), balsam of Peru, rubber chemicals in shoes, and poison ivy.

Effects of Strong Topical Corticosteroids in Children

Table 5.2 lists complications from the prolonged use of strong topical corticosteroids in children. Diffuse "wasting" of the skin on the diaper area may occur (36). Occasionally, instead of general atrophy of the skin, atrophic striae may be formed in the inguinal area (37). On the face, so-called perioral dermatitis or a more diffuse rosacea-like eruption may occur (38).

Large Granulomas in Diaper Area from Topical Corticosteroids

In recent years, a new entity in the diaper area has been observed. Firm, angioma-like, painless swellings appear on the buttocks, inner thighs, and occasionally the lower abdomen. These large, symmetrical, round or oval nodules are oriented along the axis of the buttock folds, reaching the size of a cherry or plum, and are sharply demarcated, slightly protruding, and bluish-red or maroon in color. The infants are otherwise in good health, and the condition resolves spontaneously in several months with no treatment and without sequelae. This condition was first reported by Tappeiner and Pfleger (39), who called it "granuloma gluteale infantum." The cause of this disorder is not entirely clear, but all reported patients have been on rather prolonged application of fluorinated corticosteroids for preexisting diaper eruption, and all cases cleared slowly on discontinuation of treatment (40).

Japanese investigators reported five cases of Kaposi's sarcoma–like granuloma occurring on the lesion of diaper dermatitis (41). The common characteristic features of the clinical findings in these cases are summarized, with discussion of the similarities and differences between Kaposi's

TABLE 5.2. *Complications of Strong Topical Fluorinated Corticosteroids*

Diaper area
  Diffuse atrophy
  Atrophic striae
  Granulomas
Face
  Rosacea-like dermatitis

sarcoma and the granulomas. In their cases, the lesions were in the genitocrural region, the thigh, and the penile region and were not observed on the gluteal region. Thus, the name "granuloma gluteale infantum" is not suitable. The investigators described their cases under the title of "Kaposi sarcoma–like granuloma on diaper dermatitis."

> **Prolonged use of topical fluorinated corticosteroids in the occluded diaper area may produce large granulomatous lesions that subside spontaneously when the topical corticosteroid is no longer used.**

Georgouras and Kocsard (42) described a case of a 13-year-old boy who had a diffuse facial micropapular eruption with a granulomatous histology. The diagnosis is consistent with perioral dermatitis of the Gianotti type (43). It is postulated that bubble gum was the cause of the condition. The most likely ingredients responsible for the problem were the essential oils in the gum, which may actually be selectively absorbed by the follicle to produce a follicular granulomatous reaction. We have added yet another cause for perioral dermatitis. Histologically, a granulomatous infiltrate with "sarcoid-like" appearance was present in some cases. Table 5.3 shows the numerous ingredients of chewing gum.

TABLE 5.3. *Chewing Gum Additives*[a]

BHA (butylated hydroxyanisole)
BHT (butylated hydroxyaluene) as antioxidant
Butadiene styrene rubber
Butyl rubber
Chewing gum base, which includes:
Chicle, chicuibal, crown gum, gutta hand kang, massaranduba balata, massaranduba chocolate, nespero, rosidinba, Venezuelan chicle, jelutong leche caspi, pendara, perilla, leche devaca, niger gutta, tunu, chilte, natural rubber
Chilte
Glycerine ester of partially hydrogenated wood resin
Glycerin ester of polymerized resin
Isobutylene-isoprene capolymer
Isobutylene resin
Lanolin
Latex (butadiene styrene rubber)
Paraffin wax
Polyvinyl acetate (molecular weight 2,000 minimum)
Resin, polymerized, partially hydrogenated, and/or partially dimerized, glyceral esters
Rubber (natural), smoked sheet, and latex solids
Sodium sulfate
Sodium sulfide
Terpene resin (synthetic polymers of B-pinene and natural polymers of A-pinene)

[a]Compiled by Stephen D. Lockey, Sr., M.D., 60 North West End Avenue, Lancaster, PA 17603.

> **Bubble gum may produce a fine granulomatous "sarcoid-like" dermatitis of the face.**

Contact Dermatitis in Elderly Patients

If we arbitrarily define an elderly person as one who is entitled to Medicare, then the most common causes of allergic dermatitis among such persons are topical medications applied to stasis ulcers (44,45).

Sensitizing topical agents used in the treatment of stasis ulcers produce widespread and even generalized eruptions (Table 5.4). Particularly in the elderly, "autosensitization" plays a prominent role in the development of serious eruptions from injudicious treatment of varicose ulcers and stasis eczema. A combination of sensitization to bacteria, the absorption of modified protein from inflamed or ulcerated skin, and topical medications are potential causes of autosensitization.

> **Topical medications applied to stasis ulcers and eczemas are common causes of allergic contact dermatitis in the elderly.**

Sensitizing Topical Medications Applied to Stasis Ulcers

Neomycin

This antibiotic sensitizes 30% of persons when it is applied to stasis ulcers (46). Erythromycin base in petrolatum has proved a safe, nonsensitizing antibiotic to apply to infected stasis ulcers.

Nitrofurazone

This antiseptic, a favorite of some surgeons for ulcers and burns, is a potent sensitizer. In addition, the polyethylene glycols used as a vehicle for nitrofurazone can cause allergic contact dermatitis (47).

TABLE 5.4. *Common Sensitizers in Topical Agents Applied to Stasis Ulcers*

Ethylenediamine hydrochloride
Lanolin
Neomycin
Nitrofurazone
Paraben preservatives
Vitamin E creams

Vehicle Ingredients

Lanolin and the parabens are rather rare sensitizers except when applied to stasis eczema and stasis ulcers (48).

Other Causes of Allergic Contact Dermatitis in the Elderly

As far as the older age group is concerned, Fisher felt that the common potent sensitizers, such as paraphenylenediamine, nickel, the dichromates, poison ivy, and rubber compounds, produce as many instances of contact dermatitis with strongly positive patch test reactions in patients over age 65 as in younger age groups. The experience of the North American Contact Dermatitis Group showed that, indeed, a wide variety of common sensitizers are regularly identified in patients age 80 and older (25).

> **Poison ivy, poison oak, poison sumac, ragweed, paraphenylenediamine, nickel, the dichromates, and rubber compounds are common sensitizers in the elderly.**

Aside from dermatitis owing to topical medications and poison ivy dermatitis, the following are not infrequently encountered in elderly persons.

Hair-Dye Dermatitis

Allergic eczematous contact dermatitis owing to paraphenylenediamine hair dyes is not uncommon in elderly women. In 30 persons sensitive to it, 10 were over 60 years of age (49). Furriers, occupationally sensitized to paraphenylenediamine, show positive patch test reactions long after they have retired, even if they are no longer in contact with paraphenylenediamine (50).

Wearing-Apparel Dermatitis

A dermatitis due to the finishes and dark dyes of clothes is facilitated in menopausal women because of hyperhidrosis. "Widow's dermatitis" or "mourner's dermatitis" may be produced by allergic sensitivity to the black dyes in clothing worn for the first time when the patient is in mourning. Obesity in older age groups can be a factor in producing wearing-apparel dermatitis.

Industrial Dermatitis

In industry, a severe allergic contact dermatitis can develop suddenly in older workers who have handled certain substances in their occupation for decades without difficulty. This is likely to occur in cement workers, painters, tile setters, and bakers. Even prompt retirement and the avoidance of irritants or specific allergens do not necessarily prevent the dermatitis or keep it from becoming generalized. Such widespread involvement may be due to increased nonspecific irritability of the entire skin surface, which becomes hyperreactive to many irritants and even to bland substances (45).

> **Industrial allergic contact dermatitis can erupt suddenly in older workers owing to chemicals they have handled for decades without difficulty. Retirement and avoidance of contactants will not necessarily prevent dermatitis or generalization.**

Ragweed Dermatitis

Ragweed dermatitis is caused by ragweed oleoresin, in contrast to ragweed rhinitis and asthma, which are caused by the protein fraction of ragweed pollen. Ragweed dermatitis is almost exclusively a male dermatitis, occurring most commonly in farmers age 40 to 75 (51). However, people in other occupations and in suburban areas frequently become sensitized to ragweed oil. Even "city folk" can acquire ragweed dermatitis because ragweed pollen contaminated with the sensitizing oleoresin can be airborne for long distances and can be confused easily with a photodermatitis.

Photodermatitis

Photodermatitis, owing to aftershave lotion containing musk ambrette and actinic reticuloid, is encountered in the elderly.

Dryness of the skin in elderly persons may be aggravated through normal use of toilet soaps and detergents, predisposing the elderly to allergic contact sensitization. To relieve the dryness, the patient may use lubricants and bath oils containing lanolin products or surfactants that may be sensitizers.

In tracking down the cause of contact dermatitis in the older age group, not only must the physician question the patient concerning new contactants, but a thorough investigation must also be made of substances to which the patient has been exposed for decades. It is surprising how frequently the older patient becomes sensitized to a contactant to which he or she has been exposed intermittently throughout life without any previous reaction (52). Properly performed patch tests are reliable in finding the causative agents in allergic contact dermatitis in persons of this age group.

Systemic Eczematous Contact Dermatitis in the Elderly

Elderly persons may take one or more drugs that are chemically related to topical sensitizers. Eczematous drug eruptions may closely resemble allergic contact dermatitis. Usually an eczematous drug eruption is more widespread and symmetrical than an "external" contact eruption.

Table 5.5 lists drugs that may produce an eczematous drug reaction in which the initial sensitization may have been induced by a topically applied medication chemically related to the drug. In such instances, patch testing may be valuable in detecting the offending drug.

Features of Contact Dermatitis in Elderly Patients

In older people, the disease, even during the acute stage, may show relatively little vesiculation or inflammation.

TABLE 5.5. *Topical Sensitizers and Immunochemically Related Drugs That Can Cause an Eruption upon Systemic Administration*

TOPICAL SENSITIZERS
Hydrazine hydrobromide
Para-amino compounds
   Ethyl aminobenzoate (benzocaine)
   Paraphenylenediamine

Balsam of Peru
Neomycin sulfate
Resorcinol (Resorcin)
Organic and inorganic mercurials
Metallic mercury
Cobalt
Thiamine
Ethylenediamine hydrochloride

Formaldehyde

Thiram and disulfiram
Halogenated hydroxyquinolones
Chlorobutanol
Iodine
Caladryl, diphenhydramine (Benadryl Cream)

IMMUNOCHEMICALLY RELATED DRUGS
Isoniazid, hydralazine (Apresoline), phenelzine sulfate
Para-aminobenzoic acid (PABA)
Azo dyes in foods and drugs
   Dymelor, Orinase, Diabinese, sulfonamides,
   chlorothiazide (Diuril), hydrochlorothiazide (HydroDiuril),
   hydroflumethiazide (Saluron), polythiazide (Renese),
   para-aminosalicylic acid (PAS)
Cinnamon
Streptomycin, kanamycin
Hexylresorcinol (Crystoids, Caprokol)
Mercurial diuretics
Calomel
Vitamin B_{12}
Coenzyme B (cocarboxylase)
Aminophylline, antazoline (Antistine), tripelennamine
   (Pyribenzamine), thonzylamine (Neohetramine),
   piperazine, hydroxyzine (Atarax, Vistaril), methenamine
   (Urotropin), methenamine mandelate (Mandelamine),
   urised disulfiram (Antabuse)
Iodochlorhydroxyquin (Vioform), iodoquinol (Diodoquin)
Chloral hydrate
Iodides, iodinated organic compounds
Diphenhydramine (Benadryl)

Scaling is regularly a prominent feature in all phases of dermatitis in the elderly. Thickening, hyperpigmentation, and lichenification take place readily, and itching is usually pronounced. Both allergic and irritant eruptions tend to persist and be more resistant to therapy in the aged than in younger persons.

If the older patient is managed improperly or reexposed to irritants or sensitizers, the eruption readily becomes widespread and intractable, particularly if intercurrent disease is present.

Finally, in all cases of intractable contact dermatitis, serious systemic disease or internal malignancy may be suspected (53). In addition, many elderly patients have persistent eczematous dermatoses that resemble contact dermatitis clinically and histopathologically and are in reality a form of mycosis fungoides (54).

> **Presumably "intractable" contact dermatitis in reality may be due to systemic or internal malignancy. Early mycosis and the Sézary syndrome may resemble chronic contact dermatitis histopathologically and clinically.**

Use of Patch Tests in Drug Eruptions

In general, aside from the use of patch tests in certain types of eczematous eruptions, skin tests have not as yet proved to be of predictable value.

Table 5.5 lists drugs that can produce a systemic contact-type drug eruption in patients who have been sensitized originally to the drug or to a related chemical by topical application. This type of drug reaction is usually eczematous. The patch test is valuable in confirming the identity of the offending drug (55).

Felix and Comaish (56) emphasized that, apart from clinical challenge, there is no consistently reliable test to confirm that a drug is the cause of an adverse systemic reaction. One of their patients had an eczematous reaction to diazepam and *positive patch tests,* although *intradermal* tests were negative. Another patient had two anaphylactoid reactions to meprobamate, indicating a type-1 (immediate hypersensitivity) reaction. Skin testing in this patient, however, was more in keeping with a type-4 (delayed) reaction (positive patch test).

If patch tests are positive in a patient and negative in an adequate number of controls, this finding may be considered important whenever a clinical systemic reaction has occurred.

Korbitz (57) treated a patient with quinine-induced thrombocytopenic purpura, which proved to be caused immunochemically by an IgG quinine-dependent platelet antibody. A successful "petechial" patch test of quinine was obtained using Telfa gauze pledgets saturated with a quinine solution. Parafilm was placed over the gauze, and a gauze pad was also placed on top, resulting in petechiae at 48 hours that persisted for several days.

Aside from quinidine, a patch test with a solution of carbromal or apronalide (Sedormid) may induce a petechial reaction in patients with purpura caused by these drugs. If no purpura develops spontaneously at the test site, the arm may be congested with the sphygmomanometer cuff, and the test site inspected for hemorrhages. A positive purpuric patch test may be significant, but a negative test does not exonerate the drug.

Houwerzijl et al. (58) observed an epileptic patient treated with carbamazepine and phenytoin (diphenylhydantoin) who developed an extensive erythematous, maculopapular rash and generalized lymphadenopathy. Positive patch tests were obtained for 1% and 5% carbamazepine but not for the phenytoin.

Patch tests may occasionally be positive in eczematous drug eruptions; they are less likely to be positive in purpuric reactions.

Van Ketel (59) tested 247 patients with a history of drug reactions. Ninety-three of these patients had had a skin reaction to penicillin. Patch testing of the 93 patients revealed that 21 showed positive delayed patch test reactions to one or more penicillins. Except possibly in one case, no patients were sensitized by the patch test procedure.

Penvy and Schroepl (60) stated that patch tests with drugs must be read with great caution because many drugs produce irritant reactions. The authors carried out epicutaneous control tests with 44 psychopharmaceutic agents in the pure state on 40 nonallergic persons. All subjects showed at least one positive epicutaneous reaction. It was concluded that tablets, either coated or uncoated, are unsuitable for epicutaneous testing.

In fixed drug eruption, the patch may occasionally be of some help. Thus, phenolphthalein, tested 2% powder in aqueous solution left on for several days, may sometimes reproduce a fixed drug eruption. There is a greater chance that the test will be positive if the test site was part of the initial eruption. In a recent report, a generalized eruption to the antiarrhythmia agent mexiletine hydrochloride was positive at 6.25%, 12.5%, and 25% in petrolatum *only* on previously involved skin. Patch tests and scarified patch tests of noninvolved skin were negative (61).

THE ROLE OF SEX IN CONTACT DERMATITIS

There is very little difference in susceptibility to allergic contact dermatitis due to sex. Leyden and Kligman (62) have reported that bona fide sex differences in prevalence rates of response to contact allergens reflect the intensity of past exposure. Nickel sensitivity occurs predominantly in women, as would be expected from their greater contact

with jewelry. Likewise, allergy to perfumes is far more frequent in women. These disparities may change as men increasingly adopt practices that were formerly the province of women. On the other hand, men predominate in chromium allergy because of occupational exposures such as those in the cement industry.

The prevalence of sensitization to particular allergens reflects past exposure and is not due to sex differences. Thus, ear piercing and jewelry exposure make nickel dermatitis more common in women, whereas industrial exposure to chromates makes chrome dermatitis more common in men.

Björnberg (63) was unable to demonstrate any difference between men and women in skin reactions to primary irritants.

Connubial and Consort Contact Dermatitis

Wilkinson (64), in describing two cases of connubial contact dermatitis, stated that contact dermatitis or photodermatitis in a patient may be due to the work or household activities of the spouse or to medicaments the patient is receiving. He warns us not to neglect patients' spouses when tracking down the cause of contact dermatitis.

In this day and age, however, investigation of contact with a spouse without considering other partners sometimes fails to detect many cases of contact dermatitis. The old-fashioned term "consort," which includes not only a spouse but also a companion or partner, seems to fit the present situation more accurately. In consort contact dermatitis, whether or not it is connubial, the dermatitis is not necessarily produced by sexual exposure (65).

Connubial Propylene Glycol Dermatitis (K-Y Jelly Dermatitis)

A 55-year-old man had previously experienced a severe allergic contact dermatitis after using halcinonide (Halog cream). Patch test procedures had proved that the patient was allergic to the propylene glycol in the preparation. One year later, 24 hours after having intercourse with his wife, the patient developed a severe pruritic dermatitis of the penis and scrotum with marked erythema, edema, slight scaling, and crusting.

It was ascertained subsequently that his wife had for the first time used K-Y Jelly as a vaginal lubricant prior to intercourse. After 48 hours, patch tests gave positive results to the K-Y Jelly and to 5% and 10% aqueous solutions of propylene glycol. In five controls, patch tests gave negative results to K-Y Jelly. This finding was the first reported instance of connubial K-Y Jelly dermatitis (66,67).

Feminine Hygiene Dermatitis

A 30-year-old man stated that he believed he was allergic to one of his girlfriend's secretions because each time they had intercourse he acquired a dermatitis of his penis, scrotum, and lower abdomen. Relations with other women did not produce this dermatitis. After routine patch testing, results showed a positive patch reaction only to balsam of Peru. This finding suggested the possibility of an allergic reaction to a perfume (68). After further questioning, it was discovered that this girlfriend used a feminine hygiene spray prior to intercourse.

Positive results were obtained when this feminine hygiene spray was patch tested. Patch tests to three other feminine sprays gave positive results to two of them and negative results to the third. The patient's girlfriend is now using a feminine hygiene spray that does not produce dermatitis, and the patient no longer acquires dermatitis after intercourse (69).

Connubial and consort contact dermatitis may occur from propylene glycol in K-Y Jelly as well as from feminine hygiene sprays, perfumes, contraceptives, hair dyes, and benzoyl peroxide in acne preparations.

Benzoyl Peroxide Dermatitis

A 20-year-old woman believed that she was allergic to her boyfriend because an eruption developed on her face, neck, and occasionally her arms each time they had intercourse. Examination revealed a patchy, eczematous eruption on her face and neck. Patch tests to the "screening" patch test tray and the patient's cosmetics gave negative results.

Further investigation revealed that her consort used a 5% benzoyl peroxide preparation for a facial acneform eruption. Patch tests of the benzoyl peroxide preparation and of a 1% benzoyl peroxide in petrolatum gave positive results. After the boyfriend changed the benzoyl peroxide preparation to a topical antibiotic, the patient's eruption subsided.

This case of consort contact dermatitis is quite similar to a case of connubial dermatitis reported by Caro (70), whose patient was a physician who developed a pruritic erythematous eruption localized on the right side of the neck and the right anterior axillary fold. The patient had recently given his wife a preparation containing 5% benzoyl peroxide for mild acne on her back. Patch tests with 1% benzoyl peroxide in petrolatum also gave positive results.

Caro ascertained that the patient slept on the left side of the bed; the right side of his neck and the interior axillary fold on the right were thus in contact with the bedding, which could be contaminated by benzoyl peroxide applied to his wife's back just before she retired (70). The wife dis-

continued using the preparation, and the physician has had no further dermatitis.

Consort Sunscreen Dermatitis

A young woman developed a diffuse follicular eruption of the upper arms, anterior trunk, inner thighs, and buttocks that resembled recurrent and disseminated infundibulofolliculitis of Hitch and Lund. This eruption cleared when her fair-skinned boyfriend left town and reappeared some months later upon his return. The couple frequently spent their weekends at the beach, where he applied a homosalate-containing sunscreen (Coppertone Lotion), but the woman, who was olive-complexioned, used no topical products. The physical contact that occurred following their beach excursions explained the distribution of the eruption, which occurred only on the woman. She was patch test positive to both Coppertone Lotion and 2% homosalate in petrolatum (71). The patch test produced a typical eczematous reaction, but the clinical picture resembled a folliculitis most likely due to small amounts of material transferred by skin-to-skin contact through follicular diffusion shunts.

A follicular or folliculitis-like pattern of dermatitis may be a morphologic clue to consort contact dermatitis.

Consort Seminal Fluid Reactions

There are several reports of severe pruritus, urticaria, and even anaphylaxis owing to reactions in women who proved to have allergic hypersensitivity to seminal fluid (72–77). These cases, about equally divided between connubial and nonconnubial exposure, are exquisite examples of allergic "consort" contact reactions.

Seminal fluid can produce contact urticaria and anaphylaxis in sensitized women.

Rubber Diaphragm Dermatitis

Rubber-sensitive women may acquire vulvitis and vaginitis from contraceptive rubber diaphragms. Male rubber-sensitive partners may similarly acquire balanitis from contact with such diaphragms.

Condom Dermatitis

Because allergic hypersensitivity to rubber condoms occurs occasionally, rubber-sensitive men and women should be informed that nonrubber condoms such as Fourex (Schmidt) and Lambskin (Youngs Rubber) made of processed sheep's intestine are available.

For proper disease prophylaxis, it is necessary to apply a rubber condom with the nonrubber devices. Depending on which partner is rubber sensitive, the nonrubber condom will be worn either over or under the nonrubber type (78).

Dermatitis Due to Sensitizers in Contraceptive Spermicides

Such sensitizers include phenylmercuric acetate, oxyquinoline sulfate, quinine hydrochloride, and hexylresorcinol.

Contraceptive diaphragms, rubber condoms, and spermicides may produce allergic contact dermatitis in sensitized men and women.

Connubial Work Clothes Dermatitis

Fiberglass Dermatitis

A 36-year-old woman and her husband had been treated for "scabies" for 3 months without results. The husband had marked folliculitis, papular urticaria, and linear erosions in the creases. The wife had a milder, pruritic follicular eruption. It was revealed that the husband recently had become employed in a fiberglass factory and had brought home his fiberglass-contaminated work clothes, which his wife washed together with her own clothes. Because it was believed this might be the cause of the eruption, the husband was instructed to liberally apply talcum powder to his entire body just before he put on his work clothes, and the wife was instructed to wash her husband's work clothes separately from her own. One week after this procedure was instituted, the eruption on both husband and wife subsided completely.

Fisher and Warkentin (79) also reported a case of fiberglass dermatitis in a husband and wife who washed their fiberglass curtains in the same washing machine as their clothing.

Connubial Chloracne

A persistent follicular acneiform eruption developed on the forearms of a 40-year-old woman. She then revealed that her husband delivered fuel oil and had acquired a widespread chloracne. The patient inquired whether her husband's eruption was "contagious." She also stated that before putting her husband's oil-soaked clothing in the washing machine, her forearms often came in contact with the clothing.

The patient was instructed to place the soiled work clothes in the washing machine with a long forceps. The acneiform eruption subsided completely 3 weeks after the patient started using this procedure.

Work clothes contaminated with fiberglass or oil may produce irritant or chloracne connubial dermatitis.

Irritant and Traumatic Dermatitis

This type of dermatitis is usually characterized by redness, swelling, and a burning sensation. The history may reveal unusual "gymnastic" sexual maneuvers. Patients should also be asked whether they have cleansed the skin with strong soaps or detergents or have vigorously used rough towels.

Traumatic sexual dermatitis should be suspected when abrasions, fissures, erosions, or ulcers are present on the genitalia and perirectal area. Anal sexual eroticism is a fact of modern life, playing a major role in homosexual relationships. Skin injury from various manipulations and contact with "erotic" objects must be considered in both homosexual and heterosexual exposure.

Not infrequently, traumatic contact dermatitis is complicated by a superimposed allergic reaction due to the application of various medications. Ask the patient, "What medicine did you apply to your skin?" The most common causes of allergic contact dermatitis superimposed upon traumatic dermatitis are benzocaine, neomycin, and thimerosal (merthiolate).

Patients do not always readily admit the origin of penile ulcers caused by human bites. In addition to biting, a sexual partner may produce ulcers of the penis by scratching, by burning the penis with a lighted cigarette, or by injuring the penis with some instrument.

Various instruments, human bites, and lighted cigarettes may produce wounds and burns of the genitalia.

Marked swelling of the penis in circumcised persons may occur several hours after repeated vigorous intercourse with a passive partner. The involved area may be tender. A correct diagnosis is based on the history of a young vigorous male having intercourse with a sexually nonparticipating partner. There is absence of abrasions, ulcerations, adenopathy, or urethral discharge. There is no significant incubation period, and rapid recovery occurring after sexual abstinence is the rule without any particular therapy.

Balanoposthitis, inflammation of the membrane covering the glans penis and prepuce, occurs most frequently in uncircumcised men. The amount and type of involvement depend on the presence or absence of redundant prepuce, the degree of phimosis, and the severity of the irritation.

Irritant balanitis is usually mild, but it can progress to erosive balanitis with edema, hyperemia, and bleeding of the glans. The patient should be cautioned to avoid excessive trauma and irritation from strenuous intercourse or fellatio (80–83).

The management of contact balanoposthitis consists of retraction of the foreskin two or three times daily for careful cleansing with soap and water. The prepuce must not be left in the retracted position because paraphimosis may result. The penis is soaked for 15 minutes three times daily in Burow's solution diluted 1 to 10 in water; 1% hydrocortisone cream or lotion is then applied.

Edema of the penis and irritant balanitis can occur from "rough" intercourse or fellatio.

Hemorrhagic Changes of Oral Mucosa Due to Fellatio

Worsaae and Wanscher (80) reported a 34-year-old white woman who presented with a circular hemorrhagic lesion located on the soft palate caused by fellatio. The lesion consisted of erythema, petechiae, dilated blood vessels, and vesicles. It healed in a few days. No evidence of the major clinical alternatives, such as thrombocytopenia, venereal disease, or candida infection, were found. Injuries due to fellatio must be considered as an etiologic factor of hemorrhagic changes of the oral mucosa; patients with a positive history can be spared other investigations.

Contact Dermatitis in Homosexual Men

Contact dermatitis due to self-administered medications is quite common in gay men. One type of contact dermatitis, "poppers' dermatitis," is seen occasionally in gay men.

"Poppers' Dermatitis"

This dermatitis results from the inhalation of amyl or butyl nitrite, which is popularly known as "popping," to obtain a sexual "high," a common practice among gay men. The inhalation of the nitrites produces a warm sensation, dizziness, a flushing of the skin, and a "rush" as the blood vessels dilate, the heartbeat quickens, and the blood rushes to the brain.

Inhaled amyl and butyl nitrites are "recreational" drugs used frequently by male homosexuals.

This use of amyl or butyl nitrite is related to several unconventional sexual practices in gay men. These nitrites, perhaps more than any other illicit drugs currently in use, have a specifically sexual function: They are inhaled immediately before sexual climax. In the homosexual community in particular, use of nitrites to intensify orgasm is widespread. A guide to homosexual lovemaking states that the use of amyl nitrite "has passed into every corner of gay love" (84).

Although the nitrites are used widely by homosexual men, allergic contact dermatitis rarely occurs.

Nature and Uses of the Volatile Nitrites

Lowry (84) writes that the inhaled volatile nitrites are among the most widely used sexual "enhancers" in the United States today; moreover, their use is growing.

Two volatile nitrites are most commonly used as recreational drugs: amyl nitrite ($C_5H_{11}NO_2$) and isobutyl nitrite ($CH_3(CH_2)_3ON$). Amyl nitrite is a prescription drug approved by the Food and Drug Administration for the diagnosis and treatment of heart diseases. Isobutyl nitrite is not listed as a drug but is marketed as a "room odorizer."

Amyl nitrite is a clear, yellowish, volatile, flammable liquid with a peculiarly ethereal and fruity odor. This prescription item is available from two pharmaceutical manufacturers: as Aspirols (Lilly) and as Vapolole (Burroughs Wellcome). Amyl nitrite is supplied in fragile 0.3-mL glass containers enclosed in a gauze jacket of woven absorbent covering, which can readily be crushed between the fingers and held to the nostrils for inhalation. The noise made when the bottle is crushed gives rise to the street names, "popper" and "snapper."

Isobutyl nitrite, usually distributed in a 12-mL bottle with a screw cap, does not require a prescription and is less expensive than amyl nitrite. On the street, isobutyl nitrite is sold under various names (Table 5.6) and in such places as record shops, "radical" or "erotic" boutiques, "head" shops, adult book stores, and "specialty" shops as a "personal" product, "liquid scent," or "room odorizer." One manufacturer alone is currently producing 4 million bottles a year. A conservative extrapolation would yield a nationwide annual production of 250 million recreational doses of volatile nitrites.

TABLE 5.6. *Street Names for Isobutyl Nitrite*

Aroma of men	Hi Baller
Black Jac	Krypt Tonight
Bolt	Lockaroma
Bullet	Locker Room
Cat's Meow	Mama Popperer's Olde Fashioned
Climax	Fragrance
Discorama	Oz
Dr. Bananas	Rush
The Blues	Satan's Scent
Hardware	

Use of Nitrites among Homosexuals

Thirty years ago, amyl nitrite was widely used by heterosexual and homosexual persons in New York City's artistic and theatrical colony. Today, the nitrites, especially isobutyl nitrite, are most widely used among homosexuals. Perhaps this is because of visible social clustering of homosexuals at clubs, discos, and baths, whereas heterosexual users are a more diffuse group that is hard to locate, measure, or identify (85).

Goode and Troiden (86) interviewed 150 homosexual men to determine the relationship between the use of amyl nitrite and certain aspects of homosexual practice. These investigators found that the nitrites, perhaps more than any other illicit drug currently in use, have specifically sexual functions. Thus, the volatile nitrites can be inhaled either during foreplay (producing floating sensations, increased skin perception, and loss of inhibitions) or just before orgasm. In the latter instances, users report that the climax is intensified and prolonged.

Adverse reactions from the volatile nitrites. Mild transitory headache, rapid pulse, dizziness, and flushing of the face are common among all users of nitrites. The following adverse reactions may occur in susceptible patients: nausea, vomiting, weakness, restlessness, pallor, cold sweat, involuntary passing of urine and feces, tachycardia, hypotension, syncope, and collapse. Excessively high doses of amyl nitrite may cause methemoglobinemia.

Pearlman and Adams (87) call special attention to the fact that the nitrites may also produce a transient elevation of intraocular pressure. Thus, ophthalmologists should be aware of this fact when they examine young patients who complain of pain about the eyes and intense headache and in whom increased intraocular pressure may be found. These physicians must be aware of the possibility of amyl nitrite abuse in this younger age group. Recognizing the source of their symptoms and findings can largely remove the need for a more extensive glaucoma evaluation unless the intraocular pressure remains elevated for a prolonged period. The use of nitrites, however, might also harm persons with proved glaucoma.

Effects on the skin and mucosa from inhaling the nitrites. In persons who inhale nitrites, marked vasodilation of the blood vessels in the skin is present, particularly in the "blush" zone of the head, neck, and clavicular area. In some instances, nasotracheal irritation and sinusitis develop (88,89).

> **Severe reactions due to "popping" include vomiting, incontinence, syncope, and increased intraocular pressure.**

Patch testing with nitrites. The volatile nitrites are irritants under a closed patch. "Open" testing in one patient

who had dermatitis revealed a marked eczematous reaction that did not occur in three control subjects. A yellowish dermatitis can be a clue to nitrites as a cause of dermatitis. Three patients had facial dermatitis characterized by crusts with a distinctive yellowish tint (88,89). Fregert et al. (90) have a possible explanation for this yellowish color. They noted that certain factory workers exposed to nitric acid or nitrites acquired a yellow stain on their palms. These authors state that the yellow stain caused by nitric acid or nitrites in an acid environment is known as the xanthoprotein reaction, which is presumed to arise by nitration of the aromatic nuclei of certain amino acids incorporated into the protein chain.

Finally, because some butyl nitrite preparations contain a fragrance, the possibility that an allergic reaction may develop in addition to an irritant reaction has to be considered during examination of a perfume-sensitive person.

Traumatic Penile Ulcers

Dequalinium, a quaternary ammonium compound with antimicrobial and antifungal properties, is a recognized cause of penile ulcerations. Most cases have been recognized in Europe, but the antiseptic may be acquired by travelers abroad and brought into this country. The patients are usually uncircumcised men who have been treated with dequalinium because of preexisting balanitis. The resultant ulcers may be deep and necrotic, with sites of predilection on the glans and prepuce.

Unexplained ulcers of the penis that do not correspond to well-defined disease may be of factitial origin. Patients have produced ulcers of the penis with lighted cigarettes, razor blades, and a range of objects that demonstrate a remarkable degree of resourcefulness.

Traumatic Sclerosing Lymphangitis of the Penis

Male homosexuals may exhibit a specific type of edema of the glans penis and coronal area that is doughy and plastic, appearing 24 to 48 hours after intercourse.

Lymphocele

This condition may occur following excessive sexual intercourse or masturbation. The lymphatics in the coronal sulcus temporarily become blocked. Clinically, the patient has wormlike translucent masses, in contrast to the purplish, nontranslucent lesions of sclerosing lymphangitis.

CONTACT DERMATITIS IN BLACK PATIENTS

McDonald (91) compared the disease incidence in a random sampling of patients from a private dermatology practice, in which most patients were white, with the disease incidence in a random sampling of black patients from

> **"Pomade acne" or "Vaselinoderma," a form of acne venenata, and acneiform eruption due to tar are common dermatoses in black patients.**

Kaidbey and Kligman (96) compared the results of continuous occlusive application of 25% crude coal tar to the backs of young black and adult white males for 3 weeks, which regularly induced an acneiform eruption. In blacks, the eruption consisted of a monomorphous crop of comedones that were of the open variety from the very start. In whites, the first lesions were papulopustules resulting from toxic disorganization of the follicular epithelium. This inflammatory phase was followed by the development of comedones.

This study demonstrated racial differences in follicular reactivity. The follicles of white subjects responded early with rupture of the wall and an outpouring of follicular contents into the dermis. This led to an inflammatory papule and was attributed to the cytotoxicity of the tar. Later, hyperkeratosis became pronounced. In black subjects, the first response was a proliferative one with excessive production and retention of coherent horny cells. The "fragility" of follicles in white subjects supports the clinical observation that the more severe manifestations of inflammatory acne are more common in whites. Pomade acne in blacks is also principally a noninflammatory comedonal disease. In black persons, the sebaceous follicles are evidently sturdier and more likely to respond with hyperkeratosis than with disintegration.

Verhagen (97) confirmed the findings of Plewig et al. (95) that black skin is prone to the development of pomade acne. He also confirmed the demonstration by Kaidbey and Kligman (96) that artificially induced coal tar acne in blacks differed from that in whites because it was hardly inflammatory.

Verhagen and coworkers (98) also reported that Vaselinoderma was so common in Kenya that they saw 41 cases in 2 years because of the widespread practice of treating the faces of African children with petroleum jelly (Vaseline), frequently up to twice daily. In the great majority, lesions consisted only of open comedones with minute inflammation. There were, however, a few exceptions to this rule. Almost all cases were in children between the ages of 1 and 12 years. This demonstrates the susceptibility of black skin to monomorphic comedo acne in response to acne-inducing substances. Moreover, this condition not only exists in adulthood but also can begin at an age when acne vulgaris is very rare.

Black patients readily acquire allergic contact dermatitis from such contactants as paraphenylenediamine, nickel, chromates, and mercaptobenzothiazole. Such dermatitis is often complicated by hyperpigmentation and lichenifica-

tion unless it is treated early and vigorously with systemic corticosteroids. Patch testing is reliable on black skin.

Andersen and Maibach (99) concluded that a review of the literature on differences between black and white human skin emphasizes the alleged importance of factors other than the obvious, that is, skin color. Physicochemical differences and differences in susceptibility to irritants and allergens suggest that black skin is more resistant than white skin. Differences exist in the frequency with which several skin diseases occur among blacks and whites. A striking feature in this literature is the disagreement between authors. Much of this information is difficult to interpret because of socioeconomic influences and other environmental factors. Pigmentation rather than race was identified as a factor in barrier function. Men and women with type II/III skin were compared with skin type V/VI. Darkly pigmented skin was found to have a more resistant barrier and recovered more rapidly than skin of individuals with lighter pigmentation (100). This was independent of race (white vs Asian) or gender.

Industrial Dermatitis in Blacks

Schwartz et al. (101) and Shelley (102) state that black persons resist chemical and ultraviolet light irritation better than light-skinned persons. Marshall et al. (103), who as early as 1919 used 1% dichloroethylsulfide in mineral oil on the arms of whites and blacks to produce dermatitis, found erythema in 15% of black subjects compared to 59% of white subjects.

> **Studies reporting that black skin may be more resistant to irritation than white skin are questionable because erythema is more difficult to detect in black skin.**

Weigand and Mershon (104) noted that black skin was more resistant than white skin by measuring the minimal perceptible erythema (MPE) using quantitative patch test exposures to o-chlorobenzylidene malononitrile, a lacrimator. Weigand and Gaylor (105) determined the MPE in both black and white volunteers by applying increasing amounts of dinitrochlorobenzene (DNCB) to the skin of the back. The investigators reported that white subjects tended to have MPEs at lower concentrations of DNCB than did black subjects. On stripped skin, reactivity was more homogeneous. Tests were read in a room with artificial lighting indicating that, because of constant reading conditions, the differences were not due to perceptual error in reading of erythema because a dose-response curve was made for each subject and the differences were not observed on stripped skin. The possible protective effect of melanin granules in black skin was discussed, but it was concluded that melanin

TABLE 5.7. *Complications of Contact Dermatitis in Black Skin*

Acne venenata
Hyperpigmentation
Hypopigmentation
Lichenification

several health centers. He concluded that the occurrence of the most common dermatologic diseases, such as atopic eczema, dermatitis (including contact dermatitis), and acne, is quite similar in black and in white skin. Table 5.7 lists the common complications of contact dermatitis in black skin.

COMPLICATIONS OF CONTACT DERMATITIS IN BLACK SKIN

Hypopigmentation

Contact vitiligo, which may be due to chemicals, such as the phenolic detergents (paratertiary butylphenol, paratertiary amylphenol, paratertiary butylcatchol), alkylphenols, and monobenzylether of hydroquinone, is distressing, particularly to patients who have dark skin (92). Several black hospital workers who acquired severe contact vitiligo from the use of phenolic detergents were observed (93).

Hyperpigmentation

McDonald (91) stressed that, in many cases, hyperpigmentation in black patients is the end result of the most innocuous irritant. Thus, acneiform lesions, in the process of either formation or regression, can cause persistent spotty hyperpigmentation. Keratolytics and other irritants used in acne therapy often cause such deep and distressing hyperpigmentation that many black patients voluntarily terminate therapy. In many instances, unless forewarned, the patients do not return for additional care because they prefer the disease to the hazards of therapy. Tretinoin may cause transient hyper- or hypopigmentation in deeply pigmented persons. In such cases, pigmentation recedes 3 to 6 months after removal of the irritant. In these situations, it cannot be overemphasized that the patient must be warned of both the potential for and the temporary nature of this type of hyperpigmentation. Constant reassurance is necessary during the course of active therapy.

Lichenification

Black skin appears to be especially predisposed to lichenification. This clinical entity, which in its most easily recognizable form consists of thickened, indurated, hyperpigmented plaques of skin, with accentuated normal skin markings, is usually associated with pruritic diseases of the

skin. In most affected persons, licheni early as clusters of tiny papules in skin th jected to vigorous, prolonged rubbing These papules coalesce very readily to form acteristically observed plaquelike skin lesior

Apparently, the papular state of lichenifid occurs earlier in black skin but persists late i of pruritic dermatoses, such as atopic eczema matitis, and localized neurodermatitis. Freque fied papules in black skin occur singly rather ters and are often confused clinically with the polygonal papules of lichen planus.

Acne Venenata in Black Skin

"Pomade acne" or "Vaselinoderma" is very cc black patients because of the extensive use of such tions as Vaseline petroleum jelly, Noxzema skin crea root Cream Oil hair dressing, mineral oil (heavy Royal Crown hair dressing, and Dixie Peach pomad

Plewig et al. (95) studied a total of 735 black m used scalp creams and oils daily. About 70% of th term users of pomades displayed a recognizable acn eruption of the forehead and temples that consisted of rather uniform closed comedones with occasional lopustules. The more elaborate formulations (Nox Dixie Peach, and Wildroot) induced pomade acne more quently and more intensively than simpler preparati such as mineral oil and Vaseline.

Application of five pomades to black skin under conti ous occlusion for 8 weeks produced microscopic signs early comedo formation. Histologically, pomade acne w indistinguishable from acne vulgaris. Plewig et al. (95) fu ther stressed that although individual lesions may mimi acne vulgaris clinically and histologically, pomade acne is a quite distinctive condition. Its features include localization to the forehead and temples, uniform and often numerous closed comedones with a few scattered papulopustules in more extensive cases, and a history of long-term daily use of greasy or oily hair grooming preparations. Finally, pomade acne is primarily a disease of black patients.

The chief ingredients of the pomades are high-melting hydrocarbons that are not chemically defined. Mineral oil itself comes in a great many grades, and probably no two samples are entirely alike, no matter how much they are refined. It seems very likely that the acnegenic components reside mainly in these hydrocarbons and not in some minor, potent acnegen that is inadvertently added or is not eliminated during processing.

Because the pomades are weak acnegens, it generally takes a year or more of daily use to produce the eruption. Moreover, the lesions rarely go beyond the closed comedo stage. This is in contrast to industrial acnegens, such as chloronaphthalenes, that produce huge open comedones and marked inflammatory lesions resembling acne conglobata.

could not be the main protectant because it is distributed mainly below the removed stratum corneum. Frosch and Kligman (106) found that black subjects were less susceptible to irritants than were white subjects, but no data were presented.

The use of laser Doppler velocimetry and transepidermal water loss measurements showed that black skin was more sensitive to sodium lauryl sulfate than white skin when water loss was considered. However, only minimal blood flow changes were noted in response to this irritant when black subjects were compared to white subjects, even with the laser Doppler instrument (107).

Most studies evaluated irritancy using erythema as the endpoint in equating white versus black responses. This procedure is questionable because erythema is difficult to detect in black skin, so the differences in irritancy response between the two races might be less pronounced than reported.

REFERENCES

1. Fisher AA. Childhood allergic contact dermatitis. *Cutis* 1975;15:635.
2. Epstein E. Contact dermatitis in children. *Pediatr Clin North Am* 1971;18:839.
3. Honigman, J. Bubble bath dermatitis in children. *Cutis* 1966;2:406.
4. Leyden JJ, Katz S, Stewart R, Kligman AM. Urinary ammonia and ammonia-producing microorganisms in infants with and without diaper dermatitis. *Arch Dermatol* 1977;113:1678.
5. Berg RW. Etiologic factors in diaper dermatitis: a model for development of improved diapers. *Pediatrician* 1987;14(Suppl 1):27.
6. Berg RW, Buckingham KW, Stewart RL. Etiologic factors in diaper dermatitis: the role of urine. *Pediatr Dermatol* 1986;3:102.
7. Buckingham KW, Berg RW. Etiologic factors in diaper dermatitis: the role of feces. *Pediatr Dermatol* 1986;3:107.
8. Brown CP, Wilson FH. Diaper region irritations: pertinent facts and methods of prevention. *Clin Pediatr* (Phila) 1964;3:409.
9. Montes LF, et al. Microbial flora of infant's skin: comparison of types of microorganisms between normal skin and diaper dermatitis. *Arch Dermatol* 1971;103:400.
10. Leyden JJ, Kligman AM. The role of microorganisms in diaper dermatitis. *Arch Dermatol* 1978;114:56.
11. Lane AT, Rehder PA, Helm K. Evaluations of diapers containing absorbent gelling material with conventional disposable diapers in newborn infants. *Am J Dis Child* 1990;144:315.
12. Fergusson AG, Fraser NG, Grant PW. Napkin dermatitis with psoriasiform "Ide": a review of fifty-two cases. *Br J Dermatol* 1966;78:289.
13. Andersen SL, Thomsen K. Psoriasiform napkin dermatitis. *Br J Dermatol* 1971;84:316.
14. Gibson WB. Sweaty sock dermatitis. *Clin Pediatr* (Phila) 1963;2:175.
15. Verbov JL. Atopic dermatitis and the forefoot. *Br Med J* 1978;11:962.
16. Jepsen LV. Dermatitis plantaris sicca: a retrospective study of children with recurrent dermatitis of the feet. *Acta Derm Venereol* (Stockh) 1979;59:257.
17. Epstein WL. Contact-type delayed hypersensitivity in infants and children: induction of rhus sensitivity. *Pediatrics* 1960;187:1130.
18. Hjorth N. Contact dermatitis in children. *Acta Derm Venereol* 1981[Suppl]; 95:36.
19. Edwards EK. Contact urticaria to cow's milk. *Cutis* 1981;28:450.
20. Lecks HE. Anaphylaxis from milk protein in diaper ointment [Letter]. *JAMA* 1980;244:1560.
21. Kekki OM, Turjanmaa K, Isolauri E. Differences in skin-prick and patch-test reactivity are related to the heterogeneity of atopic eczema in infants. *Allergy* 1997;52:755.
22. Isolauri E, Turjanmaa K. Combined skin prick and patch testing enhances identification of food allergy in infants with atopic dermatitis. *J Allergy Clin Immunol* 1996;97:9.
23. Rasanen L, et al. Allergy to ingested cereals in atopic children. *Allergy* 1994;49:871.
24. Veien NK, Hattel T, Justesen O, Nörholm A. Contact dermatitis in children. *Contact Dermatitis* 1982;8:373.
25. Rietschel RL, Rosenthal LE, the North American Contact Dermatitis Group. Standard patch test screening series used diagnostically in young and elderly patients. *J Am Contact Derm Soc* 1990;1:53.
26. Rademaker M, Forsyth A. Contact dermatitis in children. *Contact Dermatitis* 1989;20:104.
27. Roul S, Ducombs G, Taieb A. Usefulness of the European standard series for patch testing in children: a 3-year single-centre study of 337 patients. *Contact Dermatitis* 1999;40:232.
28. Giordano-Labadie F, et al. Frequency of contact allergy in children with atopic dermatitis: results of a prospective study of 137 cases. *Contact Dermatitis* 1999;40:192.
29. Brasch J, Geier J. Patch test results in schoolchildren: results from the Information Network of Departments of Dermatology (IVDK) and the German Contact Dermatitis Research Group (DKG). *Contact Dermatitis* 1997;37:286.
30. Sevila A, Romaguera C, Vilaplana J, Botella R. Contact dermatitis in children. *Contact Dermatitis* 1994;30:292.
31. Romaguera C, Vilaplana J. Contact dermatitis in children: 6 years' experience (1992–1997). *Contact Dermatitis* 1998;39:277.
32. Levy A, Hanau D, Foussereau, J. Contact dermatitis in children. *Arch Dermatol* 1963;87:378.
33. Peltonen L. Nickel sensitivity in the general population. *Contact Dermatitis* 1979;5:27.
34. Prystowsky SD, et al. Allergic contact hypersensitivity to nickel, neomycin, ethylenediamine, and benzocaine: relationship between age, sex, history of exposure, and reactivity to standard patch tests and use tests in a general population. *Arch Dermatol* 1979;115:959.
35. Fisher AA. Prevention of shoe dermatitis by controlling hyperhidrosis with tannic acid. *Cutis* 1973;12:493.
36. Johns AM, Bower BD. Wasting of the napkin area after repeated uses of fluorinated steroid ointment. *Br Med J* 1970;1:347.
37. Miara RH. Atrophic striae following topical fluocinolone therapy. *Br J Dermatol* 1964;76:481.
38. Savin JA, Alexander S, Marks R. A rosacea-like eruption of children. *Br J Dermatol* 1972;87:425.
39. Tappeiner J, Pfleger L. Granuloma glutaeale infantum. *Hautarzt* 1971;22:383.
40. Grupper C, Bensoussan L, Duprepaire R. Granuloma facial infantile apres corticoides fluores locaux. *Bull Soc Fr Derm Syph* 1975; 82:337.
41. Uyeda K, Nakayasu K, Takaishi Y, Sotomatsu S. Kaposi sarcoma–like granuloma on diaper dermatitis: a report of five cases. *Arch Dermatol* 1973;107:605.
42. Georgouras K, Kocsard E. Micropapular sarcoidal facial eruption in a child: Gianotti-type perioral dermatitis. *Acta Derm Venereol* 1978;58:433.
43. Gianotti F. Cutaneous benign histiocytoses in childhood. In: *Pediatric dermatology: modern problems in pediatrics*. Basel: Karger. 71:193.
44. Breit R. Allergen change in stasis dermatitis. *Contact Dermatitis* 1977;3:309.
45. Coenraads PJ, Bleumink E, Nater JP. Susceptibility to primary irritants: age dependence and relation to contact allergic reactions. *Contact Dermatitis* 1975;1:377.
46. Angelini G, Rantuccio F, Meneghini CL. Contact dermatitis in patients with leg ulcers. *Contact Dermatitis* 1975;1:81.
47. Fisher AA. Contact urticaria due to polyethylene glycol. *Cutis* 1977;19:409.
48. Fisher AA. The paraben paradoxes. *Cutis* 1977;12:830.
49. Fisher AA, Pelzig A, Kanof NB. The persistence of allergic eczematous sensitivity and the cross-sensitivity pattern to para-phenylenediamine. *J Invest Dermatol* 1958;30:9.
50. Reiss F, Fisher AA. Is hair dyed with paraphenylenediamine allergenic? *Arch Dermatol* 1974;109:221.
51. Fisher AA. Some immunologic phenomena in treatment of and patch testing for ragweed oil dermatitis. *J Invest Dermatol* 1952;19:271.
52. Smith JG Jr, Kiem IM. Allergic contact sensitivity in the aged. *J Gerontol* 1961;16:118.

53. Tindall IP, Smith JG. Skin lesions of the aged and their association with internal changes. *JAMA* 1963;186:1039.
54. Fisher AA. Drug eruptions in geriatric patients. *Cutis* 1976;18:402.
55. Fisher AA. Systemic eczematous "contact-type" dermatitis medicamentosa. *Ann Allerg* 1966;24:406.
56. Felix RH, Comaish JS. The value of patch and other skin tests in drug eruptions. *Lancet* 1974;1:1017.
57. Korbitz BC. Patch tests for quinine allergy. *Arch Environ Health* 1973;27:409.
58. Houwerzijl J, de Gast GC, Nater JP. Patch tests in drug eruptions. *Contact Dermatitis* 1975;1:100.
59. Van Ketel WG. Patch testing in penicillin allergy. *Contact Dermatitis* 1975;1:253.
60. Penvy ME, Schroepl F. Toxic skin reactions in patch testing with tricyclic psychotropic drugs. *Hautarzt* 1974;25:430.
61. Kikuchi K, Tsunoda T, Tagami H. Generalized drug eruption due to mexiletine hydrochloride: topical provocation on previously involved skin. *Contact Dermatitis* 1991;25:70.
62. Leyden JL, Kligman AM. Allergic contact dermatitis: sex differences. *Contact Dermatitis* 1977;3:333.
63. Björnberg A. Skin reactions to primary irritants in men and women. *Acta Derm Venereol* (Stockh) 1975;55:191.
64. Wilkinson DS. Connubial photodermatitis. *Contact Dermatitis* 1975;1:58.
65. Fisher AA. Consort contact dermatitis. *Cutis* 1979;24:595.
66. Fisher AA, Brancaccio RR. Allergic contact sensitivity to propylene glycol in a lubricant jelly. *Arch Dermatol* 1979;115:1451.
67. Fisher AA. Propylene glycol dermatitis. *Cutis* 1978;21:166.
68. Fisher AA. The clinical significance of positive patch test reactions to balsam of Peru. *Cutis* 1974;13:909.
69. Fisher AA. Allergic reaction to feminine hygiene sprays. *Arch Dermatol* 1973;108:801.
70. Caro I. Connubial contact dermatitis to benzoyl peroxide. *Contact Dermatitis* 1976;2:362.
71. Rietschel RL, Lewis CW. Contact dermatitis to homomenthyl salicylate. *Arch Dermatol* 1978;114:442.
72. Fisher AA. Urticarial and systemic reactions to contactants varying from hair bleach to seminal fluid. *Cutis* 1977;19:715.
73. Levine BB, Siraganian RP, Schenkein I. Allergy to human seminal plasma. *N Engl J Med* 1973;288:894.
74. Schultz KH, Schirren C, Kueppers I. Allergy to seminal fluid [Letter]. *N Engl J Med* 1974;290:916.
75. Levine BB. Allergy to seminal fluid [Letter]. *N Engl J Med* 1974;290:916.
76. Frankland AW, Parish WE. Anaphylactic sensitivity to human seminal fluid. *Clin Allergy* 1974;4:249.
77. Mikkelsen EJ, et al. Allergy to human seminal fluid. *Ann Allergy* 1975;34:239.
78. Fisher AA. Condom conundrums: part 1. *Cutis* 1991;48:359.
79. Fisher BK, Warkentin JD. Fiberglass dermatitis. *Arch Dermatol* 1969;99:717.
80. Worsaae N, Wanscher B. Oral injury caused by fellatio. *Acta Derm Venereol* (Stockh) 1978;58:187.
81. Wide H, Canby JP. Penile venereal edema. *Arch Dermatol* 1973;108:263.
82. Wright RA, Judson FN. Penile venereal edema. *JAMA* 1979;241:157.
83. Gorlick G. Chronic rash of the glans penis: a differential diagnosis. *JAMA* 1979;242:469.
84. Lowry TP. Nitrite inhalants for sex—the quest for the ultimate orgasm. *Sex Med Today* 1980(July):34.
85. Louria DB. Sexual use of amyl nitrite. *Med Aspects Hum Sexuality* 1970;4:89.
86. Goode E, Troiden RR. Amyl nitrite use among homosexual men. *Am J Psychiatry* 1979;136:1067.
87. Pearlman JT, Adams GL. Amyl nitrite inhalation fad [Letter]. *JAMA* 1970;212:160.
88. Fisher AA, Brancaccio RR, Jelinek JE. Facial dermatitis in men due to inhalation of butyl nitrite. *Cutis* 1981;271:146.
89. Fisher AA, Brancaccio RR. Popper's dermatitis from sniffing butyl nitrite. *The Schoch Letter* 1979;29(October):item 142.
90. Fregert S, Poulsen J, Trulsson L. Yellow stained skin from sodium nitrite in an etching agent. *Contact Dermatitis* 1980;6:296.
91. McDonald CJ. Dermatological problems in black skin. *Prog Dermatol* 1973;4:15.
92. Kahn G. Depigmentation caused by phenolic detergent germicides. *Arch Dermatol* 1970;102:177.
93. Fisher AA. Vitiligo due to contactants. *Cutis* 1976;17:431.
94. Fisher AA. Contact dermatitis in black patients. *Cutis* 1977;20:303.
95. Plewig G, Fulton JE, Kligman AM. Pomade acne. *Arch Dermatol* 1970;101:580.
96. Kaidbey KH, Kligman AM. A human model of coal tar acne. *Arch Dermatol* 1974;109:212.
97. Verhagen AR. Pomade acne in black skin. *Arch Dermatol* 1974;110:465.
98. Verhagen AR, Koten JW, Chaddah VK, Patel RI. Skin diseases in Kenya: a clinical and histopathological study of 3,168 patients. *Arch Dermatol* 1968;98:577.
99. Andersen KE, Maibach HI. Black and white skin differences. *J Am Acad Dermatol* 1979;1:276.
100. Reed JT, Ghadially R, Elias PM. Skin type, but neither race nor gender, influence epidermal permeability barrier function. *Arch Dermatol* 1995;131:1134.
101. Schwartz L, Tulipan L, Birmingham DJ. *Occupational diseases of the skin.* 3rd ed. Philadelphia: Lea & Febiger, 1957.
102. Shelley WB. Newer understanding of ecology in dermatology. In: Rees RB, ed. *Dermatoses due to environmental and physical factors.* Springfield: Charles C Thomas Publisher, 1962:12.
103. Marshall EK Jr, Lynch V, Smith HW. Variations in susceptibility of the skin to dichloroethylsulfide. *J Pharmacol Exp Ther* 1919;12:291.
104. Weigand DA, Mershon MM. The cutaneous irritant reaction to agent *o*-chlorobenzylidene malononitrite (CS). I. Quantitation and racial influence in human subjects. *Edgewood Arsenal Technical Report* 4332. February 1970.
105. Weigand DA, Gaylor JR. Irritant reaction in Negro and Caucasian skin. *South Med J* 1974;67:548.
106. Frosch PJ, Kligman AM. The chamber-scarification for assessing irritancy of topically applied substances. In: Drill VA, Lazar P, eds. *Cutaneous toxicity.* New York: Academic Press, 1977.
107. Berardesca E, Maibach HI. Racial differences in sodium lauryl sulphate induced cutaneous irritation: black and white. *Contact Dermatitis* 1988;18:65.

CHAPTER 6

Regional Contact Dermatitis

THE EYELIDS

The eyelids are one of the most sensitive areas. Any substance used on the scalp, face, or hands may produce allergic eczematous contact dermatitis of the eyelids, whereas those primary sites remain unaltered. Airborne pollen and dust and all types of volatile agents may affect the eyelids first and exclusively. The absence of eyelid involvement is a strong argument against an airborne exposure to volatile substances unless this is explained by the use of protective eyewear. Contamination of the fingers with small amounts of allergen can result in transfer of sufficient material to the eyelids to produce dermatitis when little or no visible sign of difficulty is found elsewhere on the body. Marked edema of the eyelids is often a feature of poison ivy or hair dye dermatitis.

Contact dermatitis is the most common eruption of the eyelid. The skin of the area is very susceptible to irritants and allergens. This may be because of the thinness of the eyelid (0.55 mm as compared to the thickness of the integument of the face, measuring about 2.0 mm) or caused by rubbing the eyelid area with the hands and fingers, which become exposed to many substances.

Eyelid Dermatitis Due to Cosmetics

Contact dermatitis of the lids and periorbital area more often is caused by cosmetics applied to the hair, face, or fingernails than by cosmetics applied to the eye area. It is important to bear in mind that the sites to which some cosmetics are applied may not be affected. This is particularly true for hair dye and nail polish. Similarly, allergic and irritant reactions to face creams, makeup (foundation lotions and bases), and blushes may be limited to the eyelids (1).

> **Cosmetic eyelid dermatitis is more often a reaction to cosmetics applied elsewhere (i.e., nail polish) than to cosmetics applied directly to the eye area.**

Two principal forms of contact dermatitis attributable to eye-area cosmetics are recognized: allergic contact dermatitis and irritant (toxic) contact dermatitis (2). The morphologic features of these two forms are not always readily distinguishable. The degree of inflammation may be of the same order (usually mild to moderate), and the interval may be the same between the initial exposure and the onset of the dermatitis. Furthermore, potential irritants in eye-area cosmetics and in cosmetics in general are usually weak; repeated exposures are often required to induce a reaction. Nor do all exposed persons react as they do generally with strong irritants (3).

Patch test responses to allergens and irritants may also be indistinguishable; erythema or edema and erythema at the patch test site may be elicited by either. An eczematous vesicular reaction diagnostic of delayed allergic hypersensitivity in response to potential allergens in eye makeup is by no means the rule.

The cause of contact dermatitis of the eyelid is not always readily ascertainable. The following approach is recommended, especially when more than one cosmetic is suspect:

1. Take a detailed history of exposure, which should include inquiry about agents other than eye-area cosmetics that are known to elicit localized contact dermatitis of the eyelids, the introduction of a new product, and the renewal or refill of a previously used product. Modification or revision of formulations without a change in nomenclature or packaging is not an uncommon practice in the cosmetic industry. The method used to remove eye makeup also merits attention. Eye-area cosmetics may be removed by face creams, wet (chemically treated) facial tissues, or eye makeup removers. Use of eyelash curlers may lead to contact dermatitis from the rubber edges or nickel plating.

> **Modifications and revisions of cosmetics may make a previously nonsensitizing cosmetic become the cause of cosmetic dermatitis.**

2. When the history is not sufficiently revealing or when more than one cosmetic is involved, the use test is often helpful in pinpointing the causative agent. The use test is

often more rewarding than an open or closed patch test with the product because of the high incidence of false-positive and false-negative reactions in response to patch testing. To carry out the use test, the product is generally applied to the back of the ear or to the antecubital fossa two or three times a day for at least 4 or 5 days. Although a positive test (i.e., reproduction of the dermatitis) is significant, a negative response does not necessarily exclude the test substance as causative.

3. Patch tests with the components (open or closed, depending on the chemical nature of the ingredient) of the product(s) incriminated by the history and use test are carried out in an attempt to identify causative allergen(s). Most cosmetic companies comply with a physician's request for such materials.

> **A cosmetic "use test" may obviate the need for patch testing or may be used to confirm patch test reactions.**

Cosmetic Irritant Eyelid and Conjunctival Reactions

Stinging and burning of the eyes and lids on application of an eye-area cosmetic are the most common complaints. These subjective symptoms are usually transitory and unaccompanied by objective signs of irritation. Evaporation of volatile components, such as mineral spirits, isoparaffins, and alcohol, and the presence of potential irritants, such as propylene glycol, sunscreens, and soap emulsifiers, in eye-area formulations are among the principal causes. In some instances, tolerance increases with subsequent applications, and the offending product does not have to be discarded.

Conjunctivitis may be elicited by physical irritants (mascara flakes, eyeshadow dust, particles of eyeliner, and mascara extenders, such as nylon or rayon fibers) and by chemical irritants (e.g., solvents and soap emulsifiers), as well as by potential allergens, such as preservatives and fragrances.

Irritation Due to Mascara

Water-based mascara may contain several soap emulsifiers, such as sodium borate and ammonium stearate, formed by the interaction of stearic acid with ammonium hydroxide, which may be irritating to certain individuals who may tolerate an anhydrous, waterproof mascara.

> **Some persons who have an irritant reaction from water-based mascara owing to the presence of soap emulsifiers may tolerate an anhydrous waterproof mascara or a cake mascara.**

A person who does not tolerate waterproof mascara or waterproof eyeliner may very well tolerate water-based counterparts. In the event that neither type of mascara or eyeliner is tolerable, a cake mascara or cake eyeliner may be tried. Maybelline Cake Mascara, Lumilane Cake Mascara (Orlane), and Maybelline Ultra Liner Cake Eyeliner have only half the number of chemicals found currently in water-based and waterproof formulations. The potential for irritation is thus considerably reduced. This is not true for Chanel's Compact Mascara, which is highly complex. Similarly, persons who cannot use cream eyeshadow may tolerate pressed-powder eyeshadow, and vice versa.

Preservatives in Eye Cosmetics

With few exceptions, parabens are common to all eye-area products. These esters of parahydroxybenzoic acid not infrequently are combined with at least one other antimicrobial, such as phenyl mercuric acetate, imidazolidinyl urea (germall-115), or quaternium-15 (Dowicel 200), to ensure adequate protection against yeasts, molds, and pseudomonads, which are widely distributed in nature. Clinique's Resistant Eyeliner and Basic Eye Emphasizer are paraben-free and contain sorbic acid as a preservative.

Paraben-sensitive persons, however, do not necessarily have to avoid paraben-containing cosmetics (4). According to Fisher, patients sensitized to parabens may nevertheless tolerate paraben-containing cosmetics even on the thin skin of the eyelids, provided the product is applied to normal skin not subjected to a dermatitis in the past. This is the so-called paraben paradox.

> **The parabens are used in practically all eye cosmetics. Many paraben-sensitive persons tolerate paraben-containing eye makeup on normal eyelids—the so-called paraben paradox.**

Quaternium-15, imidazolidinyl urea, and DMDM hydantoin are formaldehyde donors. The latter is used less frequently than the other two compounds. Quaternium-15 has a more active formaldehyde releaser than imidazolidinyl urea (5). Allergic reactions may be elicited by the compound per se or by the released formaldehyde (6). Fisher (6) maintains that imidazolidinyl urea is a much safer preservative than quaternium-15 for formaldehyde-sensitive persons. Potassium sorbate is also used as a preservative in eye-area products. Sensitization to this agent has been reported (7).

Di-isopropanolamine, used in cosmetic gloss formulations to "set up" the gel, has produced allergic contact dermatitis from an eyeshadow and a "blushing" gel (8). Ditertiarybutyl hydroquinone, an antioxidant in eyeshadow, produced an eyelid dermatitis (9).

Nail Polish Dermatitis

Nail polish dermatitis is an "ectopic dermatitis" because sensitized persons acquire dermatitis not on the nails or paronychial area but elsewhere, such as on the eyelids and neck. Dry nail polish becomes polymerized and is not a sensitizer (10). The sensitizing toluene-sulfonamide formaldehyde resin in ordinary nail polish may be replaced by a "hypoallergenic" polyester resin (Clinique). Reports of airborne contact dermatitis to resins that are sticky or poorly soluble with soap and water, such as epoxy resin, may represent ectopic rather than airborne contact due to similar finger-to-eyelid transfer.

Hair Cosmetics

Hair dyes, bleaching agents containing ammonium persulfate, perfumed hair sprays, hair setting lotions, and shampoos containing formaldehyde may affect the eyelids without producing scalp or forehead dermatitis. Paraphenylenediamine sensitivity and ammonium persulfate, in particular, may produce marked edema of the eyelids.

> **Marked edema of the eyelids may be produced by hair dyes containing paraphenylenediamine and ammonium persulfate in "platinum" blond preparations.**

Conjunctival Pigmentation Due to Eyeliner

Conjunctival pigmentation caused by eyeliner is a consequence of the application of eyeliner to the conjunctival side of the lid instead of to the exterior lid just behind the lashes. Unless the upper lid is everted to bring into view the aggregates of pigment deposited along the upper margin of the tarsal conjunctiva, this complication may be missed. Twelve cases were reported by Zuckerman (11), and another was reported by Jervey (12) in 1969. Although some patients complain of discomfort, tearing, and itching, most are asymptomatic and do not require treatment.

Eyeshadow Mimicking Orbital Calcification on a Roentgenogram

A single case of bilateral curvilinear supraorbital shadow was found on X-ray examination of the skull of a patient complaining of increasing headaches. This shadow was interpreted as calcification. It was noted that the patient wore a large amount of eye makeup, making the possibility of an artifact likely. The curvilinear shadows disappeared after the eyeshadow was removed. A subsequent survey of 25 types of eye shadow showed that many were radiopaque because of bismuth, magnesium silicate, and iron oxides within the formulation (13).

> **Eyeliners may produce permanent pigmentation of the conjunctiva. Iron oxides, bismuth, and magnesium silicate in eyeshadow are radiopaque and can produce roentgenograms mimicking orbital calcification.**

Preservatives in Ophthalmic Medications

Some preservatives may produce not only conjunctivitis but also eyelid dermatitis in sensitized individuals (14). Table 6.1 lists some of the items to consider for patch testing when conjunctivitis and eyelid dermatitis coexist. Preservatives are prime suspects, especially benzalkonium chloride and thimerosal (merthiolate). Less commonly used and less frequently reported ophthalmic preservatives include chlorobutanol, chlorhexidine, phenylmercuric nitrate, and acetate. Because preservative systems may change without notice, it may be necessary to consult the package insert, label, or manufacturer to ascertain product composition.

Adhesives Used for False Eyelashes

Artificial eyelashes consist of synthetic or natural fibers, including human hair, mounted on a thin fabric strip. The adhesive is a mixture of rubber latex, cellulose gums, and casein solubilized with a very mild alkali or other resins and water. The adhesive is formulated to be nonirritating and to permit easy removal of the lashes by simply peeling them off. This rubber latex rarely irritates the eyelids.

TABLE 6.1. *Patch Test "Series"*

Topical Ophthalmic Preparations, Including Contact Lens Solutions
Acetozolamide 0.1%
Benzalkonium chloride 0.01% pet
Benzethonium chloride 0.1% aq
Chlorhexidine 1% aq
Chlorobutanol 1% aq
Epifrin 1%
Epinephrine chloride 0.1% aq
Isopto carbachol 1%
Mannitol 2% in alcohol
Paraben mix 15% (3% ea. ethyl, methyl, butyl, benzyl, propyl) pet
Phenylmercuric acetate 0.05% pet
Phenylmercuric nitrate 0.05% pet
Pilocarpine chloride 0.1% aq
Propylene glycol 10% ag
Sorbic acid 5% pet
Thimerosal 0.1% pet

Eyelash Curlers

Nickel-sensitive patients may acquire eyelid dermatitis from nickel-plated eyelash curlers and tweezers. Such curlers and tweezers should be replaced by the stainless-steel variety. Formerly, rubber-tipped eyelash curlers produced eyelid dermatitis in rubber-sensitive patients.

Paper

Facial tissues containing perfume, formaldehyde, or benzalkonium chloride may produce dermatitis in sensitized persons. Newsprint and carbon paper produce eyelid dermatitis, particularly in persons sensitized to formaldehyde.

Plants

The *Toxicodendron* genus of plants (poison ivy, poison oak, and poison sumac) in particular may produce marked swelling of the eyelids with minimum dermatitis of the face.

Airborne Contactants

Household sprays, insecticides, animal hairs, and occupational volatile chemicals can produce eyelid dermatitis.

Eyelid Dermatitis Due to Fruits

The oil of lemon peel and the dyes of Florida orange skin can cause eyelid dermatitis.

Match Dermatitis

The phosphorous sesquisulfide in "strike anywhere" matches may produce marked eyelid dermatitis (15). Affected patients should use "safety" matches or cigarette lighters. Contact urticaria of the eyelids was ascribed to the use of "strike anywhere" matches (16).

Match dermatitis usually affects the eyelids and face, particularly on the left side. The dermatitis may also affect the thighs and hands. Even nonsmokers who do not use matches may acquire dermatitis, if they are near persons who use matches, apparently because the allergen may become airborne (17).

Eyelid Dermatitis from Quinazoline Yellow Dye (D & C Yellow No. 11)

Calnan (18) reported that Yellow D & C No. 11 dye produced an eyelid dermatitis owing to the presence of this dye in an eye cream.

FACIAL CONTACT DERMATITIS

Allergens can be transferred to the face not only by direct exposure but also indirectly from airborne or hand-to-face exposure. Thus, the face is the most common and often the main site of photodermatitis. Ragweed dermatitis, which occurs predominantly in men and boys, is most marked on the face. Toxicodendron dermatitis is often most prominent in the facial area.

An airborne exposure once weekly to a fish food caused a facial eczema from a combination of immediate and delayed hypersensitivity reactions to chironomids (nonbiting flies, midges) placed in an aquarium (19).

Unilateral Facial Dermatitis

In general, cosmetic dermatitis is bilateral, with the exception of nail polish dermatitis, which may be unilateral. Connubial or consort contact dermatitis owing to hair dyes, fragrances, and topical medication used by the partner may also occur on one side of the face.

Facial dermatitis owing to an allergic reaction to phosphorous sesquisulfide (P_4S_3), the sensitizer in "strike anywhere" matches, may be unilateral and airborne and may occur in nonsmokers (15). Crushing match heads, soaking match heads in water, and transferring the resulting mushy material to the patch test paper is the most satisfactory method of applying the allergen. Patch testing may also be performed with 0.5% of phosphorous sesquisulfide in petrolatum.

> **Unilateral facial contact dermatitis may be due to nail polish, connubial or consort dermatitis, or "strike anywhere" matches. It may be airborne and may occur in nonsmokers.**

"Status Cosmeticus" Due to "Stinging" Compounds in Cosmetics

Many currently available cosmetics are free of compounds that produce most allergic hypersensitivity. However, nonspecific irritation from cosmetics still occurs. Thus, some persons appear to be in a condition of "status cosmeticus," in which every cosmetic or soap applied to the face produces itching, burning, or stinging sensations.

The condition is somewhat analogous to "status asthmaticus," in which patients acquire allergic bronchitis in response to just about every possible airborne allergen. It must be emphasized, however, that "status cosmeticus" is an irritant and not an allergic reaction (20).

Patients who have "status cosmeticus" typically have an unremarkable clinical picture initially. They may have a mild erythema of the "butterfly" area of the face with slight edema of the eyelids. Occasionally there is a follicular eruption. However, the signs are not as vivid as the patients' bitter complaints of burning, stinging sensations. These persons usually claim to have tried at least 20 different cosmetics, all of which "disagree" with them.

Results of patch tests using the various implicated cosmetics and soaps are negative, as are results of "use" tests performed on the antecubital fossa. Undoubtedly, the facial skin differs from that of other areas of the body in its irritant sensitivity to cosmetics.

A similar constellation of findings has been reported to occur in pityriasis folliculorum. Malar erythema and a prominent follicular accentuation may give a slight sandpaper-like texture to the face accompanied by stinging, burning, or itching. A skin scraping examined with oil or potassium hydroxide demonstrates many Demodex organisms often packing into follicles in tight columns. Topical lindane, pyrethrum, malathione, or sulfur may eradicate live organisms, and a follicular purge of remaining material should be performed with topical tretinoin (21).

Frosch and Kligman (22) have confirmed that "stinging" from topically applied substances occurs mainly on the face. They found that substances that cause sustained stinging can be recognized by application to the nasolabial folds and cheeks during profuse sweating. The tests were carried out on preselected persons in whom a susceptibility to stinging had been demonstrated by exposure to 5% aqueous lactic acid. A predisposition to complaints of "stinging" was greater in women than in men and greater in whites than in blacks, especially in light-complexioned persons who tan poorly. The application of 10% lactic acid to the face elicited stinging almost equivalent to that produced by the application of 5% acid on sweating skin. It should also be noted that substances with a high capacity to induce stinging can do so in the absence of sweating.

Calnan (23) described one type of nonallergenic cosmetic complaint as an immediate stinging sensation that occurred when the product was applied to the face. However, because the stinging is transient and the product can subsequently be tolerated, a customer who has this experience does not usually complain to the manufacturer. But it is a reaction commonly mentioned in consumer surveys and market research studies of individual products. In Calnan's patient, a severe, stinging sensation developed from a powder containing 2-ethoxyethyl-*p*-methoxycinnamate. This adverse sensation was enhanced by sweating when the skin surface was damaged (e.g., from sunburn or dermatitis).

TABLE 6.2. *"Stinging" Cosmetic Agents That Can Produce "Status Cosmeticus"*

Benzoic acid
Bronopol
Cinnamic acid compounds
Dowicel 200
Formaldehyde
Lactic acid
Nonionic emulsifiers
Propylene glycol
Quaternary ammonium compounds
Sodium lauryl sulfate
Sorbic acid
Urea

Lahti (24) also showed that cinnamic acid compounds used in cosmetics can produce nonspecific redness and itching when applied to human skin. This is probably related to prostaglandin synthesis and is blocked by prostaglandin inhibitors, such as indomethacin and aspirin (25,26).

> **Stinging from topical applications and cosmetics occurs principally on the face, particularly in fair-skinned persons. Some women are in such a state of "status cosmeticus" that they do not tolerate any currently available cosmetics. Pityriasis folliculorum should be considered in the differential diagnosis of these patients.**

A review of the literature and personal experience would indicate that "ideal" cosmetics would be free of the compounds shown in Table 6.2 (6,20,22–24). This is particularly true of patients who have "status cosmeticus."

The Role of Anti-Irritants in Cosmetics

Goldenberg and Safrin (27) suggested that the "stinging" effects of cosmetic irritants may be neutralized by "anti-irritants." They proposed three possible mechanisms of action by which the anti-irritants may function: (a) complexing of the irritant, (b) blocking otherwise chemically reactive sites of skin keratin, and (c) preventing complete physical contact with the skin.

The anti-irritant chemicals are grouped in the following chemical categories: carboxyl, hydroxy, and imidazole compounds (Table 6.3). Miscellaneous anti-irritant compounds are listed in Table 6.4. Ongoing investigations will determine whether the inclusion of any of these anti-irritants in cosmetics will help eliminate "stinging" and "burning" from cosmetics and will be tolerated by those with "status cosmeticus."

Pigmented Facial Contact Dermatitis

Brown or bluish pigmentation of the face has been described as a dermatosis of great cosmetic significance in Japanese women since the 1950s (28). Many of the cases resemble the melanosis described by Riehl in Vienna in

TABLE 6.3. *"Anti-Irritant" Cosmetic Compounds*

Carboxyl Compounds
Hydroxy Compounds
  Polysorbate 20
  Aloe vera gel
Imidazole Compounds
  Germall-115—imidazolidinyl urea allantoin
  Imidazoline amphoteric surfactants (used in "no tears" shampoos)

TABLE 6.4. *Miscellaneous "Anti-Irritant" Compounds*

Amine acid surfactant (acyl glutamate)
Amine oxides
Heavy mineral oils
High-molecular-weight polypropylene glycols
Lauroyl cycloimidinium amphoteric surfactants
N-lauroyl sarcosinates
Phthalate esters
Polyvinyl pyrrolidone
Protein-fatty acid condensates (amides)
Sorbitan esters
Tertiary amine oxide surfactants
Thiodiglycolic acids

1917, and the term "Riehl's melanosis" is commonly used by Japanese dermatologists for the condition (29). At the International Conference on Dermatology and Cosmetic Science in Tokyo, the subject of facial melanosis was discussed extensively. The concept of Riehl's melanosis was considered, and the condition was defined in the perspective of recent progress in contact dermatitis (30).

In Japan, where facial melanosis has been quite common, allergic contact dermatitis to scents, such as hydroxycitronella, benzyl-salicylate, ylang-ylang oil, and jasmine, as well as to bactericides such as carbanilides, has been demonstrated as the cause of the pigmentation. Most Japanese dermatologists use the term "Riehl's melanosis" for both inflammatory and noninflammatory forms (28). Brilliant Lake Red R (widely used in cheek rouges and lipsticks until 1976) has been described as a common cause of sensitization (31). A study showed that Brilliant Lake Red R, which has been described as the most important cause of Riehl's melanosis, contains Sudan 1 as a major impurity (32). Investigations on the pattern of cross-sensitivity indicated that Sudan 1 is a potent sensitizer and that Brilliant Lake Red R itself is a weak sensitizer.

> **At present, Riehl's melanosis is synonymous with facial pigmented contact dermatitis induced by cosmetic chemicals.**

The dominant symptom of Riehl's melanosis is facial hyperpigmentation, most pronounced on the forehead and in the zygomatic or temporal regions. Riehl could find no explanation for the condition but suggested that certain foods used during the war could be responsible. Riehl's melanosis later was observed in dark-complexioned persons, in whom hyperpigmentation with pigment incontinence may be the main sign of contact dermatitis caused by certain allergens.

Today Riehl's melanosis is almost synonymous with pigmented contact dermatitis of the face. The most common cause has been sensitizing chemicals in cosmetics.

Facial Dermatitis Due to Rubber Compounds

The following rubber articles have produced facial dermatitis in rubber-sensitive persons:

scuba diver face mask (33)
bathing cap
rubber cosmetic sponges (34)
rubber-edged eyelash curlers (35)
balloons (36)
flubber (children's toys) (37)

Facial Dermatitis Due to Metallic Compounds

Nickel-plated objects used on the hair, such as bobby pins and curlers, may produce facial dermatitis in nickel-sensitive persons.

Postoperative Facial Dermatitis

The use of nickel-plated objects that make contact with the face during surgery or dentistry can produce facial dermatitis. Face masks sterilized with ethylene oxide may produce severe facial dermatitis.

THE SCALP

The scalp is particularly resistant to contact dermatitis. Allergens applied to this area often produce dermatitis of the eyelids, ears, neck, and hands, whereas the scalp remains uninvolved. Persons who have exquisite sensitivity to paraphenylenediamine or glyceryl thioglycolate, however, may show a marked scalp reaction with edema and crusting. Permanent wave solutions of ammonium thioglycolate applied improperly may produce severe irritant reactions and burns of the scalp.

Cosmetic Damage to the Scalp in Black Patients

McDonald (38) pointed out that most hair care products for black people are used to change the physical appearance of hair from naturally curly to some degree of straightness. When used improperly, they may cause severe damage to the hair and scalp.

The most potent hair straighteners (relaxers) are those containing the alkali sodium hydroxide. Sodium hydroxide straighteners, unlike thioglycolates, cause irreversible changes in the hair. When used improperly at home or by inexperienced beauticians, either on hair with small, weak fibers or on hair that has previously been abused by straighteners, these sodium hydroxide straighteners can cause devastating damage to the scalp and hair. A single, prolonged application of these products to normal hair may also result in damage to hair and scalp. Hair breakage, either immediate or removed, is the most common abnormality observed after the use of hair straighteners. Often, when remotely observed 4 to 6 months after application of the straightener, the patient may not associate hair breakage with the use of hair straighteners. As the relaxer is applied excessively, pooling on the scalp provides a greater degree of damage to the disulfide bonds that give the hair shaft its resistance to breakage. As this weak area grows away from the scalp surface, it loses the added support provided by the intrafollicular support structures and becomes increasingly "weathered" by combing, shampooing, and other treatments. The frictional injury of combing is also magnified by the added leverage exerted as the hair moves away from the scalp at a rate of about 12 to 14 mm per month. Thus, breakage occurs a month or more after a treatment.

The most severe damage caused by hot comb straightening occurs after severe burns to the scalp. This type of reaction may progress beyond the simple irritant type of skin reaction seen with many hair care products, including bleaching and coloring agents. In this case, the scalp sustains severe second- and third-degree burns that heal with permanent scarring. Hair follicles are thus destroyed, and hair loss becomes permanent. Alopecia not the result of an overt burn was critically reviewed, and the original concept of it being caused by use of a hot comb was found wanting. The patchy vertex and coronal cicatricial alopecia most commonly seen in black patients has been reclassified from hot comb alopecia to follicular degeneration syndrome, which is believed to be related to loss of the internal root sheath in sharply curved hair follicles (39).

> **Hair straighteners, particularly when not used properly, can cause severe burns of the scalp and hair damage in black patients. The concept of alopecia being caused by use of a hot comb has been found to be a flawed concept and is therefore reclassified from hot comb alopecia to follicular degeneration syndrome.**

Nickel-sensitive patients may develop localized scalp dermatitis from prolonged contact with hairpins, curlers, and bobby pins. Ill-fitting wigs, as well as some adhesives used with wigs, may irritate the scalp.

The insertion of "artificial" hairs for the treatment of male alopecia has resulted in many cases of severe dermatitis, infections, and granulomas. Vioform preparation applied to the scalp may turn white or silver hair a reddish hue (40), as may Capitrol shampoo, which may produce a strawberry blond tone.

THE FOREHEAD

Pomade acne, so-called Vaselinoderma, resulting from greasy applications to the scalp, affects the forehead. Pomades are the simplest of hair straighteners. They contain primarily paraffin and petrolatum mixtures with gums and perfumes added. They are the least damaging of all hair care products, but they often cause acneiform facial lesions (pomade acne). This is a unique form of acne characterized by the presence of uniform, localized, follicular comedones and occasionally papulopustules on the forehead and temples.

> **Pomades applied to the scalp, particularly by black patients to straighten the hair, often cause pomade acne of the scalp and temples and sometimes of the entire face.**

Phylactery Dermatitis

This type of dermatitis may occur as a square dermatitis of the forehead in Orthodox Jews who place phylacteries on their foreheads during prayer. Such a phylactery is a small, black leather cube containing a piece of parchment.

Bathing caps, rubber hair nets, and hat bands can also cause forehead dermatitis.

The Hindu practice of wearing a central forehead dot of color known as a *bindi* may lead to leukoderma associated with paratertiary butylphenol resin in the adhesive, with or without a related dermatitis or positive patch test (41,42).

> **A square localized dermatitis of the forehead may be produced by the black leather cube of the phylactery applied to the forehead by Orthodox Jews, and a circular dermatitis may occur from *bindi* worn by Hindus.**

CONTACT OTITIS: A DERMATITIS OF THE EXTERNAL EAR AND CANAL

The ear, particularly the helix, may be the site of the disease due to hair sprays, shampoos, and dyes. Earlobe dermatitis is a cardinal sign of nickel sensitivity in persons wearing costume jewelry earrings. Otitis externa may be caused by sensitizing medications applied to the ear canals, particularly neomycin. Habitual insertion of metallic objects (hairpins, pens, and pencils) into the canals may produce the dermatitis in nickel-sensitive persons. The piercing of earlobes is often a precipitating factor in nickel and gold sensitivity.

> **Earlobe dermatitis may be a cardinal sign of nickel allergy.**

The auricle and external ear canal, covered entirely by skin, are subjected to contact irritants and sensitizers just as is the skin elsewhere (43,44). Furthermore, the inflamed, occluded ear canal is as readily sensitized by topical medicaments as are stasis eczemas and ulcers.

Allergic dermatitis of either the entire auricle or a portion of it may occur in sensitized individuals. Plastic helmets or bathing caps affect the entire auricle. Nail polish, on the other hand, may produce dermatitis of any portion of the ear that sensitized persons touch before the nail polish is dry. This is an example of "ectopic" cosmetic dermatitis (45).

The site where the contact otitis originates often gives a clue to the causative contactant. Arnold (46) described "sugarcane" ears, resembling cauliflower ears in workers who carry bundles of burned stalks of sugar. The lesions are unilateral, depending on whether the worker is right- or left-handed.

Earlobe Otitis

Like nickel sensitivity, gold sensitivity may similarly affect the earlobes. The piercing of earlobes is a common precipitating cause of nickel sensitivity. By having their ears pierced and then wearing nickel-containing jewelry, many persons develop a generalized nickel sensitivity that persists indefinitely. For this reason, it is advisable to insert stainless steel earrings, under sterile conditions, for 3 weeks following ear piercing (47). Injury to the skin from ear piercing followed by intimate contact with metallic nickel favors the development of allergic eczematous dermatitis, which may be complicated by infection and hepatitis (48). Other complications of earlobe dermatitis include split earlobes (49), fissured granulomas (50), cyst formation, and keloids.

> **Piercing of the ear followed by nickel dermatitis and infection of the earlobes can be complicated by hepatitis, split earlobes, fissured granulomas, cyst, and keloid formation.**

Shore and Berger (51) described a case in which large hooped earrings produced a dermatitis of the neck but not of the earlobes. Fur neck pieces and collars may also produce dermatitis of the earlobes.

Postauricular Otitis

The metal or plastic frames of eyeglasses, plastic hearing aids, and telephone operator head sets can produce dermatitis in this area. Perfume-sensitive individuals who habitually place perfume behind their ears may also produce a postauricular otitis.

Retroauricular Dermatitis and Trauma Due to Spectacles

Jirasek et al. (52) reported retroauricular dermatitis from nickel in eyeglass frames. Barnes et al. (53) stated that mechanical trauma from eyeglass frames can cause a fissured acanthoma behind the ear.

Contact Otitis of the Helix

Allergenic preparations applied to the scalp or hair, such as hair dyes, sprays, and shampoos, may primarily affect the helices. Many persons who have mild hypersensitivity to hair dyes may acquire allergic dermatitis of the helices and eyelids without affecting the scalp or other facial areas. Earmuffs and hair nets may also produce dermatitis, principally of the helices.

External Canal Otitis

The habitual insertion of metallic objects, such as hairpins, pens, and pencils, into the canals may produce dermatitis in nickel-sensitive persons. Hearing aid inserts may also produce allergic reactions of the canal.

Once the canal becomes inflamed, occluded, and excoriated by scratching, the stage is set for ready sensitization to topical therapeutic agents, such as neomycin, benzocaine, sulfonamides, mercurials, the parabens, and even corticosteroid preparations.

The combination of dermatitis and infection may produce an infectious eczematoid contact otitis similar to that which occurs following middle ear and mastoid surgery. A chronic discharge accompanied by severe pruritus and edema of the external canal are cardinal signs of this condition.

Otitis externa is one of the most frequent conditions with which neomycin sensitivity is associated; therefore, the use of this antibiotic should be avoided in ear canal therapy (54). Unlike benzocaine dermatitis, which may be quite explosive, neomycin sensitivity is often subtle, consisting merely of an exacerbation of the otitis externa for which the neomycin was applied.

Antiseptics and antibiotics containing erythromycin (Ilotycin ointment), Terramycin, or Betadine are much less sensitizing than neomycin.

> **The inflamed, occluded external ear canal is as readily sensitized to neomycin, benzocaine, and the parabens as are stasis eczemas and ulcers.**

Local anesthetic topical agents containing xylocaine (Lidocaine) may be used instead of benzocaine.

"Sulfa" topical medication should also be avoided in benzocaine-sensitive persons because cross-reactions may occur.

McKelvie and McKelvie (55) stated that it is not unusual for patients to use match heads for cleaning or scratching their ears, and otitis externa caused by a contact dermatitis from a "strike anywhere" match head may occur.

Hearing Aid Dermatitis

Guill and Odom (56) reported a patient who developed a dermatitis from a cold-cured, acrylate hearing aid but tolerated a heat-cured variety. Jordan and Dahl (57) described retroauricular dermatitis due to resorcinol monobenzoate in a component of a patient's hearing aid. Hearing aids may be made of the following plastics: acrylate, vinyl, polyethylene, and silicone (see Chapter 20).

THE NECK

The neck, like the eyelids and genitalia, is a very reactive site. Cosmetics or topical acne medications applied to the face, scalp, or hair often initially affect the neck. Berlocque and nail polish dermatitis also commonly involve this area.

Nickel-sensitive patients may acquire dermatitis from necklaces, zippers, and the metallic neck pieces of stethoscopes. Necklaces made of various woods may also produce dermatitis. Tanita and Tagami (58) described a bizarre linear granuloma around the neck in a child who had placed a rubber band in the area. The neckline of tight leotards may produce a fine linear dermatitis of the neck, as can rubber hair nets. Rough-starched collars may also produce a dermatitis. Permanent wave solutions applied on the scalp and spilled accidentally on the neck have produced instances of allergic and irritant dermatitis of the neck.

Fiddler's Neck

"Fiddler's neck" is a common occupational mark among violin and viola players. It is an area of localized lichenification of the skin on the left side of the neck, just below the angle of the jaw, where the chin rest of the violin is in contact with the side of the neck. Additional signs are erythema, scaling, cyst formation, and papules or pustules within the area.

Lachapelle et al. (59) stated that a worsening of pseudofolliculitis of the beard has not been described as a clinical sign of "fiddler's neck."

THE CHEST

Medallions, crosses, zippers, nickel-plated buttons, and wires in brassiere cups have all produced dermatitis of the chest and breast. Perfume dermatitis of the upper chest and breast area is not uncommon. Sensitizing medications applied to eczematous nipples may produce an infiltrated dermatitis resembling a malignancy.

Lactating women may use herbal remedies for nipple eczema, and oil of chamomile contained in such remedies has caused contact dermatitis, which may exacerbate after the patient drinks chamomile tea (60).

THE BELTLINE

Many men develop dermatitis at the tops of their underwear shorts. This dermatitis is an allergic reaction to either a rubber chemical or an oxidized chlorine-bleached chemical. In either case, the patient may purchase rubber-free men's boxer shorts that are fastened with a button and free of elastic (Whitehall Mfg. Co., 180 Madison Avenue, New York, NY 10016).

THE UMBILICUS

Nickel-sensitive persons may acquire periumbilical dermatitis from metallic buttons of blue jeans.

Dermatitis of the Raw Umbilical Stump

Antiseptics, such as thimerosal (merthiolate), and antibiotics, such as neomycin, applied soon after the cord is tied may produce allergic contact dermatitis.

Umbilical Granulomas

Treatment of the raw umbilical stump with talc or starch may produce granulomas (61).

The Umbilical Stone

Ehring (62) stated that, in rare instances, a hard, smooth, almost black bolus "omphalolith" is found in the umbilicus, resembling a malignant melanoma. After removal by tweezers, it reveals on its backside a colorless lamellar epithelium. Microscopic examination shows it also consists of stratified corneocytes. Differential diagnosis of the omphalic stone includes the so-called umbilical cholesteatoma, an accumulation of crumbling, fetid masses in the umbilicus, often accompanied by seborrhea, that may lead to abscess formation.

THE TRUNK, PERIAXILLARY REGION, AND ANTECUBITAL SPACES

The trunk, periaxillary region, and antecubital spaces may be the sites of perfume dermatitis or a symmetrical type of dermatitis owing to the finishes and dyes in clothing.

AXILLAE

Deodorants, antiperspirants, and perfumes may cause contact dermatitis. "Consort" contact dermatitis may occur from resting of the head on the axilla when the consort has fresh-dyed hair or brilliantines on the scalp. Unilateral axillary dermatitis from zippers may occur in nickel-sensitive patients.

> **Irritant dermatitis from shaving and depilatories is not uncommon.**

THE FOREARMS

The forearms also may be the site of dermatitis due to sensitizers that splash above protective gloves. It must not be forgotten that loose bracelets may have considerable excursion on the forearm and thereby can produce dermatitis from the wrist to the antecubital spaces.

THE THIGHS

Gomez-Orbaneja et al. (63) reported that two men, sensitized by the striking surfaces of match boxes, developed thick, indurated plaques, first on the thighs, then on the face and other sites. These plaques fluctuated in severity and were initially identified clinically and histologically as mycosis fungoides. Another two men had patches confined to the thighs. Patch testing revealed that the four men tested positive to the striking surface of match boxes that they kept in their pockets.

Other objects in pockets that may cause thigh dermatitis include coins and keys. Police officers have acquired an irritant dermatitis of the thighs from leaking "mace" canisters used in antiriot maneuvers.

VULVITIS DUE TO CONTACTANTS

Douches, feminine hygiene sprays, cleansers, deodorants, and medications used on the vulva and in the vagina may be possible causes of contact vulvitis. In addition, medications, cosmetics such as nail polish, and other sensitizers may be conveyed by the hands to the vulva. Frequently, sensitizing medications or douches well tolerated by the vaginal mucosa produce vulvitis and dermatitis of the thighs (64).

Irritants and Sensitizers in Douches

Most over-the-counter douches are prepared by the user. Douches containing acid or alkalis that are not properly diluted may produce an irritant vulvitis. The principal acid irritants are alum, citric acid, and lactic acid. Alkalis, such as sodium bicarbonate or sodium borate, in too high a concentration may also produce vulvitis.

Britz and Maibach (65) have shown that the vulvar skin is more readily irritated than the forearm. Often low-grade erythema of the vulva is not readily apparent because of pigmentation of the skin of the vulva. The patient may complain of burning and stinging of the vulva, but examination may not readily reveal dermatitis.

> **Vulvar skin is more readily irritated than the vagina and skin on the trunk and the extremities.**

Table 6.5 lists the principal causes of allergic vulvitis from douches, as proved by positive patch test reactions. Because practically all douches are irritants under a closed patch test, testing should be performed with the individual ingredients of the douche.

Vulvitis from Feminine Hygiene Sprays (Deodorant Sprays)

Feminine hygiene sprays consist of perfume, an emollient, and a propellant. With the ban on hexachlorophene, most sprays no longer contain any antibacterial agents. Allergic reactions to spray ingredients are rare, usually occurring in patients who have miliaria, intertrigo, moniliasis, or seborrheic eczema in the inguinal or perineal area. Two cases of allergic reactions to the bacteriostat benzethonium chloride were encountered. Perfume in one instance and the emollient (isopropyl myristate) in another produced an allergic contact vulvitis (66).

Preservatives and antibacterial agents in medications, as well as in feminine hygiene sprays, may produce allergic reactions (67–70).

Irritant reactions from the chilling effect of fluorinated hydrocarbon propellants due to application too close to the vulvar area are much more common than reactions of the allergenic variety (71–73). Such allergic reactions appear to occur particularly on skin that has been previously injured by some type of nonallergic dermatitis, such as miliaria, seborrheic dermatitis, or moniliasis.

TABLE 6.5. *Sensitizers in Douches*

Aromatics (perfumes)
Benzethonium chloride
Methyl salicylate
Oil of eucalyptus
Oxyquinoline
Phenylmercuric acetate
Thymol

Vulvitis from feminine hygiene sprays may be due to an allergic reaction to the perfume or an irritation from the propellant of the spray applied too close to the vulva.

Chemical Contraceptives

Vaginal spermicides rarely irritate the vulva but may occasionally produce allergic vulvitis. Table 6.6 is a list of the principal sensitizers in vaginal spermicides.

Patch tests with chemical contraceptives must be interpreted with care because some contain soapy substances that may show nonspecific irritant reactions under a closed patch. A positive patch test reaction should be followed by testing with the individual ingredients of the product.

Many vaginal spermicides contain foaming agents and emulsifiers that may be irritating. Contact urticaria and anaphylaxis occur as a response to exposure to seminal fluid (see Chapters 5 and 33). Severe irritant dermatitis of the vulvar and suprapubic area may occur with the use of depilatories.

Rubber Products Producing Vulvitis

Rubber Support Pessaries and Contraceptive Diaphragms

Vaginitis and vulvitis may be produced by such rubber articles in rubber-sensitive individuals. For rubber-sensitive persons, plastic pessaries and contraceptive devices are now available as substitutes.

Rubber Condoms

These products may produce an acute dermatitis of the vulva and inner aspect of the thighs in a rubber-sensitive woman.

A rubber condom used by a man may produce dermatitis in a rubber-sensitive woman.

Miscellaneous Causes of Vulvitis

1. *Nickel-plated* objects (pins, fasteners, zippers, and clasps) on sanitary napkins may produce vulvitis in nickel-sensitive persons.
2. *Cosmetics* may be the cause of vulvitis. For example, nail polish dermatitis will, on occasion, manifest itself on the vulvar or anal area because of contact with fingernails on which the nail polish is not yet dry. The vulva may also be the site of perfume dermatitis from perfume or perfumed toilet tissue.

TABLE 6.6. *Sensitizers in Vaginal Spermicides*

Hexylresorcinol
Nonoxyl
Oxyquinoline sulfate
Phenylmercuric acetate and borate
Quinine hydrochloride

3. *Medicated soaps* containing sensitizing antiseptics can cause vulvitis.
4. *Wearing apparel.* Dyes and synthetic resins in underclothing may produce dermatitis in sensitized women. The wearing of close-fitting undergarments, such as panty hose, panty girdles, and tight sanitary napkins, may produce vulvar irritation.
5. *Bubble baths.* Prolonged immersion in bubble baths, particularly in children, may produce an irritant vulvitis.
6. *Medications.* Neurodermatitis of the vulva is often complicated by an allergic reaction to sensitizing medications, particularly benzocaine.
7. *Urine.* Incontinent patients, whether adults or infants, may acquire an ammoniacal vulvitis from the irritant effect of ammonia in the urine.

VULVAR DERMATITIS, PRURITUS, AND DYSESTHESIA

The value of patch testing patients with vulvar symptoms versus signs and symptoms has been investigated. Vulval itching without rash was investigated with patch testing in a group of 69 such patients (74). One or more allergic reactions were noted in 45 (65%), of which 40 (58%) were relevant. Most of the relevant substances were medications. Of the 69 patients, 31 (45%) had either complete resolution or significant improvement by avoiding the identified allergen. Lewis et al. (75) extended their series in a 1997 report. They tested 121 patients with vulvar pruritus without signs of skin disease and 32 patients with other vulvar dermatoses. The researchers found that 56 (46%) had relevant positive reactions. Medications and excipients were the most frequent source of difficulty. Seven of 16 lichen sclerosis et atrophicus patients had positive patch tests, and 6 of these benefited from avoiding the identified allergen. Overall 67 (55%) improved.

In contrast to pruritus vulvae, vulvodynia is a burning rather than an itching sensation. Erythema or signs of dermatitis are absent. In a study of 18 vulvodynia patients, no relevant allergens were found by patch testing (76). Vulval vestibulitis is part of the vulvodynia complex; the condition is characterized by burning, stinging, and dyspareunia. Patch tests in 30 women with this diagnosis were also unrewarding, as no relevant reactions were found (77). The presence of visible skin changes appears to be important in whether patch testing will be valuable. Patch tests were conducted on 201 women with a variety of anogenital symptoms, of which eczema was the most common, followed by unknown diagnosis, then psoriasis, lichen planus, vestibulitis, and lichen sclerosis. One or more positive patch tests were noted in 79 (39%) of the women. Of the group, 56 (28%) had relevant patch test reactions. If the signs and symptoms were confined to the vulva only, 19% of patients had relevant reactions. If the reactions were confined to perianal skin, 33% had relevant reactions, but if both vulva and perianal skin were involved, 43% of the reactions were relevant (78).

Patch tests were conducted on 44 women with vulval lichen simplex chronicus; 12 (27%) had relevant reactions (79). However, routine screening allergens were not particularly helpful. Medicaments and excipients were the most frequently encountered allergens. In a study of vulval dermatitis, nickel allergy was overrepresented (80). However, avoidance of nickel or a low nickel diet was felt to be helpful, leading the authors to recommend that if dermatitis is present and a positive nickel patch test is found as well, relevance might be present. Other studies have suggested that nickel is not relevant in this setting. If no dermatitis was present (vulvodynia rather than dermatitis), patch tests were not helpful (80).

CONTACT BALANITIS

The glans penis and prepuce may acquire contact dermatitis from douches, contraceptive jellies, feminine hygiene sprays, and other medicaments used by a sexual partner.

After intercourse, some men may cleanse the genital area with strong detergents that may produce severe irritant dermatitis and even superficial erosions. Traumatic balanitis may occur from certain sexual practices (see Chapter 5).

Poison ivy may cause a severe balanitis and produce such marked swelling of the foreskin as to cause urinary retention. Numerous other exposures in work and play may also be factors in producing balanitis.

Sensitizing topical applications for dermatoses, such as psoriasis and lichen planus, may produce a superimposed contact balanitis.

Rubber Condoms

These are popularly called "sheaths," "French letters," "prophylactics," "protectives," "rubbers," "skins," and "safes."

Edema of the prepuce may be the first sign of an allergic rubber condom reaction. The eruption may spread to the shaft of the penis, the scrotum, inguinal areas, and inner aspects of the thighs. Occasionally, the reaction is confined to the glans penis.

Rubber condom dermatitis is usually due to sensitivity to one or more rubber antioxidants or accelerators or natural rubber latex. Occasionally, a preservative powder dusted onto the condom is the actual cause of the dermatitis. In one instance, the powder contained 10% monobenzyl ether of hydroquinone (agerite alba), which produced balanitis, penile dermatitis, and eventually leukoderma.

Some men have found by trial and error that only certain brands of rubber condoms produce reactions, whereas others are well tolerated.

Patch Tests for Rubber Condom Sensitivity

Patch tests should be performed with the actual condom suspected of producing the reaction. If a powder or lubricant is present on the condom, tests should also be performed with these substances.

Patients allergic to tetramethyl thiuram in a rubber condom may develop a violent reaction and widespread dermatitis when given disulfuram for treatment of alcoholism.

If natural rubber latex sensitivity is suspected, prick tests or RAST rather than patch tests are indicated. In such cases, symptoms of itching and swelling are usually immediate (i.e., within minutes of skin contact).

Nonrubber Condoms

Fourex and Lambskin, which are made of processed lamb cecum, are available for persons who cannot tolerate any rubber contraceptives. Such preparations are popularly called "fishskins."

Polyurethane condoms have become available for men under the name Avanti by Durex (81). Female condoms have also become available under names such as Femidom, Reality, Bikini condom, and Woman's Choice. The Reality condom is polyurethane (82).

Female Contraceptives

Contact with rubber diaphragms, douching solutions, and feminine hygiene sprays may produce balanitis in sensitized males.

Balanitis may be produced from both male and female topical contraceptives.

Scrotum

A 69-year-old man developed redness and edema confined to the scrotum and sparing the thighs and inguinal folds. Patch testing indicated he was allergic to disperse orange 3, paraphenylenediamine, and para-aminoazobenzene. When he followed the advice to wear only white cotton underwear, his formerly recalcitrant eruption dramatically improved (83).

The Penile Tourniquet Syndrome

Swelling of the penis may be caused by infection, allergy, trauma, or entrapment by a foreign body. In children, the latter may be due to human hair wrapped around the penis.

Garty et al. (84) reported a 2½-year-old boy who had been circumcised and presented with discoloration and severe swelling of the penis of 6 weeks' duration. The child had had difficulties in voiding and cried while urinating. The swelling of the penis had been attributed to allergy and later to infection, and he was treated with various antihistamine drugs, antibiotics, and warm baths but without any improvement.

Physical examination showed constriction at the proximal part of the penis, whereas its distal part was swollen and erythematous. Several hairs buried under the epithelium caused the constriction and were removed using fine forceps and scissors. Questioning of the parents failed to reveal the circumstances under which the hair had become wrapped around the penis. Healing was complete within 15 days.

Entrapment of the penis by hair is an example of the tourniquet syndrome, which may also affect the fingers, toes, or clitoris (85–87). Foreign bodies, such as thread, metal rings, rubber bands, and hair, are usually involved in this condition. The penis becomes swollen, and difficulties in urination might arise, but surprisingly, the pain may not be severe. When the entrapment is caused by hair, as in the case reported, it may be buried under the skin and covered with epithelium. This phenomenon is attributed to the stretchable quality of moist hair. In cases of swelling of the penis in children, careful inspection for buried objects, sometimes under mild sedation, is indicated. The hair may remain undetected for a long time, and a delay of several weeks in the diagnosis is not unusual. In some cases, late diagnosis can be associated with serious sequelae, such as partial or complete transection of the urethra, deformity of the penis, or amputation of the glans (88,89). In other patients, recovery is without serious complications despite the delay. This is most likely due to the multiple blood supply of the penis and the slow progression of constriction, which allows the development of deep collateral circulation. Entrapment of the penis is usually accidental; however, the possibility of child abuse should be investigated because such cases have been reported to be caused by parents in attempts to prevent nocturnal enuresis (90).

THE BUTTOCKS

Prolonged contact with wet bathing suits may produce a follicular-type dermatitis on the buttocks. There is also that unpleasant experience for swimmers commonly referred to as "bikini bottom" and scientifically known as occlusive folliculitis. This condition, marked by the development of annoying wet blisters all over the buttocks, can be caused by wearing a swimsuit all day.

THE ROLE OF CONTACTANTS IN PRURITUS ANI AND PROCTITIS

In patients with pruritus ani or proctitis, a list of all medicaments the patient has used in the past should be made, and particular inquiry should be focused on the use of sensitizers, such as benzocaine, neomycin, and balsam of Peru. Patch tests with these topical remedies may help rule out a contact dermatitis superimposed upon the original pruritus.

The presence of hemorrhoids or fissures should lead one to inquire about special treatments used and to determine whether such treatments produced contact dermatitis. If the patient is using medicated dressings for anal hygiene, such as Tucks, medicated rectal wipes, or Balneol, one must be certain these preparations do not contain agents to which the patient is sensitized. In such instances, the patient who prefers a cooling, drying agent may use witch hazel, whereas the patient who prefers an oily cleanser may use cold mineral oil.

Perfumed and colored toilet paper should be avoided because of the remote possibility that the dyes or essences in it may be sensitizers.

The ingestion of spices, food with seeds, antibiotics, or laxatives that cause a slow leakage of oil or paraffin products may cause anal itching.

Foreign bodies inserted into the rectum and rectal intercourse may produce anal irritation that may be made worse by the use of anesthetic medications containing benzocaine.

THE LEGS

The most common cause of allergic contact dermatitis of the legs is application of sensitizing medications to stasis eczemas and ulcers (see also Chapter 17).

CONTACTANTS PRODUCING ONYCHIA AND NAIL DISCOLORATION

Ronchese (91) stated that nails are more important than teeth or hair. Thinness, fragility, splitting, separation into layers, detachment from the nail bed, and long-standing infections are serious handicaps to jewelers, weavers, metal platers, and printers. Occupational chemicals and trauma are common causes of onychia, koilonychia, nail dystrophy, and discoloration of the nail (see Table 6.7).

Occupational Koilonychia

Spoon-shaped deformity of the nails may be produced by organic solvents (thinners) in cabinetmakers and by motor oils (92,93). Trauma can produce koilonychia of the toenails in barefoot rickshaw pullers (94).

Occupationally induced nail changes, such as koilonychia, traumatic onycholysis in poultry pluckers, and broadening and shortening of the nail plate in association with acro-osteolysis in workers exposed to vinyl-chloride

TABLE 6.7. *Variety of Nail Discolorations Produced by Topical Agents*

Orange-Brown Nails
Anthralin
Arning's tincture
Burnt sugar
Chromium salts
Chrysarobin
Dinitrotoluene
Dithranol
Formaldehyde
Glutaraldehyde
Henna
Hydroquinone
Iodohydroxyquinolene
Iron
Mepacrine
Nicotine
Paraquat
Pecans
Picric acid
Potassium permanganate
Pyrogallol
Resorcin combined with nail lacquer
Rivanol
Roasted coffee
Thermal injury
Vioform
Walnuts

Yellow Nails
Amphotericin
Amphotericin B
Dinitro-orthocresol
Dinubuton
Fluorescein
Hatter's chemicals
Hydrofluoric acid

Gray-Blue Nails
Ammoniated mercury
Mercuric chloride (plus sunshine)

Purple Nails
Gentian violet

Red Nails
Carbol-fuchsin paint

Dark Blue Nails
Oxalic acid
Silver and cyanide (galvanizers)

Black Nails
Photographic developers (phenol sulfate hydroquinone)
Red wine
Silver nitrite

Green Nails
Chlorophyll (prophylline)
Copper salts

monomer indicate that nail abnormalities as manifestations of occupational injury are not uncommon (95).

Food handlers may develop contact urticaria to food, such as garlic, tomato, eggplant, chicory, kiwi fruit, egg yolk, bean, wheat flour, onion, and figs. Nine of 20 food handlers with contact urticaria of the proximal nail fold had a chronic paronychia (96).

> **Occupational nail dystrophy may result from trauma, solvents, motor oils, and permanent wave solutions used by hairdressers.**

Acute Onycholysis from Chemicals

Hydrofluoric burns have an apparent predilection for subungual tissues (97,98). Acute onycholysis can also occur from detergent enzymes (99). Hair cosmetics, such as dicyandiamide (especially useful to restore split and thin hair), depilatories, and thioglycolates used by hairdressers for permanent waving may produce occupational onychia.

Trauma to the nails on the job accompanied by quaternium-15 sensitivity (but not formaldehyde) leads to onycholysis without proximal nail fold changes. The quaternium-15 exposure was to an industrial liquid soap, and the nails returned to normal in 4 months (100).

"Athletic" Nails

Scher (101) reviewed the subject of the "athletic nail." Nail changes occurring either in professional athletes or in those who participate occasionally in weekend sports activities have not been described extensively. Ronchese (102) spoke of the "worn down" fingernails of the frequent bowler, and Pardo-Costello and Pardo (103) referred to wearing down of the nails of the third and fourth fingers and black discoloration of the nails in riflemen and hunters. Samman (104) mentioned periodic shedding of the great toenails of football players as a result of repeated minor injuries even in the absence of hematoma. Schwartz et al. (105) alluded to traumatic injuries sustained by amateur fishermen from fish scales and hooks, as well as to paronychia secondary to frequent water contact. Nail changes also have been reported to be associated with tennis and jogging (106–109), and splinter hemorrhages were reported in cricket players in England (110).

Scher (101) attributed a case of leukonychia to karate. The mechanism of formation of the white nail bed is not well understood. DeNicola et al. (111), however, attribute it to a temporary anemia of this site. Because this may result from both systemic and local causes, it is conceivable that the vigorous trauma of karate, secondary to a period of hypoxia, could produce the transverse whiteness of the nail bed observed in this patient.

Subungual Hematoma (Jogger's Toe, Tennis Toe, and Soccer Toe)

Subungual hematoma has many causes, including both local and systemic (112–114). This discussion focuses only on local traumatic factors that produce hemorrhage beneath the nail plate in specific athletes. Examples include tennis and soccer players as well as joggers. In all three, the toes hit persistently against the shoe and the ground. In the runner or jogger, the hitting is constant and tends to involve the fourth and fifth toes predominantly. On the other hand, the tennis player's intermittent stopping and going, with sudden short stops and sprints, tends to produce subungual hematoma mainly in the big toe. Finally, in the soccer player, who kicks the ball close to and somewhat distal to the instep area, the second and third digits tend to be the ones that blacken.

It must be stated, however, that all variations of these patterns occur, so that the toe involved is not a pathognomonic indication of the sport involved. Likewise, these changes seem to be more likely to occur in persons whose second toe is longer than the first—approximately 25% of the population. This configuration apparently increases the incidence of subungual hematoma of the great toe, although, in other cases, it also renders the second toe more susceptible.

In all of these cases, acral lentiginous melanoma must always be considered in the differential diagnosis. Therefore, it is incumbent upon the physician to prove that the blackness is due to blood, not to melanin. This is usually a simple matter, but occasionally the diagnosis may be more difficult, requiring partial or complete avulsion or histologic examination by nail biopsy (115).

Microbiological studies are also required to rule out both fungal and bacterial causes. Therapy for these patients is difficult, although keeping the nails cut short and wearing better fitting shoes may be of some benefit.

> **Athletic trauma may result in leukonychia of the fingernail associated with karate or black discoloration of the fingernails in riflemen and of the toenails in tennis players, joggers, and soccer players.**

Reactions to "Sculptured" Acrylate Nails

"Sculptured" artificial nails are a popular method of improving the cosmetic appearance of natural nails. They are made by mixing a liquid monomer with a powder polymer, then molding this acrylic compound onto the natural nail.

The first reported case of a severe reaction to acrylic "sculptured" nails described a dermatologist with a severe, disfiguring onychomycosis of all his fingernails in the days before griseofulvin was available (116). In an attempt to improve the appearance of his nails, he applied a mixture of methyl methacrylate monomer and acrylic polymer and fashioned artificial nails. An excruciatingly painful onychia and paronychia of all his fingers developed, requiring strong opiates. The pain and discomfort persisted for several weeks.

The United States Food and Drug Administration received so many complaints of severe reactions to methyl methacrylate monomer from consumers that, after litigation, on July 3, 1974, the District Court in Chicago issued an injunction prohibiting the further manufacture or interstate shipment of a product called Long Nails, which contained a methyl methacrylate monomer (117).

In order to comply with this injunction, the manufacturers of artificial nail products are now using ethyl or isobutyl methacrylate monomers. One preliminary study seemed to indicate that these "newer" monomers did not cross-react with the methyl methacrylate. However, Marks et al. (118) have shown that cross-reactions definitely do occur among the various methacrylate monomers.

The newer reformulated artificial nail products seem likely to cause as many problems as the old methyl methacrylate–containing formulations, because it has been shown in animals and in humans that various acrylate monomers used in nail products are sensitizers that may cross-react.

Fisher (119) reported permanent loss of fingernails from sensitization and reactions to acrylic monomer in a preparation designed to make artificial nails. There was marked erythema, edema, and pain of the eponychial and paronychial tissues with persistent paresthesia of the fingertips. Gradual destruction of the nail plates developed, and, because no regrowth of the nails resumed in 10 years, the loss of the fingernails was permanent.

> **Allergic sensitization to "sculptured" acrylate nails may cause severe onychia and paronychia, with permanent destruction of the nails.**

Reactions to "Nail Hardeners" Containing Formaldehyde

Although formaldehyde is still used in Canada as a "nail hardener," it is rarely used in the United States for this purpose at present. The United States Food and Drug Administration received so many complaints of reactions from this chemical that such nail hardeners were mostly withdrawn from the market.

Ronchese (91) reported a case of onycholysis due to a nail hardener imported from Canada and correctly predicted that, "with tighter limitations on nail hardener production in the United States, this foreign production might be the only source of this agent in the future."

Although Mitchell's (120) patient suffered only a simple onycholysis without inflammation, other reports detail much more severe reactions from the formaldehyde component of "nail hardeners." Such reactions include subungual hemorrhages, discoloration of the nail plate, subungual hyperkeratosis, and even lip hemorrhages in nail biters (121–125).

Some so-called nail hardeners now available in the United States may contain various types of "protein," collagen, nylon acetates, toluene, and nitrocellulose.

> Although most "nail hardeners" in the United States no longer contain formaldehyde, some "hardeners" may contain formaldehyde-releasing agents.

PREFORMED PLASTIC NAILS

Preformed plastic nails are made with completely cured plastic and do not cause allergic reactions. The adhesives used to allow adhesion of the plastic nails to the nail plate, however, may produce changes similar to those produced by "nail hardeners."

Stick-on Nail Dressings ("Press-on Nails")

These nail dressings consist of thin, colored synthetic film with an adhesive that makes them adhere to the nail. Nail dressings, such as "press-on nails," may produce onycholysis, paronychia, and loss of the cuticle.

Nail Wrapping

The free edge of the nail is splinted with cotton, wool, or plastic film and fixed with nitrocellulose glues. After drying, the edge is shaped and the nail coated with enamel. Nail damage can occur if the entire nail is occluded.

> "Preformed plastic nails," "press-on nails," and "nail wrapping" may occasionally produce onychia and paronychia.

Contact Chromonychia

Color changes in the nails may occur with or without inflammatory changes from exposure to certain contactants.

Discoloration and Nail Damage from Insecticides and Weed Killers

Weed killers and insecticides, paroquat, diquats, and dinitrocresol may produce nail damage that may be preceded by several weeks of a noninflammatory distinctive nail discoloration in which the proximal part of the nail plate becomes yellow or whitish (125,126).

Several grades of severity of nail damage were recognized:

Grade 1. Localized discoloration of transverse band of white discoloration affecting nail plate only.
Grade 2. Transverse bands of white discoloration affecting two or more nails (the most common lesions).
Grade 3. Nail deformity of the nail surface; irregularity of surface; transverse ridging and furrowing.
Grade 4. Grossly irregular deformity of nail plate, loosening, or both and beginning onycholysis.
Grade 5. Loss of nail.

> Weed killers and insecticides may produce nail discoloration that precedes onychia and deformity of the nails.

Chromonychia from Thermal Injury

Brodkin and Bleiberg described nail changes from exposure to heat from a microwave oven (127).

Table 6.7 lists the various colors that local agents can produce on the nails. As a rule, the range of color changes in the nail is wider than the primary colors. For example, ochreous discoloration induced by the chromium salts is intermediate between yellow and brown.

Discoloration of the Nails from Nail Enamels and Nail Hardeners

Nail enamels are responsible for a yellow-brown discoloration of the nail plate surface. This discoloration does not seem to be due to the coloring agents of the enamel but to a pigment deposit that penetrates the nail plate. It does not disappear when the varnish is washed off by a solvent and gradually disappears while the nail is growing.

Nail hardeners may be responsible for a discoloration varying in color from yellow to red-blue and brown affecting the extremity of the nail, associated with small punctate subungual hemorrhages, subungual hyperkeratosis, and distal onycholysis. A formaldehyde component of the hardener might be particularly responsible.

Rycroft (128) described nail dystrophy and dermatitis of the nail fold with discoloration of the nails in a patient who became allergic to paratertiary butylphenol resin in an artificial nail adhesive used to affix artificial nails to the fingers.

Nail Staining Due to Hydroquinone

Mann and Harman (129) reported nail staining due to hydroquinone skin-lightening creams. They reported two cases of women in whom brown discoloration developed after the use of cosmetic skin-lightening creams containing hydroquinone and for actinic lentigines of the hands.

This seemingly paradoxical nail darkening from bleaching creams was reported by Arndt and Fitzpatrick (130) in three patients who had discolored fingernails following the use of 2% and 5% hydroquinone-containing creams in the treatment of vitiligo, chloasma, freckles, and postinflammatory hyperpigmentation. Garcia et al. (131) noted diffuse orange-brown nail staining after the use of Esoterica cream by several patients. These investigators suggested that the color change was due to the oxidation products of hydroquinone and that a similar color change could be seen on the surface of the cream after exposure to air.

Hydroquinone is readily oxidized to quinone, a yellow compound, and quinone subsequently undergoes oxidation to hydroxyquinone. The oxidation of quinone is a photosensitive reaction. Hydroxyquinone, another yellow compound, is unstable and polymerizes to products that are dark brown. This reaction is also photosensitive. These oxidation and polymerization products are also probably the cause of the brown pigmentation that affects the cornea and conjunctiva of workers involved in the manufacture of hydroquinone, in which quinone is an intermediate (132).

> **Bleaching creams containing hydroquinone may produce yellowish-brown discoloration of the fingernails.**

Orange-Brown Iron Nail Pigmentation from Well Water

Olsen and Jatlow (133) reported that an orange-brown chromonychia developed on the toenails of a woman from exposure to rural well water. Samples of the water and qualitative and quantitative examination of nail clippings confirmed that the source of the discoloration was contact exposure to elemental iron. Installation of water purification equipment resulted in resolution of the nail stain over a 6-week period.

A positive Prussian blue stain following the traumatic removal of the patient's nails and the results of quantitative iron analysis of the various nail clippings confirmed the diagnosis. Although the Prussian blue iron stain cannot provide precise quantitative data, its ease of application and usage should be emphasized in clinical situations in which the clinician is looking for the presence of tissue iron.

Exogenous versus Endogenous Chromonychia

Zais (134) stressed that gross inspection of the nail plate sometimes permits the clinician to separate an exogenous from an endogenous source. Chromonychias, following the shape of the lunula, tend to be endogenous in origin, whereas discolorations following the proximal nail fold indicate a contact environmental source. Ionizing radiation, however, may produce longitudinal red streaks beginning in the lunula.

> **Chromonychia following the shape of the lunula tends to be endogenous except when caused by ionizing radiation. Discolorations that follow the proximal nail fold usually indicate an external contactant.**

Daniel and Osment (135) suggest that several important points concerning examination of abnormal nails are worthy of mention. One should study the nails with the fingers completely relaxed and not pressed against any surface. Failure to do so may alter nail hemodynamics and change the appearance of the nail. The observer should then blanch the fingertip to see if the pigmented abnormality is grossly altered. This may help differentiate discoloration of the nail plate from that of the nail vascular bed. In addition, one may illuminate the nail by placing a penlight against the finger pulp and shining it up through the nail. If the discoloration is in the vascular bed, it usually disappears. If it is in the matrix or soft tissue, the exact position can be more easily identified. Furthermore, if scraping the nail plate surface, local cleansing, or using a solvent, such as acetone, removes the discoloration, a topical agent is likely to be the cause. If the substance is impregnated more deeply into the nail or subungually, the use of potassium hydroxide preparations, nail composition studies, special stains, or examination of a biopsy specimen with a light microscope or possibly an electron microscope may be indicated.

> **Examination of the nails should take place with the fingers relaxed and with no pressure on the fingertips.**

REFERENCES

1. Pascher F. Adverse reactions to eye area cosmetics and their management. *J Soc Cosmet Chem* 1982;33:249.
2. Mathias TCG, Maibach HI. Cutaneous irritation: factors influencing the response to irritants. *Clin Toxicol* 1978;13:333.
3. Mohajerin AH. Common cutaneous disorders of the eyelids. *Cutis* 1972;10:279.
4. Fisher AA. The paraben paradoxes. *Cutis* 1973;12:830.
5. Jordan WP Jr, Sherman WI, King SE. Threshold responses in formaldehyde-sensitive subjects. *Am Acad Dermatol* 1979;1:44.
6. Fisher AA. Allergic contact dermatitis from germall-115: a new cosmetic preservative. *Contact Dermatitis* 1975;2:126.
7. Fisher AA. Cutaneous reactions to sorbic acid and potassium sorbate. *Cutis* 1980;25:350.
8. Cronin E. Di-isopropanolamine in an eyeshadow. *Contact Dermatitis Newsletter* 1973;13:364.
9. Calnan CD. Ditertiarybutyl hydroquinone in eyeshadow. *Contact Dermatitis Newsletter* 1973;13:368.
10. Fisher AA. Allergen replacements in allergic dermatitis. *Int J Dermatol* 1977;16:319.
11. Zuckerman BD. Conjunctival pigmentation due to cosmetics. *Am J Ophthalmol* 1966;62:672.
12. Jervey JH. Mascara pigmentation of the conjunctiva. *Arch Ophthalmol* 1969;81:124.

13. Forman WG, McDowell RV, Shivers JA, Steele JR. Cosmetic eye shadow mimicking orbital calcification [Letter]. *JAMA* 1977; 235:2695.
14. van Ketel WG, Melzer-van Riemskijk FA. Conjunctivitis due to soft lens solutions. *Contact Dermatitis* 1980;6:321.
15. Steele MC, Ive FA. Recurrent facial eczema in females due to "strike anywhere" matches. *Br J Dermatol* 1982;106:477.
16. Burge SM, Powell SM. Contact urticaria to phosphorus sesquisulphide. *Contact Dermatitis* 1984;10:424.
17. Ive FA. Studies in Contact Dermatitis XXI: matches. *Trans St Johns Hosp Dermatol Soc* 1967;53:135.
18. Calnan CD. Quinazoline yellow SS in cosmetics. *Contact Dermatitis* 1975;2:160.
19. Brasch J, Bruning H, Paulke E. Allergic contact dermatitis from chironomids. *Contact Dermatitis* 1992;26:317.
20. Fisher AA. Cosmetic actions and reactions: therapeutic, irritant and allergic. *Cutis* 1980;26:22.
21. Dominey A, et al. Pityriasis folliculorum revisited. *J Am Acad Dermatol* 1989;21:81.
22. Frosch PJ, Kligman AM. A method for appraising the stinging capacity of topically applied substances. *J Soc Cosmet Chem* 1977;28:197.
23. Calnan CD. Stinging sensation from ethoxyethylmethoxy cinnamate. *Contact Dermatitis* 1978;4:294.
24. Lahti A. Skin reactions to some antimicrobial agents. *Contact Dermatitis* 1978;4:302.
25. Lahti A, et al. Prostaglandins in contact urticaria induced by benzoic acid. *Acta Derm Venereol* (Stockh) 1983;63:425.
26. Lahti A, Vaananen A, Kokkonen EL, Hannuksela M. Acetylsalicylic acid inhibits non-immunologic contact urticaria. *Contact Dermatitis* 1987;16:133.
27. Goldenberg RL, Safrin L. Reduction of topical irritation. *J Soc Cosmet Chem* 1977;28:667.
28. Sugai T, Takahashi Y, Takagi T. Pigmented cosmetic dermatitis and coal tar dyes. *Contact Dermatitis* 1977;3:249.
29. Nakavama H, Hanaoka H, Ohshiro A. *Allergen controlled system (ACS).* Tokyo: Kanehara Shuppan Co., 1974.
30. Rorsman H. Riehl's melanosis. *Int J Dermatol* 1982;21:75.
31. Kozuka T, et al. Brilliant Lake Red R as a cause of pigmented contact dermatitis. *Contact Dermatitis* 1979;5:297.
32. Kozuka T, et al. Pigmented contact dermatitis from azo dyes. *Contact Dermatitis* 1980;6:330.
33. Maibach HI. Scuba diver facial dermatitis: allergic contact dermatitis to *N*-isopropyl-*N*-phenylparaphenylenediamine. *Contact Dermatitis* 1975;1:330.
34. Furman D, Fisher AA, Leider M. Allergic eczematous contact-type dermatitis caused by rubber sponges used for the application of cosmetics. *J Invest Dermatol* 1950;15:223.
35. Curtis GH. Contact dermatitis of eyelids caused by an anti-oxidant in rubber fillers of eyelash curlers. *Arch Dermatol* 1945;52:262.
36. Gaul LE. Results of patch testing with rubber antioxidants and accelerators. *J Invest Dermatol* 1957;29:105.
37. Sauer GC. Flubber dermatitis. *Arch Dermatol* 1965;91:465.
38. McDonald CJ. Special requirements in cosmetics for people with black skin. In: Frost P, Horwitz SN, eds. *Principles of cosmetics for the dermatologist.* St. Louis: Mosby, 1982:302.
39. Sperling LC, Sau P. The follicular degeneration syndrome in black patients. "Hot comb alopecia" revisited and revised. *Arch Dermatol* 1992;128:68.
40. Bandmann HJ, Speer U. Red hair after application of chinoform. *Contact Dermatitis* 1984;10:113.
41. Mathur AK, Srivastava AK, Singh A, Gupta BN. Contact depigmentation by adhesive material of *bindi*. *Contact Dermatitis* 1991;24:310.
42. Bajaj AK, Gupta SC, Chatterjee AK. Contact depigmentation from free paratertiary-butylphenol in *bindi* adhesive. *Contact Dermatitis* 1990;22:99.
43. Fisher AA. Contact otitis: a dermatitis of the external ear and canal. *Cutis* 1975;15:311.
44. Jones EH. Allergy of the external ear canal. In: *Allergy in otorhinolaryngology.* Philadelphia: WB Saunders, 1974:735.
45. Fisher AA. Unique features of nail polish sensitization. *Cutis* 1974;14:327.
46. Arnold HK. In: Ronchese F, ed. *Occupational marks and other physical signs.* New York: Grune & Stratton, 1948:116.
47. Gaul LE. Development of allergic nickel dermatitis from earrings. *JAMA* 1967;200:176.
48. Johnson CJ, et al. Clinical notes; ear piercing and hepatitis: nonsterile instruments for ear piercing and the subsequent onset of viral hepatitis. *JAMA* 1974;227:1165.
49. Munro-Ashman D, MacDonald A, Feiwel M. Split ear lobe syndrome. *Contact Dermatitis* 1975;1:393.
50. Ayala F. Granuloma fissurato dell'orecchio associato a dermatite da contatto dan nichel. *Giornale Italiano Dermatol Minerva Dermatol* 1976;111:581.
51. Shore RN, Berger BJ. Earring dermatitis sparing the ears. *Arch Dermatol* 1974;109:95.
52. Jirasek L, Kobikova M, Jiraskova M. Retroauricular eczema caused by the nickel of celluloid-rimmed spectacles. *Cesk Dermatol* 1976; 51:369.
53. Barnes HM, Calnan CD, Sarkany I. Spectacle frame acanthoma (granuloma fissuratum). *Trans St John's Hosp Dermatol Soc* 1974; 60:99.
54. Jensen CO, Allen HJ, Mordecai LR. Neomycin contact dermatitis superimposed on otitis externa. *JAMA* 1966;195:175.
55. McKelvie M, McKelvie P. Some aetiological factors in otitis externa. *Br J Dermatol* 1966;78:227.
56. Guill MA, Odom RB. Hearing aid dermatitis. *Arch Dermatol* 1978;114:1050.
57. Jordan WP, Dahl MV. Contact dermatitis from cellulose ester plastics. *Arch Dermatol* 1972;105:880.
58. Tanita Y, Tagami H. Pericervical granuloma in a child due to constricting rubber bands [Letter]. *Arch Dermatol* 1984;120:709.
59. Lachapelle JM, Tennstedt D, Cromphaut P. Pseudofolliculitis of the beard and "Fiddler's Neck." *Contact Dermatitis* 1984;10:247.
60. McGeorge BCL, Steele MC. Allergic contact dermatitis of the nipple from Roman chamomile ointment. *Contact Dermatitis* 1991;24:139.
61. McCallum DI, Hall GFM. Umbilical granulomata with particular reference to talc granuloma. *Br J Dermatol* 1970;83:151.
62. Ehring F. The umbilical stone. *Hautarzt* 1979;30:494.
63. Gomez-Orbaneja J, Inglesias Diez L, Sanchez Lozano JL, Conde Salazar L. Lymphatoid contact dermatitis. *Contact Dermatitis* 1976; 2:139.
64. Fisher AA. Vulvitis due to contactants. *Cutis* 1974;13:725.
65. Britz MB, Maibach HI. Human cutaneous vulvar reactivity to irritants. *Contact Dermatitis* 1979;5:375.
66. Fisher AA. Allergic reaction to feminine hygiene sprays. *Arch Dermatol* 1973;108:801.
67. Fisher AA, et al. Allergic contact dermatitis due to ingredients of vehicles. *Arch Dermatol* 1971;104:286.
68. Fisher AA, Stillman MA. Allergic contact sensitivity to benzalkonium chloride. *Arch Dermatol* 1972;106:169.
69. Shmunes E, Levy EJ. Quaternary ammonium compound contact dermatitis from a deodorant. *Arch Dermatol* 1972;105:91.
70. Ljunggren B, Moller H. Eczematous contact allergy to chlorhexidine. *Acta Derm Venereol* (Stockh) 1972;52:308.
71. Kaye BM. Hazards of feminine hygiene sprays for women. *JAMA* 1970;212:2121.
72. Davis BA. Irritancy from feminine hygiene sprays. *Obstet Gynecol* 1970;36:812.
73. Gowdy JM. Feminine deodorant sprays. *N Engl J Med* 1972; 287:203.
74. Lewis FM, Harrington CI, Gawkrodger DJ. Contact sensitivity in pruritus vulvae: a common and manageable problem. *Contact Dermatitis* 1994;31:264-265.
75. Lewis FM, Shah M, Gawkrodger DJ. Contact sensitivity in pruritus vulvae: patch test results and clinical outcome. *Am J Contact Dermat* 1997;8:137.
76. Petersen CS. Lack of contact allergy in consecutive women with vulvodynia. *Contact Dermatitis* 1997;37:46.
77. Nunns D, Ferguson J, Beck M, Mandal D. Is patch testing necessary in vulval vestibulitis? *Contact Dermatitis* 1997;37:87.
78. Goldsmith PC, et al. Contact sensitivity in women with anogenital dermatoses. *Contact Dermatitis* 1997;36:174.
79. Virgili A, Corazza M, Bacilieri S, Califano A. Contact sensitivity in vulval lichen simplex chronicus. *Contact Dermatitis* 1997;37:296.
80. Lucke TW, Fleming CJ, McHenry P, Lever R. Patch testing in vulval dermatoses: how relevant is nickel? *Contact Dermatitis* 1998; 38:111.

81. Fisher AA. The new female and male polyurethane condoms. *Cutis* 1995;56:82.
82. Bounds W. Female condoms. *Eur J Contracept Reprod Health Care* 1997;2:113.
83. Lucke TW, Fleming CJ, McHenry P. Clothing dye dermatitis of the scrotum. *Contact Dermatitis* 1998;38:224.
84. Garty BZ, Mimouni M, Varsano I. Penile tourniquet syndrome. *Cutis* 1983;31:431.
85. Alpert J, Filler RJ, Glaser H. Strangulation of an appendage by hair wrapping. *N Engl J Med* 1965;273:866.
86. Quinn N. Toe tourniquet syndrome. *Pediatrics* 1971;48:145.
87. Press S, Schachner L, Paul P. Clitoris tourniquet syndrome. *Pediatrics* 1980;66:781.
88. Thomas A, Timmons J, Perlmutter A. Progressive penile amputation: tourniquet injury secondary to hair. *Urology* 1977;9:42.
89. Farah R, Cerny J. Penis tourniquet syndrome and penile amputation. *Urology* 1973;2:310.
90. Kerry R, Chapman DD. Strangulation of appendages by hair and thread. *J Pediatr Surg* 1973;8:23.
91. Ronchese F. Occupational nails. *Cutis* 1965;5:164.
92. Ancona-Alayon A. Occupational koilonychia from organic solvents. *Contact Dermatitis* 1975;1:367.
93. Dawber R. Occupational koilonychia. *Br J Dermatol* 1974;91:10.
94. Bentley-Phillips B, Bayles AH. Occupational koilonychia of the toe nails. *Br J Dermatol* 1971;85:140.
95. Moulin G, et al. Aspects sclerodermiques de l'acro-osteolyse professionnelle (polymerisation du chlorure de vinyle). *Ann Dermatol Syphil* 1974;101:33.
96. Tosti A, et al. Role of foods in the pathogenesis of chronic paronychia. *J Am Acad Dermatol* 1992;27:706.
97. Shewmaker W, Anderson BG. Hydrofluoric acid burns: a report of a case and review of the literature. *Arch Dermatol* 1979;115:593.
98. Baran R. Acute onycholysis from rust-removing agents. *Arch Dermatol* 1980;116:382.
99. Hodgson G, Mayon-White RT. Acute onychia and onycholysis due to an enzyme detergent. *Br Med J* 1971;3:352.
100. Marren P, de Berker D, Dawber RPR, Powell S. Occupational contact dermatitis to quaternium 15 presenting as nail dystrophy. *Contact Dermatitis* 1991;25:253.
101. Scher RK. The athletic nail. *Dermatology* 1981;21:49.
102. Ronchese F. *Occupational marks and other physical signs.* New York: Grune & Stratton, 1948.
103. Pardo-Costello V, Pardo OA. *Diseases of the nails.* Springfield, IL: Charles C Thomas Publisher, 1960.
104. Samman PD. *The nails in disease.* London: Heinemann Medical Books, 1978.
105. Schwartz L, Tulipan L, Birmingham DJ. *Occupational diseases of the skin.* Philadelphia: Lea & Febiger, 1957.
106. Gibbs RC. Tennis toe. *Arch Dermatol* 1973;107:918.
107. Gibbs RC. *Skin diseases of the feet.* St. Louis: Warren H. Green, 1974.
108. Scher RK. Jogger's toe. *Int J Dermatol* 1978;17:719.
109. Yaffee HS. Jogging some more. *Int J Dermatol* 1979;18:319.
110. Monk BE. The prevalence of splinter hemorrhages. *Br J Dermatol* 1980;103:183.
111. DiNicola P, Morisiani M, Zavagli G. *Nail diseases in internal medicine.* Springfield, IL: Charles C Thomas Publisher, 1974.
112. Levine N. Dermatologic aspects of sports medicine. *J Am Acad Dermatol* 1980;3:415.
113. Shuster RO. Foot types and the influence of environment on the foot of long distance runners. *Ann NY Acad Sci* 1977;301:881.
114. Resnick SS, Lewis LA, Cohen BH. The athlete's foot. *Cutis* 1977;10:351.
115. Scher RK. Punch biopsy of nails: simple, valuable procedure. *J Dermatol Surg Oncol* 1978;4:528.
116. Fisher AA, Frank A, Glicks H. Allergic sensitization of the skin and nails to acrylic plastic nails. *J Allergy* 1957;28:84.
117. *UC v CEB Products, Inc.*, 380 F. Suppl. 664 (N.D. Ill., 1974).
118. Marks JF Jr, Bishop ME, Willis WP. Allergic contact dermatitis to sculptured nails. *Arch Dermatol* 1979;215:100.
119. Fisher AA. Permanent loss of finger nails from sensitization and reaction to acrylic in a preparation designed to make artificial nails. *J Dermatol Surg Oncol* 1980;6:70.
120. Mitchell JC. Non-inflammatory onycholysis from formaldehyde-containing nail hardener. *Contact Dermatitis* 1981;7:173.
121. Danto JL. Allergic contact dermatitis due to a formaldehyde finger nail hardener. *Can Med Assoc J* 1968;98:652.
122. Lazar P. Reactions to nail hardeners. *Arch Dermatol* 1966;94:446.
123. Donsky HJ. Onycholysis due to nail hardener. *Can Med Assoc J* 1967;96:1375.
124. March CH. Allergic contact dermatitis to a new formula to strengthen nails. *Arch Dermatol* 1966;93:270.
125. Baran RL. Nail damage caused by weed killers and insecticides. *Arch Dermatol* 1974;110:467.
126. Hearn CED, Keir W. Nail damage in spray operators exposed to paraquat. *Br J Ind Med* 1971;28:399.
127. Brodkin RH, Bleiberg R. Microwave injury to the nails. *Acta Dermatol Venereol* 1973;53:50.
128. Rycroft RJG. *Contact sensitization to p-tertiary butylphenol (PTBP) resin in artificial nail adhesive.* Paper presented at the Fifth International Symposium on Contact Dermatitis, Barcelona, Spain, March 1980.
129. Mann RI, Harman RRM. Nail staining due to hydroquinone skin-lightening creams. *Br J Dermatol* 1983;108:363.
130. Arndt KK, Fitzpatrick TB. Topical use of hydroquinone as a depigmenting agent. *JAMA* 1965;194:965.
131. Garcia RK, White JW, Willis WF. Hydroquinone nail pigmentation. *Arch Dermatol* 1978;114:1402.
132. Sterner JH, Oglesby FL, Anderson B. Quinone vapours and their harmful effects. *J Ind Hygiene Toxicol* 1947;29:60.
133. Olsen TG, Jatlow P. Contact exposure to elemental iron causing chromonychia. *Arch Dermatol* 1984;120:102.
134. Zais N. *The nail in health and diseases.* 1st ed. New York: Spectrum Publications, 1980;19:188.
135. Daniel CR, Osment LS. Nail pigmentation abnormalities. *Cutis* 1980;25:595.

CHAPTER 7

Noneczematous Contact Dermatitis

Irritant or allergic contact dermatitis usually begins as an eczematous process characterized by itching, redness, edema, and a tendency toward oozing and crusting. Occasionally, however, it may be noneczematous with urticarial, granulomatous, acneiform, lichen planus-like, or dry, hyperkeratotic lesions. In addition, erythema multiforme and purpuric eruptions may result from exposure to contact allergens. Pigmented contact dermatitis resembling Riehl's melanosis and the actinic reticuloid syndrome may occur. Contact dermatitis may be complicated by lymphangitis and persistent edema. Various types of acneiform eruptions owing to contactants are discussed here and in Chapter 27.

ERYTHEMA MULTIFORME–LIKE ERUPTIONS FROM CONTACT ALLERGENS

Various exotic tropical woods and certain chemicals can produce erythema multiforme–like eruptions (Table 7.1).

Tropical Woods

Holst et al. (1) described three carpenters who, after working for a short time with tropical woods, Rio rosewood (*Dalbergia nigra*), pao ferro (*Mackerium scleroxylon*), and eucalyptus saligna, developed erythema multiforme–like eruptions. The antigen of pao ferro (the ironwood tree of Brazil) is R-3,4-dimethoxy-dalbergione, and the antigen of Rio rosewood is R-4-methoxy-dalbergione. They are both quinones and are closely related.

Fisher and Bikowski (2) reported a male who had an erythema multiforme eruption from an allergic reaction on the neck and presternal area from a wooden cross. A patch test with the cross was strongly positive after 48 hours. A patch test with sawdust from the cross showed a marked reaction within 6 hours. Both reactions were eczematous.

The wood in the cross was identified as *Dalbergia nigra* by the Center of Wood Anatomy Research (U.S. Forest Products Laboratory, Madison, WI). A search of the available literature revealed that all previous reports of allergic contact dermatitis from *Dalbergia nigra* have been concerned with occupational exposures in carpenters, foresters,

and cabinetmakers. This is apparently the first report of "nonoccupational" dermatitis from *Dalbergia*.

> **Tropical woods and certain plants can produce "contact" erythema multiforme eruptions.**

Martin et al. (3) reported a case of erythema multiforme–like eruption from Brazilian rosewood in a 35-year-old carpenter who initially developed rhinitis and conjunctivitis. This eruption was succeeded by a generalized erythema multiforme–like eruption. A patch test with the wood dust produced a strong positive eczematous reaction, as did R- and S-methoxy-dalbergione. Table 7.2 lists some common names for *Dalbergia nigra*.

With regard to plants other than tropical woods, Hjorth (4) reported an erythema multiforme eruption from an allergic reaction to primula. Other plants and plant substances, such as *Artemesia* (5,6), poison ivy (7), and terpenes, can produce such eruptions (8). The initial dermatitis may resemble a traditional eczematous morphologic pattern with a subsequent distant, noncontacted area demonstrating erythema multiforme morphologic patterns. This was the case with a patient who applied an aqueous solution of Saint John's wort to treat a buttocks eczema only to subsequently develop distant erythema multiforme (9). The allergen was Hypercin from the *Hypericum erectum* (Thunb).

Other plants or plant materials have caused contact dermatitis that evolved into erythema multiforme. A homemade dressing using tincture of capsicum caused an erythema multiforme–like eruption in a 65-year-old woman who applied this to her knee for arthritis (10). Application of an "herbal bag" to the chest as a folk treatment for back pain led to eczema followed by an erythema multiforme–like eruption 2 weeks later (11). The *Inula helenium* present in the bag was found responsible, and both sesquiterpene lactone mix and alantolactone were positive. Application of Thuja essential oil for hemorrhoids was followed by an erythema multiforme–like reaction (12). Thuja oil is a distillate of *Thuja occidentalis* and contains

TABLE 7.1. *Contact Allergens Producing Erythema Multiforme*

Tropical Woods Plants
  Capsicum
  Inula helenium
  Poison ivy
  Primula
  Pyrethrum
  Saint John's wort (*Hypericum erectum*)
  Terpenes
  Thuja essential oil
Laboratory Chemicals
  Brominated compounds
  Dinitrochlorobenzene
  Diphenylcyclopropenone
  N-hydroxyphthalamide
  Phenyl sulfone derivatives
Medications
  Budesonide
  Bufexamac
  Chloramphenicol
  Econazole
  Ethylenediamine
  Idoxuridine
  Iodochlorhydroxyquin (Vioform)
  Ketoprofen
  Lincomycin
  Mafenide acetate
  Mephenesin
  Mephenesin (Europe)
  Mofebutazone
  Neomycin
  Phenylbutazone
  Povidone-iodine solution
  Proflavin
  Promethazine
  Pyrrolnitrin
  Scopolamine
  Sulfonamides
  Triamcinolone acetonide
  Vitamin E
Miscellaneous Compounds
  Disperse blue 124
  Epoxy resin
  Formaldehyde
  Hair dyes
  Oxybenzone
  Paratertiary butylphenol formaldehyde resin
  Soap
  Spray cologne
  Trichloroethylene

TABLE 7.2. *Common Names for* Dalbergia nigra

Bahia rosewood
Brazilian rosewood
Caviuana
Jacaranda (pardo)
Palissandre bresic
Rio rosewood

fenchone, thujic acid, pinene, pinipicrine, borneol esters, and tannins.

Halogenated and Miscellaneous Chemical Compounds

De Feo (13) and Powell et al. (14) reported that chemists exposed to dimethyl allyl bromide and other brominated compounds, particularly 9-bromofluorene, acquired an erythema multiforme–type reaction. Roed-Petersen (15) stated that a 22-year-old male chemistry student's eruption started when he had to synthesize a new phenylsulfone derivative compound in the laboratory. Fregert et al. (16) reported that *N*-hydroxyphthalimide produced an erythema multiforme by contact. When 7.5% povidone-iodine aqueous solution was applied to an operative wound, a dermatitis at the application site was followed by a distant erythema multiforme (9). Similarly, a 2% dinitrochlorobenzene (DNCB) solution applied to the entire scalp for 4 days to treat alopecia areata produced an erythema multiforme reaction pattern on the back, arms, and hands. A patch test of 0.1% DNCB in acetone produced an eczematous response; 0.01% was negative (17).

Magnusson and Gilje (18) stated that alkyl ether sulfates contaminated dishwashing detergents, and Bjornberg and Mobacken (19) found that benzene compounds can produce erythema multiforme–like contact dermatitis.

Nethercott et al. (20) reported that four men manufacturing printed circuit boards were exposed to palladium chloride, copper sulfate, formaldehyde, epoxy fiberglass, lead trichloroethylene, and ammonium persulfate. They developed erythema multiforme major after 6 to 12 weeks of exposure. Liver involvement was documented in three cases. On the basis of positive patch tests in two of the four workers, formaldehyde was presumed to cause the reactions.

Phoon et al. (21) reported five cases of Stevens-Johnson syndrome (erythema multiforme major) owing to exposure to trichloroethylene. All of these patients had liver involvement.

Vincenzi et al. (22) add to the list of erythema multiforme–causing agents disperse blue 124, hair dyes, and paratertiary butylphenol formaldehyde resin.

Oxybenzone produced an erythema multiforme–like eruption 1 week after the initial photoallergic contact dermatitis in a 44-year-old woman from Japan (23). Photopatch tests showed oxybenzone to be the sunscreen ingredient responsible.

A pyrethrum insecticide caused an airborne erythema multiforme–like eruption in a Spanish farmer detected by a 2% pyrethrum in petrolatum patch test (24). No cross reactivity to lichens or sesquiterpene lactones was found.

> **Exposure to formaldehyde and trichloroethylene has been implicated as the cause of erythema multiforme major (Stevens-Johnson syndrome and liver disease).**

The following contactants have been implicated as the cause of contact erythema multiforme: insecticides (25), spray colognes (26), metals (27,28), and soaps (29).

Medications

Degreef et al. (30) described five patients (all using a mephenesin-containing ointment) who had acute contact dermatitis with an idlike spread and features resembling erythema multiforme. Patch tests were performed in four patients, and because mephenesin was the common allergen in each case, the investigators assumed this allergen was also the cause of the erythema multiforme–like lesions.

In Europe, mephenesin is taken orally as a muscle relaxant and is applied locally. It is used primarily by young people after injuries from sports. With local application, a vasodilating agent (methyl nicotinate and glycol salicylate) is usually added to promote skin penetration. This agent can cause hyperemia and sometimes even purpura. The increased permeability of the skin seems to contribute to sensitization to other materials (e.g., rubber in elastic bandages, dyes, and shoe materials) and promotes an idlike spread that can take on the aspect of exudative erythema multiforme.

Meneghini and Angelini (31,32) reported that the following topical medications produced erythema multiforme: ethylenediamine, neomycin, promethazine, iodochlorhydroxyquin (Vioform), and pyrrolnitrin. Other topical medications that have produced contact erythema multiforme include mafenide acetate (33), scopolamine (34), and sulfonamides (35,36).

Saperstein et al. (37) stated that topical use of vitamin E on scar tissue resulted in a generalized erythema multiforme reaction in two patients. Patch tests with vitamin E oil showed positive local reactions in both patients.

Topical use of a phenylbutazone-containing cream caused an erythema multiforme–like eruption, which was patch test positive to 2% phenylbutazone in petrolatum (38). No reaction was seen with oxyphenbutazone at 5% in petrolatum.

An erythema multiforme–like eruption may follow localized allergic contact dermatitis to bufexamac. This nonsteroidal anti-inflammatory drug (NSAID) has been used to treat a variety of disorders, including atopic dermatitis and localized leg lesions and ulcers. No epidermal necrosis was seen in four cases, as might be expected in true erythema multiforme (39).

Mofebutazone is closely related to phenylbutazone. Its use topically and then orally resulted in a severe drug eruption (40). This was documented by positive prick and patch tests to mofebutazone. This agent is used to treat thrombophlebitis in Germany and is known under the trade name Vasotonin.

More widespread erythema multiforme–like lesions in two cases reported from Italy followed use of topical budesonide to treat contact dermatitis (41). In one case the administration of oral triamcinolone was thought to have caused extension of the eruption.

Intra-articular injection of triamcinolone acetonide was followed by an erythema multiforme–like eruption, which was treated with budesonide with acute worsening (42). Resolution was achieved with 3% boric acid dressings. The only corticosteroids positive on patch testing were triamcinolone acetonide 1% in petrolatum and budesonide 1% in petrolatum.

It appears that erythema multiforme–like reactions are not allergen specific but rather a biological response to delayed-type hypersensitivity to topical agents. Erythema multiforme is commonly seen as a sequela of herpes simplex infections.

In an effort to understand the difference between erythema multiforme from herpes simplex virus and contactants, a study was undertaken of cytokine expression in three cases of the former and two cases of the latter (43). Epidermal expression of intercellular adhesive molecule (ICAM-1) was more prominent in the erythema multiforme–like contact dermatitis, and a greater percentage of cells in the inflammatory infiltrate was CD4+. There was a lower percentage of CD69+ cells in the cases caused by contactants.

PURPURIC CONTACT DERMATITIS

Purpura in patients with normal blood counts may be from various textile fabrics, rubber and antioxidants, other chemicals, or pressure. Some physicians recommend rubbing cocoa butter into scars to produce an improved cosmetic outcome; this concept is also endorsed in some folklore. The solid blocks of cocoa butter rubbed over lower-leg scars can produce a pressure-induced, nonallergic purpuric eruption.

Clothing Purpura

Petechial and purpuric eruptions from woolen garments have been described (44). So-called pigmented purpuric eruptions of the lower extremities, including Schamberg's disease, often occur in areas exposed to woolen underwear, but the role of these garments is unclear.

In addition, a water-soluble formaldehyde urea finish applied to woolen khaki shirts worn by British soldiers has been implicated as the cause of a purpuric eruption. The sedatives apronalide (Sedormid) and carbromal, both of which are capable of producing purpuric dermatitis medicamentosa, are also urea compounds (45).

Contact with fiberglass may produce purpura, telangiectasia, folliculitis, urticaria, and linear erosions in the skin creases. Clothing washed with fiberglass curtains may become contaminated with the particles and produce a purpuric contact dermatitis in the wearer (46).

Osmundsen (47) described a dermatitis of epidemic proportions that appeared in Europe from an optical whitener in washing powders. The eruption, a reticulate pattern of faint red-brown spots with a few petechiae and dilated small vessels, may suggest a reticulosis.

> **Clothing purpura may occur from wool, textile finishes, fiberglass, optical whiteners in washing powders, and pressure.**

Flexural areas treated with clioquinol (Vioform) may develop a distinctive reticulated red-purple eruption with little scale. Patch tests in such cases are negative, and it is felt that this is an irritant contact dermatitis (48).

Pants Pressure Purpura

Petrozzi and Lockshin (49) stated that mechanical trauma may produce purpuric eruptions in young patients. Explanation of the problem occurred only after the patient disclosed he had slept overnight in a pair of tight-fitting dungarees. The instructive element in this case was the degree of trauma necessary to produce the purpura. It could not be reproduced under an inflated blood pressure cuff, nor did the number of petechiae distal to the cuff increase.

Rubber Purpura

Rubber or elasticized underwear may produce an allergic contact eczematous dermatitis associated with a secondary eruption resembling lichenoid pigmented dermatitis, eczematoid purpura, or a variant of pigmented purpuric dermatitis (49).

Calnan and Peachey (50) reported that isopropylaminodiphenylamine, an antioxidant used in the manufacture of some types of rubber, can cause an allergic contact dermatitis. Some cases are associated with a widespread purpuric capillaritis similar to the eruption produced by sensitivity to carbromal and meprobamate.

Fisher (51) reported reactions in three patients involving a rubber diving suit, elasticized shorts, and a rubberized support bandage for the leg, respectively. All had itching petechial and purpuric eruptions at the sites of contact with a rubber article containing *N*-isopropyl-*N*-phenylparaphenylenediamine (IPPD), a rubber antioxidant. One patient had previous dermatitis underneath the elastic portions of her undergarments. It was determined that IPPD is added to elastic material used in some elastic strips on undergarments in the United States. All patients had positive patch tests to IPPD. Fisher reported that IPPD is manufactured by five American companies under the trade names Cyzone, Eastozone, Fleezwx, Flexazone 3C, and Santoflex 36. It is of interest that the substance also has been listed as a stabilizer in a Japanese insecticide formulation. Romaguera and Grimalt (52) similarly confirmed a pruritic purpuric erup-

tion in a woman in the pattern of her brassiere. She was patch-test positive to IPPD (0.1% pet) with purpura.

Shmunes (53) described a 59-year-old saleswoman of black hats who had a severe purpuric eruption on the exposed areas of the face, neck, and arms. Patch testing to paraphenylenediamine produced a purpuric test reaction.

> **The rubber antioxidant *N*-isopropyl-*N*-phenyl-paraphenylenediamine (IPPD) and para-phenylenediamine, a hair and fur dye, have produced allergic contact purpura.**

Wool Dust and Wool Residues Purpura

Agarwal (54) reported that a patient acquired purpura from collecting raw wool from sheep breeders and selling it to textile mills. Although a patch test was negative, the application of wool dust on the patient's body reproduced the eruption. Agarwal emphasized that contact allergens can lead to purpura without systemic involvement and that a more vigilant search might reveal more contact allergens in the pathogenesis of intractable cases of allergic purpura. Romaguera et al. (55) implicated formaldehyde resins in wool residues as causing purpura in a man who was in charge of a special section for the recovery of the wool residues obtained from other sections of the same factory. In this case, the wool was not pure but was mixed with synthetic fibers.

Purpuric Eruption from Topical Oxyquinoline

A purpuric eruption on the extremities following application of medication containing oxyquinoline has also been reported (56).

Purpuric Patch Test Reactions

Apronalide (Sedormid) and quinidine have produced purpuric patch test reactions in persons with purpuric drug eruptions from ingestion of these medicaments (57). Apronalide (Sedormid) was tested as a saturated solution in propylene glycol. The patch test with quinidine consisted of a paste made of a crushed tablet of quinidine sulfate in a small volume of water. The material was left in contact with the patient's arm or back for 24 to 48 hours. The reaction is considered positive if the area of contact shows numerous small petechial hemorrhages.

Cobalt

Schmidt et al. (58) stated that a total of 132 patch-tested patients reacted with petechial reactions to 1% cobalt chloride in petrolatum; 23 patients were retested with various concentrations of cobalt. In about 60% of those retested, the petechial reaction could be reproduced. A histopathologic examination showed slight perivascular-lymphocytic infiltration, swollen endothelium, and extravasation of erythrocytes but no signs of vasculitis. About 5% of patients tested with 1% cobalt chloride in petrolatum show this petechial hemorrhage, which has been localized to the acrosyringium.

Patients who have purpuric eruptions from apronalide (Sedormid) or quinidine may show purpuric patch test reactions to these drugs.

PIGMENTED CONTACT DERMATITIS

Pigmented contact dermatitis may occur from optical whiteners in washing powders and from azo dyes (59).

Optical Whiteners

The term "pigmented contact dermatitis" was used by Osmundsen (60), who, in a series of excellent observations and investigations, has contributed more than anyone else to our understanding of melanosis as a feature of contact dermatitis. In light of Osmundsen's studies and the observations of others, all types of Riehl's melanosis can be comprehended as a single disease entity. Osmundsen (47) described an epidemic in Copenhagen caused by optic whiteners in washing powder. The chemical responsible was a mixture of two pyrazoline derivatives that seem to have a marked tendency to induce pigmented contact dermatitis. Pigmentation developed at the site of several patch tests with the compounds responsible.

Optical whiteners in washing powders containing pyrazoline compounds produced pigmentation of the skin with or without previous dermatitis. Some patch tests became pigmented.

In another epidemic of contact dermatitis from optical whiteners of the same type, Pinol-Aguade et al. (61) reported strong hyperpigmentation in nearly half of their patients. Some had pigmentation compatible with Riehl's melanosis. The different genetic conditions for pigment formation in the Spanish and Danish populations probably explain the much higher incidence of hyperpigmentation in the Spanish material, in which the heaviest pigmentation occurred in patients who had dark complexions.

Azo Dyes

A study of occupational pigmented contact dermatitis in a textile mill from an azo dye–coupling component (62) has further stressed the importance of the pigment-genetic predisposition for the development of pigmented contact dermatitis. Hyperpigmentation was most pronounced in persons with dark complexions, whereas more fair-skinned patients also showed "classic" eczematous symptoms, including pruritus.

Kgzuka et al. (63) reported that pigmented contact dermatitis in 23 patients was caused by cosmetics containing Brilliant Lake Red R. A strong allergen in all patients was 1-phenylazo-2-naphthol, but no patients showed a positive reaction to azobenzene.

Azo dyes in the textile industry and in cosmetics may produce pigmented contact dermatitis.

Pigmentation from Fragrances and Bactericides

In Japan, where facial melanosis has been quite common, allergic contact dermatitis from scents, such as hydrocitronellal, benzylsalicylate, ylang-ylang oil, and jasmine, and from bactericides, such as carbanilides, has been demonstrated to be the cause of pigmentation (64).

Mathias (65) studied a patient who experienced repeated episodes of facial dermatitis with subsequent development of facial hyperpigmentation. A positive patch test to potassium dichromate strongly implicated chromium hydroxide, used as a pigment in a commercial toilet soap, as the contact allergen.

Pigmented cosmetic dermatitis may result from repeated episodes of facial inflammation owing to contact allergy from cosmetics.

Riehl's Melanosis—a Variant of Pigmented Contact Dermatitis

Melanosis with incontinence of pigment may be the result of many inflammatory reactions in the skin. There are three subdivisions: (a) pigment abnormalities as an effect of irradiation, (b) pigment abnormalities after mechanical and chemical irritation, and (c) hyperpigmentation after exanthemas. Riehl's melanosis falls into Group 2 and is similar to melanodermatitis toxica caused by tar or oils. Riehl's melanosis, as originally described, was a pigmented contact dermatitis in which the inflammatory component was slight in many cases. These studies suggest that a pigmented variant of contact dermatitis is most common in persons with strong pigmentation (60,61).

It also seems that hyperpigmentation may be the only macroscopic sign of a dermatitis. Persons with dark complexions who have a tendency to react with hyperpigmentation seem less likely than fair people to develop typical eczematous changes when exposed to certain chemicals.

Hyperpigmentation is not a common feature of contact dermatitis, and marked pigment-forming capacity is not the only explanation for the appearance of a pigmented contact dermatitis. Photo-contact dermatitis more often leads to hyperpigmentation, but abnormal pigmentation may also be absent.

At present, Riehl's melanosis is usually considered synonymous with pigmented contact dermatitis, mostly from sensitizing fragrances and chemicals in cosmetics. When the skin is darker, the pigment is deeper and the eczematous reaction is smaller.

ROLE OF CHRONIC CONTACT DERMATITIS IN ACTINIC RETICULOID SYNDROME (PERSISTENT LIGHT REACTORS)

Addo et al. (66) stated that contact allergic sensitivity to allergens, such as plants of the Compositae family, is a feature of the chronic skin reaction seen in the photosensitivity dermatitis with actinic reticuloid syndrome. In 50 patients who have this syndrome, an increased incidence of contact allergic sensitivity to some common fragrance materials was demonstrated. Evidence is also presented, from in vitro and in vivo studies, that indicates a phototoxic mechanism is involved. The relevance of continued exposure to common allergens and their involvement in photosensitization mechanisms has been a theory for the state of "persistent light reaction."

These allergens include Compositae and allied compounds, rubber factors, and potassium dichromate. It therefore seems probable that the persistence of the skin reaction throughout the year is in part due to the perennial presence of such contact allergens. It also is possible that the pseudolymphomatous changes found in association with maximum skin reactivity may be explained by persistent antigen stimulation. Fragrance materials are also common environmental contactants (67,68).

The persistence of chronic dermatitis year-round in many affected subjects is thus not simply from an ability to react to a broad-action spectrum of radiation present at any time of the year, but also (and this may be an important feature) from perennial exposure to relevant contact allergens. In addition, results indicate that some of these same allergens may involve photosensitivity mechanisms and that repeated phototoxic responses are therefore also likely to be an important feature in the chronicity of the reaction.

Chronic actinic dermatitis, which includes actinic reticuloid, was studied in 86 patients by du Peloux et al. (69), who reported at the European Contact Dermatitis Society in Brussels, October 1992, that 74% of such patients had a positive patch or photopatch test: Twenty percent were fra-

grance sensitive, 20% colophony sensitive, 14% rubber sensitive, and 36% allergic to a mixture of sesquiterpene lactones (SLs). These investigators from St. John's Institute of Dermatology in London found only about 22% of SL-sensitive patients to be photosensitive. Most of the 114 relevant SL-allergic patients had hand (36%) or hand and face eczema (36%), whereas 20% had generalized dermatitis. This would indicate that multiple environmental allergens may account for persistent eczematous states. Because a reliable SL patch test allergen was not available previously, it is easy to understand how difficult it can be to exclude other environmental antigens when treating an ongoing eczema. The responsible allergen would simply go undetected.

Perennial exposure to contactants causing persistence of chronic dermatitis year-round may be a feature of the photosensitive actinic reticuloid syndrome.

POSSIBLE ROLE OF CHRONIC CONTACT DERMATITIS IN MYCOSIS FUNGOIDES

Prevalence of Nickel and Other Contact Allergies among Patients with Mycosis Fungoides

Schlenzka et al., at the International Contact Dermatitis Symposium in East Berlin in 1983, stated that 20 patients with the clinical and histologic diagnosis of mycosis fungoides were subjected to patch tests with chromate, nickel, and cobalt between 1971 and 1982. Positive results occurred in 12 patients (60%). The prevalence of such contact allergies is consequently much higher than among other people tested in recent years. These results could support the hypothesis that mycosis fungoides is an "immunoma."

Case-controlled studies have not verified an association between occupational exposures or chronic antigen stimulation and cutaneous T-cell lymphoma, despite these interesting observations (70).

LICHENOID CONTACT DERMATITIS

Lichenoid Eruptions from Contact with Film Developers

Certain substituted paraphenylenediamine (PPDA) compounds used as color film developers can produce a lichenoid eruption on skin that comes in contact with these chemicals (71). In affected persons, acute or subacute allergic eczematous or papular dermatitis appears, fades, and is replaced by an eruption identical to that of lichen planus (72). It subsides after several weeks, leaving marked pigmentation. Sensitization in exposed workers is fairly high and may take 1 month to 3 years to develop.

Patch test reactions to color developers, such as CD2 (2-amino-5-diethylamino-toluene monohydrochloride), are positive in sensitized persons who acquire lichenoid eruptions (73). Patch tests with CD2 should be performed with a 1% aqueous solution. The same chemicals used in color development are also used in high-speed, black-and-white film processing and may cause lichen planus eruptions (74).

The lichen planus eruption caused by color developers does not usually affect the buccal mucosa or the tongue, although lesions occasionally appear in the mouth (75).

Color film developer chemicals based on PPDA are associated with lichenoid tissue reactions. This has not been commonly associated with PPDA itself. However, four cases of lichenoid dermatitis were traced to PPDA in hair dyes (76).

Patch Testing for Lichenoid Contact Dermatitis

The closed patch technique is the most convenient method of testing for lichenoid contact dermatitis. The patch is removed after 24 hours, and the underlying skin is washed gently with an acid-type cleanser. This removes excess chemical, which, because of its ability to become fixed to epidermal cells, might lead to sensitization. Skin reactions are read after 1 hour and again 24 and 48 hours after removal of the patch. Evolution of the lesion over the next few days produces the typical lichenoid eruption. The brownish stain remaining on the skin after removal of the patch and subsequent washing should not be confused with a positive skin reaction.

Patch tests with color developers are not always positive in patients with lichenoid eruptions. A positive reaction that is eczematous may later become lichenoid.

Lichen planus eruptions from photographic color developers rarely affect the oral mucosa.

PPDA does not produce this type of lichenoid eruption and does not seem to cross-react with the substituted PPDA used as a color developer.

Lichen Planus Eruptions from Metals

Frykholm et al. (77) reported that a patient allergic to metallic copper developed lichen planus of the buccal mucosa and tongue. Replacement of the copper-containing amalgam fillings in her teeth eliminated the lichen planus lesions. Lombardi et al. (78) stated that a lichenoid dermatitis was caused presumably by nickel salts in a nickel-sensitive person.

Epoxy resin has also been reported to cause dermatitis that is histologically lichen planus (79). It is common for the patch test to be eczematous, whereas the clinical eruption is lichen planus–like with epoxy, metallic mercury, metallic copper, nickel salts, and even color film developer.

Oral Lichen Planus–like Changes and Mercury

Of 18 patients with oral lichenoid lesions near amalgam fillings, 15 were found to be mercury sensitive, and partial or complete removal of the amalgam improved 13 of the 15 (80). Five patients had partial amalgam removal, and all showed incomplete resolution; 7 of 10 who had complete amalgam removal had complete resolution of signs and symptoms. Lichenoid changes were frequently adjacent to amalgam fillings.

ACNEFORM ERUPTIONS FROM CONTACTANTS

It is widely believed that cosmetics may aggravate or precipitate acne and that this can be easily evaluated by the rabbit ear assay for comedogenicity. This belief and conventional wisdom have led to the concept that oil-containing cosmetics are bad and oil-free cosmetics are good. These beliefs are incorrect and have largely been discredited by a recent consensus conference of knowledgeable dermatologists and industry representatives (81).

Two separate adverse effects of topical agents fall under the category of acnegenesis. The first is a slow process over several months' time that results in a true comedo or formation of new comedones in acne-prone persons. The second occurs within weeks and is a form of follicular irritation morphologically manifested as papules and pustules. Both events are believed to be uncommon with most available cosmetics save for some hair pomades.

In the occupational setting, more severe acnegens may be encountered (Table 7.3). Halogenated hydrocarbons and coal tar are the standard categories of chemicals associated with acne, particularly chloracne. Cosmetic products have not been associated with chloracne. Lists of individual chemicals previously have been published as a way for clinicians to check products for their acnegenic potential (81). Unfortunately, both the lists and the concept that checking for individual ingredients will provide accurate information for patient instruction are incorrect. The consensus panel noted that the acnegenic potential of individual ingredients is modified by their concentrations and vehicle components, which can increase or decrease the actual acnegenic potential of a given product (81). Meaningful patient information comes only from testing with the finished product. Furthermore, oiliness alone does not predict whether a product will aggravate acne. The features of acne-genesis are found in Table 7.4.

POMADE ACNE

Pomades used as hair straighteners contain primarily a paraffin and petrolatum mixture with gums and perfumes added. They often produce acneiform facial lesions characterized by uniform, localized papulopustules and follicular papulopustules on the forehead and temples. Such

TABLE 7.3. *Causes of Occupational Acne*

1. Petrolatum and its derivatives
   Crude oil and fractions
   Cutting oils
2. Coal-tar products
   Coal-tar oils
   Creosote
   Pitch
3. Chloracne
   Chlorobenzenes
      Crude trichlorobenzene
      Crude benzene hexachloride
      3,4,3′,4′-tetrachloroazoxybenzene
      2,4,3′,4′-tetrachloroazobenzene
   Chloronaphthalenes
   Contaminants of chlorophenols
      2,3,7,8-tetrachlorodibenzo-*p*-dioxin (TCDD)
      Hexachlorodibenzo-*p*-dioxin
      Tetrachlorodibenzofuran
   Polychlorinated dibenzofurans (PCFs)—especially tri-,
      tetra-, penta-, and hexachlorodibenzofuran
   Polychlorobiphenyls (PCBs)*
4. Miscellaneous
   Asbestos
   DDT
   Frictional acne
   Halothane?
   Heavy water distillate
   Tropical acne in soldiers

*The polychlorodibenzofurans and hexachloronaph-
thalenes may occur as contaminants and may actually be
the chloracnegens in some PCBs.

acneiform eruptions are common in people with black
skin (82).

Occupational Acne

According to Taylor (83), the chemicals listed in Table 7.3
are the principal causes of occupational acne.

Occupational acne is a type of acne venenata in which
contact with a wide variety of substances can produce an
acneiform and follicular eruption. Outbreaks of severe,
generalized acne occurred in certain manufacturing plants
in the 1920s and 1930s. In the intervening years, although

TABLE 7.4. *Acnegenic Responses to Topical Agents*

Acnegenic response	Time course	Morphologic features	Potential sources
Mild	Months	True comedone increase	Cosmetics and medications
Mild	Weeks	Papules and pustules (follicular irritation)	Cosmetics and medications
Severe	Weeks/days	Comedones and straw-colored cysts	Coal-tar chlorinated hydrocarbons

advances have been made in industrial hygiene and acnegenic chemicals can be identified by the rabbit's ear test,
sporadic epidemics of acne (especially chloracne) have occurred. Most recent reports (84) have come from Europe,
because many U.S. firms are unwilling to release or publish
data on outbreaks among their employees.

> **In general, chloracne lesions look the same re-
> gardless of the causative chemical. Typical straw-
> colored cysts are almost pathognomonic. Come-
> dones, however, often abound and involve every
> follicular orifice in affected areas. Inflammatory
> pustules and abscesses also occur, as in acne
> vulgaris.**

Among the known causative agents of occupational acne
are components of crude petrolatum, cutting oils, coal tar
and some of its products, chlorinated aromatic chemicals,
and various miscellaneous agents. Workers in oil fields and
refineries who have prolonged skin contact with crude oil or
the heavier oil fractions may develop the spectrum of acne
lesions. By far, the most common sources of acneiform
eruptions are cutting oils employed in machine tool operations. The insoluble (straight) oils and semisynthetic fluids
are the most frequent culprits. Oil acne seems to start as an
inflammatory folliculitis, especially in areas in contact with
contaminated clothing. Comedones are also present.

Coal-tar oils, creosote, and pitches can produce extensive
acneiform eruptions in coal-tar plant workers, roofers, and
road building and construction workers. Comedones are
typical of this form of acne. Phototoxic reactions may complicate the picture and produce coal-tar melanosis and exacerbations of the acne.

> **Although chloracne occurs typically after external
> cutaneous contact with a chloracnegen, ingestion
> or inhalation may be important in some cases.**

Chlorinated aromatic hydrocarbon compounds are among
the most potent acnegenic materials known. These chemicals produce chloracne, an extremely refractory form of
acne venenata that may be accompanied by serious systemic toxicity. The cutaneous eruption is characterized by
straw-colored cysts and closed comedones, but inflammatory cysts and open comedones may abound. Chloracne
serves as a marker of the medical and environmental impact
of contamination of technical-grade chemicals with highly
toxic extraneous intermediates. Several new outbreaks of
chloracne have occurred from exposure to two chloroben-

zene compounds and from contaminants of chlorophenol compounds.

> **Chloracne lesions may continue to appear after all exposure to the inciting chemical has ceased. This persistence of lesions may result from release of dioxin or polychlorinated biphenyls (PCBs) from fat or hepatic stores.**

PUSTULAR ALLERGIC CONTACT DERMATITIS

Burkhart (85) presented a case of acute allergic dermatitis in which the predominant lesions were pustules developing in a patient after the application of a topical antibiotic cream containing nitrofurazone.

The pustules noted in the patient were clinically similar to those from a reaction to heavy metals; however, the erythema and pruritus displayed by the patient were not features of such a reaction. The predominantly lymphocytic pustules characteristic of an ammonium-fluoride reaction are analogous histologically to the pathologic findings in this case; however, the acantholysis and ballooning degeneration associated with a pustular patch test reaction to ammonium fluoride were not features in this case.

In a study performed by Stone and Johnson (86), 5% nickel sulfate was patch tested on patients who were not sensitive to nickel on areas previously injected with heat-killed *Corynebacterium acnes* organisms. As a result, multiple, small, asymptomatic pustules developed at the patch test sites. Histologically, the pustules contained equal parts of mononuclear cells and neutrophils. The investigators concluded that nickel sulfate produced this reaction by enhancing preexisting inflammation caused by the injection of heat-killed bacteria. Thus, they believed the reaction was an enhancement phenomenon of prior inflammation rather than an irritant or allergic reaction.

Pustules usually are associated with irritant reactions, but pustular allergic reactions have been reported to metals, nitrofurazone, and topical fluorouracil (87). A woman who used 2% minoxidil solution (Lacovin) developed a mixture of vesicles and pustules on her forehead. Histologically, perifollicular lymphocytes, histiocytes, and eosinophils were found. Her patch test reaction was 2+ and consisted of a mixture of vesicles and pustules.

Pustular contact dermatitis has also been reported from isoconazole nitrate (88). The patch test was strongly eczematous.

Pustular Patch Test Reactions

Hjorth (89) stated that such reactions are most likely to occur in atopic persons. Fisher et al. (90) found that metallic salts, particularly nickel, copper, arsenic trioxide, and mercuric chloride, produced such reactions, which usually dry promptly before disappearing completely. Pustular patch test reactions are usually irritant in nature but may sometimes accompany allergic reactions (91).

Pustular reactions to standard patch tests with nickel sulfate (5%) were found to be the rule when patients with atopic dermatitis were tested on skin bearing follicular papules, erythema, or lichenification or when the skin integrity was disturbed by minor trauma, such as a pinprick (92). This further supports the nonallergic (irritant) nature of the phenomena.

> **Allergic pustular dermatitis is rare. Pustular patch test reactions are common with metals and are irritant in nature but may accompany true allergic patch test reactions. They are more common among atopic persons.**

DYSHIDROSIFORM CONTACT DERMATITIS

In a personal communication, Martin, Piette, Boegoend, Huriez, and Desmons of France were concerned with the following questions: (a) Do dyshidrotic eczemas related to a contact allergy exist? and (b) Can dyshidrotic lesions be reproduced by patch tests?

Their study covered five patients affected by dyshidrotic eczema that had been developing for at least 4 years. Having obtained positive test results on the back, they reproduced the lesions by applying selected allergens to the palm in patch tests. These allergens were potassium dichromate (two cases), PPDA (two cases, of which one also was tested on the soles), and mercaptobenzothiazole (MBT, one case, with a sole test also positive).

Patients were tested as follows: (a) In a cement worker who since 1971 had dyshidrotic eczema of the palm with positive chromate and cobalt patch test results, patch testing of the palm and the back was positive for chromium but not for cobalt. (b) In a concrete worker with eczema on the backs of the hands who was allergic to dichromate and who had severe dyshidrotic dermatitis on the heels related to an allergy to rubber in his shoes, patch testing on the back was positive for MBT. Results of patch tests with MBT on the soles were also positive. (c) In a window cleaner with pompholyx of the palms and soles who was "intolerant" of rubber gloves and shoes, a patch test to PPDA on his back was positive. Patch testing on the palm with PPDA produced a positive reaction resembling a dyshidrotic eruption.

In this study, the allergen concentrations were identical for the patch tests on the back and on the palms or soles. These authors believed that perhaps penetration of the allergen is made easier by changes in the palms or soles in persons affected by dyshidrotic eczema, even after an apparent cure.

> **Contact allergens may play a role in dyshidrotic eczema.**

These authors commented that contact allergy is seldom proposed as a precursor of dyshidrotic eczema. They cited investigators (93) who claim that, in patients with allergy to nickel and pompholyx, intimate contact with nickel objects in no case induces an exacerbation of the hand eruption. However, some authentic cases of dyshidrotic eczema of the palm and sole appear to improve when an "external" contact with nickel is removed. Fisher and Shapiro (94) cited positive results of patch tests on the palms with nickel.

Dyshidrotic eczema or pompholyx might better be thought of as a reaction pattern with many possible causes. Internal and external allergies have been capable of producing this pattern of eczema, as noted in the references cited. Irritant contact dermatitis induced by metal-working fluids has also produced dyshidrotic eczema in workers who had neither an atopic diathesis nor positive patch tests (95). Therefore, it seems that the morphologic pattern associated with pompholyx is not specific for a route of exposure or a currently well-understood mechanism. Pompholyx is probably not a disease sui generis.

CONTACT "HALOGENOSIS" FROM TOPICAL, FLUORINATED, OR "STRONG" CORTICOSTEROIDS

In the past, the fluorinated corticosteroids have been implicated in the etiology of certain cases of perioral dermatitis, rosacea-like eruptions in both children and adults, and skin atrophy (96,97). More recently, European and Japanese dermatologists (98–100) have reported apparently new entities under such terms as "granuloma gluteale infantum" and "Kaposi's sarcoma–like granulomatous diaper dermatitis," in which fluorinated topical corticosteroids may be causative factors.

Malkinson and Pearson (101) posed the following question: Should these cases of infantile gluteal granuloma or Kaposi-like sarcomas occurring in the diaper area be considered as contact dermatitis vegetans or infant halogenosis? A brief description of these new entities complicating diaper dermatitis follows.

Granuloma Gluteale Infantum

Tappeiner and Pfleger (98) reported an apparently new entity, granuloma gluteale infantum, in six infants. All infants had painless firm nodules that resembled large angiomas or hematomas initially. The lesions were on the buttocks and the inner aspect of the thighs and consisted of symmetrical, round, or oval plum-sized, bluish-red or maroon nodules. The surrounding skin was normal. The infants were otherwise normal, as were their blood studies and X-ray examinations. The nodules resolved spontaneously in several months without sequelae.

The histologic examination did not correspond with any known dermatologic condition. No evidence of infection was present. Although the cause remained obscure, some "exogenous noxious factor" was considered the most likely.

> **Granulomas and Kaposi-like lesions may occur in the infantile diaper area from fluorinated or "strong" corticosteroids. These lesions disappear spontaneously.**

"Vegetating" Halogenosis

Bazex et al. (99) reported a 3-month-old boy, seen because of a diaper rash, who had been treated with eosin, permanganate baths, and Mycolog Cream. The eruption disappeared in about 1 month, but 1 month later violet nodules resembling hematomas of traumatic origin appeared on the inside of the thighs and pubis. The hypothesis of "vegetating bromidism" was considered, but the infant had received no bromide treatment. The nodules disappeared spontaneously without treatment after approximately 1 month without sequelae.

Kaposi's Sarcoma–like Granulomatous Diaper Dermatitis

Uyeda et al. (100) in Japan described five cases of Kaposi's sarcoma–like granuloma occurring in areas of diaper dermatitis in infants age 2 to 8 months, who had worn paper diapers. These infants had had diaper dermatitis, and in each case, synthetic corticosteroid hormones were applied topically.

The granulomas appeared in the genitocrural region, the lower abdomen, and the inner thighs and bore a clinical and histologic resemblance to the early stage of Kaposi's sarcoma. No evidence of infection was present. The lesions of diaper dermatitis disappeared, but the granulomas remained for several months, then cleared spontaneously and never recurred.

The authors, referring to the report of Tappeiner and Pfleger (98), stated that the clinical features and histologic findings of granuloma gluteale infantum were similar to their Japanese cases, except that the gluteal region was not affected. The lesions were instead in the genitocrural region, the thigh, and the penile region. Thus, because the Japanese investigators believed the term "granuloma gluteale infantum" would be unsuitable, they described their cases as "Kaposi's sarcoma–like granuloma on diaper dermatitis."

Malkinson and Pearson (101) stated that the suggestion by Bazex et al. (99) that this condition may be associated with halogen is supported to some extent by the histologic changes; however, beyond that, the evidence is very thin and highly speculative. These authors believed it was more reasonable that, rather than being directly related to the halogen contents in corticosteroids, the condition is secondary to the great potency of these corticosteroids, even though the pathogenic mechanism is obscure. A somewhat analogous situation is present in perioral dermatitis, in which some patients acquire the characteristic eruption after using potent fluorinated corticosteroids.

A recent report of Kaposi-like acroangiodermatitis from the friction and negative pressure of a suction prosthesis may shed light on a feature overlooked in the previously cited cases (102). This patient with this condition was patch test negative to the prosthesis, had no arteriovenous fistula, and was negative for human immunodeficiency virus (HIV). A lighter, larger prosthesis was therapeutic. Most cases of granuloma gluteale infantum and Kaposi's sarcoma–like granuloma have occurred in areas of friction, which may be a cofactor in their development.

Rosacea-like Eruption of Children and Adults

Although the etiology of perioral dermatitis remains controversial, many observations and reports in the literature continue to implicate strong topical corticosteroids, particularly the fluorinated variety. Savin et al. (103) reported 11 cases of children who had strong corticosteroids applied to the face; a bright malar flush was produced that was accompanied at times by small superficial papules, pustules, and scaling. The clinical picture was variable, sometimes closely resembling rosacea and sometimes perioral dermatitis, taking an average of 1 year to clear. Seven of the 11 children had a family history of atopy, and 2 had a family history of rosacea. These authors stated that potent topical corticosteroids may have played a role in the cause of these rashes and, on withdrawal, a pustular exacerbation was sometimes present. They speculated that a relationship exists between rosacea and perioral dermatitis.

> **Prolonged use of "strong" topical corticosteroids may produce a rosacea-like eruption in children and adults.**

"Topical Drug Addiction"—Adverse Effects of Fluorinated Corticosteroid Creams and Ointments

Under this eye-catching title, Burry (104) discussed the adverse effects that the anti-inflammatory powers of topical fluorinated corticosteroids have on acne rosacea, seborrheic complexions, and tinea infections of the skin as illustrated by eight cases. They stated that these steroids cause local atrophy, purpura, telangiectasia, and ulceration by interfering with skin-collagen metabolism, and that many patients are afraid to stop using locally applied corticosteroids because of the uncomfortable rebound inflammation that follows their withdrawal. Both the skin and the patient can therefore become readily "hooked" on these topical drugs.

Almeyda and Burt (105) concurred with Burry, stating it is now recognized that topically administered fluorinated compounds are just as likely to cause unwanted side effects as are systemically administered compounds.

Earlier, Sneddon (106) had drawn attention to the effects of fluorinated compounds on patients with rosacea, who seem to become addicted because corticosteroids initially suppress the soreness and inflammatory papular and pustular lesions. Each time application is stopped, however, the eruption exacerbates acutely, tempting the patient to apply more corticosteroid. With prolonged application, there is loss of dermal connective tissue, which exposes the subpapillary venous plexus and causes increasing erythema and telangiectasia. The process is slow, and the patients do not notice the deterioration in their appearance for some time. Weber (107) agreed that the rosacea-like condition and perioral dermatitis may well result from the use of fluorinated corticosteroids on the face.

Addiction to topical steroids can cause a chronic red face or eyelid dermatitis that can only be cured by withdrawal of the corticosteroid. However, a severe and prolonged rebound of facial erythema and edema is part of the pathway to a cure. This complication of topical steroid use has been detailed by Rapaport and Rapaport (108).

> **Many patients become "hooked" on strong topical corticosteroids, because when they stop applying these agents, they develop a severe rebound of facial dermatitis.**

Epstein et al. (109) pointed out that potent topical corticosteroids can produce striae and extensive bruising and ecchymoses with minor trauma owing to wasting of dermal connective tissue. Extreme soft tissue atrophy in the diaper area in an infant treated for diaper rash with fluorinated steroids for some months has also been reported by Johns and Bower (110). Growth of vellus hair, delayed healing of ulcerated areas, and systemic absorption with depression of endogenous corticosteroid secretions have all been observed with use of potent fluorinated steroids (111,112).

> **Strong topical corticosteroids can produce many of the effects of systemic administration.**

CONTACT EPILATING FOLLICULITIS

The popular depilatories include the thioglycolates, the sulfides, and the mechanical depilatories. These agents may produce a marked follicular reaction with a pustular reaction when they are not used properly (113).

A similar type of folliculitis is produced by the penetration of sharp needles of sugarcane bark into the hair follicles of sugarcane workers (114). An inflammatory, follicular, pustular eruption is produced, particularly on the extremities. The borders of the scalp, the pubic area, and the chest and back may also be involved. Pruritus is severe, and the involved follicle atrophies, causing permanent hair loss.

CONTACT GRANULOMAS

Certain chemicals elicit a local sarcoid granuloma when introduced within the skin. Zirconium, talc, stearate, silica, magnesium, and beryllium may produce granulomas once they pierce the skin (115). In addition, the pigments of tattoos, particularly chrominum oxide, may cause a granulomatous reaction in sensitized individuals.

Zirconium, beryllium, chromium, and aluminum may produce allergic granulomas. Talc, zinc, stearate, silica, and magnesium may produce irritant granulomas.

Allergic Contact Granulomas

Zirconium Granuloma

This skin lesion, seen originally following use of zirconium compounds in deodorants, continues to occur following use of these compounds for the treatment of *Toxicodendron* dermatitis (116).

The lesions usually appear 4 to 6 weeks after initial use of the zirconium preparation and are limited to the sites of contact. They appear as persistent, firm, shiny, erythematous papules the color of flesh or apple jelly, and they may be solitary, grouped, or coalescent. Eczematous changes are also usually present. Pruritus is minimal or absent. The histologic picture may be indistinguishable from sarcoid.

Any defect in the protective layer of the skin enhances the development of hypersensitivity (117–119).

In the axillae, minute abrasions from shaving as well as from excess friction and sweating enhance penetration of the zirconium salts in deodorants. The preparations containing zirconium salts used to treat *Toxicodendron* dermatitis readily penetrate acutely inflamed skin, denuded areas, vesicles, and bullae (120).

Zirconium granulomas, composed of epithelioid cells, represent an acquired, delayed-type allergic reaction to zirconium in sensitized individuals (121).

The granulomas produced by soluble zirconium salts usually disappear within a few months, whereas those produced by insoluble salts may last indefinitely. Intralesional injections of corticosteroids may be effective in resolving these granulomas.

Tests for Zirconium Hypersensitivity

Either patch or intracutaneous testing may be employed to determine allergic hypersensitivity to zirconium salts (122).

Patch Test

The zirconium preparation suspected of causing a granulomatous reaction may be rubbed into a test site previously prepared by multiple scratches or denuding with a dermal curet. The test site is then covered with an occlusive dressing for 2 days. In sensitized persons, a positive reaction is the development of reddish-brown papules in about 4 weeks. Such papules show a sarcoid granulomatous infiltrate histologically.

Intracutaneous Test

A small wheal is produced by intracutaneous injection of a 1:10,000 dilution of sodium zirconium lactate. A positive reaction consists of a discrete papule that appears in 8 to 14 days. In about 1 month, the papule clinically and histologically resembles a sarcoid lesion. The papule may persist for 6 to 24 months.

Prognosis of Zirconium Granulomas

Axillary granulomas produced by the soluble zirconium lactate in deodorants usually disappear within a few months. Lesions produced by the insoluble zirconium oxide preparations used for poison ivy (*Toxicodendron*) dermatitis usually remain unchanged for several months to years and are refractory to therapy. Temporary improvement is obtained with corticosteroids administered systemically or intralesionally.

Testing for allergic granulomatous sensitivity to zirconium salts may be performed on scarified skin or intradermally. At least three controls should be used.

Aluminum Granulomas

Patients may occasionally become allergic to aluminum, which can be detected by reactions at all Finn chamber sites owing to their aluminum construction or by testing with 2% aqueous aluminum hydroxide. Vaccination with diphtheria-pertussis-tetanus vaccine is a potential problem for such allergic persons (usually children) because aluminum hydroxide is a component of the vaccine and has caused granulomas at the vaccination sites that can last for more than 1 year (123). Of 21 cases followed, 5 cleared, 11 improved, and 5 remained unchanged. Aluminum was demonstrated in the granulomas by X-ray defraction analysis.

Nonallergic Contact Granulomas

Sodium Stearate

The granulomatous response to sodium stearate is not based on allergic reactivity. It can be contrasted with the allergic granulomatous responses in patients who have zirconium deodorant granulomas and who are prepared immunologically as a result of their allergic hypersensitivity to zirconium. Thus, relatively few people develop granulomas after skin tests with zirconium salts.

Large quantities of sodium stearate are required to elicit the granulomatous response, whereas unusually dilute preparations of zirconium produce it in susceptible individuals. Often even 0.0001-ML solutions of zirconium salts stimulate formation of a granuloma in an allergic person. Concentrations of sodium stearate or sodium palmitate more dilute than 0.1 ML do not induce such reactions.

Stearate granulomas resolve clinically within a few weeks, but allergic granulomas usually reach their peak at 3 to 6 weeks and persist for months to years. In general, allergic granulomas are still evolving when stearate granulomas have completely resolved.

Talc Granulomas

McCallum and Hall (124) stated that treatment of the raw umbilical stump can produce pyogenic granulomas and umbilical polyps. They recommend that treatment with talc or starch should be discontinued and replaced by a nonirritant, sterile substance.

Tye et al. (125) described hundreds of talc granulomas of the skin that developed in a 45-year-old woman. It is postulated that the talcum powder gained entrance through the skin at the sites of draining or incised furuncles.

Oil Granulomas

Bergeron and Stone (126) observed two cases of multiple perifollicular granulomas of the scalp produced by Egyptian Oil, a proprietary hair conditioner. Upon discontinuation of the hair conditioner, the lesions regressed in both patients.

Granuloma Fissuratum

Chronic irritation from eyeglasses or dentures can produce granulomas at sites of pressure from the hard object. Such granulomas usually have a crease down the middle of the lesion.

DRY, LICHENIFIED, OR HYPERKERATOTIC CONTACT DERMATITIS

Airborne allergens and dust tend to form dry, lichenified eruptions.

Airborne Allergens and Irritants

Contact dermatitis from prolonged, repeated exposure to relatively small quantities of airborne allergens, such as pollens, dusts, and vapors, produces diffuse, dry, and lichenified eruptions with vesiculation. The exposed portions of the body as well as wrinkles and folds are most markedly involved.

Ragweed Dermatitis

This type of dermatitis rarely is frankly vesicular unless the patient actually comes in contact with the plant. Exposure to the oleoresin through airborne pollen may result in a dry, leathery dermatitis with skin so infiltrated that a cutaneous lymphoma is suspected.

Dermatitis from Dust

Dusts and their contents may produce mechanical effects, primary irritant eruptions, and allergic reactions (127).

Dust that contains glass fibers can produce cuts from sharp glass fragments. Exposed surfaces may sustain an intensely pruritic, papular eruption. The penetrating spicules of asbestos, a fibrous, silicate mineral, are mechanical irritants that can produce asbestos "corns," particularly on the palmar aspects of the fingers. Coal, rock, and stone dust have an abrasive effect on the skin and can produce a lichenified, papular eruption that may be complicated by folliculitis. Dust collecting about a collar, belt line, or sleeve end may be rubbed into the skin by friction, producing lichenified eruptions.

The dust from relining a blast furnace has been found to cause an irritant dermatitis with frequently follicular patterns. Hydroxides of calcium, sodium, and potassium were found to produce a pH of approximately 12, and skin moisture was sufficient to exacerbate the problem (128).

> Pollens, chemical dusts, and sawdust usually produce dry, lichenified dermatitis.

Dermatitis from cement dust is also dry and lichenified, primarily because of its alkalinity, hygroscopic properties, and abrasive effects. In addition, even when cement dermatitis results from allergic hypersensitivity to the chromium or cobalt content, the eruption tends toward dryness rather than frank vesiculation.

Sawdust from teak, redwood, mahogany, and rosewood may contain sensitizers that produce a dry dermatitis, particularly on the face, penis, and scrotum among carpenters and woodworkers. A lichenified eruption may also appear on the penis and scrotum when sawdust falls inside the clothes or is conveyed to these areas by the hands.

Other chemical dusts, fumes, and vapors produce eruptions similar to sawdust dermatitis. In addition, dust and air pollutants containing pitch or tar produce follicular, keratotic, and acneiform eruptions, as well as melanosis and photosensitivity reactions.

A dermatitis resembling ichthyosis caused by a quaternary ammonium compound in an ointment has been reported in Japan (129). The compound implicated is alkyl benzyl trimethyl ammonium chloride.

CONTACT HYPERKERATOTIC ERUPTIONS OF THE FINGERS, PALMS, AND SOLES

The thick, horny layer of the fingers, palms, and soles modifies the appearance of allergic contact dermatitis by minimizing the eczematous element. The dry, fissured eruptions may resemble those from primary irritants, psoriasis, hyperkeratotic fungal infections, or atopic dermatitis. In dentists, allergic contact dermatitis from procaine hydrochloride (Novocain) or acrylic monomer is scaly, thickened, and fissured. Affected nails may become thickened, dystrophic, and separated from the nail bed.

> **Contact dermatitis of palms and soles may produce dystrophic nails and must be differentiated from psoriasis, atopic dermatitis, and hyperkeratotic dermatophytosis.**

So-called tulip bulb fingers (seen both with tulip bulbs and with *Alstromeria* contact among florists), in which the affected skin is dry, fissured, and hyperkeratotic, may resemble procaine hydrochloride (Novocain) and acrylic dermatitis. Onions, garlic, and formaldehyde and its resins may produce similar eruptions on the palms and palmar surfaces of the fingers.

In nickel-sensitive persons, pressure and prolonged contact with nickel-plated handlebars or door handles may produce dry, fissured eruptions of the palm. Similarly, nickel-plated arch supports may produce such changes on the soles.

"CONTACT" PSORIASIS: KOEBNER PHENOMENON

Fisher (130) showed that pressure, trauma, and friction from occupational procedures may produce psoriasis of the hands, particularly the palms and volar surfaces of the fingers. This psoriasis, called Koebner phenomenon, occurred in a pharmacist (from the pressure of opening and closing containers with child-resistant caps), a surgeon, a dentist (from the pressure of various instruments), a bus driver (from the pressure of the steering wheel), and an office worker (from pounding a stapler), a bartender, a seamstress, an optician, a paperhanger, a pushcart peddler, and a cellist.

Stable psoriasis may become pustular when contact dermatitis is superimposed on the stable plaque-type disease. This occurred in a patient with scalp psoriasis who became sensitive to the shampoo ingredient zinc pyrithione (131). Only areas of contact dermatitis developed the pustular form of the disease.

Often the patient does not show obvious psoriasis elsewhere. One may have to examine the scalp carefully and the intergluteal area to discover if the patient has psoriasis.

Adams (132) believed that the fact that fresh lesions of psoriasis appear following trauma from scratching, abrasions, lacerations, folliculitis, and acne has led many workers to press for compensation in the belief that the disease was caused or brought to activity by their occupation. If a "Koebnerized" lesion is followed quickly by a severe flare of the disease, the idea of occupational causation seems even more likely to the worker. Trauma undoubtedly may incite the development of new lesions of psoriasis, but this occurs only in persons who already have the disease, if only in latent form. For this reason, careful consideration should be given to the job placement of persons with active psoriasis and even to those with a history of the disease. Thus, the Koebner phenomenon is medicolegally important when it follows industrial injuries.

> **Trauma in work or play may produce psoriasis, particularly of the hands, in patients who have minimal psoriasis elsewhere on the body. Koebner phenomenon is medicolegally significant.**

IRRITANT DERMATITIS WITHOUT ERYTHEMA

At the 1983 International Contact Dermatitis Symposium in East Germany, Nakayama et al. discussed "nonerythematous irritant reactions detected by the microscopic relief method." They stated:

Erythema has been regarded as a necessary sign in irritant dermatitis. Chronic irritant dermatitis, however, provoked by repeated contact to diluted detergents often shows a scaly rough skin without accompanying marked erythema. Linear alkylbenzene sulfonate and sodium lauryl sulfate have been known to produce erythema and edema when closed patch tested at 2% in aqueous solution for 48 hours. The reactions were negative macroscopically when closed patch tested at less than 1% for 24 hours. Then, didn't these irritants actually produce a reaction under such conditions?

Even though erythema was not discernible, the reliefs of the patch-tested skin surfaces were found to have been markedly disturbed when the replicas of the reliefs were taken and microscopically examined. The replicas were taken using celluloid plates (1.5 cm in diameter) whose surfaces were dissolved by painting *n*-butyl acetate before pressed on the patch-tested sites for two minutes.

The most striking findings obtained by this method were the disappearance of normal triangle skin furrow patterns. They were replaced by rounded, flattened, or deepened skin furrows at the sites where these irritants had been applied.

FRICTIONAL CONTACT DERMATITIS

In 1993, at the International Contact Dermatitis Symposium in East Germany, Torkil Menné of Copenhagen reported as follows:

> Experimentally, friction in the palms may give rise to callosities, bullae or dermatitis-like changes. For the development of frictional dermatitis the following factors are important; individual, intensity of frictional trauma and architecture of the surfaces. The skin changes are confined to the thenar or hypothenar region and the fingertips. The lesions may heal by changing irregular surfaces to smooth ones.

CONTACT LYMPHANGITIS AND LYMPHEDEMA

Many solvents entering a fissure or abrasion may produce a "chemical" lymphangitis, distinguishable from bacterial lymphangitis by the lack of constitutional symptoms. In addition, lymphangitis and lymphedema may follow allergic contact dermatitis (133).

Worm et al. (134) reported that two patients with allergic contact dermatitis developed gross edema of the upper and lower extremities following recurrent bacterial infections. It is unlikely that the specific allergens responsible for the dermatitis have had any influence on the development of edema, because patients described previously with edema of the hands had positive patch tests to other allergens. In cases of severe dermatitis, leakage of plasma proteins from the vessels of the involved skin is abnormally increased (135). Increased drainage of lymphatic protein from the interstitium of involved skin can compensate for this leakage and thus counteract edema formation.

In the cases described, many years elapsed in which the lymphatics compensated for the increased leakage of microvascular protein without resulting edema. Recurrent bacterial skin infections, however, may have compromised the lymphatic function, causing an increased extravascular concentration of plasma proteins. We therefore suggest that a local increase in the volume of interstitial fluid in the skin elicited by colloid osmotic forces can explain the clinically manifest edema in our and in similar patients.

Benzo-pyrones diminish edema from experimentally induced protein-rich rat leg (136). The mechanism by which this occurs is probably increased proteolysis, which facilitates the removal of proteins from the interstitial space. Theoretically, therefore, this treatment should have an effect in the patients described. However, a more exact characterization of the protein content of edema fluid before and during such treatment is mandatory to evaluate the clinical and the physiologic response.

> **Solvents can produce a nonbacterial "chemical" lymphangitis. Various contact allergens can produce allergic dermatitis complicated by bacterial lymphangitis and lymphedema.**

PRURIGO NODULARIS

There have been reports of contact dermatitis to the oral antibiotic nifuroxazide, which is used to treat acute and chronic diarrhea (137). A Polish pharmaceutical worker was exposed to nifuroxazide in a packaging operation, but her lesions resembled prurigo nodularis rather than contact dermatitis. She was sensitive to this antibiotic from 1% to 0.001% aqueous and cleared when not occupationally exposed. She did not cross-react to nitrofurazone.

ERYTHEMA DYSCHROMICUM PERSTANS

A study in Panama of banana plantation workers with an erythema dyschromicum perstans–like eruption found that almost all were sensitive to a 0.001% chlorothalonil patch test (138). This finding was present in 34 of 39 such cases. Chlorothalonil is a fungicide, which is widely used on banana plantations. None of 41 controls showed a reaction. Although not proof of cause and effect, the strong possibility that sensitivity to chlorothalonil is responsible for some cases of erythema dyschromicum perstans remains.

PYODERMA GANGRENOSUM

Contact dermatitis to rubber components of an ostomy bag produced peristomal dermatitis in a patient who had undergone proctocolectomy for ulcerative colitis (139). He had been in remission with no active colitis, but the dermatitis around his stoma ulcerated and took on the characteristics typical of pyoderma gangrenosum. There was no flare of underlying bowel disease in this case, and he responded to oral minocycline combined with intralesional triamcinolone.

DESQUAMATIVE GINGIVITIS

Inflammation of both the free and attached gingiva was seen in a 27-year-old woman evaluated at a dental school in Scotland (140). A clinical diagnosis of desquamative gingivitis was made. However, the woman was extremely sensitive to the nail polish ingredient tosylamide/formaldehyde resin, and she was a nail-biter. She was cured by changing to a nail polish without the allergen.

LYMPHOCYTOMA CUTIS

Persistent lower lip dermatitis that histologically proved to be lymphocytoma cutis was traced to a dental metal (141). The patient had a strong positive reaction to zinc chloride 2% aqueous that was present in one rusted filling. Zinc was confirmed to be present in the filling. Lymphocytoma cutis and urticaria, lichen planus, stomatitis, and generalized dermatitis are forms of dental metal allergy.

Lymphocytoma cutis of the earlobes has also been reported due to contact dermatitis resulting from gold and nickel earlobe exposure (142).

PERSISTENT URTICARIAL PLAQUES

Persistent urticaria, rather than transient urticaria or chronic dermatitis, as seen in the contact urticaria syndrome, is another morphologic presentation for contact dermatitis. A persistent urticarial axillary eruption was reported due to an emulsifier in a deodorant (143). The emulsifier, commercially known as Eumulgin L, had not previously been reported to be an allergen. Patch tests were strongly positive at 30% in petrolatum and weakly positive at 1% aqueous. This compound is also known as cetyl stearyl alcohol 2 (OP) 9(OE). No cross-reactivity was found to cetyl stearyl alcohol+sodium cetyl stearyl sulfate (Lanette N) or cetyl alcohol (Lanette 16).

ANAPHYLAXIS

Anaphylaxis usually does not result from topical allergen exposure to intact skin. Mucosal surfaces, abraded skin, or skin ulceration is more fertile ground for anaphylactoid reactions.

Skin contact has resulted in anaphylaxis from latex, black rubber mix, carba mix, bacitracin, neomycin, streptomycin, cephalosporin, rifamycin, chlorhexidine, mercurochrome, Emulgade F (an emulsifying agent), chlorothalonil, formaldehyde, lidocaine, milk, rice mechlorethamine, and labetalol (Table 7.5) (144).

TABLE 7.5. *Causes of Anaphylaxis from Topical Exposure*

Natural rubber latex
Rubber antioxidants: black rubber mix
Rubber accelerators: carba mix
Antibiotics: bacitracin, neomycin, streptomycin, cephalosporin, rifamycin
Antiseptics: chlorhexidene, mercurochrome
Foods: milk, rice
Anesthetics: lidocaine
Other medications: mechlorethamine, labetalol
Miscellaneous chemicals: chlorothalonil, formaldehyde, Emulgade F

REFERENCES

1. Holst R, Kirby J, Magnusson B. Sensitization to tropical woods giving erythema multiforme–like eruptions. *Contact Dermatitis* 1976; 2:295.
2. Fisher AA, Bikowski J. Allergic contact dermatitis due to a wooden cross made of *Dalbergia nigra*. *Contact Dermatitis* 1981;7:45.
3. Martin P, Bergoend H, Piette F. *Erythema multiforme–like eruption from Brazilian rosewood.* Paper presented at the Fifth International Symposium on Contact Dermatitis, Barcelona, March 28, 1980.
4. Hjorth N. Primula dermatitis. *Trans St John's Hosp Dermatol Soc* 1966;52:207.
5. Kurz G, Rapaport MJ. External/internal allergy to plants (*Artemesia*). *Contact Dermatitis* 1979;5:407.
6. Moschella SL. Erythema multiforme. In: *Dermatology*. Vol. 1. Philadelphia: WB Saunders, 1975:387.
7. Shelley W. The Duhring conferences: poison ivy with marked edema. *Skin and Allergy News,* November 2, 1979, p. 30.
8. Kirby JS, Darley CR. Erythema multiforme associated with a contact dermatitis to terpenes. *Contact Dermatitis* 1978;4:238.
9. Torinuki W. Generalized erythema multiformae–like eruption following allergic contact dermatitis. *Contact Dermatitis* 1990;23: 202.
10. Raccagni AA, Bardazzi F, Baldari U, Righini MG. Erythema-multiforme-like contact dermatitis due to capsicum. *Contact Dermatitis* 1995;33:353.
11. Mateo MPG, Velasco M, Miquel FJ, de la Cuadra J. Erythema-multiforme-like eruption following allergic contact dermatitis from sesquiterpene lactones in herbal medicine. *Contact Dermatitis* 1995; 33:449.
12. Puig L, Alomar A, Randazzo L, et al. Erythema multiform like reaction caused by topical application of Thuja essential oil. *Am J Contact Dermat* 1994;5:94.
13. DeFeo CP Jr. Erythema multiforme bullosum caused by 9-bromofluorene. *Arch Dermatol* 1966;94:545.
14. Powell EW, et al. Skin reactions to 9-bromofluorene. *Br J Dermatol* 1968;80:491.
15. Roed-Petersen J. Erythema multiforme as an expression of contact dermatitis. *Contact Dermatitis* 1975;1:270.
16. Fregert S, Gustafsson K, Trulsson L. Contact allergy to *N*-hydroxyphthalimide. *Contact Dermatitis* 1983;9:84.
17. Viraben R, Labrousse JL, Bazex J. Erythema multiforme due to DNCB. *Contact Dermatitis* 1990;22:179.
18. Magnusson B, Gilje O. Allergic contact dermatitis from a dishwashing liquid containing lauryl ether sulphate. *Acta Derm Venereol (Stockh)* 1973;53:136.
19. Bjornberg A, Mobacken H. Sensitization to benzene compounds. *Berufsdermatosen* 1972;21:245.
20. Nethercott JR, et al. Erythema multiforme exudativum linked to the manufacture of printed circuit boards. *Contact Dermatitis* 1982;8: 314.
21. Phoon WH, et al. Stevens-Johnson syndrome associated with occupational exposure to trichloroethylene. *Contact Dermatitis* 1984;10: 270.
22. Vincenzi C, Stinchi C, Guerra L, et al. Erythema multiforme–like contact dermatitis: report of 4 cases. *Am J Contact Dermat* 1994;5: 90.
23. Zhang XM, Nakagawa M, Kawai K, Kawai K. Erythema-multiforme–like eruption following photoallergic contact dermatitis from oxybenzone. *Contact Dermatitis* 1998;38:43.
24. Garcia-Bravo B, Rodriguez-Pichardo A, de Pierola SF, Camacho F. Airborne erythema-multiforme-like eruption due to pyrethrum. *Contact Dermatitis* 1995;33:433.
25. Bhargave RK, Singh V, Soni V. Erythema multiforme resulting from insecticide spray. *Arch Dermatol* 1977;113:686.
26. Thompson JA, Wansker BA. A case of contact dermatitis, erythema multiforme and toxic epidermal necrolysis. *J Am Acad Dermatol* 1981;6:666.
27. Cook LJ. Associated nickel and cobalt contact dermatitis presenting as erythema multiforme. *Contact Dermatitis* 1982;8:280.
28. Calnan CD. Nickel dermatitis. *Br J Dermatol* 1956;68:229.
29. Agrup G, Cronin E. Contact dermatitis (X). *Br J Dermatol* 1970;82: 428.

30. Degreef H, Bonamie A, van Derheyden D, Dooms-Goossens A. Mephenesin contact dermatitis with erythema multiforme features. *Contact Dermatitis* 1984;10:220.

31. Meneghini CL, Angelini G. Secondary polymorphic eruptions in allergic contact dermatitis. *Dermatologica* 1981;163:63.

32. Meneghini CL, Angelini G. Contact dermatitis from pyrrolnitrin. *Contact Dermatitis* 1982;8:55.

33. Yaffee H, Dressler DP. Topical application of mafenide acetate: its association with erythema multiforme and cutaneous reactions. *Arch Dermatol* 1969;100:277.

34. Guill MA, et al. Erythema multiforme and urticaria: eruptions induced by chemically related ophthalmic anticholinergic agents. *Arch Dermatol* 1979;115:742.

35. Gottschalk HR, Stone OJ. Stevens-Johnson syndrome from ophthalmic sulfonamide. *Arch Dermatol* 1976;112:513.

36. Rubin Z. Ophthalmic sulfonamide-induced Stevens-Johnson syndrome. *Arch Dermatol* 1977;113:235.

37. Saperstein H, Rapaport M, Rietschel RL. Topical vitamin E as a cause of erythema multiforme–like eruption. *Arch Dermatol* 1984;120:906.

38. Kerre S, Busschots A, Dooms-Goossens A. Erythema-multiforme–like contact dermatitis due to phenylbutazone. *Contact Dermatitis* 1995;33:213.

39. Koch P, Bahmer FA. Erythema-multiforme-like, urticarial papular and plaque eruptions from bufexamac: report of 4 cases. *Contact Dermatitis* 1994;31:97.

40. Walchner M, Rueff F, Przybilla B. Delayed-type hypersensitivity to mofebutazone underlying a severe drug reaction. *Contact Dermatitis* 1997;36:54.

41. Stingeni L, et al. Erythema-multiforme-like contact dermatitis from budesonide. *Contact Dermatitis* 1996;34:154.

42. Valsecchi R, et al. Erythema-multiforme-like lesions from triamcinolone acetonide. *Contact Dermatitis* 1998;38:362.

43. Puig L, et al. Erythema-multiforme-like eruption due to topical contactants: expression of adhesion molecules and their ligands and characterization of the infiltrate. *Contact Dermatitis* 1995;33:329.

44. Greenwood K. Dermatitis with capillary fragility. *Arch Dermatol* 1960;81:947.

45. Hellier FF. Dermatitis purpura after contact with textiles. *Hautarzt* 1960;11:173.

46. Abel RR. Washing machine and fiberglass. *Arch Dermatol* 1966;93:78.

47. Osmundsen PE. Contact dermatitis from an optical whitener in washing powders. *Cutis* 1972;10:59.

48. Beck MH, Wilkinson SM. A distinctive irritant contact reaction to Vioform (clioquinol). *Contact Dermatitis* 1994;31:54–5.

49. Petrozzi JW, Lockshin NA. Pants pressure purpura. *Cutis* 1974;13:799.

50. Calnan CD, Peachey RDG. Allergic contact purpura. *Clin Allergy* 1971;1:287.

51. Fisher AA. Allergic petechial and purpuric rubber dermatitis: the PPP syndrome. *Cutis* 1974;14:25.

52. Romaguera C, Grimalt F. PPPP syndrome. *Contact Dermatitis* 1977;3:102.

53. Shmunes E. Purpuric allergic contact dermatitis to paraphenylenediamine. *Contact Dermatitis* 1978;4:225.

54. Agarwal K. Contact allergic purpura to wool dust. *Contact Dermatitis* 1982;8:281.

55. Romaguera C, Grimalt F, Lecha M. Occupational purpuric textile dermatitis from formaldehyde resins. *Contact Dermatitis* 1981;7:152.

56. Ackroyd JF. The role of sedormid in the immunological reaction that results in platelet lysis in sedormid purpura. *Clin Sci* 1954;13:409.

57. Friedman AL, Brody EA, Barr PS. Immunothrombocytopenic purpura due to quinidine: report of four new cases with special observations on patch testing. *J Lab Clin Med* 1956;48:205.

58. Schmidt H, Larsen FS, Larson PO, Sogaard H. Petechial reaction following patch testing with cobalt. *Contact Dermatitis* 1980;6:91.

59. Rorsman H. Riehl's melanosis. *Int J Dermatol* 1982;21:76.

60. Osmundsen PE. Pigmented contact dermatitis. *Br J Dermatol* 1970;83:296.

61. Pinol-Aguade J, et al. Dermatitis por blanquedores opticos. *Med Cutan* 1971;5:249.

62. Ancona-Alayon A, et al. Occupational pigmented contact dermatitis from Naphthol AS. *Contact Dermatitis* 1976;2:129.

63. Kgzuka T, et al. Pigmented contact dermatitis from azo dyes. I. Cross-sensitivity in humans. *Contact Dermatitis* 1980;6:330.

64. Nakayama H, Hanaoka H, Ohshiro A. *Allergen controlled system* (ACS). Tokyo: Kanehara Shuppan Co., 1974.

65. Mathias CGT. Pigmented cosmetic dermatitis from contact allergy to a toilet soap containing chromium. *Contact Dermatitis* 1982;8:29.

66. Addo HA, Ferguson J, Johnson BE, Frain-Bell W. The relationship between exposure to fragrance materials and persistent light reaction in the photosensitivity dermatitis with actinic reticuloid syndrome. *Br J Dermatol* 1982;107:261.

67. Frain-Bell W, Johnson BE. Contact allergic sensitivity to plants and the photosensitivity dermatitis and actinic reticuloid syndrome. *Br J Dermatol* 1979;101:503.

68. Ive FA, Magnus IA, Warin RP, Jones EW. "Actinic reticuloid"; a chronic dermatosis associated with severe photosensitivity and the histological resemblance to lymphoma. *Br J Dermatol* 1969;81:469.

69. Ross JS, du Peloux Menage H, Hawk JL, White IR. Sesquiterpene lactone contact sensitivity: clinical patterns of Compositae dermatitis and relationship to chronic actinic dermatitis. *Contact Dermatitis* 1993;29:84–87.

70. Abel EA. Mycosis fungoides and occupational exposures: is there an association? *Derm Clin* 1990;8:169.

71. Buckley WR. Lichenoid eruptions following contact dermatitis. *Arch Dermatol* 1958;78:454.

72. Canizares O. Lichen planus–like eruption caused by color developer. *Arch Dermatol* 1959;80:81.

73. Mandel EH. Lichen planus–like eruptions caused by a color-film developer. *Arch Dermatol* 1960;81:516.

74. Roed-Peterson J, Menne T. Allergic contact dermatitis and lichen planus from black and white photographic developing. *Cutis* 1976;18:699.

75. Knudsen EA. Lichen planus–like eruption caused by color developer. *Arch Dermatol* 1964;89:357.

76. Sharma VK, Mandal SK, Sethuraman G, Bakshi NA. Para-phenylenediamine-induced lichenoid eruptions. *Contact Dermatitis* 1999;41:40.

77. Frykholm KO, et al. Allergy to copper derived from dental alloys as a possible cause of oral lesions of lichen planus. *Acta Derm Venereol* (Stockh) 1969;49:268.

78. Lombardi F, Campolmi P, Sertoli A. Lichenoid dermatitis caused by nickel salts? *Contact Dermatitis* 1983;9:520.

79. Lichter M, Drury D, Remlinger K. Lichenoid dermatitis caused by epoxy resin. *Contact Dermatitis* 1992;26:275.

80. Laine J, Kalimo K, Forssell H, Happonen RP. Resolution of oral lichenoid lesions after replacement of amalgam restorations in patients allergic to mercury compounds. *Br J Dermatol* 1992;126:10.

81. Strauss JS, Jackson EM. American Academy of Dermatology Invitational Symposium on Comedogenicity. *J Am Acad Dermatol* 1989;20:272.

82. Plewig G, Fulton JE, Kligman AM. Pomade acne. *Arch Dermatol* 1974;101:580.

83. Taylor JS. Chloracne—a continuing problem. *Cutis* 1974;13:585.

84. Taylor JS. Environmental acne: update and review. *Ann NY Acad Sci* 1979;320:295.

85. Burkhart CG. Pustular allergic contact dermatitis: a distinct clinical and pathological entity. *Cutis* 1981;27:630.

86. Stone OJ, Johnson DA. Pustular patch test—experimentally induced. *Arch Dermatol* 1967;95:618.

87. Sanchez-Motilla JM, et al. Pustular allergic contact dermatitis from minoxidil. *Contact Dermatitis* 1998;38:283.

88. Lazarov A, Ingber A. Pustular allergic contact dermatitis to isoconazole nitrate. *Am J Contact Dermat* 1997;8:229.

89. Hjorth N. Diagnostic patch testing. In: Marzulli F, Maibach HI, eds. *Dermatoxicology and pharmacology.* New York: John Wiley and Sons, 1977:344.

90. Fisher AA, Chargin L, Fleischmajer R, Hyman A. Pustular patch test reactions: with particular reference to those produced by ammonium fluoride. *Arch Dermatol* 1959;80:742.

91. Wahlberg JE, Maibach HI. Sterile cutaneous pustules—a manifestation of primary irritancy? *J Invest Dermatol* 1981;76:381.

92. Uehara M, Takahashi C, Ofuji S. Pustular patchtest reactions in atopic dermatitis. *Arch Dermatol* 1975;111:1154.

93. Christensen OB, Moller H. External and internal exposure to antigen in hand eczema of nickel allergy. *Contact Dermatitis* 1975;1:136.

94. Fisher AA, Shapiro A. Allergic eczematous contact dermatitis due to metallic nickel. *JAMA* 1956;161:717.

95. de Boer EM, Bruynzeel DP, van Ketel WG. Dyshidrotic eczema as an occupational dermatitis in metal workers. *Contact Dermatitis* 1988;19:184.

96. Fisher AA. Contact halogenosis due to fluorinated corticosteroids. *Cutis* 1975;15:475.

97. Fisher AA. Facial papular dermatitis due to topical fluorinated steroids (so-called perioral or rosacea-like dermatitis). *Cutis* 1972; 10:459.

98. Tappeiner J, Pfleger L. Granuloma gluteale infantum. *Hautarzt* 1971;22:383.

99. Bazex A, et al. Vegetating granulomas in childhood. *Ann Derm Syph* (Paris) 1972;99:121.

100. Uyeda K, et al. Kaposi sarcoma–like granuloma on diaper dermatitis. *Arch Dermatol* 1973;107:605.

101. Malkinson FD, Pearson RW. Infantile gluteal granuloma (Tappeiner and Pfleger: Should it be considered as "contact dermatitis vegetans or infant halogenosis?"). In: *The Yearbook of Dermatology*. Chicago: Year Book Medical Publishers, 1973:26.

102. Santucci B, et al. Kaposi-like acro-angiodermatitis of amputation stump caused by suction socket prosthesis. *Contact Dermatitis* 1992; 27:131.

103. Savin JA, Alexander S, Marks R. A rosacea-like eruption of children. *Br J Dermatol* 1972;87:425.

104. Burry JN. Topical drug addiction: adverse effects of fluorinated corticosteroid creams and ointments. *Med J Aust* 1973;1:393.

105. Almeyda J, Burt BW. Double-blind controlled study of treatment of atopic eczema with a preparation of hydrocortisone in a new drug delivery system versus betamethasone 17—valerate. *Br J Dermatol* 1974;91:579.

106. Sneddon I. Adverse effect of topical corticosteroids in rosacea. *Br Med J* 1969;1:671.

107. Weber G. Rosacea-like dermatitis: contraindication or intolerance reaction to strong steroids. *Br J Dermatol* 1972;88:253.

108. Rapaport MJ, Rapaport V. Eyelid dermatitis to red face syndrome to cure: clinical experience in 100 cases. *J Am Acad Dermatol* 1999; 41(3 Pt 1):435–442.

109. Epstein NN, Epstein WL, Epstein JB. Atrophic striae in patients with inguinal intertrigo. *Arch Dermatol* 1963;87:450.

110. Johns AM, Bower BD. Wasting of napkin area after repeated use of fluorinated steroid ointment. *Br Med J* 1970;1:347.

111. Scoggins RB, Kligman AM. Relative potency of percutaneously absorbed corticosteroids in suppression of pituitary-adrenal function. *J Invest Dermatol* 1965;45:347.

112. Feiwel M, James VHT, Barnett ES. Effect of potent topical steroids in plasma-cortisol levels of infants and children with eczema. *Lancet* 1969;1:485.

113. Foussereau J, Beneczra C. *Les eczemas allergiques professionals.* Paris: Masson et Cie, 1970.

114. Pardo-Castello V. Epilating folliculitis. *Derm Trop* 1965;2:235.

115. Shelley WB, et al. Intradermal tests with metals and other inorganic elements in sarcoidosis and anthraco-silicosis. *J Invest Derm* 1958; 31:301.

116. Sheard G. Granulomatous reactions due to deodorant sticks. *JAMA* 1957;164:1085.

117. Rubin L. Granulomas of axillae caused by deodorants. *JAMA* 1956; 162:953.

118. Williams RM, Skipworth GB. Zirconium granulomas of glabrous skin following treatment of rhus dermatitis. *Arch Dermatol* 1959; 80:273.

119. Epstein WL, Allen JR. Granulomatous hypersensitivity after use of zirconium-containing poison oak lotions. *JAMA* 1964;190:162.

120. Baler GR. Granulomas from topical zirconium in poison ivy dermatitis. *Arch Dermatol* 1965;91:145.

121. Shelley WB, Hurley HJ. Allergic origin of zirconium deodorant granuloma. *Br J Dermatol* 1958;70:75.

122. LoPresti PJ, Hambrick GW. Zirconium granuloma following treatment of rhus dermatitis. *Arch Dermatol* 1965;92:188.

123. Kaaber K, Nielsen AO, Veien NK. Vaccination granulomas and aluminum allergy: course and pronostic factors. *Contact Dermatitis* 1992;26:304.

124. McCallum DI, Hall GFM. Umbilical granulomata—with particular reference to talc granuloma. *Br J Dermatol* 1970;83:151.

125. Tye MJ, Hashimoto K, Fox F. Talc granulomas of the skin. *JAMA* 1966;198:120.

126. Bergeron JR, Stone OJ. Multiple granulomas of the scalp of exogenous origin. *Cutis* 1969;5:57.

127. Sneddon I B. Dust and the skin. *Med Presse* 1958;21:1102.

128. Rycroft RJG, Calnan CD. Irritant dermatitis during the relining of a blast furnace. *Contact Dermatitis* 1977;3:75.

129. Skevi M, Mizuno F. Unusual cornification in ichthyosis-like dermatitis. *Arch Dermatol* 1970;50:388.

130. Fisher AA. Occupational palmar psoriasis due to safety prescription container caps. *Contact Dermatitis* 1979;5:56.

131. Nielsen NH, Menne T. Allergic contact dermatitis caused by zinc pyrithione associated with pustular psoriasis. *Am J Contact Dermat* 1997;8:170.

132. Adams BM. *Occupational contact dermatitis.* Philadelphia: JB Lippincott Co., 1969.

133. Lynde CW, Mitchell JC. Unusual complication of allergic contact dermatitis of the hands—recurrent lymphangitis and persistent lymphoedema. *Contact Dermatitis* 1982;8:279.

134. Worm A-M, Staberg B, Thomsen K. Persistent oedema in allergic contact dermatitis. *Contact Dermatitis* 1983;9:516.

135. Worm A-M. Exchange of macromolecules between plasma and skin interstitium in extensive skin disease. *J Invest Dermatol* 1981; 76:489.

136. Piller NB, Casley-Smith JR. The effect of coumarin on protein and PVP clearance from rat legs with various high protein oedemas. *Br J Exp Pathol* 1975;56:439.

137. Kiec-Swierczynska M, Krecisz B. Occupational contact allergy to nifuroxazide simulating prurigo nodularis. *Contact Dermatitis* 1998; 39:93.

138. Penagos H, et al. Chorothalonil, a possible cause of erythema dyschromicum perstans (ashy dermatitis). *Contact Dermatitis* 1996; 35:214.

139. Lenane P, McKenna D, Murphy GM. Pyoderma gangrenosum secondary to allergic contact dermatitis from rubber. *Contact Dermatitis* 1998;38:238.

140. Staines KS, Felix DH, Forsyth A. Desquamative gingivitis, sole manifestation of tosylamide/formaldehyde resin allergy. *Contact Dermatitis* 1998;39:90.

141. Komatsu H, et al. Lymphocytoma cutis involving the lower lip. *Contact Dermatitis* 1997;36:167.

142. Zemtsov A, Cameron GS, Montalvo-Lugo V. Nickel-induced lymphocytoma cutis of the earlobe. *Contact Dermatitis* 1997;36:266.

143. Corazza M, Lombardi AR, Virgili A. Non-eczematous urticarioid allergic contact dermatitis due to Eumulgin L in a deodorant. *Contact Dermatitis* 1997;36:159.

144. Skinner SL, Fowler JF Jr. Contact anaphylaxis: a review. *Am J Contact Dermat* 1995;6:133.

CHAPTER 8

Systemic Contact-Type Dermatitis

Allergic eczematous contact dermatitis is produced ordinarily by external exposure of the skin to an allergen. Occasionally, however, in sensitized individuals a systematically administered allergen may reach the skin through the circulatory system and produce a hematogenous contact-type dermatitis. Although the eczematous condition is produced by systemic administration, the first sensitizing exposure to the allergen may have been by topical application. In such instances, an eczematous contact type of eruption may be produced not only by the sensitizing allergen but also by allergens that are related immunochemically (1).

Ingestion of an allergen by a person sensitized previously by contact may result in a variety of reactions. Most frequent reactions are focal flares at sites of previous dermatitis or occasionally dyshidrotic eruptions, but generalized eruptions may occur. Sometimes such flares may occur also from *inhalation* of the allergen.

This type of endogenic contact eczema from ingestion or systemic administration of an allergen may be accompanied occasionally by systemic effects.

> **Systemic or endogenic allergic contact dermatitis may be accompanied by systemic effects.**

In relation to positive oral provocation with nickel and medicaments, general symptoms, such as headaches, fever, and malaise, may occur. In neomycin- and chromate-sensitive patients, oral provocation with hapten may produce nausea, vomiting, and diarrhea (2).

TYPES OF SYSTEMIC CONTACT DERMATITIS

> **Morphologic patterns that are seen with systemically administered allergens include vesicular hand eczema, flexural dermatitis, the baboon syndrome, vasculitis-like lesions, and morbilliform erythema. Associated symptoms may include headache, malaise, arthralgia, diarrhea, and vomiting (3).**

Pompholyx, Dyshidrotic Hand Eczema

This consists of recurring itching eruptions with deeply seated vesicles with some or no erythema, localized on the palms, volar aspects, and sides of the fingers. Exacerbations come at weekly to monthly intervals without obvious, external reasons. Patch testing may not be the best predictive test to identify all the patients who have dyshidrosiform hand dermatitis related to ingested materials. Veien (4) studied 202 patients with vesicular hand eczema and negative patch tests and found 58 to be reactive to oral provocation tests to substances, such as nickel (2.5 mg), cobalt (1 mg), and chromate (2.5 mg). However, oral provocation tests were more frequently positive when patch tests were also positive.

Flare-ups of Earlier Patch Test Reactions

This phenomenon has been observed experimentally in provocation studies with nickel and chromium in patients sensitized to these metals, medicaments, and poison ivy. The specificity with which skin reacts to topical and systemic exposure can be seen in the case of a patient with a fixed drug eruption to ibuprofen reported by Kuligowski et al. (5). Systemic exposure to ibuprofen produced several lesions of a fixed drug eruption pattern. A 1% petrolatum patch test to one prior lesion flared all the other prior lesions, but a 10% patch test on normal skin produced no reaction (4).

Generalized Maculopapular-Vesicular Rash

This rash consists of a symmetric eruption localized to the elbow flexures, axillae, eyelids, side of the neck, and genital area. This pattern seems characteristic of the systemic, contact dermatitis reaction.

Erythema Multiforme and Vasculitis

Dissemination of allergic contact dermatitis in the form of erythema multiforme, such as purpura and vasculitis, has been observed in patients sensitive to topically applied drugs (6). An example of the value of patch testing in suspected vasculitis can be found in the report of the benzodiazepine tetrazepam that caused a leukocytoclastic vasculitis of the legs and was patch test positive to a 1% petrolatum concentration (7).

Unusual routes of exposure occasionally have been associated with induction of erythema multiforme patterns, and Hayakawa et al. (8) reported a patient who had been sensitized to amlexanox (2-amino-7-isopropyl-5-oxo-5H-[1] benzopyrano [2,3-b]-3-carboxylic acid) in an ophthalmic solution. Oral ingestion of 50 mg of amlexanox subsequently for otitis media produced an erythema multiformae–like eruption. Occupational exposure to ethyl ethyoxymethylene cyanoacetate (EEMC), which is an intermediate in the synthesis of allopurinol, caused contact dermatitis (9). Subsequent exposure to vapors of EEMC produced an erythema multiformae–like eruption in the sites of former dermatitis, and a 0.01% petrolatum patch test of EEMC was eczematous (9). Contact allergens associated with erythema multiformae have been summarized by O'Donnell and Tan (Table 8.1) (10).

Circular excoriations on the back, buttocks, and thighs have been observed in nickel-sensitive women (11). Similar excoriations have been noticed in two nickel-sensitive patients treated with a nickel-chelating drug. Histopathology shows superficial allergic vasculitis.

> **Practically all patients who have systemic contact dermatitis have positive patch test reactions to a contact allergen. It is claimed that even patients who have negative patch tests to chromate and nickel will have a flare of dyshidrotic eczema when the metals are ingested.**

Urticaria and Anaphylaxis

Eczematous systemic contact dermatitis may be accompanied occasionally by urticaria. Rapid absorption through either intact skin or open wounds may rarely lead to anaphylaxis. Such was the case when rifamycin SV was applied on gauze to a leg ulcer. Contact urticaria outlined the shape of the gauze, and anaphylaxis and shock followed in 40 minutes (12). The patient recovered, and a 0.05% aqueous open test was positive at 20 minutes, as was a Prausnitz-Küstner test, suggesting the reaction was IgE mediated. A patch test has rarely been reported to cause anaphylaxis. The nonselective beta adrenergic blocking agent labetalol tested at 0.1% aqueous solution caused anaphylaxis within 90 to 150 seconds without contact urticaria (13).

> **Systemic contact dermatitis may take the following patterns: eczematous, dyshidrosis, flare of patch test reactions, symmetrical maculopapular and urticarial reactions, and rarely erythema multiforme or vasculitis.**

TABLE 8.1. *Contact Allergens Producing Erythema Multiforme*

Tropical woods
Plants
  Poison ivy
  Primula
  Terpenes
  Saint John's wort *(Hypericum erectum)*
Pyrethrum
Inula helenium
Thuja essential oil
Capsicum
Laboratory chemicals
  Brominated compounds
  N-hydroxyphthalamide
  Phenyl sulfone derivatives
  Dinitrochlorobenzene
  Diphenylcyclopropenone
Medications
  Ethylenediamine
  Iodochlorhydroxyquin (Vioform)
  Mephenesin (Europe)
  Promethazine
  Scopolamine
  Sulfonamides
  Povidone-iodine solution
  Vitamin E
  Mofebutazone
  Budesonide
  Triamcinolone acetonide
  Bufexamac
  Chloramphenicol
  Econazole
  Idoxuridine
  Ketoprofen
  Lincomycin
  Mafenide acetate
  Mephenesin
  Neomycin
  Proflavin
  Pyrrolnitrin
  Phenylbutazone
Miscellaneous compounds
  Epoxy resin
  Formaldehyde
  Soap
  Spray cologne
  Trichloroethylene
  Oxybenzone
  Disperse blue 124
  Hair dyes
  Paratertiary butylphenol formaldehyde resin

PATCH TESTING IN SYSTEMIC CONTACT DERMATITIS

Patch testing with the chemicals mentioned in this chapter may be valuable not only in determining the cause of an allergic contact dermatitis, but also in serving as a warning that the systemic administration of a related drug may produce an eczematous contact-type dermatitis medicamentosa. In addition, the epidermal contact type of sensitivity may be accompanied by the urticarial, anaphylactoid variety, particularly when penicillin is the cause. A positive patch test reaction to penicillin usually precludes its systemic use. Occasionally, the reactions to patch tests with penicillin and other drugs are positive when the scratch and intracutaneous test reactions are negative.

It is much safer to perform a patch test with a drug suspected of producing an eczematous dermatitis medicamentosa than to readminister even a tiny fractional dose of the drug to prove that it is the culprit. Such proof may result in a widespread, disabling eruption.

In evaluating the significance of a positive patch test reaction to a medication, one must have knowledge of immunochemically related agents. Such considerations may explain an allergic (contact-type), eczematous eruption after an exposure to one or more compounds to which an individual has never previously been exposed. The cross-reaction phenomenon may also explain the persistence of allergic reactions in some patients long after the original agent has been avoided.

Ingestion or systemic administration of an allergen that gives a positive patch test reaction can cause both dermatitis and systemic effects.

When several drugs have been administered concurrently or in combination and the patient has experienced an eczematous flare-up, patch tests may be of value in discovering the culprit. For example, if the patient develops an eruption following the administration of a penicillin-streptomycin combination, the drug that causes a positive patch test reaction would be implicated. Such patch tests are safer than scratch or intracutaneous tests.

MECHANISM OF SYSTEMIC CONTACT DERMATITIS

The clinical observation of rapid onset (within hours) of the effect of oral exposure to haptens in sensitized individuals suggests that mechanisms other than an allergic type 4 reaction are involved. It is not unusual for the nickel-sensitive patient who is provoked with nickel to develop a systemic eruption within hours, and after 12 to 48 hours to exhibit a flare in hand dermatitis. There is evidence that the systemic reaction to ingested haptens can be mediated by both a type 3 and a type 4 immunologic reaction. The immunologic reactivity, judged from a rise in the lymphocytic transformation test, can be maintained by oral ingestion of a hapten (14).

Systemic contact dermatitis may be mediated by both a type 3 and a type 4 mechanism.

MEDICAMENTS

Systemic contact dermatitis resulting from medicaments has been reviewed by Fisher (15) and Cronin (16). Usually, sensitization has taken place by topical application of the drug; later on, the patient has a systemic reaction when the drug or immunochemically related allergen is taken orally or parenterally. The opposite situation can occur in which a patient first has an exanthema owing to an antibiotic and later develops a localized dermatitis when the drug is applied topically. Pirila (17) termed this phenomenon "primary endogenic contact eczema."

At the European Contact Dermatitis Society Meeting in Brussels in 1992, Bruynzeel and Camarasa (18) reported that their highest yield in patch testing drug eruptions actually came from testing morbilliform and even urticarial patterns rather than eczematous dermatitis cases. They recommend testing 6 to 12 weeks after the eruption clears, preferably with a pure drug in powder form with a concentration of 1% to 5% in a vehicle known to solubilize the drug. This later information is available in pharmaceutical texts. Tablets or capsules can be used when pure drugs are not available. They also found the best concentration for penicillin, amoxicillin, aminoglycocides, and cephalosporins to be 20%. A safe way to proceed is to perform a 20-minute open test, then a 48-hour closed test (18).

ANTIBIOTICS

Topical use of penicillin and streptomycin should be avoided because of the high sensitization potential (19). Although neomycin has been reported to produce many instances of allergic contact dermatitis, it is still used widely. The other antibiotics, such as the tetracyclines, erythromycin, and chloramphenicol, rarely produce allergic contact dermatitis.

Penicillin

Topical use of penicillin is largely avoided at present because many individuals would develop contact sensitivity to the drug. Allergic contact dermatitis from penicillin occurs particularly in physicians, nurses, and pharmacists who handle this antibiotic. Systemic administration of penicillin to such "externally" sensitized individuals may produce an eczematous, contact-type dermatitis, which may be accompanied by urticarial, anaphylactic sensitivity. Penicillin in milk was the cause of attacks of eczema in two patients, both of whom were sensitive to penicillin on patch testing (20).

Among the antibiotics, penicillin, neomycin, and streptomycin have the highest potential as topical sensitizers. The other antibiotics rarely cause allergic contact dermatitis or eczematous contact-type dermatitis medicamentosa.

Streptomycin

Although topical application of streptomycin is now avoided, members of the medical, nursing, and pharmaceutical professions who handle the drug readily become sensitized, and subsequent systemic administration may produce a severe eczematous contact-type dermatitis medicamentosa. Because streptomycin may cross-react with neomycin, systemic administration of streptomycin may produce the eczematous contact-type dermatitis in individuals who had become sensitized to neomycin but had never been exposed to streptomycin. Streptomycin may also cross-react with kanamycin sulfate (Kantrex).

Streptomycin may be administered alone or in combination with penicillin in preparations such as Strep-Combiotic (Pfizer), Bivillimycin (Wyeth), and Wycillin (Wyeth). Desensitization procedures by subcutaneous injection of streptomycin may be accompanied by urticaria or flares of dermatitis.

> **Topical sensitization to streptomycin is a hazard to members of the medical, nursing, and pharmaceutical professions.**

Neomycin Sulfate

Not only is this antibiotic present in a host of ointments, creams, and other topical medications, but it also has been added to cosmetics, soaps, and deodorants (21). It has a significant capacity to produce allergic contact sensitivity (22). Once sensitization to neomycin from topical exposure has been established, systemic administration of either streptomycin or kanamycin, both of which may cross-react with neomycin, may cause an eczematous contact-type dermatitis medicamentosa (23).

In addition, although neomycin and bacitracin are not related chemically, in many instances there is a combined sensitivity to these two drugs. Such occurrences represent coincidental simultaneous sensitization rather than true cross-sensitivity (24).

Pirilä and Rantanen (25) gave an account of repeated eruptions in a patient sensitive to neomycin and bacitracin because of their topical use on an amputation stump. Later, the patient developed a severe stomatitis from throat tablets containing bacitracin and from a paste containing both antibiotics used to fill an infected root canal. Oral administration of neomycin produced diarrhea and dermatitis. Ekelund and Moller (26) also produced dermatitis by the oral administration of neomycin in sensitized patients. Previous patch test sites flared.

Neomycin may be administered systemically in Bacimycin, Cremomycin, Kaomycin, Mycifradin, Paremycin, Prednicidin, Sorboquel with Neomycin, and Sulfacidin.

Neomycin shows strong cross-sensitization with paromomycin and ambutyrosin (CL-642) because of the presence of neosamine sugars in all three (W. Schorr, personal communication).

> **Systemic contact dermatitis in neomycin-sensitive patients may occur from administration of streptomycin and kanamycin, with which neomycin cross-reacts.**

Tetracyclines

These antibiotics are safe to apply topically, because allergic contact dermatitis occurs rarely from such usage. Eczematous eruptions of the fixed type do result occasionally from systemic administration (27). Furthermore, cross-fixed drug eruptions from systemic use of chlortetracycline (Aureomycin), tetracycline (Achromycin), and oxytetracycline (Terramycin) have been described (28).

In rare instances in which allergic contact dermatitis does occur from use of Aureomycin or Achromycin ointment, the sensitizer may be the parabens added as preservatives or the certified azo dyes.

Erythromycin (Ilotycin, Ilosone, Erythrocin, and Pediamycin)

Topical sensitization to this antibiotic is rare. Ilotycin ointment does not contain parabens or coloring matter.

Chloramphenicol

The report by Schwank and Jirasek (29) that there was cross-sensitization between 2,4-dinitrochlorbenzene and chloramphenicol was not confirmed by Palacios et al. (30). Dr. J. E. Rasmussen (personal communication) has also failed to find such cross-sensitization.

Bacitracin

Roupe and Strannegard (31) stated that a case of anaphylactic shock followed topical administration of an ointment containing bacitracin and neomycin. Antibacitracin reagins were demonstrated in sera from the patient who had atopic dermatitis. There is strong evidence that the anaphylactic shock was due to hypersensitivity to bacitracin.

Cephalosporins

A morbilliform eruption was traced to cefuroxime by patch testing with 0.1 mL of a 100 mg/mL solution in normal saline. The same concentrations of cephalothin and cephaloridine were also positive (32). There was no sign of immediate hypersensitivity to cephalosporins or either major or minor penicillin determinants. Bruynzeel and Camarisa (18) report that in their experience cross-reactions among cephalosporins are infrequent.

SULFONAMIDES

Cross-reactions can occur between the antibacterial sulfonamides and chemically related sulfonamides used as diuretics, oral hypoglycemics, and sweetening agents. Topical application of a sulfonamide may sensitize the patient, and subsequent systemic administration of a sulfonamide may produce eczematous contact-type dermatitis medicamentosa (33).

Sulfanilamide

The systemic administration of this older sulfonamide preparation has largely been discarded. Exposure to sulfanilamide, however, may still take place from topical application of the medications shown in Table 8.2.

Compounds containing sulfanilamide may be sensitizers and photoallergic agents and may cross-react with chemicals with a para-amino group and with diuretics such as hydrochlorothiazide (hydro-diuril) and thiazide antihypertensive drugs, which may be photosensitizers (34).

The Role of Sulfonamide Drugs in Diabetics

Many adult diabetics receive oral "para-amino" hypoglycemic sulfonyl-urea drugs, such as tolbutamide (Orinase) and chlorpropamide (Diabinese). These diabetic patients may become sensitized to widely used topical para-amino compounds, such as hair dyes, particularly paraphenylenediamine, sunscreens containing para-aminobenzoic acid (PABA) or its esters, and local anesthetics, such as benzocaine. In addition, sensitization to the less widely used topical para-amino sulfanilamide compounds poses the threat of a systemic contact dermatitis to the ingestion of the closely related antidiabetic drugs and sulfonamide-sweetening agents (Tables 8.3 and 8.4).

Thus, a patient sensitized to a topical sulfanilamide cream may acquire a systemic contact dermatitis from tolbutamide (Orinase) or other oral sulfonamide hypoglycemic drugs or by sulfonamide-sweetening agents. It should be noted that all of the oral hypoglycemic compounds and sweetening agents are para-amino sulfonamide compounds (Tables 8.3 and 8.4).

It has long been known that topical agents containing an amino group in the para position of the benzene ring are

TABLE 8.2. *Sulfanilamide Topical Agents Still in Use*

AVC Cream (Merrell-National)
AVC Suppositories (Merrell-National)
Cervex Vaginal Cream (Medics)

TABLE 8.3. *Sulfonamide Oral Hypoglycemic Agents*

Carbutamide (Nadisan)*
Diabinese (chlorpropamide)
Orinase (tolbutamide)

*Still used in Europe.

sensitizers. Such agents include paraphenylenediamine, PABA and its esters, certain local anesthetics (e.g., benzocaine), and sulfanilamide.

These para-amino compounds may cross-react with one another and with azo and aniline dyes. Allergic contact dermatitis may occur readily from exposure to paraphenylenediamine in hair and fur dyes. Of the topical anesthetics in this group, benzocaine is the most notorious sensitizer. The salts of para-aminobenzoic acid used in sunscreens occasionally sensitize, but the acid is not as potent a sensitizer as its esters. Although sulfanilamide is used sparingly as a topical medication at present, exposure to the topical agents shown in Table 8.2 may still take place.

Once a diabetic patient is sensitized to a topical sulfanilamide medication or other para-amino compound, the systemic administration of sulfanilamide-containing compounds, such as tolbutamide (Orinase) and chlorpropamide (Diabinese), may produce a systemic contact dermatitis. Tolbutamide [Orinase; 1-butyl-3-(p-tolysulfonyl) urea] and chlorpropamide [Diabinese; 1-(p-chlorophenylsulfonyl)-3-propylurea], are widely used hypoglycemic drugs that are photosensitizers (35–37). The fact that they can produce a systemic contact dermatitis in patients sensitized to topical para-amino compounds is not so well known (38).

Angelini and Meneghini (39) reported that a group of 34 patients who had contact allergy to para-amino compounds (sulfanilamide, paraphenylenediamine, and benzocaine) underwent a series of peroral tests using the structurally related substances sulfonyl ureas (carbutamide, tolbutamide, and chlorpropamide), diaminodiphenylsulfone, saccharin, and salicylazosulfapyridine. They found that these sulfonyl urea drugs given orally produced a widespread dermatitis in 11 subjects who had contact sensitivity to sulfanilamide, but not in those sensitized to paraphenylenediamine and benzocaine.

The positive results in 11 of 34 inpatients who reacted were as follows: (a) itching in all 11 patients, (b) the reappearance of erythema and vesicles at the site of the primary contact dermatitis in six patients, and (c) the relapse of the primary contact dermatitis with a moderate secondary vesicular eruption together with a reactivation of the

TABLE 8.4. *Sulfonamide Sweetening Agents*

Calcium cyclamate
Saccharin
Sodium cyclamate
Sucaryl
Sweeta

patch test reaction in five patients. The provocative oral tests were considered positive when at least one of the following was produced: pruritus with recurrence of the primary dermatitis, spread of eczematous lesions, or reactivation of the patch test reactions.

In Italy, where topical sulfanilamide is apparently still used on leg ulcers and wounds, it was found that patients who were sensitized to such topical application had a positive response to the oral provocative tests with the hypoglycemic drugs, whereas those who were sensitized to other substances of the para-amino group, such as paraphenylenediamine and benzocaine, did not react.

Angelini and Meneghini (39) state that none of the patients who were sensitized to sulfanilamide, paraphenylenediamine, or benzocaine reacted to the ingestion of saccharin. Although the sweetening agents shown in Table 8.4 are all sulfanilamide compounds, there are as yet no reports of "systemic" contact dermatitis in individuals using these agents who have been sensitized to topically applied para-amino compounds.

Diabetic patients sensitized by topical medication combining such para-amino compounds as sulfanilamide and benzocaine can acquire a widespread eczematous "systemic" contact dermatitis from the oral administration of such para-amino sulfonamide hypoglycemic drugs as tolbutamide (Orinase) and chlorpropamide (Diabinese).

Nystatin

Oral nystatin is generally regarded as an oral agent that is not absorbed. However, fixed drug eruption and generalized systemic contact dermatitis have occurred with oral ingestion, and as little as 125,000 IU can cause generalized dermatitis (40). A patch test with 30,000 IU in polyethylene glycol was positive in a patient after oral ingestion of nystatin, and no cross-reaction was found to amphotericin B.

PHENOTHIAZINES

All phenothiazines are potential photosensitizers. Medical and nursing personnel who inject these drugs and those handling the compounds in the pharmaceutical industry readily acquire allergic eczematous contact dermatitis from such exposure. Often a photoallergic reaction occurs in combination with the contact dermatitis (41). Systemic administration of the phenothiazine drugs may produce an eczematous contact-type dermatitis medicamentosa in individuals sensitized by topical application. Cross-reactions take place readily between phenothiazines and related antihistamines such as promethazine (Phenergan), isothipendyl (theruhistin), and pyrathiazine (Pyrrolazotte). Methylene blue, a phenothiazine dye, is also a powerful photosensi-

tizer. Nurses sensitized to chlorpromazine have been desensitized by taking the drug orally. Positive patch test reactions have been reported to become negative after such procedures (42).

Because chlorpromazine in particular is excreted almost unchanged in the urine, sensitized hospital personnel who handle urine-contaminated bed linen unprotected may acquire allergic contact dermatitis.

Cross-Reactions between the Phenothiazine Antihistamines and Other Phenothiazine Compounds

The phenothiazine drugs listed in Table 8.5 are all capable of cross-reacting with the phenothiazine antihistamines, and all of these compounds are potential sensitizers. Often a photoallergic reaction occurs in combination with allergic eczematous contact dermatitis. The systemic administration of the phenothiazine drugs shown in Table 8.5 may produce an eczematous contact-type dermatitis medicamentosa in individuals sensitized by such topical exposure. Cross-reactions take place readily between these phenothiazines and the related antihistamines.

The phenothiazine group of drugs can produce allergic contact dermatitis, photoallergic reactions, and eczematous contact-type dermatitis and may cross-react with certain antihistamines and phenothiazines, such as chlorpromazine (Thorazine) and prochlorperazine (Compazine).

BENZODIAZEPINES

A generalized dermatitis occurred in two patients as a result of ingestion of tetrazepam given as a muscle relaxant. A 1% aqueous patch test to pure powder proved positive in both patients and negative in 30 controls (43). Similarly, clobazepam was suspected of causing a generalized drug eruption. A crushed tablet in petrolatum caused a positive patch test and 36 hours later a generalized eruption (44).

TABLE 8.5. *Phenothiazine Antihistamines*

Generic name	Trade name
Methdilazine hydrochloride	Tacaryl
Promethazine hydrochloride	Phenergan
Trimeprazine tartrate	Temaril
Drugs That Cross-React with Phenothiazine Antihistamines	
Generic name	Trade name
Chlorpromazine	Thorazine
Prochlorperazine	Compazine
Trifluoperazine hydrochloride	Stelazine
Trifluopromazine	Vesprin
Trimeprazine tartrate	Temaril

SALICYLATES AND ASPIRIN

Acetylsalicylic acid is a rare contact sensitizer. One patient sensitized to methyl salicylate developed a systemic contact dermatitis when treated with aspirin. A patch test with aspirin was negative but was positive with sodium salicylate. Hindson (45) suggests that the common intermediate metabolite was the cause of the systemic reaction.

Piroxicam

The nonsteroidal anti-inflammatory drug piroxicam causes photosensitivity. Animals sensitized to thimerosal develop both contact and photocontact dermatitis on exposure to piroxicam alone or piroxicam plus ultraviolet A (UVA) light, respectively (46). Because piroxicam photosensitivity begins rapidly after ingestion, it was initially thought to be a phototoxic drug. Later it was learned that the rapid onset of photodermatitis could be explained by a cross-reaction to thimerosal (47). Studies found that no new photo product was produced when piroxicam was exposed to light, but when L-cysteine was added to piroxicam and UVA light, a product capable of causing a positive patch test in those patients clinically photosensitive to piroxicam was produced (47). The thiosalicyclate portion of thimerosal, as well as thimerosal itself, produces positive reactions in patients with clinical piroxicam photodermatitis, and it is felt that these are photoallergic reactions (48).

Corticosteroid

Although covered elsewhere in this book, it is helpful to remember that erythroderma has been produced by as little as 1 mg of several corticoids: hydrocortisone sodium phosphate, hydrocortisone butyrate, and budesonide (49). In this case, adrenocorticotrophic hormone (ACTH) did not reproduce the systemic reaction.

HALOGENATED HYDROXYQUINOLINES

These therapeutic agents include iodochlorhydroxyquin (Vioform), iodoquinol (Diodoquin), chlorquinaldol (Sterosan), and halquinol (Quinolor). Such preparations are commonly used topical agents. In addition, Vioform and Diodoquin may be administered systemically. Cross-sensitization between these compounds may exist. Vioform and Diodoquin administered orally may lead to an eczematous dermatitis medicamentosa in patients sensitized by topical application of any one of this group of compounds (50).

Vioform, Diodoquin, Sterosan, and Quinolor may cross-react. Oral Vioform and Diodoquin can produce eczematous contact-type dermatitis medicamentosa in persons topically sensitized to these halogenated quinolines.

Quinolor Compound

This ointment consists of chlorhydroxyquinoline, benzoyl peroxide, menthol, methyl salicylate, and eugenol in Plastibase vehicle. When dermatitis occurs from its use, the chlorhydroxyquinoline is not necessarily the culprit, because the benzoyl peroxide, eugenol, and Plastibase, which is a polyethylene compound related to Carbowax, can all cause allergic reactions.

RESORCINOL (RESORCIN)

Individuals sensitized to resorcin are usually also sensitized to resorcinol monoacetate (Euresol), which is present in Ar-Ex RMS Lotion and Scalp Lotion, Resulin-F, and Sulforcin Lotion.

Hexylresorcinol, which may cross-react with resorcinol (51) (resorcin), is present in ST37, Sucrets, Tetrazets, Caprokol, and Crystoids Anthelmintic. The ingestion of Crystoids or Caprokol could produce a contact-type dermatitis in patients sensitized to topical application of resorcin or hexylresorcinol. Some troches, including Iso-Thirium, Listerine, and Nymore, also contain hexylresorcinol.

CHLORAL HYDRATE

Sensitization to chloral hydrate in topical medications may occur from exposure to hair tonics and other scalp medications. Rectules and Calmitol Ointment contain chloral hydrate. Chlorbutanol (chlorbutol), a local anesthetic and preservative for parenteral solutions, is a chloral derivative. Chloral hydrate is also used in the manufacture of DDT, which is 1,1,1-trichloro-2–2-bis(p-chlorophenyl)ethane.

Chloral hydrate may be administered as a sedative in Aquachloral Supprettes, Beta-Chlor, EnChlor, Fello-Sed, Felsules, Loryl, Noctagetic, Noctec, and Somnos.

The ingestion of chloral hydrate by patients sensitized to it by topical exposure may result in an eczematous contact-type dermatitis medicamentosa (52,53). Placidyl (ethchlorvynol), a condensation product of chloral hydrate, may produce a fixed drug eruption, with a flare-up upon patch testing with the drug (54).

CARDIOVASCULAR AGENTS

Nitroglycerin

Nitroglycerin is another example of a medicament that when employed systemically (sublingually) did not produce any allergic reaction. Its recent use topically, however, has resulted in allergic contact dermatitis in several patients sensitized to topical nitroglycerin. Sublingual or oral use of nitroglycerin may produce an allergic systemic contact dermatitis (55,56).

> **Systemic nitroglycerin is not a sensitizer. Topical nitroglycerin, however, may sensitize. Such topically sensitized individuals may react with a systemic contact dermatitis by oral or sublingual nitroglycerin.**

Mexiletine Hydrochloride

The antiarrhythmia agent mexiletine hydrochloride produced a drug eruption that was confirmed by patch tests at 6.25%, 12.5%, and 25% in petrolatum. These tests were positive only on skin that initially developed dermatitis and were negative or equivocal on noninvolved normal or even noninvolved scarified skin at the same concentrations (57).

Captopril

The ACE inhibitor captopril produced a drug eruption confirmed by a 10% aqueous patch test, whereas patch tests to other ACE inhibitors were negative (58).

Pseudoephedrine

Two days after a patient took oral vasoconstrictor containing pseudoephedrine, an eczematous dermatitis of the neck, arms, and trunk occurred. Patch tests of skin previously involved in the rash were positive by day 4 to 1% and 3% concentrations of pseudoephedrine with concomitant cross-reactions to ephedrine and phenylephrine (59).

Salbutamol

Salbutamol used in a nebulizer to treat chronic obstructive pulmonary disease caused central facial dermatitis with systemic spread of dermatitis to the arms and legs (60). This compound is an adrenergic agent that selectively stimulates beta-receptors. A 5% concentration in petrolatum was positive in the patient but negative in 30 controls.

THIAMINE HYDROCHLORIDE (VITAMIN B₁, BETABION HYDROCHLORIDE, AND ANEURIN HYDROCHLORIDE)

Hypersensitivity to various vitamins has been reported, with thiamine accounting for the largest number of such cases (61). Allergic contact dermatitis may occur in workers who fill vials during its manufacture (62). The injection or ingestion of this vitamin in such sensitized individuals may produce an eczematous relapse in the form of a contact-type dermatitis (63,64).

Thiamine may cross-react with coenzyme B (diphosphothiamin) and cocarboxylase.

VITAMIN B₅

Dexpanthenol is a component of topical products such as hair care cosmetics, baby lotions, sunscreens, and topical medications. It is an alcoholic derivative of pantothenic acid, which is better known as vitamin B_5. Sensitization topically about the face and scalp margin was traced to use of a baby lotion in a 33-year-old woman (65). She subsequently developed a flare of this dermatitis and a nummular eczema pattern of systemic dermatitis after ingesting a capsule containing Ca-D-pantothenate. A diet low in vitamin B_5 was found helpful, whereas a diet high in vitamin B_5 caused worsening of face and hand eczema within 1 week.

VITAMIN B₁₂ (COBIONE AND BERUBIGEN)

Young et al. (66) reported a case of sensitivity to B_{12} concentrate in which there was a delayed tuberculin-type reaction to the intradermal injection of B_{12}. Subcutaneous and intramuscular injections did not produce a flare-up of the dermatitis.

Fisher (67) observed a patient with cobalt sensitivity who acquired a pruritic eruption at the site of injection of vitamin B_{12} (Berubigen, cyanocobalamin). This area flared when vitamin B_{12} was taken orally. The patient had a strongly positive patch test reaction to cobalt chloride and a delayed positive scratch and intradermal test reaction to vitamin B_{12} (Berubigen). Most surprising of all, the patient had a positive patch test reaction to vitamin B_{12} (Berubigen) alone.

HYDRAZINE HYDROBROMIDE

A large percentage of individuals who are exposed to this compound in solder flux become sensitized (68). It is the parent chemical of isoniazid (INH, Niconyl, Nydrazid, Rimifon, Tyvid), hydralazine (Apresoline), and phenelzine (Nardil), an antidepressant drug. The systemic administration of these drugs in individuals sensitized to hydrazine hydrochloride may produce eczematous contact-type dermatitis medicamentosa.

PRESERVATIVES

Parabens

Fourteen patients who were sensitive to paraben mixture took oral capsules containing 100 mg of methyl-*p*-hydroxybenzoate and 100 mg of propyl-*p*-hydroxybenzoate in a study to determine whether oral parabens can cause systemically induced dermatitis (69). Only two patients reacted, and both exhibited vesicular hand eruptions. One had a flare of a previous paraben patch test. A low paraben diet was of no value to these two individuals, and therefore oral challenge testing of paraben-sensitive patients was not recommended.

Sorbic Acid

Perianal and buttock dermatitis was traced to sorbic acid ingestion in a 50-year-old man in whom the positive patch test seemed irrelevant until his dietary intake of sorbic acid was restricted (70). The presentation was "baboon syndrome" like, and this morphology has repeatedly been linked to systemic reactions. A low sorbic acid diet restricts:

Fruits: chestnuts, plums, prunes, strawberries, currants, cranberries
Candies: almond base, jellied candy, chocolates, ice cream and sherbet made with the above noted fruits
Dairy products: margarine and light butter, cheese spreads, fruit yogurt
Drinks: grape and apple flavored beverages
Other: refrigerated salads with meats or shellfish

Thimerosal

Nummular eczema and dyshidrosiform eczema occurred in two children who were repeatedly exposed to oral and intranasal vaccines preserved with thimerosal (71).

Phenoxyethanol

The DPT (diphtheria-pertussis-tetanus) vaccine was administered to an 18-month-old child on several occasions, and each time the child experienced generalized eczema (72). A patch test to 2-phenoxyethanol 2% in petrolatum was the only reaction seen from testing of the vaccine ingredients (Infanrix). Use of a thimeros preserved vaccine (Merioux) was successful. This preservative is a component of Eurxyl K 400 that also contains methyldibromoglutaronitrile.

FLAVORING AGENTS

Cinnamon Oil

This oil is used for flavoring foods, cakes, toothpaste, chewing gum, tobacco, vermouth, aperitifs, bitters, and beverages of the cola type. Cassia oil is a type of Chinese cinnamon. Occupational dermatitis from oil of cinnamon may occur in bakers, candy makers, cooks, and housewives.

Cinnamon may cross-react with balsam of Peru.

Ingestion of oil of cinnamon may produce an eczematous contact-type flare-up in individuals previously sensitized by contact with the oil (73).

Fisher (67) observed a patient sensitized to cinnamon in a toothpaste whose dermatitis flared after drinking vermouth containing cinnamon.

Other Flavorings

Hjorth (74) reported two children who were sensitive to balsam of Peru and orange peel and whose eczema flared after eating fruits and ices. Hjorth (75) also described a man with a severe hand eczema who was allergic to balsam of Peru and whose eczema flared when he ate some orange marmalade. After he avoided perfumes, cola drinks, vermouth, throat tablets, and cinnamon, his hand eczema cleared. Eating vanilla sugar has also caused a flare of eczema in a patient sensitive to balsam of Peru (17). It is possible that garlic may also have this effect (76). Veien (4) reported that 47% of patients placed on a low-balsam diet reported long-term improvements.

> **Dermatitis due to sensitization to balsam of Peru may flare with ingestion of cinnamon, oranges, and other flavors.**

Balsam of Peru

Oral challenges of patients who were patch test positive to balsam of Peru were carried out in double-blind, placebo-controlled fashion by Niinimaki (77). Spices such as clove, cinnamon, Jamaica pepper, and vanilla, as well as balsam of Peru, were used for challenges. The only adverse reaction observed from the challenges was an increase in the number of palmar vesicles. This occurred with active as well as placebo challenges, although it was more common with the active challenges. Neither the challenges nor the patch tests were predictive of who might benefit from an avoidance diet.

Garlic

Contact dermatitis to garlic has been associated with finger-tip dermatitis but caused a pompholyx pattern of dermatitis when ingested orally as a commercially available garlic extract to treat hyperlipidemia (78). A 5% aqueous patch test to garlic extract was positive. Cooked garlic did not cause a reaction, as this denatures the allergens diallyldisulfide, allylpropyldisulfide, and allicin.

DISULFIRAM (ANTABUSE, TETRAETHYLTHIURAM DISULFIDE)

Antabuse is used as adjunctive treatment in alcoholism to help the patient remain in the state of self-imposed sobriety. When on Antabuse therapy, patients ingesting even small amounts of alcohol experience a highly unpleasant reaction, consisting of flushing, palpitations, dyspnea, hyperventilation, tachycardia, nausea, and vomiting. Antabuse *implants* are being used in the treatment of alcoholism (see Chapter 20).

Antabuse (disulfiram) and thiram (tetramethylthiuram) are used as rubber accelerators and may show cross-reactions. Thiram is used widely as an insecticide and germicide and is present in Rezifilm (Squibb), a surgical wound dressing.

Sensitization by contact with thiram may make the patient susceptible to an eczematous dermatitis medicamentosa if Antabuse is given (76).

A patient sensitized to dipentamethylene thiuram disulfide from a rubber condom developed a violent reaction and a widespread eczema when given Antabuse (tetraethylthiuram disulfide) for the treatment of alcoholism (79). A similar patient was described by Pirila (80). The reaction occurred within 4 hours, and a thiuram patch test reaction that had faded was reactivated.

QUININE AND QUINIDINE

It has long been known that quinine can sensitize the skin, particularly when inflammation is present. Topical sensitization may take place from hair preparations containing quinine. Quinamm (National) contains quinine sulfate, as do many over-the-counter cold and headache remedies. The ingestion of such remedies and even quinine water may produce eczematous contact-type dermatitis in sensitized individuals. Quinidine contact dermatitis has been reported in a patient who worked in the pharmaceutical industry and whose exposure resulted from grinding the drug (81). Quinidine and quinine apparently do not cross-react (82).

HYDROXYZINE

Cross-reactivity between hydroxyzine and ethylenediamine has been reported. Ash and Scheman (83) encountered a patient who was patch test positive to ethylenediamine and on oral challenge with hydroxyzine on three occasions developed pruritus and abdominal rash within 2 days. The ethylenediamine patch test did not flare, and the patient was completely clear after discontinuing hydroxyzine.

5-FLUOROURACIL

Extensive topical use of 5-fluorouracil led to allergic contact dermatitis due to this agent (84). When the patient developed adenocarcinoma, intravenous 5-fluorouracil was administered. Within 1 day the patient developed severe head and neck erythema and edema that ultimately led to discontinuation of intravenous use of 5-fluorouracil.

FLUORIDES

Shea et al. (85) reported seven individuals who had urticaria, exfoliative dermatitis, atopic dermatitis, stomatitis, and gastrointestinal and respiratory allergy apparently due to fluorides in a fluoride-containing toothpaste and vitamin preparations. One individual had a positive patch test reaction to fluoride.

METALS THAT CAUSE SYSTEMIC CONTACT DERMATITIS*

The role of dietary restriction of metal salts such as nickel, cobalt, and chromate, as well as oral balsams, has been investigated in Denmark (4). Of 7,887 patients evaluated for eczema, oral challenge led to a final diagnosis in 122 (1.5%). Of 675 patients on diets restricting metal salts, balsams, and food allergens in general, 262 reported improvement. Seventy percent of those available for a follow-up questionnaire reported long-term benefit from diets of this type (144 of 206). Atopic patients with vesicular hand eczema were more likely to benefit (4).

Exposure of the oral cavity to dental metals can result in recurrent vesicular hand eczema (86). Patch tests did not accurately predict all the patients who would benefit from removal of the dental metal. Rather, oral provocation with 2.5 mg of nickel and 1 mg of cobalt caused the dermatitis to flare. Of the five patients studied, one was chromate sensitive and one nickel sensitive by patch test, but four of the five had a positive oral challenge to either chromate, nickel, or cobalt. Two of the cases had features of atopic dermatitis, as well as hand eczema. Oral symptoms were present in only one case.

In a related study of chromate-sensitive patients, oral challenge proved provocative in 17 of 30 subjects who did not react to placebo. Most had hand and foot eruptions (87). Veien et al. (87) used 2.5 mg of chromate for the oral challenge.

REFERENCES

1. Fisher AA. Allergic dermatitis medicamentosa: the "systemic contact-type variety." *Cutis* 1976;18:637.
2. Menne T, Hjorth N. Reactions from systemic exposure to contact allergens. *Semin Dermatol* 1982;1:15.
3. Menne T, et al. Systemic contact dermatitis. *Am J Dermatitis* 1994; 5:1.
4. Veien NK. Systemically induced eczema in adults. *Acta Derm Venereol* (Stockh) 1989[Suppl];147:1.
5. Kuligowski ME, Chang A, Rath A. Multiple fixed drug eruption due to ibuprofin. *Contact Dermatitis* 1991;25:259.
6. Meneghini CL, Angelini G. Secondary polymorphic eruptions in allergic contact dermatitis. *Dermatologica* 1981;163:63.
7. Collet E, et al. Tetrazepam allergy once more detected by patch test. *Contact Dermatology* 1992;26:281.
8. Hayakawa R, Ogin Y, Aris K, Matsunaga K. Systemic contact dermatitis to amlexanox. *Contact Dermatitis* 1992;27:122.
9. Hsu C-K, et al. Systemic contact allergy from occupational contact with ethyl ethoxymethylene cyanoacetate. *Contact Dermatitis* 1992; 27:58.
10. O'Donnell BF, Tan CY. Erythema multiforme reaction to patch testing. *Contact Dermatitis* 1992;27:230.
11. Hjorth N. Nickel vasculitis. *Contact Dermatitis* 1976;2:356.
12. Mancuso G, Masara N. Contact urticaria and severe anaphylaxis from rifamycin SV. *Contact Dermatitis* 1992;27:124.
13. Bause GS, Kugelman LC. Contact anaphylactoid response to labetalol. *Contact Dermatitis* 1990;23:51.
14. Veien NK, Svejgaard E, Menne T. In vitro lymphocyte transformation to nickel: a study of nickel-sensitive patients before and after epicuta-

*See also Chapter 34.

neous and oral challenge with nickel. *Acta Derm Venereol* (Stockh) 1979;59:447.

15. Fisher AA. Allergic reactions due to metals used in dentistry. *Cutis* 1974;14:797.

16. Cronin E. Contact dermatitis XVII: reactions to contact allergens given orally or systemically. *Br J Dermatol* 1972;86:104.

17. Pirila V. Endogenic contact eczema. *Allerg Asthma* 1970;16:15.

18. Rietschel RL. Selected highlights of the European Contact Dermatitis Society Meeting, Brussels, Belgium, October 8–10, 1992. *Am J Contact Dermatitis* 1993;4:66.

19. Rees BR. Cutaneous reactions to antibiotics. *JAMA* 1964;189:685.

20. Vickers HR, Bagratuni L, Alexander S. Dermatitis caused by penicillin milk. *Lancet* 1978;61:351.

21. Shelley WB, Cahn MM. Effect of topically applied antibiotic agents on axillary odor. *JAMA* 1957;159:1736.

22. Epstein S. Dermal contact dermatitis from neomycin: observations on forty cases. *Ann. Allergy* 1958;16:268.

23. Epstein S, Wenzel FJ. Cross-sensitivity to various "mycins": neomycin, kanamycin, streptomycin, and bacitracin: an experimental study. *Arch Dermatol* 1962;86:183.

24. Epstein S, Wenzel FJ. Sensitivity to neomycin and bacitracin, cross sensitization or coincidence? *Acta Derm Venereol* (Stockh) 1963;43:1.

25. Pirilä V, Rantanen AV. Root canal treatment with bacitracin-neomycin as cause of flare-up of allergic eczema. *Oral Surg Oral Med Oral Pathol* 1960;13:589.

26. Ekelund AG, Moller H. Oral provocation in eczematous contact allergy to neomycin and hydroxy-quinolines. *Acta Derm Venereol* (Stockh) 1969;49:422.

27. Welsh AL. The fixed eruption: a possible hazard of modern drug therapy. *Arch Dermatol* 1961;84:1004.

28. Welsh AL, Ede H. Cross-fixed drug eruption from three antibiotics. *Arch Dermatol* 1955;71:521.

29. Schwank R, Jirasek L. Contact allergy to chloramphenicol with special reference to group sensitization. *Hautarzt* 1963;14:24.

30. Palacios J, Nemuth MG, Blaylock WK. Lack of cross sensitization between 2,4-dinitrochlorbenzene and chloramphenicol. *South. Med. J.* 1968;61:243.

31. Roupe G, Strannegard O. Anaphylactic shock elicited by topical administration of bacitracin. *Arch Dermatol* 1969;100:450.

32. Romano A, et al. Delayed hypersensitivity to cefuroxime. *Contact Dermatitis* 1992;27:270.

33. Sulzberger MB, et al. Sensitization by topical application of sulfonamides. *J Allergy* 1947;18:92.

34. Harber LC, Lashinsky AM, Baer RL. Photosensitivity due to chlorothiazide and hydrochlorothiazide. *N Engl J Med* 1959;261:1378.

35. Seale E. Saccharin-A factor in sunlight sensitivity: current news in dermatology. *The Schoch Letter*, Dallas, Texas, July 1965.

36. Hitselberger JF, Fosnaugh RP. Photosensitivity due to chlorpropamide. *J Am Acad Dermatol* 1962;180:62.

37. Kennedy B, et al. Phototoxic and photoallergic skin reactions resulting from modern drug therapy. *J La State Med Soc* 1961;113:367.

38. Fisher AA. Systemic contact dermatitis from Orinase and Diabinese in diabetics with para-amino hypersensitivity. *Cutis* 1982;29:551, 556, 565 passim.

39. Angelini G, Meneghini CL. Oral tests in contact allergy to para-amino compounds. *Contact Dermatitis* 1981;7:311.

40. Quirce S, et al. Generalized dermatitis due to oral nystatin. *Contact Dermatitis* 1991;25:197.

41. Epstein S. Allergic photocontact dermatitis from promethazine (Phenegran). *Arch Dermatol Syphilol* 1960;81:175.

42. Morris-Owen RM. "Cover-dose" management of contact sensitivity to chlorpromazine. *Br J Dermatol* 1963;75:167.

43. Camarasa JG, Serra-Baldrich E. Tetrazepam allergy detected by patch test. *Contact Dermatitis* 1990;22:246.

44. Machet L, et al. Patch testing with clobazepam: relapse of generalized drug eruption (published erratum appears in *Contact Dermatitis* 1992;27:351). *Contact Dermatitis* 1992;26:347.

45. Hindson C. Contact eczema from methyl salicylate reproduced by oral aspirin (acetyl-salicylic acid). *Contact Dermatitis* 1977;3:348.

46. Kitamura K, et al. Cross-reactivity between sensitivity to thimerosal and photosensitivity to piroxicam in guinea pigs. *Contact Dermatitis* 1991;25:30.

47. Cirne de Castro JL, et al. Sensitivity to thimerosal and photosensitivity to piroxicam. *Contact Dermatitis* 1991;24:187.

48. Ikezawa Z, et al. Photosensitivity to piroxicam is induced by sensitization to thimerosal and thiosalicylate. *J Invest Dermatol* 1992;98:918.

49. Wilkinson SM, Smith AG, English JS. Erythroderma following the intradermal injection of the corticosteroid budesonide. *Contact Dermatitis* 1992;27:121.

50. Leifer W, Steiner K. Studies in sensitization to halogenated hydroxyquinolines and related compounds. *J Invest Dermatol* 1951;17:233.

51. Caron GA, Calnan CD. Studies in contact dermatitis: XIV: resorcin. *Trans St John's Hosp Dermatol Soc* 1962;48:149.

52. Baer RL, Sulzberger MB. Eczematous dermatitis due to chloral hydrate (following both oral administration and topical application). *J Allergy* 1938;9:519.

53. Christianson HB, Perry HO. Reactions to chloral hydrate. *Arch Dermatol* 1956;74:232.

54. Auerbach R. Fixed drug eruption: ethchlorvynol: report of a case. *Arch Dermatol* 1965;92:184.

55. Chandraratna PAN, O'Dell RE. Allergic reactions to nitroglycerin ointment: report of five cases. *Curr Ther Res* 1979;25:481.

56. Sausker WF, Frederick FD. Allergic contact dermatitis secondary to topical nitroglycerin [Letter]. *JAMA* 1978;239:1743.

57. Kikuchi K, Tsunoda T, Tagami H. Generalized drug eruption due to mexiletine hydrochloride: topical provocation on previously involved skin. *Contact Dermatitis* 1991;25:70.

58. Cnudde F, Leynadier F, Dry J. Cutaneous reaction to captopril: value of patch tests. *Contact Dermatitis* 1990;23:375.

59. Tomb RR, et al. Systemic contact dermatitis from pseudoephedrine. *Contact Dermatitis* 1991;24:86.

60. Smeenk G, Burgers JA, Teunissen PC. Contact dermatitis from salbutamol. *Contact Dermatitis* 1994;31:123.

61. Combes FC, Groopman J. Contact dermatitis due to thiamine: report of 2 cases. *Arch Dermatol Syphilol* 1950;61:858.

62. Dalton JE, Peirce JD. Dermatological problems among pharmaceutical workers. *AMA Arch Dermatol Syphilol* 1951;64:667.

63. Neils H. Contact dermatitis from vitamin B_1 (thiamine). *J Invest Dermatol* 1958;30:261.

64. Hjorth N. Contact dermatitis from Vitamin B_1 (thiamine): relapse after ingestion of thiamine: cross-sensitization to cocarboxylase. *J Invest Dermatol* 1958;30:261.

65. Hemmer W, et al. Maintenance of hand eczema by oral pantothenic acid in a patient sensitized to dexpanthenol. *Contact Dermatitis* 1997;37:51.

66. Young WC, Ulrich CW, Fouts PJ. Sensitivity to vitamin B_{12} concentrate. *JAMA* 1950;143:893.

67. Fisher AA. *Contact Dermatitis*. 3rd ed. Philadelphia: Lea & Febiger, 1986.

68. Wheeler CE Jr, Penn SR, Cawley EP. Dermatitis from hydrazine hydrobromide solder flux. *Arch Dermatol* 1965;91:235.

69. Veien NK, Hattel T, Laurberg G. Oral challenge with parabens in paraben-sensitive patients. *Contact Dermatitis* 1996;34:433.

70. Giordano-Labadie F, Pech-Ormieres C, Bazex J. Systemic contact dermatitis from sorbic acid. *Contact Dermatitis* 1996;34:61.

71. Zenarola P, Gimma A, Lomuto M. Systemic contact dermatitis from thimerosal. *Contact Dermatitis* 1995;32:107.

72. Vogt T, Landthaler M, Stolz W. Generalized eczema in an 18-month-old boy due to phenoxyethanol in DPT vaccine. *Contact Dermatitis* 1998;38:50.

73. Leifer W. Contact dermatitis due to cinnamon: recurrence of dermatitis following oral administration of cinnamon oil. AMA *Arch Dermatol Syphilol* 1951;64:52.

74. Hjorth N. *Eczematous allergy to balsams, allied perfumes and flavoring agents.* Copenhagen: Munkgaard, 1961:134.

75. Hjorth N. Allergy to balsams. *Spectrum* 1971;8:97.

76. Burks JW Jr. Classic aspects of onion and garlic dermatitis in housewives. *Ann Allergy* 1954;12:592.

77. Niinimaki A. Double-blind placebo-controlled peroral challenges in patients with delayed-type allergy to balsam of Peru. *Contact Dermatitis* 1995;33:78.

78. Burden AD, Wilkinson SM, Beck MH, Chalmers RJ. Garlic-induced systemic contact dermatitis. *Contact Dermatitis* 1994;30:299.

79. Shelley WB. Golf-course dermatitis due to thiram fungicide. *JAMA* 1961;198:415.

80. Pirila V. Dermatitis due to rubber. *Proc 11th Int Cong Derm* 1957;2:252.

81. Klaschka F. Discussion of high grade quinine contact-allergy. *Derm Wschr* 1964;149:4.

82. Fernstrom AI. Occupational quinidine contact dermatitis: a concept apparently not yet described. *Acta Derm Venereol* (Stockh) 1965;45: 129.

83. Ash S, Scheman AJ. Systemic contact dermatitis to hydroxyzine. *Am J Contact Dermatitis* 1997;8:2.

84. Nadal C, et al. Systemic contact dermatitis from 5-fluorouracil. *Contact Dermatitis* 1996;35:124.

85. Shea JJ, et al. Allergy to fluoride. *Ann Allergy* 1967;25:388.

86. Veien NK, Borchorst E, Hattel T, Laurberg G. Stomatitis or systemically-induced contact dermatitis from metal wire in orthodontic materials. *Contact Dermatitis* 1994;30:210.

87. Veien NK, Hattel T, Laurberg G. Chromate-allergic patients challenged orally with potassium dichromate. *Contact Dermatitis* 1994; 31:137.

CHAPTER 9

Contact Dermatitis in Atopic Persons

"Atopic dermatitis is (at least in some cases) characterized by a susceptibility to start to itch (and persist in itching) when omnipresent, usually harmless, substances in the stratum corneum meet and react with specific circulating antibodies, presumably IgE" (1,2).

Antigen-presenting cells of both the epidermis and dermis express IgE on their surfaces in atopic dermatitis to a significantly ($p = .001$) greater degree than patients with either irritant or allergic contact dermatitis (3). The penetration of antigen through the stratum corneum to the epidermis would be sufficient to elicit a reaction. It is the peculiarity of atopy that ordinarily harmless antigens elicit harmful reactions in certain selected shock tissues. There is some evidence suggesting that substances from the horny layer (including its own constituents, soil, and products of microorganisms that colonize it, e.g., staphylococci) may elicit reactions in persons who have atopic skin.

Extracts of human dander produced wheal reactions in most atopic persons but did so in only a minority of persons with nonatopic skin. Thus, the human dander test can help to diagnose atopy and to divide a population roughly between the atopic reactors and the nonatopic nonreactors. These wheal reactions are based on an immunologic mechanism and can be passively transferred—that is, IgE mediates them.

It is also well known that atopic persons experience reactions to skin tests with house dust, a mixture that must contain a substantial amount of desquamated human horny material. Furthermore, urticarial skin reactions occur after prick tests or intradermal injections of feathers, wool, and substances that may well contain antigenic groups in common with human stratum corneum.

Often the first signs of atopic dermatitis in the infant are itching and rubbing of the scalp and then of the cheeks. A large amount of stratum corneum material is present in young infants, exemplified by conditions such as physiologic desquamation, cradle cap, and increased scaling of the scalp. Moreover, infant skin, as well as the skin of patients who have atopic dermatitis, allows penetration of many substances more easily than does the skin of normal adults. It is an appealing hypothesis that patients who have atopic dermatitis itch when stratum corneum antigens penetrate to

the superficial vessels—the shock tissue—and that scratching and rubbing enhance this penetration.

> In atopic individuals, usually harmless substances in the stratum corneum may react with IgE, which produces itching.

The incidence of allergic contact dermatitis superimposed on atopic dermatitis, however, is still controversial (4–6). Some patients who have atopic conditions, such as allergic asthma and rhinitis, never suffer from atopic dermatitis. Regardless of whether atopic dermatitis is present, however, atopic individuals may acquire a contact dermatitis, which may be either the irritant or the allergic variety, or both. Atopic eczema renders the skin vulnerable to nonspecific irritants, such as heat, humidity, perspiration, dust, strong soaps, detergents, and wool.

The literature is divided on whether atopic individuals have skin that is more easily irritated than normal individuals or not. Gallacher and Maibach (7) reviewed studies supporting both points of view. They point out that most of the epidemiological data that suggest patients with atopic dermatitis are more prone to irritant dermatitis relate to hand eczema, but studies of such cases rarely test the hands. Rather, those studies are done on the forearm, back, or thigh. Variables they identified that in part account for the different positions expressed in the literature include the definition of atopic dermatitis, the definition of normal, sex, race, age, anatomic site, whether the tests were patch tests or open tests, the nature of the irritant studied, and the method of assessment.

In a carefully controlled study of sodium lauryl sulfate irritant reactions, atopic and nonatopic patients were found to react similarly with, if anything, a slightly lesser amount of reaction among the atopic patients (8). At the time of the study, the atopic dermatitis patients had no active eczema at the test site. Assessment was visual, chromometric, laser Doppler flowmetric, and by transepidermal water loss.

> **An international study revealed that individuals who have atopic dermatitis are no more likely to develop allergic contact dermatitis than are patients who have other types of eczema.**

When controlled exposures to a new antigen are compared between atopic subjects and nonatopic subjects, fewer atopic subjects become sensitized. This proved the case with dinitrochlorobenzene (DNCB) (9). The induction phase of contact dermatitis seems more susceptible to disruption by experimental inflammation even when nonatopic individuals are studied with DNCB as the potent allergen (10). The presence of inflammatory mediators in atopic dermatitis may inhibit the acquisition of new contact allergy or delayed hypersensitivity. This down-regulating effect does not provide absolute protection against the acquisition of delayed hypersensitivity, and patch tests are useful in detecting the elicitation phase of the hypersensitivity. The elicitation phase is more difficult to affect experimentally than is the induction phase. Although several studies found patients with atopic dermatitis less likely to sensitize to strong allergens such as DNCB and poison ivy extract, several other studies have shown that contact dermatitis is prevalent in patients with atopic dermatitis and frequently related to medications used to treat the dermatitis (11). In a study of 74 atopic dermatitis patients with persistent facial dermatitis (12), 39.2% were found to have one or more positive patch tests, and 31 of the 40 such patients were female. The female predominance has been found by other authors (12).

PATCH TESTING

When diagnostic patch tests were investigated prospectively in atopic and nonatopic patients, positive tests were seen in 37% of atopic patients versus 57% of nonatopic patients (13).

In a study of 410 patients with chronic eczematous dermatitis, it was found that atopics were just as likely as nonatopics to have allergic contact dermatitis and benefit from patch testing (14). Furthermore, atopic dermatitis patients had significantly more positive tests (2.7 vs 2.0) when compared with nonatopic dermatitis patients. Fifty-four percent of atopic patients had definite relevant positive patch tests. In this study, the more positive patch tests occurred, the more reactions of doubtful meaning were found. The authors refer to these as irritant reactions, but they likely represent the Janus phenomena discussed in Chapter 2.

In a similar study of 122 English atopic dermatitis patients, 60 (49%) were found to have one or more positive patch tests (15). The patch test reactions were deemed relevant in 44% of the cases. These findings underscore the value of patch testing atopic dermatitis cases.

When screening patch tests were used in a study of 137 children with atopic dermatitis (16), the value of patch testing in this group was confirmed. Contact sensitization was found in 43% of all children with atopic dermatitis tested. The most common allergen category was metals (19%), then fragrance (4%) and balsam of Peru (3%), lanolin (4%), and neomycin (3%).

REACTION INDEX

In a study of 15,553 patients patch tested by 18 dermatology departments, the reaction index was calculated from the number of allergic, questionable, and irritant reactions using 13 standard screening allergens (17). A history of atopic dermatitis did not have a consistent influence on the reaction index.

> **Exposure of atopic dermatitis skin to new potential contact allergens is less likely to result in acquisitions of contact dermatitis than would the skin of normal individuals.**

Although atopic dermatitis does not seem to render the patient particularly susceptible to allergic contact dermatitis, a search for the presence of contactants in all instances of persistent atopic dermatitis is important in the management of atopic individuals (4). This is especially necessary when the atopic dermatitis is not responding to therapy or when the eruption suddenly flares. In an effort to allay the itching, many individuals who have atopic dermatitis are exposed to sensitizing topical medications that produce a superimposed allergic contact dermatitis.

The prompt recognition and removal of irritating and sensitizing contactants may prevent the atopic dermatitis from becoming widespread. It is surprising how often the detection and elimination of offending contactants markedly alleviate an otherwise intractable atopic dermatitis.

Allergic contact dermatitis superimposed on atopic eczema usually appears as an insidious aggravation of the eczema rather than as an acute, easily recognized epidermal eczematous contact dermatitis. The reason may be that many patients who have atopic eczema receive topical or systemic corticosteroid therapy, which can modify the appearance of the dermatitis. Patients whose atopic eczema is not responding well to therapy, therefore, should be investigated for the possibility of a superimposed contact dermatitis from topical applications, particularly neomycin.

Aside from being modified by corticosteroid therapy, a superimposed contact dermatitis may not appear typical in atopic individuals because the so-called dermal type of contact dermatitis is especially likely to develop in such patients. Clinically, the lesions are edematous and erythematous rather than papulovesicular and may closely resemble the papular, dry form of atopic dermatitis. The allergens reported as producing "dermal" contact sensitivity include neomycin, formaldehyde, nickel, and ragweed oleoresin (18).

PATCH TESTING IDIOSYNCRASIES IN ATOPIC INDIVIDUALS

As in nonatopic individuals, the proof of allergic contact dermatitis often consists of obtaining a positive patch test reaction with a suspected contactant. There is usually a normal incidence of typical eczematous reactions to patch tests performed on patients who have atopic dermatitis (2). Atopic individuals, however, may have unique patch test reactions, such as pustular reactions and specific and non-specific patch test responses to protein substances.

> **Patch testing with topical medications and their preservatives is indicated in many chronic cases of atopic dermatitis.**

Pustular Patch Test Reactions

There is a high incidence of papulopustular reactions to patch tests with nickel sulfate, the halogens, and sodium arsenate that probably represent some form of irritation. In contrast to true allergic patch test reactions, pustular eruptions rarely itch, do not spread beyond the patch test site, and usually heal within 24 hours after the patch has been removed (19). Although pustular patch test reactions, particularly to nickel sulfate, are more common in atopic individuals, such reactions occur in the nonatopic patient and are not diagnostic evidence of the atopic state.

Nonspecific Patch Test Reactions to Protein Substances

When tested with simple chemicals, the atopic individual may show either an eczematous or a pustular reaction. In addition, atopic individuals who are patch tested with certain protein substances, such as feathers, silk, and foods, may show nonspecific reactions characterized by closely aggregated, discrete, pinpoint vesicles and occasionally pustules (20,21). There is no exudation and no crusting. Erythema and itching are minimal and are localized to the patch test site. The reaction reaches its greatest intensity in 4 to 5 days. This response has been noted in atopic individuals with or without atopic dermatitis. If dermatitis is present, a positive reaction is not associated with a flare-up of the dermatitis, and the spontaneous flare phenomenon is absent.

Atopic individuals may also have a nonspecific reaction to the tuberculin patch test that is similar to that described for feathers, silk, and foods. A specific, positive reaction to a tuberculin patch test consists of a group of tiny vesicles and papules on a reddened, indurated area. False-positive reactions to the tuberculin test may appear as vesicles and pustules with minimal erythema and no induration.

> **Nonspecific pustular patch test reactions to metals and halogens and pseudo-reactions to protein and tuberculin patch tests are common in atopic individuals.**

These nonallergic patch test reactions are probably due to an irritable skin and indicate that the atopic individual may react nonspecifically to many protein substances. Such reactions must be distinguished carefully from true allergic changes, which are characterized by itching and a spread of the reaction beyond the borders of the test site.

Specific Allergic Patch Test Reactions to Protein Substances

Atopic individuals may rarely react in a specific manner to patch tests with molds, feathers, dander, and wool. Allergic patch test reactions to the defatted pollen protein of grasses and ragweed are also occasionally obtained in atopic individuals. The specific allergic reaction to these substances differs from the nonspecific atopic patch test reaction in that the former is characterized by erythema, vesiculation, exudation, and crusting. Furthermore, the reaction may spread beyond the patch test site and may be associated with a flare-up of the existing dermatitis. Such positive reactions would seem to signify that inhalation of or external contact with protein substances may cause a flare-up of atopic dermatitis. Patch testing with protein substances is not a routine procedure, and the clinical significance of the reactions is uncertain even when they seem specific.

RELATIONSHIP OF CONTACT DERMATITIS TO EXPOSURE TO SPECIFIC PROTEIN ALLERGENS IN THE ATOPIC INDIVIDUAL

Contact dermatitis can be prolonged and aggravated by the intranasal, subcutaneous, or surface application of specific protein allergens to which an atopic individual has been shown by scratch tests to be sensitive. For example, poison ivy dermatitis in an atopic individual may be made worse by the prophylactic injection of ragweed pollen extract or intradermal testing with protein antigens. Such injections on occasion render the atopic skin more irritable, and a concentration of a chemical that is usually innocuous may produce contact dermatitis. Furthermore, in atopic individuals who have contact dermatitis, external exposure to proteins in foods, pollens, and molds can produce exacerbations (22,23). These observations indicate that there is a mechanism by which specific antigens can produce a flare-up of an existing, etiologically unrelated contact dermatitis in certain susceptible individuals, regardless of whether the antigen reaches the skin by contact, ingestion, inhalation, or injection.

> **During acute phases of dermatitis, atopic individuals should not receive hay fever, asthma, or other protein-desensitizing injections.**

It would therefore be advisable for atopic individuals who have contact dermatitis to avoid desensitization procedures or other injections with protein substances while the dermatitis is in the acute or subacute phase.

INHALATION AND AIRBORNE CONTACTANTS IN ATOPIC DERMATITIS

Occasionally, inhalation of pollens, dusts, and animal hairs causes either a flare-up of atopic dermatitis or an apparent superimposed contact dermatitis. In some instances, these airborne allergens may produce positive patch test reactions.

Champion (24) reported five patients who had atopic dermatitis in which exacerbations were provoked both by inhalation and by direct contact with algae. These patients also reacted to lichens, which contain algae in symbiosis with fungi. All of the patients had allergic rhinitis or asthma, often very mild in relation to the severity of the skin symptoms. Three of them also had a delayed hypersensitivity contact dermatitis from lichens but not from algae.

It is important to investigate patients who have suspected sensitivities to lichens and algae both by patch testing and by prick testing, because specific desensitization may help those with immediate wheal reactions.

Mold allergens were implicated in the dermatitis experienced by a 25-year-old who had childhood atopic dermatitis (25). Face and neck dermatitis were accompanied by cough, rhinitis, and conjunctivitis when she was in her apartment but improved in other living quarters. Her apartment had mold on the ceiling, and several species of fungi were cultured. Positive patch tests were obtained with *Fusarium, Cladosporium, Pullularia, Rhizopus,* and *Penicillium* aeroallergens. Prick tests were positive to these also. Moving to a new apartment was curative.

Airborne contact dermatitis correlated with harvest season for a 42-year-old rural worker (26). The eruption had been seasonal for 10 years. A mite associated with grain storage facilities was found to be the source of the eruption. A positive RAST and a positive patch test to the mite *Tyrophagus putrescentiae* was found. The mite can be found in pastures, as well as in grain storage areas.

Champion (24) also stated that immediate *contact* wheal reactions may occur in atopic patients handling eggs or being licked by dogs.

The aeroallergens routinely used for prick and scratch tests have been used to complement the diagnostic armamentarium in an effort to narrow the list of potential environmental sources thought to be responsible for generalized atopic dermatitis (27). The clinical benefits described in reports, such as those of Clark (27), demonstrate the utility of selective use of these allergens for patch test purposes, even though standardized procedures for their use are not yet agreed upon.

Dust Mites

Patch tests can be performed with allergen extracts commonly used for prick tests. Sometimes relevant reactions occur with only patch tests, at other times only prick tests, and at times both types of tests are positive.

A 49-year-old atopic dermatitis patient who was known to have IgE antibodies to *Dermatophagoides pteronyssinus* by RAST was patch tested to a variety of allergens, including the dust mite antigen (28). His only reaction was to *D. pteronyssinus,* and he experienced a generalized flare of his dermatitis following this positive patch test. This would either be a coincidence or a specific immunologic event that relates to the cause of his dermatitis. He was advised to keep his home free of dust mites.

The dust mites *D. pteronyssinus* and *D. farinae* have been implicated in causing atopic dermatitis based on various patch test observations. A study was undertaken using equal amounts of purified adult bodies from the two species in a 20% concentration in petrolatum (29). Patch tests were performed on normal skin of the back and read on day 2 and day 3. The same tests were done on 52 control subjects. About half (47.8%) of the atopic patients, and only 15.3% of normal subjects reacted. Of the 22 atopic patients with positive patch test reactions, only 15 were also positive to a prick test with the mites.

Manzini et al. (30) studied 313 atopic dermatitis patients and 100 healthy controls with three different commercially prepared dust mite patch test allergens. Patch test reactions did not correlate with prick test reactions to dust mite antigens. Thirty-eight percent of atopic dermatitis cases reacted to one or more dust mite patch test material, but only 13% of normal individuals reacted. One source of patch test material produced positive reactions in 54% of atopics, another in 51%, and a third source in only 20%.

To further establish a link between dust mites and dermatitis, 23 patients with atopic dermatitis and a positive patch test to *D. pteronyssinus* were studied in vitro by incubating peripheral blood mononuclear cells with the mite antigen (31). This led to the production of cytokines typical of delayed hypersensitivity reactions rather than immediate hypersensitivity reactions. Marked secretion of IL-2 and INF-gamma but not IL-4 was observed.

Similar studies have been conducted in children with atopic dermatitis. When aeroallergens are used as patch test material and compared with the standard use as prick test allergens, there is some agreement and disagreement between the results in atopic patients. In a group of children with well-defined atopic dermatitis, 29% had at least one positive patch test and 54% had at least one positive prick test (32). Patch and prick test results corresponded in 8 of 17 patients. The most commonly positive aeroallergens were *D. pteronyssinus* and *D. farinae* in 27% of patients, then trees in 12%, plantain in 10%, and timothy grass, mugwort, and damp area trees at 5% each. The significance of these findings is uncertain.

SUBSTANCES THAT CAN PRODUCE BOTH ALLERGIC CONTACT DERMATITIS AND ATOPIC MANIFESTATIONS

Theoretically, there is no absolute difference between agents that cause eczematous allergy and those that engender urticarial (atopic-anaphylactoid) allergy. Under actual conditions, however, some agents generally cause eczematous allergy but rarely or never cause urticarial allergy. Many other agents generally cause urticarial allergy but rarely or never cause eczematous allergy. A small group of agents may cause both forms of hypersensitivity at the same time (33).

> **Penicillin, quinine, sulfonamides, mercury, and arsenic can produce delayed contact reactions and immediate anaphylaxis.**

Some allergens alternately produce asthma and contact dermatitis. Among the drugs, penicillin, quinine, sulfonamides, mercurials, and arsenicals produce both allergic contact and atopic reactions in the same individual. These drugs can produce an eczematous contact dermatitis when applied topically and, in addition, can cause asthma, urticaria, or even anaphylactic shock when ingested or injected (34). Fortunately, procaine (Novocain), which not infrequently produces allergic eczematous hypersensitivity, rarely produces an anaphylactic reaction in atopic individuals or even in those who have epidermal hypersensitivity to the anesthetic (35).

Paraphenylenediamine can produce both an allergic eczematous contact dermatitis and asthma in furriers. Allergic rhinitis has been described from the inhalation of epoxy resins and the amine hardeners in a patient who also had a contact dermatitis from processing these resins (36).

ALLERGIC CONTACT DERMATITIS IN ATOPIC INDIVIDUALS

Allergic contact dermatitis in atopic individuals may appear as an eczematous eruption. If the patient is receiving topical or systemic corticosteroid therapy for an atopic dermatitis, however, the superimposed contact dermatitis may appear as an erythematous, papular, noneczematous eruption simulating the original atopic dermatitis. An allergic contact der-

matitis to a topical medication, therefore, may not be suspected.

> **Superimposed contact dermatitis may make an atopic eczema appear to be intractable.**

Features of the "Dermal" Type of Allergic Contact Dermatitis in the Atopic Individual

Aside from being modified by corticosteroid therapy, a superimposed contact dermatitis may appear to be atypical in atopic individuals because the so-called dermal type of contact dermatitis is most likely to develop in these patients (37).

In Fisher's (38) experience, patch tests with sensitizing contactants in atopic individuals yield positive reactions similar to those in nonatopic patients, and it is not necessary to perform intracutaneous tests, as advocated by Epstein (37).

> **Allergic contact dermatitis in atopic individuals may closely mimic atopic eczema.**

Most cases of contact dermatitis in atopic individuals seem to be a combination of eczematous and dermal sensitivity. Usually one can demonstrate both a positive eczematous patch test reaction and a positive dermal intracutaneous test reaction in the atopic skin with superimposed allergic contact dermatitis. It is claimed, however, that occasionally the patch test reaction is negative, and only an intracutaneous test reveals the dermal contact reaction (39).

Diagnostic Features of Allergic Contact Sensitivity to Neomycin

Some investigators report that most individuals investigated for allergic contact hypersensitivity to neomycin had atopic dermatitis (40,41).

Wereide (42) states that this study does not support the view that the atopic state (as it occurs in atopic dermatitis patients) predisposes to neomycin sensitivity. Patients who had stasis dermatitis of the lower part of the leg had a significantly higher incidence of neomycin sensitivity than did any other groups with eczematous dermatitis.

> **In atopic dermatitis, neomycin sensitivity is often obscured by a topical neomycin-corticosteroid preparation and is usually detected only by routine patch tests.**

Both the classic form of allergic contact dermatitis with vesiculation and eczematization and the papular, erythematous "dermal" type of sensitivity may occur in patients who have neomycin sensitivity and atopic eczema. Because neomycin is frequently prescribed in a mixture with a corticosteroid preparation, the corticosteroid may modify the appearance of the superimposed neomycin dermatitis. When an individual treated with a neomycin-containing preparation fails to improve or the eruption becomes worse, neomycin sensitivity should be suspected (42).

In order to prove the neomycin sensitivity, the patient should be patch tested with the suspected topical neomycin preparation. In some instances in which allergic contact sensitivity is present, a typical positive patch test reaction is obtained with the preparation or only with a 20% aqueous solution of neomycin. When the reaction to a neomycin preparation is negative, it may be worthwhile to perform an intradermal skin test with a 1:1,000 solution of neomycin sulfate. A positive reaction consists of a delayed indurated papule present 48 hours after testing. Intradermal testing has rarely been necessary.

When neomycin sensitivity has been demonstrated, the patient should avoid exposure to streptomycin and kanamycin, which may cross-react with neomycin and with bacitracin, which may co-react with neomycin.

Precautions in Testing Atopic Individuals for Allergic Contact Sensitivity to Nickel

Allergic contact dermatitis due to nickel may occasionally take the "dermal" form and closely mimic atopic dermatitis. Although most cases of nickel dermatitis occur in the nonatopic population, nickel sensitivity superimposed on atopic eczema may not be readily recognized (43).

> **Nickel dermatitis may often be dry and closely resemble the eruption of atopic dermatitis.**

Patch testing for nickel sensitivity in atopic individuals may also present the difficulty of properly interpreting pustular patch test reactions, which occur frequently in this group.

Wahlberg and Skog (44) reported that in eczematous patients who had nickel allergy, immunoglobulin E (IgE) and the threshold of sensitivity were determined by patch testing with dilutions of nickel sulfate ($NiSO_4$). In four of the 47 patients investigated, the IgE value increased. The occurrence of atopic disease in nickel-sensitive patients was 9% and, among relatives, 38%.

Although not all investigators agree, several groups have found a higher prevalence of atopy among nickel-sensitive patients (45). However, McDonagh et al. (46) did not find either increased or decreased susceptibility to nickel among atopic patients undergoing diagnostic patch testing. Instead, atopic patients reported more jewelry dermatitis but were frequently negative to notorious jewelry allergens. When atopic dermatitis has been long-standing, sensitization to contact allergens has been found more commonly (47). The most frequently encountered allergens have been nickel, fragrance mix, balsam of Peru, and neomycin. These same investigators (47) found that a 50% dilution of test allergens did not reduce the number of irritant patch test reactions.

> **Jewelry reactions are commonly reported among atopics, but patch tests to notorious jewelry allergens are negative.**

Relationship of Allergic Contact Ragweed Oil Sensitivity to the Atopic State

Ragweed oil dermatitis may mimic a generalized atopic eczema, particularly the seasonal type (48). Ragweed oil dermatitis is due to an oil-soluble oleoresin, whereas ragweed rhinitis, asthma, and possibly certain cases of atopic dermatitis are due to the water-soluble protein fraction of the pollen.

In Fisher's (49) experience, most patients who had ragweed dermatitis had no atopic dermatitis or evidence of the atopic state.

> **Ragweed rhinitis and asthma are due to atopic sensitivity to the protein fraction of the plant; ragweed dermatitis is nonatopic and is due to the oil-soluble fraction.**

Wool as an Irritant and Sensitizer in Patients Who Have Atopic Dermatitis

The mechanism by which wool produces dermatitis, particularly in atopic individuals, is still controversial. Some investigators (50) feel that the inhalation of wool is an important factor. Contact with wool, including house dust, which may be largely wool fibers, may readily irritate the atopic skin (51). Although wool is usually a weak allergen, on rare occasions the degree of sensitivity is so great that mere contact of wool with the skin can produce urticaria.

> **Contact with woolen objects and dust exacerbates atopic dermatitis.**

Apart from allergic sensitization, wool is irritating to many individuals, particularly those with atopy.

Atopic Dermatitis Confined to the Hands or Feet

Atopic dermatitis confined to the hands may be precipitated by household or occupational irritants and sensitizers. In other instances, particularly in children, primary irritant reactions from friction, perspiration, and tight shoes are factors in a recurrent dermatitis of the feet in atopic individuals (52). Such atopic dermatitis may resemble shoe dermatitis. Occasionally, only the dorsal aspect or the large toe is involved.

> **Atopic dermatitis confined to the feet may be mistaken for allergic shoe dermatitis.**

Fredriksson and Faergemann (53) found, in a retrospective survey of 1,112 patients who had atopic dermatitis, that lesions localized to the lower gluteal and posterior femoral regions reached their peak in patients age 7 to 8 years. These investigators speculate that this is due to sweat retention caused by prolonged sitting when these individuals start school.

In another study of 1,385 subjects who had hand eczema in the prior 12 months, it was learned that the most important predictive factor was childhood eczema, followed by being female. Additional factors of lesser importance were occupation, asthma, and/or hay fever (54).

ATOPIC DERMATITIS AND OCCUPATION

Occupation

Atopy has been said to be a risk factor for occupational skin disease. However, studies in Singapore and Taiwan did not support this (55). Rather, nonatopic individuals were found to be at highest risk of occupational skin disease.

JUVENILE PLANTAR DERMATOSIS AND ATOPIC CONDITION

Verbov (56–58) states that juvenile plantar dermatosis (JPD) is a characteristic dermatosis of infancy and childhood localized to the distal soles, including the toes, particularly the big toe but sparing the toe spaces. He believes that JPD describes not only a true localized atopic dermatitis but also a frictional contact dermatitis to which those with an atopic condition are prone but which may occur in susceptible nonatopic persons. His series, dating from 1973, has reached 72 patients, of whom 33 (46%) have had a personal or family history of atopy. The criteria for a diagnosis of atopy are a personal or family history of asthma, hay fever, perennial rhinorrhoea, or typical eczema of atopic type. Using similar criteria, Jepsen (59) also found a high incidence of atopy.

> **Juvenile plantar dermatosis is often a manifestation of atopic dermatitis.**

ATOPICS AND BEER

Beer

Three atopic patients developed urticaria after drinking beer (60). Prick tests to grains showed immediate hypersensitivity to malt, wheat flour, barley flour, maize flour, and rice flour. Fresh cereal preparations rather than commercial products were recommended for testing. In contrast, beer was not a problem when ingested for a maltworker who became sensitive to barley malt (61). Patch tests were positive to barley residues (as is and 10% in petrolatum), malt radicle, and malt residues at the same concentrations. A prick test to barley was negative.

ATOPIC CHILDREN AND GRAINS

Children with atopic dermatitis may be allergic to grains such as barley, oats, rye, and wheat. Oral provocation with these cereals can provoke dermatologic, gastrointestinal, and oropharyngeal reactions that can be either immediate or delayed. Prick tests with these grains were performed on atopic children who had positive oral challenges to the grains (62). Prick tests, RAST, or histamine release test detected the allergen in 8 of 8 children who had immediate reactions and in 9 of 14 who had delayed reactions. Five children had allergens identifiable only with patch tests to the cereals or by lymphocyte proliferation assay. Wheat was the most common cereal allergen and antibodies to gliadin of IgE, IgA, and IgG classes were found.

ATOPIC CHILDREN AND COW'S MILK

Oral challenges with cow's milk may provoke atopic dermatitis especially in children under the age of 2 years. A study of 113 infants 2 to 24 months old found a positive oral cow's milk challenge in 54 (63). Of these 54, immediate reactions were documented in 36 and delayed reactions in 18. Prick tests were useful to detect the immediate reactions, and patch tests to cow's milk detected the delayed reactions. The detection of cow's milk allergy was possible only by patch tests 26% of the time. The authors define immediate reactions as pruritus, urticaria, and/or exanthema, and delayed reactions were eczematous (64).

REFERENCES

1. Dahl MV. Forum discussion: some aspects of atopic dermatitis. *Arch Dermatol* 1983;119:237.
2. Sulzberger MB, Witten VH. Atopic dermatitis. In: Lowenthal LJA, ed. *The enzymes.* Edinburgh: E. & S. Livingstone, 1954:78.
3. Ward KA, et al. A comparison of expression of surface-bound immunoglobulin E on antigen-presenting cells in cutaneous tissue between patients with allergic, irritant and atopic dermatitis. *Contact Dermatitis* 1991;25:115.
4. Epstein S, Mohajerin AH. Incidence of contact sensitivity in atopic dermatitis. *Arch Dermatol* 1964;90:284.
5. Baer R, Witten V. Editorial comment. In: *Year book of dermatology and syphilography.* Chicago: Year Book Medical Publishers, 1955: 414.

6. Fisher AA. Contact dermatitis superimposed on atopic eczema. *Dermatol Digest* 1966;5:45.

7. Gallacher G, Maibach HI. Is atopic dermatitis a predisposing factor for experimental acute irritant contact dermatits? *Contact Dermatitis* 1998;38:1.

8. Basketter DA, Miettinen J, Lahti A. Acute irritant reactivity to sodium lauryl sulfate in atopics and non-atopics. *Contact Dermatitis* 1998; 38:253.

9. Rees J, Friedmann PS, Matthews JN. Contact sensitivity to dinitrochlorobenzene is impaired in atopic subjects. *Arch Dermatol* 1990; 126:1173.

10. Rietschel RL, Klemm J, Jones HE. Chronic irritant dermatitis interferes with induction of dinitrochlorobenzene (DNCB) sensitization. *Clin Res* 1982;30:915A.

11. Lever R, Forsyth A. Allergic contact dermatitis in atopic dermatitis. *Acta Derm Venereol Suppl* (Stockh) 1992;176:95.

12. Tada J, Toi Y, Arata J. Atopic dermatitis with severe facial lesions exacerbated by contact dermatitis from topical medicaments. *Contact Dermatitis* 1994;31:261.

13. de Groot AC. The frequency of contact allergy in atopic patients with dermatitis. *Contact Dermatitis* 1990;22:273.

14. Klas PA, et al. Allergic and irritant patch test reactions and atopic disease. *Contact Dermatitis* 1996;34:121.

15. Lewis FM, Shah M, Gawkrodger DJ. Contact sensitivity in atopic dermatitis. *Am J Contact Dermatitis* 1995;6:150.

16. Giordano-Labadie F, et al. Frequency of contact allergy in children with atopic dermatitis: results of a prospective study of 137 cases. *Contact Dermatitis* 1999;40:192.

17. Brasch J, Geier J, Henseler T. Evaluation of patch test results by use of the reaction index: an analysis of data recorded by the Information Network of Departments of Dermatology (IVDK). *Contact Dermatitis* 1995;33:375.

18. Epstein S. Contact dermatitis from neomycin due to dermal delayed (tuberculin-type) sensitivity: report of 10 cases. *Dermatologica* 1956; 113:191.

19. Fisher AA, et al. Pustular patch-test reactions. *AMA Arch Dermatol* 1959;80:742.

20. Fisher AA. Management of atopic dermatitis. *NY J Med* 1966;66:236.

21. Baer RL. Conference on infantile eczema: history, definitions, concepts. *J Pediatr* 1965;66:248.

22. Strauss JS, Kligman AM. The relationship of atopic allergy and dermatitis. *AMA Arch Dermatol* 1957;75:806.

23. Jadassohn W. Contact dermatitis versus atopic eczema. *Int Arch Allergy* 1957;11:20.

24. Champion RH. Atopic sensitivity to algae and lichens. *Br J Dermatol* 1971;85:551.

25. Kanny G, Becker S, de Hauteclocque C, Moneret-Vautrin DA. Airborne eczema due to mould allergy. *Contact Dermatitis* 1996;35:378.

26. Vidal C, Rial A. Airborne contact dermatitis from *Tyrophagus putrescentiae*. *Contact Dermatitis* 1998;38:181.

27. Clark RAF, Adinoff AD. Aeroallergen contact can exacerbate atopic dermatitis: patch tests as a diagnostic tool. *J Am Acad Dermatol* 1989; 21:863.

28. Stinco G, de Francesco V, Frattasio A, Patrone P. A dermatitis flare after patch testing with *Dermatophagoides pteronyssinus* in an atopic patient. *Contact Dermatitis* 1997;37:52.

29. Gaddoni G, Baldassari L, Zucchini A. A new patch test preparation of dust mites for atopic dermatitis. *Contact Dermatitis* 1994;31:132.

30. Manzini BM, Motolese A, Donini M, Seidenari S. Contact allergy to *Dermatophagoides* in atopic dermatitis patients and healthy subjects. *Contact Dermatitis* 1995;33:243.

31. Kubota Y, Koga T, Imayama S, Hori Y. Mite-antigen-stimulated cytokine production by peripheral blood mononuclear cells of atopic dermatitis patients with positive mite patch tests. *Contact Dermatitis* 1994;31:217.

32. Cabon N, et al. Contact allergy to aeroallergens in children with atopic dermatitis: comparison with allergic contact dermatitis. *Contact Dermatitis* 1996;35:27.

33. Mayer RL. Contact dermatitis versus atopic dermatitis. *Int Arch Allergy* 1957;11:1.

34. Fisher AA. Recent developments in the diagnosis and management of drug eruptions. *Med Clin N Am* 1959;43:1.

35. Fisher AA, Sturm H. Procaine sensitivity: the relationship of the allergic eczematous contact type sensitivity to the urticarial, anaphylactoid variety. *Ann Allergy* 1958;16:593.

36. Morris GE. Allergic rhinitis acquired during the processing of epoxy resins. *Ann Allergy* 1959;17:74.

37. Epstein S. Contact-dermatitis due to nickel and chromate: observations on dermal delayed (tuberculin-type) sensitivity. *Arch Dermatol* 1956;73:236.

38. Fisher AA. *Contact dermatitis.* 3rd ed. Philadelphia: Lea & Febiger, 1986.

39. Baer RL. Allergic eczematous sensitization in man. *J Invest Dermatol* 1964;43:223.

40. Jillson OF, Curwen WL, Alexander BR. Problems of contact dermatitis in the atopic individual: with reference to neomycin and ragweed oil sensitivity. *Ann Allergy* 1959;17:215.

41. Patrick J, Panzer JD, Derbes VL. Neomycin sensitivity in the normal (nonatopic) individual. *Arch Dermatol* 1970;102:532.

42. Wereide K. Neomycin sensitivity in atopic dermatitis and other eczematous conditions. *Acta Derm Venereol* (Stockh) 1970;50:114.

43. Fisher AA, Shapiro A. Allergic eczematous contact dermatitis due to metallic nickel. *JAMA* 1956;161:717.

44. Wahlberg IE, Skog E. Nickel allergy and atopy threshold of nickel sensitivity and immunoglobulin E determinations. *Br J Dermatol* 1971;85:97.

45. Motolese A, Truzzi M, Seidenari S. Nickel sensitization and atopy. *Contact Dermatitis* 1992;26:274.

46. McDonagh AJ, Wright AL, Cork MJ, Gawkrodger DJ. Nickel sensitivity: the influence of ear piercing and atopy. *Br J Dermatol* 1992; 126:16.

47. Lammintausta K, Kalimo K, Fagerlund VL. Patch test reactions in atopic patients. *Contact Dermatitis* 1992;26:234.

48. Fromer IL, Burrage WS. Ragweed oil dermatitis. *J Allergy* 1953;24: 425.

49. Fisher AA. Some immunologic phenomena in treatment of and patch testing for ragweed oil dermatitis. *J Invest Dermatol* 1952;19:271.

50. Osborne ED, Murray PF. Atopic dermatitis: a study of its natural course and of wool as a dominant factor. *AMA Arch Dermatol Syphilol* 1953;68:619.

51. Hambly EM, Levia L, Wilkinson DS. Wool intolerance in atopic subjects. *Contact Dermatitis* 1978;4:240.

52. Silvers SH, Glickman FS. Atopy and eczema of feet in children. *Am J Dis Child* 1968;116:400.

53. Fredriksson T, Faergemann J. The atopic thigh: a "starting-school" symptom? *Acta Derm Venereol* (Stockh) 1981;61:452.

54. Meding B, Swanbeck G. Predictive factors for hand eczema. *Contact Dermatitis* 1990;23:154.

55. Sun C-C, Cheng C-S. Frequency and determinants of occupational contact dermatitis in 2793 consecutively-investigated patients. *Contact Dermatitis* 1998;38:230.

56. Verbov JL. Atopic dermatitis and the forefoot. *Br Med J* 1978;11:962.

57. Verbov JL. Atopic eczema localized to the forefoot: an unrecognized entity. *Practitioner* 1978;220:465.

58. Verbov JL. Skin problems in childhood. *Practitioner* 1976;217:403.

59. Jepsen LV. Dermatitis plantaris sicca: a retrospective study of children with recurrent dermatitis of the feet. *Acta Derm Venereol* (Stockh) 1979;59:257.

60. Santucci B, et al. Urticaria from beer in 3 patients. *Contact Dermatitis* 1996;34:368.

61. Pereira F, Rafael M, Lacerda MH. Contact dermatitis from barley. *Contact Dermatitis* 1998;39:261.

62. Rasanen L, et al. Allergy to ingested cereals in atopic children. *Allergy* 1994;49:871.

63. Kekki OM, Turjanmaa K, Isolauri E. Differences in skin-prick and patch-test reactivity are related to the heterogeneity of atopic eczema in infants. *Allergy* 1997;52:755.

64. Isolauri E, Turjanmaa K. Combined skin prick and patch testing enhances identification of food allergy in infants with atopic dermatitis. *J Allergy Clin Immunol* 1996;97:9.

CHAPTER 10

Reactions to Selected Medications and Medical Care

ALUMINUM AND ITS SALTS

Aluminum compounds are used extensively in cosmetic and medicinal preparations. In these preparations, advantage is taken of their astringent, antacid, antibacterial, and antiperspirant properties. The irritant effect of aluminum salts on the skin varies considerably; the chloride and nitrate have greater irritant properties than the chlorhydrate, allantoin, and citrate. Aluminum salts are also used as styptic agents for hemostasis and for aluminum-precipitated allergens.

Allergic Contact Sensitivity

Sensitivity reactions to aluminum are rare. Desensitization of hay fever patients who have an aluminum-precipitated allergen, however, has been found to cause contact sensitivity to aluminum (1). When such sensitivity occurs, the patients may show an allergic reaction to the aluminum-disc Finn Chamber used for patch testing. Fischer and Rystedt (2) pointed out that if all patches in a Finn Chamber test show red, infiltrated papular rings, contact sensitivity to aluminum ought to be suspected; irritant factors, however, may also be the cause of the reactions.

The patient of Fischer and Rystedt (2) had an axillary dermatitis that cleared up when she stopped using an antiperspirant stick. This was followed by attacks of more widespread eczema while she was receiving desensitizing, hay fever injections made up in an aluminum vehicle. There were no local eczematous reactions, but the eczema disappeared when the injections stopped. On patch testing, she reacted to the rims of the aluminum Finn Chamber and later was strongly positive (+++) to aluminum sulfate (2% aq), aluminum chloride (2% aq), and aluminum subacetate (1% aq). An intradermal test with 0.05 mL aluminum hydroxide in 0.5% sodium chloride was also positive.

> Reaction to the aluminum discs of Finn Chamber may occur from aluminum allergy. Testing with mercury salts in a Finn Chamber may give irritant reactions owing to a mercury-aluminum complex.

It was not certain whether she was sensitized by the deodorant or the injections.

Allergic Aluminum Hydroxide Granulomas from Vaccines

Slater et al. (3) described three children in whom painful subcutaneous nodules developed 1 to 2 years after the injection of absorbed diphtheria-pertussis-tetanus (DPT) vaccine. The diagnosis of aluminum hydroxide granuloma was established by ultrastructural examination with X-ray microanalysis.

Vaccination with aluminum hydroxide containing DPT in patients allergic to aluminum (as confirmed by reactions to Finn Chamber or 2% aq aluminum chloride) can produce granulomas lasting more than 1 year (4). Aluminum was confirmed in the granulomas by X-ray defraction analysis, and of 21 such cases followed, 5 cleared, 11 improved, and 5 remained unchanged.

False-Positive Reactions When Testing Mercury Salts on Aluminum Discs

Dr. K. J. Kalveram and G. Forck of Munster, Germany, at the Fifth International Symposium on Contact Dermatitis, Barcelona, March 1980, reported nonspecific skin irritant reaction when using the aluminum Finn Chamber to patch test mercury salts. They explained the irritation as being due to a chemical reaction between the aluminum of the Finn Chamber and the tested mercury salt solution.

> Aluminum hydroxide in vaccine may produce granulomas.

ALLANTOIN

Certain cosmetics and many over-the-counter topical medications, particularly those advocated for use in psoriasis, contain allantoin as one of their ingredients (5).

Nature of Allantoin

Allantoin (5-ureido-hydantoin), a uric acid derivative known chemically as the diureide of glyoxylic acid, is a product of purine metabolism. It is prepared synthetically by the oxidation of uric acid with alkaline potassium permanganate with dichloroacetic acid.

The Safety of Allantoin

The Food and Drug Administration reported that a search of the literature has not produced any reports of adverse reactions to the topical use of allantoin (6,7). Moreover, the Schwartz patch test on 200 persons has shown that allantoin is nontoxic, nonirritating, and nonallergenic. The Draize technique in rabbits has shown that allantoin is nonirritating even when applied to the conjunctival sac of the eye. The repeated insult test on 12 human subjects has shown that allantoin is not a primary skin irritant or a primary sensitizer.

> **There are currently no reports of allergic hypersensitivity to allantoin.**

ANTHRALIN (DITHRANOL)

This topical medication used for psoriasis may sensitize occasionally (8,9).

Anthralin Cream is available at present as Dithocreme (American Dermal Company) and Anthra-Derm (Dermik). Staining of clothes, skin, nails, and hair is frequent. An unusual cutaneous anthralin-like staining of the perineum may follow the use of danthron as a laxative. Danthron (1,8-dihydroxyanthroquinone) is reduced in the bowel to 1,8-dihydroxyanthron, which is the purgative, and can produce an irritant contact dermatitis (10). Anthralin ointment is a strong irritant when covered. Covered patch tests may be made with 1/30 strength in petrolatum.

BENZYL BENZOATE

Wranicz and Czernielweski (11) reported a 79-year-old female patient who was treated for scabies with Novoscabin, which contains 30% benzyl benzoate. She developed an erythematous-bullous eruption on the sites to which the drug had been applied. The presence of circulating antibodies and of antibodies bound to the basement membrane could be demonstrated immunologically. The authors discussed the possibility of provoking "pemphigoid" by topical application of Novoscabin.

PHENYLBUTAZONE (BUTAZOLIDIN)

This medication is not used topically to any extent in the United States. It may cause dermatitis from its use as a cream (12), as an ointment (13), and in suppositories (14). Cross-reactions may occur with phenylbutazone.

DIETHYLSTILBESTROL

This hormone is present in such proprietary medications as Aquarant "E" (Webster), Furestrol suppositories (Eaton), and Diethylstilbestrol Suppositories (Lilly) and is used as pellets in veterinary medications. It may cross-react with dienestrol, hexestrol, bisphenol A, monobenzylether of hydroquinone, eugenol, stilbene benzophenone, and benzestrol (15,16).

EPINEPHRINE (ADRENALIN)

Several investigators have reported allergic contact reactions to epinephrine with positive patch tests from its use in ophthalmic solutions and as a spray treatment for asthma (17–20).

Inasmuch as Aaronson and Jamamoto (21) reported circulating antibodies to epinephrine following ocular hypersensitivity, an opinion as to the safety of injectable epinephrine was sought in those patients who had a delayed type of allergic contact hypersensitivity. The following communication from Dr. Philip S. Norman (Baltimore, MD) is helpful:

> The question calls attention to several reports of contact reactions to topically applied epinephrine preparations usually in the form of eyedrops. Although it is possible that some of the reactions reported were due to preservatives or chemicals in the vehicle, at least some of the reactions were reproduced with crystalline epinephrine dissolved in water. Such reactions are unlikely to have much relation to immediate systemic symptoms after injection of epinephrine, although the subject has not of course been thoroughly explored. While one might look for an alternative to epinephrine in the treatment of asthma in individuals with a history of contact dermatitis after exposure to epinephrine solutions, I would not withhold epinephrine in an emergency such as systemic anaphylaxis.

> **The injection of epinephrine has been deemed safe in an emergency, such as systemic anaphylaxis, in patients who have allergic contact sensitivity to epinephrine.**

EPHEDRINE

A systemic eruption of the trunk and arms due to ephedrine HCl in a cough medicine was reported (22). A 5% aqueous solution of ephedrine HCl was used for diagnosis.

PHENYLEPHRINE

Phenylephrine has usually been reported to cause contact dermatitis from an ophthalmic product, but it has also been reported from an eardrop (23). There was a positive reaction to a 5% petrolatum concentration of phenylephrine.

CROTAMITON (EURAX)

Crotamiton (Eurax) used topically as a scabicide and antipruritic is a rare sensitizer (24,25). However, allergic contact dermatitis was reported from crotamiton (Eurax) after 6 days of an application three times per day. A 5% petrolatum concentration was used for diagnosis. Other cases have usually been from use on chronic eczemas, such as stasis dermatitis (26).

ICHTHAMMOL (ICHTHYOL)

Ichthammol, a sulfonated bitumen, is derived from mineral deposits containing the remains of fish, consisting of sulfur (about 10%), ammonium sulfate (5 to 7%), hydrocarbons, nitrogenous bases, acids, and derivatives of thiophene. It has slight antiseptic and analgesic properties. Ichthammol is a weak antigen. A few scattered reports from Europe indicate allergic reactions to this medication (27–30).

SULFUR

Sensitivity to sulfur, particularly when used as a topical agent, is rare. There are two reports in the literature of allergic hypersensitivity to sulfur (31,32).

WHITFIELD'S OINTMENT

This ointment, containing 6% salicylic acid, 12% benzoic acid in petrolatum, is a rare sensitizer. The benzoic acid occasionally may produce a nonallergic contact urticaria that may cause a stinging sensation, particularly in the intertriginous areas. Such stinging sensations may become less evident if the Whitfield's ointment is mixed with equal parts of zinc oxide ointment.

> **The benzoic acid in Whitfield's ointment occasionally may produce a nonallergic contact urticaria that can cause a stinging, irritant reaction, especially in the body folds.**

HALOGENATED HYDROXYQUINOLINES

These therapeutic agents include iodochlorhydroxyquin (Vioform, Clioquinol), iodoquinol (Diiodohydroxyquinoline, Diodoquin), chlorquinaldol (Sterosan), and chlorhydroxyquinoline (Quinolor). Such preparations are commonly used topical agents. In addition, Vioform and Diodoquin may be administered systemically (33). Cross-sensitization between these compounds may exist (34). Vioform and Diodoquin administered orally may lead to an eczematous dermatitis medicamentosa in patients sensitized by topical application of any one of this group of compounds.

> **Vioform, Diodoquin, Sterosan, and Quinolor may cross-react; oral Vioform and Diodoquin can produce eczematous contact-type dermatitis medicamentosa in persons topically sensitized to these halogenated quinolines.**

Quinolor Compound

This ointment consists of chlorhydroxyquinoline, benzoyl peroxide, menthol, methyl salicylate, and eugenol in Plastibase vehicle. When dermatitis occurs from the use of quinolor compound, chlorhydroxyquinoline is not necessarily the culprit, because the benzoyl peroxide, eugenol, and Plastibase, which is a polyethylene compound related to Carbowax, can all cause allergic reactions.

Kero et al. (35) reported irritant dermatitis from Vioform, particularly in men in the inguinal and scrotal areas. The topical use of Vioform and Diodoquin, iodine-containing compounds, may increase the protein-bound iodine of the blood. Such an increase may be mistaken for thyroid disease (36,37).

> **Vioform and Diodoquin are iodine-containing compounds whose topical use may increase the protein-bound iodine of the blood.**

SODIUM PERBORATE

Vilanova and Camarasa (38) found that this oxidizing agent was a common sensitizer in Spain. In the United States, it is a rare sensitizer. Sodium perborate is present in Kleenite (Vick), a denture-cleansing preparation.

Sodium perborate, like other oxidizing agents, is a strong irritant (39). Fisher (40) noted irritant stomatitis in which Kleenite is not thoroughly washed off a denture before it is inserted into the mouth.

SILVER NITRATE

Gaul and Underwood (41) described a man who developed a vesicular reaction to the 10% silver nitrate used for marking patch tests. On patch testing, he reacted to 5% and 10% aged silver nitrate but not to 10% fresh silver nitrate; a test with silver foil was positive, but one with silver chloride powder was negative.

Silver nitrate is kept in an amber bottle because on exposure to air and light it decomposes, forming small amounts of nitric acid, silver nitrite, and colloidal silver, which liberate silver ions. The ionized silver was considered the sensitizer in this patient, and its effect explained the discrepancy between the results of testing with old and fresh solutions.

Marcussen (42) stated long ago that silver nitrate, used therapeutically, occasionally sensitized.

The prolonged use of topical silver nitrate can lead to systemic argyria (43).

> **Silver nitrate, a rare sensitizer, becomes an irritant when aged or exposed to light. Prolonged use may produce argyria.**

PHENOL

Irritant and Toxic Effects of Phenol

The inclusion of phenol in such medications as Castellani's (Carbol-fuchsin) paint, Carbolated Vaseline, P & S Liquid, and Panscol Lotion has proved to be an irritant in certain persons (44).

Rogers et al. (45) proved that phenol was toxic in infants when it was applied in the form of magenta (Carbol-fuchsin) paint.

Irritation from Phenol in Castellani's (Carbol-Fuchsin Paint) Natural Formula 13

This original Carbol-fuchsin paint has caused irritant dermatitis in so many individuals, particularly when used in the intertriginous areas, that several years ago it was decided at the New York Skin and Cancer Unit of New York University to remove the phenol and use the formula shown in Table 10.1. Removal of the phenol has not impaired the efficacy of the paint.

> **Topical phenol in very dilute solutions may be an irritant, particularly in the diaper area and in skin folds.**

It has been observed that children who have fair complexions or those who have applied paint immediately after bathing become mildly shocked and drowsy.

Estimations of phenol and methyl alcohol in the urine in 16 infants who had seborrheic eczema treated with magenta (Castellani's) paint BPC were made by Rogers et al. (45) to determine the degree of absorption. Phenol was detected in four patients and methyl alcohol in none.

Lack of Allergic Sensitivity to Phenol

There has been only a single report of allergic dermatitis to phenol in the past three decades (46).

TABLE 10.1. *Phenol-Free Modified Carbol-Fuchsin Solution*

	cc
Combine	
Alcohol	20.0
Fuchsin	2.6
Water	190.0
Filter and add	
Boric acid	2.0
Let stand 2 hours and add	
Acetone	10.0
Resorcinol (resorcin)	20.0
Filter solution	

*NY Skin and Cancer Formulary. This paint has proved useful in chronic intertriginous dermatitis, otitis externa, stasis ulcers, and eczema.

Irritant Dermatitis from Phenol in Carbolated Vaseline

Carbolated Vaseline contains 0.2% phenol and 0.5% para-chloro-meta-xylenol (PCMX) in a petrolatum base.

Rubin and Pirozzi (47) reported that Carbolated Vaseline, a widely employed self-medication in the black community, is used to acquire a "shiny" complexion. In their study of 28 patients who had dermatitis from Carbolated Vaseline, acute reactions occurred in eight (28%) patients, all of whom had an underlying eczematous dermatitis. These reactions were due either to allergic contact sensitization to PCMX (four patients) or to a primary irritant response to phenol (four patients). Chronic reactions occurred in 20 (72%) patients and developed over a period of weeks. A low-grade primary irritant reaction to phenol was responsible for the chronic reactions.

Precautions in the Use of P & S Liquid

P & S Liquid is a specially prepared mixture of liquid paraffin, oil, sodium chloride, and phenol, less than 1%. It is stated that "P & S Liquid provides safe and effective management of scaling conditions of the scalp resulting from psoriasis or seborrhea." There is a warning, however, stating that P & S Liquid should not be applied to large portions of the body.

> **Phenol (carbolic acid), a nonsensitizer, can cause toxic effects in dilute solutions if used over a wide area of skin and can cause gangrene if not diluted.**

SALICYLIC ACID

Salicylic acid is used widely in prescribed medications and in over-the-counter medications.

It is used for wart removal as a 2% to 20% solution in collodion or as a 10% to 40% plaster for plantar warts and plantar hyperkeratosis, in a salicylic acid soap for tinea versicolor, and as a 6% salicylic acid preparation in a 60% propylene gel for hyperkeratotic diseases. Low concentrations of salicylic acid are in shampoo and other medications in which they would be used to cause desquamation.

Whitfield's ointment with 6% salicylic acid and 12% benzoic acid in wool fat and petrolatum is used occasionally for desquamation and as a nonspecific antifungal agent. Gels with 8.7% choline salicylate have been used for symptomatic relief of painful aphthous ulcers. Topical salicylates are bacteriostatic and photo-protective.

Salicylic acid–mercury combinations may form bichloride of mercury or other severe mercury irritants, particularly under a closed patch test.

The Use of Salicylic Acid in Psoriasis

Goldsmith (48) states that psoriatic patients receiving topical salicylates and methotrexates are at potential risk of methotrexate toxicity. Taylor and Halprin (49) state that Keralyt (6 salicylic acid, 20% alcohol in 60% propylene glycol) is safe to use under occlusion over widespread areas of the body for psoriasis. Soyka and Soyka (50), however, report that salicylate intoxication can occur as a result of the Keralyt-occlusive regimen.

Birmingham et al. (51) studied the systemic absorption of salicylic acid in humans following topical application. Drug absorption was minimal following application to intact skin. Experimentally, measurable salicylate plasma levels were obtained, however, if the stratum corneum was removed before the salicylic acid was applied. This finding indicates that the use of salicylic acid in psoriasis is safe.

Allergic Reactions to Salicylic Acid

Although allergic reactions to salicylic acid are rare, Rudzki and Koslowska (52) reported five patients who had allergic reactions to salicylic acid. In four cases, the source of salicylic acid was 2% salicylic acid in alcohol. Three patients themselves noticed that the use of this preparation was responsible for the reactions. In none of the patients did aspirin cause exacerbation or relapses of the dermatitis.

> **Salicylic acid, a rare sensitizer, can be toxic if used under occlusion.**

RESORCINOL (RESORCIN)

Allergic reactions to resorcinol are rare and have been reported mainly from its use in Castellani's Carbol-fuchsin paint (53).

Discoloration from Resorcinol

Unless alcoholic solutions of resorcinol and resorcinol monoacetates are kept in dark bottles, they may produce a yellow-orange discoloration of the fingernails. In addition, the discolored resorcinol may act as an irritant.

Toxic Effect of Resorcinol

Acute resorcinol poisoning is rare. The application of an ointment containing 12.5% resorcinol to the diaper area of an infant produced dusky cyanosis, a maculopapular eruption, hemolytic anemia, and hemoglobinuria.

Resorcinol has an antithyroid activity similar to that of methyl thiouracil. The continued application to large leg ulcers of ointment containing resorcinol has given rise to myxedema, which may be associated with ochronosis. Hydroquinone, which is an isomer of resorcinol, can also produce ochronosis (54).

Resorcinol in Acne Preparations

In the United States, the most common exposure to resorcinol is probably in its use in acne preparations as a keratolytic agent and mild antiseptic. Table 10.2 lists acne preparations containing resorcinol. Because such preparations are usually applied to noneczematous skin, allergic reactions to resorcinol from such therapy are rare.

Resorcinol in Cosmetics

In eyedrops, skin "fresheners," freckle creams, hair "tonics," hair dyes, and certain lipsticks, as Caron and Calnan (55) point out, resorcinol allergic contact dermatitis is a very uncommon occurrence.

Resorcinol in Suppositories

In 1933, Mitchell (56) reported the first case of anal dermatitis from resorcinol in Anusol suppositories.

Other Therapeutic Agents That Contain Resorcinol

Table 10.3 lists resorcinol-containing products that also contain benzocaine, a common and potent sensitizer.

TABLE 10.2. *Acne Preparations Containing Resorcinol*

Acne Dome Creme and Lotion (Dome)
Acnomel Cream and Cake (Menley and James)
Bensulfoid Lotion (Poythress)
Exzit Medicated Creme and Lotion (Dome)
Rezamid Acne Lotion (Dermik)

TABLE 10.3. *"Anti-itch" Preparations Containing Resorcinol and Benzocaine*

Bi Cozene Creme (Creighton Products)
Lanacane Medicated Creme (Combe)
Vagisil Feminine Itching Medication (Combe)

Industrial Exposure to Resorcinol

Resorcinol (*m*-dihydroxybenzene, $C_6H_6O_2$) is an important compound in the preparation of numerous dyestuffs, especially those of the azo, fluorescein, and oxazine series. Styphnic acid (2,4,6-trinitroresorcinol) is used, like picric acid, as an explosive, as well as for the separation and characterization of organic bases, which frequently form well-crystallized styphnates. Table 10.4 lists the industrial uses of resorcinol.

Resorcinol Cross-Reactions

Caron and Calnan (55) studied cross-sensitivity reactions to resorcinol and found that the most clinically significant cross-reactions were to resorcinol monoacetate (Euresol) (Table 10.5) and to hexylresorcinol (Table 10.6). Keil (57) reported that "milder" cross-reactions are occasionally encountered between resorcinol, pyrocatechol, hydroquinone, phenol, pyrogallol, and hydroxyhydroquinone, and orcinol.

Relation of Resorcinol to Orcinol (5-Methylresorcinol)

Orcinol, a homologue of resorcinol, is a constituent of many substances occurring in lichens of the *Rocella* and *Lecanora* series. It is obtained synthetically from P-toluidine. Orcinol becomes blue-violet in the presence of ferric chloride. With chloroform and alkali it becomes red, and, when then diluted with water, it becomes yellow with a green fluorescence.

Orcinol is the parent substance of the orseille and litmus dyes and is used in chemistry as a reagent for pentoses, lignin, beet sugar, saccharoses, and arabinose.

PETROLATUM

Very few cases have been reported of allergic hypersensitivity to petrolatum, which is a rare sensitizer (58–61).

TABLE 10.4. *Industrial Exposures to Resorcinol*

Celluloid manufacturers
Duplicating fluid
Dyes and dye intermediates
Explosives
Mildew-proofing agents
Photocopy machines
Photographic developers
Plastic manufacture
Rubber additives
Tanning agents

TABLE 10.5. *Resorcinol Monoacetate (Eurosol) Products That May Cross-React with Resorcinol*

AR-EX-RMS Scalp Lotion (AR-EX)
Hil Cortac Lotion (Hill Dermaceuticals)
Resulin-F (Schiefflien)
Sulforcin Lotion (Texas Pharmacal)

The Nature of Petrolatum (Soft Paraffin)

Petrolatum (C_nH_{2n+2}), a mixture of semisolid hydrocarbons chiefly of the methane series, is a colloidal system of nonstraight-chain solid hydrocarbons and high-boiling liquid hydrocarbons. Petrolatum is also known as petroleum jelly, paraffin jelly, vasoliment, Vaseline, Saxoline, Cosmoline, and stonolene. Its various trade names are listed in Table 10.7.

There are three types of petrolatum. The first type, natural petrolatum, is a purified mixture of semisolid hydrocarbons obtained from petroleum. The purification is usually done with sulfuric acid and percolation through bone black or adsorptive clays. This removes odors and modifies the color. The second type, artificial petrolatum, is manufactured by mixing natural hydrocarbon waxes with refined mineral oils. It is also purified by the aforementioned process. The third type, synthetic petrolatum, is made of synthetic hydrocarbons obtained by hydrogenation.

White versus Yellow Petrolatum

White petrolatum is prepared in the same manner as yellow petrolatum. The only difference is that the purification process is extended until practically all of the yellow color is removed. Fisher (58) had a patient allergic to both white and yellow petrolatum. Malten's (59) patient reacted only to yellow petrolatum, and the patient of Grimalt and Romaquera (60) was allergic to both the white and yellow varieties.

Dooms-Goossens and Degreef (61) reported on two patients who were allergic to yellow petrolatum but not to the white variety. These authors tested their patients with several brands of yellow petroleum, and two of these tests gave positive results. Further patch testing with white soft paraffins and related products, such as liquid paraffin, ozokerite, ceresin, and hard paraffin, yielded negative results. The authors concluded that

1. Natural petrolatum is a biological product whose chemical composition may vary greatly. If yellow petrolatum is considered as an ideal vehicle for patch testing, then a

TABLE 10.6. *Hexylresorcinol-Containing Products That May Cross-React with Resorcinol*

Oil-O-Sol Liquid (Health Care)
S.T. 37 (Beecham Products)
Sucret Lozenges (Beecham Products)

TABLE 10.7. *Trade Names for Petrolatum*

Amber (Penreco)
Amojell Petrolatum Cream (Amoco)
Amojell Petrolatum Snow White (Amoco)
Cream White (Penreco)
Extra Amber (Penreco)
Fonoline (Witco)
Fybrene (Witco)
Lilly White (Penreco)
Mineral Jelly (Penreco)
Pennsoline (Penreco)
Penreco White (Penreco)
Peffecta (Witco)
Petrolatum Snow White (Penreco)
Protopel (Witco)
Sonojell (Witco)
Ultima White (Penreco)

thoroughgoing standardization must be implemented as regards both its purity and the use of additives. In any event, it seems always necessary to test the vehicle.

2. White petrolatum should be used as a vehicle instead of yellow petrolatum because it is purer.

3. Synthetic petrolatum might be better than natural petrolatum because a synthetic mixture of hydrocarbons is controlled more easily.

4. If contact allergic reactions to a topical preparation occur, patch tests should be performed with the same quality of ingredients that the patient has used.

Petrolatum as a Therapeutic Agent

Penneys et al. (62) reported that petrolatum preparations that contain no known pharmacologically active ingredients frequently produce partial or complete resolution of skin inflammation and burns. The beneficial effects, however, of a commonly applied "banal" substance, such as petrolatum, are difficult to explain. Clinical improvement has been ascribed generally to the physical effect of removing scale, crust, and debris and giving protection from irritants, thus allowing natural recuperative functions to operate. It also seems likely that complex biochemical mixtures, such as petrolatum, lanolin, and mineral oil from organic sources, would contain fractions that are active in various biochemical systems. Ghadially et al. (63) found that petrolatum enhanced recovery of human skin from acetone-induced irritation. This was accomplished by petrolatum occupying the intercellular spaces during recovery of barrier function.

Irritation, Acne, and Pigmentation in Black Skin from Petrolatum

Maibach (64) reported on a black patient who acquired a chronic dermatitis and hyperpigmentation from white and yellow petrolatum, and Plewig et al. (65) studied 735 black men who had allergic reactions to scalp creams and oils.

About 70% of these long-term users of pomades had a recognizable acneiform eruption of the forehead and temples. This eruption consisted mainly of uniformly closed comedones with occasional papulopustules. The more elaborate formulations (Noxzema, Dixie Peach, and Wildroot) induced pomade acne more frequently and more intensively than simpler preparations, such as mineral oil and petrolatum. Moreover, the application of five pomades to black skin under continuous occlusion for 8 weeks produced microscopic signs of early comedone formation. Pomade acne was indistinguishable histologically from acne vulgaris.

"Vaselinomas" and "Paraffinomas" Due to Injection of Petrolatum

Aronete and Grupper (66) issued a warning against intralacrimal injections of medication with pure petrolatum. Such injections are likely to cause complications manageable only by complicated surgical procedures. In the past, certain so-called dermatologic institutes have injected the skin with paraffin or petrolatum to remove wrinkles, form dimples, and otherwise change the normal contour of the face to suit the fancy of the patient. Tumors following such injections may occur as late as 3 years after the original injection.

Petrolatum as a Patch Test Vehicle

Generally, it is agreed that petrolatum (USP), also known as Vaseline or yellow soft paraffin, is the best vehicle for most test substances used in patch tests. Petrolatum is nonsensitizing, nonirritating, and so occlusive that it is possible to fix the patch test with nonocclusive, nonirritant adhesive tape. In many cases, this prevents adhesive reactions from interfering with test readings. In addition, test substances dissolved in petrolatum remain allergenic for at least 1 year.

When solvents are used instead of petrolatum as vehicles, there is the possibility they may evaporate, making the dissolved allergens irritant in nature. Because formaldehyde and propylene glycol do not dissolve well in petrolatum, they are tested in aqueous solution. In general, Fisher (58) found metals, such as nickel, cobalt, dichromates, and gold, present better patch test results when dissolved in aqueous solutions than when dissolved in petrolatum. Alcohol, acetone, methyl ethyl ketone, and butyrolactone have to be used as vehicles for patch testing organic chemicals, liquid resins, and resin components.

> **Petrolatum, a rare sensitizer, remains the best vehicle for most patch test allergens. Prolonged use of petrolatum can produce acneiform eruptions, irritation, and pigmentation. Injections of petrolatum into the skin can form tumors.**

Most recently, Dooms-Goossens and DeGreef (67), using several chromatographic and spectrometric procedures, established that the allergens present in pharmaceutical and cosmetic petrolatums are probably polycyclic aromatic hydrocarbons. These substances are impurities, and the quantity present is largely a function of the source of the petrolatum and the purification procedures. Because the aromatic portion in petrolatum is a complex and unstable mixture of chemically related agents, only two out of the several possible allergens present could be identified; they were most probably phenanthrene derivatives with molecular weights of 230 and 244.

OLIVE OIL

Van Joost et al. (68) state that sensitization to olive oil is seldom reported in the literature. By use of epicutaneous tests, a delayed type of hypersensitivity to pure, freshly prepared olive oil could be demonstrated in two patients. Patch tests with certain major constituents of olive oil, the methyl ester of linoleic acid, the glyceryl ester of palmitic acid, the glyceryl ester of stearic acid, glyceryl trioleate, and glycerides of arachidic acid, appeared to be negative. In one patient, a weak reaction to balsam of Peru was found. It is concluded that sensitization to olive oil must be taken into consideration, especially when it is used as a vehicle in patch testing.

SESAME OIL

"Immediate" urticarial reactions may occur from this oil (69). Several patients who applied a zinc oxide "liniment" to stasis ulcers were sensitized to sesame oil (70).

The principal allergens of sesame oil are sesamin and sesamolin (71). Patch testing may be done with sesame oil 100% "as is."

Sesame oil, a rare sensitizer, can produce allergic contact dermatitis when used on stasis ulcers.

CASTOR OIL

This oil may be used in cosmetics, particularly lipsticks, and may rarely produce allergic contact dermatitis (72,73).

LINDANE (KWELL)

This gamma benzene hexachloride product is used for scabies and pediculosis. The toxic effects from topical application have been reviewed by Matsum (74). No reports of allergic contact sensitivity have appeared.

Lindane (Kwell) may be toxic, but apparently it is not a sensitizer.

METHYL SALICYLATE

Methyl salicylate, the active ingredient in oil of wintergreen, is present in many over-the-counter liniments used for the treatment of muscle aches and bursitis but is usually not formulated into prescription drugs (Table 10.8). Hindson (75) reported that an ointment containing methyl salicylate sensitized a man whose eruption flared when he took aspirin.

Patients who have topical sensitization to methyl salicylate may flare when aspirin is ingested.

CERUMENEX (XERUMENEX)

This solvent preparation to dissolve ear wax contains 10% triethanolamine polypeptide condensate, which may produce allergic contact dermatitis (76,77).

VITAMIN A ACID (TRETINOIN, RETINOIC ACID)

Tretinoin produces an irritant dermatitis and scaling in most individuals, particularly in high concentrations. Several instances of allergic reactions have been reported (78–81).

Jordan et al. (81) found that two men on patch testing were sensitive to transretinoic acid. They were positive to 0.05% in petrolatum base and to 0.00625% in the commercial lotion diluted with alcohol. A cross-sensitivity was presumed, because neither man had had previous exposure, but the primary allergen was not identified.

TABLE 10.8. *Uses of Methyl Salicylate*

Ben-Gay External Analgesic Products (Leeming)
Bensulfoid Lotion (Poythress)
Black-draught Syrup (Chattem)
Deep-down Pain Relief Rub (JB Williams)
Heet Analgesic Liniment (Whitehall)
Heet Spray Analgesic (Whitehall)
Icy Hot Balm (Searle Consumer Products)
Icy Hot Rub (Searle Consumer Products)
Listerine Antiseptic (Warner-Lambert Co.)
Mentholatum Deep Heating Lotion (Mentholatum)
Mentholatum Deep Heating Rub (Mentholatum)
Panalgesic (Poythress)
Sinex Decongestant Nasal Spray (Vicks)
Soltice Quick-Rub (Chattem)
Vatronol Nose Drops (Vicks)
Vicks Inhaler (Vicks Health Care)
Vicks Sinex Decongestant Nasal Spray (Vicks)
Vicks Vatronol Nose Drops (Vicks)

Nordqvist and Mehr (78) reported a woman who had been sensitized by Retin-A liquid 0.05%, which she had used to treat a folliculitis of her legs.

Patch testing with tretinoin may be performed 0.05% in petrolatum or 0.01% in alcohol.

Tosti et al. (82) reported the sudden development of facial erythema and swelling after 1 year of Retin A cream 0.05% use. Patch tests were positive to tretinoin at 0.1% in petrolatum and 0.005% in alcohol.

Balato et al. (83) used tretinoin 0.05% in petrolatum and ethanol to identify sensitization to this retinoid best known for its irritant properties. Ten control subjects were negative, and they found nine other case reports in the literature.

VITAMIN A ACETATE

Exposure to vitamin A manufacturing led to contact dermatitis to retinyl acetate or vitamin A acetate (84). Patch tests were positive from 10% down to 0.1% in petrolatum. Retinol palmitate has previously been reported to cause contact dermatitis in cosmetics.

THIAMINE HYDROCHLORIDE (VITAMIN B$_1$, BETABION HYDROCHLORIDE, AND ANEURINE HYDROCHLORIDE)

Hypersensitivity to various vitamins has been reported, with thiamine accounting for the largest number of such cases. Allergic contact dermatitis may occur in workers who fill vials in its manufacture. The injection or ingestion of this vitamin in such sensitized individuals may produce an eczematous relapse in the form of a contact-type dermatitis (85,86).

Thiamine hydrochloride may cross-react with coenzyme B (diphosphothiamin) and cocarboxylase.

In the past, workers who filled vials with vitamin B$_1$ became sensitized to the vitamins. Such workers can acquire a "systemic" contact dermatitis on ingestion of the vitamin.

VITAMIN B$_6$

Vitamin B$_6$ is actually three different substances: pyridoxine, pyridoxal, and pyridoxamine. When a disulfide bridge joins two molecules of pyridoxine, the compound pyritinol is formed. Pyritinol has been reported to cause pemphigus-like eruptions, lichen planus–like eruptions, and photosensitive and erythema multiforme–like eruptions. Contact dermatitis from pyritinol can occur during its manufacture. It is marketed in Europe as Encephabol tablets, which have also caused airborne contact dermatitis (87).

VITAMIN B$_{12}$ (COBIONE AND BERUBIGEN)

When a patient has an allergic reaction to B$_{12}$, there are two possibilities: (a) The patient is allergic to vitamin B$_{12}$ itself, as reported by Young et al. (88), who described a case of sensitivity to Cobione, a B$_{12}$ concentrate, in which there was a delayed tuberculin-type reaction to the intradermal injection of B$_{12}$; and (b) the reaction is due to cobalt sensitivity. In one patient Fisher (89) studied, a positive patch test reaction to cobalt was correlated with an allergic reaction to vitamin B$_{12}$ in injectable Berubigen (1 mL of Berubigen contains 43.4 µg of cobalt). This cobalt-sensitive patient gave a positive patch reaction to 2% aqueous solution of cobalt chloride and to the vitamin B solutions in strengths of 100 and 1,000 µg/mL. In addition, there were positive delayed scratch and intradermal reactions to the vitamin B$_{12}$ solutions. The patient noted that after each injection of vitamin B$_{12}$, the injected area became red, tender, and pruritic but not eczematous. Oral ingestion of vitamin B$_{12}$ produced similar flares in the sites of previous injections. She also has an intractable hand eczema.

Rostenberg and Perkins (90) reported that a sensitive patient injected intradermally with crystalline vitamin B$_{12}$ gave a tuberculin-type action.

Vitamin B$_{12}$ sensitivity may be due to the vitamin itself or to cobalt.

VITAMIN D$_3$

The use of $1,25(OH)_2D_3$ for psoriasis is increasing. A report of a positive patch test noted only at the day 4 (delayed) reading with a negative test to the vehicle confirmed allergic contact dermatitis to this medicament (91).

The irritant properties of calcipotriol make it a challenging substance to evaluate for delayed hypersensitivity. De Groot (92) reported what he believes is the third clearly identified case of allergic contact dermatitis to this vitamin D$_3$ derivative. He used both 10 and 2 µg/mL in isopropanol for patch testing and had reactions at both concentrations. Studies of controls found 3 of 26 had transient weak reactions to the 10 µg concentration. Frosch and Rustemeyer (93) endorsed the 2 µg/mL calcipotriol patch test in isopropanol as the most suitable for identifying true allergy to this vitamin D derivative.

Contact sensitivity to calcipotriol was noted after 18 months of uneventful use in a patient with palmoplantar psoriasis (94). Positive patch tests were found down to 0.4 µg/mL. This patient was not sensitive to the closely related tacalcitol, which is another vitamin D derivative. Cross-reaction between tacalcitol and calcipotriol has been reported, but apparently it is not obligate.

VITAMIN E (ALPHA-TOCOPHEROL)

Vitamin E acts as an antioxidant. The natural vitamin E$_1$ obtained from plants such as germ oil and synthetic vitamin E (alpha-tocopherol) is incorporated into many cosmetics. There are several reports of allergic reactions to the vitamin in cosmetics and deodorants (95–97).

A vitamin E aerosol deodorant produced so many instances of widespread allergic dermatitis that it had to be withdrawn from the market. Many women pierce vitamin E capsules to rub the vitamin oil into their faces to "improve" the skin. Many such patients have had an allergic contact dermatitis from this procedure.

Topical vitamin E (alpha-tocopherol) is a potent sensitizer that can produce both "delayed" allergic contact dermatitis and "immediate" allergic urticaria.

Mitchell (98) reported that severe contact urticaria occurred in siblings who had been treated with a vitamin E preparation for burns.

A generalized dermatitis was caused by vitamin E in a soapy oats lotion. One percent tocopherol acetate in aqueous solution produced a positive reaction (99).

Thus, vitamin E is another product that practically never produces allergic reactions when ingested; when applied to the skin, it frequently produces allergic contact dermatitis and urticaria.

VITAMIN K

Two types of adverse cutaneous reactions occur with vitamin K$_1$ (phytomenadione or phytonadione). The more common reaction consists of erythematous plaques at the injection sites that resolve in a few weeks after the injection. Scleroderma-like lesions known as Texier's syndrome can develop without antecedent inflammation. In a report by Guidetti et al. (100), the sclerodermatous plaque developed over the buttock injection site, and patch tests with vitamin K$_1$ were negative while an intradermal test with 0.1 mL of vitamin K$_1$ was positive. Results of the intradermal test were negative in 10 control patients, suggesting that delayed hypersensitivity was involved in the scleroderma-like lesion.

In a review of the literature on vitamin K reactions, Bruynzeel et al. (101) found 52 cases and reported 2 more of their own. Reactions were not dose related and occurred with or without the presence of liver disease.

A 9-year-old child developed vesicular dermatitis of the buttock at the site of intramuscular vitamin K injections (10 mg/mL). Phytomenadione (vitamin K) at 10% and the injectable preparation both produced positive patch tests, whereas vitamins K$_2$ and K$_3$ were negative. Interestingly,

sublingual administration of 10 drops per day of the 10 mg/mL intramuscular preparation was tolerated without side effects (102).

SELENIUM SULFIDE

Various "Selsun" preparations, which are used for seborrhea and tinea versicolor, contain this compound. No allergic reaction to this compound has been reported. Toxic effects, however, may occur if use is prolonged on acutely inflamed areas of the scalp (103,104).

Selsun suspension is not a sensitizer but may cause a toxic reaction if used for prolonged periods on inflamed skin.

CAPTAN (N-TRICHLOROMETHYLTHIO-4-CYCLOHEXENE-1,2-DICARBOXIMIDE)

Captan derived from the mercaptans is used in over 300 products, particularly as a fungicide for agricultural crops, house plants, and nursery businesses. Captan is also used extensively in veterinary shampoos to treat animals for ticks and fleas.

In aqueous solutions, the captans release sulfur-containing compounds. Captan is also used as a bacteriostat in cosmetic formulations, especially for the hair, including Selsun, Selsun Blue, Vancide 89, and Vancide 89 RE. Captan is present in Dangard, used almost exclusively by barbers and hairdressers. Table 10.9 shows the numerous uses of Captan.

Marzulli and Maibach (105), using a concentration of 1%, both for induction and for challenge, sensitized 9 of 205 subjects (4.4%). Fregert (106) described a farmer who had allergic contact dermatitis from Captan.

Epstein (107) reported an instance of photoallergic contact dermatitis due to Dangard, which is a trade name for the antimicrobial-antiseborrheic ingredient used in Q.E.D. Hair Groom and Q.E.D. Shampoo, which are sold exclusively by barbers. Dangard is a trade name for Vancide 89 RE, which is used in cosmetic and pharmaceutical preparations.

TABLE 10.9. *Exposure to Captan*

Agricultural antifungal agent
Barbers and hairdressers
   Dangard
   Q. E. D. Shampoo
Cosmetic bacteriostat in shampoos
   Selsun
   Selsun Blue
   Vancide
Veterinary medicine
   Ticks and fleas

> **Captan, used widely as an agricultural fungicide and in veterinary medicine, is also used in such shampoos as Selsun, Vancide 89, and Dangard and by barbers in Q.E.D. Shampoo and Q.E.D. Hair Groom.**

COAL TAR

Coal tar used as a topical therapeutic agent is a rare cause of allergic contact dermatitis and skin cancer (108).

Tar and pitch (the residue after the distillation of tar) are phototoxic agents, which, in industry, can produce diffuse burning and erythema of the exposed skin. Edema and hyperpigmentation may develop later. "Tar itch" produces pruritus, folliculitis, and comedones on the trunk from oil-soaked clothes.

Emmett et al. (109) found that roofers working with coal-tar pitch develop a phototoxic keratoconjunctivitis that is enhanced markedly by ultraviolet exposure. Photosensitizing chemicals present in tar include anthracene, acridine, methylanthracene, pyrene, fluoranthene, and 3,4-benzpyrene.

As exposure to tar continues, poikilodermatous changes appear on the skin that are manifested by irregular areas of atrophy, loss of pigment with patch areas of hyperpigmentation, and diffuse telangiectasis on the neck, cheeks, and scrotum. Tar warts and multiple keratoacanthomas may develop (110–112).

> **Topical medicinal tar is a rare cause of allergic contact dermatitis or skin cancer. Industrial workers who are near tar or pitch may acquire conjunctivitis, tar "warts," and phototoxic dermatitis resulting in pigmentation, poikiloderma, and folliculitis.**

FLUOROURACIL

Efudex and Fluoroplex are used widely as chemotherapeutic agents for the treatment of solar keratoses and superficial basal-cell carcinomas.

Efudex solutions and creams are topical preparations containing the fluorinated pyrimidine 5-fluorouracil (5-FU), an antineoplastic antimetabolite. Efudex Solution consists of 2% or 5% fluorouracil (Roche) compounded with propylene glycol, tris (hydroxymethyl) aminomethane, hydroxypropyl cellulose, parabens, and edetate disodium (disodium edetate). Efudex Cream contains 5% fluorouracil in a vanishing cream base consisting of white petrolatum, stearyl alcohol, propylene glycol, polysorbate 60, and parabens.

> **Topical 5-FU preparations may contain propylene glycol, benzyl alcohol, and parabens, which may be sensitizers rather than the 5-FU itself.**

Fluoroplex 1% topical cream has the following formula: fluorouracil (1.0%), benzyl alcohol (0.5%), ethoxylated stearyl alcohol, mineral oil, isopropyl myristate, sodium hydroxide, and purified water. Fluoroplex 1% solution in a clear propyleneglycol base has the following formula: fluorouracil (1.0%), propylene glycol, sodium hydroxide, and hydrochloric acid.

Allergic Reactions to Fluorouracil

Leyden and Kligman (113) evaluated 1% and 5% formulations of 5-FU in the Kligman maximization procedure for inducing contact sensitization, and they were unable to induce contact allergy to 5-FU. On the basis of these experiments, they concluded that contact allergy to 5-FU is unlikely to be as common as suggested by others, and they classified 5-FU as a weak sensitizer at best.

Mansell et al. (114) and Sams (115) have reported allergic responses to 5-FU. Goette et al. (116) describe several patients who have acquired allergic contact dermatitis owing to 5-FU. Because irritant reactions are common with 5-FU, Goette et al. (116) suggested the following criteria for one differentiation of an allergic from an irritant contact dermatitis to topical fluorouracil: (a) development of a severely pruritic eczematous eruption at the site of contact with a topical fluorouracil preparation, (b) development of a widespread pruritic dermatitis away from the treated area during fluorouracil treatment or the occurrence of a flare phenomenon at a site exposed previously to the drug, (c) development of a positive epicutaneous skin test reaction to preservative-free test materials of fluorouracil in concentrations of 5% or 10%, (d) development of a pruritic indurated erythema with papules or vesicles at the site of the intracutaneous injections (0.1-mL injections of 50 mg/mL, 25 mg/mL, 10 mg/mL of fluorouracil in sterile water), (e) excellent correlation of the intracutaneous and epicutaneous reactions, and (f) compatible histologic findings (116).

The development of a severely pruritic eczematous dermatitis at the site of fluorouracil application in a fluorouracil-experienced patient should alert the clinician to the possibility of an acute allergic contact dermatitis to the drug. The simple testing methods outlined in this article can readily confirm or negate this diagnosis.

Ecdysis Due to Fluorouracil

Yaffee and Grots (117) found that the use of fluorouracil in three patients who had basal-cell carcinoma was followed by a peculiar necrosis, which, when curetted, shelled out completely like a snake skin. They have termed this "ecdysis."

Histologic examination revealed tumor necrosis, leukocytes, and fibrin. There have been no recurrences to date.

Yaffee and Grots (117) commented that the appearance of a swollen, discolored lesion in the site of the original basal-cell tumor is alarming. It contrasts with the usual erythematous and necrotic reaction seen in the response of basal-cell carcinoma to topical fluorouracil. It may be reassuring to the clinician to recognize the "ecdysis" of the necrotic tumor, which casts out the entire noxious lesion.

> **Allergic reaction may occur in reaction to fluorouracil accompanied by a severe, pruritic eczematous reaction and flare of previous treatment sites.**

Nonallergic Adverse Reactions to Fluorouracil

The most frequently encountered local reactions are pain, pruritus, hyperpigmentation, and burning at the site of application. Other local reactions include scarring, soreness, tenderness, suppuration, scaling, and swelling. Also reported are alopecia, insomnia, stomatitis, irritability, medicinal taste, photosensitivity, lacrimation, telangiectasia, and urticaria.

TOPICAL NITROGLYCERIN

Nitroglycerin administered sublingually or systemically almost never produced allergic reactions. Because nitroglycerin has become available in ointment form, however, there are several reports of allergic reactions to nitroglycerin administered in this form (118–120). Most individuals tolerate sublingual nitroglycerin after having been sensitized by the ointment.

Contact dermatitis among those who are engaged in the manufacture of nitroglycerin has been reported (121). Chandraratna and O'Dell (119) reported that one patient experienced an anaphylactoid reaction with oral mucosal and conjunctival edema within 6 hours of cutaneous application. Because of the possibility of a nitroglycerin withdrawal reaction, sublingual nitrate therapy should be instituted before discontinuing nitropaste treatment.

> **Sensitization to topical nitroglycerin does not usually preclude sublingual use. Application of a potent topical corticosteroid at the site of the application may minimize the allergic reaction.**

Hendricks and Dec (118) reported that topical nitroglycerin ointment is among the most effective long-acting vasodilators currently available. They reported two cases of contact dermatitis in which patch testing showed allergy to nitroglycerin-containing compounds. The severity of this dermatitis necessitated the discontinuation of topical nitroglycerin therapy in both patients. A potent corticosteroid cream applied once to previous nitroglycerin application sites prevented or minimized this dermatitis and enabled continuation of topical nitroglycerin therapy.

Topical nitroglycerin is now available in a transdermal system in which the nitroglycerin is incorporated into a disc. Three types are available: (a) Nitro-Dur (Key). This transdermal system contains nitroglycerin in a gel-like matrix composed of glycerin, water (purified), lactose, polyvinyl alcohol, providene, and sodium citrate to provide a continuous source of the active ingredient. Each unit is sealed in a polyester-foil-polyethylene laminate. The bandage portion consists of a medical-grade nonwoven, heat-sealable, microporous tape, which contains an acrylate adhesive. (b) Nitrodisc (Searle). Contains nitroglycerin (on lactose) polyethylene glycol, water, silicone, rubber, plasticizers, aluminum foil laminate, polyethylene foam, and acrylic adhesive. (c) Transderm-Nitro (CIBA). This system comprises four layers. Proceeding from the visible surface toward the surface attached to the skin, these layers are (i) a tan-colored backing layer (aluminized plastic) that is impermeable to nitroglycerin; (ii) a drug reservoir containing nitroglycerin adsorbed on lactose, colloidal silicon dioxide, and silicone medical fluid; (iii) an ethylene-vinyl acetate copolymer membrane that is permeable to nitroglycerin; and (iv) a layer of hypoallergenic silicone adhesive. Before use, a protective peel strip is removed from the adhesive surface.

Two patients were observed who were allergic to acrylate adhesive in the disc. In such cases, the silicon adhesive may be used (40).

Adverse cutaneous reactions to transdermal therapeutic systems (TTS) of nitroglycerin are said to occur in 10% to 70% of users. A prospective study (122) found that 15% of nitroglycerin TTS patients experienced an irritant reaction, which was transient. None of the 33 patients studied developed allergic contact dermatitis, and none had to stop treatment. A 0.5% aqueous or 2% petrolatum concentration was recommended for nitroglycerin patch testing to identify the allergic cases.

> **Nitroglycerin "transderm discs" may contain an acrylate adhesive to which some patients are allergic. Transderm-Nitro (CIBA) contains a silicon adhesive that may be substituted.**

GLUTARALDEHYDE (PENTANEDIAL)

The Nature of Glutaraldehyde

Glutaraldehyde (1,5-pentanedial), an aliphatic dialdehyde that forms colorless crystals, is soluble in water, alcohol, ether, and similar organic solvents. It is available most frequently as a 50% aqueous solution. It is used in a 2% water solution as a cold sterilizer, especially in hospital-medical work for sterilizing instruments, bronchoscopes, cystoscopes, and anesthetic equipment; in renal dialysis units for sterilizing forceps; and by patients at home for sterilizing their artificial kidney.

Relation of Cidex to Glutaraldehyde

Cidex is a 2% acidic glutaraldehyde, which is stable for long periods if stored in a cool place. When the buffering agent sodium bicarbonate is added, the resultant alkaline solution undergoes polymerization and loses its antimicrobial activity within 2 to 3 weeks. This alkaline Cidex is more active and quicker to take effect than the acidic glutaraldehyde.

Unbuffered solutions of glutaraldehyde are stable for long periods of time, have a mildly acid pH, and a negligible odor, and are not potently antimicrobial; however, when Cidex becomes buffered to an alkaline pH of 7.5 to 8.0 upon the addition of sodium bicarbonate, glutaraldehyde is "activated" and its antimicrobial (sporocidal, bactericidal, viricidal, fungicidal) activity is greatly enhanced for periods of up to 14 days (123).

Activated glutaraldehyde (Cidex) retains skin-sensitizing properties of pure glutaraldehyde. Furthermore, the relatively strong irritant effect of pure glutaraldehyde on the eyes, nasal passages, upper respiratory tract, and skin is enhanced slightly when this dialdehyde is activated.

> **Glutaraldehyde is used for treating warts, dermatophytosis, bullous disease, and hyperhidrosis. It is too irritating to use in the axillae and is an occasional sensitizer.**

Glutaraldehyde as a Therapeutic Agent

The Use of Glutaraldehyde as an Antifungal Agent

Glutaraldehyde has been shown to have antifungal properties. Jordan et al. (124) reported a case of acute contact dermatitis in a man who used glutaraldehyde for onychomycosis.

Glutaraldehyde in Waterless Hand Cleaners

Waterless hand cleaners are commonly used by machinists. Storrs (125) reported hand dermatitis among machinists from glutaraldehyde found in several brands of waterless hand cleaners.

Glutaraldehyde as a Therapeutic Agent for Warts

The use of glutaraldehyde for warts has occasionally been marked by irritation, but apparently no allergic reactions have been encountered from such use.

Glutaraldehyde as a Therapeutic Agent for Bullous Disease

Comaish (126) reported that topical glutaraldehyde decreased skin friction and enhanced resistance to friction injury produced at a given load in short-term experiments. A single application produces a detectable effect for up to 31 days. These observations partly explain glutaraldehyde's known antiperspirant action; however, similar observations have been made with dead skin in vitro. It is suggested that glutaraldehyde and similar substances may be useful when a reduction in friction trauma is necessary, such as in the case of epidermolysis bullosa and porphyria cutanea tarda.

Des Grosseilliers and Brisson (127) stated that in two patients who had localized epidermolysis bullosa (recurrent bullous eruption of the hands and feet or Weber-Cockayne syndrome), experimentally induced blisters were studied histopathologically. The blisters showed cleft formation in the suprabasal layers of the epidermis. Therapy with topically applied 10% glutaraldehyde was beneficial, but the irritant and skin-sensitizing side effects of this chemical proved a limiting factor for its use.

These authors concluded that the therapeutic use of topical glutaraldehyde presents three general shortcomings: (a) the solution causes brown discoloration of the soles; (b) because of its chemical composition and instability, the preparation must be kept refrigerated in order to remain therapeutically effective for a 1-month period, and a new supply of the solution must be prepared every month; and (c) glutaraldehyde is an irritant and a potential skin sensitizer, and the development of an allergic contact dermatitis in a patient precludes further extensive use of therapy.

Gordon (128), in commenting on Des Grosseliers and Brisson's article, stated that because allergic reactions to glutaraldehyde are quite rare, and because there is no specific treatment for localized bullous epidermolysis, the treatment with glutaraldehyde should not be discarded. Furthermore, the brown discoloration can be minimized by use of a 2% solution of glutaraldehyde, and three baths will remove the stain.

Gordon (129) has also advocated the use of glutaraldehyde for herpes zoster and simplex and pseudomonas infections. Gordon stated that he has received many requests for information on where to get glutaraldehyde and commented: "Any large hospital with an inhalation therapy department may be using buffered glutaraldehyde, (Cidex), as a sterilant" (130). Union Carbide, Ethicon, and the Arbrook Companies provide it. It is supplied as a 25% solution, by Matheson, Coleman, Bell, in 1-kg volume bottles, to which sodium bicarbonate is added to a pH of 7.5, as reported by London (131).

The fumes from glutaraldehyde may act as an irritant to the bronchial and laryngeal mucous membranes, and prolonged exposure could produce localized edema and symptoms suggestive of an allergic response.

The Use in Hyperhidrosis of the Soles

Maibach and Prystowsky (132) found that glutaraldehyde is effective for hyperhidrosis of the soles. A usage test was performed on the soles and antecubital fossae of six previously documented glutaraldehyde-sensitive subjects. All subjects had negative-usage test reactions when 25% glutaraldehyde was applied to the soles. But when tested on the antecubital fossae with 2.5% glutaraldehyde, these same patients developed severe dermatitis within 48 hours. These data demonstrate a striking variation by which glutaraldehyde-sensitive patients tolerate or react to its use in two diverse anatomic sites. Glutaraldehyde is not recommended for axillary hyperhidrosis.

Jordan et al. (124) reported on a man who developed an allergic contact hypersensitivity from the use of glutaraldehyde for hyperhidrosis of the soles.

Allergic Glutaraldehyde Dermatitis in the Medical and Allied Professions

Table 10.10 shows the exposure to glutaraldehyde in medical and allied professions. Certain X-ray film developing solutions contain glutaraldehyde. Fisher (133) reported allergic contact dermatitis in radiologists and technicians handling such films.

There are several reports of nurses who acquired allergic glutaraldehyde dermatitis from handling instruments sterilized with this compound (134–136). Also, a technician handling a renal dialysis unit and an inhalation therapy assistant acquired allergic contact dermatitis from contact with glutaraldehyde used as a cold sterilizing agent.

The Safety of Glutaraldehyde-Tanned Leather Shoes

There are no reports of shoe dermatitis developing from glutaraldehyde-tanned leather shoes. Jordan et al. (124) studied three patients who had allergic hypersensitivity to glutaraldehyde. Although all of them had positive patch test reactions to glutaraldehyde-tanned leather, none of them had shoe dermatitis. Even the patient who had hyperhidrosis was not sensitized by the use of glutaraldehyde.

Does Glutaraldehyde Cross-React with Formaldehyde?

In a report by Neering and van Ketel (137), test results with formaldehyde were negative in all of the glutaraldehyde-sensitive patients but one, a renal dialysis assistant who was in contact with both formaldehyde and glutaraldehyde and had positive reactions on patch testing. Maibach (138) found that 20 patients with positive patch test reactions to 1% aqueous glutaraldehyde all had negative reactions to 2% aqueous formaldehyde.

Glutaraldehyde is prone to irritant reactions even when tested at 1% in petrolatum; 9 of 13 reactions were found to be irritant when evaluated by Hansen and Menné (139). They further studied 0.1% in petrolatum and detected allergy in 2 of 884 but could not speculate on how many other cases might have been missed. They did not conclude what the ideal patch test concentration for glutaraldehyde should be.

Garcia (140) reported on a man who had positive reactions to both glutaraldehyde and formaldehyde. This was not unusual, because he was exposed extensively to formaldehyde in his work as a prosecutor's assistant; apparently, however, he had never been exposed to glutaraldehyde.

Glutaraldehyde Rarely Cross-Reacts with Formaldehyde

Belani and Priedklans (141) described an "epidemic" of serious laryngeal injury associated with endotracheal intubation. Glutaraldehyde used for sterilization was suspected. Since the introduction of single-use disposable endotracheal tubes, there have been no further cases of "pseudomembranous laryngotracheitis."

Effect of Glutaraldehyde Vapors

Zach (142) suspects that several radiologists and X-ray technicians have developed asthma and laryngeal edema from the inhalation of the glutaraldehyde present in certain X-ray film emulsions.

Hansen (143) has emphasized that glutaraldehyde used as a hospital disinfectant is an occupational hazard. Table 10.11 lists industrial exposures to glutaraldehyde.

TABLE 10.10. *Exposure to Glutaraldehyde in Medical and Allied Professions*

Buffered (Cidex)
  Renal dialysis
  Pulmonary apparatus
Cold sterilizing solutions
Embalming
Tissue fixative
X-ray solution

TABLE 10.11. *Industrial Exposure to Glutaraldehyde*

Clothing
Hardening of photographic gelatin
Increase in water resistance in wallpaper
Intermediate in resin and dyes
Liquid fabric softener
Tanning of leather

> **Medical and allied professionals, including X-ray film handlers, may be exposed to glutaraldehyde.**

CANTHARIDIN (SPANISH FLY)

Spanish fly, or cantharides, is a powder derived from certain crushed beetles that contain cantharidin, which is a vesicant and a potent irritant to the gastrointestinal and genitourinary mucosa (144). The local application of cantharidin is used for treatment of resistant plantar and periungual warts (Cantharone, Cantharone Plus, Verr-Canth, and Verrusol). Two patients seen by Dilaimy developed a severe reaction with edema, redness, and tenderness accompanied by lymphangitis (145). The reaction started about 30 hours after therapy. According to the author, this reaction is not uncommon.

> **Cantharidin, a powerful vesicant, may produce lymphangitis.**

BORIC ACID

Although most cases of borism are due to accidental ingestion of boric acid, many have been traced to its topical application. Valdes-Dapena and Arey (146), in a review of the literature on boric acid poisoning, found that 53 of 172 patients had been treated externally for burns, wounds, or an eruption. A detailed account of boric acid intoxication via a transcutaneous route appeared in the *Archives of Dermatology* some years ago (147). A dusting powder, with an undisclosed concentration of boric acid but nevertheless advertised as "safe for baby's sensitive skin," was applied several times daily to a 3-year-old boy who had diaper rash. Edema of the eyelids, exfoliation of the axillary areas, and bullae with exfoliation of the suprapubic area and along the inner aspect of the thighs appeared after 3 months of use. The child was febrile, restless, and irritable. Culture showed no bacterial growth. The diagnosis of borism was confirmed by the finding of high levels of boron in the blood (5.4 mg/dL as compared to a norm of 0.08 mg/dL). The findings suggest toxic epidermal necrolysis resulting from percutaneous absorption of the drug.

Topically applied drugs that have associated systemic effects are shown in Table 10.12.

MECHLORETHAMINE (NITROGEN MUSTARD)

Contact Allergic Dermatitis

Approximately 50% of patients who apply topical mechlorethamine develop cutaneous sensitization of the delayed cell-mediated type. The sensitization is much less frequently of the immediate anaphylactoid (urticarial) type (148–150). The probability of a delayed hypersensitivity reaction depends on many factors, including age of the patient, type and extent (stage) of disease, and previous or concurrent administration of immunosuppressant agents (148). Attempts to prevent allergic sensitization by administering preliminary small doses of mechlorethamine (HN_2) intravenously for induction of specific immunologic tolerance or by administering ultraviolet radiation with or without psoralen for their inhibitory effects on Langerhans cell function have been incompletely successful (151,152).

Contact allergic dermatitis usually develops between 2 and 4 weeks after initiation of topical therapy and may rarely manifest initially at lesion sites only or as an eczematous hand dermatitis. Distinction from a simple irritant dermatitis may be clinically difficult, and open patch testing may be required to clarify the nature of the reaction. For this purpose, fresh HN_2 solution, which is diluted to provide 10 mg in 0.1 mL, is applied uniformly over a 3 × 5-cm area of normal skin, usually on the back. For patients who have positive skin tests, both topical and systemic procedures have been used for desensitization.

Contact Irritant Dermatitis

Substantial irritation from the usual dose of HN_2 (10 mg/50 mL applied once daily) may be encountered in some patients, particularly in those who have generalized erythroderma or atrophic skin from advanced age or prior radiotherapy. In such sensitive patients, the concentration or frequency of topical HN_2 applications may be reduced temporarily until the skin becomes "hardened" to the irritant effects. Concurrent administration of a topical corticosteroid

TABLE 10.12. *Topical Drugs and Associated Systemic Effects*

Boric acid	Bullae, exfoliation
Corticosteroids	Adrenocortical suppression
? Gamma benzene hexachloride	Neurotoxicity
Hexachlorophene	Neurotoxicity
	Vacuolar encephalopathy
Lomustine	Pancytopenia
Mercurials	Acrodynia
	Nephrotic syndrome
Phenol	Dizziness, collapse
Podophyllin	Coma, acute toxicity
Resorcinol	Chronic myxedema
	Exogenous ochronosis
	Hemoglobinuria
	Hemolytic anemia
	Methemoglobinemia
Salicylic acid	Deep, rapid breathing
	Dizziness, tinnitus
	Purpura
	Scarlatiniform rash
? Selenium sulfide	Tremor, GI distress
	Garlic breath

preparation also is useful in this circumstance. Optionally, the physician may prepare the HN_2 in a water-free vehicle (153).

Drying Effect

Daily applications of aqueous solutions of HN_2 to the skin may aggravate preexisting xerosis and cause pruritus. This effect can usually be counteracted by adding 1 to 3 tsp of an emulsified bath oil or propylene glycol to the HN_2 mixture. If necessary, additional emollient preparations may be applied to the skin after the HN_2 solution has dried.

Hyperpigmentation

Lesion sites heal frequently with hyperpigmentation, but normal skin also may darken dramatically, indicative of a direct melanogenic influence. Such pigmentation is reversible and decreases gradually in most patients even if topical therapy is continued.

Epidermal Carcinogenesis

This remains a potential risk as with other therapeutic modalities used to treat mechlorethamine. In patients treated for extended periods of time, an increased frequency (10%) of squamous cell carcinomas and keratoacanthomas has been noted on sun-exposed areas in whites, indicating at least a promoting activity of HN_2 on epidermal neoplastic development. Therefore, patients who have clinical evidence of solar damage and patients previously treated with ultraviolet or ionizing radiation should be monitored carefully. In addition, a few patients have developed epidermal neoplasms in areas not usually associated with solar-induced cancer, particularly the genital skin, indicating that HN_2 has initiating as well as promoting activity. These observations are quite consistent with animal studies that show topically applied HN_2 to be a potent carcinogen. No apparent increase has been made in the frequency of malignant melanomas, internal malignancies, or any demonstrable mutagenic effect on the reproductive system of patients treated with topical HN_2.

Conclusions

After a quarter century of use, topical HN_2 chemotherapy for mycosis fungoides has been shown to have an excellent therapeutic profile (benefit/risk ratio) that compares favorably with other treatment modalities. The major issues that must be addressed in the future concern the mechanism of action on malignant lymphoid infiltrates in the skin, the determination of the curative potential of topical HN_2 chemotherapy in mycosis fungoides, and the modification of existing therapeutic procedures to minimize potential adverse effects, particularly epidermal carcinogenesis.

Price et al. (153) state that the use of topical mechlorethamine hydrochloride in the treatment of skin disease has been restricted because of the frequent development of contact dermatitis. A series of 24 patients who had mycosis fungoides in stages 1A (8 patients), 1B (15 patients), and 2 (1 patient) were treated with ointment-based mechlorethamine prepared by an anhydrous method. This preparation was therapeutically effective. Complete clearing occurred in 15 of 18 patients who had the active disease over evaluation periods of up to 27 months, and 1 patient had partial clearing. Two patients showed a partial relapse during their evaluation periods. The incidence of contact dermatitis was very low: 8% in individuals who had a history of hypersensitivity to mechlorethamine and 0% in patients who were exposed to the medication for the first time. This new preparation is effective therapy for mycosis fungoides. Patient use is associated with minimal side effects.

> The treatment of mycosis fungoides with ointment-based nitrogen mustard has been reported as lowering the incidence of contact dermatitis.

Thomsen and Mikkelsen (154) stated that rubber gloves do not protect nurses who apply nitrogen mustard to patients. They found that one type of glove made of polyvinyl chloride (PVC) protected the nurse against penetration of nitrogen mustard. Rubber gloves did not give protection, and a polyethylene glove also permitted penetration of nitrogen mustard.

> Nitrogen mustard frequently produces allergic contact dermatitis. Desensitization procedures are difficult and hazardous. Contact urticaria and anaphylaxis may also occur. Heavy-duty vinyl gloves, but not rubber gloves, protect medical personnel who apply nitrogen mustard to patients.

Fisher (40) observed several dermatologists who became allergic to nitrogen mustard, which they applied to patients while wearing rubber gloves.

COUMARIN

The coumarins are used in over 300 products in the United States in acne preparations, fungal solutions, antiseptics, deodorants, "skin fresheners," hair dyes, and shampoos. They encompass a large class of synthetics, as well as naturally occurring substances. Exposure to these agents is common. Coumarin itself is present in several plants and essential oils (e.g., balsam of Peru) and has been in extensive use as a fragrance commonly incorporated into soaps, detergents, toiletries, cosmetics, sunscreens, and perfumes.

Other coumarin derivatives, such as limettin (5,7-dimethoxycoumarin), occur naturally in bergamot oil. Several other coumarin derivatives have been synthesized for use as optical bleaches and as fragrances.

Allergic contact dermatitis was reported in a patient who applied a coumarin-containing ointment to a foot ulcer (155).

Kaidbey and Kligman (156) report that coumarin and several of its derivatives were investigated for their photosensitizing properties. With a few exceptions, the coumarins are potentially strong photocontact sensitizers but do not evoke phototoxic reactions. Substitution at the six or seven positions of the benzopyrone ring confers photoallergic capability, whereas hydrogenation abolishes activity. Photo cross-reactions among closely related derivatives can develop.

Kwong et al. (157) reported that the systemic administration of warfarin may produce generalized erythema. Schleicher and Fricker (158) reported that necrosis of the skin developed soon after the initiation of coumarin therapy in an elderly woman. Inadvertent rechallenge resulted in similar lesions. Coumarin necrosis has been found to relate to low levels of protein C rather than an allergic mechanism and is reversed by protein C concentrate administration (159).

> **Topical coumarins may produce allergic contact dermatitis and photoallergic reactions. Systemic coumarins may produce generalized erythema or local necrosis.**

HEPARIN

There are several types of heparin and related anticoagulants. Unfractionated heparin refers to high molecular weight heparins such as Liquemin N 25000 and Thrombophob 25000. Fractionated heparins refer to low molecular weight heparins that have once a day dosing for easier patient use. Examples of low molecular weight heparins include dalteparin (Fragmin), enoxaparin (Lovenox), reviparin (Clavarine), andeparin (Normiflu), and nadroparin (Fraxiparine). Heparinoids include danaparoid (Orgaran) and pentosan polysulfate (Fibrezym). Hirudin is an anticoagulant derived from leeches and is available in a recombinate form: lepirudin (Refludan).

Although heparin allergy is rare, one patient with such an allergy who developed an eczematous reaction to subcutaneous heparin was able to tolerate 2,600 units of anti-factor Xa low-molecular-weight heparin when coadministered with 250 mg of methylprednisolone and 2 mg of clemastine hydrogen fumarate. The patient also tolerated subcutaneous glycosaminoglycan polysulfate. This treatment was not recommended for skin necrosis patients (160).

> **Eczematous plaques rather than skin necrosis are the hallmark of allergy to heparin.**

Eczematous plaques can occur around sites of subcutaneous injection of heparin due to delayed hypersensitivity. Topical application of low-molecular-weight heparin in gel form can also cause contact dermatitis. Cross-reactions between fractionated and nonfractionated heparins have occurred (161). Moreau et al. (162) reported a case of delayed hypersensitivity to three low-molecular-weight heparins and unfractionated subcutaneous calcium heparin but not to intravenous sodium heparin.

Koch et al. (163) reported a case of heparin sensitivity in a patient in whom pentosan polysulfate had to be used as an alternative due to broad cross-reactivity among various types of heparin. Even this agent became problematic and required simultaneous administration of topical corticosteroids to the injection sites as reactions occurred after about 2 weeks of use. Eczematous plaques rather than skin necrosis are the hallmark of allergy to heparin. In their case, unfractionated heparins from three suppliers and low-molecular-weight heparins from four companies all produced reaction. The latter group included dalteparin-sodium, enoxaparin-sodium, and reviparin-sodium. Even the heparinoid, danaparoid-sodium, was positive on patch and intradermal testing. Contrary to the experience in the case of Koch et al., tolerance of intravenous heparin and heparinoid in the face of cutaneous reactions to subcutaneous injections of heparins was reported by Boehncke et al. (164).

The need for heparin in patients who are developing adverse subcutaneous reactions led to a study of the safety of intravenous (IV) heparin in this setting. Eight patients who tested positive to either high- or low-molecular-weight heparin were given IV Liquemin N 25000 without any adverse reactions. The high-molecular-weight heparins Liquemin N 25000 and Thrombophob 25000 and the low-molecular-weight heparins Fragmin P, Fraxiparine, and the heparinoid Orgaran, as well as sodium pentosan polysulfate (Fibrezym), were the agents that had caused the subcutaneous reactions (165).

Allergy to the heparin alternative pentosan polysulfate was found in a patient who was positive to multiple heparins but had never had exposure to pentosan polysulfate. This patient was sensitive to certoparin, dalteparin, enoxaparin, nadroparin, and reviparin, all proven by patch tests. She was also sensitive to danaparoid, heparin-calcium, and heparin-sodium by intracutaneous testing. In this case, hirudin was tolerated (166).

HIRUDIN

A hirudin-containing ointment was used to treat hemorrhoids, but a 64-year-old man applied it to thrombophlebitis of his arm and developed contact dermatitis. A positive patch test produced by 20% raw hirudin in ethanol was confirmed with recombinant hirudin. Hirudin is the anticoagulant-antiinflammatory agent extracted from leeches. Twenty controls did not react to hirudin, and in vitro tests were also positive (167).

LANOLIN

Lanolin (wool fat, wool grease, wool wax, wool alcohol, and adeps lanae anhydrous) and its various esters, fatty acids, and aliphatic alcohols are used in many topical medicaments and cosmetics.

Lanolin is a natural product obtained from the fleece of sheep, and its constituents vary from time to time and place to place.

Composition

Lanolin contains sterols, fatty alcohols, and fatty acids. The lanolin sterols (lanolin alcohols or wool alcohols) include principally cholesterol, lanosterol, and agnesterol and are built from one or more benzene rings.

Commercially, these wool alcohols are called Cerolan, Type HO, Hartolan, Golden Dawn, and Nimco. Cholesterol is the major ingredient of lanolin alcohol, and commercial lanolin products list the cholesterol content. Further studies are required to establish whether these lanolin alcohols are the sole or main sensitizers in lanolin (168).

The fatty alcohols are long-chained and include the closely related stearyl and cetyl alcohols. The fatty acids, the other ingredients of lanolin, have not been found to be sensitizers.

Modifications

Acetylated lanolin (Modulan), according to Cronin (168), is less of a sensitizer than plain lanolin. Dewaxed lanolin (Lantrol), formed by a solvent crystallization process, is also claimed to cause less sensitization than lanolin.

Another modification is hydrogenated lanolin. Vollum (169) reported that it is being used more frequently in the pharmaceutical and cosmetic industry because it is colorless, odorless, free from tackiness, and more hydrophilic than lanolin.

Hydrogenation is carried out by heating lanolin with a catalyst to 330°C at a pressure of 180 atmospheres. The absorption of hydrogen is complete within a half hour, and the hydrogenated lanolin contains dihydrocholesterol, other hydrogenated steroids, and some saturated alcohol. It was hoped originally that hydrogenated lanolin, or a modification, could be used in cases of lanolin sensitivity, but some patients show a marked sensitivity to hydrogenated lanolin and not to the plain lanolin. Dermatitis owing to hydrogenated lanolin may be missed if patients are patch tested with wool alcohols or plain lanolin and not the hydrogenated variety.

Patch Tests for Lanolin Sensitivity

Many investigators routinely test with 30% wool alcohol in petrolatum, but because it may not be the sensitizing substance in lanolin, patch testing should be performed with lanolin. Thune's (170) investigation indicates that the addition of salicylic acid to lanolin or Eucerin may cause false-positive reactions. Patch tests for wool fat sensitivity should be performed with lanolin without the addition of salicylic acid.

Newcomb (171) emphasizes that lanolin is a complex natural material, which is never completely identified because of the wide variations in purity. The development of new derivatives and further purification may contribute to lowering the incidence of skin reactions to this emollient (172).

> **Patch test results with lanolin alcohols should be verified by testing natural lanolin from several sources.**

Oleffe et al. (173) emphasized that lanolin is a complex mixture of esters and polyesters of 33 alcohols with high molecular weights and 36 fatty acids. He made the following points: (a) The response of tested patients varies greatly; thus, a patient may react to one brand of lanolin and not to another. (b) The lanolin alcohols are plainly responsible for allergy to lanolin. (c) The Trolab wool alcohol test is reliable for detecting lanolin allergy. (d) A positive reaction to wool alcohols should prompt the dermato-allergist to test the patient with the lanolin preparation he or she actually will use. (e) The hydrogenated lanolin that was tested had a very slight allergenic capacity, whereas in Japan, hydrogenated lanolin appears to be a strong sensitizer.

The exact allergenic fraction awaits clarification. It is still unknown whether or not lanolin-sensitive patients can tolerate modified or purified lanolin and its derivatives.

> **Lanolin is a natural product that is an important sensitizer. The exact sensitizing component has not been isolated. Lanolin-sensitive patients can sometimes tolerate one lanolin preparation but not another.**

The results of Giorgini et al. (174) confirm the sensitizing action of lanolin alcohols and the fact that acetylation, ethylenation, and transesterification eliminate the allergenic activity of lanolin.

One must stress, however, that the various chemical treatments capable of reducing the sensitizing potential of lanolin may prejudice its use as an excipient and that Sulzberger et al. (175) pointed out that a considerable reduction in the emulsifying powers of acetylated derivatives compromises their usefulness in pharmaco-cosmetic preparations.

> **Chemical treatments to reduce the allergenicity of the lanolin alcohols may reduce the usefulness of lanolin as an excipient.**

Sensitizing Potential of Lanolin

The incidence of lanolin sensitivity is a controversial subject. Kligman (176) concludes that "[l]anolin is an extremely weak sensitizer. Its reputation as an allergen has been vastly inflated by reports emanating from European clinics where patients with chronic eczema have been treated with lanolin-based medicaments for many years. In the healthy population, the incidence is vanishingly small. Lanolin exposure takes place in many ways besides skin care products" (refer to Table 10.13). "I was not able to discover a single reported case among workers engaged in recovering wool wax, in refining it, in transporting it, or among wool sorters."

There is general agreement, however, that lanolin frequently produces allergic contact dermatitis when applied to stasis eczemas and ulcers.

> **Lanolin sensitivity is very low in noneczematous skin, moderate in atopic and other eczema dermatoses, and high in stasis eczema and ulcers.**

Breit and Bandmann (177) found that 13.2% of 326 cases of leg eczema were sensitive to wool alcohols. Of the 43 Eucerin-positive patients of Bandmann and Reichenberger (178), about 70% had stasis eczemas. Thus, stasis dermatitis patients are at unusually high risk.

Lanolin allergy is rare in patients who have chronic skin diseases that are not of the eczematous type (e.g., psoriasis, lichen planus, and bullous diseases).

Cronin et al. (179) showed that the proportion of atopic patients reacting to wool alcohols was comparable to that of

TABLE 10.13. *Lanolin: Noncosmetic and Industrial Exposure*

Fur
Furniture polishes
Leather
Metallic corrosion preventatives
Paper
Printing inks
Shoe polishes
Textile finishes

other eczematous patients, except those patients who had stasis eczema.

> **Allergic reactions to Eucerin may be due to its content of lanolin alcohols or to methylchloroisothiazolinone/methylisothiazolinone (MCI/MI), the present preservative in Eucerin Cream.**

TRANSDERMAL ESTROGEN

The Estraderm TTS delivers 0.05 mg of estrogen per 24 hours. About 17% of patients have cutaneous reactions, but only about 2% stop because of the reaction. The exact nature of the adverse reactions has been difficult to pinpoint (180). Ethanol was incriminated in some cases (181) and estrogen (estradiol) in others (182). Robert Adams (personal communication) observed patients who could tolerate the Estraderm TTS if they let about 1 minute elapse between opening the patch and placing it on the skin.

Most reactions to transdermal estradiol are irritant, but allergies to the adhesive, hydroxypropyl cellulose and ethanol, as well as one case of allergy to estradiol itself, have been reported (1990). A second case due to 17-beta-estradiol proven by a positive patch test to 4% in ethanol was reported by Boehncke and Gall (183). Their patient was tolerant of the oral use of this agent before and after contact sensitization, as has been seen with clonidine and occasionally other agents.

Not all estradiol sensitive patients induced by Estraderm TTS are tolerant of oral estrogen. Two such cases were reported from Portugal (184). Diffuse morbilliform erythema occurred 5 to 16 days after resumption of oral estrogen therapy. As the eruption is not life threatening, a trial of oral estrogen was not considered to be contraindicated when cutaneous sensitization is proven.

TRANSDERMAL TESTOSTERONE

Contact dermatitis to transdermal testosterone patch (Andropatch) was traced to a positive patch test reaction to testosterone propionate 1% in ethanol 90% (185). The patient also reacted to progesterone and testosterone undecenoate, the latter of which was tested at 2.5% in oil. He tolerated intramuscular injections of a preparation containing testosterone propionate (Sustanon 250).

Jordan (186) compared the testosterone patch (Androderm, SmithKline Beecham) with a scrotal system (Testoderm Testosterone Transdermal System, Alza Corp.) and found less topical irritation with the scrotal system. His patients had reactions using the nonscrotal system, but no reaction was seen when they switched to the scrotal system. This suggested that testosterone was not the responsible substance.

TRANSDERMAL NICOTINE

In addition to nicotine itself causing contact dermatitis in transdermal systems, a variety of acrylates may be present in these patches and can cause allergic contact dermatitis (187).

About 7% of patients using a nicotine TTS experience skin reactions. A 10% aqueous nicotine base concentration can be used for patch test purposes. Fourteen patients intolerant of the device were evaluated; 5 proved allergic, and 9 acquired irritant dermatitis (188).

Although allergy to nicotine can be a cause for adverse reactions to the transdermal nicotine patches, von Bahr and Wahlberg (189) point out that vasodilation is a normal pharmacological effect of nicotine that can be confused with allergy. In their patient it occurred at from 10% to 30% nicotine levels but not at lower levels.

NICOTINIC ACID ESTERS

Nicotinic acid esters have been used as topical rubefacients and generally produce erythema lasting from 2 to 4 hours. Benzyl nicotinate and bitoxyethyl nicotinate produced delayed (72-hour) reactions confirmed by 2.5% concentrations as patch tests in petrolatum (190).

MITOMYCIN C

Instillation of mitomycin C, an antineoplastic antibiotic produced by *Streptomyces caespitosus,* into the bladder is followed by an acral eruption that may also affect genital or buttocks skin. A 0.1% concentration in petrolatum is used for patch testing (191,192). Up to 9% of patients receiving the treatment may experience this side effect, which usually follows five to eight bladder instillations (193).

MINOXIDIL

Topical minoxidil at 2% concentration in a vehicle of propylene glycol, ethanol, and water has been used to partially reverse androgenetic alopecia in men and women. Allergic contact dermatitis (35 cases) and photoallergic contact dermatitis (1 case) have been reported from an occupational exposure (194). Patient use for alopecia has also been associated with allergic contact dermatitis. In some cases, patch tests in petrolatum were negative and were only found positive with the addition of propylene glycol to facilitate percutaneous absorption (195,196).

OPHTHALMIC TOPICAL PRODUCTS

Cycloplegics

An ophthalmic preparation used before eye examinations to dilate the pupil was found to cause contact dermatitis (197). The agent was cyclopentolate hydrochloride 0.5%. Patch tests with this concentration were positive in the patient and negative in 20 controls.

The mydriatic tropicamide is used diagnostically at a 1% concentration. It is sold under the name Mydriacyl and is used to obtain mydriasis and cycloplegia. Boukhman and Maibach (198) had no trouble eliciting a positive patch test to 1% tropicamide in petrolatum, and this was negative in 20 controls. The patient had experienced dermatitis of the face, eyelids, and periorbital skin after this agent had been used for diagnostic purposes.

Eyelid and facial dermatitis occurred in a 43-year-old woman who applied eyedrops to patients in an ophthalmology clinic in her capacity as a nurse (199). Homatropine 1% aqueous was strongly positive on patch testing. This cycloplegic is a semisynthetic tertiary amine antimuscarinic. The patient also reacted to phenylephrine 10% aqueous, which was also a component of eyedrops that she instilled in patients' eyes.

Beta-blockers

Contact dermatitis has been reported from the following beta-blockers: practolol, timolol, metoprolol, oxprenolol, metipranolol, befunolol, levobunolol, betaxolol, and propranolol (200).

Beta-adrenergic receptor antagonists (beta-blockers) are used to treat glaucoma. These ophthalmic preparations cause dermatitis of the eyelids and periorbital areas. Koch (201) reported three such cases. In two of the cases the sensitizer was timolol maleate, and in one both levobunolol and pilocarpine. No cross-reactivity to other beta-blockers was seen. Skin stripping before patch testing was helpful in identifying these cases.

Alpha 2-Adrenergic Agents

Eyedrops of apraclonidine, a selective alpha 2-adrenergic agent, are used to treat glaucoma in patients who are intolerant of beta-blockers. Adverse reactions to topical 0.5% and 0.1% apraclonidine range from 21% to 48%, and two cases with positive patch tests reported from Spain support the mechanism as being delayed hypersensitivity (202).

Mydriatics

In a study of mydriatic eyedrops (phenylephrine, tropicamide, and cyclopentolate hydrochloride), it was determined that patch tests were not as sensitive as direct instillation into the conjunctival sac in the detection of allergy (203). In 31 subjects studied, 94% were sensitive to phenylephrine. Patch tests detected only 68% of those allergic using 1% and 10% concentrations in both aqueous and petrolatum vehicles. Twenty-four percent of phenylephrine-allergic subjects were detected only by conjunctival challenge.

Carbonic Anhydrase Inhibitors

Carbonic anhydrase inhibitors are used for glaucoma therapy. A topical carbonic anhydrase inhibitor, dorzolamide, has caused eyelid dermatitis when used to treat glaucoma. Dorzolamide is a sulfonamide, and conjunctivitis and lip eczema are estimated to occur in about 4% of users (204).

Miscellaneous Ophthalmics

Ketotifen fumarate used as an eyedrop to treat allergic conditions has caused contact dermatitis of the periorbital skin (205).

Pilocarpine produced both allergic and photoallergic conduct allergy, and on patch testing the reaction was first noticed at day 7, which is quite late. A use test took 3 weeks to become positive. Pilagan 2% (pilocarpine nitrate) and Pilocar 4% (pilocarpine HCl) may be used for patch testing (206).

Rubidium iodide is thought to interact with lens opacification and is used to prevent cataracts. Contact dermatitis was reported and confirmed with a 1% concentration in petrolatum (207).

To prevent fibrosis of the cornea after chemical trauma, topical d-penicillamine was used. This can cross-react with penicillin and cause contact dermatitis, even in the absence of penicillin allergy. This was confirmed with 1% and 3% aqueous patch tests in a patient who used d-penicillamine eyedrops (208).

ß-Interferon eyedrops produced contact conjunctivitis and dermatitis at a 1:32 dilution. There was a prior report of allergy to interferon-a 2 C, but the ß-interferon patient did not cross-react with α- or γ-interferon (209).

Hard contact lenses that were cleaned with Aersolv produced eyelid dermatitis due to cocamidopropyl betaine present at 1.8%. A 1% concentration in petrolatum was positive, as was the product tested as is (210).

Herbst and Maibach (211) reviewed the many reports of ophthalmic sensitivity and suggested the patch test concentrations given in Table 10.14.

To their list of ophthalmic allergens Herbst and Maibach added prednisolone, diclofenac, tetracaine, ketotifen

TABLE 10.14. Potential Ophthalmologic Contact Allergens*

Class	Compound	Patch test concentration (%)	Vehicle
Preservatives	Benzalkonium chloride	0.1	aq
	Benzethonium chloride	1.0	aq
	Chlorhexidine gluconate	1.0	aq
	Cetalkonium chloride	0.1	aq
	Sodium EDTA	1.0	aq
	Sorbic acid	2.5	pet
	Thimerosal (Merthiolate)	0.1	pet
Beta-blocking Agents	Befunolol	1.0	aq
	Levobunolol HCl	1.0	aq
	Metipranolol	2.0	aq
	Metoprolol	3.0	aq
	Timolol	0.5	aq
Mydriatics	Atopine sulfate	1.0	aq
	Epinephrine HCl	1.0	aq
	Phenylephrine HCl	10.0	aq
	Scopolamine hydrobromide	0.25	aq
Antibiotics	Bacitracin	5.0	pet
	Chloramphenicol	5.0	pet
	Gentamycin sulfate	20.0	pet
	Kanamycin	10.0	pet
	Neomycin sulfate	20.0	pet
	Polymixin B sulfate	20.0	pet
Antiviral drugs	Idoxuridine	1.0	pet
	Trifluridine	5.0	pet
Antihistaminics	Chlorpheniramine maleate	5.0	pet
	Sodium cromoglycate	2.0	aq
Anesthetics	Benzocaine	5.0	pet
	Procaine	5.0	pet
	Oxyburprocaine	0.5	aq
	Proxymetacaine	0.5	aq
Enzymatic cleaners	Papaine	1.0	pet
	Tegobetaine	1.0	aq
Miotics	Pilocarpine	1.0	aq
	Tolazoline	10.0	aq
	Echothiophate iodine	1.0	aq
Other	Epsilon-amino caproic acid	1.0	aq

*From Ref. 211. Used with permission.

fumarate, resorcinol, tobramycin sulfate, dipivalyl epinephrine hydrochloride, cyclopentolate hydrochloride, and betaxolol (212).

INTERFERON

Reactions to injections of interferon (α and β) are common and may occur in up to 65% of patients. Erythema and infiltration are most common, but necrosis can also occur. Injection of less than 200,000 IU/mL are used to try to check for allergy with β-interferon. Depth of injection appears to be the prime determinant of whether a reaction will occur, with deeper reactions being less problematic (213).

SPIRONOLACTONE

Topical spironolactone has been used to treat androgenetic alopecia, hirsutism, and acne. In this form, contact dermatitis has occurred with concentrations ranging from 2% to 5% solutions or creams. The onset of dermatitis usually occurs within 1 month of starting the application (214).

ALPHA-ADRENERGIC BLOCKING AGENTS

The alpha-adrenergic blocking agent phenoxybenzamine hydrochloride is used to treat hypertension. Nurses who mix the injectable medication may become sensitized. Contamination of work surfaces is another route of exposure. The correct patch test concentration is 0.1% aqueous (215).

BENZODIAZEPAMS

A mother rendering care to her daughter with cerebral paralysis was required to handle powdered forms of several medications, including diazepam, and developed fingertip dermatitis (216). A positive patch test to diazepam was observed with a 1% aqueous patch test. A positive test was also found to tetrazepam but not to lorazapam.

TETRAZEPAM

Photosensitivity to tetrazepam occurred from systemic administration and was proven by photopatch testing (217). In this case, no cross-reaction to diazepam was seen.

PIROXICAM AND THIMEROSAL

A link has been established between allergy to thimerosal and photosensitivity to piroxicam. The link is strongest for those thimerosal-sensitive patients who are allergic to the thiosalicylate portion of the molecule. In one study (218), the overall cross-reactivity between thimerosal allergy and piroxicam photosensitivity was found to be only 8%. A form of piroxicam with enhanced bioavailability is used in Portugal: piroxicam-β-cyclodextrin (219). Photosensitivity was commonly found with this form of piroxicam and attributed

in part to a high sensitization rate to thimerosal in Portugal. A nonphotosensitizing oxicam, tenoxicam, is recommended as an alternative drug. Another study of thimerosal-sensitive patients found that 45% were sensitive to thiosalicylic acid and thus at risk for photosensitivity to piroxicam (220).

Ampiroxicam, the prodrug of piroxicam, is available in Japan. It is metabolized to piroxicam and causes photosensitivity in individuals who are also thimerosal sensitive. The same restrictions that apply to the thimerosal-piroxicam story are appropriate for ampiroxicam (221). Additional cases of ampiroxicam photosensitivity were confirmed by Toyohara et al. (222).

8-METHOXYPSORALEN

The drug 8-methoxypsoralen has been used to treat alopecia areata, psoriasis, vitiligo, and chronic dermatitis, and reports of contact dermatitis or photocontact dermatitis have occurred in each setting. The commercially available 1% solution can be diluted 1:100 to 1:1,000 for patch test purposes. Protection from inadvertent light exposure is necessary to assess contact dermatitis as opposed to phototoxic reactions. These reactions are thought to be rare (223).

CHOLESTEROL-LOWERING AGENTS

Nummular eczematous plaques developed on a 59-year-old man who was taking multiple medications (224). The medications were pulverized and applied as patch tests. A positive reaction to pravastatin occurred; this same procedure in 20 controls was negative. A prick test was also positive with pulverized pravastatin in a drop of saline. This same method for prick testing pravastatin was negative in 10 controls. Simvastatin has previously been associated with generalized dermatitis.

Photosensitivity in the ultraviolet A (UVA) range was detected in a 50-year-old woman treated with simvastatin to treat hypercholesterolemia (225). A 10% simvastatin in petrolatum exposed to 4.5 J/cm² gave a positive photopatch test. Persist photosensitivity with a lowered minimal erythema dose to ultraviolet B (UVB) over 7 months after stopping simvastatin was found as a form of chronic actinic dermatitis in a Spanish man (226). His minimal erythema dose (MED) was decreased within 5 days of taking simvastatin, but his photopatch test with UVA was negative. When the photopatch test with simvastatin (Zocor) was repeated with UVB light at suberythemagenic doses, a photopatch test was positive at 24 hours.

CONTACT DERMATITIS FROM AGENTS USED TO CARE FOR PATIENTS

Respiratory Agents and Gases

Tiopronin [N(2-mercaptopropionyl)glycine] is a sulfhydryl compound used in aerosol therapy as a mucolytic. It has caused contact dermatitis, erythema multiforme, and lichen planus–like eruptions, and the similar sulfhydryl, stepronin, has also caused contact dermatitis. The eruption is usually in the perioral region due to the mask worn during administration (227).

Airborne dermatitis resulted from exposure to metaproterenol (Alupent) used by a respiratory therapist to treat patients (228). A 2.5% aqueous concentration was used for patch testing, and 50 controls were negative.

Sleep apnea is treated with nasal continuous positive air pressure (CPAP). The device is secured with elastic bands around the scalp and lateral aspects of the face. Bands containing thiourea compounds produced eczematous changes in a patient allergic to diethylthiourea (229). These lesions were eczematous on the face and in the scalp. However, in the scalp, circular patches of alopecia followed the eczema, and this was accompanied by the regrowth of depigmented hair. It was not clear if the contact dermatitis had triggered alopecia areata, but because contact dermatitis is used to correct alopecia areata, this seems less likely. Alternatively, depigmentation may have been a sequelae of the thiourea allergy and unique for scalp melanocytes, as no pigment alteration occurred on the face.

An anesthetist who had worked in that capacity for 25 years developed dermatitis on exposed surfaces when using isoflurane (Halothane) anesthesia (230). Open applications repeated five times produced a nummular erythematous patch. This test was negative in 10 controls.

Contact dermatitis can occur from volatile gases such as ethyl chloride, which is used as a local anesthetic. Cross-reactivity with dichlorodifluoromethane (CFC 12) has been seen in such cases (231). Patch tests with volatile gases requires a ventilated chamber, and Bircher et al. (231) constructed a device of a 16-mm pad covered by a plastic membrane on silk tape (Leukotest) that was punctured several times with a thick injection needle.

Hydrocolloid Dressing

Hydrocolloid dressings are a popular form of wound management. One such device is known as DuoDERM CGF, or in the United Kingdom, Granuflex E. One component of this dressing has been identified as a cause of dermatitis: pentaerythritol ester of rosin. This allergen is tested at either 10% or 20% in petroleum (232).

Hydrocolloid dressings sold under the name DuoDERM E, as well as DuoDERM CGF, contain pentaerythritol ester of hydrogenated rosin, to which colophony-sensitive patients will react (233). The same dressing is available under the names Granuflex E and Verihesive E.

Polyisobutylene has been found to be a potential source of allergic contact dermatitis in hydrocolloid dressings. This material is also found in chewing gum, insulating tapes, and wound plasters. However, in a series of eight cases, most of the dermatitis cases were patch test negative, raising the possibility that the reactions were either irritant or unpolymerized contaminants (234).

Contrast

Nonionic contrast medium used for coronary angiography can produce delayed reactions 1 to 2 days after a procedure. The delay makes some physicians suspect causes other than the contrast. Systemic symptoms of nausea, flulike illness, asthma, or abdominal pain have been part of these delayed reactions, and patch tests can produce positive reactions in these individuals. Iopromid is an example of one such substance proven to give positive patch test reactions (235).

Technetium

Bone scans with technetium Tc 99m may be followed by an eruption beginning from 4 to 24 hours after the injection. Previously it was thought that methylene diphosphonate, which is part of the preparation, was responsible, but Mooser et al. (236) demonstrated that it is the technetium Tc 99m that is at fault. Intravenous methylene diphosphonate was negative in their patient, and a patch test to technetium 99m was positive after 2 and 3 days.

TENS Gel

Patch test reactions that occur to TENS units have been traced to the gels that are placed in the electrical field between the skin and electrode. Patch testing with the individual ingredients in these gels has frequently been negative, whereas a reaction occurs to either the finished product or the gel only after subjected to electrical stimulation by the TENS device. The cause for these reactions remains elusive, and some authors have invoked compound allergy to try to explain the phenomena (237).

Photodynamic Therapy

Use of topical delta aminolevulinic acid (d-ALA) produced dermatitis that was a spreading reaction beyond the area of application (238). The application was to the vulva as part of photodynamic therapy for Bowen's disease. A photoprotected patch test to a 20% aqueous preparation was positive in the patient to d-ALA and negative in 10 controls.

Devices

ID Bands

Identification bands placed on all patients admitted to the hospital are usually constructed of polyvinyl chloride. Tung and Taylor (239) had a patient who reacted to three of four types of these bands and also to resorcinol monobenzoate and benzoyl peroxide. They were unable to confirm the presence of these additives in the bands.

Pens

Fluorescent marking pens are commonly used to highlight the location of patch tests, as the ink can be seen under black light examination. Such use can sometimes lead to contact dermatitis if the patient is allergic to any of the ingredients in the marking pen. Triethanolamine has been identified as a cause of marking pen reactions (240).

Adhesive Remover

Adhesive remover contact dermatitis occurred around the stoma of two patients who used ConvaCare stoma bag adhesive remover (241). In one of the cases sensitivity to *d*-limonene was demonstrated, and this sensitizer was found to be present in the adhesive remover.

Gowns

Fiber gowns used to provide a barrier against water or blood are treated with epoxy-based materials to bind the waterproof plastic film to the fibers. Use of such gowns can result in unexpected exposure to epoxy allergens in a medical setting. Contact dermatitis to this processing was discovered in the production of such gowns. In the case reported by Tarvainen et al. (242), an epoxy hardener rather than resin was the allergen. Isophoronediamine (IPDA) was the epoxy hardener found responsible, and a 1% patch test concentration was positive. IPDA is also known as 3-amino-methyl-3,5,5-trimethylcyclohexylamine and is considered a cycloaliphatic epoxy resin hardener. IPDA has also caused occupational asthma and contact dermatitis in epoxy floor-laying, painting, tennis racket manufacture, and floor coatings.

Grounding Plate

Acrylates are being used to adhere grounding plates for electrosurgical devices to skin. Both 2-hydroxyethyl acrylate and 2-hydroxyethyl methacrylate are confirmed to be present in the pressure-sensitive adhesive of these devices (243,244).

Cedar Oil

Oil is used with dermatoscopic examination of skin lesions. Three days after her dermatoscopic examination, a woman with atypical nevi developed discs of eczema, which were traced to cedarwood oil (245). This oil has the same refractive index as glass and is derived from *Juniperus mexicana* and *virginiana*.

Plaster of Paris

Reactions to plaster of paris are rare and almost always due to benzalkonium chloride present in the plaster of paris. The lining material of plaster casts has been another potential source of contact dermatitis due to dioctyl sodium sulfosuccinate in the lining material (246).

Stoma Bags

Stoma-related contact dermatitis reactions have been reported from epoxy resin and stoma adhesive, as well as rubber. The hydrocolloid used to make the bags adhere is polyisobutylene, which proved to be the source of dermatitis in a 48-year-old woman (247).

Insulin Pump

Acrylates used to attach infusion needles for insulin pumps, commonly known as butterfly catheters, have caused contact dermatitis at the site of skin introduction (248). Epoxy resins have also caused problems in this setting. The Pureline Basic®, also known as the Disetronic Plus®, has been recommended as an alternative because the needle is attached by heat rather than glue.

Cannula

Epoxy resin can cause reactions around hemodialysis cannulas, and this presents as dermatitis over the shunt used for vascular access (249).

REFERENCES

1. Clemmensen O, Knudsen HE. Contact sensitivity to aluminum in a patient hyposensitized with aluminum precipitated grass pollen. *Contact Dermatitis* 1980;6:305.
2. Fischer T, Rystedt R. Case of contact sensitivity to aluminum. *Contact Dermatitis* 1982;8:343.
3. Slater DN, et al. Aluminum hydroxide granulomas: light and electron microscopic studies and X-ray microanalysis. *Br J Dermatol* 1982;107:103.
4. Kaaber K, Neilsen AO, Veien NK. Vaccination granulomas and aluminum allergy: course and prognostic factors. *Contact Dermatitis* 1992;26:304.
5. Fisher AA. Allantoin: a non-sensitizing topical medication: therapeutic effect of the addition of 5% allantoin to Vaseline. *Cutis* 1981; 27:5.
6. Mecca SB. The function and applicability of the allantoins. *Proc Scientific Section Toilet Goods Association* 1963;39:7.
7. Mecca SB. Allantoin and the newer allantoinates. *Proc Scientific Section Toilet Goods Association* 1959;31:31.
8. Lawlor P, Hindson C. Allergy to dithranol. *Contact Dermatitis* 1982; 8:137.
9. DeGroot AC, Nater JP. Contact allergy to dithranol. *Contact Dermatitis* 1981;7:5.
10. Harland CC, Mortimer PS. Laxative-induced contact dermatitis. *Contact Dermatitis* 1992;27:268.
11. Wranicz A, Czernielweski A. Pemfigoid sprowokowany nowoskabina. *Preg Dermatitis* 1974;61:693.
12. Krook G. Contact sensitivity to oxyphenbutazone (Tanderil) and cross sensitivity to phenylbutazone (butazolidin). *Contact Dermatitis* 1975;1:385.
13. Thormann J, Kaaber K. Contact sensitivity to phenylbutazone ointment (Butazolidin). *Contact Dermatitis* 1978;4:235.
14. Valsecchi R, et al. Drug reaction from oxyphenbutazone. *Contact Dermatitis* 1983;9:419.
15. Fregert S, Rorsman H. Hypersensitivity to diethylstilboestrol. *Acta Derm Venereol* (Stockh) 1960;40:206.

16. Fregert S, Rorsrnan H. Hypersensitivity to diethylstilbestrol with cross-sensitization to Benzestrol. *Acta Derm Venereol* (Stockh) 1962;42:290.

17. Romaguera C, Grimalt F. Contact dermatitis from epinephrine. *Contact Dermatitis* 1980;6:364.

18. Gibbs RC. Allergic contact dermatitis to epinephrine. *Arch Dermatol* 1970;101:92.

19. Alani SD, Alani MD. Allergic contact dermatitis and conjunctivitis from epinephrine. *Contact Dermatitis* 1976;2:147.

20. Colldahl H, Fagerberg E. Conjunctivitis and eyelid eczema due to hypersensitiveness to adrenalin solution employed by spray treatment for asthma. *Acta Allergy* 1956;10:77.

21. Aaronson SB, Jamamoto EA. Ocular hypersensitivity to epinephrine. *Invest Ophthalmol Vis Sci* 1960;5:75.

22. Audicana M, et al. Sensitization to ephedrine in oral anticatarrhal drugs. *Contact Dermatitis* 1991;24:223.

23. Bardazzi F, et al. Phenylepherine in eardrops causing contact dermatitis. *Contact Dermatitis* 1991;24:56.

24. Bereston ES. Contact dermatitis due to *N*-ethyl-o-crotonotoluide ointment (Eurax). *Arch Dermatol* 1952;65:100.

25. van Dijk E, Manen K. Allergic contact dermatitis from Eurax. *Contact Dermatitis Newsletter* 1972;12:334.

26. Baptista A, Barros MA. Contact dermatitis to crotamiton. *Contact Dermatitis* 1992;27:59.

27. Bandmann H-J. Ichthyol dermatitis. *Contact Dermatitis Newsletter* 1971;10:224.

28. Calnan CD. Ichthyol. *Contact Dermatitis Newsletter* 1971;9:218.

29. Cooke MA, Hocken Robertson DE. Ichthammol dermatitis. *Contact Dermatitis* 1981;7:335.

30. Lawrence CM, Smith AG. Ichthammol sensitivity. *Contact Dermatitis* 1981;7:335.

31. Schneider HG. Allergy to sulphurs. *Hautarzt* 1978;29:340.

32. Wilkinson DS. Sulphur sensitivity. *Contact Dermatitis* 1975;1:58.

33. Ekelund A, Moeller H. Oral provocation in eczematous contact allergy to neomycin and hydroxyquinolines. *Acta Derm Venereol* (Stockh) 1969;49:422.

34. Van Ketel WG. Cross-sensitization to 5.7-di-bromo-8-hydroxy quinoline (D.B.O.) (a compound of Synalar + D.B-O- Cream). *Contact Dermatitis* 1975;1:385.

35. Kero M, Hannuksela M, Sothman A. Primary irritant dermatitis from topical clioquinol. *Contact Dermatitis* 1979;5:115.

36. Boe A, Knut W. Increased protein-bound iodine in the serum from the topical use of iodochloro-hydroxy-quinoline (Vioform). *Acta Dermatol* 1970;50:397.

37. Hodgson-Jones IS. Clioquinol (Vioform) and iodine metabolism. *Trans St Johns Hosp* 1970;56:53.

38. Vilanova S, Camarasa G. Present importance of the so-called cutaneous tests in the diagnosis of contact eczema. *Acta Derm Venereol* (Stockh) 1959;50:243.

39. Phillips B. Occupational dermatitis. *Practitioner* 1954;172:531.

40. Fisher AA. *Contact dermatitis*. 3rd ed. Philadelphia: Lea & Febiger, 1986.

41. Gaul LE, Underwood GB. The effect of aging a solution of silver nitrate on its cutaneous reaction. *J Invest Dermatol* 1948;11:7.

42. Marcussen PV. Variations in the incidence of contact hypersensitivities. *Trans St John's Hosp Dermatol Soc* 1962;48:40.

43. Marshall JP, Schneider BP. Systemic argyria secondary to topical silver nitrate. *Arch Dermatol* 1977;113:1077.

44. Fisher AA. Irritant and toxic reactions to phenol in topical medications. *Cutis* 1980;26:363.

45. Rogers SCF, Burrows D, Neill D. Percutaneous absorption of phenol and methyl alcohol in magenta patient BPC. *Br J Dermatol* 1978;98:559.

46. Baer RL, Serri F, Weissenbach-Vial C. Studies on allergic sensitization to certain topical therapeutic agents. *Arch Dermatol* 1955;72:19.

47. Rubin MB, Pirozzi DJ. Contact dermatitis from carbolated Vaseline. *Cutis* 1973;12:52.

48. Goldsmith LA. Salicylic acid. *Int J Dermatol* 1979;18:38.

49. Taylor RP, Halprin RM. Percutaneous absorption of salicylic acid. *Arch Dermatol* 1975;111:740.

50. Soyka P, Soyka L. Absorption of salicylic acid. [Letter]. *JAMA* 1980;224:7.

51. Birmingham BK, Greene DS, Rhodes CT. Systemic absorption of topical salicylic acid. *Int J Dermatol* 1979;18:228.

52. Rudzki E, Koslowska A. Sensitivity to cylic add. *Contact Dermatitis* 1976;2:178.

53. Fisher AA. Resorcinol-A rare sensitizer. *Cutis* 1982;29:331.

54. Findlay GH, DeBeer HA. Chronic-hydroquinone poisoning of the skin from skin lightening cosmetics: a South African epidemic of ochronosis of the face in dark-skinned individuals. *S Afr Med J* 1980;57:187.

55. Caron GA, Calnan CD. Studies in contact dermatitis: 14. Resorcin. *Trans St Johns Hosp Dermatol Soc* 1962;48:149.

56. Mitchell JH. Resorcin anal dermatitis due to resorcin in anusol suppositories. *JAMA* 1933;101:1067.

57. Keil H. Group reactions in contact dermatitis due to resorcinol. *Arch Dermatol* 1962;86:212.

58. Fisher AA. Cutaneous reactions to petrolatum. *Cutis* 1981;28:23.

59. Malten KE. A case of contact eczema to yellow soft paraffin. *Contact Dermatitis* 1978;4:62.

60. Grimalt F, Romaquera C. Sensitivity to petrolatum. *Contact Dermatitis* 1978;4:377.

61. Dooms-Goossens A, Degreef H. Sensitization to yellow petrolatum used as a vehicle for patch testing. *Contact Dermatitis* 1980;6:146.

62. Penneys NS, Eaglestein W, Ziboh V. Petrolatum: interference with the oxidation of arachidonic acid. *Br J Dermatol* 1980;103:257.

63. Ghadially R, Halkier-Sorensen L, Elias PM. Effects of petrolatum on stratum corneum structure and function. *J Am Acad Dermatol* 1992;26:387.

64. Maibach H. Chronic dermatitis and hyperpigmentation from petrolatum. *Contact Dermatitis* 1978;4:62.

65. Plewig G, Fulton JE, Klisman AIM. Pomade acne. *Arch Dermatol* 1970;101:580.

66. Aronete J, Grupper C. Vaselinoma of the eyelid (second reported case). *Bull Soc Fr Dermatol Syphiligr* 1970;77:808.

67. Dooms-Goossens A, Degreef H. Contact allergy to petrolatums: attempts to identify the nature of the allergens. *Contact Dermatitis* 1983;9:247.

68. Van Joost R, Sillevis Smitt JH, Van Ketel WG. Sensitization to olive oil *(olea europea)*. *Contact Dermatitis* 1981;7:309.

69. Tomsey PJ. Hypersensitivity to sesame seed. *J Allergy* 1964;35:514.

70. Van Dijk E, Neering H, Vitanyi BEJ. Contact hypersensitivity to sesame oil in patients with leg ulcers and eczema. *Acta Derm Venereol* (Stockh) 1973;53:133.

71. Neering H, et al. Allergens in sesame oil contact dermatitis. *Acta Derm Venereol* (Stockh) 1975;55:31.

72. Brandle I, Boujnah-khouadja A, Foussereau J. Allergy to castor oil. *Contact Dermatitis* 1983;9:121.

73. Sais I. Contact dermatitis to castor oil in a lipstick. *Contact Dermatitis* 1983;9:75.

74. Matsum LY. Convulsions following application of gamma benzene hexachloride. *J Am Acad Dermatol* 1981;5:98.

75. Hindson C. Contact eczema from methyl salicylate reproduced by oral aspirin (acetyl salicylic acid). *Contact Dermatitis* 1977;3:348.

76. Grice K, Johnson CL. Contact dermatitis from Xerumenex. *Br Med J* 1972;1:508.

77. Boxlev JD, Dawber RPR. Contact dermatitis from one ingredient in Xerumenex Ear Drops. *Contact Dermatitis* 1976;2:233.

78. Nordqvist B, Mehr K. Allergic contact dermatitis to retinoic acid. *Contact Dermatitis* 1977;3:55.

79. Romaguera C, Grimalt F. Sensitization to benzoyl peroxide, retinoic acid and carbon tetrachloride. *Contact Dermatitis* 1980;6:442.

80. Rudzki E, Grzywa A. Dermatitis from retinoic acid. *Contact Dermatitis* 1978;4:305.

81. Jordan WP, Higgins M, Dvorak J. Allergic contact dermatitis to all-trans-retinoic acid: epicutaneous and leukocyte migration inhibition testing. *Contact Dermatitis* 1975;1:306.

82. Tosti A, Guerra L, Morelli R, Piraccini BM. Contact dermatitis due to topical retinoic acid. *Contact Dermatitis* 1992;26:276.

83. Balato N, et al. Allergic contact dermatitis from retinoic acid. *Contact Dermatitis* 1995;32:51.

84. Heidenheim M, Jemec GBE. Occupational allergic contact dermatitis from vitamin A acetate. *Contact Dermatitis* 1995;33:439.

85. Dalton IE, Pierce ID. Dermatological problems among pharmaceutical workers. *Arch Dermatol Syphilol* 1951;64:667.

86. Hjorth N. Contact dermatitis from vitamin B (thiamine): relapse after ingestion of thiamine cross-sensitization to co-carboxylase. *J Invest Dermatol* 1958;30:261.

87. Wigger-Alberti W, Elsner P. Occupational contact dermatitis due to pyritinol. *Contact Dermatitis* 1997;37:91.
88. Young WC, Ulrich CW, Fouts PI. Sensitivity to B$_{12}$ concentrate. *JAMA* 1950;143:893.
89. Fisher AA. Contact dermatitis at home and abroad. *Cutis* 1972;10:719.
90. Rostenberg A, Perkins AJ. Nickel and cobalt dermatitis. *J Allergy* 1952;22:466.
91. Yip J, Goodfield M. Contact dermatitis from MC 903, a topical vitamin D$_3$ analog. *Contact Dermatitis* 1991;25:139.
92. de Groot AC. Contact allergy to calcipotriol. *Contact Dermatitis* 1994;30:242.
93. Frosch PJ, Rustemeyer T. Contact allergy to calcipotriol does exist: report of unequivocal case and review of the literature. *Contact Dermatitis* 1999;40:66.
94. Zollner TM, et al. Delayed-type reactivity to calcipotriol without cross-sensitization to tacalcitol. *Contact Dermatitis* 1997;37:251.
95. Aeling JL, Panagotacos PJ, Andreozzi RJ. Allergic contact dermatitis to vitamin E aerosol deodorant. *Arch Dermatol* 1973;108:579.
96. Brodkin RH, Bleiberg J. Sensitivity to topically applied vitamin E. *Arch Dermatol* 1965;92:76.
97. Minkin W, Cohen HJ, Frank SB. Contact dermatitis from deodorants. *Arch Dermatol* 1973;107:774.
98. Mitchell J. Contact urticaria from a vitamin E preparation (vitamin E–vegetable oil) in two siblings. *Int J Dermatol* 1975;14:246.
99. Garcia-Bravo B, Mozo P. Generalized contact dermatitis from vitamin E. *Contact Dermatitis* 1992;26:280.
100. Guidetti MS, Vincenzi C, Papi M, Tosti A. Sclerodermatous skin reaction after vitamin K$_1$ injections. *Contact Dermatitis* 1994;31:45.
101. Bruynzeel I, Hebeda CL, Folkers E, Bruynzeel DP. Cutaneous hypersensitivity reactions to vitamin K: 2 case reports and a review of the literature. *Contact Dermatitis* 1995;32:78.
102. Pigatto PD, et al. Allergic dermatitis from parenteral vitamin K. *Contact Dermatitis* 1990;22:307.
103. Pascher F. Systemic reactions to topically applied drugs. *Int J Dermatol* 1978;17:269.
104. Ransome JW, Scott NM, Knoblock EC. Selenium sulfide intoxication. *N Engl J Med* 1961;264:384.
105. Marzulli FN, Maibach HI. Antimicrobials: experimental contact sensitization in man. *J Soc Cosmet Chem* 1973;24:399.
106. Fregert S. Allergic contact dermatitis from the pesticides captan and phaltan. *Contact Dermatitis Newsletter* 1967;2:28.
107. Epstein S. Photoallergic contact dermatitis—report of case due to Dangard. *Cutis* 1968;4:856.
108. Jacobs PH, Farber EM, Nall ML. Psoriasis and skin cancer. In: Farber EM, Cox A, eds. *Second International Symposium on Psoriasis.* New York: Yorke Medical Books, 1977:350.
109. Emmett EA, Stetzer L, Taphorn B. Phototoxic keratoconjunctivitis from coal tar pitch volatiles. *Science* 1977;198:841.
110. Goetz H. Tar keratosis. In: Andrade R et al, eds. *Cancer of the skin.* Philadelphia: WB Saunders, 1976:495.
111. DeMoragas JM. Multiple keratoacanthomas: relation to jamarsan therapy of pemphigus foliacens. *Arch Dermatol* 1966;93:679.
112. Colomb DJ, Descos L, Gauthier D. Multiple keratoacanthomas and coal tar disease. *Rev Lyon Med* 1966;15:449.
113. Leyden JJ, Kligman AM. Studies on the allergenicity of 5-fluorouracil. *J Dermatol Surg Oncol* 1977;3:518.
114. Mansell PWA, Litwin MS, Ichinose H, Krementz ET. Delayed hypersensitivity to 5-fluorouracil following topical chemotherapy of cutaneous cancers. *Cancer Res* 1975;35:1288.
115. Sams WM. Untoward response with topical fluorouracil. *Arch Dermatol* 1968;97:14.
116. Goette DK, Odom RB, Owens R. Allergic contact dernatitis from topical fluorouracil. *Arch Dermatol* 1977;113:196.
117. Yaffee HS, Grots I. "Ecdysis" secondary to 5-fluorouracil. *Cutis* 1980;25:649.
118. Hendricks AA, Dec GW Jr. Contact dermatitis due to nitroglycerin ointment. *Arch Dermatol* 1979;115:853.
119. Chandraratna PAN, O'Dell RE. Allergic reactions to nitroglycerin ointment: report of five cases. *Curr Ther Res Clin Exp* 1979;25:481.
120. Zugerrnan C, Zheutlin T, Giacobetti R. Allergic contact dermatitis secondary to nitroglycerin in Nitro-Bid ointment. *Contact Dermatitis* 1979;5:270.
121. Bressler RR. Nitroglycerin reactions among pharmaceutical workers. *Ind Med Surg* 1949;18:519.
122. Vaillant L, et al. Skin acceptance of transcutaneous nitroglycerine patches: a prospective study of 33 patients. *Contact Dermatitis* 1990;23:142.
123. Stonehill AA, Krop S, Borick MP. Buffered glutaraldehyde a new chemical sterilizing solution. *Am J Hosp Pharm* 1963;20:458.
124. Jordan WP, Dahl MV, Albert HL. Contact dermatitis from glutaraldehyde. *Arch Dermatol* 1972;105:94.
125. Storrs FJ. Technical and ethical problems associated with patch testing. *Clin Rev Allergy Immunol* 1996;14:185.
126. Comaish S. Glutaraldehyde lowers skin friction and enhances skin resistance to acute friction injury. *Acta Derm Venereol* (Stockh) 1973;53:455.
127. Des Grosseilliers JP, Brisson P. Localized epidermolysis bullosa: report of two cases and evaluation of therapy with glutaraldehyde. *Arch Dermatol* 1974;109:70.
128. Gordon HH. Glutaraldehyde therapy for epidermolysis bullosa. [Letter]. *Arch Dermatol* 1974;110:297.
129. Gordon HH. Herpes zoster and simplex: local therapy with glutaraldehyde. *Cutis* 1973;12:918.
130. Gordon HH. Pseudomonas infections. *Arch Dermatol* 1974;109:261.
131. London ID. Buffered glutaraldehyde solution for warts. *Arch Dermatol* 1971;104:96.
132. Maibach HL, Prystowsky SD. Glutaraldehyde (pentanedial) allergic contact dermatitis. *Arch Dermatol* 1977;113:170.
133. Fisher AA. Reactions to glutaraldehyde with particular reference to radiologists and X-ray technicians. *Cutis* 1981;28:113.
134. Sanderson KV, Cronin E. Glutaraldehyde and contact dermatitis. *Br Med J* 1968;3:820.
135. Skog E. Sensitivity to glutaraldehyde. *Contact Dermatitis Newsletter* 1968;4:79.
136. Lyon TC. Allergic contact dermatitis due to Cidex. *Oral Surg* 1971;32:895.
137. Neering H, van Ketel WG. Glutaraldehyde and formaldehyde allergy. *Contact Dermatitis* Newsletter 1874;16:518.
138. Maibach H. Glutaraldehyde: cross reaction to formaldehyde. *Contact Dermatitis* 1975;1:326.
139. Hansen EM, Menné T. Glutaraldehyde: patch test, vehicle and concentration. *Contact Dermatitis* 1990;23:369.
140. Garcia RL. Delayed hypersensitivity reaction to glutaraldehyde and formaldehyde. *Bull Assoc Military* 1972;21:11.
141. Belani KG, Priedklans J. An epidemic of pseudomembranous laryngotracheitis. *Anaesthesia* 1977;47:530.
142. Zach RG. How prevalent is glutaraldehyde sensitivity? *Consultant* 1980(May):116.
143. Hansen KS. Glutaraldehyde occupational dermatitis. *Contact Dermatitis* 1983;9:81.
144. Presto AJ III, Muecke EC. A dose of Spanish fly. *JAMA* 1970;214:592.
145. Dilaimy M. Lymphangitis caused by cantharidin. *Arch Dermatol* 1975;111:398.
146. Valdes-Dapena MA, Arey JB. Boric add poisoning: three fatal cases with pancreatic inclusions and a review of the literature. *J Pediatr* 1962;61:531.
147. Skipworth GB, Goldstein N, McBrite WP. Boric acid intoxication from "medicated talcum powder." *Arch Dermatol* 1967;95:83.
148. Vonterheid EC, Van Scott EJ, Grekin DA. Topical chemotherapy and immunotherapy of mycosis fungoides: intermediate-term results. *Arch Dermatol* 1977;133:454.
149. Daughters D, Zackheim H, Maibach H. Urticaria and anaphylactoid reactions after topical applications of mechlorethamine. *Arch Dermatol* 1973;107:429.
150. Grunnet E. Contact urticaria and anaphylactoid reaction induced by topical application of nitrogen mustard. *Br J Dermatol* 1976;94:101.
151. Leshaw S, Simon RS, Baer BL. Failure to induce tolerance to mechlorethamine hydrochloride. *Arch Dermatol* 1977;113:1406.
152. Monk BE, Vollum DI, Du Vivier AWP. Combination nitrogen mustard and photochemotherapy for mycosis fungoides: effects on sensitization and treatment. *Br J Dermatol* 1982;107(Suppl 22):25.
153. Price NM, Deneau DG, Hoppe RT. The treatment of mycosis fungoides with ointment based mechlorethamine. *Arch Dermatol* 1982;228:234.
154. Thomsen K, Mikkelsen HI. Protective capacity of gloves used for handling of nitrogen mustard. *Contact Dermatitis* 1975;1:268.
155. van Ketel WG. Allergy to coumarin and coumarin derivatives. *Contact Dermatitis Newsletter* 1972;13:355.

156. Kaidbey C, Kligman, A. Photocontact allergy to coumarins. *Arch Dermatol* 1981;217:259.
157. Kwong P, Roberts P, Prescott SM, Tikoff G. Dermatitis induced by warfarin. *JAMA* 1978;239:1884.
158. Schleicher SM, Fricker MP. Coumarin necrosis. *Arch Dermatol* 1980;116:444.
159. Schramm W, et al. Treatment of coumarin-induced skin necrosis with a monoclonal antibody purified protein C concentrate. *Arch Dermatol* 1993;129:753.
160. Koch P, Bahmer FA, Schäfer H. Tolerance of intravenous low-molecular-weight heparin after eczematous reaction to subcutaneous heparin. *Contact Dermatitis* 1991;25:205.
161. Krasovec M, Kammerer R, Spertini F, Frenk E. Contact dermatitis from heparin gel following sensitization by subcutaneous heparin administration. *Contact Dermatitis* 1995;33:135.
162. Moreau A, et al. Delayed hypersensitivity at the injection sites of a low-molecular-weight heparin. *Contact Dermatitis* 1996;34:31.
163. Koch P, Hindi S, Landwehr D. Delayed allergic skin reactions due to subcutaneous heparin-calcium, enoxaparin-sodium, pentosan polysulfate and acute skin lesions from systemic sodium-heparin. *Contact Dermatitis* 1996;34:156.
164. Boehncke WH, Weber L, Gall H. Tolerance of intravenous administration of heparin and heparinoid in a patient with delayed-type hypersensitivity to heparins and heparinoids. *Contact Dermatitis* 1996;35:73.
165. Trautmann A, Brocker EB, Klein CE. Intravenous challenge with heparins in patients with delayed-type skin reactions after subcutaneous administration of the drug. *Contact Dermatitis* 1998;39:43.
166. Hunzelmann N, Gold H, Scharffetter-Kochanek K. Concomitant sensitization to high and low molecular-weight heparins, heparinoid and pentosanpolysulfate. *Contact Dermatitis* 1998;39:88.
167. Zollner TM, Gall H, Volpel H, Kaufmann R. Type IV allergy to natural hirudin confirmed by in vitro stimulation with recombinant hirudin. *Contact Dermatitis* 1996;35:59.
168. Cronin E. Lanolin dermatitis. *Br J Dermatol* 1966;78:617.
169. Vollum DI. Sensitivity to hydrogenated lanolin [Letter]. *Arch Dermatol* 1969;100:774.
170. Thune P. Allergy to wool fat: the addition of salicylic acid for patch test purposes. *Acta Derm Venereol* (Stockh) 1969;49:282.
171. Newcomb EA. Lanolin allergy. *J Soc Cosmet Chem* 1966;17:149.
172. Peter C, Schropl F, Franzwa H. Experimental investigation regarding allergenic effects of wool wax alcohols. *Hautarzt* 1969;20:450.
173. Oleffe JD, Blondeel A, Boschmans L. Patch testing with lanolin. *Contact Dermatitis* 1978;4:233.
174. Giorgini S, Melli MC, Sertoli A. Comments on the allergenic activity of lanolin. *Contact Dermatitis* 1983;9:425.
175. Sulzberger MB, Warshaw T, Herrmann F. Studies of skin hypersensitivity to lanolin. *J Invest Dermatol* 1953;20:33.
176. Kligman AM. Lanolin allergy: crisis or comedy. *Contact Dermatitis* 1983;9:99.
177. Breit R, Bandmann H-J. Dermatitis from lanolin. *Br J Dermatol* 1973;88:414.
178. Bandmann H-J, Reichenberger M. Beobachtungen und Untersuchungen zur Frage der durch Eucerin Bedingten seltenen Allergies. *Hautarzt* 1957;8:11.
179. Cronin E, et al. Contact dermatitis in the atopic. *Acta Derm Venereol* (Stockh) 1970;50:183.
180. McBurney EI, Noel SB, Collins JH. Contact dermatitis to transdermal estradiol system. *J Am Acad Dermatol* 1989;20:508.
181. Pecquet C, Pradalier A, Dry J. Allergic contact dermatitis from ethanol in a transdermal estradiol patch. *Contact Dermatitis* 1992;27:275.
182. Carmichael AJ, Foulds IS. Allergic contact dermatitis from oestradiol in oestragen patches. *Contact Dermatitis* 1992;26:194.
183. Boehncke WH, Gall H. Type-IV hypersensitivity to topical estradiol in a patient tolerant to it orally. *Contact Dermatitis* 1996;35:187.
184. Goncalo M, et al. Allergic and systemic contact dermatitis from estradiol. *Contact Dermatitis* 1999;40:58.
185. Buckley DA, Wilkinson SM, Higgins EM. Contact allergy to a testosterone patch. *Contact Dermatitis* 1998;39:91.
186. Jordan WP Jr. Allergy and topical irritation associated with transdermal testosterone administration: a comparison of scrotal and nonscrotal transdermal systems. *Am J Contact Dermat* 1997;8:108.
187. Dwyer CM, Forsyth A. Allergic contact dermatitis from methacrylates in a nicotine transdermal patch. *Contact Dermatitis* 1994;30:309.
188. Bircher AJ, Howald H, Rufli T. Adverse skin reactions to nicotine in a transdermal therapeutic system. *Contact Dermatitis* 1991;25:230.
189. von Bahr B, Wahlberg JE. Reactivity to nicotine patches wrongly blamed on contact allergy. *Contact Dermatitis* 1997;37:44.
190. Audicana M, Schmidt R, Fernandez de Corres L. Allergic contact dermatitis from nicotinic acid esters. *Contact Dermatitis* 1990;22:60.
191. Giorgini S, Martinelli C, Sertoli A. Delayed type sensitivity reaction to mitomycin. *Contact Dermatitis* 1991;24:378.
192. Arregui MA, et al. Dermatitis due to mitromycin C bladder instillations: study of 2 cases. *Contact Dermatitis* 1991;24:368.
193. de Groot AC, Conemans JM. Systemic allergic contact dermatitis from intravesical instillation of the antetumor antibiotic mitromycin C. *Contact Dermatitis* 1991;24:201.
194. Veraldi S, Benelli C, Pigatto PD. Occupational allergic contact dermatitis from minoxidil. *Contact Dermatitis* 1992;26:211.
195. Whitmore SE. The importance of proper vehicle selection in the detection of minoxidil sensitivity. *Arch Dermatol* 1992;128:653.
196. Rietschel RL. The patch test as an exercise in cutaneous pharmacokinetics. Does compound allergy exist? [Editorial; comment]. *Arch Dermatol* 1992;128:678.
197. Camarasa JG, Pla C. Allergic contact dermatitis from cyclopentolate. *Contact Dermatitis* 1996;35:368.
198. Boukhman MP, Maibach HI. Allergic contact dermatitis from tropicamide ophthalmic solution. *Contact Dermatitis* 1999;41:47.
199. Marcos ML, et al. Occupational allergic contact dermatitis from homatropine and phenylephrine eyedrops. *Contact Dermatitis* 1997;37:189.
200. Valsecchi R, et al. Occupational contact dermatitis from propranolol. *Contact Dermatitis* 1994;30:177.
201. Koch P. Allergic contact dermatitis due to timolol and levobunolol in eyedrops, with no cross-sensitivity to other ophthalmic beta-blockers. *Contact Dermatitis* 1995;33:140.
202. Armisen M, et al. Allergic contact dermatitis from apraclonidine. *Contact Dermatitis* 1998;39:193.
203. Villareal O. Reliability of diagnostic tests for contact allergy to mydriatic eyedrops. *Contact Dermatitis* 1998;38:150.
204. Aalto-Korte K. Contact allergy to dorzolamide eyedrops. *Contact Dermatitis* 1998;39:206.
205. Niizeki H, et al. Contact dermatitis from ketotifen fumarate eyedrops. *Contact Dermatitis* 1994;31:266.
206. Helton J, Storrs FJ. Pilocarpine allergic contact and photocontact dermatitis. *Contact Dermatitis* 1991;25:133.
207. Cameli N, Bardazzi F, Morelli P, Tosti A. Contact dermatitis from rubidium iodide in eyedrops. *Contact Dermatitis* 1990;23:377.
208. Conraads PJ, Woest TE, Blanks LJ, Houtman WA. Contact allergy to d-penicillamine. *Contact Dermatitis* 1990;23:371.
209. Pigatto PD, et al. Allergic contact dermatitis from beta-interferon in eyedrops. *Contact Dermatitis* 1991;25:199.
210. Cameli N, Tosti G, Venturo N, Tosti A. Eyelid dermatitis due to cocamidopropyl betaine in a hard contact lens solution. *Contact Dermatitis* 1991;25:261.
211. Herbst RA, Maibach HJ. Contact dermatitis caused by allergy to ophthalmic drugs and contact lens solution. *Contact Dermatitis* 1991;25:305.
212. Herbst RA, Maibach HI. Allergic contact dermatitis from ophthalmics: update 1997. *Contact Dermatitis* 1997;37:252.
213. van Rengen A, Goossens A. Local reactions after subcutaneous injections of β-interferon. *Contact Dermatitis* 1998;39:209.
214. Fernandez-Vozmediano JM, et al. Contact dermatitis due to topical spironolactone. *Contact Dermatitis* 1994;30:118.
215. Sommer S, Wilkinson SM. Contact dermatitis caused by phenoxybenzamine hydrochloride. *Contact Dermatitis* 1998;38:352.
216. Garcia-Bravo B, Rodriguez-Pichardo A, Camacho F. Contact dermatitis from diazepoxides. *Contact Dermatitis* 1994;30:40.
217. Quinones D, et al. Photodermatitis from tetrazepam. *Contact Dermatitis* 1998;39:84.
218. Stingeni L, Lapomarda V, Lisi P. What risk of piroxicam photodermatitis in thimerosal-positive patients? *Contact Dermatitis* 1996;34:60.
219. Varela P, et al. Piroxicam-β-cyclodextrin and photosensitivity reactions. *Contact Dermatitis* 1998;38:229.

220. Goncalo M, Figueiredo A, Concalo S. Hypersensitivity to thimerosal: the sensitizing moiety. *Contact Dermatitis* 1996;34:201.
221. Kurumaji Y. Ampiroxicam-induced photosensitivity. *Contact Dermatitis* 1996;34:289.
222. Toyohara A, et al. Ampiroxicam-induced photosensitivity. *Contact Dermatitis* 1996;35:101.
223. Korffmacher H, et al. Contact allergy to 8-methoxypsoralen. *Contact Dermatitis* 1994;30:283.
224. de Boer EM, Bruynzeel DP. Allergy to pravastatin. *Contact Dermatitis* 1994;30:238.
225. Morimoto K, et al. Photosensitivity to simvastatin with an unusual response to photopatch and photo tests. *Contact Dermatitis* 1995;33:274.
226. Granados M, de la Torre C, Cruces MJ, Pineiro G. Chronic actinic dermatitis due to simvastatin. *Contact Dermatitis* 1998:38:294.
227. Romano A, et al. Contact allergy to tiopronin: a case report. *Contact Dermatitis* 1995;33:269.
228. Fung MA, Geisse JK, Maibach HL. Airborne contact dermatitis from metaproterenol in a respiratory therapist. *Contact Dermatitis* 1996;35:317.
229. Reynaerts A, Bruze M, Erikstam U, Goossens A. Allergic contact dermatitis from a medical device, followed by depigmentation. *Contact Dermatitis* 1998;39:204.
230. Caraffini S, Ricci F, Assalve D, Lisi P. Isoflurane: an uncommon cause of occupational airborne contact dermatitis. *Contact Dermatitis* 1998;38:286.
231. Bircher AJ, et al. Allergic contact dermatitis from ethyl chloride and sensitization to dichlorodifluoromethane (CFC 12). *Contact Dermatitis* 1994;31:41.
232. Mallon E, Powell SM. Allergic contact dermatitis from Granuflex hydrocolloid dressing. *Contact Dermatitis* 1994;30:110.
233. Sasseville D, Tennstedt D, Lachapelle JM. Allergic contact dermatitis from hydrocolloid dressings. *Am J Contact Dermat* 1997;8:236.
234. Schliz M, Rauterberg A, Weiss J. Allergic contact dermatitis from hydrocolloid dressings. *Contact Dermatitis* 1996;34:146.
235. Schick E, Weber L, Gall H. Delayed hypersensitivity reaction to the non-ionic contrast medium iopromid. *Contact Dermatitis* 1996;35:312.
236. Mooser G, Gall H, Peter RU. Delayed-type allergy to technetium Tc 99m. *Contact Dermatitis* 1998;39:269.
237. Dwyer CM, Chapman RS, Forsyth A. Allergic contact dermatitis from TENS gel. *Contact Dermatitis* 1994;30:305.
238. Gniazdowska B, Rueff F, Hillemanns P, Przybilla B. Allergic contact dermatitis from delta-aminolevulinic acid used for photodynamic therapy. *Contact Dermatitis* 1998;38:348.
239. Tung RC, Taylor JS. Contact dermatitis from polyvinyl chloride identification bands. *Am J Contact Dermat* 1998;9:234.
240. Hamilton TK, Zug KA. Triethanolamine allergy inadvertently discovered from a fluorescent marking pen. *Am J Contact Dermat* 1996;7:164.
241. Lazarov A, Trattner A. Allergic contact dermatitis from the adhesive remover wipe of stoma bags. *Contact Dermatitis* 1998;39:48.
242. Tarvainen K, Jolanki R, Henriks Eckerman ML, Estlander T. Occupational allergic contact dermatitis from isophoronediamine (IPDA) in operative-clothing manufacture. *Contact Dermatitis* 1998;39:46.
243. Miranda-Romero A, et al. Allergic contact dermatitis from the acrylic adhesive of a surgical earthing plate. *Contact Dermatitis* 1998;38:279.
244. Jagtman BA. Contact dermatitis from acrylates in an electrosurgical earthing plate. *Contact Dermatitis* 1998;38:280.
245. Franz H, Frank R, Rytter M, Haustein UF. Allergic contact dermatitis due to cedarwood oil after dermatoscopy. *Contact Dermatitis* 1998;38:182.
246. Stanford D, Georgouras K. Allergic contact dermatitis from benzalkonium chloride in plaster of paris. *Contact Dermatitis* 1996;35:371.
247. Parslew R, Evans S, King CM. Allergic contact dermatitis from polyisobutylene in stoma bags. *Contact Dermatitis* 1996;35:178.
248. van den Hove J, Jacobs MC, Tennstedt D, Lachapelle JM. Allergic contact dermatitis from acrylates in insulin pump infusion sets. *Contact Dermatitis* 1996;35:108.
249. Ng PPL, Leow YH, Ng SK, Goh CL. Allergic contact dermatitis to epoxy resin in a hemodialysis cannula. *Am J Contact Dermat* 1998;9:55.

CHAPTER 11

Medications from Plants

BALSAM OF PERU

Balsam of Peru is used widely in topical medicines for wounds, burns, hemorrhoids, and scabies and in sunscreening agents (Tables 11.1 and 11.2). It is an effective capillary-bed stimulant used to increase circulation in a wound-site area. Also, balsam of Peru has a mild, bacteriocidal action; toothpastes, medicated cough lozenges, dental cements, and liquids may also contain this balsam (1).

Exposure to Balsam of Peru in Infancy and Childhood

The following "baby care" medicaments containing balsam of Peru have produced dermatitis in infants: Balmex Baby Powder, Emollient Lotion and Ointment, Diaprex Ointment, and A and D Pediatric Ointment. This reaction to balsam of Peru in infants is described in a report by Fregert and Möller (2), who tested 101 children under age 15 and found that 24% reacted to balsam of Peru 25% in petrolatum, which was much higher than the 6% found in more than 2,000 adults tested. This sensitization was thought to occur by exposure to compounds related to balsam of Peru in medicaments.

In addition, Ebner (3) tested 51 patients under age 20 who had contact allergy. Balsam of Peru was the most frequent cause of contact allergy in children and young persons attending the clinic.

> Exposure and sensitization to balsam of Peru can occur at any age, including infancy. Nonallergic contact urticaria from balsam of Peru is not uncommon.

About 30% of persons who apply balsam of Peru medicaments obtain an immediate red flare, which lasts about 1 hour. Such a flare is a nonspecific, urticarial-type reaction (4,5).

Olholm-Larsen and Heydenreich (6) stated that the increased use of perfumes produces an increasing allergy to balsam of Peru and wood tars. Veien et al. (7) reported that certain patients with chronic eczema were challenged by administration of two capsules containing 450 mg of balsam of Peru. Several patients had flares of eczema after ingesting the substance. Later, 45 of 210 patients with various eczemas were found to have flares after challenge with oral balsam of Peru (8). In further studies of 64 patients placed on a diet restricting oral sources of balsams, 37 derived long-term benefit. Generally, benefit was evident by 1 to 2 months. While a 1-g oral challenge was used to evaluate some cases, this was not found to be a reliable predictor of the benefits of a dietary restriction of balsam of Peru (9). The restricted foods are listed in Table 11.3.

In further studies, Veien et al. (10) extended their work with 1-g oral challenges of balsam of Peru. They did not find the oral challenge sufficiently predictive of who might benefit from a low-balsam diet to recommend such testing. However, the diet did provide long-term benefit to 28 of 46 patients. The foods most often identified as causing dermatitis were wine, candy, chocolate, cinnamon, citrus fruit, and flavorings. Personal observations (Robert L. Rietschel) on this type of diet suggest that usually only one or two items are critical, and the rest of the restrictions are unnecessary. Identifying the critical item requires some trial and error.

> Balsam of Peru and many of its ingredients are primary urticariogenic agents. Dietary restriction of balsams improves some chronic eczemas.

TURPENTINE

Turpentine is the ingredient in many "liniments," cold remedies, and veterinary medications. Some of these "liniments" and "rubs" for human use are listed in Table 11.4.

Turpentine oil is regarded as a local irritant. Medically, it is used externally as a counterirritant. Cronin (11) reported that turpentine oil has become an infrequent allergen because of its replacement by the petroleum product white spirit and its deliberate exclusion from industrial products, and because the balsam oils used now do not contain the sensitizer α-carene.

TABLE 11.1. *Trade Names of Products That May Contain Balsam of Peru*

Product	Product
A and D Hemorrhoidal Suppositories with Hydrocortisone	Kurlene (eyelash pomade)
Anusol Suppositories	Manhatten Drug Rectal Ointment
Benzoin (Tincture of)	Marlock Hemorrhoidal
Bonaseptic Foot Lotion	M-D-C Rectal Ointment
Bonate Suppositories	Medicone Rectal Suppositories
B.Q.R. (for colds)	Medicone Rectal Unguent
Calmol 4 Suppositories	Moava Rectal Suppositories
Carson Scarlet Wound Spray	Nap-ol Ointment (for nipples during nursing)
Castroid Inj. Unguentum	N.J.F. Hemorrhoidal Suppositories
Chap Balm	Obtundia Calamine Lotion
Codallate Suppositories	Obtundia Cream
Consin Rectal Suppositories	Obtundia Liniment
Derma Zemo Ointment	Obtundo bulbs (analgesic)
Dermo-o-creme	Obtundorrhoid (for hemorrhoids)
Desitin Hemorrhoidal	Pad Kote—astringent (external veterinary)
Diaprex Ointment	Palmer's Antiseptic Lotion
Doctient Suppositories	Pearsons Suppositories
Ergozide (for boils and burns)	Pilodyne Ointment
Ferol Rectal Ointment	Recreo Powder Plain (dusting)
Fort Dodge Scarlet Oil (wound dressing)	Rectodyne Ointment
Granulex	Rectone Improved Suppositories
Hance Improved Rectone Suppositories	Resicaine Suppositories
Hemasthesia Ointment (for hemorrhoids)	Soothe Salve
Hemasthesia Suppositories	Thoroughbred Heel Ointment (veterinary)
Hemoid Ointment	TO-NE-KA Brand Ointment
Husk Dressing (antiseptic)	Tuf-foot (for tender feet of dogs)
Itchybalm (antiseptic veterinary)	Wyanoid Suppositories (for hemorrhoids)

Dooms-Goossens et al. (12) reported a case of turpentine-induced hypersensitivity to peppermint oil owing to the sensitizing properties of three ingredients, d-pinene, limonene, and phellandrene. These compounds are also found in turpentine oil.

Peppermint oil is used widely for its aromatic properties in confections (chewing gum, candies), cosmetics, toothpaste, and pharmaceutical products such as mouthwashes. Fisher (13) and Andersen (14) have reported contact allergy to peppermint oil from certain toothpastes.

> **Industrial exposure to turpentine is somewhat less frequent, but medicinal exposure is still high.**

ROSIN (COLOPHONY)

This natural resin is used widely in topical medications, particularly the veterinary variety. A list of these medications is shown in Table 11.5.

TABLE 11.2. *Balsam of Peru in Sunscreening Agents*

Beach Party Tanning Cream
Bronze Lustre Moisturizing Tan Cream
Bronze Lustre Moisturizing Tan Gelee
Glamomour Tan Sun Cream
Golden Gaby Suntan Lotion
Hypoallergic Suntan Lotion
Moon Drops Bronze Lustre Moisturizing Tanning Lotion and Gelee
Rvpaque
Sundare Lotion
Sun Foam
Sun Lo
Sunbath Moisturizing Tanning Lotion
Sunbath Spray with Insect Repellent
Suntan Glee

TABLE 11.3. *Low-Balsam Diet: Foods to Be Restricted*

Products containing the peel of citrus fruits (oranges, lemons, grapefruit, bitter oranges, tangerines, mandarin oranges, etc.), for example, marmalade, juice, baked goods, cocktails
Products flavored with essences, for example, baked goods, candy, chewing gum
Perfumed products, for example, perfumed teas, tobacco
Various types of cough medicine and lozenges
Ice cream
Cola and other spiced soft drinks
Spices such as cinnamon, cloves, vanilla, curry (and products made with these spices), for example, tomato ketchup, chili sauce, chutney, pickled herring, pickled vegetables such as beets and cucumbers, baked goods, liver paste, paté, vermouth, bitters, and other similarly spiced beverages

TABLE 11.4. *Turpentine in Over-the-Counter Preparations*

Cloverine Salve
Johnson's Anodyne
Mentholatum
Minard Liniment
Penetro Analgesic Rub
Sloan's Liniment
Vicks Vaporub

In dentistry, rosin in chloroform solution has been used as a varnish for pulp protection in deep cavities. It has been added to zinc oxide or to eugenol as an ingredient of pulp-capping preparations, surgical packs, impression pastes, dental and periodontal dressings, dental cement, and liquid and cavity varnishes, and as an antiseptic for sealing pulp canals. Denture adhesive powder may also contain rosin. Such dental exposure to rosin can produce stomatitis (15,16).

Rasmussen and Fisher (17) reported two patients in whom allergic eczematous contact dermatitis developed to salicylic acid plaster used to treat plantar warts. Both patients were shown subsequently to be allergic to dehydroabietic acid present in the rosin contained in the plaster.

Hambly and Wilkinson (18) described a dermatitis from physiotherapy wax "contaminated" with rosin. Ducombs (19) reported a patient who was allergic to many adhesive tapes because of his allergic hypersensitivity to rosin. He had a cross-reaction to a lubricant prepared from pine resin used on the leather belts of an electric saw.

Newer adhesives such as Dermicel, Scanpor, and Blenderm are free of rosin.

> **Nonindustrial dermatitis from rosin may occur from topical medications in dentistry, adhesives, salicylic acid plasters, and yellow laundry soap.**

TABLE 11.5. *Rosin in Topical Medications*

Ace Adherent
Amlab Drawing Salve
Boilex Drawing Salve
Drawex Salve
Dr. Daniels Hoof Ointment and Softener
Dr. Naylor's Red-Kote
Falk's Nu Salve
Gilkey's Blister
Griswold's Family Salve
Larson's Podiatry Pre-tape, Formula JC-6
Larson's Trainer's Pre-tape, Formula JC-4
Legulo
Mollimentus
Severa's First Aid Ointment
Udderkream
Wonderful Dream Brand Salve

Yellow soft laundry soap owes its consistency to the presence of rosin.

TIGER BALM

Tiger balm is a popular Chinese proprietary ointment now used in the United States. Three patients Fisher (20) observed acquired contact dermatitis from this ointment. They all had cross-reactions to balsam of Peru.

> **"Oriental" tiger balm cross-reacts with balsam of Peru. "Bavarian" tiger balm cross-reacts with rosin.**

Agathos (21) stated, "Tiger balm seems to be an allergen of increasing importance. In Bavaria, a similar ointment is used; we have occasionally seen severe allergic contact dermatitis to this substance, which is sold by a 'healer' on written demand." Agathos's patient had a positive reaction to rosin.

An additional Chinese herbal medicine is known as musk and tiger bone plaster. It is used as a medical plaster for treatment of rheumatic disease, arthralgias, neuralgias, aches, and sprains. The contents include musk, tiger bone, evodia fruit, bornelone, rhizome, monkshood, kusnezoff monkshood, camphor, menthol, and zinc resinate. Zinc resinate is a mixture of zinc oxide and colophony and thus is more akin to "Bavarian" tiger balm in this respect (22).

Benzoin Tincture (Gum Benzoin)

Benzoin tincture contains 10% benzoin in alcohol, whereas the compound formulation also contains 2% aloes, 8% storax (styrax), and 4% tolu balsam in alcohol. Benzoin may be present in adhesives, water-repellent barrier creams, lozenges, benzoinated lard, and cosmetics.

Spott and Shelley (23) reported that a student developed acute eczematous contact dermatitis in response to the application of benzoin tincture to the skin under a cast. This finding was followed within 48 hours by the appearance of a generalized, noneczematous exanthem. Analysis led to the conclusion that absorption of benzoin through the skin was responsible for both the contact dermatitis and the exanthem. Patch tests demonstrated an eczematous reaction to benzoin with cross-sensitivity extending to the gums of myrrh, locust, galbanum, gamboge, and oblibanum.

Cullen et al. (24) reported a patient who had allergic contact dermatitis to compound benzoin-tincture spray under a cast.

Coskey (25) had one patient who developed allergic contact dermatitis after applying benzoin tincture for pruritus ani. Another patient developed dermatitis from applying the tincture to his leg.

Cross-reactions may occur to balsam of Peru, storax (styrax), eugenol, vanilla, pinene, benzyl alcohol, and benzyl cinnamate. Many athletes apply benzoin tincture to toughen various parts of their skin, particularly the feet, in order to prevent the formation of blisters.

In a personal communication, Dr. W. D. James (Walter Reed Army Medical Center, Washington, DC) reported that five military cadets acquired allergic dermatitis from benzoin tincture. All five were allergic to storax (styrax). Mastic also proved to be a much less potent sensitizer than benzoin tincture.

Medications Related to Benzoin

Arning's Tincture

This compound contains benzoin, ammonium tumenol, anthrarobin, and ether.

Mastic (Mastisol, Balsam Tree, Pistachia Galls, Mastiche, Mastix, and Lentisk)

Mastic is a resin derived from certain varieties of *Pistacia lentiscus* trees growing in Mediterranean countries. It is used in dentistry to secure surgical dressings and in chewing gums, incense, and varnish.

Contact dermatitis from Mastisol, which contains gum mastic, styrax liquid, methyl salicylate, and alcohol, was reported by Mitchell and Dupuis (26). The patient reacted to styrax 2% in petrolatum, benzoin 10% in ethanol, and balsam of Peru 10% in petrolatum.

> **Benzoin tincture cross-reacts with balsam of Peru and Arning's tincture. Mastic (Mastisol) has proved to be a less potent sensitizer than benzoin tincture.**

Smith's Cremolia Cream

This British preparation, which contains benzoin, produced allergic contact dermatitis, as reported by Mann (27).

Greasepaint Makeup

One patient acquired allergic contact dermatitis from benzoin in a makeup (28).

Storax (Styrax)

Storax is the purified balsam from the Turkish tree *Liquidambar orientalis*; it is a component both of benzoin inhalation and compound benzoin tincture and has been used as a parasiticide. Storax may cross-react with benzoin, balsam of Peru, and styrene, which is used in polyester resins. Storax is present in Plexoderm in a 6% concentration with 1% allantoin and 1% salicylic acid.

Fregert and Rorsman (29) reported that a woman sensitive to diethylstilbestrol also reacted to storax and balsam of Peru.

WOOD TARS

The wood tars include pine tar, beech tar, juniper tar (oil of Cade), and birch tar (oleum rusci). They are present in shampoos, deodorants, cough syrups, counterirritant veterinary liniments, pyorrhea and tooth pulp treatments, tooth powders, disinfectants, and insecticides.

Hjorth (1) stated that of 230 patients sensitive to balsam of Peru, 79 (34%) had positive reactions to wood tar and 37 (16%) had positive reactions to coal tar. Some of these patients were sensitive to both wood tar and coal tar. Positive reactions to coal tar and wood tar are much more frequent among patients sensitive to balsam of Peru than among other patients with eczema. Patients sensitive to balsam of Peru have positive reactions to wood tars twice as frequently as they have positive reactions to coal tar.

> **Many patients with hypersensitivity to balsam of Peru cross-react to tars, particularly wood tars.**

Van Andel et al. (30) found that 9% of 650 persons tested positive to wood tar, whereas 7% reacted to coal tar. Many had cross-reactions to balsam of Peru, rosin (colophony), and turpentine. Juniper tar was the most active sensitizer.

Olholm-Larsen and Heydenreich (6) believed that this increase in positive reactions to balsam of Peru and wood tars may indicate an increased frequency of allergy to perfumes in toilet soaps and cosmetics in Denmark.

In Spain, Alomar et al. (31) found that in 10.3% of patients the wood tars produced an irritant response with mild erythema and edema at 48 hours, which disappeared at 96 hours. The reactions were considered allergenic in only 1.8% of patients.

Juniper Tar (Oil of Cade)

Mathias et al. (32) suspected that juniper extract is an irritant in many instances and probably should be tested at half its commercial strength or possibly at a lower concentration.

Rothe et al. (33) reported a case of contact dermatitis and asthma from occupational exposure to oil of juniper, which is used for spicing sausage and as a smoking additive. The allergy to oil of juniper was proved by patch tests, intracutaneous tests, and a respiratory allergen test.

Pine Oil

Pine oil is a mixture of terpene alcohols, hydrocarbons, and ethers. Products containing pine oil include Breath-O-Pine Disinfectant, Black Flag Disinfectant, Go-Fecto Disinfectant, Pinuseptol, West Pine Deodorant, Whitepine Disinfectant, and Wilbert's Fresh Pine Deodorant. This oil is capable of producing serious toxic effects if ingested or aspirated.

Pine and juniper tar oil may be strong irritants. Birch may produce contact urticaria.

Birch Tar Oil, Empyreumatic (Oleum Rusci)

Lahti and Hannuksela (34) reported that fresh sap and crushed leaf of birch *(Betula verrucosa)* were tested with the scratch-chamber method in 117 atopic persons, 74 of whom were allergic and 43 of whom were nonallergic to birch pollen.

Immediate positive reactions to birch sap were seen in 39% of the patients, and positive reactions to birch leaf were seen in 28% of the patients allergic to birch pollen. These investigators stated that birch leaves may cause contact urticaria in Finnish saunas, where bath whisks made of birch sprigs are traditionally used.

Rothenborg and Hjorth (35) found that positive patch test reactions to a mixture of wood tars consisting of pine, juniper, beech, and birch often produce false-positive reactions. When a mixture of wood tars is positive, each tar should be tested individually.

Testing with mixtures of wood tars may produce false-positive reactions. Patch testing should be controlled with testing reactions to individual wood tars.

Relationship of Wood Tars to Coal Tars

Whereas wood tars and coal tars may cross-react occasionally, it must be emphasized that, although coal tars are phototoxic, wood tars are not.

Wood tars may cross-react with coal tars, but unlike coal tars, they are not phototoxic. Coal tars are rare sensitizers.

Rothenborg and Hjorth (35) stated that most patch test reactions to coal tars are irritant reactions and that allergic reactions are rare. Rudzki and Grzywa (36) reported that a pharmacist who prepared coal-tar ointments became allergic to coal tar.

The solution of coal tar (Liquor Carbonis Detergens), which consists of coal tar, quilla bark, and alcohol, is probably the least phototoxic coal-tar preparation (37).

Precautions Regarding Use of Medicinal Coal Tar

All patients using coal-tar products (with the possible exception of shampoos) should be cautioned that their exposure to the sun should be limited. No more than 15 minutes of direct exposure to midday summer sun should be tried the first time. Exposure can be increased gradually as patients define their own responses. All patients using tar products should be warned of the carcinogenic potential of tar used alone and in combination with the sun (38).

PODOPHYLLUM RESIN

Podophyllum resin remains a common treatment for condylomata acuminata (venereal warts). As a rule, an intense inflammatory reaction occurs that may become quite painful for a few days. The treatment is usually successful, and no local or systemic sequelae occur. Occasionally, however, severe systemic and local reactions do occur (39).

Systemic Effects from Topical Use of Podophyllum Resin

Although many dermatologists have used topical podophyllum resin for many years without encountering systemic reactions in their patients, a review of the literature reveals several reports of severe systemic reactions. Among the various systemic effects that have been reported from the use of topically applied podophyllum resin are the following: paresthesia, polyneuritis, paralytic ileus, pyrexia leukopenia, thrombocytopenia, coma, and death.

Grabbe (40) described a 19-year-old female patient who developed weakness and polyneuritis of the legs 2 days after a single application of a 25% podophyllum solution. On the sixth day she developed a paralytic ileus. The patient recovered after approximately 10 weeks. An 18-year-old female patient studied by Ward et al. (41) became comatose approximately 24 hours after the application of 25% podophyllum ointment on vulvar warts. She died 8 days later.

Schirren (42) observed a 25-year-old man whose extensive condylomata acuminata on the prepuce and perianal area was treated with a 16% solution of podophyllum in alcohol. Two hours after treatment, the patient vomited and became unconscious and cyanotic. It should be mentioned that this patient had consumed a large amount of alcohol immediately after the local treatment. According to

Schirren, this may have increased the absorption of podophyllum.

Cormaine (43) reported a 20-year-old woman who was treated for extensive condylomata acuminata of the labia majora, labia minora, and vaginal mucosa. A 10% podophyllum solution in collodion was applied with a tampon and left in place for 6 hours. The patient became febrile and experienced paresthesia and weakness of the toes and fingers. The paresis from polyneuritis disappeared after 14 days.

Hasler and Standish (44) stated that vomiting and an acute confused state occurred from the use of podophyllum in the treatment of hairy tongue. Chamberlain et al. (45) described a case of severe intoxication in a woman in the 32nd week of pregnancy who had subsequent delivery of a stillborn infant. According to the authors, podophyllum resin should never be used during pregnancy or in circumstances in which the genital warts are either florid with a large surface area or so hemorrhagic that absorption of the toxin resin is probable.

> **Podophyllum resin may produce toxic effects and should not be used over extensive areas on the buccal mucosa or during pregnancy.**

Larsson (46) reported two patients who developed urticaria and transient fever after the use of podophyllum resin. Stoehr et al. (47) observed a case of leukopenia and thrombocytopenia resulting from podophyllum-resin treatment of condylomata acuminata. Montaldi et al. (48) and Balucani and Zellers (49) stated that systemic toxicity may produce nausea, vomiting, respiratory stimulation, peripheral neuropathy, fever, acute confused states, tachycardia, oliguria, anuria, adynamic ileus, coma, and death.

Prevention of Systemic Reactions to Podophyllum Resin

Stoehr et al. (47) stated that systemic toxicity from local podophyllum treatment occurred when the drug was applied to extensive areas or was allowed to remain in contact with the skin for an extended period. To avoid toxicity, they recommend that applications be limited to small areas of intact skin. Although most dermatologists allow the podophyllum to remain on the skin for 4 to 6 hours, Stoehr et al. recommend that the drug should be allowed to remain in contact with the skin for no longer than 1 hour.

Schirren (42) suggested that because ingestion of alcohol shortly after local therapy may increase the absorption of podophyllum, alcoholic beverages should be avoided by patients for several hours following this treatment. Also, the use of podophyllum resin on the buccal mucosa or tongue and during pregnancy should be avoided (44,45,50).

Unusually Severe Local Reactions to Topical Podophyllum Resin

Usually the application of podophyllum resin causes an acute inflammatory reaction and the subsequent development of yellowish necrosis over the treated area. The drug induces arrest of mitosis in metaphase and epithelial cell death. Vacuolation, nuclear degenerations, and swelling of the cell give rise to the podophyllum cell. The cytotoxic principles in podophyllum resin are podophyllotoxin and its derivatives.

Sullivan and King (51) were among the first to warn that podophyllum can produce "bizarre forms of epithelial cells" that can be mistaken for carcinoma cells. Maxwell and Lamb (52) described a hyperplastic infiltrated reaction to the application of podophyllum, simulating epithelioma in two patients.

Wade and Ackerman (53) stated that it has been suggested that podophyllum can induce changes in condylomata acuminata that are indistinguishable from those of squamous cell carcinoma in situ. These investigators have shown that these two conditions can be differentiated histologically. They found that podophyllum induces necrosis and mitosis in keratinocytes, but not cytologic atypia or multinucleated cells. Cytologic atypia is the sine qua non for squamous cell carcinoma in situ.

Fisher (20) became aware of severe necrosis and scarring of the anogenital area in two patients from the use of podophyllum resin. In one instance, a fistula-in-ano developed. Additional local reactions to podophyllum resin include paraphimosis requiring circumcision and pseudoepitheliomatous hyperplasia.

The Prevention of Local Complications from Podophyllum Resin

The United States Pharmacopeia (USP) podophyllum-resin topical solution is 25% podophyllum resin and benzoin in alcohol. Although the USP calls for the use of "native" American podophyllum resin, in actual practice it has been found that the practitioner may be using a mixture of the American and Indian resins. The Indian resin is stronger and more irritating than the American variety (see Table 11.6). In addition, some resins on the market are contaminated with guaiacium wood, which may be a sensitizer (54).

> **American podophyllum resin is less toxic than Indian podophyllum resin.**

ARNICA TINCTURE

This volatile oil obtained from the composite plant *Arnica montana* is applied as a rubefacient for sprains, bruises, and painful swellings. Self-medication with arnica tincture has

TABLE 11.6. *Differences between American and Indian Podophyllum*

	American	Indian
Scientific name	*Podophyllum pelatatum*	*Podophyllum emodi*
Common name	May apple, Mandrake	
Habitat	Eastern US	Tibet, Afghanistan
Resin content	2% to 8%	6% to 12%
Podophyllotoxin	20%	36% to 39%
Reaction to copper acetate	Bright green color	Brown color
Addition of alcohol and potassium hydroxide	Does not gelatinize	Gelatinizes

produced many cases of allergic contact dermatitis (55). The sequiterpene lactones (helanalin) and methacrylate esters have proved to be the primary sensitizers (56).

Hausen (57) stated that arnica tincture is a strong sensitizer that has caused dermatitis in hundreds of persons.

PSORALEN

Topical 8-methoxypsoralen is phototoxic and may also occasionally be photoallergic (58). In addition, ordinary allergic contact dermatitis may occur from its topical use. Thus, Weissmann et al. (59) reported that a 20-year-old male patient was treated topically with 8-methoxypsoralen and long-wave ultraviolet light (UVA) for alopecia areata. He developed contact allergy to 8-methoxypsoralen after the sixth treatment (day 17), which was verified by patch testing and histopathology.

> **Topical psoralen may be phototoxic or photoallergic and may produce a nonphoto type of allergic contact dermatitis.**

ALOE VERA

The gelatinous material inside the leaf of aloe vera has been recommended from ancient times for the alleviation of inflammatory changes in the skin. More recently, it has been advocated in the treatment of radiodermatitis and leg ulcers (60–62).

Aloes consist of a variable mixture of aloin, aloe-emodin, and other substances. Aloin is an anthraquinone that may be regarded as a potential sensitizer. Cross-reactions may occur with benzoin and balsam of Peru.

At present, Dermaide Aloe Ointment is listed as an over-the-counter product (Dermaid Research Corporation). Dermaide Aloe Ointment has as an active ingredient 70% gel of the aloe vera plant in a special white, homogenous base of mineral oil, stearic acid, petrolatum, triethanolamine, beeswax, synthetic spermaceti, propyl-paraben, methyl paraben, and fragrance.

Morrow et al. (63) described a case of hypersensitivity to aloe manifested by generalized nummular eczematous and papular dermatitis, and presumably by contact urticaria, that developed in a 47-year-old man after 4 years' use of oral and topical aloe. Patch tests for aloe were positive in this patient.

> **Aloe vera is a rare sensitizer. The preservatives may be sensitizers when incorporated in topical medications.**

PROPOLIS (BEE GLUE) AND BEESWAX

Propolis (bee glue) is a dark yellow-brown adhesive resin that bees mix with wax to form a cementing substance in their hives. The purified wax from the honeycomb, beeswax, is used widely in cosmetics. Beeswax may be used as cera alba (bleached) or as cera flava (unbleached).

Propolis (Bee Glue)

Propolis (bee glue), derived mainly from poplar and other tree resins, contains, among other things, well-known sensitizers such as cinnamic acid and vanillin. It may cross-react with balsam of Peru. Allergic contact dermatitis from propolis is an occupational hazard for beekeepers (64,65). In rare instances, a beekeeper may be allergic to beeswax. Beekeepers who have dermatitis may be tested with the contactants shown in Table 11.7.

Propolis is sold in many health food stores in various forms for ingestion as a "cure-all" for numerous diseases and as a topical agent in ointments, powders, and cosmetic creams. Solid propolis, which can be chewed, may produce a perioral dermatitis and stomatitis. Thus, Wanscher (66) described two patients who had contact dermatitis and stomatitis from chewing so-called natural propolis products, which are sold without prescription as tablets or as solid propolis in large or small chunks.

Petersen (67) predicted that, with the increasing employment of propolis for self-medication, a growing number of cases of allergic contact eczema from exposure to this preparation should be anticipated.

TABLE 11.7. *Beekeepers Patch Test Series*

Allergens	Test
Balsam of Peru	25% pet
Pine balsam	10% pet
Pine bud	As is
Poplar resin	10% pet
Propolis (bee glue)	As is
Wax (beeswax)	As is

Propolis (bee glue), which may cross-react with balsam of Peru, may also produce allergic contact dermatitis not only in beekeepers but also in the general population from increasing self-medication with this product.

Beeswax

Beeswax is secreted by bees. Camasara (68) reported a woman who was employed in molding art objects from beeswax who developed chronic palmar dermatitis. A strongly positive patch test to natural beeswax was obtained. A beekeeper described by Rothenborg (65) reacted to raw, unpurified beeswax but not to purified beeswax. The raw wax was considered contaminated by poplar tree resins, to which he was sensitive.

Beeswax, secreted by bees and used in cosmetics, is a rare sensitizer unless contaminated with propolis (bee glue).

Honey is a saccharin substance deposited in the honeycomb by the honeybee. It is used as an excipient, as a flavor in gargles and cough medicine, and as a food.

CHAMOMILE (CAMOMILE)

Chamomile is a yellow dye extracted from the dried flower heads of *Chamaemelum nobile* (Roman source) and *Matricaria recutita* (German source), both of which are of the Asteraceae family. The Roman product is thought to be more allergenic (69).

Chamomile is used in shampoos, hair rinses, and as a vegetable hair dye. Allergic contact dermatitis has occurred in persons who have handled the plant or who have used compresses of chamomile or chamomile ointment (70,71). Chamomile may cross-react with the *Compositae* group of plants. Oil of chamomile has been added to nipple eczema cream used by nursing mothers, and contact dermatitis has been confirmed with 0.1% in petrolatum of the oil of chamomile. Drinking chamomile tea was found to flare the original contact dermatitis (69).

German Chamomile

Allergy to chamomile is most commonly reported from Roman chamomile *(Anthemis nobilis)*, but Pereira et al. (72) had a patient who used chamomile tea compresses to treat an eczema of the forearms and became sensitive to both Roman and German chamomile *(Matricaria chamomilla)*. The allergen in the German chamomile is sesquiterpene lactone desacetyl matricarin.

German chamomile tea used to treat a facial dermatitis resulted in contact dermatitis to the tea (73). In this case, sesquiterpene lactone mix was positive and Roman chamomile negative. Subsequent ingestion of German chamomile tea caused flare-up of the facial dermatitis, as well as eczema of the arms and trunk and anal pruritus.

Arnica and chamomile may cross-react with the ragweed group of plants. Ingestion of chamomile tea may flare areas of previous dermatitis from tropical products that contain chamomile.

TANNIN

Some hemorrhoid ointments contain up to 10% tannin, a rare sensitizer. Two cases from hemorrhoid ointments were reported by van Ketel and Bruynzeel (74), which brings to four the number of reported cases of tannin sensitivity. A 1% to 10% petrolatum or aqueous tannin patch test is positive.

NATURAL OILS

Jojoba Oil

Jojoba oil is a liquid-wax ester extracted from the jojoba bush, which grows wild in the southwestern United States and in northern Mexico. It is now grown commercially in the United States and Israel.

The oil is used in cosmetics as a skin lubricant, hair conditioner, and wrinkle "remover." Jojoba oil was first reported as a sensitizer by Markin (75) and later by Scott (76).

Tea Tree Oil

Topical use of tea tree oil has been a source of allergic contact dermatitis. De Groot (77) reported a patient who developed facial dermatitis from vapors of tea tree oil used to treat bronchitis. He noted that while the allergen most frequently sited in tea tree or melaleuca oil is *d*-limonene, the sensitizing components include aromadendrene, alpha terpinene, 1,8-cineole (eucalyptol), terpinen-4-ol, *p*-cymene, and alpha-phellandrene.

Black Cumin Oil

Therapeutic use of black cumin *(Nigella sativa)* oil, which is promoted in Germany for skin diseases of many divergent types, has led to contact dermatitis (78). The oil is sold as an herbal remedy under the name Schwedenkreuther, or Swedish herbs. A 1:200 dilution in olive oil can be used for patch testing.

VEGETABLE GUMS

These gums are resinous plant exudates. Karaya, acacia, and tragacanth are probably the most common sensitizers among them (79). They may be used "as is" for patch tests.

Karaya is an ingredient in many cosmetics, particularly hair-waving lotions. It is used in toothpastes, powders, adhesives, and cement substances to make ileostomy and colostomy bags adhere to the skin. Fasteeth, a denture adhesive, contains karaya gum, sodium borate, and peppermint flavoring.

Acacia (gum arabic) is used in cosmetics and in offset sprays in the printing industry.

Gum tragacanth (tragacanth), an insoluble vegetable gum that absorbs water to form a jelly, may cross-react with acacia. Tragacanth is used in cosmetics, particularly gumbased hair dressings, and in troches, toothpastes, depilatories, and other topical medications. Exposure may take place from contact with textile finishes and sizing papers or in printing operations or enameling.

Gum resins are naturally occurring mixtures of gum, oil, and resin. There is probably wider exposure to benzoic gum resin than to other gum resins. Acacia (gum arabic), which is used in adhesives, may be a sensitizer (80). Other gums (plant exudates consisting of high-polymer polysaccharides, some with a low nitrogen content) such as karaya, acacia (gum arabic), and gum tragacanth, may act occasionally as sensitizers.

ERGOT

The principal medical use of ergot is via systemic administration; however, nicergoline (1,6-dimethyl-8-β-5-bromonicotinyl-oxymethyl-10-α-methoxyergoline) is used in the manufacture of a calcium channel blocker derived from ergot. Nicergoline caused an airborne contact dermatitis in a factory worker exposed to the product. A 7% concentration in ethyl alcohol produced a positive patch test (81).

RUE

In some parts of the world, members of the Rutaceae family are used as folk remedies and to protect against mosquito bites. Unfortunately, this leads to photocontact dermatitis and intense hyperpigmentation, as members of this family contain 5- and 8-methoxypsoralen. Reports of this type of reaction include *Ruta montana, R. graveolens,* and *R. chalenpensis* (82).

VERBENA

An "omelette" made from *Verbena officinalis* (wild verbena) and egg whites is used as a folk medicine for sinusitis, bronchitis, ocular diseases, and dermatitis (83). This mixture may facilitate contact dermatitis, as the allergenic fraction of the plant is thought to be oil soluble, and mere handling of the plant was not sufficient to cause dermatitis.

KRAMERIA

Krameria triandra is also known as Peruvian rhatany, red rhatany, rhatanhia, and rhatania. It is a member of the Krameriaceae family and is a low shrub native to South America. It has been used as a botanical medication due to astringent, antidiarrheic, and anti-inflammatory properties. When compounded into an antihemorrhoidal gel, it caused allergic contact dermatitis, proven by a positive patch test to rhatany tincture 1% in petrolatum (84).

ELECAMPANE

Elecampane is the common name of an herb used systemically and topically as a supplement in phytotherapy. The scientific name is *Inula helenium,* a member of the *Compositae* family, which contains both isoalantolactone and alantolactone. This herb was added to a massage liniment and caused contact dermatitis in a woman who had taken this herb orally 1 year previously (85). Although on the oral form of this botanical, she experienced facial dermatitis.

CENTELLA

Slow-healing wounds and chronic ulcers are treated with a cream containing the triterpenic fraction of *Centella asiatica,* a member of the Umbelliferae family. This is commercially available as Centelase cream. The plant is thought to be of low sensitization potential based on guinea pig tests of the sensitizing constituents: asiaticoside, asiatic acid, and madecassic acid (86).

ROSEMARY

Use of rosemary leaves as a topical anti-inflammatory plaster caused contact dermatitis, confirmed by patch testing with the leaves (87). Rosemary *(Rosmarinus officinalis L.)* is a member of the Labiatae family. Other members of Labiatae include thyme, origanum, and mint. Patch tests to these three plants were negative.

SANDALWOOD

Traditional sandalwood is *Santalum album,* whereas red sandalwood is *Pterocarpus santalinus.* Red sandalwood bark is used as a folk remedy in India to treat postacne scarring and when used this way has caused allergic contact dermatitis. The allergens are santalin A (9,10,12-tri-o-methylsantalin) and santalin B (9,10,12,4′-tetra-o-methylsantalin), and the allergens in *S. album* are alpha and beta santalol (88).

GINKGO BILOBA

Dietary supplements containing *Ginkgo biloba* are popular for cerebral function enhancement. Because these are similar to *Toxicodendron*, the possibility of systemic contact dermatitis exists. Hausen (89) attempted to quantify the risk that these supplements hold. He found that pure ginkgolic acids could sensitize guinea pigs but that extracts of the *Ginkgo biloba* leaves could not. He found that leaf extracts up to 1,000 ppm of ginkgolic acids would be safe.

BURDOCK

Burdock *(Arctium lappa)* is used as an herbal supplement in the United States, and it is applied topically in Spain as burdock root plasters for an anti-inflammatory effect. Burdock is a member of the Compositae family, and three cases of contact dermatitis to the plasters were reported from Spain (90).

GOLDENROD

Oral ingestion of a medication (Urodyn) that contains goldenrod resulted in a systemic contact dermatitis (91). Patch tests confirmed reactions to goldenrod *(Herba solidaginis)* and related Compositae tansy and yarrow.

REFERENCES

1. Hjorth N. Eczematous allergy to balsams. *Acta Dermatol Venereol Suppl* (Stockh) 1961;41:34.
2. Fregert S, Möller H. Contact allergy to balsam of Peru in children. *Br J Dermatol* 1963;75:218.
3. Ebner H. Contact allergy to Peru balsam in children and adolescents. *Tagl Prax* 1976;17:155.
4. Rudzki E, Grzywa Z. Immediate reactions to balsam of Peru, cassia oil and ethyl vanillin. *Contact Dermatitis* 1976;2:360.
5. Forsbeck M, Skog E. Immediate reactions to patch tests with balsam of Peru. *Contact Dermatitis* 1977;3:201.
6. Olholm-Larsen P, Heydenreich G. Allergy to balsam of Peru and wood tars: an increasing problem? *Contact Dermatitis* 1976;2:293.
7. Veien N K, Hattel T, Justesen O, Norholm A. Oral challenge with balsam of Peru in patients with eczema: a preliminary study. *Contact Dermatitis* 1983;9:75.
8. Veien N K, Hattel T, Justesen O, Norholm N. Oral challenge with balsam of Peru. *Contact Dermatitis* 1985;12:104.
9. Veien N K, Hattel T, Justesen O, Norholm N. Reduction of intake of balsams in patients sensitive to balsam of Peru. *Contact Dermatitis* 1985;12:270.
10. Veien N K, Hattel T, Laurberg G. Can oral challenge with balsam of Peru predict possible benefit from a low-balsam diet? *Am J Contact Dermatitis* 1996;7:84.
11. Cronin E. Oil of turpentine—a disappearing allergen. *Contact Dermatitis* 1979;5:30.
12. Dooms-Goossens A, Degreef H, Holvoet C, Maertens M. Turpentine induced hypersensitivity to peppermint oil. *Contact Dermatitis* 1977;3:304.
13. Fisher A A. Contact stomatitis, glossitis, and cheilitis. *Otolaryngol Clin North Am* 1971;7:82.
14. Andersen K E. Contact allergy to toothpaste flavors. *Contact Dermatitis* 1978;4:195.
15. Lysell L. Contact allergy to rosin in a periodontal dressing: a case report. *J Oral Med* 1976;31:24.
16. Dawson T J. Colophony sensitivity in dentistry. *Contact Dermatitis* 1977;3:342.
17. Rasmussen I E, Fisher A A. Allergic contact dermatitis to a salicylic acid plaster. *Contact Dermatitis* 1976;2:237.
18. Hambly E M, Wilkinson D S. Dermatitis from contaminated physiotherapy wax. *Contact Dermatitis* 1975;1:53.
19. Ducombs G. Allergy to colophony. *Contact Dermatitis* 1978;4:118.
20. Fisher A A. *Contact dermatitis.* 3rd ed. Philadelphia: Lea & Febiger, 1986.
21. Agathos M. Bavarian tiger balm. *Contact Dermatitis* 1982;8:215.
22. Barbaud A, Mougeoll J M, Tang J Q, Protois J C. Contact allergy to colophony in Chinese musk and tiger bone plaster. *Contact Dermatitis* 1991;25:324.
23. Spott D A, Shelley W B. Exanthem due to contact allergen (Benzoin) absorbed through skin. *JAMA* 1970;214:1881.
24. Cullen S I, Tonkin A, May F E. Allergic contact dermatitis to compound tincture of benzoin spray. *J Trauma* 1974;14:348.
25. Coskey R J. Contact dermatitis owing to tincture of benzoin. *Arch Dermatol* 1978;114:128.
26. Mitchell I C, Dupuis G. Allergic contact dermatitis from storax (styrax). *Contact Dermatitis Newsletter* 1972;11:274.
27. Mann R J. Benzoin sensitivity. *Contact Dermatitis* 1982;8:263.
28. Hoffman T E, Adams R M. Contact dermatitis to benzoin in greasepaint makeup. *Contact Dermatitis* 1982;4:379.
29. Fregert S, Rorsman H. Hypersensitivity to diethylstilbestrol with cross-sensitization to benzestrol. *Acta Derm Venereol* (Stockh) 1962;42:290.
30. Van Andel P, Bleumink E, Nater I P. The significance of positive patch tests to wood tars. *Trans St Johns Hosp Dermatol Soc* 1974;60:94.
31. Alomar A, Camarasa J G, Garcia Perez A, Pascual M. Wood tar patch test. *Contact Dermatitis* 1977;3:220.
32. Mathias C G T, Maibach H I, Mitchell I C. Plant dermatitis—patch test results (1975–1978). *Contact Dermatitis* 1979;5:336.
33. Rothe A, Heine A, Rebohle E. Oil of juniper as an allergenic substance for skin and respiratory tract. *Berufsdermatosen* 1973;21:11.
34. Lahti A, Hannuksela M. Immediate contact allergy to birch leaves and sap. *Contact Dermatitis* 1980;6:464.
35. Rothenborg H W, Hjorth N. Allergy to perfumes from toilet soaps and detergents in patients with dermatitis. *Arch Dermatol* 1968;97:417.
36. Rudzki E, Grzywa A. Occupational dermatitis partly elicited by coal tar. *Contact Dermatitis* 1877;3:54.
37. Kaidbey K H, Kligman A M. Clinical and histological study of coal tar phototoxicity in humans. *Arch Dermatol* 1977;123:592.
38. Rasmussen J E. The crudeness of coal tar. *Prog Dermatol* 1978;12:23.
39. Fisher A A. Severe systemic and local reactions to topical podophyllum resin. *Cutis* 1981;28:233.
40. Grabbe W. Gefahren bei der Behandlung spitzer Kondylome mit Podophyllin beigleichzeitiger Neosalvarsan-Therapie. *Hautarzt* 1951;2:325.
41. Ward J W, et al. Fatal systemic poisoning following podophyllin treatment of condyloma acuminatum. *South Med J* 1954;47:1204.
42. Schirren C G. Schwere Allgemeinvergiftung nach ortlicher Anwendung von Podophyllin-Spiritus bein spitzen Kondylomen. *Hautarzt* 1966;17:321.
43. Cormaine R H. Condylomata acuminata en podofyllin. *Ned Tijdschr Geneeskd* 1968;112:2305.
44. Hasler J F, Standish S M. Podophyllin treatment of hairy tongue: a warning. *J Am Dent Assoc* 1969;78:563.
45. Chamberlain M J, Reynolds A L, Yoeman W B. Toxic effect of podophyllum application in pregnancy. *Br Med J* 1972;3:391.
46. Larsson L G. Podophyllin treatment of skin carcinomas. *Acta Derm Venereol* (Stockh) 1952;32:56.
47. Stoehr G P, Peterson A, Taylor W J. Systemic complications of local podophyllin therapy. *Ann Intern Med* 1978;89:362.
48. Montaldi D H, Giambrone J P, Courey N G, Taefi P. Podophyllin poisoning associated with the treatment of condyloma acuminatum: a case report. *Am J Obstet Gynecol* 1974;119:1130.
49. Balucani M, Zellers D D. Podophyllum resin poisoning with complete recovery. *JAMA* 1964;189:639.
50. Nelson L M. Use of podophyllin (podophyllum resin) in dermatology. *Arch Dermatol Syphilol* 1953;67:488.
51. Sullivan M, King L S. Effects of resin of podophyllum on normal skin: condylomata acuminata and verrucae vulgaris. *Arch Dermatol Syphilol* 1947;56:30.
52. Maxwell T B, Lamb J H. Unusual reaction to application of podophyllum resin. *Arch Dermatol Syphilol* 1954;70:510.

53. Wade T, Ackerman A B. The effects of resin of podophyllin on condyloma acuminatum. *Am J Dermatopathol* 1984;6:109.
54. Mitchell J, Rook A. *Botanical dermatology—plants and plant products injurious to the skin.* Vancouver: Greengrass, 1979:720.
55. Rudzki E, Grzywa Z. Dermatitis from *Arnica montana. Contact Dermatitis* 1977;3:281.
56. Hausen B M, Herman H D, Willuhn G. The sensitizing capacity of *Composite* plants *(Arnica). Contact Dermatitis* 1978;4:3.
57. Hausen B M. Identification of the allergens of *Arnica montana. Contact Dermatitis* 1978;4:308.
58. Plewig G, Hofmann C, Braun-Falco O. Photoallergic dermatitis from 8-methoxy psoralen. *Arch Dermatol Res* 1978;261:201.
59. Weissmann I, Wagner G, Plewig G. Contact allergy to 8-methoxypsoralen. *Br J Dermatol* 1980;102:113.
60. Gjerstad G, Riner T D. Current status of aloe as a "cureall." *Am J Pharm* 1968;140:58.
61. El Zawahry M, Hegazy M R, Helal M. Use of Aloe in treating leg ulcers and dermatoses. *Dermatol Int* 1973;12:68.
62. Wright C S. Aloe vera in treatment of roentgen ulcers and telangiectasis. *JAMA* 1936;106:1363.
63. Morrow D M, Rapaport MJ, Strick A. Hypersensitivity to aloe. *Arch Dermatol* 1980;116:1064.
64. Bunney M H. Contact dermatitis in beekeepers due to propolis (bee glue). *Br J Dermatol* 1968;80:17.
65. Rothenborg H W. Occupational dermatitis in a beekeeper due to poplar resins in beeswax. *Arch Dermatol* 1967;95:381.
66. Wanscher B. Contact dermatitis from propolis. *Br J Dermatol* 1976;94:451.
67. Petersen H O. Allergy to propolis (bee glue) in patients with eczema. *Ugeskr Laeger* 1977;139:2331.
68. Camasara G. Occupational dermatitis from beeswax. *Contact Dermatitis* 1975;1:124.
69. McGeorge B C, Steele M C. Allergic contact dermatitis of the nipple from Roman chamomile ointment. *Contact Dermatitis* 1991;24:139.
70. Mitchell J C, Rook A. *Botanical dermatology.* London: Henry Kimpton, 1979:187.
71. Beetz D, Cramer H J, Mehlhorn C H. Zur Haufigkeit der Epidermalen Allergie gegenuber Kamille in Kamillenhaltigen Arzneimitteln und Kosmetica. *Dermatol Monatsschr* 1971;157:505.
72. Pereira F, Santos R, Pereira A. Contact dermatitis from chamomile tea. *Contact Dermatitis* 1997;36:307.
73. Rodriguez-Serna M, Sanchez-Motilla J M, Ramon R, Aliaga A. Allergic and systemic contact dermatitis from *Matricaria chamomilla* tea. *Contact Dermatitis* 1998;39:192.
74. van Ketel W G, Bruynzeel D P. Contact sensitivity to tannin. *Contact Dermatitis* 1991;25:75.
75. Markin L E. Boxwood sensitiveness. *J Allergy* 1930;1:346.
76. Scott M J. Jojoba oil. *J Am Acad Dermatol* 1982;6:545.
77. De Groot A C. Airborne allergic contact dermatitis from tea tree oil. *Contact Dermatitis* 1996;35:304.
78. Steinmann A, Schatzle M, Agathos M, Breit R. Allergic contact dermatitis from black cumin *(Nigella sativa)* oil after topical use. *Contact Dermatitis* 1997;36:268.
79. Nilsson D S. Sources of allergenic gums. *Ann Allergy* 1960;18:518.
80. Cooke M A, Wilkinson J F. Formalin sensitivity in gum arabic. *Contact Dermatitis Newsletter* 1973;13:379.
81. Fumagalli M, Bigardi A S, Legori A, Pigatto P D. Occupational contact dermatitis from airborne nicergoline. *Contact Dermatitis* 1992;27:256.
82. Ortiz-Frutos F J, et al. Photocontact dermatitis from rue *(Ruta montana L.). Contact Dermatitis* 1995;33:284.
83. Del Pozo M D, et al. Allergic contact dermatitis from *Verbena officinalis L. Contact Dermatitis* 1994;31:200.
84. Goday Bujan J J, et al. Allergic contact dermatitis from *Krameria triandra* extract. *Contact Dermatitis* 1998;38:120.
85. Pazzaglia M, Venturo N, Borda G, Tosti A. Contact dermatitis due to a message liniment containing *Inula helenium* extract. *Contact Dermatitis* 1995;33:267.
86. Danese P, Carnevali C, Bertazzoni M G. Allergic contact dermatitis due to *Centella asiatica* extract. *Contact Dermatitis* 1994;31:201.
87. Fernandez L, et al. Allergic contact dermatitis from rosemary *(Rosmarinus officinalis L.). Contact Dermatitis* 1997;37:248.
88. Sandra A, Shenoi S D, Srinivas C R. Allergic contact dermatitis from red sandalwood *(Pterocarpus santalinus). Contact Dermatitis* 1996;34:69.
89. Hausen B M. The sensitizing capacity of ginkgolic acids in guinea pigs. *Am J Contact Dermatitis* 1998;9:146.
90. Rodriguez P, et al. Allergic contact dermatitis due to burdock *(Arctium lappa). Contact Dermatitis* 1995;33:134.
91. Schatzle M, Agathos M, Breit R. Allergic contact dermatitis from goldenrod *(Herba solidaginis)* after systemic administration. *Contact Dermatitis* 1998;39:271.

CHAPTER 12

Antiseptics and Disinfectants

Antiseptics are chemicals applied to living tissue that kill or prevent the growth of microorganisms. They must retain their activity in the presence of body fluids without being harmful locally or systemically.

Disinfectants, on the other hand, are used on inanimate objects. They must be effective in the presence of organic materials, such as blood, feces, and sputum, but nondestructive to the materials they contact, such as surgical instruments or counter tops. In this chapter, the following antiseptics and disinfectants are discussed:

1. mercurials
2. iodine
3. chlorinated compounds
4. hexachlorophene and dichlorophene
5. triclosan (irgasan DP 300)
6. TEGO
7. benzoyl peroxide
8. quaternary ammonium compounds
9. antiseptic dyes

THIMEROSAL (MERTHIOLATE)

This compound, sodium ethylmercurithiosalicylate, is used as an antiseptic and a preservative in topical medicaments, cosmetics, and vaccines (Table 12.1).

Solution no. 45 Merthiolate is formulated to contain sodium borate in the current formulation but is colored with two dyes, fluorescein (D & C Yellow no. 70) and eosin yellowish-(YS) (D & C Red no. 22) (1).

> **Merthiolate solution contains sodium borate, whereas tincture of Merthiolate is colored with fluorescein and eosin dyes and contains ethylenediamine.**

The Nature of Sensitization to Thimerosal (Merthiolate)

It should be noted that thimerosal contains two distinct radicals: an organic mercury compound and a thiosalicylate. The allergic reactions may be from either compound. Ellis (2) and Gaul (3) were among the first to show that the thiosalicylate compound is a strong sensitizer. More recently, Takino (4) reported that almost all of 23 Japanese thimerosal-sensitive persons were allergic to the thiosalicylate radical.

Reports of cross-sensitivity of thimerosal with other mercury compounds are confusing because the investigators did not state whether they had tested the thimerosal-sensitive persons to both the mercury and the thiosalicylic acid radicals. Epstein (5) stated that one of his five thimerosal-sensitive patients had cross-reactions to ammoniated mercury. Sertoli et al. (6) reported that a thimerosal-sensitive person had cross-reactions to phenylmercuric nitrate, whereas Fisher et al. (7) found that none of their thimerosal-sensitive patients had cross-reactions with organic mercury compounds. In addition, Möller (8) states that cross-sensitization occurs to a few organic mercurials, but not to inorganic and metallic mercury in thimerosal-sensitive persons.

Patients sensitive to thimerosal (Merthiolate) can be divided into three groups: (a) positive to thimerosal but negative to other mercurials and to thiosalicylic acid, (b) positive to thimerosal and to some other mercurials but negative to thiosalicylic acid, and (c) positive to thimerosal and to thiosalicylic acid but negative to other mercurials.

> **Patients sensitive to thimerosal (Merthiolate) may be allergic to either the organic mercurial molecule or the thiosalicylic acid.**

Thimerosal (Merthiolate) as a Sensitizer in Eye Preparations

There are numerous reports of allergic contact sensitization to thimerosal (Merthiolate) in various eye preparations and contact lens solutions. The allergic reaction may produce conjunctivitis alone or a combination of conjunctivitis and eyelid dermatitis. In one instance, a sensitized person had dermatitis of the hands without conjunctivitis.

Fregert and Hjorth (9) stated that allergic reactions to eyedrops often produce both conjunctivitis and eyelid

TABLE 12.1. *Partial List of Agents Containing Thimerosal (Merthiolate)*

Adapettes	Jenkins Nasal Spray
Adapt	Lauro Eye Wash
Adsorbonac (2% and 5%)	LC-65 Daily Contact Lens Cleaner
Aeroaid	Loridine Cephaloridine
Aerocauticals Aerosol Merthiolate	McKesson's IBath and IDrops
Allerest Eye Drops	Merthiolate (also contains ethylenediamine, fluorescin, and
Allergex (Concentrate)	eosin dyes)
Amertan	Metycaine with Merthiolate Ophth.
Amlab Brite Eye Lotion and Eye-Care Drops	Munichem Mycobac
Biomydrin Nasal Spray/Drops	Murine
BoilnSoak	Mycostatin Cream
Bonmiotin	Neosporin Ophthalmic Solution, Sterile
Collyrium and Collyrium with Ephedrine	Ocusol Eye Drops
Coly-Mycin S Otic	Paredrine 1% with Boric Acid Ophthalmic Solution
Contact Nasal Mist	Phenspray Nasal Spray
Cortisporin Ophthalmic Suspension	Polyspectrin Ophthalmic Solution
Cortisporin Otic Suspension	Preflex
Del Staph 600	Prefrin-Z Liquifilm
Drilitol Spraypak & Solution	Pyocidin-Otic Solution
Dristan Nasal Mist and Children's Dristan Mist	Quotane
Econochlor	Rexall Eye Drops
Elase Ointment	S.A.C. Nasal Spray
Elase-Chloromycetin Ointment	Soaclens
Elcide	Soltice Nasal Spray
Eppy 1/2%	Soothe Eye Drops
Esromiotin 1/4%	Stoxil Ophthalmic Ointment and Ophthalmic Solution
Estivin	Sulfa-Statin
Eye Drop Liquid	Sulf-10 Dropperette Ophthalmic Solution
Eye-Gene	Sulf-10 Ophthalmic Solution
Eyelo Eyedrops	Surfacaine
Florotit	Triscocort Spraypak
4-Way Long Acting Nasal Spray	20/20 Eye Drops
4-Way Mentholated Long Acting Nasal Spray	Vapocyn II Nasal Spray
4-Way Mentholated Nasal Spray	Vasocort Spraypak
4-Way Nasal Spray	Vicks Sinex Nasal Spray
Fungicin	Va-tro-nal Nose Drops
Impact Nasal Spray	V12
Isotogen Ear Drops	

dermatitis, whereas van Ketel and Melzer-van Riemsduk (10) pointed out that thimerosal, present as a preservative in many soft-lens solutions, produced allergic conjunctivitis but no eyelid dermatitis in three of their patients. Pedersen (11) also described conjunctivitis without eyelid dermatitis.

Sertoli et al. (6) reported that a patient who had allergic thimerosal sensitization developed allergic contact dermatitis on the fingers and palms; however, when this same solution was applied to the eyes, it did not produce conjunctivitis or eyelid dermatitis. The patient in this case, a 20-year-old woman, had two small patches of dyshidrosiform vesicles which merged into blisters and contained clear fluid; one patch of vesicles was located in the center of the right palm, and the other was on the tip of the left index finger. She had worn soft contact lenses for 1 month before the eruption began. When not worn, the lenses were kept in a lens container with a preserving liquid; they were taken out for use individually using the tip of the left index finger, put on the right palm, and there washed with a liquid

again using the tip of the left index finger before being put into the eyes.

Rietschel and Wilson (12) reported that soft contact lenses cleaned and stored in thimerosal-containing solutions may produce an ocular inflammatory process and, if untreated, corneal neovascularization. They examined 38 patients who were using soft contact lenses and found that 31 had positive ocular provocation test results to a thimerosal-preserved, artificial-tears solution. Delayed hypersensitivity to thimerosal was demonstrated by positive patch tests in 27 patients. Avoidance of thimerosal and the use of unit-dose sterile saline solutions resulted in complete resolution of ocular symptoms.

> **Many ophthalmic solutions, including various "eyedrops," "eye lotions," sprays, and contact lens solutions, contain thimerosal (Merthiolate).**

> **Thimerosal (Merthiolate) preservative sensitivity in biological testing solutions may confuse the evaluation of results.**

Life-Threatening Reactions to Thimerosal (Merthiolate)

Maibach (13) reported a case of marked reaction to thimerosal after treating a patient's slightly sore throat with a thimerosal first-aid spray. The next day, because of continued discomfort, he repeated the treatment. Laryngeal obstruction followed within hours. Emergency tracheotomy produced prompt improvement. Patch testing revealed an extreme spreading reaction to thimerosal. It was believed that the acute laryngeal obstruction developed as a delayed hypersensitivity reaction to this first-aid spray.

Patch Test with Thimerosal (Merthiolate)

At present, most testing is done with 0.1% thimerosal in petrolatum. Although there has been controversy as to whether positive patch test reactions to thimerosal are irritant or allergic in nature, allergy is the most likely explanation because provocative product use tests are positive in most subjects who have patch test reactions to thimerosal. Occasionally, however, mercury salts may produce a false-positive reaction when the patch test is performed in a Finn chamber, because a chemical reaction between the aluminum of the chamber with the tested mercury salt may occur (Kalveram, K.J., and Forck, G., Munster, Germany, personal communication).

Thimerosal (Merthiolate) as a Sensitizer in Injectable, Biological Solutions

Thimerosal (Merthiolate) is used as a preservative in vaccines, antitoxins, parenteral medications, and diluting fluids used for preparations of antigens for scratch or intradermal testing.

Epstein (5) observed five patients within 1 year who showed consistently delayed-type reactions to intradermal tests with multiple antigens. The diluting fluid of these extracts contained thimerosal; all five patients were allergic to this preservative.

Reisman (14), in the course of routine allergy investigation, found ten patients who had delayed hypersensitivity reactions to the thimerosal preservative in the testing solutions. Three patients had previous contact dermatitis from thimerosal. Five patients may have been sensitized through either direct contact or parenteral injections, and the mode of sensitization in at least two patients was unknown. Reisman stated that the availability of phenol, which rarely if ever sensitizes, indicates there is no reason to continue to use thimerosal as a preservative in allergy extracts.

Rietschel and Adams (15) reported that thimerosal was a limiting factor in Heptavax immunization against hepatitis B. Two patients, both working in the medical field, had intense local reactions to as little as 0.1 mg of intradermal Heptavax from the thimerosal preservative (15). All current hepatitis B vaccines in the United States contain thimerosal.

Hansson and Möller (16) stated that thimerosal gives a high frequency of positive reactions when tested epicutaneously and intracutaneously in young adults. Thimerosal is added as a preservative to Swedish old tuberculin (OT). The reactions to intracutaneously injected OT thimerosal and purified protein derivative (PPD) have been compared in 412 healthy young adults, and a positive reaction to thimerosal was recorded in 15%. Thimerosal influenced the reactions in 63 of the 163 positive OT tests. Consequently, it was concluded that thimerosal should not be added to intracutaneous test solutions because this additive may interfere with the evaluation of positive reactions.

Although thimerosal is commonly found in vaccines such as hepatitis, tetanus, and meningoencephalitis, reports of significant adverse reactions to this type of exposure are rare. Only 10% of thimerosal sensitive patients reported slight to moderate adverse reactions to thimerosal-containing vaccines consisting mainly of painful swelling at the injection site (17).

Worldwide Incidence of Thimerosal (Merthiolate) Sensitivity

The North American Contact Dermatitis Research Group reintroduced thimerosal in the "standard" or "screening" patch test tray because preliminary results indicate that thimerosal is a fairly common cause of allergic contact sensitization in the United States.

Möller (18) stated that, from laboratories in which patch testing is performed with a standard series including thimerosal, quite different figures emerge from the incidence of contact allergy to this compound. Apparently, there is a geographic variation. High figures of 8% to 15% have been reported from the United States and Brazil, whereas moderate figures of 3% to 4% have been reported from Denmark and Sweden.

When thimerosal was used as a disinfectant and sold over the counter for self-medication, a high degree of sensitization was recorded in several countries, including the United States and Brazil. A particular problem arose when remarkably high figures of thimerosal allergy (15% to 25%) were reported among healthy young Swedes from subpopulations of military recruits, nursing students, and medical students. The occurrence could not be explained on the basis of self-medication, because thimerosal had never been sold over the counter in Sweden, and the agent was no more available than in low-allergy countries. A national campaign against tuberculosis in Sweden, however, had suggested repeated tuberculin testing in children and young people. It was shown that the thimerosal contained in the tuberculin could sensitize when injected intracutaneously. This iatrogenic sensitization, however, did not induce any skin disease or other clinical manifestation (19).

Also in Sweden, Hansson and Möller (20) reported that patch test results were positive in 16% of healthy young military service recruits tested with 0.1% thimerosal in petrolatum and in 15% tested intracutaneously with 0.01% thimerosal in saline. These reactions to thimerosal caused false-positive responses to tuberculin because thimerosal was present as a preservative in the tuberculin solution.

On the basis of their results, the authors stressed that thimerosal (Merthiolate) should not be used as a preservative in solutions for the detection of delayed-type hypersensitivity; however, if it is present, a control test with thimerosal should be included in the investigation.

In Japan, Takino (4) found 23 cases of thimerosal sensitivity in a 2-year period. In Czechoslovakia, Novak and Kvicalova (21) reported 38 positive thimerosal patch test results in 316 patients examined. These investigators found it difficult to correlate the patch test reactions with the clinical picture. The authors did not exclude the possibility that the reactions were caused by subcutaneous or intramuscular injections of biological preparations containing thimerosal (Merthiolate). This shows the importance of a search for thimerosal (Merthiolate) in the environment.

The significance of thimerosal allergy has expanded because it has been learned that piroxicam photosensitization occurs regularly in thimerosal-sensitive individuals (22). Furthermore, animals sensitized to thimerosal develop contact and photocontact dermatitis on exposure to piroxicam (Feldene) alone or piroxicam plus ultraviolet A (UVA), respectively (23). See Chapter 10 for additional information.

> **Thimerosal (Merthiolate) preservatives in allergy-testing solutions may produce false-positive tests. Intradermal control tests with thimerosal (Merthiolate) should be performed.**

MERBROMIN (MERCUROCHROME, FLAVUROL)

This organic mercurial antiseptic may cross-react with inorganic mercurials. There are several reports of allergic contact dermatitis to merbromin (24).

Camarasa (25) reported a man with injuries treated with merbromin who developed a violent, local reaction, a generalized eruption, and facial and laryngeal edema of such severity that he required treatment in an intensive care unit. Patch tests revealed that he was strongly positive to thimerosal (Merthiolate) (0.1% aqueous) and to mercuric chloride (0.05% aqueous). The response to Mercromina, containing 2% aqueous solutions of the sodium salt of dibromohydroxy mercuric resorcinolphthalein, precipitated

an erythroderma and laryngeal edema that necessitated his return to the intensive care unit.

A similar case was reported by Pelaez Hernandez et al. (26). Minutes after applying Mercurochrome, a 51-year-old man developed anaphylaxis consisting of generalized urticaria, dyspnea, dysphonia, and dizziness. His evaluation revealed both immediate and delayed hypersensitivity to Mercurochrome. He was prick test positive, PK test positive (but negative with serum heated to 56°C to destroy IgE antibodies), patch test positive to multiple mercury compounds, but patch test negative to thimerosal.

Merbromin may be tested "as is," undiluted.

Mercurochrome and Merthiolate are not the same compound and will not cross-react unless the patient is sensitive to the Mercurial component of Merthiolate (thimerosal) (27).

> **Inorganic mercury may cross-react with organic mercurial compounds.**

PHENYLMERCURIC SALTS (ACETATE, NITRATE, BROMIDE, AND BENZOATE)

Phenylmercuric salts may be present in the products shown in Table 12.2. The U.S. Food and Drug Administration (FDA) allows these salts in eye solutions and cosmetics used about the eyes because they are effective against pseudomonad infections.

Phenylmercuric Acetate

Morris (28) reported that a woman's vulva itched and burned when she used a contraceptive jelly containing 0.02% phenylmercuric acetate. A patch test with 0.06% phenylmercuric chloride was positive. Although Hjorth and Trolle-Lassen (29) indicated that patch tests with a 0.1% concentration of phenylmercuric acetate may give false-positive irritant reactions, such reactions did not occur in our experience. In sensitized persons, however, patch test reactions may be obtained in concentrations from 0.01% to 0.16% in petrolatum.

Not infrequently, cross-reactions occur between organic mercury compounds, such as phenylmercuric acetates, and the inorganic salts, such as ammoniated mercury and bichloride of mercury. Moreover, an allergic eczematous dermatitis from external sensitization by a mercurial compound may be exacerbated or reproduced by *systemic* administration of medication containing mercury, such as metalluride (Mercuhydrin), in sensitized persons.

TABLE 12.2. *Phenylmercuric Salts*

Contraceptives	Ophthalmic solutions
Cosmetics	Shampoos
Emulsion paints	Shoe linings

> **To avoid irritant reactions, phenylmercuric salts should be tested 0.05% in petrolatum, not in aqueous solutions.**

An allergic contact dermatitis from phenylmercuric acetate and phenylmercuric oleate was reported by Hartung (30) in a worker who sewed tarpaulin treated with these chemicals. Three such patients were patch tested with each of these chemicals in concentrations of 0.025% and 0.026%, and all three reacted to both.

Phenylmercury Borate (Phenylmercuric Borate)

In Germany, phenylmercury borate is used for tinea pedis and preoperatively on the skin. Breit and Bandmann (31) reported that it was the cause of dermatitis in 116 of 1,094 patients sensitized by a topical medicament, and many of these patients had cross-sensitivity to other mercury compounds used as preservatives in creams and ointments. The use of phenylmercury borate as thermometer disinfectant also caused allergic contact dermatitis.

Phenylmercuric Nitrate

This preservative contains 65% mercury. Morris (28) reported two patients sensitized by phenylmercuric nitrate. The first patient developed a contact dermatitis on his legs after putting a weed-killer powder containing this chemical on his lawn. A woman developed dermatitis of the face from the acetate in an ointment. Both patients reacted to patch tests with a 0.06% solution of phenylmercuric nitrate.

RELATIONSHIP OF ORGANIC AND INORGANIC MERCURY COMPOUNDS

The organic mercurials used as antiseptics include thimerosal (Merthiolate), merbromin (Mercurochrome), nitromersol (Metaphen), and mercocresol (Mercresin). The inorganic mercurials include metallic mercury, ammoniated mercury, yellow oxide of mercury, and the phenylmercuric salts (acetate, nitrate, bromide, and borate). Cross-reactions between metallic mercury and the organic and inorganic mercurial compounds may occur. Sidi and Casalis (32) reported a case of chronic eczema of the face and arms of a patient who had positive patch test reactions to dental amalgam, inorganic mercury, and merbromin (Mercurochrome). Hjorth and Trolle-Lassen (29) stated categorically, however, that "the mercury ion does not cross-sensitize to the organic compounds." In Fisher's experience (33), three patients who had mercury sensitivity reacted to metallic mercury, as well as the organic and inorganic compounds. Furthermore, in patients who had allergic contact sensitivity to mercury, the skin lesions may be exacerbated or reproduced by systemic administration of mercurial compounds (34).

Van Ketel and Roeleveld (35) reported a case of cross-reactions among the following mercurial compounds: mercuric oxycyanide, thimerosal (Merthiolate), phenylmercuric nitrate, ammoniated mercury, and metallic mercury.

> **The inorganic mercurials such as metallic mercury and ammoniated mercury may cross-react with the organic mercurials such as thimerosal, merbromin, and the phenylmercuric salts.**

Mercuric Chloride

Other names for mercuric chloride are mercury bichloride, mercury perchloride, and corrosive sublimate. This mercury compound may be found in some antiseptic hair "tonics," such as Elm's Hair and Scalp Treatment, Scalpo Ointment, and Bar Soap, and is also used in embalming fluids.

Mercuric chloride is a strong sensitizer that may produce a nonspecific, pustular reaction or an irritant patch test reaction even when diluted to 0.05% solution (36,37).

Mercurous Chloride (Calomel)

Calomel, used in the past as an antiseptic, is still occasionally used at present as a laxative. In mercury-sensitive persons, the ingestion of Calomel may produce "systemic" contact dermatitis (33).

Para-Chloromercuriphenol

This organic mercurial is used occasionally in soaps or topical medications as a disinfectant. Mathias et al. (38) reported a case of dermatitis of the hands and forearms from a woman's allergic hypersensitivity to this mercury compound used to treat her baby's diaper rash. There was a cross-reaction to phenylmercuric acetate but not to thimerosal (Merthiolate).

MISCELLANEOUS ANTISEPTIC AND DISINFECTANT MERCURY COMPOUNDS

Table 12.3 lists several other mercury compounds used as antiseptics, disinfectants, fungicides, and wood preservatives. Table 12.4 lists the numerous antiseptic topical skin preparations that at one time have contained mercury compounds other than thimerosal (Merthiolate), merbromin (Mercurochrome), or nitromersol (Metaphen).

The tables list other categories of topical preparations that have contained mercury compounds: Table 12.5, acne preparations; Table 12.6, fungicides; Table 12.7, eye, ear, nose, and throat preparations; Table 12.8, vaginal medications and "prophylactic kits"; Table 12.9, plant fungicides and antiseptics.

TABLE 12.3. *Mercury Compounds*

Mercuric chloride
Mercuric cyanide
Mercuric dimethyldithiocarbamate
Mercuric lactate
Mercuric oleate
Mercuric stearate
Mercurous chloride
Phenylmercuric acetate
Phenylmercuric benzoate
Phenylmercuric chloride
Phenylmercuric ethanolammonium acetate and lactate
Phenylmercuric hydroxide
Phenylmercuric lactate
Phenylmercuric naphthenate
Phenylmercuric nitrate
Phenylmercuric oleate
Red mercuric oxide
Yellow mercuric oxide

TABLE 12.4. *Topical Skin Preparations Containing Mercury Compounds*

Antiseptic and first-aid
  AAA Paste
  Bag Balm
  Dermacol Liquid
  Dermato Ointment
  Hermesol
  Kay-Sen
  Lanacane
  Lubafax
  Marsa
  Massengill's Tanic Acid. Jelly, and Benzocaine
  Mazon
  Mercoseptic
  Mertok
  Metaphen
  Mystacin Cream
  Palmer's Antiseptic Lotion
  Phillips Corona Ointment
  Purepas Blue Ointment
  Raleigh's Ointment
  Rexall Skin Antiseptic
  Sperti Ointment
  Unguentine
Veterinary preparations
  Bag Balm
  McClellan's Eyelid Ointment
  Mulrilicare
  Stevens Ointment

TABLE 12.5. *Acne Preparations Containing Mercury Compounds*

Derma-Teen Skin Soap
Derma-Tone
Teen-Ac

TABLE 12.6. *Fungicides Containing Mercury Compounds*

Amber Liquid
Athlete Ointment
Epidex
Gebauer's PMC Spray
Maseda Foot Powder
Melsan
Phe-Mer-Nite
Phytox-ointment

TABLE 12.7. *Mercury Compounds in Ear, Nose, Eye, and Throat Preparations*

Ear preparations
  Clopane
Nasal preparations (drops and spray)
  Neotrol
  Otall Drops
  Privine
  Vasefrin
  Vasohist
Eye preparations
  Blinx Eye Wash
  Clean-N' Soak
  Coloptin
  Noxmol
  Wetting Solution
  Yellow Mercuric Oxide Ointments
Throat lozenges
  B & R Homeopathic Tablets no. 195A
  Phe-Mer-Caine
  Phe-Mer-Nite
  Thantis

TABLE 12.8. *Mercury Compounds in Vaginal Medications and Prophylactic Kits*

Prophylactic kits
  Dough-Boy
Vaginal jellies, tablets, and douches
  Baculin
  Dorana
  Koromex
  Lorophyn
  Merpertogel
  Norforms
  Nylmerate
  Phe-Mer-Nite
  Servex
  Southern Pharmacal
  Tricho-San
  Triserts
  Vagagill

TABLE 12.9. *Mercury Compounds in Plant Fungicides and Antiseptics*

Seed fungicides, protectants, and disinfectants	*Herbicides (crabgrass and weed killer)*
Amacene	Blitz
Gallotox	Dynaside Homelawn Crabgrass Killer
Gy-Treet SQS	PMAS
Isotox Seed Treater	Puraturf
Merc-O-Dent	*Insecticides*
Mergamma "C"	Green Cross
Merlane Dust	Hubbard Cabbage Maggot Dust
Merlane Liquid	Magic Brand Bug Killer
Panodrin	Mergamma
Panogen	P & P Cabbage Maggot Destroyer
Pantirra	Real-Kill Bug Killer
Parson's Seed Saver Dust	Real-Kill Moth Bomb
Semesan	Setrete Mist
Turf fungicides and disinfectants	*Root, bulb, and grain treatments*
Calocine	Mercan
Caloclor	Merfendel 41
Calogreen	Merfenel 51
Coromerc	Merfenelope
Corrosive sublimate	Merlane Dust
Mersolite-8	Mer-Sol 48
Mersolite-10	Mer-Sol 51
Phenylmercuric acetate Phix	*Soil conditioners*
PM Grain Protectant	*Fertilizers*
PMN Germicide	
Semesan	
Plant fungicides	
Orchard Brand Mercury Spray	
Puratized Agricultural Spray	
Puratized Apple Spray	
Semesan Fungicide	

IODINE

Iodine USP is 2% iodine and 2.4% sodium iodide in alcohol, whereas strong iodine tincture NF is 7% iodine and 5% potassium iodide in alcohol.

Tincture of iodine is a primary irritant that should be tested by the "open" method. Old solutions of iodine are particularly irritating. Povidone-iodine (Betadine), iodine in a base of polyvinyl pyrrolidine, is not as irritating as tincture of iodine and may be tested "as is" by the usual patch test method. The irritancy of several antiseptics was evaluated in an open application 30 minutes' exposure time twice a day for 4 days (39). Normal use concentrations were studied. Sodium hypochlorite 0.25% and 1% iodine in 70% ethanol were both too irritating to complete the study. In this method 4% chlorhexidine, 0.5% chlorhexidine in 70% ethanol, and ethanol 70% were deemed nonirritating.

Povidone-iodine (Betadine) may produce allergic contact dermatitis (40,41). Two recent cases of povidone-iodine contact dermatitis were positive at 10% concentration in petrolatum (42).

Prolonged skin contact with povidone-iodine saturated drapes can occur during surgery, and the surgical team may be unaware of the pooling of povidone-iodine prep solution in this manner (43). After 3 to 4 hours of exposure in this fashion, a chemical burn–like skin change can result. These reactions are commonly mistaken for electrical burns. A direct toxic effect is thought to be responsible.

Povidone-iodine is a rare cause of allergic contact dermatitis and has also caused irritant and systemic reactions (44). A 10% aqueous solution of povidone-iodine is used for patch test purposes.

Hjorth (45) reported that 1,3-di-iodo-2-hydroxypropane, a "white tincture of iodine" used in Denmark for first aid, caused contact dermatitis in one patient. He had a strong positive patch test, whereas 20 control subjects were negative.

Iodine may cross-react with iodoform, which is insoluble in water but readily soluble in alcohol and with thymol iodide. Both of these iodide preparations may be tested 25% in petrolatum. They may cross-react with radiopaque iodine and iodides in medications. Thus, cross-reactions with the organic and inorganic iodides may occur.

> **Topical inorganic iodine preparations such as povidone-iodine (Betadine) are rare sensitizers that may cross-react with injectable radiopaque iodine.**

Patch tests with iodine and potassium iodide may result in a nonspecific, papulopustular reaction that must be differentiated from a contact allergic response. Patch tests with potassium iodide have been used in the diagnosis of dermatitis herpetiformis (DH) but are nonspecific.

A positive patch test reaction to iodine may mean that the patient may react adversely if an iodine-containing contrast material is administered. Lieberman et al. (46), however, stated that a review of the literature involving anaphylactoid reactions to iodinated contrast material suggests that the reactions are nonantibody-mediated but that a complex activation of inflammatory mediators occurs. Histamine release or complement activation has been demonstrated in experimental systems both in vitro and in vivo. It appears that pretreatment of selected cases (patients with a previous anaphylactoid reaction) with antihistamine and corticosteroids is effective in reducing the frequency and severity of subsequent reactions when readministration is necessary.

Rothe et al. (47), reporting a case of contact dermatitis from a radiopaque iodine used in angiography and renography, stated that a difficulty with iodine-containing contrast material is the lack of a consistently reliable in vitro test or a safe in vivo test to predict whether a given patient is likely to have an adverse reaction. The generally adopted practice today is to regard all patients who have highly allergic backgrounds or histories of adverse reactions to contrast media as being at greater than average risk.

> There appears to be no reliable in vitro or in vivo test to predict adverse reactions to intravenous iodine-contrast compounds.

CHLORINE AND CHLORINATED PRODUCTS

Chlorinated Water

Neering (48) described a patient who acquired contact urticaria whenever he swam in chlorinated, swimming pool water disinfected with sodium hypochlorite. This patient also developed contact urticaria from contact with a cleansing powder containing Chlorox. Closed patch tests were negative, but a scratch test produced a strongly positive reaction.

> Chlorinated swimming pool water may produce contact urticaria to be distinguished from aquagenic urticaria.

Sodium Hypochlorite

This chlorinated product is present in the following products in the United States: eau de Javelle, Chlorox, Dazzle, and Dakin's Solution. Osmundsen (49) reported a case of severe allergic contact dermatitis from sodium hypochlorite in a patient who had avoided swimming pools for years because the heavy smell of chlorine made her feel ill. After an abortion in which chloramine-T (chloramine) was used, she developed severe dermatitis in the genital area. Osmundsen performed patch testing with a popular bleaching agent, 10% in water, corresponding to about 0.5% sodium hypochlorite. The patch test elicited a more than palm-sized, red, vesicular, strongly edematous, and infiltrated reaction.

Suspected contact dermatitis to bleach (sodium hypochlorite) can be tested with a 1% aqueous solution using 17 to 20 μL volume in the Finn chamber, provided that the concentration of sodium hydroxide in the bleach is not more than 1% (50). The concentration of sodium hydroxide in bleach varies with different manufacturers and may cause irritant reactions.

Bromine

Bromine-based disinfectants are used in pools and hot tubs to maintain water purity. Three cases of dermatitis were traced to bromine in the form of Halobrome, which is 1-bromo-3-chloro-5,5-dimethylhydantoin (51). Patch tests with 0.1% aqueous were positive.

Chloramine-T (Chloramine)

Chloramine is used commonly as a sterilizer, disinfectant, and chemical reagent. It has been described as an occupational hazard for pharmaceutical workers, nurses, butchers, cleaners, and brewers (52).

Dooms-Goossens et al. (53) reported a case of contact urticaria from chloramine. Over several months, the patient had recurrent attacks of edema of the eyelids accompanied by dyspnea, rhinitis, and a tingling sensation in her mouth and occasionally in her fingers whenever she came in contact with chloramine powder, which she frequently (two to three times a week) had to dissolve in water to make 0.5% solutions to disinfect bedpans. The symptoms appeared 15 to 20 minutes after contact with the chloramine powder and sometimes lasted for several days despite local treatment with a corticosteroid cream. She also had minor reactions after coming in contact with 0.5% chloramine solutions. An open test with chloramine "as is" on the patient's forearm yielded erythema and wheal formation after 20 minutes. A closed patch test with a 0.2% solution produced erythema and wheal formation at the 48-hour patch test reading, which disappeared by the 96-hour reading.

There are several reports of asthma produced by chloramine in industrial use (54–57). Kramps et al. (57) demonstrated the presence of specific IgE antibodies in the serum of asthmatic chloramine-allergic patients. Bourne et al. (54) stated that it is advisable to open chloramine powder under water or in a glove box or else with the operator fully protected by an air-fed hood or suit or a properly fitting, appropriate filter-type mask, preferably pressurized.

Chloramine-T (chloramine) can produce delayed allergic contact dermatitis, contact urticaria, and asthma.

Chlorhexidine

Chlorhexidine (1.1-hexamethylenebis [5(P chlorophenyl) biguanide]) is an antibacterial compound active against gram-positive and gram-negative bacteria even in the presence of body fluids. The chlorhexidine salts used most frequently in medicine are digluconate, acetate, and diacetate. The use of chlorhexidine as an antiseptic has increased in recent years at the expense of quaternary ammonium compounds. Chlorhexidine is used clinically for disinfection of hands and operation sites in the treatment of burns and scalds, in urology and gynecology, and by dentists in the treatment of caries and periodontitis.

Mobacken and Wengstrom (58) have suggested that, pending further knowledge, chlorhexidine be used with caution on wounds caused by disturbed circulation where additional tissue injury may be dangerous, and on tissue structures with function that may be restricted by excessive scar tissue, for example, exposed tendons and tendon sheaths. Occlusive dressings may increase penetration into the tissues and contribute consequently to the development of untoward effects.

Although chlorhexidine is used widely, allergic reactions are rare (59–61). Ljunggren and Möller (60) described a case of contact dermatitis resulting from the antiseptic chlorhexidine. The allergic nature of the reaction was proved by epicutaneous and intracutaneous testing with various salts and solvents. False-negative patch tests were obtained when chlorhexidine was applied in petrolatum, because chlorhexidine for physicochemical reasons is biologically and allergologically active in aqueous solutions only. Surfactants incorporated in emulsions may also interfere with the patch test response. Use of a chlorhexidine preparation for insertion of an intrauterine device (IUD) resulted in urticaria and dyspnea (62). Prick tests to both diacetate (0.5% aq) and digurconate (0.5% aq) were positive.

The ideal test for chlorhexidine is uncertain. Acetate at 1% produces more reactions than gluconate at 1%, but many reactions are irritant (63). Thirteen percent of patients with leg ulcers are sensitive to chlorhexidine; therefore, it is not recommended for use with such patients. A 0.05% aqueous concentration of acetate is probably acceptable for screening purposes (63).

Application of chlorhexidine antiseptic to the buttocks led to anaphylactic shock in a 33-year-old man who had irritation after a riding lesson (64). Prick tests were positive

to 0.2% chlorhexidine in the patient and negative in three controls. Prior reports of anaphylaxis from chlorhexidine involved mucosal exposure or catheter insertion.

Patch tests of chlorhexidine in petrolatum are not reliable. Aqueous solution, however, may produce irritant reactions in test controls.

Cetrimide

At times patients use antiseptics improperly by applying them undiluted to skin disease. A series of 18 such patients used a product containing 3% cetrimide and 0.3% chlorhexidine (65). Within 1 to 4 weeks dermatitis was seen principally in the genital region and antecubital fossa. Patch tests revealed irritant reactions to cetrimide at 0.5%, 1%, or 2% aqueous. The morphology of the reactions was xerotic or chemical burn–like, and the histology showed ortho and parakeratosis without spongiosis.

Chloroxine

Chloroxine is a dichloro-hydroxyquinoline antiseptic compound that readily forms colored complexes with polyvalent metal ions but is not a sensitizer. This antiseptic, present in Capitrol shampoo, may produce a yellow tint on white or light-colored hair. Individuals working with Capitrol may acquire yellow skin on the hands and fingers. This discoloration disappears usually within 24 hours (Levy, J., Westwood Pharmaceuticals, Inc., personal communication).

It is known that greenish discoloration of light-colored hair has been traced to the use of copper-containing algaecides used in swimming pools and the presence of copper eluted from copper plumbing (66,67). Because chloroxine complexes with copper, the use of Capitrol shampoo could increase the chance of greenish discoloration of the hair (68).

Chloroxine, a nonsensitizer present in Capitrol shampoo, may enhance the greenish discoloration of light-colored hair when exposed to the copper in swimming pools and in water eluted from copper plumbing.

Although Bhat et al. (69) have said that shampooing does not remove the green color, an acidic cream rinse or a "vinegar" rinse does readily remove the greenish color. A 3% solution of peroxide also removes the color.

Chloroxylenol

This chlorinated phenol antiseptic is also known as parachlorometaxylenol (PCMX), *p*-chloro-*m*-xylenol, 4-chloro-3,5,-xylenol, ottasept, and benzytol.

Table 12.10 shows the products that may contain chloroxylenol. The related chlorinated phenols, 4-chloro-*m*-cresol (chlorocresol) and parachlorometaxylenol, are used as preservatives in betamethasone cream, electrocardiogram paste, and in more than 30 over-the-counter products. Contact allergic eczema does occur sporadically. The two compounds may cross-react (70,71).

According to Calnan (59), chloroxylenol ranked second in his list of antibacterial agents (excluding antibiotics) in the incidence of allergic sensitivity produced. Of 220 cases of contact allergy to antibacterial agents, 53 were caused by chloroxylenol. Only mercury (60 cases) caused more disease than chloroxylenol. Hjorth and Trolle-Lassen (72) demonstrated cross-sensitization between chlorocresol and chloroxylenol in three patients. This finding means that the chemical structure of these two compounds is so close the human body cannot tell them apart. As a result, a patient allergic to one compound may react to both.

4-Chloro-*m*-cresol (4-Chloro-3-Methylphenol, Ottafect, Ottawa, Parachlorometacresol, PCMC, Phenol, Chloro-3-Methyl)

Incidence of Sensitivity

Clinically, chlorocresol is an infrequent sensitizer. Of 1,000 patients who had contact dermatitis analyzed by Burry et al. (73) in southern Australia, only 11 reacted to chlorocresol.

TABLE 12.10. *Products Containing Parachloro-Metaxylenol**

Absorbine Junior (W.F. Young)
Acne Aid (Steifel)
Aveeno Baby Powder (Cooper)
Carbolated Vaseline
Cebum Shampoo (Dermik)
Cenathesin (Central)
Chloroxylenol (British Pharmacopea)
Desitin Baby Powder (Leeming)
Enden Shampoo Cream & Lotion (Curtis)
Natural Wonder Alive & Well Transparent Face Color (Revlon)
Natural Wonder Oil Free Makeup (Revlon)
Nu-Flow Shampoo
Nullo Foot Cream (De Pree)
Redux ECG Paste
Rezamid, Rezamid Cream, and Rezamid Lotion (Dermik)
Stopette Deodorant Roll-on Clear (Helene Curtis)
Top Brass (Revlon)
Unburn Spray (Leeming)
Unguentine Plus (Norwich)
Unguentine Spray (Norwich)
Vaseline Medicated First Aid Petroleum Jelly
Zeasorb Powder
Zetar Shampoo (Dermik)

*Also in some contraceptive douches.

Causes of Sensitivity

Dermatitis from chlorocresol in betamethasone creams was reported in 13 patients in Australia by Burry et al. (73). Many were thought to have been primarily sensitized by chloroxylenol because, on patch testing, although all were positive to chloroxylenol, only eight were additionally positive to chlorocresol. It was suggested that, in the negative reactors, absorption of chlorocresol was dependent upon its incorporation into the corticosteroid cream. A woman who had been sensitized, possibly by betamethasone cream, was described by Park (74) in New Zealand. Oleffe et al. (75) also reported an allergic reaction to chlorocresol in a steroid cream.

> **Chlorocresol dermatitis may occur from cortico-steroid creams in which chlorocresol is used as a preservative.**

Chlorocresol is used as a preservative in Valisone Cream and some cosmetics. It is also present in Royal Bond Pre-injection fluid. In veterinary medicine, it is used in pesticides and fungicides. Certain embalming fluids contain this antiseptic.

HEXACHLOROPHENE (G-11, AT-7, K-34)

This halogenated phenolic antiseptic closely related to dichlorophene was once widely used in cosmetics, soaps, and pharmaceutical vehicles as an antiseptic. At present, hexachlorophene is present in pHisoHex and Burdeo (Hill). The results of testing with a vehicle series show that hexachlorophene is a rare sensitizer. Irritant reactions of the scrotum and the face from pHisoHex, which contains a soluble from hexachlorophene, have been reported, but in none was hexachlorophene implicated as a sensitizer (76).

The FDA restriction of the use of hexachlorophene is related to toxic brain damage and not to marked skin toxicity or sensitivity.

Epstein (77) found cross-sensitivity between dichlorophene and hexachlorophene. Fisher et al. (7) found no such cross-reactions. Fregert and Hjorth (78) reported a sensitization index of 0.3% in 660 patients, although acute primary irritant contact dermatitis occurred more frequently, especially in areas with susceptible skin, such as the scrotum (79). Positive patch tests believed to be cross-reactions to hexachlorophene were found in patients who had allergy to tetrachlorosalicylanilide, bithionol, and dichlorophene.

Cross-Reactions

Hexachlorophene may cross-react to such halogenated photosensitizers as tetrachlorosalicylanilide and bithionol (80). (Bithionol is not used in the United States.)

> Hexachlorophene is a rare sensitizer but may be an irritant and toxic in high concentrations; it cross-reacts with halogenated photosensitizers.

DICHLOROPHENE (G-4, CUNIPHEN)

Dichlorophene is a fungicide and bactericide used in dentifrices, shampoos, antiperspirant and deodorant creams, powder, toilet waters, and preparations for dermatophytosis of the foot. Compound G-4 is used extensively as a mildewcide to treat and preserve cotton fibers, various fabrics, paper, synthetic leather lattices, and some adhesive tape backings.

Allergic stomatitis and cheilitis owing to G-4 in dentifrices have been reported, and it is now used rarely in such products (81,82). Gaul and Underwood (83) reported allergic dermatitis from G-4 used as a fungicide. This compound is still present in numerous over-the-counter preparations for "athlete's foot."

> Dichlorophene is a more potent sensitizer than hexachlorophene. Although closely related chemically, they rarely cross-react. The U.S. Food and Drug Administration has restricted greatly the use of hexachlorophene for its possible toxic, but not allergic, effect.

Schorr (84) reported instances of allergic contact dermatitis from the presence of G-4 in Duke Gelocast Bandage for treatment of stasis ulcers. [*Note:* The Primer Medicated Bandage (Glenwood) contains glycerin, acacia, zinc oxide, white petrolatum, and amylum in a vegetable oil base and is free of preservatives.] Schorr also found instances of allergic dermatitis from the presence of G-4 in Jergens Lotion.

THE IRGASANS

Two popular "Irgasans" are chemically unrelated to each other:

1. Triclosan (irgasan DP 300), a diphenyl ether (2,4,4′-trichloro′-2″-hydroxydiphenyl ether). Table 12.11 lists some products that have contained irgasan DP 300. There are reports of allergic contact dermatitis from a deodorant foot powder, a deodorant, and an antiperspirant spray (85,86). Wahlberg (87) also reported an allergic reaction to irgasan DP 30 during routine screening. Irgasan DP 300 incorporated into such footwear as men's hosiery and insoles of shoes are called "odor-eaters" because it is claimed that this chemical can suppress the odor produced by foot organisms. Such hosiery and insoles may produce "odor-eater" dermatitis (88).

2. Cluflucarban [irgasan CF 3(4,4′-dichloro-3-(trifluoromethyl) carbanilide)] is a carbanilide unrelated chemically to irgasan DP 300. Safeguard soap, marketed in the United States, contains irgasan CF 3.

> Irgasan DP 300, used widely as an antiseptic in soaps and as a "deodorant," can produce "odor-eater" dermatitis of the feet when used in insoles and men's hosiery.

TRICLOCARBAN (TCC)

This antiseptic is used in several antiseptic soaps. Maibach et al. (89) found that the potential for allergic contact dermatitis was minimal following use of bar soap containing triclocarban. Freeman and Knox (90) studied photocontact dermatitis caused by the halogenated salicylanilides and related compounds, and found only one patient positive on photopatch testing to TCC alone. Triclocarban, however, has been described as a contact allergen from certain antiperspirants marketed in Europe (91,92).

TEGO

TEGO (dodecylic aminomethyl glycine hydrochloride, Nisson Anon, and Ampholyt G) is an antiseptic detergent used abroad in hospitals, food industries, and public baths and for cleaning machinery. Several cases of allergic dermatitis have occurred in hospital operating room personnel (93–95). Positive patch tests were obtained to 1:1000 and 1:100 aqueous solutions.

The workers cleaning milk tanks with TEGO 51 developed hand eczema and were patch test positive to 0.05% and 1% aqueous solutions, although ten control subjects were negative (96). TEGO 51 is derived from glycine. Cleaning pipes in the milk industry with TEGO Diocto S® (97) similarly caused contact dermatitis. This product is a blend of dioctyl-trioctyl-diethylenetriamine alcohol, acetic acid, and polyethylene glycol trioleate, and it may cross-

TABLE 12.11. *Irgasan DP 300*

Bacterio Polyvinyl Gloves (Europe)
Calgon
Calm
Colgate P300
Commercial laundry products
Deodorant antiperspirant spray
Deodorant Foot Powder (Durope) (Cosmea)
Dial Soap
Disposable paper products
Irish Spring Soap
"Odor Eaters" Latex Insole (Combe)
"Odor Eaters" Men's Hose (Burlington Mills)
Palmolive
Paper linings for rodent cages
Right Guard

react with triethanolamine. A 1% petrolatum concentration of TEGO Diocto S® had been used.

BENZOYL PEROXIDE

Exposure to benzoyl peroxide may occur from its use in the products shown in Table 12.12.

Topical Acne Preparations

Whereas mild irritant reactions to benzoyl peroxide are common, allergic reactions are rare (98–102). Caro (103) reported that a physician acquired a "connubial" contact dermatitis to benzoyl peroxide, which his wife used for acne. Bushkell (104) stated that benzoyl peroxide used on the bearded area can bleach black hair to a "patchy orange."

> **Benzoyl peroxide in acne preparations is a rare sensitizer. It may bleach facial hair. It is a sensitizer when used on ulcers.**

Benzoyl Peroxide Used for Leg Ulcers

The use of benzoyl peroxide for the treatment of leg ulcers may be accompanied by sensitization dermatitis (105,106).

Benzoyl Peroxide as an Activator of Acrylic Bone Cement

Jager and Balda (107) reported loosening of a total hip prosthesis due to an allergic reaction to benzoyl peroxide in the acrylic bone cement.

Benzoyl Peroxide as a Cause of Baker's Dermatitis

On rare occasions, benzoyl peroxide has been used to bleach flour. Fisher (108) has reported allergic hand dermatitis in a baker owing to such flour.

Benzoyl Peroxide as an Airborne Contactant

Benzoyl peroxide is used to bleach candles white. Intense exposure to burning candles in a church has caused facial dermatitis. The patch test was positive to benzoyl peroxide at 0.5% in petrolatum (109).

TABLE 12.12. *Benzoyl Peroxide*

Acne preparations
Additive to self-curing acrylic
Bleach for flour and oils
Quinilor ointment
Stasis ulcer treatments
Unguentum benzoyl peroxide

QUATERNARY AMMONIUM COMPOUNDS

These compounds are the active ingredient in disinfectants and sanitizers for homes, farms, offices, and public transportation vehicles. They are also used as algaecides and slimicides for swimming pools, industrial water reservoirs, and farm ponds. They are included in the last rinse in laundering by some hospitals, diaper services, and various institutions.

Quaternary ammonium compounds are also used as surface active agents. These compounds are strongly absorbed by many substances. The positive charge imparts antistatic properties to wool, cotton, and other cellulosic fibers, as well as certain synthetic fibers. The compounds are used in hair conditioners, as softeners for textiles and paper products, and as pigment dispersers. It was for this latter reason that the manufacturer included a quaternary ammonium compound in a roll-on deodorant, which produced dermatitis in a patient reported by Shmunes and Levy (110).

Even in solutions as dilute as 0.1%, the quaternary ammonium compounds are irritants under the closed patch technique. Several controls must always be used when a "positive" patch test reaction is obtained with a patch test procedure. In addition, the "use" test should be used to confirm patch test findings (111).

> **The quaternary ammonium compounds are irritants under the "closed" patch test procedures even in dilute solutions.**

Benzalkonium Chloride

Benzalkonium chloride (BZK), a mixture of alkyl dimethyl benzyl ammonium chlorides, is a quaternary ammonium cationic detergent. It is used widely as a preoperative skin disinfectant, for disinfecting surgical instruments, and in the treatment of burns, ulcers, wounds, and infected dermatoses. It is also present in many cosmetics, deodorants, mouthwashes, dentifrices, lozenges, and ophthalmic preparations. It is used industrially in the fabrication of textiles and dyes and in metallurgy and agriculture.

BZK is present in such products as Zephiran Chloride, Zephirol, BTC, Rocca, Benirol, Enuclen, Germitol, Drapolene, Drapolex, Cequartyl, Paralkan, Germinol, Rodalon, and Osvan. It has produced allergic contact dermatitis in medical personnel from exposure to instruments soaked in it (112,113) and from its use in the treatment of ulcers, burns, and cutaneous infections (114,115).

A bizarre ichthyosis-type dermatitis was reported in Japan to be caused by an ointment containing alkyl benzyl trimethylammonium chloride (116), which differs from BZK only by an additional methyl group. Pandos et al. (117) reported an instance of combined cutaneous and mucous membrane allergic contact reaction from BZK that complicated a tracheotomy procedure.

> **Benzalkonium chloride (Zephiran Chloride), a widely used antiseptic and preservative, is a rare sensitizer.**

Theodore and Schlossman (118) stated that BZK in ophthalmic preparations may produce allergic reactions, but they did not cite specific cases with confirming patch test proof. Fisher and Stillman (119) reported that one of the authors (M. A. Stillman) developed conjunctivitis from acquired hypersensitivity to BZK in an ophthalmic medicament, which was then made worse when an unsuspecting ophthalmologist prescribed another preparation containing BZK.

Dabiez et al. (120) pointed out that the primary preservative of most contact lens soaking solutions is BZK, and in a personal communication Dabiez suggested the ophthalmic preparations shown in Table 12.13 for BZK-sensitive persons.

Huriez et al. (121) reported that allergic contact sensitivity to topically applied quaternary ammonium compounds is common in France, and that generalized reactions may result from systemic administration of chemically related drugs. Such medications include the cholinergic medicaments, hypotensive drugs (2 γ-tetraethylammonium chloride), neuromuscular blocking agents (e.g., decamethonium bromide), and heparin antagonists (hexadimethrine bromide).

Ocular inflammation was suspected to be caused by airborne exposure to a quaternary ammonium compound (Lofarma) and a lauryl alkyl sulfonate (Firma) in an Italian nurse. The patch tests to 0.1% aqueous solutions of both compounds produced a vesicular reaction increasing at day 3 and 4 of the patch test readings.

Lovell and Staniforth (122) reported an unusual case of allergic contact dermatitis owing to the presence of benzalkonium chloride in plaster of paris. Moreover, this patient showed cross-reactions to cetrimonium bromide (cetrimide), another quaternary ammonium compound.

Benzoxonium Chloride

Benzoxonium chloride is used in Spain in Cohortant® cream and antibiotic. It is also known as D-301, dodecylbenzyldihydroxyethylammonium chloride, dodecyldi-(betaoxethyl) benzylammonium chloride, and benzyldodecyl-

TABLE 12.13. *Ophthalmic Preparations Free of Benzalkonium Chloride*

Soaclens (Alcon)
Vasocon (Cooper)

bis (2-hydroxyethyl) ammonium chloride. Topical use for seborrheic dermatitis led to scalp, forehead, and retroauricular dermatitis (123). A patch test of 0.1% aqueous was positive, and no cross-reactivity to benzalkonium chloride was seen.

Dequalinium Chloride

Dequalinium chloride is an ingredient of Micrin and Gargilon, a rare sensitizer, but this quaternary ammonium compound has been reported as a cause of necrotic ulcers on the penis, in the vulva, the perineum, and the body folds (124). Allergic hypersensitivity to this compound has been reported (125).

> **Dequalinium chloride, a rare sensitizer, can produce necrotic ulcers on the genitals and in the body folds.**

Dental wipes used to disinfect equipment have caused contact dermatitis due to N-benzyl-N,N-dihydrosyethyl-N-cocsalkyl-ammonium chloride (126). This quaternary ammonium compound is also found in dental mouthwashes used to reduce plaque and treat gingivitis. No cross-reactivity to benzalkonium chloride was found.

A hospital worker became sensitive to a disinfectant used on the job and was relocated to another area. She was exposed to a room cleaned with the disinfectant and had a flare of her dermatitis even though 7 months had passed since the initial eruption. The allergens in the disinfectant were quaternary ammonium compounds: didecyldimethylammonium chloride, which was positive at 0.01% aqueous, and bis-(aminopropyl)-laurylamine, which was positive at 0.1% aqueous. Didecyldimethylammonium chloride is used as a wood preservative against termites, as an algicide in swimming pools, and as a fungicide for wood (127).

Cetyl pyridinium chloride (CPC) is a quaternary ammonium compound that is present in Biogel® latex gloves. It was found to be a cause of contact dermatitis in eight nurses in Norway who had positive patch test reactions to their gloves but negative latex prick tests and use tests (128). CPC is used in cosmetics, antiseptics, and disinfectants. Biogel® gloves without CPC were tested and found negative in seven of the eight cases; in the remaining case only a doubtful reaction was encountered (128).

ANTISEPTIC TRIPHENYL METHANE DYES

Triphenylmethane dyes such as gentian violet, crystal violet, methyl violet, rosaniline, malachite green, brilliant green, chrysoidine, and eosin are weak sensitizers. Sensitization to these dyes occurs especially when they are applied to statis ulcers or eczematous skin.

Bielicky and Novak (129) observed 11 patients who had eczema mainly on the legs due to allergic sensitization to brilliant green. A simultaneous sensitivity to gentian violet and crystal violet was found in eight patients and to malachite green in six patients. Patch tests with various triphenylmethane dyes have shown the possibility of cross-sensitization between crystal violet (contained in gentian violet), brilliant green, and malachite green. The probable determinant groups of sensitization are $N(CH_3)_2$ or $-N(C_2H_5)_2$ in the para position of the benzene-ring structure. Cross-reactions are limited only to substances with amino groups substituted with at least two alkyl groups. The test reactions to pararosaniline were all negative.

Bjornberg and Mobacken (130) described three patients in whom a necrotic, painful, and slowly healing skin reaction developed after topical treatment with 1% gentian violet in aqueous solution. The reaction could be reproduced in stripped but not in nonstripped skin in normal humans and in guinea pigs with both gentian violet and brilliant green. These adverse reactions to triphenylmethane dyes may be diagnosed erroneously as exacerbations of the underlying skin disease for which treatment was given. Treatment with 1% aqueous solutions of these dyes is not as harmless as supposed.

Epstein (131) studied a patient who was treated for a resistant stasis dermatitis of the lower part of her right leg. After a period of time, gentian violet seemed to irritate the skin. Patch tests with this drug were negative, but an intradermal test with 0.5 mL of a 1:5,000 dilution produced a positive delayed tuberculin-type reaction.

Gentian violet is also known as pyoctanin, and previous reports of contact dermatitis to this dye often blurred the irritant and allergic qualities of the weak and very rare sensitizer. Although some have patch tested with 1% to 2% concentration of gentian violet, 0.0025% to 0.05% is considered preferable to eliminate any toxicity issues and distinguish allergy from irritation. Two such cases were reported from Germany (132).

Antiseptic therapeutic dyes such as gentian violet and brilliant green are weak sensitizers except when used on ulcers and eczematized skin.

Triphenylmethane dyes have produced anaphylactic reactions when used topically and during lymphography (133). Thus, patent blue (PB), a triphenylmethane dye, is in common use for the visualization of the lymphatic vessels before lymphography. Severe complications in association with PB injections have been reported in 0.1% to 2.8% of procedures; these complications include hypersensitivity reactions from urticaria to cardiovascular collapse (134). Inhalation of these dyes may produce asthma (135).

TABLE 12.14. *Patch Test Concentrations for Dyes*

Brilliant green (2% in water)
Crystal violet (2% in water)
Gentian violet (2% in water)
Malachite green (2% in water)
Pararosaniline (saturated solution)
Rosaniline or basic fuchsin (2% in water)
Triphenylmethane (1% in petrolatum)

The most widely used of these dyes, gentian violet, may produce not only allergic contact dermatitis but also necrosis in the intertriginous areas (136,137). The concentration of dyes for patch testing are given in Table 12.14.

In instances in which the erythematous patch test reaction is obscured by the color of the tested dye and papules or vesicles are not evident, an intradermal test with 0.05 mL of a 1:500 dilution of the dyes may be performed. A delayed tuberculin-type reaction indicates sensitivity.

Acriflavine (Acridine) Dyes

Acriflavine and proflavine dihydrochloride, rarely used at present, have been reported in the past as the causes of allergic contact dermatitis (138,139). Patch testing may be done with a 0.1% concentration in petrolatum.

Acriflavine is an acridine derivative of proflavine and is bacteriostatic against gram-positive and some gram-negative organisms. It is sold over the counter in the tropics and developing countries and has been reported to be a potent sensitizer. Purpuric and erythema multiformae–like eruptions have also been seen (140). A 0.1% aqueous concentration has been used for patch testing. Proflavine at 0.5% aqueous concentration has also been incriminated (140).

Eosin

Formerly a lipstick allergen in the 1950s, and tested at 50% in petrolatum, eosin is occasionally used as an antiseptic. It should be patch tested at the use concentration of 1% to 2% aqueous or alcoholic solution. A contaminant is suspected to be the true sensitizer (141).

Disinfectants and Gloves

Gloves made of latex, vinyl, and polyethylene are not impermeable to disinfectants, such as PCMX and glutaraldehyde. Gloves of these types generally provide about 60 minutes of protection against permeation. The structural integrity of these glove types is lost in less than 10 minutes on exposure to ethanol and isopropanol (142).

Alcohol

Alcohol can produce a variety of adverse topical reactions ranging from subjective irritation to irritant contact dermatitis and contact urticaria. In ten cases of contact urticaria from alcohol identified by patch test concentrations ranging from 0.5% to 100%, oral provocation was also positive in some of the cases. Allergic contact dermatitis to alcohol has also been reported and identified with patch test concentrations down to 1%. The allergen in alcohol has been found to be ethanol itself, impurities, or aldehyde metabolites. It is not common for primary alcohols to cross-react with secondary or tertiary alcohols (143).

REFERENCES

1. Fisher A A. Allergic reactions to Merthiolate (thimerosal). *Cutis* 1981;27:580.
2. Ellis F A. The sensitizing factor in Merthiolate. *J Allergy* 1947;18:212.
3. Gaul L E. Sensitizing component in thiosalicylic acid. *J Invest Dermatol* 1958;31:91.
4. Takino C. Thiomersal contact dermatitis (Japanese). *Jap J Clin Dermatol* 1971;25:1175.
5. Epstein S. Sensitivity to merthiolate: a cause of false delayed intradermal reactions. *J Allergy* 1963;35:225.
6. Sertoli A, et al. Allergic contact dermatitis from thimerosal in a soft contact lens wearer. *Contact Dermatitis* 1980;6:292.
7. Fisher A A, Pascher F, Kanof N B. Allergic contact dermatitis due to ingredients of vehicles. *Arch Dermatol* 1971;204:286.
8. Möller H. Merthiolate allergy: a nationwide iatrogenic sensitization. *Acta Derm Venereol* (Stockh) 1977;57:509.
9. Fregert S, Hjorth H. Contact Dermatitis. In: Rook AJ, Wilkinson DS, Ebling JFG, eds. *Textbook of dermatology.* Oxford: Blackwell, 1972.
10. van Ketel W G, Melzer-van Riemsduk F A. Conjunctivitis due to soft lens solutions. *Contact Dermatitis* 1980;6:321.
11. Pedersen N B. Allergic conjunctivitis from Merthiolate in soft contact lenses. *Contact Dermatitis* 1978;4:165.
12. Rietschel R L, Wilson L A. Ocular inflammation in patients using soft contact lenses. *Arch Dermatol* 1982;118:147.
13. Maibach H I. Acute laryngeal obstruction presumed secondary to thiomersal (Merthiolate) delayed hypersensitivity. *Contact Dermatitis* 1975;1:221.
14. Reisman R E. Delayed hypersensitivity to Merthiolate preservative. *J Allergy* 1969;43:245.
15. Rietschel R L, Adams R M. Reactions to thimerosal in hepatitis B vaccines. *Dermatol Clin* 1990;8:161.
16. Hansson H, Möller H. Intracutaneous test reactions to tuberculin containing Merthiolate as a preservative. *Scand J Infect Dis* 1971;3:169.
17. Wantke F, Demmer C M, Gotz M, Jarisch R. Contact dermatitis from thimerosal: 2 years' experience with ethylmercuric chloride in patch testing thimerosal-sensitive patients. *Contact Dermatitis* 1994;30:115.
18. Möller H. Why thimerosal allergy? *Int J Dermatol* 1980;19:29.
19. Mannuksela M, et al. Merthiolate hypersensitivity and vaccination. *Contact Dermatitis* 1980;6:241.
20. Hansson H, Möller H. Patch test reactions to Merthiolate in healthy young subjects. *Br J Dermatol* 1970;83:349.
21. Novak M, Kvicalova E. The problem of contact reactions to Merthiolate. *Cesk Dermatol* 1978;53:313.
22. Cirne de Castro J L, et al. Sensitivity to thimerosal and photosensitivity to peroxicam. *Contact Dermatitis* 1991;24:187.
23. Kitamura K, et al. Cross-reactivity between sensitivity to thimerosal and photosensitivity to piroxicam in guinea pigs. *Contact Dermatitis* 1991;25:30.
24. van Ketel W G. Sensitization to mercury from Mercurochrome. *Contact Dermatitis* 1980;6:499.
25. Camarasa G. Contact dermatitis from Mercurochrome. *Contact Dermatitis* 1976;2:120.
26. Pelaez Hernandez A, et al. Mercurochrome allergy: concurrence of 2 hypersensitivity mechanisms in the same patient. *Contact Dermatitis* 1994;30:48.
27. Bardazzi F, et al. Mercuochrome-induced allergic contact dermatitis. *Contact Dermatitis* 1990;23:381.
28. Morris G E. Dermatoses from phenylmercuric salts. *Arch Environ Health* 1960;1:53.
29. Hjorth N, Trolle-Lassen C. Skin reactions to preservatives in cream with special regard to paraben esters and sorbic acid. *Am Perf* 1962;77:43.
30. Hartung J. Phenyl-Quecksilberacetate und Phenyl-Quecksilberoleat in textilien. *Berufs-dermatosen* 1965;13:116.
31. Breit R, Bandmann H-J. The wide world of antimycotics. *Br J Dermatol* 1973;89:657.
32. Sidi E, Casalis F. Les intolérances de la muqueuse buccale. *Presse Med* 1951;59:730.
33. Fisher A A. Recent developments in the diagnosis and management of drug eruptions. *Med Clin North Am* 1959;43:787.
34. Foussereau J, Laugier P. Allergic eczema from metallic foreign bodies (tooth fillings and denture alloys). *Clin Dermatol* 1966;52:221.
35. van Ketel W G, Roeleveld C G. A curious case of allergy to mercuric compounds. *Contact Dermatitis* 1977;3:106.
36. Baer R L, Ramsey D L, Biondi E. The most common contact allergens. *Arch Dermatol* 1973;108:74.
37. Epstein E. Mercury allergy and patch testing. *Arch Dermatol* 1974;109:98.
38. Mathias C G T, Maibach H I, Chappler R R. Contact dermatitis to para-chloromercuriphenol. *Contact Dermatitis* 1981;7:117.
39. Tupker R A, Schuur J, Coenraads P J. Irritancy of antiseptics tested by repeated open exposures on the human skin, evaluated by non-invasive methods. *Contact Dermatitis* 1997;37:213.
40. Feldtman R W, Andrassy R I, Page C P. Povidone iodine skin sensitivity observed with possibly altered immune status. *JAMA* 1979;242:239.
41. Marks J G, Jr. Allergic contact dermatitis to povidone-iodine. *J Am Acad Dermatol* 1982;6:473.
42. Tosti A, et al. Allergic contact dermatitis due to povidone-iodine. *Contact Dermatitis* 1990;23:197.
43. Corazza M, Bulciolu G, Spisani L, Virgili A. Chemical burns following irritant contact with povidone-iodine. *Contact Dermatitis* 1997. 36:115.
44. Mochida K, et al. Skin ulceration due to povidone-iodine. *Contact Dermatitis* 1995;33:61.
45. Hjorth N. Contact dermatitis from 1,3-di-iodo-2-hydroxypropane. *Contact Dermatitis Newsletter* 1972;12:322.
46. Lieberman P, Siegle R L, Raylor W W, Jr. Anaphylactoid reactions to iodinated contrast material. *J Allergy Clin Immunol* 1978;62:174.
47. Rothe A, Yousif S H, Zschunke E. Allergic contact eczema from sodium amidotrizoate—a radiopaque substance in angiography and renography. *Contact Dermatitis* 1977;3:284.
48. Neering H. Contact urticaria from chlorinated swimming pool water. *Contact Dermatitis* 1977;3:279.
49. Osmundsen P. Contact dermatitis due to sodium hypochlorite. *Contact Dermatitis* 1978;4:177.
50. Hostynek J J, et al. Irritation factors of sodium hypochlorite solutions in human skin. *Contact Dermatitis* 1990;23:316.
51. Fitzgerald D A, et al. Spa pool dermatitis. *Contact Dermatitis* 1995;33:53.
52. Key M. Some unusual allergic reactions in industry. *Arch Dermatol* 1961;83:57.
53. Dooms-Goossens A, et al. Allergic contact urticaria to chloramine. *Contact Dermatitis* 9:319, 1983.
54. Bourne M, Flindt M, Walker J. Asthma due to industrial use of chloramine. *Br Med J* 1979;7:10.
55. Charles T. Asthma due to industrial use of chloramine. *Br Med J* 1979;4:334.
56. Dijkman J, Vooren P, Kramps J. Occupational asthma due to inhalation of chloramine-T: 1. Clinical observations and inhalation-provocation studies. *Int Arch Allergy Appl Immunol* 1981;64:422.
57. Kramps J, et al. Occupational asthma due to inhalation of chloramine-T: 2. Demonstration of specific IgE antibodies. *Arch Allergy Appl Immunol* 1981;64:428.
58. Mobacken H, Wengstrom C. Interference with healing of rat skin incisions treated with chlorhexidine. *Acta Derm Venereol* (Stockh) 1974;54:29.
59. Calnan C D. Contact dermatitis from drugs. *Proc R Soc Med* 1962;55:39.

60. Ljunggren B, Möller H. Eczematous contact allergy to chlorhexidine. *Acta Derm Venereol* (Stockh) 1972;52:308.
61. Muston H L, Boss J M, Summerly R. Dermatitis from Ammonyx 1.0, a constituent of Hibiscrub. *Contact Dermatitis* 1977;3:347.
62. Wong W K, Goh C L, Chan K W. Contact urticaria from chlorhexidine. *Contact Dermatitis* 1990;22:52.
63. Knudsen B B, Avnstorp C. Chlortrexidine gluconate and acetate in patch testing. *Contact Dermatitis* 1991;24:45.
64. Autegarden J E, et al. Anaphylactic shock after application of chlorhexidine to unbroken skin. *Contact Dermatitis* 1999;40:215.
65. Lee J Y, Wang B J. Contact dermatitis caused by cetrimide in antiseptics. *Contact Dermatitis* 1995;33:168.
66. Nordlund J J, Hartley C, Fister J. On the cause of green hair. *Arch Dermatol* 1977;113:1700.
67. Lampe R M, Hendersen A L, Hansen G H. Green hair. *JAMA* 19:2092, 1977.
68. Goette D K. Swimmers' green hair [Letter]. *Arch Dermatol* 1978;114:128.
69. Bhat G R, et al. The green hair problem: a preliminary investigation. *J Soc Cosmet Chem* 1979;30:1.
70. Burry J N, et al. Chlorocresol sensitivity. *Contact Dermatitis* 1975;1:41.
71. Storrs F. Para-chloro-meta-xylenol allergic contact dermatitis in seven individuals. *Contact Dermatitis* 1975;1:211.
72. Hjorth N, Trolle-Lassen C. Skin reactions to ointment bases. *Trans St John Hosp Derm Soc* 1963;49:127.
73. Burry J N, et al. Environmental dermatitis: patch tests in 1000 cases of allergic contact dermatitis. *Med J Aust* 1973;2:681.
74. Park R G. Chlorocresol sensitivity. *Contact Dermatitis Newsletter* 1970;7:152.
75. Oleffe J A, Blondeel A, de Coninck A. Allergy to chlorocresol and propylene glycol in a steroid cream. *Contact Dermatitis* 1979;5:53.
76. Baker H, Ive F A, Lloyd M J. Primary irritant dermatitis of the scrotum due to hexachlorophene. *Arch Dermatol* 1969;99:663.
77. Epstein E. Dichlorophene allergy. *Ann Allergy* 1966;24:437.
78. Fregert S, Hjorth N. Results of standard patch tests with substances abandoned. *Contact Dermatitis Newsletter* 1969;5:85.
79. Morikawa F, et al. Some problems on the appraisal of the skin safety of hexachlorophene. *J Soc Cosmet Chem* 1974;25:113.
80. Epstein J H, Wuepper K D, Maibach H I. Photocontact dermatitis to halogenated salicylanilides and related compounds. *Arch Dermatol* 1968;97:236.
81. Fisher A A, Lipton M. Allergic stomatitis due to "BAXIN" in a dentifrice. *Arch Dermatol* 1951;64:640.
82. Fisher A A, Tobin L. Sensitivity to compound G-4 ("Dichlorophene") in dentifrices. *JAMA* 1953;151:998.
83. Gaul L E, Underwood G B. The cutaneous toxicity of dihydroxy-dichlordiphenylmethane: a new fungicide for athlete's foot. *J Indian Med Assoc* 1949;42:22.
84. Schorr W F. Dichlorophene (G-4) allergy. *Arch Dermatol* 1979;102:515.
85. Roed-Petersen J, Auken G, Hjorth N. Contact sensitivity to irgasan DP 300. *Contact Dermatitis* 1975;1:293.
86. Hindson T C. Irgasan DP 300 in a deodorant. *Contact Dermatitis* 1975;1:328.
87. Wahlberg J E. Routine patch testing with Irgasan DP 30D. *Contact Dermatitis* 1976;2:292.
88. Fisher A A. Irgasan DP 300 and Irgasan CF3. *Contact Dermatitis Newsletter* 1974;14:416.
89. Maibach H I, et al. Triclocarban: evaluation of contact dermatitis potential in man. *Contact Dermatitis* 1978;4:283.
90. Freeman R G, Knox J M. The action spectrum of photocontact dermatitis. *Arch Dermatol* 1968;97:130.
91. Agren-Jonsson S, Magnusson B. Sensitization to propanitheline bromide, trichlorocarbanilide and propylene glycol in an antiperspirant. *Contact Dermatitis* 1976;2:79.
92. Osmundsen P E. Concomitant contact allergy to propantheline bromide and TCC. *Contact Dermatitis* 1975;1:251.
93. Foussereau J, Samsoen M, Hecht M T. Occupational dermatitis to Ampholyt G in hospital personnel. *Contact Dermatitis* 1983;9:233.
94. Lachapelle J M, Reginster J P. Occupational contact dermatitis from an ampholytic soap (TEGO). *Contact Dermatitis* 1977;3:211.
95. Suhonen R. Contact allergy to do-ecyldi-(aminoethyl) glycine-Desimex I. *Contact Dermatitis* 1980;6:290.
96. Valsecchi R, Leghissa P, Pazzolla S. TEGO allergy in the food industry. *Contact Dermatitis* 1990;23:188.
97. Piraccini B M, et al. Occupational contact dermatitis due to the disinfectant TEGO Diocto S[reg]. *Contact Dermatitis* 1991;24:228.
98. Vena G A, Angelini G, Meneghini C L. Contact dermatitis to benzoyl peroxide. *Contact Dermatitis* 1981;7:137.
99. Lindemayr H, Drobil M. Contact sensitization to benzoyl peroxide. *Contact Dermatitis* 1981;7:137.
100. Rietschel R L, Duncan S H. Benzoyl peroxide reactions in an acne study group. *Contact Dermatitis* 1982;8:323.
101. Romaguera C, Grimalt F. Sensitization to benzoyl peroxide, retinoic acid and carbon tetrachloride. *Contact Dermatitis* 1980;6:442.
102. Cunliffe W J, Burke B. Benzoyl peroxide: lack of sensitization. *Acta Dermatol* 1982;62:458.
103. Caro I. Connubial contact dermatitis to benzoyl peroxide. *Contact Dermatitis* 1976;2:362.
104. Bushkell L L. Bleaching-benzoyl peroxide [Letter]. *Arch Dermatol* 1974;110:465.
105. Angelini G, Rantuccio F, Meneghini C L. Contact dermatitis in patients with leg ulcers. *Contact Dermatitis* 1975;1:81.
106. Jensen O, Petersen S H, Vesteroger L. Contact sensitization to benzoyl peroxide following topical treatment of chronic leg ulcers. *Contact Dermatitis* 1980;6:179.
107. Jager M, Balda B R. Loosening of a total hip prosthesis at contact allergy due to benzoyl peroxide. *Arch Orthop Traumat Surg* 1979;94:175.
108. Fisher A A. Hand dermatitis-A "Baker's Dozen." *Cutis* 1982;29:214.
109. Bonnekoh B, Merk H F. Airborne allergic contact dermatitis from benzoyl peroxide as a bleaching agent of candle wax. *Contact Dermatitis* 1991;24:367.
110. Shmunes E, Levy E J. Quaternary ammonium compound contact dermatitis from a deodorant. *Arch Dermatol* 1972;105:91.
111. Norrlind R (cited by Wahlberg J E). Two cases of hypersensitivity to quaternary ammonium compounds. *Acta Derm Venereol* (Stockh) 1962;42:230.
112. Huriez C, et al. L'allergie aux sels d'ammonium quaternaire. *Semin Hop* (Paris) 1965;41:230.
113. Garcie-Perez A, Moran M. Dermatitis from quaternary ammonium compounds. *Contact Dermatitis* 1975;1:316.
114. Afzelius H, Thulin H. Allergic reactions to benzalkonium chloride. *Contact Dermatitis* 1974;5:60.
115. Wahlberg J E. Two cases of hypersensitivity to quaternary ammonium compounds. *Acta Derm Venereol* (Stockh) 1962;42:239.
116. Seiji M, Mizuno F. Unusual cornification in ichthyosis-like dermatitis. *Acta Dermatol* 1970;50:338.
117. Pandos E, Horowitz I D, Wunder G. Contact dermatitis complicating tracheostomy. *Am J Dis Child* 1965;109:90.
118. Theodore F H, Schlossman A. *Ocular allergy*. Baltimore: Williams & Wilkins, 1958.
119. Fisher A A, Stillman M A. Allergic contact sensitivity to benzalkonium chloride (BAK): cutaneous, ophthalmic and general medical implications. *Arch Dermatol* 1972;106:169.
120. Dabiez O H, Naugle B S, Reich L. Evaluation of a stronger concentration of preservative (benzalkonium chloride) in contact lens soaking solution. *Eye, Ear, Nose, Throat Monthly* 1966;45:78.
121. Huriez C, et al. Frequences des sensibilisations aux ammoniums quaterniers. *Bull Soc Franc Derm Syph* 1965;72:106.
122. Lovell C R, Staniforth P. Contact allergy to benzalkonium chloride in plaster of paris. *Contact Dermatitis* 1983;7:343.
123. Diaz-Ramon L, Aguirre A, Raton-Nieto J A, de Miguel M. Contact dermatitis form benzoxonium chloride. *Contact Dermatitis* 1999;41:53.
124. Coles R B, Wilkinson D S. Necrosis and dequalinium: 1. Balanitis. *Trans St. John Hosp Derm Soc* 1965;51:46.
125. Wilkinson D S. Durch Dequalinium hervogerufene hautnergrosen. *Hautarzt* 1970;21:114.
126. Placucci F, Benini A, Guerra L, Tosti A. Occupational allergic contact dermatitis from disinfectant wipes used in dentistry. *Contact Dermatitis* 1996;35:306.
127. Dejobert Y, et al. Contact dermatitis from didecyldimethylammonium chloride and bis-(aminopropyl)-lauryl amine in a detergent-disinfectant used in hospital. *Contact Dermatitis* 1997;37:95.

128. Steinkjer B. Contact dermatitis from cetyl pyridinium chloride in latex surgical gloves. *Contact Dermatitis* 1998;39:29.

129. Bielicky T, Novak M. Contact-group sensitization to triphenylmethane dyes-gentian violet, brilliant green and malachite green. *Arch Dermatol* 1969;100:540.

130. Bjornberg A, Mobacken H. Necrotic skin reactions caused by 1 per cent gentian violet and brilliant green. *Acta Derm Venereol* (Stockh) 1972;52:55.

131. Epstein S. Dermal contact dermatitis. *Dermatologica* 1958;117:291.

132. Schoppelrey H P, Mily H, Agathos M, Breit R. Allergic contact dermatitis from pyoctanin. *Contact Dermatitis* 1997;36:221.

133. Koehler P R. Complications of lymphography. *Lymphology* 1968;1:116.

134. Kalimo K, Saarni H. Immediate reactions to patent blue dye. *Contact Dermatitis* 1983;7:171.

135. Keskinen H, Wagar G. Occupational asthma due to ECG ink. Presented at the annual meeting of the European Academy of Allergology and Clinical Immunology, Helsinki, 1979 (abstract).

136. Meurer M, Konz B. Necrotic skin reactions after treatment with crystal violet. *GFR Hautarzt* 1977;28:94.

137. Lawrence C M, Smith G. Ampliative medicament allergy: concomitant sensitivity to multiple medicaments including yellow soft paraffin, white soft paraffin, gentian violet and Span 20. *Contact Dermatitis* 1982;8:240.

138. Beare J M. Generalized skin sensitivity following local application of acriflavine: report of case. *Lancet* 1947;1:410.

139. Mitchell J C. Contact dermatitis from proflavine dihydrochloride. *Arch Dermatol* 1972;106:294.

140. Lim J, Goh C L, Lee C T. Perioral and mucosal oedema due to contact allergy to proflavine. *Contact Dermatitis* 1991;25:195.

141. Tomb R R. Allergic contact dermatitis from eosin. *Contact Dermatitis* 1991;24:27.

142. Mellström G A, Lindberg M, Boman A. Permeation and destructive effects of disinfectants on protective gloves. *Contact Dermatitis* 1992;26:163.

143. Ophaswongse S, Maibach H I. Alcohol dermatitis: allergic contact dermatitis and contact urticaria syndrome: a review. *Contact Dermatitis* 1994;30:1.

CHAPTER 13

Reactions to Topical Antimicrobials

NEOMYCIN

Neomycin, the most widely used topical antibiotic in the United States, has become the most sensitizing of all topical antibacterial preparations since the use of topical penicillin was banned (1). It has been found that 30% of persons who have stasis ulcers, 15% of patients who have chronic otitis externa, and 5% of those who have various chronic eczematous conditions become sensitized by treatment with neomycin (2–4).

Wereide (3) did not find that atopic dermatitis predisposes patients to neomycin sensitivity when compared with other eczematous conditions. Patrick et al. (4), however, stated that, in their study, the occurrence of neomycin sulfate sensitivity in the normal population was less than in a population of patients who have atopic dermatitis or those who have nonatopic dermatoses.

Leyden and Kligman (5) concluded that the intermittent use of neomycin on minor cuts and wounds is not associated with an excessive rate of sensitization. Prystowsky et al. (6) found that the prevalence of neomycin patch test sensitivity in the general population is approximately 1%. Such positive patch tests correlate closely with "use tests." These authors suggest wisely that the package instructions for topical neomycin-containing products should carry warnings to the effect that (a) people who have previously used products containing neomycin on inflammatory dermatoses, such as leg ulcers or otitis externa, for extended periods of time have an increased chance of experiencing an allergic reaction; and (b) failure of acute minor lesions to heal or chronic lesions to improve within 7 days after treatment with such products indicates that the medication should be discontinued until the advice of a physician is sought.

> **Neomycin is sensitizing, particularly when used on stasis ulcers, in chronic otitis externa, and on chronic eczematous conditions.**

In general, ointment vehicles are less sensitizing than creams or lotions because they do not usually contain preservatives, emulsifying agents, or solvents (7,8). Hjorth and Thomscn (9), however, stated that neomycin ointments are the major cause of sensitization to this antibiotic, and they recommended that neomycin should not be prescribed in ointments. The risk of inducing sensitization with neomycin in creams, lotions, or powders appears to be significantly less, according to these investigators.

Cross-Reactions with Neomycin

There is general agreement that the drugs shown in Table 13.1 cross-react with neomycin (10–12). Tobramycin (Nebcin) is an aminoglycoside antibiotic for prescription ophthalmologic use in the United States. Schorr and Ridgway (13) stated that tobramycin (ophthalmic) should not be used to treat known neomycin-allergic patients without first testing the patient with 20% tobramycin in white petrolatum. Cross-reactions to neomycin among aminoglycosides have been evaluated, and Table 13.2 (14) lists the frequency of cross-reactions.

Neomycin Systemic Contact Dermatitis

The administration of a cross-reacting drug, such as streptomycin, to a neomycin-sensitive person can produce a severe "systemic eczematous contact-type dermatitis." Also, Ekelund and Möller (15) have shown that the oral administration of neomycin sulfate to neomycin-sensitive persons may cause a flare-up of the original neomycin dermatitis in addition to a "toxicodermic" type of drug eruption. A flare-up of the positive patch test reaction to neomycin may occur infrequently. These authors stress that neomycin may be used occasionally in the treatment of hepatic cirrhosis and in preparative therapy for bowel surgery. Neomycin is given in daily doses of 6 to 8 g (and with good renal function 1% to 3% oral neomycin is excreted in the urine).

Panzer and Epstein (16) found that no percutaneous absorption was detected using a bioassay method sensitive to 0.033 µg/mL for serum following topical application of neomycin sulfate ointment in groups of normal male volunteers who had neomycin sulfate ointment applied to their bodies and that very little absorption has been found with neomycin sulfate administered orally. In fact, it is used

TABLE 13.1. *Neomycin Cross-Reactors*

Butirosin (ambutylosin)
Gentamicin (Garamycin)*
Kanamycin
Neomycin (framycetin)
Paromomycin
Spectinomycin
Streptomycin
Tobramycin (Nebcin)†

*Topical preparation.
†Ophthalmic preparation.

frequently as a bowel preparation before gastrointestinal surgery because of its poor absorption from the bowel. According to Ekelund and Möller (15), however, sufficient neomycin is absorbed to produce a systemic contact-type reaction in neomycin-sensitive persons.

Co-Reactions with Bacitracin

Although bacitracin and neomycin are not related chemically, it is not unusual for patients to become sensitized to both antibiotics simultaneously from the use of Neosporin ointment. Thus, Polysporin ointment, free of neomycin, but containing bacitracin, is not a safe alternative for neomycin-sensitive persons.

> **Although neomycin and bacitracin are not related chemically, they often "co-react." Neomycin-sensitive individuals thus may react to such neomycin-free preparations as Polysporin ointment, which contains bacitracin.**

Pirila and Rouhunkosky (17) reported that all 99 patients who had positive patch tests to bacitracin also had positive neomycin patch tests. Bjorkner and Möller (18), who patch tested 1,000 patients who had suspected contact dermatitis, found three patients allergic to bacitracin, all of whom also had positive tests to neomycin. Binnick and Clendenning (19) further point out that because bacitracin and neomycin are not chemically related, positive reactions are left to represent coincidental sensitization rather than cross-sensitiza-

TABLE 13.2. *Neomycin Cross-Reactions*

Substance	% Cross Reacting
Gentamycin	40–66
Paromomycin	66–97
Tobramycin	25–65
Kanamycin	43–60
Sisomycin	50
Amikacin	33
Amino sydin	91
Streptomycin	0

tion. This lack of cross-sensitization is also borne out by Epstein and Wenzel's (20) guinea pig studies showing that animals sensitized to neomycin did not react to bacitracin, and vice versa. However, within a 1-year period, Fisher and Adams (1) observed nine cases of bacitracin sensitivity without coexistent neomycin sensitivity and recommended that the North American Contact Dermatitis Group begin routinely screening for bacitracin allergy. Within the first year of routine patch testing with bacitracin ointment, this author (RLR) observed three cases of bacitracin allergy with negative reactions to neomycin, all relevant to the current dermatitis. It would appear that bacitracin is capable of inducing sensitization without co-reactivity, contrary to the report of Binnick and Clendenning (19).

Pirila and Rantanen (21) gave an account of repeated eruptions in a patient sensitive to neomycin and bacitracin because of their topical use on an amputation stump. Later, the patient developed a severe stomatitis from throat tablets containing bacitracin and from a paste containing both antibiotics used to fill an infected root canal. Oral administration of neomycin produced diarrhea and dermatitis.

Table 13.3 lists topical medicaments containing neomycin that should be avoided in neomycin-sensitive persons. As alternatives to the medicaments in Table 13.3, Table 13.4 lists those free of neomycin, bacitracin, and polymyxin. Van Ketel (22) reported a patient who was allergic to both bacitracin and polymyxin and concluded that the sensitization to polymyxin and bacitracin may be cross-sensitization because both antibiotics are obtained from *Bacillus subtilis*. It would, therefore, be wise to use the numerous bacitracin-polymyxin topical medications with caution in neomycin-sensitive persons because of the possibility of "co-reactors" between these antibiotics.

TABLE 13.3. *Topical Medicaments Containing Neomycin*

Alba-3 Ointment (Alba)
Bacimycin (Merrell-National)
Biotres Ointment (Central Pharmacal)
BPN Triple Antibiotic Ointment (Norwich-Eaton)
Cortisporin Cream and Ointment (Burroughs Wellcome)
Mycifradin Powder (Upjohn)
Myciguent Antibiotic Ointment (Upjohn)
Mycitracin Antibiotic Ointment (Upjohn)
Mycolog Cream and Ointment (Squibb)
Mycotriacet Cream and Ointment (Premo)
Mytrex Cream and Ointment (Savage)
Neo-Cortef Cream and Ointment (Upjohn)
Neo-Medrol Ointment (Upjohn)
Neo-Oxylone Ointment (Upjohn)
Neo-Polycin (Dow Pharmaceuticals)
Neosporin Aerosol (Burroughs Wellcome)
Neosporin G.U. Irrigant (Burroughs Wellcome)
Neosporin Powder and Ointment (Burroughs Wellcome)
Neosporin-G Cream (Syntex)
Neo-Synalar Cream and Ointment (Syntex)
Nyst-olone Cream (Schein)
Septa Ointment—Triple Antibiotic Ointment (Circle)

TABLE 13.4. *Alternative Antibiotics for Neomycin-Sensitive Persons*

Betadine Solution and Ointment (Purdue Frederick)
Bactroban Ointment
Ilotycin Ointment (Dista)

These ointments may be combined with Nystatin Cream or ointment for candida infections.

Table 13.5 lists otic preparations that should be avoided by neomycin-sensitive persons. Table 13.6 lists alternative otic preparations that can be used by neomycin-sensitive persons. It should be noted that several of these alternative otic preparations contain acetic acid, which has proved quite effective for the treatment of otitis externa in neomycin-sensitive persons (23–25). When all other different treatments of otitis externa fail, Fisher (26) has found that half-strength Carbol-fuchsin paint often succeeds in controlling the condition.

Table 13.7 shows ophthalmic preparations that should be avoided by neomycin-sensitive persons. It should be noted that ophthalmic preparations containing tobramycin may cross-react with neomycin. Table 13.8 lists ophthalmic preparations free of neomycin that can be used as alternatives in neomycin-sensitive persons. It has been found that the proper application of antibiotic ophthalmic ointments gives results superior to that of an aqueous vehicle, and that by placing the ophthalmic ointment on the fingertip and applying it medially and laterally to the lids and lashes, the medication can thus reach the conjunctival sac. This medication has an antibacterial effect lasting for several hours (27).

Table 13.9 lists some miscellaneous methods by which individuals are exposed to neomycin. Neomycin-sensitive persons may acquire an allergic contact dermatitis from handling such products.

PENICILLIN

The topical use of penicillin is largely avoided at present because many individuals would develop contact sensitivity to the drug. Allergic contact dermatitis from penicillin occurs particularly in physicians, nurses, pharmacists, and veterinarians who handle this antibiotic. Allergic sensitization to penicillin may be initiated by external contact with

TABLE 13.5. *Neomycin Otic Preparations to Be Avoided by Neomycin-Sensitive Persons*

Coly-Mycin S Otic with Neomycin and Hydrocortisone (Parke-Davis)
Cortisporin Otic Solution (Burroughs Wellcome)
Cortisporin Otic Suspension (Burroughs Wellcome)
Otobione Otic Suspension (Schering)
Otocidin Otic Drops (Marin)
Otocort Ear Drops (Lemmon)

TABLE 13.6. *Alternative Otic Preparations for Neomycin-Sensitive Persons*

Castellani's Paint (Pedinol Pharmacal, Inc.)
Chloromycetin Otic (Parke-Davis)
  Chloramphenicol in Propylene Glycol*
Lidosporin Otic Solution (Burroughs Wellcome)
  Polymyxin B Sulfate,† Lidocaine Hydrochloride, Propylene Glycol*
Orlex Otic Solution (Baylor)
  Acetic Acid Propylene Glycol*
Orlex HC Otic Solution (Baylor)
  Acetic Acid, Hydrocortisone, Propylene Glycol*
Otic Domeboro Solution (Dome)‡
  Acetic Acid in Aluminum Acetate (Modified Burow's) Solution
VoSOL and VoSOL-HC Otic Solution (Wallace)
  Acetic Acid in Propylene Glycol,* Propylene Glycol Diacetate Hydrocortisone

*Propylene glycol may be a sensitizer.
†The polymyxin may rarely "co-react" with neomycin.
‡A nonsensitizing preparation.

various forms of penicillin, and dermatitis may be produced in sensitized individuals by contact with penicillin used for injections or by cleaning syringes contaminated with it. Allergic contact sensitivity to penicillin is usually combined with the immediate anaphylactic variety. Inhalation of penicillin from powder, aerosols, or molds may produce asthma and anaphylactoid shock in individuals who have contact sensitivity. In Malaysia, where penicillin medicaments are available over the counter, penicillin is the most frequent cause of contact dermatitis from antibiotics (28). The systemic administration of penicillin to such "externally" sensitized individuals may produce an eczematous contact-type dermatitis, which may be accompanied by urticarial anaphylactic sensitivity.

Girard (29) reported a patient who applied penicillin topically on a varicose ulcer. Two days later, a severe contact dermatitis developed around the ulcer. The immunologic investigations, which were done a few days later, failed to reveal specific IgG or IgE antibodies. The RAST test was

TABLE 13.7. *Ophthalmic Preparations to Be Avoided by Neomycin-Sensitive Persons*

Cortisporin Ointment Ophthalmic (Burroughs Wellcome)
NeoDECADRON Sterile Ophthalmic Ointment (Merck Sharp & Dohme)
NeoDECADRON Sterile Ophthalmic Solution (Merck Sharp & Dohme)
Neo-Hydeltrasol Sterile Ophthalmic Ointment (Merck Sharp & Dohme)
Neo-Hydeltrasol Sterile Ophthalmic Solution (Merck Sharp & Dohme)
Neosporin Ophthalmic Ointment (Burroughs Wellcome)
Neosporin Ophthalmic Solution (Burroughs Wellcome)
Tobramycin* Solution (benzalkonium chloride) (Alcon)*

*Tobramycin (Nebcin) may cross-react with neomycin.

TABLE 13.8. *Alternative Ophthalmic Preparations Free of Neomycin*

Achromycin Ophthalmic Ointment (Lederle)
Achromycin Ophthalmic Suspension 1% (Lederle)
Chloromycetin Ophthalmic Ointment 1% (Parke-Davis)
Gantrisin Ophthalmic Ointment (Roche)
Gantrisin Ophthalmic Solution (Roche)
Garamycin Ophthalmic Ointment—Sterile (Schering)
Garamycin Ophthalmic Solution—Sterile (Schering)
Ilotycin Ophthalmic Ointment (Dista)
Metimyd Ophthalmic Ointment—Sterile (Schering)
Metimyd Ophthalmic Suspension (Schering)
Sodium Sulamyd Ophthalmic Ointment (Schering)
Sodium Sulamyd Ophthalmic Solution (Schering)
Terra-Cortril Ophthalmic Suspension (Pfizer)

negative, but the lymphocyte transformation test was highly positive.

> **Exposure to penicillin in sensitized individuals may result not only in delayed eczematous reactions but also in immediate, urticarial, and anaphylactic reactions.**

Desensitization of penicillin sensitivity is hazardous and should be attempted with great caution.

Hjorth (30) stated that occupational dermatitis in veterinary surgeons is common and that in six veterinarians the dermatitis had been provoked or aggravated by penethamate hydriodide (benzyl-penicillin β-diethylaminoethyl ester hydriodide), used for local treatment of mastitis in cows. Penethamate is used as a 25% suspension in oil injected into the teat of the udder. In Denmark, it is the drug usually used for mastitis, not only because it achieves a high concentration but also because it is rapidly eliminated from the milk. Penethamate is a base, whereas benzyl penicillin is an acid.

Although the six patients were all sensitive to penethamate, only three had positive patch test reactions to benzyl penicillin, indicating that patch tests should also be per-

TABLE 13.9. *Miscellaneous Exposure to Neomycin*

In dentistry
  Tooth root canal work
In deodorants
  Hi and Dry
  Top Brass
In pet foods
In veterinary use
  Growth promoter in feeds (particularly for poultry)
  Systemic (Calf Drench)
  Topical medicaments

formed with penethamate. This finding may explain why some patients who have a definite history of reaction after treatment with one penicillin have tolerated later treatment with another type of penicillin. Thus, the different types of penicillin do not necessarily cross-react when it comes to allergic contact sensitivity. Some individuals may be allergic to ampicillin, some to penicillin G, some to oxicillin, and some to dicloxacillin. One must not take for granted that cross-sensitivity occurs.

> **The various types of penicillin do not necessarily cross-react. Patch tests should be performed with the specific penicillin to which the patient had been exposed.**

Reports with Positive Penicillin Patch-Test Reactions

Blanton and Blanton (31) reported that patch tests may be performed with penicillin powder, ointment (500 units/g), or topical medications. The usual positive reaction occurs in 24 to 48 hours. In sensitive individuals, however, an immediate reaction consisting of an erythematous wheal, sometimes with pseudopods, may occur within a half hour.

A positive patch test reaction of the delayed type may be significant, because the allergic eczematous contact sensitivity is accompanied frequently by the immediate anaphylactic reaction. If there is a compelling need for penicillin in a patient who had a positive test reaction to it, scratch and intracutaneous tests must be performed to determine the presence or absence of the immediate type of sensitivity before systemic administration is attempted.

Valsecchi et al. (32) stated that a 14-year-old boy who had acute tonsillitis was treated for 1 week with ampicillin. The treatment was then stopped because of a widespread urticarial eruption with mucous membrane edema and itching. When treated again with ampicillin, the patient showed the same generalized cutaneous eruption and was hospitalized.

Patch tests to ampicillin and cephalexin gave positive reactions. The patient had not had any previous known contact with topical compounds containing ampicillin or cephalexin. This finding indicates the value of patch testing in the diagnosis of adverse drug reactions and supports a possible cross-reaction between penicillin, its derivatives, and cephalosporins; the latter compounds have the same antigenic determinant, namely the β-lactam ring.

The utility of patch tests to evaluate β lactams was undertaken in 101 patients who had either intentional or accidental reexposure to the drug to which they were sensitive (33). Therefore, confirmation of allergy was established by systemic means. In this group of patients, patch, prick, and intradermal tests were conducted. Patch tests were conducted with amoxicillin in 25%, sodium penicillin G 5%, ampicillin 25%, bacampicillin 25%, aztreonam 20%, and ceftriazone 20% all in petrolatum. The type of systemic reactions experienced when challenged had been urticaria, angioedema, morbilliform eruptions, and anaphylactic shock. Intradermal tests were the most sensitive, and about half of the patients had one or more positive test. Patch tests were positive in 31% of morbilliform eruptions, 20% of urticarial/angioedematous eruptions, and none of the anaphylactic shock cases.

Vickers et al. (34) reported that penicillin in milk from cows treated for mastitis caused dermatitis in two patients. Both patients had positive patch tests. One reacted to penicillin at 200,000 units/mL and the other to procaine penicillin at 100,000 units/mL.

Ampicillin sensitivity is an occupational hazard among nurses. A 5% aqueous solution may be used for patch tests. Hand dermatitis developed in a nurse and continued for a 20-year period as vesiculation and erythema of the sides of the fingers of the right hand (35). This was associated with handling ampicillin or amoxicillin vials for parenteral use. Patch tests with 50 mg/mL aqueous ampicillin and amoxicillin were strongly positive, whereas sodium benzylpenicillin at 100 U/mL aqueous was negative. Oral challenge with 250 mg of phenoxymethylpenicillin was negative. The difference in structure between these antibiotics is an aminogroup on the benzene ring. This minor difference in β-lactam side chains led to a very different immunologic response.

Schulz et al. (36) described 62 cases of occupational eczema occurring among members of the medical and allied professions. Sixty-one had an allergic contact dermatitis, principally from drugs. Ampicillin was the most frequent allergen, being the sensitizer in 24 of the patients, most of whom were nurses exposed occupationally. Patch tests revealed positive reactions to ampicillin 5% aqueous solution.

Inappropriate application of cloxicillin to the skin from vials intended for intravenous use led to contact dermatitis in two women (37). No cross-reactivity to other β-lactam antibiotic was found in these two cases, which is consistent with animal studies showing no cross reactivity.

STREPTOMYCIN

Streptomycin produced by actinomycetin *Streptomyces griseus* has its greatest application in the treatment of tuberculosis and may be administered alone or in combination with penicillin in preparations such as Wycillin (Wyeth).

Desensitization procedures by subcutaneous injection of streptomycin are dangerous and may be accompanied by urticaria or flares of dermatitis. Furthermore, such desensitization is rarely successful.

Although topical application of streptomycin is now avoided, members of the medical, nursing, and pharmaceutical professions who handle the drug readily become sensi-

tized, and subsequent administration may produce a severe eczematous contact-type dermatitis medicamentosa. Because streptomycin may cross-react with neomycin, systemic administration of streptomycin may produce the eczematous contact-type dermatitis in individuals who had become sensitized to neomycin and had never been exposed to streptomycin. However, this was not observed by Menendez-Ramos et al. (14). Streptomycin may also cross-react with kanamycin sulfate (Kantrex).

Medical, nursing, and pharmaceutical professionals handling streptomycin may readily become sensitized and show cross-reactions to neomycin and kanamycin.

This drug is an important occupational hazard to nurses and a frequent cause of allergic contact sensitization. The allergic dermatitis may first be noted at the tips of the thumb and the index and middle fingers, where there is contact with streptomycin from a leaking syringe or needle. Prolonged contact in the sensitized individual may produce deep fissures and hyperkeratoses with superimposed eczematization.

For patch test purposes, a 2.5% aqueous solution of streptomycin is used. In most instances, sensitized individuals show a strongly positive patch test reaction. The reaction is negative occasionally, but a scratch test may produce an urticarial wheal within 15 minutes, which may remain for an hour or so and may be replaced by a papule or vesicle after 24 to 48 hours. Although scratch testing with streptomycin is a relatively safe procedure, the intracutaneous test is hazardous and may cause a generalized urticaria and anaphylactoid shock. Desensitization to streptomycin is dangerous and usually fails.

Contact dermatitis among nurses giving streptomycin to patients who have tuberculosis was first reported by Strauss and Warring (38). Four of 12 nurses working in a sanatorium developed dermatitis of their hands and eyelids, and each had a positive patch test to 2% streptomycin. In a study of 18 sensitized nurses, Wilson (39) reported that the hands, arms, and eyelids were affected most frequently; 17 nurses had positive patch tests to streptomycin 5% in aqueous solution, and 1 reacted only to an intradermal injection. It was found that, on wards where gloves and masks were worn for giving injections, nurses escaped sensitization, whereas on other wards where nurses were not so protected, dermatitis occurred.

Adams (40) states that streptomycin is used to control bacterial disease, such as fire blight of pears, apples, begonias, roses, and other flowers. The streptomycin is often combined with tetracycline, and allergic contact dermatitis from such exposure to streptomycin may take place.

> **Streptomycin may be sprayed onto plants to control gram-negative bacterial disease.**

CEPHALOSPORINS

Nursing can also lead to cephalosporin exposure and occupational contact dermatitis. A 24- year-old nurse was found reactive to cefazolin, cefoxitin, ceftriaxon, and cedfazidime on patch testing, and this explained her hand, forearm, and facial dermatitis (41).

Ceftiofur

Ceftiofur sodium is a third-generation veterinary cephalosporin used in chicks to control *E. coli*. Chicken vaccinators are at risk for contact dermatitis to this agent, and two cases have been reported (42). Other contact allergens seen in chicken vaccinators include tylosin, spectinomycin, and lincomycin. Other cephalosporins reported to cause contact dermatitis are listed in Table 13.10.

BACITRACIN

Bacitracin is a sensitizer. Topical application may produce anaphylactic shock. Comaish and Cunliffe (43) reported that soon after a woman applied bacitracin to a statis ulcer, she complained that she had a pricking sensation and swelling of her face, generalized itching, sweating, dyspnea, and hypotension. She then collapsed. Later, she remembered that twice in the past she had had urticaria after her ulcer had been treated with other preparations containing bacitracin. Three months later, because a prick test with bacitracin 1/1,000 was negative, 0.03 mL of the bacitracin 1/1000 (2.3 units) was injected intradermally, and within 4 minutes she suffered severe anaphylactic shock and lost consciousness.

It was stressed that the concentration for intradermal testing should be 1,000-fold less than that for prick tests.

Roupe and Strannegard (44) described a 14-year-old atopic girl who collapsed with anaphylactic shock after an ointment containing bacitracin was applied to her atopic dermatitis. Two months previously, a similar application had caused irritation and swelling of her lip. Prausnitz-Kustner tests done on monkeys and one human were positive.

At the 1992 meeting of the American Contact Dermatitis Society, Dr. William James reported another case of anaphylactic shock in response to bacitracin. The patient was a healthy adolescent (his son) who applied bacitracin to an abrasion. James's case was subsequently reported by Farley et al. (45). They collected nine cases from the literature and added two of their own. They recommended prick testing with 0.1 U/mL and if no reaction occurred, then increasing the concentration tenfold.

Van Ketel (22) stated that a woman who had contact dermatitis of her feet had positive patch test reactions to polymyxin B sulfate and bacitracin. It was thought these might be cross-reactions rather than independent sensitizations.

> **Bacitracin is a rare sensitizer that can produce anaphylaxis by topical application.**

Although bacitracin and neomycin are not chemically related, they often "co-react" because the patients may have become sensitized simultaneously to both antibiotics when they are used in combination in such preparations as Neo-Polycin and Neosporin (Table 13.11). At a meeting of the North American Contact Dermatitis Group (NACDG) in the mid-1980s, Alexander Fisher presented his experience with bacitracin sensitivity and suggested that it might be more prevalent than neomycin sensitivity, but, because routine testing for bacitracin was not done at that time, the issue was unanswerable. The NACDG began testing bacitracin after that presentation. A study of leg ulcer patients found Fisher's concern to be legitimate, as bacitracin was the most common antibiotic allergen among leg ulcer patients, slightly exceeding neomycin (46). This was attributed to the widespread use of a polymyxin/bacitracin mixture for the management of leg ulcers at the institution.

Thus, Bjorkner and Möller (18) patch tested 1,000 patients who had suspected contact dermatitis and found only 3 allergic to bacitracin, all of whom also had positive tests to neomycin. After intracutaneous injection of bacitracin, the three patients showed a delayed eczematous reaction. A strong, immediate wheal and flare reaction was induced by intracutaneously injected bacitracin. This was inhibited by

TABLE 13.10. *Cephalosporins Reported to Cause Contact Dermatitis*

Cephalexin	Cefoxitin
Cefuroxime	Ceftriaxone
Cephaloridine	Cefodizime
Cephamandol	Ceftazidime
Cephazolin	Cedfazidime
Cephazoline	Cephotaxime
Cefotiam	Ceftizoxime

TABLE 13.11. *Bacitracin-Containing Antibiotics*

Baciguent Antibiotic Ointment (Upjohn)
Bacitracin Ointment (American Pharm.)
Bacitracin Topical Ointment (Pfipharmecs)
BNP Ointment (Norwich-Eaton)
Cortisporin Ointment (Burroughs Wellcome)
Mycitracin Antibiotic Ointment (Upjohn)
Neo-Polycin (Merrell Dow)
Neosporin Aerosol, Ointment, Powder (Burroughs Wellcome)
Norwich Bacitracin Ointment (Norwich Eaton)
Polysporin Ointment (Burroughs Wellcome)

a simultaneous, local injection of the antihistamine mepyramine, which also abolished the vascular response to histamine and to the histamine liberator polymyxin B. Depletion of cutaneous histamine by pretreatment with polymyxin B diminished the wheal and flare induced by bacitracin. The vascular effects of bacitracin in human skin are due apparently to a release of histamine.

> **Bacitracin may "co-react" with neomycin and may be a histamine-releasing agent.**

Binnick and Clendenning (19) reported a patient who had allergic contact dermatitis owing to bacitracin. As noted in the discussion of neomycin cosensitivity, isolated bacitracin sensitivity has been found increasingly when looked for by members of NACDG.

POLYMYXIN

Polymyxin is used widely in topical medications, often in combination with neomycin and bacitracin (Table 13.12).

Van Ketel (22) pointed out that polymyxin B sulfate is used in patients who have ulcers of the legs contaminated with *Pseudomonas aeruginosa*. In contrast to bacitracin, which is also present in topically used preparations, polymyxin B sulfate and the related polymyxin E (Colistin) are used parenterally in cases of infection of the intestines and other organs, mainly in cases of *P. aeruginosa* infection. Thus, patients topically sensitized to polymyxin B sulfate could acquire a systemic contact dermatitis.

TABLE 13.12. *Polymyxin-Containing Antibiotics*

Aerosporin Powder (Burroughs Wellcome)
Chloromyxin (Parke Davis)
Cortisporin Cream (Burroughs Wellcome)
Cortisporin Ophthalmic Ointment and Suspension (Burroughs Wellcome)
Cortisporin Otic Suspension (Burroughs Wellcome)
Neo-Polycin (Merrell Dow)
Neosporin Aerosol and Ointment (Burroughs Wellcome)
Neosporin GU Irrigant (Burroughs Wellcome)
Neosporin Ophthalmic Ointment and Solution (Burroughs Wellcome)
Neosporin Powder and Cream (Burroughs Wellcome)
Ophthocort (Parke-Davis)
Otobiotic Sterile Otic Solution (Schering)
Otocidin Otic Drops (Marin)
Polymyxin B Sulfate (Burroughs Wellcome)
Polysporin Ophthalmic Ointment (Burroughs Wellcome)
Pyocidin-Otic Solution (Berlex)
Terramycin Ointment (Pfipharmecs)
Terramycin with Polymyxin B Sulfate Ophthalmic Ointment (Pfipharmecs)

> **Sensitization to topical polymyxin or bacitracin may cause systemic contact dermatitis if a polymyxin is then used parenterally.**

According to van Ketel (22), topical polymyxin B sulfate cross-reacts not only with Colistin (polymyxin E) but also with bacitracin, because both antibiotics are obtained from *B. subtilis*.

Möller (47) reported that patients who had stasis ulcers and eczema treated with Terramycin-polymyxin B ointment became sensitized to polymyxin B sulfate.

GENTAMICIN (GARAMYCIN, CIDOMYCIN, GENTALYN, GENTICIN, AND REFOBACIN)

The topical antibiotics listed in Table 13.13 contain this antibiotic. Cross-reactions between gentamicin (Garamycin) and neomycin have been reported several times. Thus, Pirila et al. (48) demonstrated that of 100 neomycin-sensitive individuals, 40 showed positive patch test reactions to gentamicin (Garamycin) despite lack of previous exposure to gentamicin. Bandmann and Mutzek (49), Braun and Schutz (50), and Schorr et al. (51) showed similar cross-reactions between neomycin and gentamicin. Lynfield (52) described a patient who was so sensitive to gentamicin that he gave a positive patch test reaction to a cream containing 0.1% concentration of gentamicin. This patient also cross-reacted with neomycin. Drake (53) reported that a woman developed tinnitus each time she applied Garamycin Cream 0.1% to a paronychia.

> **Gentamicin (Garamycin) frequently shows cross-reactions with neomycin.**

PRISTINAMYCIN

Cross-reactivity to pristinamycin administered orally occurred in patients who had previously been sensitized topically to virginiamycin ointment (54). Features of both immediate and delayed hypersensitivity were present in these cases reported in France.

TABLE 13.13. *Topical Garamycin (Gentamicin)*

Garamycin Cream and Ointment (Schering)
Garamycin Ophthalmic Ointment and Sterile Solution (Schering)
Gentamicin Cream 0.1% and Ointment 0.1% (Schein)

Allergic Sensitization to Topical Clindamycin

Allergic contact dermatitis owing to topical clindamycin is rare but should be suspected when patients using topical clindamycin complain of itching. Patch testing with the preparation and its separate ingredients should than be performed.

Mild, local, adverse reactions to topical clindamycin preparations, such as burning, stinging, excessive dryness, itching, and erythema, are not uncommon but are usually caused by the vehicle. Contact allergy to clindamycin seems to be rare, especially in relation to the widespread use of this antibiotic in topical formulations.

Coskey (55) and DeGroot (56) have reported positive patch test reactions and dermatitis from topical clindamycin. Conde-Salazar et al. (57) described a patient who was exposed to both systemic and topical clindamycin for an atopic dermatitis. The patient developed a superimposed contact dermatitis and showed positive reactions to both clindamycin and lincomycin. Lincomycin is an antibiotic of the *Streptomyces* genus, and clindamycin is a semisynthetic derivative used as a phosphate, chlorhydrate, or palmitate. Yokoyama et al. (58) reported clindamycin sensitivity with positive patch tests to the hydrochloride form at 0.5% aqueous and the phosphate form at 0.1% aqueous. Their patient did not react to lincomycin.

Topical clindamycin (either as the hydrochloride salt or the phosphate ester) is used widely in the treatment of acne vulgaris (59,60). Topical clindamycin has been used to treat acne for more than 20 years. Case reports of contact dermatitis to this antibiotic are rare. Vejlstrup and Menne (61) found three cases in the literature and reported one additional case of their own. They considered clindamycin to be a weak allergen.

Nonallergic Adverse Reactions to Topical Clindamycin

Several adverse reactions to topical clindamycin have been described that are similar to those described from systemic administration: diarrhea, abdominal pains, pseudomembranous colitis, migraine, and fatigue.

Feingold et al. (62), after experimental topical application of clindamycin to the backs of hamsters, state: "The possibility of colitis from topical applications of antibiotics cannot be dismissed out of hand. In these hamsters, care was taken that no clindamycin could be ingested. In patients using clindamycin on the face, it is likely that some of the drugs would enter through the mouth."

Milstone et al. (63) reported that abdominal cramping and diarrhea developed in a 24-year-old woman 5 days after she started topical therapy with 1% clindamycin hydrochloride for treatment of facial acne vulgaris. A stool specimen contained a significant titer of a toxin produced by *Clostridium difficile*. Findings from sigmoidoscopy and a colonic biopsy specimen were consistent with pseudomembranous colitis. The patient became asymptomatic after 10 days of supportive care and oral vancomycin hydrochloride therapy. This case is presented as an example of pseudomembranous colitis associated with topical application of clindamycin. Milstone et al. (63) concluded that topical clindamycin is a safe and apparently effective therapy for some forms of acne vulgaris in many patients. Pseudomembranous colitis can be fatal, however, if not recognized and treated appropriately. All patients receiving topical clindamycin should be warned that they should discontinue therapy and consult their physicians if intestinal symptoms occur.

> **Although colitis from topical clindamycin is rare, therapy should stop promptly if any significant abdominal symptoms occur.**

Percutaneous absorption does occur, however, and several other cases of associated diarrhea have been reported (64,65). Another possible unwanted effect of topical antibiotic usage is the selection of a resistant gram-positive skin flora (60), which may pose a drawback to this therapeutic approach, as the drugs used for acne are also utilized for other infections caused by gram-positive organisms. Some authors, however, consider this to be a theoretical rather than a practical problem (66).

LINCOMYCIN

Lincomycin along with spectinomycin has been implicated in causing hand and forearm rashes in chicken vaccinators. Lincomycin was tested at 5% in petrolatum and spectinomycin at 1% petrolatum (67).

ERYTHROMYCIN

Fisher's (66) experience with erythromycin base in a petrolatum ointment in more than 300 infected dermatoses and in a study of 60 patients who had infected stasis ulcers failed to produce even a single instance of sensitization. He was unable to find any reports in the literature of allergic reactions to the topical application of erythromycin base at that time.

Lombardi et al. (68) describe "delayed hypersensitivity to erythromycin." It should be emphasized that they patch tested with an erythromycin salt, erythromycin sulfate 25% in petrolatum. In addition, van Ketel (69) reported an allergic reaction to erythromycin stearate.

Although erythromycin is an extremely rare sensitizer, topical use followed by oral use caused both a local and generalized dermatitis (70). In this case, erythromycin base at 2.5% in petrolatum was positive, as was the ethylsuccinate base.

CHLORAMPHENICOL

Table 13.14 lists some topical chloramphenicol preparations. Allergic contact sensitivity to this antibiotic is rare.

Schwank and Jirasek (71) reported much sensitivity to chloramphenicol applied to stasis ulcers and eczemas. Patch tests with chloramphenicol 1% in petrolatum or in alcohol elicited reactions in all the patients, but in only 9 of 149 controls. Six further patients, who worked in a plant making chloramphenicol, developed a contact dermatitis of the face and hands. The report of Schwank and Jirasek (71), concerning cross-sensitization between 2,4-dinitrochlorbenzene and chloramphenicol, was not confirmed (72,73).

Rudzki et al. (74) attributed a positive patch test reaction to 50% chloramphenicol to a previous drug eruption from intramuscular chloramphenicol. Kozakova (75) reported that a woman who had used chloramphenicol topically in the past was given the drug by mouth. She developed anaphylactic shock with edema of the face and generalized urticaria. A week later, a patch test with 1% chloramphenicol produced the same reaction, but to a lesser degree.

Bandmann (76) attributed the small number of case reports of chloramphenicol sensitivity to the fact that this antibiotic is used rarely for eczema.

Milkowski (77) presented a patient who had two episodes of contact conjunctivitis and dermatitis of the lids after application of chloramphenicol as drops into the conjunctival sac. Chloramphenicol is available in France only in topical form as an eyedrop preparation. In this form, it caused contact dermatitis of the face and conjunctivitis (78). Cross-reactivity with thiamphenicol was observed. Wereide (79) reported that azidamphenicol used as an antibiotic showed cross-reactions with chloramphenicol.

TETRACYCLINES

Although fixed-drug eruptions from the systemic use of tetracycline are fairly commonly observed in the United States, allergic reactions to the topical application of tetracycline are rarely seen. European investigators, however, report that allergic reactions to tetracycline are not uncommon. Thus, Fontanot (80) reported in Italy that four patients were sensitized to ointments containing tetracycline compound. Bojs and Möller (81) reported in Belgium that, whereas neomycin is still the leading contact antibiotic allergen, the tetracyclines are not "harmless." They reported

TABLE 13.14. *Chloramphenicol*

Chloromycetin Cream (Parke Davis)
Chloromycetin Ophthalmic and Otic Ointment (Parke Davis)
Chloromyxin Ointment (Parke Davis)
Ophthochlor Solution (Parke Davis)
Ophthocort Ointment (Parke Davis)

three cases of eczematous contact allergy in patients using oxytetracycline. Results of patch tests with six other tetracyclines showed that cross-sensitivity to tetracycline and methacycline could be demonstrated in two of the patients.

Calnan (82) stated that a woman who had used Aureomycin ointment on a dermabraded tattoo developed dermatitis. Another patient used Aureomycin ointment to treat her varicose ulcers. Patch tests revealed that the first patient reacted to the Aureomycin ointment, chlortetracycline, and demeclocycline, but not to tetracycline. The second patient reacted to Aureomycin 0.5% (in petrolatum).

It should be emphasized that these European reports do not deal with the topical application of tetracycline in lotion form for acne.

Cosmetic Drawbacks to Topical Tetracycline

Standlee (83) emphasized that topical tetracycline preparations yellow the skin. The discoloration is noticeable, especially on patients who have fair complexions. Furthermore, patients complain about the drug's fluorescence. Standlee states, "A patient on Topicycline was slightly shocked and embarrassed when visiting a display of fluorescent minerals in a museum. To her dismay, her face fluoresced as brightly as the minerals!"

> **Topical tetracycline rarely sensitizes but may cause a yellow discoloration of the skin and fluoresce under fluorescent black lights.**

NYSTATIN

Wasilewski (84) studied a patient who was allergic to nystatin following exposure to two topical medications containing this antibiotic in combination with different ingredients. On patch testing, the patient reacted to Mycolog Cream, Nystaform-HC Ointment, and ethylenediamine. Although original Mycolog Cream contained ethylenediamine, Nystaform-HC Ointment does not. Nystatin is the only ingredient common to both preparations, and a subsequent patch test with nystatin (Mycostatin sterile powder for laboratory use) was strongly positive. The patch test material was prepared in a concentration of 100,000 units/mL (1 mg = approximately 3,000 units), and 70% ethanol was used as the vehicle. None of ten volunteers patch tested with this material showed any reaction.

Coskey (85,86) and Foussereau et al. (87) have also reported allergic contact sensitivity to nystatins.

NITROFURAZONE (FURACIN)

Topical nitrofurazone is available in the following forms:

Furacin Soluble Dressing (Norwich-Eaton), which contains 0.2% nitrofurazone (Furacin) in Solubase (a water-soluble base of polyethylene glycols 4,000, 1,000, and 300).

Furacin Soluble Powder (Norwich-Eaton), which contains 0.2% nitrofurazone (Furacin) in a water-soluble powder of polyethylene glycol 6,000.

Furacin Topical Cream (Norwich-Eaton), which contains nitrofurazone (Furacin) in a water-miscible base consisting of glycerin, cetyl alcohol, mineral oil, an ethoxylated fatty alcohol, methylparaben, propyl-paraben, and water.

Nitrofurazone is a well-known sensitizer, and many instances of severe allergic contact dermatitis occur where it is used extensively.

Hull and de Beer (88) state that patients who had stasis eczema and ulcers or injury to the skin of the leg are particularly prone to sensitization, whereas Braun and Schutz (50) reported that 58 patients (many of whom had stasis eczema or ulcers) were sensitized by medicaments containing 0.2% nitrofurazone (Furacin), and that reexposure to it had caused a generalized eczema in some patients. Sensitization has also been reported by Bleumink et al. (89) in 14 patients who had leg ulcers. A positive patch test to Furacin ointment containing 0.2% nitrofurazone was obtained in each patient.

Furacin is a potent sensitizer, particularly when used on stasis ulcers, eczemas, and burns.

Nitrofurazone (Furacin) is also used in veterinary medicine and in animal feeds. Caplan (90) reported a man who worked in a feed shop and scooped chicken feed containing Furacin from storage bins into sacks. He developed acute attacks of dermatitis. On patch testing he reacted to 1% nitrofurazone. Neldner (91) also reported contact dermatitis from Furacin added to animal feed.

Contact Dermatitis from Polyethylene Glycol in "Soluble" Furacin Preparations

Fisher (92) reported that Furacin Soluble Dressing (Eaton) applied to a second-degree burn of the leg produced a severe allergic contact dermatitis. Patch tests with Furacil Soluble Dressing, polyethylene glycol (PEG) 300 and 400, were strongly positive in the patient and negative in six controls. Patch tests to PEG 1,000 and 4,000 were negative.

A second patient was a 64-year-old man who had received cobalt radiation for carcinoma of the lung and had developed a severe second-degree burn of the irradiated skin of the chest for which he had been treated with a spray of Furacin Solution (Eaton). A severe, edematous vesicular and crusted contact dermatitis became superimposed upon the radiation burn. Patch tests with Furacin solution, PEG

400 and 300, were strongly positive. Patch tests with PEG 1,000 and 4,000 were negative.

Braun (93) studied 40 patients who showed a delayed allergic contact sensitivity to a medication containing nitrofurazone (nitrofural), which is a Furacin-like product. In 3 of 40 cases, the active ingredient nitrofurazone was not the cause of the dermatitis, but the solvent PEG 300 proved to be the culprit.

It should be emphasized that Furacin Soluble Dressing and Powder contain polyethylene glycols. Allergic reactions may occur either from Furacin or the polyethylene glycols.

The low-numbered polyethylene glycols in "soluble" Furacin preparations may produce allergic contact dermatitis.

Nifuroxazide

The oral antibiotic nifuroxazide is used to treat acute and chronic diarrhea. There have been reports of contact dermatitis to this. A Polish pharmaceutical worker was exposed to nifuroxazide in a packaging operation, but her lesions resembled prurigo nodularis rather than contact dermatitis (94). She was sensitive to this antibiotic from 1% to 0.001% aqueous and cleared when not occupationally exposed. She did not cross-react to nitrofurazone.

Furaltadone

Furaltadone is an antibiotic most commonly associated with veterinary practice or use in animal feeds. It is a component of a Spanish eardrop and along with neomycin caused contact dermatitis. The product (Panotile) contains 4.5 mg/mL of furaltadone chlorhydrate, and a 1% concentration in petrolatum was positive in the patient but negative in 20 controls (95).

THE SULFONAMIDES

Cross-reactions can occur between the various antibacterial sulfonamides and chemically related sulfonamides used as diuretics, oral hypoglycemics, and sweetening agents. In addition, cross-reactions may occur occasionally with para-amino compounds, such as paraphenylenediamine and para-aminobenzoic acid (PABA).

Sulfanilamide

The topical administration of this older sulfonamide preparation has largely been discarded. Exposure to sulfanilamide may still take place, however, from topical application of the compounds shown in Table 13.15.

In certain European countries, mafenide acetate (Sulfamylon Acetate Cream) (4-homosulfanilamide) is used particularly for burns. Bandmann and Breit (96) reported that 6.4% of the men and 5.4% of the women had positive patch tests to 10% mafenide, a popular antibiotic in Germany. Yaffee and Dressler (97) studied 400 patients treated with mafenide; although the incidence of skin complications was 9.5%, none of the 11 patients had positive patch test reactions to mafenide.

Velasco and Africk (98) reported three patients who developed an eruption at the site of application. All three reacted to mafenide acetate 8.5% and to mafenide hydrochloride 5%, but cross-reactions to sulfanilamide 8.5% or to a mixture containing sulfadiazine, sulfamerazine, and sulfamethazine did not occur.

It is of interest to note that they believe that the critical antigenic site of the mafenide molecule is the methyl group in the para position.

The various topical sulfonamides shown in Tables 13.16 to 13.20 may all cross-react with one another. Because patch testing to one sulfonamide, however, does not necessarily detect sensitivity to the whole group, the specific sulfonamide that the patient has used should be used for patch test purposes.

Sulzberger et al. (99) showed that prolonged use of topical sulfonamides can readily cause allergic sensitization. Gottschalk and Stone (100) reported a case of Stevens-Johnson syndrome from an ophthalmic sulfonamide preparation.

Sodium Fusidate

Sensitization to this antibiotic used abroad may occur from its use on stasis ulcers (101,102). De Groot (103) reported a patient who had used an ointment employing sodium fusidate on a stasis ulcer with resulting superimposed allergic contact dermatitis. Positive patch tests to the ointment and sodium fusidate 1% in petrolatum were obtained. Sodium fusidate at 0.5% in petrolatum was used to diagnose a case caused by 2% Fucidin cream (104). This drug is used widely in Europe, but not as yet in the United States.

Certain topical European antibiotics not yet introduced into the United States, such as manefid, virgiamycin, and sodium fusidate, have been reported to cause allergic contact dermatitis.

Systemic Contact Dermatitis from Sulfonamide Drugs

Topical sensitization to a sulfonamide compound may engender a systemic contact dermatitis when the following sulfonamide compounds are administered:

1. sulfonamide diuretics (Table 13.21)

TABLE 13.15. *Topical Sulfanilamides*

AVC Cream and Suppositories (Merrell Dow)
Vagimide Cream (Legere)
Vaginal Sulfa Suppositories (Schein)

TABLE 13.16. *Topical Sulfabenzamides*

Sultrin Triple Sulfa Cream (Ortho Pharmaceutical)
Triple Sulfa Vaginal Cream (Schein)
Trysul Cream (Savage)

TABLE 13.17. *Topical Sulfacetamides*

Sultrin Triple Sulfa Cream (Ortho)
Triple Sulfa Vaginal Cream (Schein)
Trysul Cream (Savage)

TABLE 13.18. *N′-Acetylsulfanilamide (Sulfacetamide Sodium)*

Sodium Sulamyd Ophthalmic Solution and Ointment (Schering)

TABLE 13.19. *Sulfisoxazole*

Cantri Vaginal Cream (Hauck)
Koro-Sulf Vaginal Cream (Youngs)
Vagilia Cream and Suppositories (Lemmon)

TABLE 13.20. *Sulfisoxazole Diolamine*

Gantrisin Ophthalmic Ointment/Solution (Roche)

TABLE 13.21. *Sulfonamide Diuretics*

Bendroflumethiazide (Naturetin)
Benzthiazide (Exna)
Chlorothiazide (Diuril)
Cyclothiazide (Anhydron)
Hydrochlorothiazide (Esidrix, Hydrodiuril, Oretic)
Hydroflumethiazide (Saluron)
Polythiazide (Renese)
Trichlormethiazide (Naqua)

TABLE 13.22. *Sulfonamide Oral Hypoglycemic Agents*

Carbutamide (Nadisan)*
Diabinese (Chlorpropamide)
Orinase (Tolbutamide)

*Still used in Europe.

2. sulfonamide oral hypoglycin agents (Table 13.22)
3. sulfonamide sweetening agents (Table 13.23)

Fisher (105) has reported that many adult diabetics receive oral "para-amino" hypoglycemic sulfonyl urea drugs, such as Orinase and Diabinese. These diabetic patients may become sensitized to widely used topical para-amino compounds, such as hair dyes, particularly paraphenylenediamine, sunscreens containing PABA or its esters, and local anesthetics, such as benzocaine. In addition, sensitization to the sulfanilamide compounds poses the threat of a systemic contact dermatitis to the ingestion of the closely related antidiabetic drugs. Thus, a diabetic person sensitized to the topical vaginal sulfanilamide cream acquired a systemic contact dermatitis from the administration of Orinase, an oral antidiabetic compound.

> **Sensitization to topical sulfonamide compounds may engender cross-sensitization to para-amino compounds, such as hair dyes, benzocaine, and PABA sunscreens.**

Angelini and Meneghini (106) reported that a group of 34 patients who have contact allergy to para-amino compounds (sulfanilamide, paraphenylenediamine, and benzocaine) underwent a series of peroral tests using structurally related substances, sulfonyl ureas (carbutamide, tolbutamide, and chlorpropamide), diaminodiphenyl sulfone, saccharin, and salicylazo-sulfapyridine. They found that these sulfonyl urea drugs given orally produced a widespread dermatitis in 11 subjects who have contact sensitivity to sulfanilamide, but not in those sensitized to paraphenylenediamine and benzocaine.

The positive results in 11 of 34 inpatients who reacted were manifest as follows: (a) itching in all 11 patients; (b) the reappearance of erythema and vesicles at the site of the primary erythema and vesicles at the site of the primary contact dermatitis in 6 patients; and (c) the relapse of the primary contact dermatitis with a moderate secondary

TABLE 13.23. *Sulfonamide Sweetening Agents*

Calcium Cyclamate
Saccharin
Sodium Cyclamate
Sucaryl
Sweeta

vesicular eruption, together with a reactivation of the patch test reaction in 5 patients.

The provocative oral tests were considered positive when at least one of the following was produced: pruritus with recurrence of the primary dermatitis, spread of eczematous lesions, and reactivation of the patch test reactions.

Angelini and Meneghini (106) state that none of the patients who were sensitized to sulfanilamide, paraphenylenediamine, or benzocaine reacted to the ingestion of saccharin. Although the sweetening agents shown in Table 13.23 are all sulfanilamide compounds, there are as yet no reports of "systemic" contact dermatitis in individuals using these agents who have been sensitized to topically applied para-amino compounds.

> **Systemic contact dermatitis in patients sensitized to topical sulfonamides may occur from the administration of many sulfonamide diuretics and oral antidiabetic agents.**

ACETARSONE

Vaginal treatment for trichomonal vaginitis with acetarsone caused vulval and inner thigh urticaria and dermatitis (107). Acetarsone is also known as acetarsol, acetphenarsine, and [3-(acetylamino)-4-hydroxyphenyl]-arsonic acid. It also can be found in toothpaste, mouthwashes, and treatments for proctitis.

METRONIDAZOLE

Facial contact dermatitis has been reported from 1% metronidazole gel (108). This is chemically an imidazole; although cross-reaction with imidazoles commonly used as antifungals has not been reported, it is a potential issue for this widely used rosacea therapy.

QUINOLONE

A drug eruption due to norfloxacin presented with a genitocrural toxicoderma that resembled the baboon syndrome (109). The quinoline mix patch test commonly included in European screening series of patch test materials was positive and resulted in a recall dermatitis in the genitocrural area 1 month after the initial rash had cleared. Because norfloxacin is a quinolone antibiotic, it may be possible to screen for this allergy with the quinoline mix.

CLOXYQUIN

Cloxyquin, which is closely related to clioquinol, caused dermatitis confirmed with a 5% patch test concentration (110). The patient also reacted to clioquinol, and it was not certain whether induction of allergy came from the former or the later.

VIRGINIAMYCIN (STAPHLOMYCIN), STAPOLIDEX, AND PRISTINAMYCIN (STAPYOCINE)

Baes (111) reported that a man sensitized to virginiamycin in a topical preparation took one tablet of pristinamycin and 4 hours later had an anaphylactic reaction with stupor, urticaria, and vomiting. Patch tests with virginiamycin, pristinamycin, and factors M and IIa, each 1% in petrolatum, were all positive. He developed transient edema of his eyes and lips and wheals adjacent to a positive patch test.

Pristinamycin, like virginiamycin, contains two fractions (Ia and IIa). Chemically, both antibiotics are very closely related, and all patients sensitized by virginiamycin have reacted to pristinamycin.

Bleumink and Nater (112,113) and Lachapelle and Lamy (114) also reported allergic contact dermatitis from these antibiotics when used for burns and other inflammatory dermatoses. Tennstedt et al. (115) state that these antibiotics are used as a food additive for pigs and poultry and pose an occupational hazard for individuals dispensing such feed.

RIFAMYCIN

Three cases of contact dermatitis due to rifamycin occurred in patients using it to treat leg ulcers. A 2.5% concentration in petrolatum was used for patch testing (116).

KITASAMYCIN AND MIDECAMYCIN

Kitasamycin is a macrolide antibiotic from *Streptomyces ketasatoensis* and very similar to midecamycin from *S. mycarofaciens*. Occupational exposure to large quantities of dust caused an airborne allergic contact dermatitis. No coreactions were observed to either erythromycin or triolendomycin (117).

MUPIROCIN

Mupirocin, a very rare sensitizer, when applied to leg ulcers, has caused contact dermatitis (118). The reaction was confirmed to be due to the active ingredient in Bactroban® by patch testing with calcium mupirocin–free base 10% in ointment base with a negative reaction to the ointment alone.

TOPICAL ANTIFUNGAL AGENTS

Tolnaftate (Tinactin)

Gellin et al. (119), reporting the first case of delayed hypersensitivity to Tinactin, stated that no other instances of tolaftate sensitivity have been reported in the past literature

despite its use by several million persons in the past decade. Soon after, Emmett and Marrs (120) reported a similar case.

Haloprogin (Halotex)

Rudolph (121) described a case of allergic contact dermatitis from Halotex. Moss (122) and Berlin and Miller (123) state that ethyl sebacate, a solubilizer in both the cream and the lotion formulations of haloprogin, has caused contact dermatitis.

Desenex Ointment

This "older" antifungal agent containing undecylenic acid rarely irritates or sensitizes.

Clotrimazole

Sensitization by a connubial exposure was assumed to have occurred due to intravaginal clotrimazole used by a 35-year-old man's wife (124). When he was instructed to use topical clotrimazole at the same time that his wife was retreated intravaginally, a genital dermatitis appeared. No cross-reaction was seen to miconazole, econazole, ketoconazole, bifonazole, or isoconazole.

A man who was known to have used only one imidazole antifungal, clotrimazole, was found to be allergic to it (125). He also reacted to croconazole and itraconazole. Although both clotrimazole and croconazole are phenylmethyl imidazoles, itraconazole is a triazole.

Sertaconazole

Sertaconazole is an imidazole used topically in Spain. Patch tests 1% and 5% in petrolatum were positive in a 26-year-old man who developed contact dermatitis from use of this product on his hand (126). Cross-reactivity with micronazole and econazole were seen but not to seven other closely related imidazoles.

Croconazole

Croconazole is promoted for both antifungal and antiinflammatory properties. It is a phenoxyethyl imidazole derivative, but it has sensitized in as little as 4 weeks of use (127). It has a distinct structure and does not cross-react with clotrimazole or bifonazole.

Lanoconazole

A new member of the imidazole family introduced into Japan caused contact dermatitis within 1 month of use on the feet of a 79-year-old man (128). The agent in this case was lanoconazole, and a 20% concentration in petrolatum was used to confirm the sensitivity. In a second report of lanoconazole, no cross-reactivity to vinyl imidazoles such as croconazole and neticonazole was observed (129).

Neticonazole

The vinyl imidazole, neticonazole, caused contact dermatitis of the feet after 6 months of use (130). This patient also reacted to econazole and sulconazole.

The Imidazole Derivatives

These antifungal agents include clotrimazole (Lotrimin) (Table 13.24), which Roller (131) reported caused an allergic reaction with a positive reaction to 1% in methyl ethyl ketone. Clotrimazole is present in Gyne-Lotrimin Vaginal Cream and Mycelex Cream and Solution, as well as Lotrimin AF.

Degreef and Verhoeve (132) reported one allergic reaction and many irritant reactions to Micatin. Such irritant reactions are most likely to occur when Micatin is applied to moist, intertriginous areas (133).

The newer topical imidazole antifungals may cross-react. Two cases of contact dermatitis due to topical ketoconazole were both found to cross-react to miconazole and sulconazole (all tested at 1% in ethanol) (134). Baes (135) reported a pattern of cross-reactivity among antifungals that were β-substituted 1-phenethyl imidazoles with an ortho-chlorine substitution and dubbed this "ortho-chloro cross-reactivity." The group of antifungal agents includes isoconazole, tioconazole, oxiconazole, and miconazole. The non-β-substituted 1-phenethyl imidazoles include econazole, sulconazole, enilconazole, and ketoconazole (136). Machet et al. (136) observed that cross-reactions within groups were common (see Table 13.25), but cross-reactions between groups occurred less frequently. Marren and Powell (137) reviewed 43 published cases of allergic contact dermatitis due to imidazoles from 1974 to 1992 and found 34 reports of cross-reactions to other imidazoles. Their own case of tioconazole allergy cross-reacted to ketoconazole but not miconazole, sulconazole, or clotrimazole. Tioconazole used on a paronychia led to contact dermatitis but without cross-reactions to other imidazoles (138), but Stubb et al. (139) found that 9 of 14 patients who were allergic to tioconazole cross-reacted with clotrimazole, econazole, miconazole,

TABLE 13.25. *Antibiotic Patch Test Series*

Ampicillin, 5% aq sol
Bacitracin, 20% in pet
Chloramphenicol, 5% in pet
Clindamycin, 1% aq
Erythromycin, 5% in pet
Furacin, 0.2% in pet
Garamycin (Gentamicin), 20% in pet
Lincomycin, 1% aq
Mafenide, 5% in pet
Neomycin, 20% in pet
Nystatin, 100,000 units/mL in alcohol
Penicillin, 100,000 units/mL
Polymyxin B, 3% in pet
Sodium fusidate, 2% in pet
Streptomycin, 2.5% aq sol
Sulfanilamide, 5% in pet
Tetracycline, 5% in pet
Tobramycin, 20% in pet

and ketoconazole. The introduction of a 28% tioconazole lotion for nail fungus was suggested as the cause for most of the recent case reports (139). Patch testing with commercial products has been said to be more satisfactory than breakdown of the formulas (136).

As an example of the somewhat unpredictable nature of cross-reactions, Jones and Kennedy (140) reported a tioconazole-sensitive onychomycosis patient who cross-reacted to ketoconazole but not miconazole, clotrimazole, or sulconazole. The pattern that has emerged does not allow for good generalizations about cross-reactions, even though the work of Baes (135) and Marren and Powell (137) attempted to place this on a chemical conceptual framework. Instead, the emerging pattern seems idiosyncratic.

Dooms-Goossens et al. (141) have reviewed the literature and their experience with 15 cases of imidazole contact dermatitis with an eye toward making sense of the cross-reaction patterns. They were able to identify three common patterns of cross-reactivity. Isoconazole, miconazole, and econazole commonly are linked, as are sulconazole, miconazole, and econazole; the third linkage was isoconazole and tioconazole. This can be remembered as I-ME, S-ME, IT. Patients with these sensitivities can be treated with non-imidazoles or alternatively with ketoconazole, clotrimazole, bifonazole, or flutrimazole.

Imidazole Intermediate

The production of azathioprine has caused occupational contact dermatitis to the finished compound, but Jolanki et al. (142) reported a patient who manufactured azathioprine but was sensitive to an intermediate rather than the final product. The intermediate was 5-chloro-1-methyl-4-nitroimidazole. This patient showed sensitivity to other imidazoles commonly used to treat fungal infections including tioconazole, econazole, and miconazole.

TABLE 13.24. *Imidazole Classes*

2,4-Dichlorophenylethyl imidazole derivatives	Chemically less similar imidazoles
Miconazole	Ketoconazole
Isoconazole	Clotrimazole
Tioconazole	
Oxiconazole	
Sulconazole	
Econazole	
Enilconazole	

Naftifine

The allylamine antifungal, naftifine, has caused contact dermatitis (143). Because the risk of sensitization is estimated to be 1 in 100,000, the frequency of case reports makes this estimate suspect. Some have suggested that it has greater sensitizing potential than the imidazoles.

Amorolfine

Amorolfine 0.5 cream is marketed in Japan as an antimycotic and has caused contact dermatitis when applied to the leg of a 29-year-old woman (144). A patch test concentration of 0.25% and 0.5% yielded positive results in the patient and negative results in 30 controls.

Nifuratel

Corazza et al. (145) reported a case of vulvar contact dermatitis caused by a vaginal cream containing nifuratel. This substance, *N*-(5-nitro-2-furfurilidene)3-amino-5-methyl-mercaptom ethyl-2-oxazolidone, is considered both antimycotic and antitrichomonal. It was tested at 1% in acetone. A man whose wife used the product Macmiror complex ointment developed a genital rash through connubial contact (146). Corazza et al. (145) cite other cases.

ANTIVIRAL TOPICAL AGENTS

Idoxuridine (5-iodo-2-deoxyuridine)

Idoxuridine, used widely for herpes simplex, is sold under the names Herplex, Stoxil, Dendrid, Emanil, Iducher, and Iduviran. Europeans or those traveling abroad may have used idoxuridine as Herpid (Britain), Iduridin (Denmark), or Zostrum and Viruquent (Germany).

Many instances of sensitivity occur from its use, particularly in genital herpes, but also in its use as eyedrops (147–154).

Cross-reactions may occur with pyrimidine analogues, such as trifluridine (trifluorothymidine) eyedrops (155). Cross-reactions, however, do not occur with 5-FU, which also has a pyrimidine structure but is a 5-fluorinated compound (149). Trifluoridine eyedrops for herpetic eye infection sensitized two patients, and patch tests at 5% and 10% petrolatum were diagnostic (156).

> **Idoxuridine is a not uncommon sensitizer that cross-reacts with trifluorothymidine eyedrops but not with 5-FU.**

Amon et al. (149) reported that idoxuridine has been used for many years in the treatment of herpes simplex infections of the eye. Ophthalmologists have noted occasional conjunctival and corneal-irritant reactions, but no true delayed cutaneous hypersensitivity has been verified. Amon et al. (149) studied four cases of allergic contact dermatitis from idoxuridine, sensitized by both eye and skin applications. Cross-reactivity to brominated and chlorinated, but not fluorinated, pyrimidine analogues was noted.

Tromantadine Hydrochloride

This synthetic antiviral compound, unrelated to idoxuridine, is used abroad in the form of Viru-Merz ointment for topical treatment of herpes simplex. Several instances of allergic sensitization have been reported (157–159).

In the search for a "cure" for herpes, several Americans used this agent, one of whom acquired an allergic contact dermatitis from its use.

Tromantadine is derived from amantadine, with which it may cross-react. A 10% petrolatum concentration was used to diagnose a patient sensitized by Viruserol (160).

Acyclovir

Topical 5% acyclovir ointment (Zovirax) has been reported to cause contact dermatitis. Concentrations of this 9-[(2-hydroxyethoxy) methyl] guanine used for patch testing include 1%, 3%, and 5% in petrolatum (161) and 5% aqueous (162).

Use of Zovirax cream produced cheilitis on sun exposure initially confused with recurrent herpes labialis (163). Photopatch tests with 9 J of UVA light and the Zivirax cream were positive, but testing with the individual ingredients proved negative (compound allergy).

REFERENCES

1. Fisher AA, Adams RM. Alternative for sensitizing neomycin topical medicaments. *Cutis* 1981;28:491.
2. Fisher AA. Prevention of contact dermatitis. *NY State J Med* 1978;78:1739.
3. Wereide K. Neomycin sensitivity in atopic dermatitis and other eczematous conditions. *Acta Derm Venereol* (Stockh) 1970;50:114.
4. Patrick J, Panzer JD, Derbes VJ. Neomycin sensitivity in the normal (nonatopic) individual. *Arch Dermatol* 1970;102:32.
5. Leyden JJ, Kligman AM. Contact dermatitis to neomycin sulfate. *JAMA* 1979;242:1276.
6. Prystowsky SD, Nonomura JH, Smith MS, Allen AM. Allergic hypersensitivity to neomycin: relationship between patch test reactions and "use" tests. *Arch Dermatol* 1979;115:713.
7. Hannuksela M, Kousa M, Pinla V. Allergy to ingredients of vehicles. *Contact Dermatitis* 1976;2:105.
8. Fisher AA, Pascher F, Kanof NB. Allergic contact dermatitis due to ingredients of vehicles: a "vehicle tray" for patch testing. *Arch Dermatol* 1971;104:286.
9. Hjorth N, Thomsen K. Differences in the sensitizing capacity of neomycin in creams and in ointments. *Br J Dermatol* 1968;80:163.
10. Pirila V, Pirila L. Sensitization to the neomycin group of antibiotics: patterns of cross sensitivity as a function of polyvalent sensitization to different portions of the neomycin molecule. *Acta Derm Venereol* (Stockh) 1966;46:489.
11. Chung CW, Carson TR. Sensitization potentials and immunologic specificities of neomycins. *J Invest Dermatol* 1975;64:158.
12. Forstrom L, Pirila V, Pirila L. Cross-sensitivity within the neomycin group of antibiotics. *Acta Derm Venereol* (Stockh) 1979;59(Suppl):67.

13. Schorr WF, Ridgway HB. Tobramycin-neomycin cross-sensitivity. *Contact Dermatitis* 1977;3:133.

14. Menendez-Ramos F, et al. Allergic contact dermatitis from tobramycin. *Contact Dermatitis* 1990;22:305.

15. Ekelund AG, Möller H. Oral provocation in eczematous contact allergy to neomycin and hydroxyquinolines. *Acta Derm Venereol* (Stockh) 1969;49:422.

16. Panzer JD, Epstein WL. Percutaneous absorption following topical application of neomycin. *Arch Dermatol* 1970;102:536.

17. Pirila V, Rouhunkosky S. On sensitivity to neomycin and bacitracin. *Acta Derm Venereol* (Stockh) 1959;39:470.

18. Bjorkner B, Möller H. Bacitracin: a cutaneous allergen and histamine liberator. *Acta Derm Venereol* (Stockh) 1973;53:487.

19. Binnick AN, Clendenning WE. Bacitracin contact dermatitis. *Contact Dermatitis* 1978;4:180.

20. Epstein S, Wenzel F. Cross-sensitivity to various "mycins." *Arch Dermatol* 1962;86:183.

21. Pirila V, Rantanen AV. Root canal treatment with bacitracin-neomycin as cause of flare-up of allergic eczema. *Oral Surg* 1960; 13:589.

22. van Ketel WG. Polymixine 8-sulfate and bacitracin. *Contact Dermatitis Newsletter* 1974;15:445.

23. Dadagian AJ, Hicks JJ, Ordonez GE, Glassman JM. Treatment of otitis externa: a controlled bacteriological-clinical evaluation. *Curr Ther Res* 1974;16:431.

24. Jenkins BH. Simplified approach to otitis externa. *Arch Otolaryngol* 1963;77:442.

25. Kremer WF. Management of external otitis. *West J Med* 1961;2:15.

26. Fisher AA. *Contact dermatitis.* 3rd ed. Philadelphia: Lea & Febiger, 1986.

27. Nom MS. Eyelid ointment penetration into the conjunctival sac. *Acta Ophthalmol* 1972;50:206.

28. Nagreh DS. Contact dermatitis from proprietary preparations in Malaysia. *Int J Dermatol* 1976;15:34.

29. Girard JP. Recurrent angioneurotic oedema and contact dermatitis due to penicillin. *Contact Dermatitis* 1978;4:309.

30. Hjorth N. Occupational dermatitis among veterinary surgeons caused by penethamate (benzyl penicillin-beta-diethylaminoethyl ester). *Berufs-Dermatosen* 1967;15:163.

31. Blanton WB, Blanton FM. Unusual penicillin hypersensitiveness. *J Allergy* 1953;24:405.

32. Valsecchi R, et al. Patch testing in adverse drug reactions to penicillin and cephalosporin. *Contact Dermatitis* 1981;7:158.

33. Lisi P, et al. Skin tests in the diagnosis of eruptions caused by beta-lactams. *Contact Dermatitis* 1997;37:151.

34. Vickers HR, Bagratuni L, Alexander S. Dermatitis caused by penicillin milk. *Lancet* 1958;61:351.

35. Gamboa P, Jauregui I, Urrutia I. Occupational sensitization to aminopenicillins with oral tolerance to penicillin V. *Contact Dermatitis* 1995;32:48.

36. Schulz KH, Schopf E, Wex O. Allergische Berufsekzeme durch Ampicillin. *Berufs-Dermatosen* 1970;18:132.

37. Gamboa P, et al. Contact sensitization to cloxacillin with oral tolerance to other beta-lactam antibiotics. *Contact Dermatitis* 1996;34: 75.

38. Strauss MJ, Warring FC. Contact dermatitis from streptomycin. *J Invest Dermatol* 1947;9:3.

39. Wilson HTH. Streptomycin dermatitis in nurses. *Br Med J* 1958; 1:1378.

40. Adams RM. *Occupational skin disease.* New York: Grune & Stratton, 1983:367.

41. Filipe P, Almeida RS, Rodrigo FG. Occupational allergic contact dermatitis from cephalosporins. *Contact Dermatitis* 1996;34:226.

42. Garcia-Bravo B, Gines E, Russo F. Occupational contact dermatitis from ceftiofur sodium. *Contact Dermatitis* 1995;33:62.

43. Comaish JS, Cunliffe WJ. Absorption of drugs from varicose ulcers: a cause of anaphylaxis. *Br J Clin Pract* 1967;21:97.

44. Roupe G, Strannegard O. Anaphylactic shock elicited by topical administration of bacitracin. *Arch Dermatol* 1969;100:450.

45. Farley M, et al. Anaphylaxis to topically applied bacitracin. *Am J Contact Dermatitis* 1995;6:28.

46. Zaki I, Shall L, Dalziel KL. Bacitracin: a significant sensitizer in leg ulcer patients? *Contact Dermatitis* 1994;31:92–4.

47. Möller H. Eczematous contact allergy to oxytetracycline and polymyxin B. *Contact Dermatitis* 1970;2:289.

48. Pirila V, Hirvonen ML, Rouhunkosh S. The pattern of cross-sensitivity to neomycin: secondary sensitization to gentamicin. *Dermatologica* 1968;236:321.

49. Bandmann H-J, Mutzek E. Contact allergy to gentamycin sulfate. *Contact Dermatitis Newsletter* 1973;13:371.

50. Braun W, Schutz R. Beitrag zur Gentamycin Allergie. *Hautarzt* 1969;20:108.

51. Schorr WF, Wenzel FJ, Hededus SI. Cross-sensitivity and aminoglycoside antibiotics. *Arch Dermatol* 1973;107:533.

52. Lynfield YL. Allergic contact sensitization to gentamicin. *NY State J Med* 1970;70:2235.

53. Drake TE. Reaction to gentamicin sulfate cream [Letter]. *Arch Dermatol* 1974;110:638.

54. Michel M, et al. Eczematous-like drug eruption induced by synergistins. *Contact Dermatitis* 1996;34:86.

55. Coskey RJ. Contact dermatitis due to clindamycin [Letter]. *Arch Dermatol* 1978;114:446.

56. De Groot AC. Contact allergy to clindamycin. *Contact Dermatitis* 1982;8:428.

57. Conde-Salazar L, et al. Contact dermatitis from clindamycin. *Contact Dermatitis* 1983;9:225.

58. Yokoyama R, et al. Contact dermatitis due to clindamycin. *Contact Dermatitis* 1991;25:125.

59. Becker LE, et al. Topical clindamycin therapy for acne vulgaris: a cooperative clinical study. *Arch Dermatol* 1981;217:482.

60. Eady EA, Holland KT, Cunliffe WJ. Topical antibiotics in acne therapy. *J Am Acad Dermatol* 1981;5:455.

61. Vejlstrup E, Menne T. Contact dermatitis from clindamycin. *Contact Dermatitis* 1995;32:110.

62. Feingold DS, Chen WC, Chou DL, Chang TW. Induction of colitis in hamsters by topical application of antibiotics. *Arch Dermatol* 1979;115:580.

63. Milstone EB, McDonald AJ, Scholhamer CE Jr. Pseudomembranous colitis after topical application of clindamycin. *Arch Dermatol* 1991; 117:154.

64. Voron DA. Systemic absorption of topical clindamycin [Letter]. *Arch Dermatol* 1978;114:798.

65. Tedesco FJ, Barton RW, Alpers DH. Clindamycin-associated colitis: a prospective study. *Ann Intern Med* 1974;81:429.

66. Fisher AA. The safety of topical erythromycin. *Contact Dermatitis* 1976;2:43.

67. Vilaplana J, Romaguera C, Grimalt F. Contact dermatitis from lincomycin and spectinomycin in chicken vaccinators. *Contact Dermatitis* 1991;24:225.

68. Lombardi P, Campolmo P, Spallanzani P, Settoli A. Delayed hypersensitivity to erythromycin. *Contact Dermatitis* 1982;8:416.

69. van Ketel WG. Immediate and delayed-type allergy to erythromycin. *Contact Dermatitis* 1976;2:363.

70. Fernandez Redondo V, Casas L, Taboada M, Toribio J. Systemic contact dermatitis from erythromycin. *Contact Dermatitis* 1994;30:43.

71. Schwank R, Jirasek L. Contact allergy to chloramphenicol with special reference to group sensitization. *Hautarzt* 1963;14:24.

72. Palacios J, Nemuth MG, Blaylock WK. Lack of cross sensitization between 2,4- dinitrochlorobenzene and chloramphenicol. *South Med J* 1968;61:243.

73. Enksen K. Cross allergy between paranitro compounds with special reference to DNCB and chloramphenicol. *Contact Dermatitis* 1978; 4:29.

74. Rudzki E, Grzywa Z, Maciejowska E. Drug reaction with positive patch test reaction to chloramphenicol. *Contact Dermatitis* 1976;2: 181.

75. Kozakova M. Sub-shock state brought on by epidermic test for chloramphenicol (in Slovak; author's translation). *Cesk Dermatol* 1976; 52:82.

76. Bandmann N-J. Sind Chloramphenikol-haltige extelna kontraindiziert. *Hautarzt* 1972;23:145.

77. Milkowski S. Contact conjunctivitis following local application of chloramphenicol. *Wiad Lek* 1971;24:695.

78. Le Coz C-J, Santinelli F. Facial contact dermatitis from chloramphenicol with cross-sensitivity to thiamphenicol. *Contact Dermatitis* 1998;38:108.

79. Wereide K. Sensitivity to azidamphenicol. *Contact Dermatitis* 1975; 1:271.

80. Fontanot S. Tetracycline compounds and responsibility for allergic dermatitis after local use. *G Ital Dermatol Venereol* 1978;113:397.

81. Bojs G, Möller H. Eczematous contact allergy to oxytetracycline with cross-sensitivity to other tetracyclines. *Berufs-Dermatosen* 1974;22:202.

82. Calnan CD. Chlortetracycline sensitivity. *Contact Dermatitis Newsletter* 1967;1:16.

83. Standlee TL. Facial fluorescence. *Schoch Lett* 1979;29:7.

84. Wasilewski C Jr. Allergic contact dermatitis from nystatin. *Arch Dermatol* 1970;102:216.

85. Coskey RJ. Contact dermatitis due to nystatin. *Arch Dermatol* 1971; 103:228.

86. Coskey RJ. Contact dermatitis due to multiple corticosteroid creams. *Arch Dermatol* 1978;114:115.

87. Foussereau J, Liman-Mestiri S, Khochnevis A, Basset A. L'Allergie a l'association therapeutique locale nystatine, neomycine et acetonide de triamcinolone. *Bull Soc Fr Dermatol Syphilol* 1971;78: 457.

88. Hull PR, de Beer HA. Topical nitrofurazone, a potent sensitizer of the skin and mucosae. *South Afr Med J* 1977;52:189.

89. Bleumink E, te Lintum JC, Nater JP. Kontaktallergie durch Nitrohrazon (Furacin) und Nihrprazin (carohr). *Huutarzt* 1974;25: 403.

90. Caplan RM. Cutaneous hazards posed by agricultural chemicals. *J Iowa Med Soc* 1969;59:295.

91. Neldner KH. Contact dermatitis from animal feed additives. *Arch Dermatol* 1972;106:722.

92. Fisher AA. Immediate and delayed allergic contact reactions to polyethylene glycol. *Contact Dermatitis* 1978;4:135.

93. Braun W. Contact allergies to polyethylene glycols. *Z Haut Geschlectskr* 1969;44:385.

94. Kiec-Swierczynska M, Krecisz B. Occupational contact allergy to nifuroxazide simulating prurigo nodularis. *Contact Dermatitis* 1998; 39:93.

95. Sanchez-Perez J, Cordoba S, del Rio MJ, Garcia-Dies A. Allergic contact dermatitis from furaltadone in eardrops. *Contact Dermatitis* 1999;40:222.

96. Bandmann HJ, Breit R. Die medikamentose allergische kontaktdermatitis. *Internist* 1974;15:47.

97. Yaffee HS, Dressler DP. Topical application of mafenide acetate: its association with erythema multiforme and cutaneous reactions. *Arch Dermatol* 1969;100:277.

98. Velasco JE, Africk JA. Contact dermatitis to mafenide acetate. *Arch Dermatol* 1971;103:61.

99. Sulzberger MD, et al. Sensitization by topical application of sulfonamide. *J Allergy* 1947;18:92.

100. Gottschalk HR, Stone OJ. Stevens-Johnson syndrome from ophthalmic sulfonamide. *Arch Dermatol* 1976;112:513.

101. Verbov JL. Sensitivity to sodium fusidate. *Contact Dermatitis Newsletter* 1970;7:150.

102. Dave VK, Main RA. Contact sensitivity to sodium fusidate. *Contact Dermatitis Newsletter* 1973;14:398.

103. de Groot AC. Contact allergy to sodium fusidate. *Contact Dermatitis* 1982;8:429.

104. Baptista A, Barros MA. Contact dermatitis from sodium fusidate. *Contact Dermatitis* 1990;23:186.

105. Fisher AA. Systemic contact dermatitis from Orinase™ and Diabinese™ in diabetics with para-amino hypersensitivity. *Cutis* 1982; 29:551.

106. Angelini G, Meneghini CL. Oral tests in contact allergy to para-amino compounds. *Contact Dermatitis* 1981;7:311.

107. Sasseville D, Carey WD, Singer MI. Generalized contact dermatitis from acetarsone. *Contact Dermatitis* 1995;33:431.

108. Vincenzi C, Lucente P, Ricci C, Tosti A. Facial contact dermatitis due to metronidazole. *Contact Dermatitis* 1997;36:116.

109. Silvestre JF, et al. Systemic contact dermatitis due to norfloxacin with a positive patch test to quinoline mix. *Contact Dermatitis* 1998; 39:83.

110. Wantke F, Gotz M, Jarisch R. Contact dermatitis from cloxyquin. *Contact Dermatitis* 1995;32:112.

111. Baes H. Allergic contact dermatitis to virginiamycin. *Dermatologica* 1974;149:231.

112. Bleumink E, Nater JP. Allergic contact dermatitis to virginiamycin. *Dermatologica* 1972;144:253.

113. Bleumink L, Nater JP. Allergic contact dermatitis to virginiamycin (Staphlomycin) and pristinamycin (Stapyocin). *Contact Dermatitis Newsletter* 1972;12:337.

114. Lachapelle JM, Lamy F. On allergic contact dermatitis to virginiamycin. *Dermatologica* 1973;146:320.

115. Tennstedt D, Dumont-Fruytier M, La Chapelle JM. Occupational allergic contact dermatitis to virginiamycin, an antibiotic used as a food additive for pigs and poultry. *Contact Dermatitis* 1978;4: 133.

116. Guerra L, et al. Contact dermatitis to rifamycin. *Contact Dermatitis* 1991;25:328.

117. Dooms-Goossens A, et al. Airborne allergic contact dermatitis from kitasamycin and midecamycin. *Contact Dermatitis* 1990;23:118.

118. Eedy DJ. Mupirocin allergy in the setting of venous ulceration. *Contact Dermatitis* 1995;32:240.

119. Gellin GA, Maibach HI, Wachs GN. Contact allergy to tolnaftate. *Arch Dermatol* 1972;106:715.

120. Emmett EA, Marrs JM. Allergic contact dermatitis from tolnaftate. *Arch Dermatol* 1973;108:98.

121. Rudolph RI. Allergic contact dermatitis caused by haloprogin. *Arch Dermatol* 1975;111:1487.

122. Moss HV. Allergic contact dermatitis due to Halotex solution [Letter]. *Arch Dermatol* 1974;109:572.

123. Berlin AR, Miller OF. Allergic contact dermatitis from ethyl sebacate in haloprogin cream. *Arch Dermatol* 1976;112:1563.

124. Valsecchi R, Pansera B, di Landro A, Cainelli T. Connubial contact sensitization to clotrimazole. *Contact Dermatitis* 1994;30:248.

125. Erdmann S, Hertl M, Merk HF. Contact dermatitis from clotrimazole with positive patch-test reactions also to croconazole and itraconazole. *Contact Dermatitis* 1999;40:47.

126. Goday JJ, et al. Allergic contact dermatitis from sertaconazole with cross-sensitivity to miconazole and econazole. *Contact Dermatitis* 1995;32:370.

127. Steinmann A, Mayer G, Breit R, Agathos M. Allergic contact dermatitis from croconazole without cross-sensitivity to clotrimazole and bifonazole. *Contact Dermatitis* 1996;35:255.

128. Nakano R, Miyoshi H, Kanazaki T. Allergic contact dermatitis from lanoconazole. *Contact Dermatitis* 1996;35:63.

129. Tanaka N, et al. Contact dermatitis from lanoconazole. *Contact Dermatitis* 1996;35:256.

130. Kawada A, et al. Contact dermatitis from neticonazole. *Contact Dermatitis* 1997;36:106.

131. Roller JA. Contact allergy to clotrimazole. *Br Med J* 1978;2:737.

132. Degreef H, Verhoeve L. Contact dermatitis to micronazole nitrate. *Contact Dermatitis* 1975;1:269.

133. Wade TR, Jones HE, Artis WA. Irritant and allergic reactions to topically applied Micatin cream. *Contact Dermatitis* 1979;5:168.

134. Santucci B, et al. Contact dermatitis from ketaconazole cream. *Contact Dermatitis* 1992;27:274.

135. Baes H. Contact sensitivity to miconazole with othro-chloro cross-sensitivity to other imidazoles. (Published erratum appears in *Contact Dermatitis* 1991;25:79.) *Contact Dermatitis* 1991;24:89.

136. Machet L, et al. Contact dermatitis and cross-sensitivity from sulconazole nitrate. *Contact Dermatitis* 1992;26:352.

137. Marren P, Powell S. Contact sensitivity to tioconazole and other imidazoles. *Contact Dermatitis* 1992;27:129.

138. Brunelli D, et al. Contact dermatitis from tioconazole. *Contact Dermatitis* 1992;27:120.

139. Stubb S, et al. Contact allergy to tioconazole. *Contact Dermatitis* 1992;26:155.

140. Jones SK, Kennedy CT. Contact dermatitis from tioconazole. *Contact Dermatitis* 1990;22:122.

141. Dooms-Goossens A, Matura M, Drieghe J, Degreef H. Contact allergy to imidazoles used as antimycotic agents. *Contact Dermatitis* 1995;33:73.

142. Jolanki R, et al. Occupational allergic contact dermatitis from 5-chloro-1-methyl-4-nitroimidazole. *Contact Dermatitis* 1997; 36: 53.

143. Willa-Craps C, Wyss M, Elsner P. Allergic contact dermatitis from naftifine. *Contact Dermatitis* 1995;32:369.

144. Kaneko K, et al. Allergic contact dermatitis from amorolfine cream. *Contact Dermatitis* 1997;37:307.

145. Corazza M, Virgili A, Mantovani L. Vulvar contact dermatitis from nifuratel. *Contact Dermatitis* 1992;27:273.

146. Di Prima TM, De Pasquale R, Nigro MA. Connubial contact dermatitis from nifuratel. *Contact Dermatitis* 1990;22:117.

147. Lombardi P, Spallanzani P, Giorgini S, Seroli A. Allergic contact dermatitis from idoxuridine. *Contact Dermatitis* 1982;8:50.

148. Thormann J, Wildenhoff KE. Contact allergy to idoxuridine: sensitization following treatment of herpes zoster. *Contact Dermatitis* 1980;6:170.
149. Amon RB, Lis AW, Hanifin JM. Allergic contact dermatitis caused by idoxuridine. *Arch Dermatol* 1975;111:1581.
150. Osmundsen PE. Allergic contact dermatitis from idoxuridine. *Contact Dermatitis* 1975;1:251.
151. Calnan CD. Contact dermatitis to idoxuridine. *Contact Dermatitis* 1976;2:58.
152. Calnan CD. Allergy to idoxuridine ointment. *Contact Dermatitis* 1979;5:194.
153. Reiffers J. Allergy to 5-iodo-2'-desoxyuridine. *Contact Dermatitis* 1981;7:125.
154. Van Ketel WG. Allergy to idoxuridine eyedrops. *Contact Dermatitis* 1977;3:106.
155. Cirkel PKS, van Ketel WG. Allergic contact dermatitis to trifluor-thymidine eyedrops. *Contact Dermatitis* 1981;7:49.
156. Millan-Parrilla F, de la Cuadra J. Allergic contact dermatitis from trifluoridine in eyedrops. *Contact Dermatitis* 1990;22:289.
157. Brandao FM, Pecegueiro M. Contact dermatitis to tromantadine hydrochloride. *Contact Dermatitis* 1982;8:140.
158. Fanta D, Mischer P. Contact dermatitis from tromantadine hydrochloride. *Contact Dermatitis* 1976;2:282.
159. Mischer P, Fanta D. Das Tomantadin-Kontaktekzem. *Hautarzt* 1978;29:337.
160. Patruno C, et al. Allergic contact dermatitis to tromantadine hydrochloride. *Contact Dermatitis* 1990;22:187.
161. Valsecchi R, Imberti G, Cainelli T. Contact allergy to acyclovir. *Contact Dermatitis* 1990;23:372.
162. Goday J, et al. Allergic contact dermatitis from acyclovir. *Contact Dermatitis* 1991;24:380.
163. Rodriguez-Serna M, et al. Photoallergic contact dermatitis from Zovirax cream. *Contact Dermatitis* 1999;41:54.

CHAPTER 14

Antihistamine Dermatitis

It must be emphasized that, although the *systemic* administration of the antihistamines rarely engenders sensitization, *topical* applications, such as antihistamines, on occasion produce allergic contact sensitivity. Once the patient is sensitized by topical application of the antihistamine, an eczematous contact dermatitis may occur from the antihistamine or from immunochemically related compounds. As a rule, the systemic administration of an antihistamine to which there has been topical sensitization will not only reproduce the original allergic eczematous contact dermatitis but at times will also produce a generalized dermatitis with a resulting exfoliative dermatitis (1,2). In some instances, "systemic" eczematous contact dermatitis is accompanied by urticarial elements. On rare occasions, systemic administration of an antihistamine can induce allergic hypersensitivity with production of urticaria, morbilliform and scarlatiniform eruptions, erythema multiforme, photosensitivity, and anaphylactic shock. In asthmatic patients, the antihistamine may lead to bronchial obstruction with anaphylactic reactions.

Eruptions from antihistaminic agents appear usually 6 to 12 hours after their ingestion. There may be an incubation period, or dermatitis may appear after ingestion of the first dose. The eruption is usually generalized and explosive. The lesions may resemble any of the acute drug eruptions. Skin tests are of little value in these reactions. The history of dermatitis occurring within 12 hours after the introduction of one of these agents suggests that the antihistamine is the cause of the eruption. Testing by readministering the drug is justifiable only in mild dermatoses and is contraindicated in severe reactions.

Systemic antihistamines are rare sensitizers, whereas topical antihistamines are common sensitizers. Once topical sensitization occurs, the systemic administration of the antihistamine produces a "systemic" contact dermatitis.

THE NATURE AND CLASSIFICATION OF THE ANTIHISTAMINES

For appropriate management of antihistamine dermatitis, knowledge of the nature and the classification of the various antihistamines is necessary. Most antihistamines are basically related at their structural core by a substituted ethylamine group that is also present in the histamine and has the following structure: $X-CH_2-CH_2-N$. This portion of the molecule presumably competes with histamine for cell receptors and thus blocks the action of histamine. To this substituted core, different arrangements of atoms can be added to make different antihistamines. X represents the element that links the ethylamine group to the rest of the compound. Depending on the nature of X, oxygen (O), nitrogen (N), or carbon (C), the antihistamine belongs to a specific class.

The two main reasons for becoming familiar with the various groups of antihistamines are the following: (a) It is generally agreed that if any antihistamine is not effective in a particular patient, the rest of the antihistamines in that group are not likely to be as effective as an antihistamine in a different group. This concept of choosing an antihistamine from a new group is one of the reasons certain pharmaceutical companies manufacture two different antihistamine compounds. (b) A patient who is allergic to an antihistamine in one group is very likely to also be allergic to every other antihistamine in that particular group. It is, therefore, important that the sensitized patient be informed of which antihistamines must be avoided and which can be used safely.

Table 14.1 lists the various classes of antihistamines. The antihistamines are useful primarily in the control of certain allergic disorders. Their effect in allergic conditions is purely palliative and largely due to the suppression of symptoms attributable to the action of histamine, which is but one of the chemicals released by the antigen-antibody reaction. In addition, they may diminish capillary permeability to substances other than histamine.

Topical antihistamine preparations are used because they are slightly antipruritic and may have a mild local

TABLE 14.1. *Classes of Antihistamines*

Carbon-linked alkylamines
Cyclizines (piperazines)
Nitrogen-linked ethylenediamines
Oxygen-linked ethanolamines
Phenothiazine antihistamines
Piperidines
Miscellaneous

anesthetic effect. Such topical antihistamines, however, are common and potent sensitizers. The use of topical antihistamines should be discouraged. Instead, topical corticosteroids or nonsensitizing local anesthetic preparations free of benzocaine, such as lidocaine (Xylocaine) and pramoxine (Pramosone), may be used to control pruritus.

THE NITROGEN-LINKED ETHYLENEDIAMINES

Table 14.2 lists the ethylenediamine antihistamines. It should be noted that ethylenediamine hydrochloride, the parent substance of this group of histamines, a component of aminophylline, and a stabilizer in the popular nystatin-neomycin sulfate-gramicidin-triamcinolone acetonide cream, has become such a common sensitizer that it is included in the "Screening" Patch Test Series of the North American Contact Dermatitis Group. (Nystatin-neomycin sulfate-gramicidin-triamcinolone acetonide *ointment* is free of ethylenediamine hydrochloride.)

Unless the sensitized patient is informed of how to avoid ethylenediamine hydrochloride and related chemicals, the ethylenediamine-sensitive individual is doomed not only to repeated attacks of dermatitis, but also to drug eruptions from the systemic administration of aminophylline and ethylenediamine-related antihistamines and from topical exposure to antihistamines derived from ethylenediamine (3,4).

The ethylenediamine-sensitive individual should be given the written instructions listed in Table 14.3. The systemic administration of these antihistamines in an ethylenediamine-sensitive individual may cause a previous dermatitis to flare and may, in addition, produce a generalized drug eruption.

TABLE 14.2. *Nitrogen-Linked Ethylenediamine Antihistamines*

Trade name	Generic name
Atarax	Hydroxyzine hydrochloride
Fiogesic	Pyrilamine maleate
Histadyl	Methapyrilene hydrochloride
Pyma	Pyrilamine maleate
Pyribenzamine	Tripelennamine hydrochloride
Vistaril (intramuscular)	Hydroxyzine hydrochloride
Vistaril (oral)	Hydroxyzine pamoate

TABLE 14.3. *Instructions for Ethylenediamine-Sensitive Patients*

Avoid the following injections, tablets, creams, capsules, or suppositories:

1. Aminophylline
2. Antihistamine tablets, capsules, or creams: tripelennamine (Pyribenzamine), Histadyl, Fiogesic, Pyma, Hydroxyzine (Atarax, Vistaril), Durrax, and piperazine antihistamines: Fedrazil, Mantadil, Migral, Marezine, Bucladin-S, Bonine Antivert
   Avoid the following creams: Mycotriocet, Pyribenzamine, Surfadil, and Allergan
   Avoid the following nose or eye solutions: Prefrin, Privine, and Vasocon-A

It should be emphasized that, fortunately, ethylenediamine hydrochloride does not cross-react with the ubiquitous ethylenediamine tetra-acetate (EDTA).

> **Ethylenediamine-sensitive patients should avoid the use of the hydroxyzines Atarax, Vistaril, and Durrax, which are ethylenediamine derivatives.**

The Asthmatic Patient and Ethylenediamine Sensitivity

The following facts must be taken into consideration by the practitioner should an asthmatic patient become sensitized to ethylenediamine hydrochloride:

1. Aminophylline is composed of theophylline and ethylenediamine.
2. Ethylenediamine renders theophylline soluble so that it can be injected.
3. The administration of aminophylline to an ethylenediamine-sensitive individual can produce a severe disabling "systemic" contact dermatitis with generalized exfoliative dermatitis (5).
4. Although there are many theophylline medications without ethylenediamine that can be given orally, in an emergency, aminophylline cannot be given intramuscularly or intravenously. Travenol Labs, Inc., Deerfield, IL, has made available intravenous preparations of theophylline that are free of ethylenediamine.
5. Ethylenediamine-free theophylline for intramuscular injection is available as dyphylline (Lufyllin) (Wallace).

> **Aminophylline contains theophylline and ethylenediamine, which renders the theophylline soluble. It should not be injected into ethylenediamine-sensitive individuals. Soluble ethylenediamine-free theophylline is now available for intramuscular and intravenous administration.**

Industrial Dermatitis from Ethylenediamine Sensitivity

In industry, ethylenediamine is used in the preparation of dyes, inhibitors, rubber accelerators, fungicides, synthetic waxes, resins, insecticides, and asphalt wetting agents. Industrial exposure, however, rarely leads to sensitization, probably because exposure is usually not prolonged or intimate, and normal rather than abnormal skin is exposed.

Epoxy Resin Dermatitis

Certain polyamines, such as triethylenetetramine, triethylenediamine, and ethanolamine, used as amine "curing" agents of "hardeners" in epoxy resin systems, may cross-react with ethylenediamine. Such cross-reactions can produce epoxy resin dermatitis in ethylenediamine-sensitive individuals (6,7).

Machine Worker's Dermatitis

Synthetic coolants used in factories producing pistons can produce eruptions on the hands of machine tool operators (8). In these cases, ethylenediamine sensitivity may be a major cause (9).

The Relationship of the Hydroxyzines to Ethylenediamine

Although the hydroxyzine ethylenediamines Atarax and Vistaril are not usually classified with the ethylenediamine antihistamines, it should be noted that the formula of Atarax (hydroxyzine hydrochloride) is 1-*p*-chlorobenzyhydryl-4,2 (2 [2-hydroxyethoxy]ethyl) *diethylenediamine dihydrochloride*. It would be prudent to avoid the use of hydroxyzine antihistamines in individuals with ethylenediamine sensitivity.

Hydroxyzine and Cetirizine

Three cases of systemic reactions to hydroxyzine allergy confirmed by patch testing were reported from France (10). In these individuals, there was no cross-reactivity to piperazine, ethylenediamine, triethanolamine, dexchlorpheniramine, loratadine, chlorpromazine, mequitazine, terfenadine, and the hydroxyzine derivative cetirizine. A 2% aqueous solution of hydroxyzine was positive. In contrast, the following case shows broad cross-reactivity.

A 70-year-old woman developed a morbilliform and urticarial eruption traced to the use of cetirizine (11). This was confirmed by a positive patch test to cetirizine at 2.5% and 5% in petrolatum. She was also sensitive to ethylenediamine dihydrochloride and diethylenediamine, which is a piperazine. It has been suggested that cross-reactions between ethylenediamine and piperazine-based antihistamines are dependent on sensitivity to diethylenediamine, which can be visualized as two molecules of ethylenedi-

TABLE 14.4. *Piperazine Antihistamines*

Trade name	Generic name
Bonine Antivert	Meclizine hydrochloride
Bucladin-S	Buclizine hydrochloride
Fedrazil, Mantadil	Chlorcyclinine hydrochloride
Marezine	Cyclizine hydrochloride
Migral	Cyclizine hydrochloride

amine glued together to make a cyclic structure that is in fact piperazine. Because she was sensitive to not only ethylenediamine but also piperazine and diethylenediamine, it is not surprising that cetirizine, which contains a piperazine ring, was also capable of causing an allergic reaction.

The Relationship of the Piperazine (Cyclizine) Antihistamines to Ethylenediamine

The piperazine (cyclizine) antihistamines are listed in Table 14.4. The piperazine antihistamines, like the hydroxyzines, are related closely to the ethylenediamine antihistamines. It is believed that, because ethylenediamine is on the metabolic pathway of both piperazine and hydroxyzine, it is advisable to avoid the use of piperazine antihistamines in ethylenediamine-sensitive individuals.

Thus, piperazine citrate used for the treatment of pinworms (threadworms) can produce an allergic drug eruption in ethylenediamine-sensitive individuals (12). Cross-reactions can occur in chemists and laboratory technicians who handle both of these chemicals (13). Price and Hall-Smith (14) reported a patient who was sensitive to ethylenediamine hydrochloride and developed a generalized erythroderma after he took piperazine phosphate for treatment of threadworm infection. The patient had been exposed previously to Triadcortyl Cream, which is an English preparation identical to the original formula Mycolog Cream. The original formula of Mycolog Cream is only available from generic suppliers, as Mycolog II has been reformulated without ethylenediamine. The original formula is no longer made by Squibb-Westwood.

THE OXYGEN-LINKED ETHANOLAMINE ANTIHISTAMINES

Table 14.5 lists these antihistamines. Of this group of antihistamines, diphenylenediamine hydrochloride has been widely used both systemically and topically for four decades. The other ethanolamines are used only systemically.

The incidence of cutaneous reactions to topically applied diphenhydramine is difficult to assess (15). In one series, 12 of 117 cases of dermatitis medicamentosa seen in England in 1 year were due to a lotion composed of diphenhydramine hydrochloride and calamine (16). All 12 were confirmed by positive patch tests, although in 10 instances, closed patch tests were positive only when performed on areas that had undergone repeated cellophane-tape strippings.

TABLE 14.5. *Ethanolamine Antihistamines*

Trade name	Generic name
Ambenyl	Diphenhydramine hydrochloride
Benadryl	Diphenhydramine hydrochloride
Benylin	Diphenhydramine hydrochloride
Clistin	Carbinoxame maleate
Decapryn	Doxylamine succinate
Diphenadril	Diphenhydramine hydrochloride
Dramamine	Dimenhydrinate
Tavist	Clemastine fumarate

Systemic "Endogenic" Contact Dermatitis from Ethanolamines

Individuals who have become sensitized by topically applied diphenhydramine can acquire a "systemic" eczematous contact dermatitis when diphenhydramine or any of the other ethanolamines listed in Table 14.5 are ingested or injected.

> **Topical ethanolamines that should be avoided by ethanolamine-sensitive patients are white diphenhydramine cream (Benadryl) and pink diphenhydramine cream (Caladryl).**

It is not generally realized that dimenhydrinate (Dramamine) is an ethanolamine (the chlorotheophylline salt of the antihistaminic agent diphenhydramine). Dimenhydrinate contains between 53% and 56% diphenhydramine and therefore should not be administered to any individual who has allergic hypersensitivity to the ethanolamine groups of antihistamines.

> **Dramamine contains ethanolamine.**

Photoallergic Dermatitis from Diphenhydramine

Antihistamine photodermatitis to the *systemic* administration of such ethanolamines as diphenhydramine and carbinoxamine and to topical ethanolamines are rare (17). Although topical promethazine therapy appears to be a relatively frequent cause of photoallergic contact dermatitis, for years a single report of photoallergy induced by topical diphenhydramine therapy was reported (15). The diagnosis was confirmed by photopatch testing. This diphenhydramine photoallergy appeared to differ from most other forms of photoallergy in that it was elicited by ultraviolet light in the 290- to 320-nm wavelength range (UVB), rather than the more usual 320- to 400-nm range (UVA). This finding may be related to the photochemical properties of diphenhydramine, which absorbs in the UVB, but not in the UVA, the UVB absorption being associated with a distinctive fluorescence.

A case of diphenhydramine photosensitivity with the more customary UVA activation wavelength was reported from Japan (18). A 1% diphenhydramine in petrolatum patch test irradiated with 4.85 J/cm2 was used to confirm the photoallergy.

THE PHENOTHIAZINES

Although topical phenothiazine antihistamine preparations, such as promethazine hydrochloride (Phenergan) cream, are no longer used in the United States, such topical antihistamine preparations are still widely used in Europe. Individuals who have become sensitized by such topical phenothiazine antihistamines often suffer a flare of the dermatitis when a phenothiazine antihistamine is taken, that is, a "systemic" eczematous contact dermatitis. In addition, many individuals acquire allergic sensitization to various phenothiazine drugs that show cross-reactions with the phenothiazine antihistamines. Table 14.6 lists the phenothiazine antihistamine compounds.

Promethazine Hydrochloride

This antihistamine is used not only in tablet form but also as suppositories. Proctitis and perianal dermatitis have occurred from the use of such suppositories in sensitized individuals. This antihistamine can also produce phototoxic and photoallergic reactions (19). In France, where Phenergan cream is used extensively as a topical antipruritic agent, many instances of photocontact dermatitis occur. Photosensitivity seems to be induced primarily by contact exposure to promethazine hydrochloride cream (20). Systemic administration without topical sensitization does not appear to induce photosensitivity (21).

TABLE 14.6. *Phenothiazine Antihistamines*

Trade name	Generic name
Phenergan	Promethazine
Tacaryl	Methdilazine
Temaril	Trimeprazine
Note: May cross-react with the following phenothiazine drugs:	
Compazine	Prochlorperazine
Stelazine	Trifluoperazine
Temaril	Trimeprazine
Thorazine	Chlorpromazine
Vesprin	Triflupromazine
Veterinary medications such as insecticides and anthelmintics	

Cross-Reactions between the Phenothiazine Antihistamines and Other Phenothiazine Compounds

The phenothiazine drugs listed in Table 14.6 are all capable of cross-reacting with the phenothiazine antihistamine, and all of these compounds are potential photosensitizers (22). Often a photoallergic reaction occurs in combination with the allergic eczematous contact dermatitis. The systemic administration of the phenothiazine drugs shown in Table 14.6 may produce an eczematous contact dermatitis medicamentosa in individuals sensitized by such topical exposure. Cross-reactions take place readily between phenothiazines and the related antihistamines (23).

Exposure of Medical and Nursing Personnel to Phenothiazines

Medical and nursing personnel who inject phenothiazine drugs or who handle phenothiazine tablets that are given to patients, as well as those who come into contact with the compounds in the pharmaceutical industry, readily acquire allergic eczematous contact dermatitis of the hands from such exposure; the dermatitis may flare when a phenothiazine antihistamine is given (24). Because chlorpromazine, in particular, is excreted almost unchanged in the urine, sensitized nurses and orderlies who handle unwashed linen may experience flares.

Exposure of Veterinarians and Farmers to Phenothiazines

The same phenothiazines or closely related compounds that are used as psychotropic drugs or as sedatives in humans are used by veterinarians and farmers as insecticides and anthelmintics for animals and birds. Table 14.7 lists some commercial phenothiazine insecticides and "wormers" used by veterinarians. Many individuals in these professions have acquired allergic contact dermatitis, photoallergic reactions, or both by spraying such phenothiazines for insect control or feeding these compounds as wormers. Such individuals must avoid using phenothiazine antihistamines because of the likelihood of producing flares of the phenothiazine dermatitis.

Exposure to Methylene Blue

Methylene blue is 3,7-bis-(dimethyl-amino) phenozathionium chloride tetramethyl thionin chloride, a phenothiazine derivative used in various ways, as shown in Table 14.8.

TABLE 14.7. *Phenothiazines Used in Veterinary Medicine*

Anthelmintics	Worm Free Eddie
	Early Bird Wormer
Insecticides	Fly Free Eddie
	Bar-Fly Feed

TABLE 14.8. *Sources of Exposure to Methylene Blue (a Phenothiazine Dye)*

Antidotes for methemoglobinemia and cyanide poisoning
Biologic stains
Blue hair dyes
Photodynamic treatment of herpes
Urinary antiseptics
   M-B tablets, Urolene Blue, TRA tablets, Urised

The administration of methylene blue urinary antiseptic produced a flare of photodermatitis in one observed individual who had acquired a photosensitivity from a phenothiazine compound (25).

Dilute mixtures of methylene blue, acid violet, and nigrosine are used as a color rinse for gray hair. Such rinses should be used with great care in those who have become sensitized to the phenothiazines.

Varieties of Allergic Reactions to Phenothiazine Compounds

Three types of allergic hypersensitivity are seen with the phenothiazine drugs. These reactions are:

1. The classical allergic contact eczematous variety, in which the covered patch test reaction is positive.
2. A photoallergic reaction, in which the *covered* patch reaction is negative but becomes positive when the patch test site is exposed to sunlight or ultraviolet radiation (25).
3. A photoallergic reaction in combination with an allergic eczematous contact sensitization, in which the patch test reaction is positive with the phenothiazine derivative alone, but a stronger response is elicited if the site is irradiated with a suberythematous dose of ultraviolet rays or exposed to strong sunlight for 20 minutes. The increase in intensity of an ordinary patch test reaction on exposure to light must be carefully interpreted, because it may be a nonspecific irritating effect.

If possible, controls should be used as on other positive patch test reactions. Whenever an allergen can produce both photoallergic and allergic eczematous contact hypersensitivity, the photoallergic reaction appears to be more intense. At times, phenothiazine, capable of producing photoallergic and ordinary allergic eczematous contact dermatitis, will produce a photoallergic reaction in areas exposed to light, whereas the same concentration of the drug that reaches the skin from systemic administration will not produce a contact dermatitis on covered areas of the body. In many instances, however, both types of reactions occur simultaneously.

A unique feature of photoallergic reactions to the phenothiazines is that the wavelengths that produce the photoallergic reactions are not always identical to those

29. Li LF, Sun XY, Li SY. Allergic contact dermatitis from cyproheptadine hydrochloride. *Contact Dermatitis* 1995;33:50.
30. Rietschel RL. Selected highlights of the European Contact Dermatitis Society Meeting: Brussels, Belgium, October 8–10, 1992. *Am J Contact Dermatitis* 1993;4:66.
31. Greenberg JH. Allergic contact dermatitis from topical doxepin. *Contact Dermatitis* 1995;33:281.
32. Taylor JS, Praditsuwan P, Handel D, Kuffner G. Allergic contact dermatitis from doxepin cream: one-year patch test clinic experience. *Arch Dermatol* 1996;132:515.
33. Aldridge RD, Main RA, Smith ME. Dyes and preservatives in oral antihistamines. *Br J Dermatol* 1980;102:545.
34. Lockey S. Reactions to hidden agents in foods and drugs can be serious. *Ann Allergy* 1975;35:239.
35. Michaëlsson G, Juhlin L. Urticaria induced by preservatives and dye additives in food and drugs. *Br J Dermatol* 1973;88:525.
36. Juhlin L, Michaëlsson G, Zetterstrum O. Urticaria and asthma induced by food and drug additives in patients with aspirin hypersensitivity. *J Allerg Clin Immunol* 1972;50:92.
37. Ros A, Juhlin L, Michaëlsson G. A follow-up study of patients with recurrent urticaria and hypersensitivity to aspirin benzoates and azo dye. *Br J Dermatol* 1976;95:19.

CHAPTER 15

Local Anesthetics and Topical Analgesics

The local anesthetics may be applied topically or by injection, and certain local anesthetics may be used in either fashion. Topical anesthetics may produce allergic contact dermatitis, whereas the injectable variety may also produce adverse reactions, some of which are allergic in nature. Such reactions may be mild or, if more serious, may produce anaphylactic shock, angioedema, urticaria, serum-sickness syndrome, or vasculitis.

Anesthetic allergy is commonly suspected when an unexplained perioperative collapse occurs. The epidemic of latex sensitivity added this concern in the setting of perioperative collapse. An investigation of 26 patients who experienced perioperative anaphylactoid reactions found that 84% were allergic to at least one anesthetic agent (1). Only 7.7% were latex sensitive, and atopy was confirmed to be a risk factor for latex sensitivity. Both RAST and skin prick tests with raw latex were performed in this investigation.

TOPICAL ANESTHETICS

The topical anesthetic drugs comprise several chemically dissimilar structures, including alkaloids related to cocaine, and aminoalcohol esters of benzoic acid related to procaine, amides, anilides, phenylalkyl alcohols, and phenols (2). Table 15.1 classifies topical anesthetics.

Because topical application may induce an allergy to a local anesthetic and a cross-reaction to related drugs, dermatologists, allergists, and dental personnel should, insofar as possible, limit topical application of local anesthetics to drugs that are not used parenterally.

Although benzocaine, which is a sensitizer, is not used systemically, it may cross-react with anesthetics of the "ester" type that are administered parenterally. It must be emphasized that the parabens are *parahydroxy* compounds, which Fisher (3) did not find cross-react with the para-amino compounds.

> **The parabens (parahydroxy) compounds do not appear to cross-react with the para-amino compounds.**

Benzocaine

Benzocaine is commonly used in many topical anesthetic compounds. The synonyms for benzocaine include ethyl aminobenzoate, Anesthesin, Anesthone, and Parathesin. Benzocaine is a para-aminobenzoic acid (PABA) derivative and is related chemically and immunologically to topical anesthetics based on benzoic acid, such as cocaine.

Because benzocaine is an effective topical anesthetic, it is used in at least 600 different products. Not only is it used in the treatment of pruritus and burns, but benzocaine also has been used as a smoke inhibitor and appetite suppressant and for the control of coughing. Benzocaine is used in every orifice of the body, including the ear, mouth (even in "teething lotions"), vagina, and rectum.

As a result of such wide exposure, benzocaine has become a common cause of allergic contact dermatitis. The International and North American Contact Research Groups have placed benzocaine on the "Screening" Patch Test Series. Benzocaine and procaine have been thought to cross-react. This finding has been disputed by Wilkinson et al. (4). In an attempt to refine the cross-reactions among benzocaine, tetracaine, and dibucaine, Sidhu et al. (5) found that a cross-reaction between benzocaine and tetracaine was uncommon (3/22 cases, or 13.6%). Cross-reactions between benzocaine and dibucaine were no more frequent. A stronger tendency was found for cross-reactions between tetracaine and dibucaine (about one in three).

> **Benzocaine is a sensitizer that is widely used not only on the skin, but also in every orifice of the body and for coughs and sore throat.**

Benzocaine-sensitized patients occasionally may suffer urticarial reactions and anaphylaxis from procaine injections. Furthermore, benzocaine may show cross-reactions with sulfonamides and certain dyes. The administration of "sulfa" drugs to a benzocaine-sensitive person may result in a widespread dermatitis, and exposure to paraphenylenediamine in hair and fur dyes may also cause a severe allergic contact dermatitis. Table 15.2 lists local anesthetics and

TABLE 15.1. *Classification of Topical Anesthetics*

Amides
  Dibucaine hydrochloride (Nupercaine)
  Lidocaine (Xylocaine)
  Lidocaine hydrochloride (Xylocaine)
Esters
 Aminobenzoate esters
    Benzocaine (Americaine)
    Benoxinate hydrochloride (Dorsacaine)
    Butamben picrate (Butesin picrate)
    Tetracaine hydrochloride (Pontocaine)
 Benzoic acid esters
    Cocaine hydrochloride
    Hexylcaine hydrochloride (Cyclaine)
    Piperocaine hydrochloride (Metycaine)
    Proparacaine hydrochloride (Alcaine, Ophthaine)
 Miscellaneous
    Cyclomethycaine (Surfacaine)
    Dimethisoquin (Quotane)
    Diperodon monohydrate (Diothane)
    Dyclonine (Dyclone)
    Pramoxine (Tronolane, Tronothane)

various medications and chemicals that may cross-react with benzocaine.

About 14% of benzocaine-sensitive individuals are also sensitive to paraphenylenediamine, the most popular of hair dyes (5). Some sunscreens containing glyceryl PABA actually contained benzocaine (6).

Hjorth et al. (7) reported that benzocaine-reactive patients were patch tested to two commercial sources of glyceryl *p*-aminobenzoate containing varying concentrations of benzocaine as a contaminant. Eleven of 20 patients reacted to the source with 0.3% benzocaine; none reacted to the source with 0.001% benzocaine.

TABLE 15.2. *Benzocaine Cross-Reactors*

Butacaine
Butethamine HCL (Monocaine)
Chloroprocaine HCL (Nesacaine)
Cocaine—topical
Isobucaine (Kinacaine)
Meapaine
Meprylcaine (Oracaine)
Metabutethamine (Unacaine)
Neo-Orthoform
Orthoform
Para-amino salicylic acid
Para-aminobenzoic acid and glyceryl PABA (sunscreens)
Paraphenylenediamine
Procainamide (Pronestyl) used for treating heart
  arrhythmias
Procaine hydrochloride (Novocain)
Propoxycaine hydrochloride (Ravocaine) with 2% procaine
Sulfonamides
Tetracaine hydrochloride (Pontocaine)

> **Benzocaine-sensitive patients should avoid sunscreens containing PABA or glyceryl PABA. Some sunscreens containing glyceryl PABA had considerable amounts of benzocaine.**

Benzocaine-sensitive patients may show cross-reactions with the following injectable local anesthetics, which are based on PABA: procaine hydrochloride (Novocain), butethamine hydrochloride (Monocaine), tetracaine hydrochloride (Pontocaine) with 2% procaine, and propoxycaine hydrochloride (Ravocaine).

Metabutethamine (Unacaine), which is based on meta-aminobenzoic acid, and meprylcaine (Oracaine), which is based on benzoic acid, may also cross-react with benzocaine.

The injection of these local anesthetics into benzocaine-sensitive persons may lead to localized swelling of the oral mucosa at the site of injection. On rare occasions, generalized urticaria or anaphylaxis will result from the injection of procaine into benzocaine-sensitive patients. Unfortunately, although many cross-reactions *may* occur, they also may not. Cross-reactions have not been predictable, and a positive test for benzocaine with a negative test for paraphenylenediamine would suggest that broad allergy is not likely to be present. Because both compounds are routinely used in patch test screening series worldwide, it is possible to let these tests assist (but not dictate) the magnitude of cross-reactions likely to occur. If both the benzocaine and the paraphenylenediamine tests are positive, the theoretical cross-reactions become more likely.

Benzocaine as a Screening Allergen

Wilkinson et al. (4) found that 5% benzocaine in petrolatum as a screen for local anesthetic allergy would have identified only 5 of 13 patients so sensitive. Among the anesthetic allergens missed were cinchocaine (2.5%) (Dibucaine) and amethocaine (2.5%) (4). Similarly, benzocaine was found not to detect allergy to butyl aminobenzoate (*n*-butyl-*p*-amino-benzoate), which in the United States is found in hemorrhoid suppositories under the names butamben picrate and butesin picrate (8).

Wilkinson's group (5) further reviewed their data over a 10-year period and found that benzocaine was an inappropriate screening allergen for local anesthetic sensitivity. Rather, tetracaine and dibucaine made up 78.1% of reactions seen. This finding is consistent with the observations of Beck and Holden (9), who found only 0.63% of patients tested reactive to benzocaine. The recommended screening allergen of Sidhu, et al.'s (5) data is a mix of 5% benzocaine, 5% tetracaine hydrochloride (amethocaine), and 5% dibucaine hydrochloride (cinchocaine).

Alternatives for Benzocaine-Sensitive Individuals

Safe *topical* anesthetics for benzocaine-sensitive individuals include lidocaine (Xylocaine), mepivacaine (Carbocaine), prilocaine hydrochloride (Citanest), pyrrocaine (Dynacaine), and pramoxine (Pramasone).

The following *injectable* local anesthetics do not cross-react with benzocaine because they are based on an "amide" structure: lidocaine (Xylocaine), mepivacaine (Carbocaine), prilocaine hydrochloride (Citanest), pyrrocaine (Dynacaine), and nupercaine (Dibucaine).

Table 15.3 lists products containing tetracaine that may need to be avoided by some benzocaine-sensitive persons. Kalveram et al. (10,11) showed that guinea pigs are readily sensitized to tetracaine and that tetracaine cross-reacts with procaine and PABA.

Benzocaine may cross-react not only with cocaine and topical and injectable anesthetics based on benzoic acid and PABA, with hair dyes (PPDA) and aniline dyes, but also with such drugs as para-aminobenzoic acid, parasalicylic acid, antidiabetic medications, and sulfonamides.

"AMIDE" LOCAL ANESTHETICS

Lidocaine (Xylocaine)

Lidocaine (Xylocaine) is an "amide" compound that does not cross-react with benzocaine. It is used widely not only as a surface anesthetic and as an injectable local anesthetic, but also intravenously for cardiac arrhythmias. Allergic reactions to lidocaine (Xylocaine) are rare, but do occur.

Lignocaine is a synonym for lidocaine. The amide group of anesthetics includes lidocaine, bupivacaine, prilocaine, and cinchocaine. Cross-reactions occur within the group but are most common between lidocaine and bupivacaine (12).

Thus, Fregert et al. (13) reported two patients who had contact allergy to lidocaine (Xylocaine) who also reacted to chemically related anesthetics of the "amide" type. One reacted to bupivacaine, mepivacaine (Carbocaine) only. The patients also reacted to the chemically nonrelated dibucaine hydrochloride (Cincaine), an anesthetic of the ester type. Reactions to lidocaine (Xylocaine) metabolites *o*-toluidine, and *m*-xylidine were negative. These authors state that the patient who reacted to all four anesthetics of the amide type should avoid being treated with the usual anesthetics (e.g., those administered by a dentist). Tetracaine, which gave a negative reaction, could be used.

The "amide" type of local anesthetics, including lidocaine (Xylocaine), dibucaine (Nupercainal), and mepivacaine (Carbocaine), are uncommon sensitizers either by topical application or by injections.

Roed-Petersen (14) reported that two patients were sensitized to an ointment containing betamethasone valerate 0.05%, metaoxedrine hydrochloride 0.1%, and lidocaine (Xylocaine) hydrochloride 2.5%. Results of a patch test in one patient showed a +2 reaction to lidocaine hydrochloride (Xylocaine).

Goransson's (15) patient suffered an anaphylactic reaction from a dental injection of the "amide" prilocaine. Black et al. (16) reported similarly that a patient sensitive to Xyloproct ointment (1% lignocaine) cross-reacted with prilocaine but not to other members of the class, including bupivacaine and mepivacaine.

Hofmann et al. (17) reported on a patient who had a generalized papular, pruritic eruption from a dental anesthetic injection of lidocaine (Xylocaine). The skin tests were performed as follows: (a) The results of patch tests with 20% lidocaine hydrochloride in petrolatum were negative at 72 and 96 hours after the test. (b) Intradermal test with 2% lidocaine hydrochloride was negative to 45 minutes. Eight hours after intradermal and patch testing, however, a papular, pruritic rash appeared on his upper extremities and shoulders.

Chin and Fellner (18) conclude that allergic hypersensitivity to lidocaine hydrochloride is rare. Only four such cases had been found in the literature in the past 18 years, and in these, symptoms ranged from urticaria to bronchospasms and hypotension with syncope. These symptoms were reversible usually with epinephrine and antihistamines. Skin testing with "as is" lidocaine has been useful in some patients but may be dangerous and is not recommended.

Allergy to lidocaine or lignocaine, as it is known in Australia, is not rare. Many of the cases of contact dermatitis

---

TABLE 15.3. *Products That Have Contained Tetracaine (Pontocaine)*

Clean 'N Treat
Icy Kool Lotion (Daniels)
Isotraine Ointment (Phillips)
PNS Suppositories (Winthrop)
Pontocaine Cream and Ointment, Ophthalmic Liquid (Winthrop)
Rectodyne Ointment (SeMed)
Tycal Lotion (Daniels)
Vanocide Lotion, Cream Foam (Daniels)
Vertussin Loz-Tablets (Warren-Teed)
Products containing both benzocaine and tetracaine
  Cetacaine Topical Anesthetic Ointment (Cetylite)
  Novol-Benzocaine-Tetracaine Solution (Novocol) in the topical, liquid, ointment and spray forms

have been reported from Australia. This has been attributed to the wide availability of lignocaine-containing preparations in Australia. A total of 49 of the 62 cases reported worldwide were from Australia, according to Weightman and Turner (19). They tested with lignocaine 15% in petrolatum and reported 29 cases seen from 1990 to 1998. For so many cases to have been found by one group would seem to suggest that the cases are not being picked up because testing for "amide" anesthetics is not routinely done.

Allergy to lidocaine was documented by intradermal patch and lymphocyte transformation tests (20). Cross-reactivity to other aminoacylamide local anesthetics was found. These cross-reacting substances include bupivacaine, mepivacaine, and prilocaine. Articaine, which has a thiophen ring instead of a methylated phenyl ring, was safe for use in this patient, as was the case in one prior patient who was found to be allergic to mepivacaine. Because of the structural difference, articaine would seem the logical alternative when any of the other aminoacylamide anesthetics becomes an issue. Alternatively, the ester anesthetics (benzocaine, procaine, tetracaine) or the aminoalkylamide cinchocaine could be considered. A patient exhibiting sensitization to both raised the possibility that lidocaine and crotamiton cross-react (21). The structural formulas are similar, as both have a butanoyl toluidine moiety in common.

Crotamiton and lidocaine may cross-react based on a common butanoyl toluidine moiety.

Some patients who are allergic to lidocaine have been found to tolerate procaine, prilocaine, or mepivacaine. Klein and Gall (22) had a patient who was allergic to both lidocaine and mepivacaine, but who was, however, able to use articaine. All the reactions were type 4 with erythema and itching 1 day after subcutaneous injection (22).

Fisher (23) reported a patient who acquired an allergic contact dermatitis from Xylocaine ointment. This patient showed a strongly positive patch test reaction to propylene glycol, which is present in the ointment. Results of patch tests with 20% lidocaine hydrochloride in petrolatum were negative.

In this connection, it should be noted that both lidocaine (Xylocaine) 5% ointment and lidocaine (Xylocaine) 2.5% ointment contain propylene glycol, but that lidocaine (Xylocaine) hydrochloride 4% solution, lidocaine (Xylocaine) hydrochloride jelly, and lidocaine (Xylocaine) hydrochloride viscous solution do not.

Soesman-van Waadenoden Kernekamp and van Ketel (24) treated a patient whose contact allergy was apparently due to lidocaine itself and not to any of the ingredients in the base.

Allergic reactions to topical anesthetics may be due to the anesthetic or to an ingredient in the vehicle.

A mixture of 2.5% lidocaine and 2.5% prilocaine in a vehicle that keeps both anesthetics in solution at room temperature (rather than crystals) has been introduced for topical anesthesia under the brand name EMLA (Astra). A patient who was allergic to lignocaine (lidocaine), prilocaine, and pseudoephedrine led Downs et al. (25) to propose that structural similarity of the three compounds could account for this. In their patient, EMLA cream was thought to be the source of the sensitization to the anesthetics. Prilocaine and lidocaine are known cross-reactants as members of the amide group of anesthetics.

The prilocaine component of EMLA caused contact dermatitis in a 78-year-old man who applied the medication to a leg ulcer. No reaction was seen to the other active ingredient, which is lidocaine (26).

Topical application of EMLA cream with Tegaderm occlusion caused purpura in five patients within 30 to 60 minutes (27). Immediate and delayed patch tests did not confirm sensitization, and a toxic effect on capillary endothelium is thought to be the explanation.

Table 15.4 lists some "injectable" "amide" local anesthetics, and Table 15.5 lists some topical anesthetics with the "amide" structure.

Dibucaine Hydrochloride (Nupercaine)

Dibucaine hydrochloride (Nupercaine), a local anesthetic, is also known as percaine, cincaine, sovcaine, and cinchocaine. Because it is a quinoline derivative, there is a possibility that it may cross-react with iodochlorhydroxyquin (Vioform), but not with the ester types of local anesthetics, because it is an "amide" anesthetic.

Wilson (28) reported several patients who had allergic contact sensitivity to this medication. Table 15.6 lists some products containing this anesthetic.

As noted earlier in this chapter, Sidhu et al. found (5) cross-reactions between dibucaine and tetracaine in about one-third of cases and between dibucaine and benzocaine

---

TABLE 15.4. *Injectable "Amide" Anesthetics*

Bupivacaine HCl [Marcaine HCl (Breon) and Sensorcaine (Astra)]
Dibucaine (Nupercainal)
Etidocaine [Duranest Solution (Astra)]
Lidocaine HCl [Lidocaine Ups (Abbott) and Xylocaine (Astra)]
Lidopen auto-injector (Survival)
Mepivacaine [Carbocaine HCl (Breon)]
Prilocaine [Citanest Solution (Astra)]

TABLE 15.5. *Topical "Amide" Anesthetics*

Dibucaine [Corticaine Cream (Glaxo)]
Lidocaine [Anestacon (Webcon)]
Lidocaine HCl [Bactine First Aid Spray (Miles)]
Lidocaine HCl [Lidosporin Otic Solution (Burroughs Wellcome)]
Lidocaine 2.5% and Prilocaine 2.5% [EMLA® (Astra)]
Lidocaine HCl [Unguentine Plus First Aid and Burn Cream (Procter & Gamble)]
Lidocaine HCl [Xylocaine Jelly and Ointment (Astra)]

about 14% of the time.

Cyclomethycaine (Surfacaine)

Cyclomethycaine (Surfacaine) is a substituted piperidine alkyl benzoate and thus is not related to para-aminobenzoic acid. It closely resembles piperocaine (Metycaine). Although cyclomethycaine (Surfacaine) is a rare sensitizer, cyclomethycaine sulfate (Jelly Surfacaine) contains propylene glycol and thimerosal.

Over the years, Fisher (3) observed three patients who were allergic to Jelly Surfacaine. One patient was allergic to propylene glycol and two patients to thimerosal.

Aside from Jelly Surfacaine, Surfadil Cream and Surfadil Lotion (Lilly), both containing cyclomethycaine, are available as surface local anesthetic agents. Cyclomethycaine is also present in Surfadil (Lilly), Surfathesin, and Topocaine.

> **Although cyclomethycaine (Surfacaine) sensitivity is rare, the base of the anesthetic (propylene glycol) or the preservative (Merthiolate) may cause allergic contact dermatitis.**

Pramoxine Hydrochloride (Tronothane)

Pramoxine hydrochloride (Tronothane), 4-[3 (*p*-butoxyphenoxy) propyl], morpholine hydrochloride, is a surface anesthetic agent different from local anesthetics of the benzoate ester type, such as benzocaine and procaine. It is *not used* by injection.

Although Schmidt et al. (29) reported the virtues of pramoxine hydrochloride (Tronothane) more than 25 years ago, this surface anesthetic is not widely used as yet by der-

TABLE 15.6. *Dibucaine Hydrochloride (Nupercaine)*

Nupercainal Cream and Ointment (Ciba)
Nupercainal Suppositories (Ciba)
Nupercaine Heavy Solution (Ciba)
Nupercaine Hydrochloride 1:200 and 1:1,500 (Ciba) (for spinal anesthesia)

matologists. These investigators stated that "Tronothane exhibits outstanding qualities as a topical local anesthetic agent. It combines high potency with low systemic toxicity. Also it possesses a low sensitizing potential and is well tolerated by tissues. Extensive laboratory and clinical testing have demonstrated the following properties of Tronothane: (1) it is equivalent to ethyl aminobenzoate in anesthetic activity; (2) its effective minimal concentration is greater than cyclomethycaine; (3) its duration of action is double that of cocaine; (4) it produces no apparent irritation to skin and mucous membranes; and (5) it possesses a low sensitizing potential."

Peal and Karp (30) confirmed the low sensitization and irritation potential in a study involving 71 adult volunteers. Several patients sensitive to other topical anesthetics showed no sensitization to Tronothane. The patch test sensitization reactions that did occur were of a mild and moderate character. The incidence of such reactions was approximately one-fifth that observed in similar tests on the same objects using cyclomethycaine.

> **Pramoxine hydrochloride (Tronothane), applied only topically, is a rare sensitizer that has long been used by obstetricians, surgeons, proctologists, and dentists. Dermatologists have found it effective in pruritic dermatoses in the form of Pramosone lotion and cream.**

The Combined Use of Pramoxine (Tronothane) with Hydrocortisone Acetate

Sladek (31) reported that a new foam preparation, containing 1% hydrocortisone acetate and 1% pramoxine hydrochloride, was clinically investigated in 118 postoperative and 5 nonsurgical proctologic patients with beneficial results. Excellent to good responses in terms of smooth and faster healing of surgical wounds and relief of discomfort were seen in 95% of patients. Eight patients showed fair to poor response to therapy. No untoward reactions were observed. This new mode of administration appears to offer significant advantages over hemorrhoidal suppositories, ointments, and other forms of therapy. Sladek (31) believed that the use of these two active ingredients was superior to either one alone. Presently, preparations containing pramoxine hydrochloride and hydrocortisone acetate together with their vehicles are available. Fisher (32) has reviewed the literature related to pramoxine and listed some available products in Tables 15.7 and 15.8.

Van Ketel (33) reported two patients who had allergic contact sensitivity to pramoxine (Tronothane) apparently from the application of a Dutch preparation called Nestosyl ointment, which reportedly contains pramoxine. This is the

TABLE 15.7. *Products Containing Pramoxine Hydrochloride*

Anugesic Ointment (Warner/Chilcott)
Anugesic Suppositories (Warner/Chilcott)
F-E-P Creme (Boots)
Otall Ear Drops (Saron)
Perifoam (Rowell)
Pramosone Lotion and Ointment (Ferndale)[a]
Prax Lotion and Cream (Ferndale)[b]
ProctoFoam/nonsteroid (Reed & Carnrick)
Tronothane Hydrochloride Cream, Jelly (Abbott)

[a]Contains pramoxine hydrochloride and hydrocortisone.
Note: Pramoxine used only for surface anesthesia and not for injections, so sensitization to this anesthetic does not entail any risk of future systemic reactions.
[b]Contains pramoxine hydrochloride alone.

only report of allergic reaction that Fisher (32) could find in the literature.

Table 15.9 lists miscellaneous topical anesthetics. Adverse reactions have been described in Chapter 10.

TESTING FOR ALLERGIC REACTIONS TO LOCAL ANESTHETICS

Patch testing for allergic contact dermatitis caused by topical anesthetics is quite reliable. The reliability of skin tests for adverse reactions to injectable anesthetics, however, leaves much to be desired.

The unreliability of skin tests to decide what local anesthetic is safe for a patient who has a history of prior adverse reactions is illustrated by the findings of Incaudo et al. (34). These investigators reported the following.

The clinical histories of 71 patients evaluated for suspected local anesthetic (LA) allergy were reviewed retrospectively. The clinical histories were classified as immediate generalized reactions (15%), localized swelling at the injection site (25%), nonspecific systemic symptoms (42%), and other histories (17%). Serial dilutional intradermal skin tests were performed in 59 patients using mepivacaine, lidocaine, and procaine. There were five skin-test positive patients, each with a positive reaction to an LA to

TABLE 15.8. *Pramoxine Hydrochloride with Hydrocortisone*

Pramosone Cream and Ointment (Ferndale)
Pramosone Lotion (Ferndale)
Proctofoam (Reed & Carnrick)

which, according to their medical history, they had never reacted before. In 50 patients when an LA was subsequently required, a subcutaneous challenge was performed, with an LA chosen for chemical nonsimilarity. No significant reactions were observed in this group. Three patients tolerated a challenge with an LA to which they were skin-test positive.

These data indicate the low incidence of reactions compatible with a systemic IgE-mediated mechanism by history in patients referred for evaluation of LA allergy, the lack of specific and clinically relevant information provided by dilutional skin tests, and the apparent safety and usefulness of careful challenge with an alternative LA.

> **Patch tests for allergic contact dermatitis to topically applied anesthetics are reliable. Intradermal skin tests for allergic reactions to injectable anesthetics are unreliable. In vitro tests have not yet been standardized. Careful challenge with an "alternative" anesthetic is useful.**

Other in vivo tests, such as nasal and conjunctival tests, are not only unreliable but also risky. Thus, Adriani (35) reported a fatal reaction to the instillation of one drop of a local anesthetic into the conjunctival sac.

In vitro testing, such as the leucocyte histamine release test and the lymphocyte transformation test, may possibly be of some value.

Lehner (36) reported positive results for four patients who had suspected allergy to local anesthetics and for whom the intradermal test was negative.

TABLE 15.9. *Miscellaneous Topical Anesthetics*

Topical anesthetics	Ingredients
Aspercreme (Thompson Medical)	Triethanolamine salicylate
Ben-Gay (Leeming)	Methyl salicylate, menthol
Chloraseptic Gel (Norwich Eaton)	Phenol, sodium phenolate
Deep Down Pain Relief Rub (Beecham)	Methyl salicylate, menthol, methyl nicotinate, camphor
Icy Hot Balm (Searle)	Methyl salicylate, menthol
Mentholatum Ointment, Rub (Mentholatum)	Methyl salicylate, menthol
Myoflex Creme (Adria)	Triethanolamine salicylate
Oraderm Lip Balm (Schattner)	Sodium phenolate, sodium tetraborate, phenol
Panalgesic (Poythress)	Methyl salicylate, aspirin, menthol, camphor
Proctodon (Rowell)	Diperodon hydrochloride
Soltice Quick-Rub (Chattem)	Menthol, methyl salicylate, camphor, eucalyptus oil
Thera-Gesic (Mission)	Methyl salicylate, menthol
Vicks Vaporub (Vicks Health Care)	Menthol, spirits of turpentine, eucalyptus oil, camphor, cedar leaf oil, thymol

MISCELLANEOUS

Proparacaine (Proxymetacaine; Ophthaine, Ophthetic)

This ophthalmic topical anesthetic, with the formula 3-amino-4-propoxybenzoic acid 2(diethylamino) ethyl ester, may produce dermatitis of the hands in sensitized ophthalmologists and allergic conjunctivitis from its presence in eye preparations (37,38).

Diperoton Hydrochloride (Proctodon)

This topical anesthetic in the form of Diperodon cream is based on dicarbanalide, and thus does not cross-react with the PABA anesthetics. Diperodon cream is used as a lubricant and anesthetic for rectal examination and to alleviate pain of postoperative bowel movements. Calnan (39) reported an allergic reaction to this anesthetic.

Phenolic Anesthetics

The phenolic anesthetic preparations are listed in Table 15.9. The accompanying literature to these preparations stresses that they are free of "caines" and are anesthetic and antiseptic. These phenolic compounds are rare sensitizers.

Propanidid

Propanidid, which is not listed in the Physicians' Desk Reference, is a derivative of eugenol used in Europe as an intravenous anesthetic instead of barbiturates. Gastelain and Piriou (40) have reported a contact dermatitis due to propanidid in an anesthetic. Sneddon and Caldwell (41) reported a similar case previously.

TOPICAL ANALGESICS

A wide variety of topical analgesic preparations are available in Europe but not the United States. Contact dermatitis and photocontact dermatitis have been reported from a variety of topical analgesic products.

Salicylates

Hydroxyethyl salicylate in topical analgesic gel has caused contact dermatitis and was detected by use of 0.1% in petrolatum (42). No cross reactivity to salicylic acid, sodium salicylate, or acetylsalicylic acid was noted.

Methyl butetisalicylate is used topically for musculoskeletal pain. It is also known as methyl diethylacetylsalicylate, and the usual use concentration is 30% in a cream base. A 40-year-old woman developed contact dermatitis to methyl butetisalicylate used to treat a painful knee (43). Oral acetylsalicylic acid (aspirin) up to 1,000 mg did not cause any reaction in this case.

Topical salicylates are rare contact allergens. Picolinamine salicylate used as a topical antiinflammatory cream in Spain was found to be a potential source of contact dermatitis (44). A patch test with 2% concentration in oil was positive.

Acetaminophen (Propacetamol)

Nurses who do not wear gloves while mixing or handling the analgesic propacetamol may develop contact dermatitis on the hands and forearms. Four such cases were reported from France, where the drug is used commonly for postoperative pain (45). The agent is a prodrug composed of diethylglycine linked to paracetamol. The patients tolerated oral paracetamol. Paracetamol is better known as acetaminophen.

Propacetamol is broken down by esterases or nonenzymatic mechanisms into acetaminophen and N,N-diethylglycine. Patch tests in propacetamol sensitive patients have found the allergenic determinant to reside in the N,N-diethylglycine, which is a phenyl ester, and these are known skin sensitizers (46).

Indomethacin

Topical indomethacin caused contact dermatitis in a 14-year-old boy within 10 days after he applied it to his right ankle (47). A patch test of 1% pure indomethacin in petrolatum was positive, and there was no cross-reaction to multiple other topical nonsteroidal anti-inflammatory drugs (NSAIDs) or to the excipients of Inacid gel.

Ketoprofen

Topical ketoprofen is sold in Italy in both cream and gel bases. It is a propionic acid derivative categorized as an NSAID. Seven cases of both contact and photocontact allergy were reported by Tosti et al. (48) and confirmed by patch testing with the 2.5% gel formula, which was positive in all seven cases. A 10% petrolatum patch test was positive in only two of seven cases, demonstrating the importance of proper vehicle selection for patch testing with ketoprofen. However, a 2.5% petrolatum patch test plus 10J of UVA light confirmed contact and photocontact dermatitis in another study (49). In this later case, cross-reactivity with ibuproxam was observed.

NSAID Cross-Reactions

An Italian study of topical NSAID cross-reactions found most of the 123 patients tested to be monosensitive, and ketoprofen was the most common problem (50). The investigators felt that a possible cross-reaction between cinnamic aldehyde and ketoprofen might exist based on a common ketonic group and the frequency of co-reactivity between fragrance mix, cinnamic aldehyde, and ketoprofen. The most common linkage between topical NSAIDs was between ketoprofen and ibuproxam (10 contact dermatitis cases and 3 photocontact dermatitis cases). There were five ketoprofen-thiaprophenic acid cases.

Le Coz et al. (51) investigated the pattern of cross-reactivity among photosensitizing NSAIDs. Ketoprofen photoallergic patients and tiaprofenic acid patients cross-reacted in 12 of 12 cases. These are arylpropionic acid derivatives. These same patients reacted to fenofibrate in 8 of 12, oxybenzone in 3 of 12, and unsubstituted benzophenone in 11 of 12 cases. Ketoprofen has an unsubstituted benzophenone moiety that appears to be the basis for the cross-reactions. In the case of tiaprofenic acid, the thiophene-phenylketone moiety is very similar to the benzophenone moiety and is the likely basis for cross-reactions. The arylpropionic moiety does not appear to be part of the cross-reaction problem.

Topical ketoprofen caused photosensitivity that recurred in the absence of reapplication but recurred from sun exposure up to 6 months after the last application of the drug (52). Cross-reactivity to benzophenone-3 was found in this patient.

Connubial contact led to photodermatitis from ketoprofen (53). A husband was using topical ketoprofen, and his wife also frequented tanning salons. After UVA exposure, a handprint on her thigh appeared due to the connubial contact.

An erythema multiforme pattern of dermatitis occurred in an 82-year-old man following application of a ketoprofen-containing gel for diffuse rheumatic pain (54). The patch test was positive to ketoprofen 1% in petrolatum at days 2 and 3.

Ibuproxam

Both ibuproxam and ketoprofen are aryl-propropionic acid derivatives that are possible but not obligate cross-reacting molecules (55). Contact dermatitis to topical ibuproxam cream has been confirmed with a 5% concentration in petrolatum (56).

Suprofen

Topical 1% suprofen ointment is sold as an NSAID in Japan and has been reported to cause photocontact dermatitis (57). In five patients, UVA elicited photoallergy in conjunction with patch tests of 0.1% to 0.01% in petrolatum. In three patients, UVB elicited photoallergy with 0.1% to 1.0% in petrolatum. All cases cross-reacted with tiaprofenic acid but not with ketoprofen, piroxicam, bufexumac, bendazac, ibuprofen piconol, or ufenamate (57).

Bufexamac

Topical NSAIDs are in widespread use in Germany, where more than 130 such products are available. Routine testing with a group of NSAIDs in 371 consecutive patients found 17 sensitized individuals (4.6%). The most frequently encountered allergen was bufexamac, which was positive in 12 (3.2%) of patients (58).

Bufexamac was found to be a common sensitizer when applied to treat eczema. Females seem more likely to be sensitized, as, in one series, 88% of the bufexamac cases were female (59).

No cross-reactivity between bufexamac and diclofenac was seen in 11 cases of bufexamac sensitivity (60). Although both have benzene rings, the different side chains (acetamide for bufexamac and acetic acid for diclofenac) probably account for the lack of cross-reactivity.

An erythema multiforme–like eruption may follow localized allergic contact dermatitis to bufexamac. This NSAID has been used to treat a variety of disorders, including atopic dermatitis and localized leg lesions and ulcers. No epidermal necrosis was seen in four cases, as might be expected in true erythema multiforme (61).

Benzydamine Hydrochloride

Topical application of the NSAID benzydamine hydrochloride caused both contact and photocontact dermatitis. The commercial ointment (Tantam) is a 5% concentration, and patch tests with 5% aqueous were positive (62).

Etofenamate

Etofenamate is 2-(2-hydroxyethoxy)-ethyl N-(ααα-trifluro-m-tolyl) anthranilate, and contact dermatitis has been reported and confirmed with 2% petrolatum (63) and 5% lanolin (64) patch tests. Application to the lumbosacral region has progressed to exfoliative erythroderma (65).

Nine cases of contact allergy to etofenamate were reported by Hergueta et al. (66), with onset of rash generally within 7 days of using the product (range 1–30 days). A 2% concentration in petrolatum identified all of the cases, with no reaction in 30 controls.

Diclofenac

This arylacetic NSAID was reported as the cause of three cases of contact allergy. A 2.5% petrolatum patch test concentration was used (67).

Diclofenac sodium and diclofenac diethylamine tested at 10% in petrolatum produced delayed positive patch test reactions (68). Diclofenac is in the arylacanoic acid group, which also includes bufexamac, mefenamic, meclofenamic, flufenamic, tolfenamic, and etofenamic acids.

Diclofenac has also caused contact dermatitis when used as an ophthalmic preparation (69). Eyelid dermatitis and conjunctivitis were produced, but cross-reactivity with bufexamac was not observed.

Cinnoxicam

Cinnoxicam, an ester of piroxicam and cinnamic acid, is used topically in Italy and has caused contact dermatitis. It was not found to cross-react with other common NSAIDs (70).

Piketoprofen

Piketoprofen is used topically in Spain and caused contact dermatitis in a 27-year-old woman who applied it to treat back pain (71). Patch tests with 1% and 5% in petrolatum were positive, and 5 controls were negative. No cross-reactions were found to oxicams, phenylacetic, indole, fenamates, or propionic acid–derived NSAIDs.

Enoxolone and Mafenide

Topical Pentalmicina produced contact dermatitis around a tracheostomy site (72). This compound is 1.5% enoxolone and 7% mafenide. Enoxolone is a topical anti-inflammatory drug from glycyrrhizinic acid and was tested at 10% in petrolatum.

Mafenide, a sulfonamide (para-amino methylbenzylsulfonamide), also tested at 10% in petrolatum. No cross-reactions between mafenide and other para-amino group compounds, such as paraphenylenediamine and sulfonanilamide, have been found (72).

Fepradinol

A topical spray of fepradinol caused two cases of contact dermatitis confirmed by 0.1% to 5% aqueous patch tests (73). Although 20 controls were negative at 5% aqueous, Izu et al. (73) do not recommend testing above 1% aqueous. No cross-reactions to other NSAIDs were found, and this agent is not chemically an NSAID. Fepradinol is used topically as an anti-inflammatory agent, although it is an adrenergic compound more closely related to ephedrine, phenylephrine, and terbutaline (74).

Two cases of contact dermatitis to fepradinol were studied to look for cross-reactivity to phenylethanolamine compounds, such as adrenergics phenylephrine, ephedrine, and terbutaline. No cross-reactivity was found (75).

Fepradinol caused allergic contact dermatitis when applied to a 12-year-old boy for treatment of myalgia (76). The application was in the form of a spray known as Flexidol. Patch tests were positive at 0.1 and 1.0% in both aqueous and petrolatum bases.

Photocontact dermatitis to fepradinol was reported from the use of a spray (Dalgen) that contained this anti-inflammatory (77).

Chlorproethazine

An ointment containing chlorproethazine was used for chronic neck pain and subsequently incriminated in producing lip and eyelid edema after sun exposure (78). Photocontact urticaria was reproduced by 0.1% patch tests for 24 hours of chlorproethazine and chlorpromazine followed by 10J of UVA light that produced immediate erythema (78).

Pyrazinobutazone

Topical use of this compound, which is an equimolar salt of piperazine and phenylbutazone, produced a dermatitis in an individual sensitized through prior pharmaceutical industry exposure. Patch tests with 5% piperazine hexahydrate and 1% phenylbutazone were positive. Oral provocation produced a hand eczema (79).

Opium Alkaloids

Occupational exposure to codeine and morphine was the cause of 11 cases of dermatitis, of which 7 reacted to para group chemicals, such as paraphenylenediamine (80). Interestingly, the neutral alkaloid piocarpine was found to cause dermatitis from an eyedrop in a patient also paraphenylenediamine sensitive (81).

Belladonna

A belladonna plaster used as a topical analgesic for back pain caused contact dermatitis traced to atropine. The product was 0.25% belladonna, and the patient was negative to a 2% hyoscine patch test and positive to a 1% atropine in petrolatum patch test (82).

REFERENCES

1. Tan BB, et al. Perioperative collapse: prevalence of latex allergy in patients sensitive to anesthetic agents. *Contact Dermatitis* 1997;36:47.
2. Mathewson HS. *Structural forms of anesthetic compounds.* Kansas City, MO: Charles C Thomas Publisher, 1961.
3. Fisher AA. *Contact dermatitis.* 3rd ed. Philadelphia: Lea & Febiger, 1986.
4. Wilkinson JD, et al. Preliminary patch testing with 25% and 15% "caine"-mixes. *Contact Dermatitis* 1990;22:244.
5. Sidhu SK, Shaw S, Wilkinson JD. A 10-year retrospective study on benzocaine allergy in the United Kingdom. *Am J Contact Dermatitis* 1999;10:57.
6. Fisher AA. The presence of benzocaine in sunscreens containing glyceryl PABA (Escalol 106). *Arch Dermatol* 1977;113:1299.
7. Hjorth N, et al. Glyceryl *p*-aminobenzoate patch testing in benzocaine-sensitive subjects. *Contact Dermatitis* 1978;4:46.
8. van Ketel WG, Bruynzeel DP. A "forgotten" topical anesthetic sensitizer: butyl aminobenzoate. *Contact Dermatitis* 1991;25:131.
9. Beck MH, Holden A. Benzocaine—an unsatisfactory indicator of topical local anesthetic sensitization of the UK. *Br J Dermatol* 1988;118:91.
10. Kalveram K, Semmelmann J, Forck G. Experimental animal study of the allergenicity of Tetracaine. *Contact Dermatitis* 1978;4:374.
11. Kalveram K, et al. Tetracaine allergy: cross-reactions with paracompounds? *Contact Dermatitis* 1978;4:376.
12. Hardwick N, King CM. Contact allergy to lignocaine with cross-reaction to bupivacaine. *Contact Dermatitis* 1994;30:245.
13. Fregert S, Tegner E, Thelin I. Contact allergy to lidocaine. *Contact Dermatitis* 1979;5:185.
14. Roed-Petersen J. Contact sensitivity to metaoxedrine. *Contact Dermatitis* 1979;5:185.
15. Goransson K. Hypersensitivity to prilocaine. *Dermatologica* 1976;152:158.
16. Black RJ, Dawson TA, Strang WC. Cross-sensitivity to lignocaine and prilocaine. *Contact Dermatitis* 1990;23:117.
17. Hofmann H, et al. Presumed generalized exfoliative dermatitis to lidocaine [Letter]. *Arch Dermatol* 1976;111:266.
18. Chin TM, Fellner MJ. Allergic hypersensitivity to lidocaine hydrochloride. *Int Soc Trop Derm* 1980;19:147.

19. Weightman W, Turner T. Allergic contact dermatitis from lignocaine: report of 29 cases and review of the literature. *Contact Dermatitis* 1998;39:265.
20. Bircher AJ, Messmer SL, Surber C, Rufli T. Delayed-type hypersensitivity to subcutaneous lidocaine with tolerance to articaine: confirmation by *in vivo* and *in vitro* tests. *Contact Dermatitis* 1996;34:387.
21. Kawada A, et al. Simultaneous contact sensitivity due to lidocaine and crotamiton. *Contact Dermatitis* 1997;37:45.
22. Klein CE, Gall H. Type IV allergy to amide-type local anesthetics. *Contact Dermatitis* 1991;25:45.
23. Fisher AA. Propylene glycol dermatitis. *Cutis* 1978;21:166.
24. Soesman-van Waadenoden Kernekamp A, van Ketel WG. Contact allergy to lidocaine (Xylocaine, Lignocaine). *Contact Dermatitis* 1979; 5:403.
25. Downs AMR, Lear JT, Wallington TB, Sansom JE. Contact sensitivity and systemic reaction to pseudoephedrine and lignocaine. *Contact Dermatitis* 1998;39:33.
26. van den Hove J, Decroix J, Tennstedt D, Lachapelle JM. Allergic contact dermatitis from prilocaine, one of the local anesthetics in EMLA cream. *Contact Dermatitis* 1994;30:239.
27. de Waard-van der Spek FB, Oranje AP. Purpura caused by Emla is of toxic origin. *Contact Dermatitis* 1997;36:11.
28. Wilson HTH. Dermatitis from anesthetic ointments. *Practitioner* 1966;197:673.
29. Schmidt JL, Blockus LE, Richards RK. The pharmacology of pramoxine hydrochloride: a new topical anesthetic. *Anesth Anal* 1953; 32:418.
30. Peal L, Karp M. A new surface anesthetic agent: Tronothane. *Anesthesiology* 1954;15:637.
31. Sladek WR. Clinical evaluation of a new product for proctologic inflammatory conditions and postoperative use. *Am J Clin Res* 1970;1:33.
32. Fisher AA. Allergic reactions to topical (surface) anesthetics with reference to the safety of Tronothane (pramoxine hydrochloride). *Cutis* 1980;25:584.
33. van Ketel WG. Allergy to pramoxine (pramocaine). *Contact Dermatitis* 1981;7:49.
34. Incaudo G, Schatz M, Patterson R. Administration of local anesthetics to patients with a history of prior adverse reaction. *J Allergy Clin Immunol* 1978;61:339.
35. Adriani J. Etiology and management of adverse reactions to local anesthetics. *Int Anesthesiol Clin* 1972;10:127.
36. Lehner T. Lignocaine hypersensitivity. *Lancet* 1971;1:1245.
37. March C, Greenwood MA. Allergic contact dermatitis to proparacaine. *Arch Ophthalmol* 1968;79:159.
38. Bandman H-J, Breit R, Mutzeck E. Allergic contact dermatitis from proxymetacaine. *Contact Dermatitis Newsletter* 1974;14:451.
39. Calnan CD. Allergy to the local anesthetic Diperodon. *Contact Dermatitis* 1980;6:367.
40. Gastelain PY, Piriou A. Contact dermatitis due to propanidid in an anesthetist. *Contact Dermatitis* 1980;6:360.
41. Sneddon IB, Caldwell RG. Contact dermatitis due to propanidid in an anaesthetist. *Practitioner* 1973;211:321.
42. Reichert C, Gall H. Contact dermatitis from hydroxyethyl salicylate. *Contact Dermatitis* 1995;33:275.
43. Valsecchi R, et al. Contact dermatitis from methyl butetisalicylate. *Contact Dermatitis* 1998;38:360.
44. Gamboa P, et al. Contact sensitization to topical salicylate. *Contact Dermatitis* 1995;33:52.
45. Szczurko C, et al. Occupational contact dermatitis from propacetamol. *Contact Dermatitis* 1996; 35:299.
46. Berl V, Barbaud A, Lepoittevin J-P. Mechanism of allergic contact dermatitis from propacetamol: Sensitization to activated N,N-diethylglycine. *Contact Dermatitis* 1998; 38:185.
47. Pulido Z, et al. Allergic contact dermatitis from indomethacin. *Contact Dermatitis* 1999;41:112.
48. Tosti A, Gaddoni G, Valeri F, Bardazzi F. Contact allergy to ketoprofen: report of 7 cases. *Contact Dermatitis* 1990;23:112.
49. Mozzanica N, Pigatto PD. Contact and photocontact allergy to ketoprofen: clinical and experimental study. *Contact Dermatitis* 1990;23: 336.
50. Pigatto P, et al. Cross-reactions in patch testing and photopatch testing of ketoprofen, thiaprophenic acid, and cinnamic aldehyde. *Am J Contact Dermatitis* 1996;7:220.
51. Le Coz CJ, et al. Photocontact dermatitis from ketoprofen and tiaprofenic acid: cross-reactivity study in 12 consecutive patients. *Contact Dermatitis* 1998;38:245.
52. Horn HM, Humphreys F, Aldridge RD. Contact dermatitis and prolonged photosensitivity induced by ketoprofen and associated with sensitivity to benzophenone-3. *Contact Dermatitis* 1998;38:353.
53. Mirande-Romero A, et al. Ketoprofen-induced connubial photodermatitis. *Contact Dermatitis* 1997;37:242.
54. Mastrolonardo M, Loconosole F, Rantuccio F. Conjugal allergic contact dermatitis from ketoprofen. *Contact Dermatitis* 1994;30:110.
55. Valsecchi R, Cainelli T. Contact dermatitis from ibuproxam: a case with cross-reactivity with ketoprofen. *Contact Dermatitis* 1990;22:51.
56. Molinini R. Contact allergy to ibuproxam. *Contact Dermatitis* 1991; 24:302.
57. Kurumaji Y, et al. Allergic photocontact dermatitis due to suprofen: photopatch testing and cross-reaction study. *Contact Dermatitis* 1991;25:218.
58. Gniazdowska B, Rucff F, Przybilla B. Delayed contact hypersensitivity to non-steroidal antiinflammatory drugs. *Contact Dermatitis* 1999;40:63.
59. Kranke B, Derhaschnig J, Komericki P, Aberer W. Bufexamac is a frequent contact sensitizer. *Contact Dermatitis* 1996;34:63.
60. Barbaud A, et al. Bufexamac and diclofenac: frequency of contact sensitization and absence of cross-reactions. *Contact Dermatitis* 1998;39:272.
61. Koch P, Bahmer FA. Erythema-multiforme-like, urticarial papular and plaque eruptions from bufexamac: report of 4 cases. *Contact Dermatitis* 1994;31:97.
62. Vincenzi C, Cameli N, Tardio M, Piraccini BM. Contact and photocontact dermatitis due to benzydamine hydrochloride. *Contact Dermatitis* 1990;23:125.
63. Guerra L, et al. Contact dermatitis due to etofenamate. *Contact Dermatitis* 1992;26:199.
64. Götze A, Teikemeier G, Goerz G. Contact dermatitis from etofenamate. *Contact Dermatitis* 1992;26:209.
65. Correia O, Barros MA. Exfoliative dermatitis with etofenamate. *Contact Dermatitis* 1990;23:264.
66. Hergueta JP, Ortiz FJ, Iglesias L. Allergic contact dermatitis from etofenamate: report of 9 cases. *Contact Dermatitis* 1994;31:60.
67. Schiavino D, et al. Delayed allergy to diclofenac. *Contact Dermatitis* 1992;26:357.
68. Gebhardt M, Reuter A, Knopf B. Allergic contact dermatitis from topical diclofenac. *Contact Dermatitis* 1994;30:183.
69. Valsecchi R, Pansera B, Leghissa P, Reseghetti A. Allergic contact dermatitis of the eyelids and conjunctivitis from diclofenac. *Contact Dermatitis* 1996;34:150.
70. Valsecchi R, Pansera B, Di Landro A, Cainelli T. Contact allergy to cinnoxicam. *Contact Dermatitis* 1995;32:63.
71. Navarro LA, Jorro G, Morales C, Pelaez A. Allergic contact dermatitis due to piketoprofen. *Contact Dermatitis* 1995;32:181.
72. Fernandez JC, Gamboa P, Jauregui I. Concomitant sensitization to enoxolone and mafenide in a topical medicament. *Contact Dermatitis* 1992;27:262.
73. Izu R, et al. Allergic contact dermatitis from fepradinol. *Contact Dermatitis* 1992;27:266.
74. Schnuch A. Fepradinol allergy: possibly a case of unnoticed cross-reaction due to misclassification. *Contact Dermatitis* 1994;30:243.
75. Goday JJ, et al. No evidence of cross-reaction between fepradinol and other phenylethanolamines. *Contact Dermatitis* 1997;36:170.
76. Gomez A, Martorell A, de la Cuadra J. Allergic contact dermatitis from fepradinol in a child. *Contact Dermatitis* 1994;30:44.
77. Rodriguez Granados T, Pineiro G, de la Torre C, Cruces Prado MJ. Photoallergic contact dermatitis from fepradinol. *Contact Dermatitis* 1998;39:194.
78. Loesche C, Dejobert Y, Thomas P. Immediate wheal after topical administration of chlorproethazine. *Contact Dermatitis* 1992;26:278.
79. Bris J MD, Montanes MA, Candela MS, Diez AG. Contact sensitivity to pyrazinobutazone (Carudol®) with positive oral provocation test. *Contact Dermatitis* 1992;26:355.
80. Conde-Salazar L, et al. Occupational allergic contact dermatitis from opium alkaloids. *Contact Dermatitis* 1991;25:202.
81. Ortiz FJ, et al. Allergic contact dermatitis from pilocarpine and thimerosal. *Contact Dermatitis* 1991;25:203.
82. Williams HC, duVivier A. Belladonna plaster—not as bella as it seems. *Contact Dermatitis* 1990;23:119.

CHAPTER 16

Reactions to Topical Corticosteroids

Reactions to topical corticosteroids or their vehicles should be suspected when the use of the topical corticosteroids either does not improve the existing dermatitis or makes it worse. One should be alerted particularly when a patient has used a topical corticosteroid with a good response but then no longer responds, or the existing dermatitis becomes worse. Superimposed contact dermatitis from the topical steroid may be due to allergic hypersensitivity to the corticosteroid itself or to one of the ingredients in the vehicle or base of the topical corticosteroid. Some patients are allergic to a single corticosteroid, whereas others may be sensitized to several corticosteroids.

THE HYDROCORTISONES

Soon after hydrocortisones were introduced, several cases of allergic contact sensitivity to these low-potency topical corticosteroids were reported (1–4).

> **Suspect hypersensitivity to a topical corticosteroid when the patient is not doing as well as expected.**

Over-the-Counter Topical Hydrocortisone Preparations

The U.S. Food and Drug Administration has approved the use of over-the-counter (OTC) preparations containing ½% and 1% hydrocortisone or hydrocortisone acetate.

It is a paradox, however, that, prescription-type corticosteroid preparations require the manufacturer to give details of the vehicles, but no such requirement is made for OTC preparations. This creates difficulty in testing persons suspected of having superimposed allergic contact dermatitis from an ingredient in the vehicle of the OTC hydrocortisone preparations.

Table 16.1 lists those OTC topical corticosteroids that contain parabens often used as preservatives. It should be noted that most prescription-type topical corticosteroids do not contain parabens; however, most OTC nonprescription-type corticosteroids do (5). Table 16.2 lists OTC topical corticosteroid creams and lotions free of parabens.

> **Sixteen OTC topical corticosteroid preparations were investigated; 12 of the 16 contained paraben preservatives, and the other 4 were paraben free.**

Table 16.3 lists preparations that contain propylene glycol. Certain manufacturers of topical corticosteroid preparations state that a 25% concentration of propylene glycol in the vehicle may have sufficient bactericidal reactions to guarantee formulation stability without any of the usual preservatives, such as parabens (6).

The only preparation sold in the United States that contains sorbic acid is Hytone Cream (Dermik), a nonprescription preparation with ½% hydrocortisone. Sorbic acid is a rare sensitizer, but, not uncommonly, it produces a slight stinging sensation and erythema in some persons (7).

> **Prescription topical corticosteroids require listing of the ingredients of their vehicles. Paradoxically, no such requirement is made for OTC hydrocortisone preparations, most of which contain parabens as a preservative.**

Several reports show that hydrocortisone sensitivity may be accompanied by hypersensitivity to more potent topical corticosteroids (2,8–10).

Hydrocortisone-17-butyrate has been reported to have produced allergic contact sensitivity in several patients in Europe (11–13). Brandao and Camarasa (11) obtained a positive patch test with 0.1% in petrolatum, whereas Soesman-van Waadenoden Kernekamp and van Ketel (12) obtained a positive patch test with 1% in petrolatum. Corticosteroid allergy has been so commonly reported that 2.9% to 4.8% of patients screened in European clinics have been found to be allergic to one or more corticosteroids (14).

The availability of corticosteroids not sold in the United States has aided in screening for hydrocortisone and other corticosteroid allergy. Tixocortol pivalate and budesonide in petrolatum (1%) detect most cases, but, just as

TABLE 16.1. *OTC Topical Corticosteroids Containing Parabens*

Nonprescription hydrocortisone ½%
  Bactine Hydrocortisone Skin Care Cream (Miles
    Laboratories)
  Caldecort Hydrocortisone Cream (Pennwalt)
  Corticaine (Glaxo)
  Delacort (Medicon)
  Prepcort Hydrocortisone Cream (Whitehall)
  Resicort Cream (Mentholatum)
Nonprescription hydrocortisone acetate ½%
  Cortaid Cream, Lotion, Ointment (Upjohn)
  Cortef Feminine Itch Cream (Upjohn)
  Cortef Rectal Itch Ointment (Upjohn)
  Gynecort Antipruritic Cream (Combe)
  Lanacort Antipruritic Cream (Combe)
  Wellcortin Cream, Lotion (Burroughs Wellcome)[a]

[a]No longer manufactured.

petrolatum is not the ideal base for delivering corticosteroids through the stratum corneum, it has not always proven to be the correct base for patch testing (14). A study of 127 patients allergic to one or more corticosteroids found that the combination of tixocortol pivalate and budesonide detected 91.3% of the cases (15). In the study, a larger group of corticoids was used for patch testing, and the frequency of reactions was as follows: tixocortol, 96; hydrocortisone butyrate, 51; budesonide, 47; betamethasone valerate, 11; clobetasone butyrate, 11; clobetasol propionate, 8. Although some investigators recommend ethanol or mixtures of ethanol, propylene glycol, and isopropanol or higher concentrations of corticosteroid (14), others have found the commercial preparations adequate for screening purposes (16,17).

Freeman (18) found that the best way to screen for corticosteroid allergy was to use the patient's corticosteroid in cream base for patch testing. This had the highest yield followed by commercially prepared corticosteroid ointment, and this was more sensitive than pure corticosteroid in either petrolatum or alcohol. Delayed positive reactions were common and required late readings for proper detection. The repeat open application test proved a simple and useful diagnostic tool.

Tixocortol pivalate (Pivalone) has been shown to be both a sensitive and specific marker for hydrocortisone allergy confirmed by intradermal skin tests with hydrocortisone (19). Pivalone was more accurate than hydrocortisone in tests with ethanol or a hydrocortisone/ethanol/-dimethylsulfoxide (DMSO) mixture (19). An intradermal skin test

TABLE 16.2. *Paraben-Free OTC Corticosteroid Lotions and Creams*

Dermolate Anti-Itch Cream (Schering)
Dermolate Scalp Itch Lotion (Schering)
Hytone Cream (Dermik)
Rhulicort Cream and Lotion (Lederle)

TABLE 16.3. *OTC Corticosteroid Preparations Containing Propylene Glycol*

Nonprescription hydrocortisone ½%
  Bactine Hydrocortisone Skin Care Cream (Miles
    Laboratories)
  Caldecort Hydrocortisone Cream, Spray, Ointment
    (Pennwalt)
  Cortef Feminine Itch Cream (Upjohn)
  Delacort (Medicon)
  Dermolate Anti-Itch Cream and Spray (Schering)

with 1 mg of hydrocortisone sodium phosphate confirms the accuracy of tixocortol pivalate, and tests with precursors and metabolites of hydrocortisone do not appear to be the allergen (20). Intradermal skin tests for corticosteroid allergy are thought to be more sensitive but less convenient than patch tests. However, this is only true for some corticosteroids. Tixocortol pivalate 1% in petrolatum detected all the cases of corticosteroid allergy to hydrocortisone that were detected by intradermal hydrocortisone succinate (21). Likewise, budesonide 1% in petrolatum was as sensitive as intradermal budesonide. But patch tests with hydrocortisone-17-butyrate missed 30% of cases due to this corticosteroid.

Corticosteroids as Haptens

The C17 position on the corticosteroid has been suggested as the site for protein binding to form a complete antigen (20).

The mechanism by which corticosteroids become complete allergens rather than haptens has focused around binding to arginine. An alternative hypothesis involving the metabolism of the corticosteroid at the 21 position to form a 21-dehydroderivative, which is then converted to an alpha-ketoaldehyde, has been proposed and partially supported by patch test observations as a potential mechanism (22).

The Effect of Concentration and Time

The standard recommended concentration for patch testing with budesonide is 0.1% in petrolatum. However, a lower dose was found to yield higher results in some patients (23). Patch test concentrations down to 0.0002% were at times more sensitive in detecting allergy than higher concentrations. It was recommended that 0.02% to 0.002% be used based on cases from Sweden and Belgium in whom this dosage range proved most effective (23).

A careful evaluation of the relationship between the pharmacological and immunological effects of the corticosteroid budesonide was undertaken to examine the time course, dose, and occlusion times on reactions (24). A range of 2% to 0.002% was studied with occlusion times of 5, 24, and 48 hours and readings at days 2, 4, and 7. High concentrations tended to produce late reactions, and lower concentrations were seen at day 2. A 48-hour occlusion time was best. A phenomenon seen with corticosteroids known as the edge effect or a rim reaction, in which erythema occurs only around the circumference of the chamber, represents true sensitization. This can be demonstrated by lowering the concentration and repeating the test. A more traditional reaction is then seen.

Isaksson et al. (25) tried to improve on our ability to identify corticosteroid allergy by using mixes and lower concentrations of three corticoids: budesonide, tixocortol pivalate, and hydrocortisone-17-butyrate. Although they found merit in the lower concentration, of more significance was the fact that all tests regardless of concentration were positive when readings were taken at day 10 rather than day 7. The value of late readings in corticosteroids appears to be confirmed.

In response to the uncertainty of optimal vehicle, concentration, route of exposure (patch test vs intradermal), and proper screening substances, Chang et al. (26) recommended testing the commercial formulas of corticosteroids in question for the patient by provocative use tests or repeated open application tests as they did in their patient who was sensitive to 23 different corticosteroids.

Corticosteroid Allergen Classes

Four classes of corticosteroids have been suggested based on the frequency of corticosteroid cross-reactivity (Table 16.4). Although these classes can be used as a guide (17), many exceptions occur, and nothing can fully substitute for testing the corticosteroid preparation directly on the patient. Sasaki (16), in a review of 18 cases of corticosteroid allergy and cross-sensitivity, found that betamethasone (Class C) types of allergy rarely cross-react with triamcinolone (Class B). An example of cross-reactivity within a class may be seen in the case of Gamboa et al. (27), who reported facial edema, nasal edema, and dermatitis from a budesonide nasal spray confirmed by a 0.2% petrolatum patch test. A cross-reaction with amcinonide was observed (both Class B). However, allergic contact dermatitis was reported from

prednicarbate (a Class D corticosteroid), and the patch test was positive at the use concentration (28). This patient cross-reacted only to 1% budesonide (Class B) but not to others, including other Class D corticosteroids.

The somewhat unpredictable nature of cross-reactions among these four classes has given rise to various recommendations for simplified corticosteroid screening. Lauerma (29) found that Classes A, B, and D cross-reacted most frequently, and he proposed tixocortol pivalate and hydrocortisone-17-butyrate as a good screening combination (29). He also found that Class C (betamethasone type) was the least common corticosteroid allergen in Finland (29). Although hydrocortisone-17-butyrate (Locoid) is available in the United States, tixocortol is not. Screening with the corticosteroids used by a patient in the commercial formula along with hydrocortisone-17-butyrate would be the reasonable alternative in the United States in the absence of tixocortol availability.

Tixocortol pivalate used as a nasal spray has produced sensitization in as little as 11 days (30). This would suggest that the greatest use of tixocortol pivalate may be in screening for contact dermatitis rather than treatment for inflammatory disorders. An example of that use can be seen in the report of a lymphoma patient who received methylprednisolone as part of a chemotherapy program and developed a generalized rash from prednisolone hemisuccinate detected by patch testing with tixocortol (31). A 5% prednisolone hemisuccinate patch test in 50/50 ethanol/DMSO was also positive.

Narrow versus Broad Corticosteroid Allergy

The four classes of corticosteroids that are based on allergen cross-reaction patterns may give the impression that cross-reactions are expected and always predictable. This is not the case. Some patients have very narrow allergy and react only to one or two corticosteroids. An example of this is found in the case of Corazza and Virgili (32), who tested a 26-year-old nurse and found her allergic to 6-alpha-

TABLE 16.4. *Four Classes of Corticosteroids Based on Frequency of Cross-Reactivity*

Class A	Class B	Class C	Class D
Hydrocortisone type	Triamcinolone type	Betamethasone type (not valerate)	Hydrocortisone-17-butyrate type
Hydrocortisone with C17 and/or C21-acetate ester	Triamcinolone acetonide or alcohol	Betamethasone and disodium phosphate	Hydrocortisone butyrate and valerate
	Amcinonide	Dexamethasone and disodium phosphate	Clobetasol propionate and butyrate
	Fluocinolone acetonide	Flucortolone	Betamethasone valerate and dipropionate
Tixocortol pivalate	Budesonide	Desoximetasone	Prednicarbate
Prednisone	Halcinonide		Fluocortolone hexanoate and pivalate
Prednisolone ± acetate	Flucinonide		Aclometasone dipropionate
	Desonide		
Methylprednisolone ± acetate			

methylprednisolone aceponate, which is allergen Class D. A positive reaction to budesonide 0.1% in petrolatum was found, and this is a known marker for Class B and D allergy. However, no other reactions were noted to members of Classes A, B, or D. Thus, this patient exhibits narrow allergy rather than broad allergy.

The difficulty of testing for corticosteroid allergy is illustrated by the case reported by Quirce et al (33). Their patient developed periocular dermatitis after use of a corticosteroid eye product containing hydrocortisone and dexamethasone. Patch tests with tixocortol and budesonide were negative, as was hydrocortisone. The patient had a systemic eczematous dermatitis when treated with prednisone 30 mg per day. A challenge with 30 mg of prednisone again caused a systemic eczema. Patch tests with prednisone powder as is and prednisone 5% in ethanol were positive, yet prednisone 10% in petrolatum was negative.

Newer corticosteroids have also caused dermatitis and produced positive patch test reactions. Prednicarbate is one such molecule, and it fits into allergen Class D. Although it is nonhalogenated, it is esterified at C17 and C21. Villas Martinez et al. (34) reported a patient who had broad corticosteroid sensitivity reacting to corticosteroids of Classes A, B, and D.

One case has been reported of contact dermatitis from flucortin butyl, detected with a 0.25% petrolatum patch test that did not cross-react with tixocortol or any of the other four corticosteroid classes (35).

Class C—The "Hypoallergenic Corticosteroids"

Although there are fewer reports of allergic reactions to Class C corticosteroids, it is unclear if desoximetasone, which is the only topical agent in Class C, is truly less reactive. It has been reported most commonly as an allergen in the setting of multiple positive corticosteroids, and it has also been a source of erythema multiforme–like eruption (36).

Paramethasone acetate is a 6-alpha-methylprednisolone 21-acetate, which is in allergen Class C. A Spanish patient with alopecia areata reacted to injections of paramethasone into the balding areas of the scalp (37). No other Class C corticosteroids reacted, but tixocortol pivalate (Class A) and hydrocortisone-17-butyrate (Class D) reacted. Paramethasone is used primarily for intralesional injections. It has also been reported to cause systemic reactions of an urticarial type.

Mometasone furoate and fluticasone propionate, which are in Class D, were found to produce fewer reactions than other tested corticosteroids in a series by Wilkinson and Beck (38). Novel substitutions at the C17 position make mometasone less likely to cross-react with other corticosteroids. In the case of fluticasone, fluorine at C6 and C9 rather than the ester at C17 are thought to be responsible for lesser cross-reactivity.

Endogenous Steroids

Glucocorticoid allergy may be a clue to reactivity to other endogenous substances. Infusion of adrenocorticotrophic hormone (ACTH) in patients with corticosteroid allergy has been shown to cause systemic dermatitis (39). This concept was carried even further in a study of 19 corticosteroid-allergic patients, 11 of whom reacted to 11-deoxycortisol and 5 of whom reacted to 17-alpha-OH-progesterone (40). This latter group of progesterone-allergic patients could express autoimmune progesterone dermatitis.

An investigation of five women with autoimmune progesterone dermatitis and one with estrogen-sensitive dermatitis was conducted to examine the relationship of sex steroid allergy to corticosteroid allergy (41). An extensive patch test evaluation failed to confirm a linkage between the two conditions; furthermore, patch testing with 17-alpha-OH-progesterone was not helpful.

Systematic patch testing with 17-hydroxyprogesterone hexanoate 1% in ethanol revealed that 19.4% of corticosteroid-sensitive patients also reacted to this progesterone (42). It had previously been reported that 26.3% of corticosteroid patients react to progesterone. This is an adrenal hormone in men and women but also has ovarian sources in women. This was felt to be a cross-reaction and was seen more commonly in the setting of allergy to multiple corticosteroid as opposed to solitary corticosteroid sensitivity. The broader the allergy, the more likely the cross-reaction to the sex steroids.

Corticosteroid allergy has produced widespread or generalized eruptions following intralesional, intra-articular, and systemic administration. Corticoids that have been reported to cause generalized eruptions include methylprednisolone, prednisone, dexamethasone, triamcinolone, acetonide, budesonide, and betamethasone (43).

SENSITIZERS IN THE VEHICLES OF TOPICAL CORTICOSTEROIDS

Table 16.5 lists the ingredients of topical corticosteroid preparations that have caused allergic contact dermatitis from their presence in the base. Use of commercial corticosteroid preparations for patch test screening leaves open the possibility that a vehicle ingredient is at fault, but testing both the ointment and the cream formulas of the positive preparations can sometimes quickly resolve this issue. At other times, only patch tests with individual ingredients

TABLE 16.5. *Excipients in Topical Corticosteroids That Have Caused Contact Dermatitis*

Benzyl alcohol
Chlorocresol
Ethylenediamine hydrochloride
Isopropyl palmitate
Parabens
Polysorbate 60
Propylene glycol
Stearyl alcohol
Dioctyl sodium sulfosuccinate
Sodium metabisulfite
1,2,6-hexanetriol

TABLE 16.6. *Topical Corticosteroids Containing Sorbic Acid*

Aristocort Cream (Lederle)[a]
Fluorone Cream (Upjohn)
Hytone Cream (Dermik)
Kenalog Cream (Squibb)
Maxiflor Cream (Herbert)
Pramosone Cream (Ferndale)[a]

[a]Contains both sorbic acid and potassium sorbate. Aristocort A cream is free of these preservatives. *Note:* Sorbitol solution, sorbitan, and polysorbate are emulsifying agents unrelated to sorbic acid.

may be able to answer the academic and practical questions regarding corticosteroid allergy.

Ethylenediamine hydrochloride was undoubtedly the most common cause of topical corticosteroid sensitivity from its presence in original Mycolog Cream, in which it was used as a stabilizer. This ingredient, the parent substance of several antihistamines, is present in aminophylline. It should be noted that original Mycolog Ointment was free of ethylenediamine hydrochloride. Currently, only generic formulations of the original Mycolog formula are available. This compound has been reformulated without ethylenediamine and has replaced the original formula from Squibb as Mycolog II cream.

The paraben preservatives produce allergic hypersensitivity, particularly in OTC preparations, which may contain this preservative. Fisher (44) saw three patients who became allergic to Cortaid Cream, an OTC preparation that contains paraben.

Lazzarini (45) described a patient allergic to triamcinolone, benzyl alcohol, and isopropyl palmitate, ingredients of certain topical corticosteroids. Black (46) reported contact dermatitis from stearyl alcohol in a fluocinonide cream. Oleffe et al. (47) described allergic reactions to chlorocresol and propylene glycol in a steroid cream.

Maibach and Conant (48) described contact urticaria from polysorbate 60, which is present in 1% hydrocortisone cream. It should be noted that polysorbate, an emulsifier, is not related chemically to sorbic acid.

NONALLERGIC COMPLICATIONS OF TOPICAL CORTICOSTEROIDS

Nonspecific Irritation for Sorbic Acid

Table 16.6 lists topical corticosteroids that contain sorbic acid. Sorbic acid is a rare sensitizer, but much more commonly it is a primary urticariogenic agent that produces temporary erythema and a stinging sensation from use of the corticosteroid creams shown in Table 16.6. Unless the stinging reaction is marked, this is not a contraindication for the use of these corticosteroid creams. Stinging and erythema are more marked on the face than elsewhere on the body (7).

Long-Term Complications from the Use of Topical Corticosteroids

These complications are listed in Table 16.7. Robertson and Maibach (49) noted transient vasodilation rather than vasoconstriction occasionally when patch testing with fluorinated corticosteroids. They also observed persistent erythema of the eyelids with repeated application of fluorinated corticosteroids.

> **Sorbic acid, a rare sensitizer, often produces stinging and erythema when used as a preservative in topical corticosteroid preparations. Such reactions are caused by a nonspecific, mild, primarily urticariogenic effect.**

CORTICOSTEROID CREAMS VS. OINTMENTS

Most topical corticosteroid ointments are free of preservatives because they do not contain water as do most creams; therefore, topical ointments are unlikely to be contaminated with mold and bacteria.

Polyethylene Glycols

These chemicals are solvent vehicles, emollients, and emulsion stabilizers. Halog Ointment, Halog Cream, and Cortaid Cream contain low-numbered polyethylene glycol sensitizers.

TABLE 16.7. *Nonallergic Complications of Topical Corticosteroids*

Atrophy
Granuloma of the diaper area
Hypertrichosis
Hypopigmentation
Masking of cutaneous infections
Perioral dermatitis
Sorbic acid, erythema, and stinging
Steroid acne
Steroid rosacea

> Low-numbered polyethylene glycols, particularly the 300 to 400 variety, are much more likely to produce allergic eczematous contact dermatitis and contact urticaria than are the higher numbered compounds.

The lower molecular weight liquid polyethylene glycols (PEGs) varying from 200 to 700 are used extensively as solvent vehicles in topical medicaments. Fisher (50,51) reported four patients who had allergic reactions to these PEGs in topical medications.

Two patients had immediate urticarial reactions to PEG 400. Two other patients had delayed allergic eczematous reactions, one to PEG 200 and one to PEG 300. Cross-reactions occurred among PEG 200, 300, and 400 but not between these liquid polyethylenes and the higher molecular weight solid polyethylenes from 1,000 to 6,000.

Maibach (52) stressed that PEGs of varying molecular weights are used extensively as vehicles in topical medicaments but are not listed as sensitizers in standard reference books.

Braun (53) studied 40 patients who had delayed allergic contact sensitivity to a medication containing nitrofural, a Furacin-like product. In 3 of 40 cases, the active ingredient, nitrofuran, was not the cause of the dermatitis, and the solvent polyethylene glycol 300 was the culprit.

BENZYL ALCOHOL

Benzyl alcohol, also known as alpha-hydroxytoluene, phenylmethanol, and phenylcarbinol, is used in topical corticosteroids as a solvent and a preservative and is also used in perfumes.

> Benzyl alcohol is aromatic, anesthetic, antiseptic, and antipruritic.

Fisher (54) found that two patients who had contact dermatitis, one from a perfume and the other from an aftershave lotion, were sensitized by benzyl alcohol. Both patients had positive patch tests to benzyl alcohol 1% in petrolatum. Neither patient had evidence of immediate-type hypersensitivity.

Schultheiss (55) reported a patient who contacted dermatitis from various flavors for drinks. The patient reacted on patch testing to benzyl alcohol 0.5% in olive oil. He had been sensitized previously to balsam of Peru. Lagerholm (56) reported benzyl-alcohol sensitivity from a vitamin B_{12} injection that had been preserved with benzyl alcohol.

Table 16.8 lists topical corticosteroid preparations that contain benzyl alcohol.

TABLE 16.8. *Topical Corticosteroids Containing Benzyl Alcohol*

Aristocort A Cream
Cordran Cream
Cyclocort Cream
Original Mycolog Cream (in the perfume)

MENTHOL

This antipruritic agent is used in Cordran Lotion. It should be noted that menthol used over a wide area of the body, particularly in elderly persons, may produce a marked chilling effect. Menthol is a rare sensitizer (57,58).

UREA

This compound is present in Alphaderm HC and in Carmol HC. Although urea does not cause contact allergies, it often produces irritation. Thus, Hannuksela (59) stated that burning and itching sensations are the most usual untoward effects of urea creams. The burning and itching disappear usually within 1 hour. Cramers and Thormann (60) stated that under occlusion, urea cream may cause irritation and that patch testing with urea cream often produces an irritant reaction, frequently in intertriginous areas.

PERFUMES

It is likely that many corticosteroid creams contain fragrances. These, however, may be so-called masking fragrances that are not listed in the ingredients of the vehicles. They are usually of such low concentration that they are unlikely to produce allergic contact dermatitis.

SODIUM BISULFITE

This antioxidant, reducing agent is present in Carmol HC Cream. Epstein (61) described a patient who was allergic to the ingredients of Veg-White Powder, which contains sodium bisulfite. Patch tests were positive to 5% and to 10% of sodium bisulfite in petrolatum. Sodium bisulfite is also used to prevent discoloration of fruits and vegetables, particularly of foods used in salads. The presence of this antioxidant in foods has been implicated as the cause of toxicity in some persons. Several controls should be tested with this substance for comparison, because patch testing with sodium bisulfite often leads to irritant patch test reactions.

SODIUM METABISULFITE

Sodium metabisulfite was also a cause of contact dermatitis in an experimental corticosteroid cream evaluated by Vestergaard and Andersen (62). They tested 1% sodium metabisulfite in petrolatum in 54 patients and found 3 doubtful positive reactions. However, their patient had a 2+ reaction to 1% and a delayed 2+ reaction to 0.2% sodium metabisulfite. No reaction was seen to sodium sulfite. Tucker et al. (63) reported contact dermatitis from sodium metabisulfate found in Trimovate cream.

Cumulative irritancy testing of OTC hydrocortisone preparations led to 2 of 50 subjects becoming sensitized to sodium metabisulfite (64). A 1% sodium metabisulfite patch test was positive in these two individuals. Higher concentrations in the range of 5% can produce transient day 2 patch test responses.

DIOCTYL SODIUM SULFOSUCCINATE

Excipients in corticosteroids that have been a cause of contact dermatitis include benzyl alcohol, chlorocresol, ethylenediamine hydrochloride, isopropyl palmitate, parabens, polysorbate 60, propylene glycol, stearyl alcohol, and dioctyl sodium sulfosuccinate (65).

I,2,6-HEXANETRIOL

Miura et al. (66) added 1,2,6-hexanetriol in fluocinonide cream to the list of excipients found in corticosteroids. This agent is used as a humectant and viscosity regulating agent. Patch tests were positive down to 0.5% in petrolatum.

LOCAL ANESTHETICS

Pramasone Lotion (Ferndale) contains hydrocortisone and the local anesthetic pramoxine hydrochloride. There is only one report in the literature of sensitization to this local anesthetic (67,68).

Corticaine Cream contains the local anesthetic dibucaine hydrochloride, which has an amide structure and does not cross-react with benzocaine.

REFERENCES

1. Sams WM, Smith GJ. Contact dermatitis due to hydrocortisone ointment. *JAMA* 1957;164:1212.
2. Kooij R. Hypersensitivity to hydrocortisone. *Br J Dermatol* 1959;71:392.
3. Burckhardt W. Contact eczema caused by hydrocortisone. *Hautarzt* 1959;10:42.
4. Wilkinson RD, McGarry EM, Solomon S. Allergic contact dermatitis to hydrocortisone. *J Invest Dermatol* 1967;43:295.
5. Fisher AA. Paraben dermatitis due to a new medicated bandage: the "paraben paradox." *Contact Dermatitis* 1979;5:273.
6. Fisher AA. The management of propylene glycol–sensitive patients. *Cutis* 1980;25:24.
7. Fisher AA. Cutaneous reactions to sorbic acid and potassium sorbate. *Cutis* 1980;25:350.
8. Alani MD, Alani SD. Allergic contact dermatitis to corticosteroids. *Ann Allergy* 1972;30:181.
9. Coskey RJ. Contact dermatitis due to multiple corticosteroid creams. *Arch Dermatol* 1978;114:115.
10. Zina G, Bonu G. Contact sensitivity to corticosteroids. *Contact Dermatitis Newsletter* 1967;2:26.
11. Brandao FM, Camarasa JM. Contact allergy to hydrocortisone-17-butyrate. *Contact Dermatitis* 1979;5:354.
12. Soesman-van Waadenoden Kernekamp A, van Ketel WG. Contact allergy to hydrocortisone-17-butyrate. *Contact Dermatitis* 1979;5:268.
13. Brown R. Allergy to hydrocortisone-17-butyrate—two more cases. *Contact Dermatitis* 1980;6:504.
14. Dooms-Goosens A, Morren M. Results of routine patch testing with corticosteroid series in 2073 patients. *Contact Dermatitis* 1992;26:182.
15. Boffa MJ, Wilkinson SM, Beck MH. Screening for corticosteroid contact hypersensitivity. *Contact Dermatitis* 1995;33:149.
16. Sasaki E. Corticosteroid sensitivity and cross-sensitivity—a review of 18 cases, 1967–1988 (published erratum appears in *Contact Dermatitis* 1991 Jul;25(1):79). *Contact Dermatitis* 1990;23:306.
17. Dunkel FG, Elsner P, Burg G. Contact allergies to topical corticosteroids: 10 cases of contact dermatitis. *Contact Dermatitis* 1991;25:97.
18. Freeman S. Corticosteroid allergy. *Contact Dermatitis* 1995;33:240.
19. Wilkinson SM, English JS. Hydrocortisone sensitivity: a prospective study of the value of tixocortol pivalate and hydrocortisone acetate as patch test markers. *Contact Dermatitis* 1991;25:132.
20. Wilkinson SM, English JSC. Hydrocortisone sensitivity: an investigation into the nature of the allergen. *Contact Dermatitis* 1991;25:178.
21. Seukeran DC, Wilkinson SM, Beck MH. Patch testing to detect corticosteroid allergy: is it adequate? *Contact Dermatitis* 1997;36:127.
22. Matura M, Lepoittevin JP, Arbez-Gindre C, Goossens A. Testing with corticosteroid aldehydes in corticosteroid-sensitive patients (preliminary results). *Contact Dermatitis* 1998;38:106.
23. Isaksson M, Bruze M, Matura M, Goossens A. Patch testing with low concentrations of budesonide detects contact allergy. *Contact Dermatitis* 1997;37:241.
24. Isaksson M, Bruze M, Goossens A, Lepoittevin JP. Patch testing with budesonide in serial dilutions: the significance of dose, occlusion time and reading time. *Contact Dermatitis* 1999;40:24.
25. Isaksson M, et al. The benefit of patch testing with a corticosteroid at a low concentration. *Am J Contact Dermat* 1999;10:31.
26. Chang YC, Clarke GF, Maibach IH. Provocative use test (PUT) [repeated open application test (ROAT)] in topical corticosteroid allergic contact dermatitis. *Contact Dermatitis* 1997;37:309.
27. Gamboa PM, Jauregui I, Antépara I. Contact dermatitis from budesonide in a nasal spray without cross-reactivity to amcinonide. *Contact Dermatitis* 1991;24:227.
28. Dunkel FG, Elsner P, Burg G. Allergic contact dermatitis from prednicarbate. *Contact Dermatitis* 1991;24:59.
29. Lauerma AI. Screening for corticosteroid contact sensitivity: comparison of tixocortol pivalate, hydrocortisone-17-butyrate and hydrocortisone. *Contact Dermatitis* 1991;24:123.
30. Bircher AJ. Short induction phase of contact allergy to tixocortol pivalate in a nasal spray. *Contact Dermatitis* 1990;22:237.
31. Fernandez de Corres L, et al. Allergic dermatitis from systemic treatment with corticosteroids. *Contact Dermatitis* 1990;22:104.
32. Corazza M, Virgili A. Allergic contact dermatitis from 6-alpha-methylprednisolone aceponate and budesonide. *Contact Dermatitis* 1998;38:356.
33. Quirce S, Alvarez MJ, Olaguibel JM, Tabar AI. Systemic contact dermatitis from oral prednisone. *Contact Dermatitis* 1994;30:53.
34. Villas Martinez F, Navarro Echeverria JA, Joral Badas A, Garmendia Goitia FJ. Prednicarbate contact allergy. *Contact Dermatitis* 1997;37:299.
35. Aguirre Martinez-Falero A, et al. Allergic contact dermatitis from fluocortin butyl. *Contact Dermatitis* 1990;22:241.
36. Stingeni L, Hansel K, Lisi P. Morbilliform erythema-multiforme-like eruption from desoxymethasone. *Contact Dermatitis* 1996;35:363.
37. Miranda-Romero A, et al. Delayed local allergic reaction to intralesional paramethasone acetate. *Contact Dermatitis* 1998;39:31.
38. Wilkinson SM, Beck MH. Fluticasone propionate and mometasone furoate have a low risk of contact sensitization. *Contact Dermatitis* 1996;34:365.
39. Lauerma A, Reitamo S, Maibach HI. Systemic hydrocortisone/cortisol induces allergic skin reactions in presensitized subjects. *J Am Acad Dermatol* 1991;24:182.
40. Schoenmakers A, et al. Corticosteroid or steroid allergy? *Contact Dermatitis* 1992;26:159.
41. Stephens CJM, McFadden JP, Black MM, Rycroft RJ. Autoimmune progesterone dermatitis: absence of contact sensitivity to glucocorticoids, oestrogen and 17-alpha-OH-progesterone. *Contact Dermatitis* 1994;31:108.
42. Wilkinson SM, Beck MH. The significance of positive patch tests to 17-hydroxyprogesterone. *Contact Dermatitis* 1994;30:302.

43. Whitmore SE. Delayed systemic allergic reactions to corticosteroids. *Contact Dermatitis* 1995;32:193.
44. Fisher AA, Cortaid cream dermatitis and the "paraben paradox." J Am Acad Dermatol 1982;6:116–7.
45. Lazzarini S. Contact allergy to benzyl alcohol and isopropyl palmitate, ingredients of topical corticosteroids. *Contact Dermatitis* 1982;8: 349.
46. Black H. Contact dermatitis from stearyl alcohol in Metosyn (fluocinonide) Cream. *Contact Dermatitis* 1975;1:125.
47. Oleffe JA, Blondeel A, DeConinch A. Allergy to chlorocresol and propylene glycol in a steroid cream. *Contact Dermatitis* 1979;5:53.
48. Maibach H, Conant M. Contact urticaria to a corticosteroid cream: Polysorbate 60. *Contact Dermatitis* 1977;3:350.
49. Robertson DK, Maibach HI. Topical corticosteroids. *Int J Dermatol* 1982;21:59.
50. Fisher AA. Contact urticaria to polyethylene glycol. *Cutis* 1977;19: 409.
51. Fisher AA. Immediate and delayed allergic contact reactions to polyethylene glycol. *Contact Dermatitis* 1978;4:135.
52. Maibach HI. Polyethylene glycol: allergic contact dermatitis potential. *Contact Dermatitis* 1975;1:247.
53. Braun W. Contact allergies to polyethylene glycols. *Zeitschrift Fuer Haut-Und Geschlechtskrankheiten* 1969;44:385.
54. Fisher AA. Allergic paraben and benzyl alcohol hypersensitivity relationship of the "delayed" and "immediate" varieties. *Contact Dermatitis* 1975;1:281.
55. Schultheiss E. Benzyl alcohol sensitivity. *Dermatologica Wochenschr* 1957;135:629.
56. Lagerholm B. Hypersensitivity to phenyl-carbinol preservative in Vitamin B_{12} for injection. *Acta Allerg* 1958;23:295.
57. Papa GM, Shelley MB. Menthol hypersensitivity. *JAMA* 1964;189: 546.
58. Camarasa G, Alomar A. Menthol dermatitis from cigarettes. *Contact Dermatitis* 1978;4:169.
59. Hannuksela M. Allergic and toxic reactions caused by cream bases in dermatological patients. *Int J Cosmetic Sci* 1979;1:257.
60. Cramers M, Thormann J. Skin reactions to a urea-containing cream. *Contact Dermatitis* 1981;7:189.
61. Epstein E. Sodium bisulfite. *Contact Dermatitis Newsletter* 1970;7: 155.
62. Vestergaard L, Andersen KE. Allergic contact dermatitis from sodium metabisulfite in a topical preparation. *Am J Contact Dermatitis* 1995; 6:174.
63. Tucker SC, Yell JA, Beck MH. Allergic contact dermatitis from sodium metabisulfite in Trimovate cream. *Contact Dermatitis* 1999;40: 164.
64. Heshmati S, Maibach HI. Active sensitization to sodium metabisulfite in hydrocortisone cream. *Contact Dermatitis* 1999;41:166.
65. Lee AY, Lee KH. Allergic contact dermatitis from dioctyl sodium sulfosuccinate in a topical corticosteroid. *Contact Dermatitis* 1998; 38:355.
66. Miura Y, et al. Allergic contact dermatitis from 1,2,6-hexanetriol in fluocinonide cream. *Contact Dermatitis* 1999;41:118.
67. van Ketel WG. Allergy to pramoxine (Pramocaine). *Contact Dermatitis* 1981;7:49.
68. Fisher AA. Allergic reactions to topical (surface) anesthetics with reference to the safety of tronothane (pramoxine hydrochloride). *Cutis* 1980;25:584.

CHAPTER 17

Allergy to Preservatives and Vehicles in Cosmetics and Toiletries

There are many allergens in topical products such as cosmetics and toiletries. As a group, the preservatives are the most common allergens, closely followed by fragrances (1). Many of the other ingredients, called excipients, can also cause allergic contact dermatis (ACD). This chapter considers the preservatives and other excipients found in cosmetics and skin care products, recognizing that the same chemicals may be found in industrial settings in coolant fluids, lubricants, and so on. Fragrance allergy is discussed in Chapter 21. In addition, some comments on the cosmetic products themselves are given. This chapter is organized into the following subsections:

1. **Formaldehyde and formaldehyde-releasing preservatives**
2. **Other common preservatives**
3. **Less common preservative allergens**
4. **Other additives in topical products**
5. **Vehicles**
6. **Cosmetics and toiletries**

FORMALDEHYDE

Formaldehyde is a common allergen and is a widely used chemical substance found in a variety of applications. A partial listing of formaldehyde-containing products is given in Table 17.1. Apart from specific occupational exposures, the most frequent sources of exposure include skin and hair care products and cosmetics, along with permanent press textiles. Extremely sensitive individuals may react to formaldehyde in paper or smoke. Certain cleaning products, disinfectants, and medications may contain formaldehyde.

The most recent data from the North American Contact Dermatitis Group (NACDG) (2) showed that formaldehyde was positive in 9.3% of 3,440 patients, ranking seventh of all 50 allergens tested.

In addition to causing ACD, formaldehyde vapors may irritate the conjunctiva and nasal mucosa. Formaldehyde may cause cutaneous irritation and contact urticaria (3).

Formaldehyde in Skin Care Products

Formaldehyde itself is rarely listed on ingredient labels as a component of cosmetics and toiletries. In fact, its direct use is forbidden in countries such as Sweden and Japan (4). However, several preservatives degrade to release formaldehyde as a partial mode of action. Formaldehyde may be present in some other ingredients as an impurity. It has been speculated that formaldehyde may be released from some plastic bottles and tubes into the product contained therein.

Some plastic tubes intended for cosmetics and hand lotions were coated on the outside with melamine or carbamide-formaldehyde resin. Examination revealed that formaldehyde was present in 39 of 113 tubes. The tubes coated with the formaldehyde resins were filled with formaldehyde-free oil in water and water in oil preparations, water, and peanut oil. After 1 or 2 months the analysis revealed that the contents in tubes coated with melamine or carbamide-formaldehyde resin contained formaldehyde (5).

Persistence of Formaldehyde Allergy

Formaldehyde allergy is common, and formaldehyde is present in many products encountered on a daily basis. Patients with formaldehyde allergy must be instructed that time and persistent treatment are necessary for clearing to occur. Perhaps more than with any other allergen, the dermatologist must remind the patient that slow resolution is expected even if the patient attempts careful allergen avoidance. To illustrate this, Agner et al. (6) reported a follow-up study of 57 patients diagnosed with ACD to formaldehyde several years previously. Twenty-eight were clear or nearly so, but 29 (51%) still had frequent or constant dermatitis. Of 709 products analyzed for formaldehyde, 25% were positive. These included cosmetics, toiletries, household cleaners, and paper.

TABLE 17.1. *Formaldehyde Uses and Exposure*

1. Clothing: wash and wear, antiwrinkle, sizing, antishrink, alkali stabilization, stabilization of casein, and mordant for dyes (occurs free or in combination with urea)
    a. wearing apparel that may contain formaldehyde resins and some free formaldehyde:
        Permanent press
        Anticling finishes
        Antistatic finishes
        Chlorine-resistant finishes
        Stiffening on lightweight nylon knits
        Anticurl or lightweight knits
        Waterproof finishes
        Perspiration-proof finishes
        Mothproof finishes
        Mildew-resistant fabrics
        Screen-printed fabrics
        Suede and chamois
    b. formaldehyde-sensitive individuals can usually wear without difficulty clothing made from a single fiber, such as 100% cotton, polyester (Dacron, Fortrel, Avlin, Trevera, and Quintesse), nylon, or acrylic (Orlon, Creslan, and Zephran)
2. Glues, papers, and wet-strength tissues made water-resistant with gelatin and starch. Library and school pastes. Rubber cements. Cements for paper cups and plywood
3. Embalming fluid and fixatives
4. Photographic plates, papers, print-flattening solutions, hypo-test solution, hardeners, and toners
5. Cosmetics and personal care products containing formaldehyde releasing preservatives
6. Fumigators—formaldehyde, para-formaldehyde, and $KMnO_4$
7. Some household cleaners—rug, tire, toilet bowl, and window
8. Some polishes—automobile, cement floor, shoe, and suede shoe
9. Certain medications:
    a. some wart remedies
    b. anhidrotics
    c. formitol mouthwash
    d. antidote for mercury poisoning (sodium formaldehyde sulfoxylate)
    e. methenamine USP (Mandelamine, Tetraiodide, Helmitol, Hexalet, Salixchin, Argolaval, Felemine, and Urised)
    f. denatured alcohol
    g. renal dialysis unit disinfectants
    h. root canal preparation disinfectant (Forno-Cresol)
10. Cellulose esters
11. Products used in the manufacture of explosives
12. Mildew preventative in some fruits and vegetables
13. Disinfectants used in dairy equipment
14. Preservative and coagulant of rubber latex
15. Some paints—primers, model toy and gloss enamels, tempera, fingerpaint, anticorrosion paint, and paint-stripping agents
16. Some tanning agents (not chrome)
17. Printing-etching materials, inks (marking), sealers for cylinder die rolls, "autoprime" used in offset printing machines
18. Canned ice
19. Reducing agent for recovery of silver and gold
20. Some dry-cleaning spotting agents
21. Coatings and adhesives—phenol, melamine, urea, sulfonamide, and cashew nutshell–type resins
22. Smoke contact and inhalation: formaldehyde is a component of smoke from burning wood, coal, charcoal, cigarettes, and cigars

Formaldehyde-Releasing Preservatives

The five commonly used formaldehyde-releasing preservatives (FRP) are listed in Table 17.2. These substances are antibacterial and antifungal in their own right. They may be used alone or in combination with other agents, such as parabens. Generally, the concentration in a commercial product varies between 0.1% and 0.2%. The free formaldehyde concentrations, therefore, would be even lower. Unfortunately, the highest safe level to avoid ACD to these agents is unknown. Presumably, even low concentrations of

an allergen, applied repeatedly to irritated or abnormal skin, may induce sensitization and expression of ACD. Accordingly, patients allergic to formaldehyde should avoid all the formaldehyde releasers.

Quaternium-15

Quaternium-15 (Q-15) is one of the most widely used topical preservatives. Shampoos and conditioners, eye makeup, foundation makeup, lotions and creams, shaving products,

TABLE 17.2. *Formaldehyde-Releasing Preservatives*

Bronopol
Diazolidinyl urea
DMDM hydantoin
Imidazolidinyl urea
Quaternium-15

bath gels, liquid soaps, and dusting powders may contain Q-15. Older names and trade names (which are not now used in labeling in the United States) include Dowicil 75, 100, or 200; *N*-(3-chlorallyl)-hexaminium chloride; and chlorallyl methenamine chloride. Q-15 is highly soluble in water, odorless, and colorless. Its antimicrobial activity is independent of the pH of the product.

Most, but not all, individuals allergic to Q-15 are also allergic to formaldehyde. Some cross- or co-reactivity occurs between Q-15 and other FRPs as well (3). Q-15 was the sixth most common allergen in a study by the NACDG between 1985 and 1989 (7). Of 4,000 patients tested, 6.2% had positive reactions to Q-15 (2% pet). The most recent ranking of Q-15 in North America is eighth, with 9.0% of 3,436 patients tested positive. It is a much more common allergen in the United States than any of the other topical preservatives (1,2,7). However, studies in Europe have shown a prevalence rate of positive tests between 1% and 3% (8). This discrepancy is likely due to different usage rates in various regions and countries.

Q-15 may be an occupational allergen, but the frequency is no greater than for the general patch test clinic population. Health care workers, hair stylists, and machine tool workers may be exposed to Q-15 in hand cleansers and lotions, hair care products, and cutting fluids (9).

Parker and Taylor (10) studied 89 patients allergic to Q-15 over a 5-year period. They found that neither atopy nor gender had any bearing on Q-15 allergy. However, there were significantly more black (10.4%) than white (5.7%) patients with Q-15 allergy. No reason for this was given. Moisturizers were by far the leading source of Q-15 exposure, occuring in 79% of the patients. Noncoloring hair care products accounted for exposure in one-third of the patients, whereas makeup accounted for about 12%. Fifty-five percent of patients were also allergic to formaldehyde, whereas reactions to other FRPs occurred in 3% to 6%.

> **Skin moisturizers are the major source of sensitization to quaternium-15.**

It should be noted that other quaternium compounds are used in some cosmetics, cleaning agents, and industrial products. Quaternium-15 is the only formaldehyde releaser and the major sensitizer. Cross-reactivity among the various quaterniums has not been shown to occur.

> **Other quaterniums may be safely used by those sensitive to quaternium-15.**

Diazolidinyl Urea

Diazolidinyl urea (DiU) is the newest of the FRPs. It was introduced in 1982 as Germall II. As with quaternium-15, it is effective at various pH levels, is soluble in water, and has a broad spectrum of activity. It is a superior biocide to imidazolidinyl urea (ImU) but is usually combined with another agent for antifungal efficacy. In 1987, DiU was ranked twentieth on the list of preservative usage compiled by the Food and Drug Administration (FDA) from voluntary reporting, but due to increasing usage, is likely higher today.

Jordan (11) found DiU to be a stronger sensitizer than ImU in human volunteers. In guinea pigs it was found to be a "mild sensitizer" (12). Unpublished data compiled by the NACDG from 1996 to 1998 showed a prevalence of positive reactions to DiU of 3.7%. This was higher than the prevalence rate for ImU, DMDM hydantoin, or bronopol but much lower than for Q-15. Cross-sensitivity between DiU and ImU is common but does not always occur.

Imidazolidinyl Urea

Imidazolidinyl urea (ImU), also known as Germall 115, is one of the most commonly used cosmetic preservatives after the parabens. It is reported to be nontoxic and nonirritating (13). This preservative is compatible with almost all cosmetic ingredients. Its water solubility is high and its oil solubility low. It is colorless, odorless, and tasteless, and is not pH-dependent. ImU is more active against bacteria than against yeast and molds. It is active against both gram-positive and gram-negative organisms. Against yeast and molds it is selectively effective (14).

A key property of ImU is its ability to act synergistically with other preservatives, particularly with the parabens, which results in a preservative system that gives not only a wider range of protection against microbial insult but also a greater preservative capacity. Rosen et al. (15) reported that a model cosmetic lotion containing 0.2% methyl paraben and 0.1% propylparaben was shown previously to be unsatisfactorily preserved, because it failed to kill *Pseudomonas aeruginosa*. The addition of 0.3% imidazolidinyl urea to the lotion gave an imidazolidinyl urea–paraben preservative system, which was effective against both an initial challenge of *P. aeruginosa* and two rechallenges.

Theoretically, ImU releases about one-eighth as much formaldehyde as Q-15 (16). In one report, only 6 of 15 ImU-sensitive patients also reacted to formaldehyde (17). Although guinea pig sensitization testing has given equivocal results, clinical patch test studies suggest ImU is a less frequent sensitizer than formaldehyde or Q-15 and slightly less frequent than DiU (2,18). Fisher (19,20) studied 30 formaldehyde-allergic patients and found that only 1 reacted to ImU, whereas 9 reacted to Q-15.

Bronopol

Bronopol (BNPD; 2-bromo-2-nitropropane-1,3-diol) has been used as a preservative, most commonly in cosmetic product formulations (21). It is an odorless, colorless, crystalline solid that is soluble in water, alcohols, glycols, and, to a lesser extent, oils (22). BNPD has a wide range of antimicrobial properties and is active against gram-positive and gram-negative bacteria, fungi, and yeasts (23–25). It is particularly effective against *P. aeruginosa* (26).

According to data from the FDA in 1987, BNPD was the thirteenth most commonly used preservative in cosmetic formulations. Most often, products contain bronopol in concentrations of less than 0.1%. The largest group consists of makeup bases, followed by hair conditioners, blushers, cleansing preparations, and eyebrow pencils. Many shampoos, moisturizers, and other cosmetics contain from 0.1% to 1% BNPD. Although BNPD is usually encountered in cosmetics, it has also been used as a preservative for milk samples (27), as well as an additive in simulated silage (28).

Peters et al. (21) reported that an analysis of patch tests performed on their patients revealed an incidence of 12.5% relevant positive results to 0.5% or 0.25% BNPD. This result reflects a history of prolonged use of BNPD-containing lubricants in their referral population of patients with different types of severe, extensive dermatitis. Contact sensitization to BNPD in this population is probably facilitated by abnormal cutaneous barrier function.

Storrs and Bell (29) described seven patients who developed acute allergic contact dermatitis after using Eucerin cream on previously dermatitic skin from 5 weeks to 2 years. In 1978, Eucerin was preserved with BNPD to assist in controlling a problem with *P. aeruginosa* contamination. All of the patients were BNPD and Eucerin patch test positive.

> **Bronopol, in Eucerin cream and lotion, which produced allergic contact dermatitis on dermatitic skin but not on normal skin, has been replaced by MCI/MI.**

In the United States the rate of positivity in patch test clinic patients has remained stable at about 2% to 3% since the late 1970s. In other countries, a range of 0.5% to 1.5% positivity is common. Possibly this discrepancy is due to different usage patterns, because test concentration in Europe was equal to or greater than the concentrations used in the United States (0.5% pet).

Microbicidal activity of BNPD is excellent. However, degradation to formaldehyde may limit the shelf life of products containing BNPD. Also, BNPD is a cutaneous irritant in concentrations as low as 0.5% to 1.0%. Whether it is due to these or other reasons, the use of BNPD by the cosmetics industry is on the decline.

Because BNPD may be an irritant, patch tests should not be done at a concentration of more than 0.5% pet.

DMDM Hydantoin

DMDM hydantoin (DMDMH) is a colorless liquid marketed under the name Glydant. It contains 0.5% to 2% free formaldehyde and over 17% combined formaldehyde (30). Accordingly, formaldehyde-allergic patients would definitely be expected to react to DMDMH both in patch testing and from clinical use. Fransway and Schmitz (9) estimate that over 200 ppm formaldehyde would be present in cosmetics preserved with DMDMH. This exceeds recommended threshold levels. DeGroot et al. (31) tested formaldehyde-allergic persons to DMDMH along with two related compounds: DMH, which does not contain formaldehyde, and MDMH, a chemical intermediate. None of the patients reacted to DMH. Seven of 21 (33%) reacted to MDMH, and 8 of 15 (57%) reacted to DMDMH.

The NACDG testing with 1% aqueous and 1% petrolatum found 1.9% and 2.6% positive, respectively (2). Testing at 3% aqueous, deGroot (32) found 1.2% of patients positive. The amount of formaldehyde present, along with the degree of usage of DMDMH, suggests that this allergen should be included on patch test (PT) screening series.

Formaldehyde and Related Agents Used in Medications

Paraformaldehyde has been used in deodorant and fumigating preparations. Hexamethylenetetramine (methenamine), which decomposes into formaldehyde, is used as a urinary antiseptic. These are covered in Chapter 10 (see Tables 17.3 and 17.4).

TABLE 17.3. *Paraformaldehyde Medicaments*

Buckley's Paraformal paste topical anesthetic and zinc oxide
Cardinal Stop mildew preventive
Cenol Foot Joy foot bath
D-Odor Tabs air freshener and deodorizer (Circle Chemicals)
Dr. Scholl's preparations
  Bromidrosis powder
  Foot Magic spray
  Foot Magic foot spray aerosol lotion
  Foot Magic foot spray deodorant
Orocide deodorant powder and preservative
Paraformal paste desensitizer for hypersensitive dentin (Crosby Labs)

TABLE 17.4. *Formaldehyde-Releasing Urinary Antiseptics*

Methavin
Methenamine
  Urised
Methenamine hippurate
  Hiprex
  Urex
Methenamine and sodium acid phosphate
  Uro-phosphate
Methenamine mandelate
Methenamine mandelate with sodium acid phosphate
  Uroquid-Acid
Methenamine mandelate with phenazopyridine
    hydrochloride
  Azo-Mandelamine
Proklar
Prosed
Trac Tabs
Uristat
Urotropin

FRPs in Metalworking Fluids

A number of FRPs are used as biocides to retard bacterial and fungal contamination of coolant and cutting oils. Machinists allergic to these may also react to formaldehyde and FRPs in skin care products. This is discussed in Chapter 25 (Table 17.5).

Formaldehyde in Clothing

Individuals may react to either formaldehyde or formaldehyde-based textile resins present in permanent press clothing. Cross-reaction with FRPs may confuse the clinical pattern and complicate therapy (see Chapter 19).

Occupational Formaldehyde Allergy

Sterilizing agents and fumigants have caused ACD in brewery workers (33), mushroom (34) and poultry farmers (35), workers making binders for paints and glues (36), newsprint workers (37), woodworkers (38), and lithoprinters (39). Formaldehyde may occur in photography-developing chemicals and steel foundry molds (40).

Contact Urticaria to Formaldehyde

Formaldehyde has been reported as a rare cause of contact urticaria (CU). Three dental patients experienced anaphy-

TABLE 17.5. *Miscellaneous Formaldehyde-Releasing Compounds*

Bakzid	Preventol D1, D2, D3
Bioban	Taurolin
Dantoin	Trisnitro
Dimethylol urea	Tryosan
Hydantoin (glycourea)	Vancide TH
Nuosept	

lactoid reactions after receiving treatment with a paraformaldehyde/cresol mix (3). Skin prick tests were negative, but serum RAST tests were positive to formaldehyde 1% aqueous.

Tests for the Presence of Formaldehyde

The chromotropic acid test, which has been used since the 1930s for the detection of formaldehyde, is limited in its usefulness by the occurrence of frequent false-positive reactions. Fregert and colleagues (41) in 1984 popularized the acetylacetone method, which follows:

Reagent: ammonium acetate 15 g; acetylacetone 0.2 ml; acetic acid (Glacial) 0.3 ml; distilled water to 100 ml.

Procedure: Add 2.5 ml of the reagent to the sample in a clean glass container. Sample size about 0.5 g. Solids and liquids are tested as is. Ointments, oils, or greasy products are mixed with a few drops of Triton X-100 (Merck), an emulsifying agent. Heat the mixture for 10 minutes at 140°F (60°C). A yellow color develops if formaldehyde is present. This is due to the formation of 3.5 diacetyl-1,4-dihydrolutidine. Positive controls (0.025% to 0.1% formaldehyde) and a negative control (distilled water) should be tested for comparison.

A comparison of this method with high-performance liquid chromatography (HPLC) showed that the acetylacetone test was positive down to about 4 ppm (42). The chromotropic acid method was not as sensitive and frequently produced a nonspecific discoloration, which obscured the test results.

The Extent of Exposure in Formaldehyde-Sensitive Patients

Flyvholm and Menné (43) performed an extensive evaluation of 11 patients with formaldehyde allergy. By using computer records, contacting manufacturers, chemically analyzing products, and so on, they studied not only skin care products but also cleaning products and other household and occupational items suspected of containing formaldehyde. The list of products containing formaldehyde is shown in Table 17.6.

TABLE 17.6. *Types of Formaldehyde-Containing Products in a Danish Study of 11 Patients*

Skin and hair care products
Cosmetics
Deodorants
Dishwashing liquid
Liquid soap
Photographic developer
Water-based paint
Laundry detergent (liquid)
Plastic bags
Paper products
Foam rubber

Source: Flyvholm and Menné (43).

Cronin (44) described 62 women with hand eczema who were allergic to formaldehyde. In 23 of the women, extensive investigations were conducted looking at personal care and household cleaning products. Twenty of the 23 had been using formaldehyde-containing products. Household products containing formaldehyde included dishwashing liquids, furniture polishes, and a window cleaner.

These studies illustrate the ubiquitous occurrence of formaldehyde in everyday usage.

Formaldehyde Reactions to Medicaments and Medical Devices

Logan and Perry (45) reported three patients with allergic contact dermatitis due to exposure to orthopedic casts. In each instance, the causative agent was considered to be free formaldehyde derived from the melamine formaldehyde resin incorporated into certain casts. All patients had positive patch tests to formaldehyde, and free formaldehyde was demonstrated in the cast material. Patch tests to the plaster itself were negative when fresh plaster was used but were positive with the use of aged plaster.

Fabry (46) cited a patient who was given two injections of antitetanus vaccine (Tetanol made by Behringwerke). Eight weeks after the second injection, he had generalized urticaria. Scratch, patch, or intradermal tests were not performed. Passive transfer PK test was positive with formalin and with Tetanol. Tetanol is an aluminum hydroxide/formol adsorption vaccine.

> **"Hidden" sources of formaldehyde exposure in medicine include certain orthopedic casts, vaccines, injectable antibiotics, and renal dialysis units.**

Renal Dialysis Units

In some renal dialysis units, 2% to 4% formaldehyde solutions are used for sterilization and for home kidney machines. Sneddon (47) reported that in one such unit, 6 of 13 staff members developed dermatitis of the eyelids, face, and hands. Patch tests showed that four people were sensitive to formaldehyde.

Abdel-Aziz and Hodgson (48) reported a man who used formaldehyde to sterilize his wife's kidney machine and who presented with extensive eczema of his hands and arms; patch testing confirmed his sensitivity to formaldehyde. Three cases of formaldehyde dermatitis occurred in the hospital's dialysis unit.

Some individuals exposed to formaldehyde to sterilize artificial kidney machines may develop asthma (49).

One Formaldehyde-Sensitive Patient's Experience

A 26-year-old woman was referred for the management of a marked formaldehyde sensitivity confirmed by a strongly positive, spreading, pruritic, vesiculopapular patch test reaction to 1% aqueous solution of formaldehyde. The patient, a textile designer and freelance artist, may have acquired her formaldehyde sensitivity in a high school biology class while dissecting animals preserved in formaldehyde.

The patient is a member of the American Association of Textile Chemists and Colorists, and by persistent inquiries and correspondence she has acquired an encyclopedic knowledge of products containing formaldehyde that must be avoided in order to control her dermatitis.

Fisher reports:

> To my chagrin, after lying on the table paper of my office examining table for a short while on her initial visit, [the patient] complained of itching on her back and arms, areas which at the time were free of dermatitis. Within an hour a diffuse, erythematous maculopapular eruption developed on the dorsal aspect of her shoulders, arms, and entire back. It was ascertained subsequently that the glossy table paper contained a formaldehyde resin and free formaldehyde. The shiny, heavy, more expensive table paper is much more likely to contain formaldehyde than is the thinner, less expensive, duller, more fragile type of paper. To be on the safe side, formaldehyde-sensitive patients should be protected from table paper with an all-cotton sheet.

The handling of most newspapers, magazines, and both hardcover and paperback books produces dermatitis in this patient. Handling glossy paper readily produces dermatitis.

This patient also acquires dermatitis from many types of paper tissues, paper towels, and paper plates and cups except Marcal brand products. It is of interest to note that, although formaldehyde is not present in the actual ingredients of Dixie brand plates and cups, there is a minute quantity of formaldehyde in the lubricants used to keep the paperboard from wrinkling during their manufacture.

The patient found that she could not tolerate any art paper used for acrylic paint or water colors, except paper with the Grumbacher label. Incidentally, she tolerates Bon-cour brand acrylic paint, but not Liquitex (50).

The following excerpts are from a letter recently obtained from Fisher's patient describing some of her trials and tribulations due to formaldehyde sensitivity:

> Avoiding formaldehyde completely is next to impossible. There is always one more product or item of clothing which is suspect. While I am free of major dermatitis at present, it is a constant battle to keep exposure to a minimum. The troublesome items and situations to avoid are books, newspapers, and magazines, formaldehyde fumes from a gas stove (confirmed by the Gas Company), and smoke from cigarettes. Most typewriter ribbons give me trouble.
>
> I have had some difficulty with permanent press upholstery in furniture and in automobiles. I find a cotton towel handy to put on chairs and in cars. I recently acquired a contact dermatitis by leaning on a neighbor's plastic tablecloth. A pollution face mask to filter dust while cleaning produced a dermatitis on my face. One must be careful that an ironing board cover does not contain any formaldehyde because ironing formaldehyde-free fabrics on such a board

will contaminate the fabrics. Also, I'm having trouble with clotheslines, and I can't use electric curlers because the heat must be vaporizing formaldehyde from the plastic.

> **Formaldehyde-sensitive individuals can acquire dermatitis from many paper products, including newspaper, magazines, books, paper towels, tissues, paper plates and cups, art paper, and photography paper.**

Formaldehyde in Paper Products and Newsprint

There are several reports describing the presence of free formaldehyde in various paper products (44,51,52). Simpson (53) reported formaldehyde dermatitis from an offset printing machine. The "autoprime" used in the machine contained formaldehyde.

In connection with paper dermatitis, Black (54) reported a formaldehyde-sensitive individual who was allergic to blank newsprint. The estimation of free formaldehyde content of the newsprint showed it to be 0.02%. A similar estimation done on paper towels used in his hospital as an "economy" measure was 0.03%.

Effect of Formaldehyde on Food

Thomsen (55) described a housewife who complained to the Association of Danish Cooperative Societies that the gelatin she bought was impossible to melt, even by prolonged boiling. The gelatin had been exposed to formaldehyde from an air cleaner. Aldehydes even in such minute concentrations can make gelatin "insoluble." Other similar complaints could be traced to formaldehyde vapor from varnish from kitchen cupboards. Sufficient formaldehyde can be released even from dry varnish without any scent of formaldehyde.

Gluten flour is deteriorated by formaldehyde. Dough made from such formaldehyde-contaminated flour will not "rise" and becomes unsuitable for consumption.

The Presence of Formaldehyde in Some SLS Preparations

A 37-year-old woman who had atopic dermatitis was informed that she was "allergic" to sodium lauryl sulfate (SLS) and would have to avoid the numerous cosmetics and topical agents containing this surfactant. The patient apparently had not been patch tested with formaldehyde.

Patch testing with a "screening" tray revealed a strongly positive patch test reaction to formaldehyde. Then, patch testing was performed with three batches of SLS (5% aq solution) from three different sources. The patient had a positive reaction to two of the SLS preparations but not to the third (56).

Although no mention is made in the dermatologic literature that formaldehyde is used as a preservative in some SLS solutions, it was suspected from the results of this patient's patch tests that formaldehyde may have been present.

The three solutions of SLS that had been used for patch testing this formaldehyde-sensitive patient were sent for qualitative chemical analyses to determine if formaldchyde was present. The two SLS solutions to which the patient had had a positive reaction were proven by qualitative chemical analyses to contain formaldehyde, whereas the SLS solution to which the patient had had a negative reaction was proven not to contain formaldehyde.

We then corresponded with the three manufacturers of the different SLS solutions and received the following replies: (a) "This is to inform you that some of our SLS products do contain formalin at a 0.1% level as a preservative"; (b) "The use of formalin as a preservative in SLS is a function of consumer demand. Shampoo manufacturers usually request preserved SLS. Certain other users request nonpreserved SLS"; and (c) "We add formalin to our SLS (liquid) on customer request."

It was learned subsequently that many major suppliers of SLS routinely add approximately 0.1% formalin (formalin is 37% wt/wt formaldehyde in water) to their bulk SLS surfactant to preserve it, and that many pharmaceutical manufacturers are not aware of this fact.

> **Certain batches of sodium lauryl sulfate (SLS) contain formaldehyde as a preservative.**

Where There's Smoke, There May Be Formaldehyde

Formaldehyde is a component of smoke from burning wood, coal, charcoal, cigarettes, and cigars. According to the Office of the Surgeon General of the United States, cigarette smoke contains 30 parts of formaldehyde per million, which is six times the safe level for industrial exposure.

One patient of Fisher's stated that her gas company has confirmed the fact that fumes from a gas stove may contain free formaldehyde. In a follow-up letter, she wrote: "Parties where a number of people are smoking and there is a wood fire burning are particularly hazardous to me. I learned to be careful of exposure time and ask for ventilation to prevent a formaldehyde 'hangover' of dermatitis, burning eyes, lethargy, and depression."

Smoked ham and fish, containing traces of formaldehyde, may have to be avoided by formaldehyde-sensitive individuals.

> **All sources of smoke, including smoked ham and fish, may contain traces of formaldehyde.**

Patch Testing with Formaldehyde

Most centers recommend patch testing with formaldehyde 1% in water. Fowler has noted occasional patients who react only to 2% in water. Trattner et al. (57), however, recommend testing at 1% because of increased irritation from the 2% solution. About half of 121 patients were positive to both concentrations, with 32% positive only to 2% and 19% positive only to 1%.

ALLERGY TO OTHER COMMON PRESERVATIVES: PARABENS, MCI/MI, MDGN/PE, AND IPBC

The Parabens

The propyl- and methylparaben esters are popular preservatives incorporated into many cosmetics and topical therapeutic agents to prevent bacterial and fungal contamination. The other paraben esters commonly used are ethyl-, butyl-, and benzylparabens. In addition, many parenterally administered medications, especially those in multidose packages, also contain parabens as preservatives. These paraben-containing parenterals include antibiotics, corticosteroids, local anesthetics, radiopharmaceuticals, vitamins, antihypertensives, diuretics, insulin, heparin, and chemotherapeutic agents. The parabens are rated second only to water as the ingredient most commonly used in cosmetic formulations (58). The parabens are more active against gram-positive than against gram-negative organisms; as such, they react poorly against *Pseudomonas*. Generally, parabens are less active against bacteria than against yeast and molds, although the properties of the individual parabens differ in this regard (59). The parabens are often used in combination with other preservatives. They are colorless, odorless, and nonvolatile. Relative insolubility in water may help explain their poor activity against *P. aeruginosa*. Lorenzetti & Weet (58) states that the parabens meet several of the criteria of an ideal preservative in that they have a broad spectrum of antimicrobial activity, are safe to use (i.e., are relatively nonirritating, nonsensitizing, and nonpoisonous), and are stable over the pH range encountered in cosmetics. In the United States, the paraben concentration in cosmetics is generally less than 0.3%, and a typical paraben preservative system contains 0.2% methyl- and 0.1% propylparaben. Parabens are inactivated by nonionic surfactants. Propylene glycol potentiates paraben activity.

Considering the volume of paraben use, incidence of allergy to them is relatively low compared to the other common preservatives. For example, the NACDG reported allergy to the paraben mix (15% pet) in 1.7% of 4,096 patients (2) . In comparison, quaternium-15 was positive in 9.0% and methylchloroisothiazolinone/methylisothiazolinone (MCI/MI) in 2.9%. Similarly, Schnuch et al. (60) reported that parabens were positive in 1.6% of over 28,000 patients tested with a screening series, the lowest of the common preservatives.

The "Paraben Paradox"

Several puzzling aspects to the use of paraben preservatives are discussed as "paradoxes" (61).

Why do the parabens in topical therapeutic agents sensitize about 1.5% of the population, whereas these identical parabens are "safe" in cosmetics so widely used by millions of individuals? Various investigators have found so many instances of sensitization to the parabens in various topical therapeutic agents that most pharmaceutical manufacturers have removed the parabens from topical therapeutic agents and have replaced them with other preservatives (62–65). No similar attempt to remove the parabens from cosmetics has been attempted or seems to be necessary. Indeed, for example, most mascara preparations on the market, including the so-called hypoallergenic variety, still contain the parabens. Why is it, then, usually safe to use paraben-containing cosmetics without any difficulty, even on the thin skin of the eyelids?

The answer to this seeming paradox is that mascara and other cosmetics are usually applied to normal skin, whereas therapeutic agents are applied to inflamed, eczematous, excoriated, or otherwise damaged skin, which is much more readily sensitized than even the thinnest skin. Indeed, some women who are allergic to the parabens can nevertheless apply paraben-containing cosmetics, providing the cosmetic is applied to skin that is normal at the time of application and has not been subjected to a dermatitis in the past. It appears that sites of healed dermatitis sometimes flare when a sensitizer is applied, whereas skin that has never been the site of dermatitis does not react in the sensitized individual. This may be due to local populations of sensitized T lymphocytes residing in the area.

> A combination of methyl- and propylparabens is the most widely used of antibacterial and antifungal preservatives in cosmetics both in the United States and in other countries.

Simpson (66) reports a rare instance of a patient with allergic hypersensitivity to parabens in several cosmetic preparations. This dermatologist agrees that most patients who have sensitivity to parabens can tolerate cosmetics in which they are contained.

Brauer (67) states that "[i]t is generally recognized by the food, drug, and cosmetic industries, by worldwide health ministries, as well as by dermatologists who have extensive experience in contact dermatitis with consumer products, that the parabens are representative of the best preservative agents. The consumer population would be ill-served were the parabens to be deleted from commercial use."

Marzulli and Maibach (68) reviewed the literature and concluded that "[t]he clinical impression reported by Fisher et al. (69) was that whereas occasional cases of paraben sensitivity occur and are important to the stricken patient's welfare, sensitization is low when the extensive use of the material is considered."

The benefit/risk ratio for the use of parabens in cosmetics is high. The cosmetic microbiologist recognizes that preservatives must be used to ensure product stability and safety and that the parabens are among the most innocuous preservatives. The parabens, therefore, are the preservatives of choice for most formulations. The widespread use of the parabens in cosmetic products made in the United States gives testimony to their safety and effectiveness.

Finally, it must be reemphasized that allergic contact dermatitis from the parabens in cosmetics is rare. Although patients who have such a rare paraben sensitivity could readily obtain paraben-free topical medications, they would have great difficulty finding paraben-free cosmetics.

Why do paraben-containing therapeutic agents, which have caused an allergic contact dermatitis in paraben-sensitive individuals, often produce false-negative patch test reactions? This situation is not unique for the parabens, because it is known that a topical medication may sometimes give a false-negative patch test reaction in a sensitized individual even though it contains chemicals that are sensitizers and have produced a severe allergic contact dermatitis in the patient.

Such false reactions may be due to the following causes: (a) A patch test is performed on normal skin. The dermatitis-producing medication, of course, is used on inflamed, eczematous, or ulcerated skin; (b) the vehicle may contain a corticosteroid that can suppress a mild allergic reaction on a patch test site, but not on abnormal skin; or (c) the concentration of the vehicle ingredient that is producing the allergic reaction is too low to produce a positive patch test reaction. For example, the parabens are used in a concentration of less than 0.5% as preservatives in vehicles, but a concentration of at least 3% is necessary to produce a positive patch test reaction on the *normal* skin in the sensitized individual where the patch test is applied.

Paraben-containing therapeutic agents, which have caused allergic contact dermatitis in paraben-sensitive patients, may produce false-negative patch reactions because the paraben concentration is too low to give a positive reaction on normal skin. A patch test with a higher concentrated "paraben mix" must be used to detect allergic hypersensitivity.

Fisher (70) reported two patients who had allergic contact sensitivity to the parabens. One patient had applied a corticosteroid cream to a stasis ulcer, with a resulting superimposed allergic contact dermatitis. The other patient had atopic dermatitis, with a superimposed allergic contact dermatitis from a corticosteroid cream containing the

parabens. Both of these individuals had strongly positive patch tests to the parabens.

These individuals showed negative reactions to scratch, intracutaneous, and subcutaneous injections of paraben-stabilized solutions containing methylparaben 0.12% and propylparaben 0.012% in saline.

Why are there conflicting reports concerning cross-reactions between the parabens and the so-called para group?

The "para" groups include para-aminobenzoic acid (PABA), whose esters form local anesthetics, and para-phenylenediamine, used in hair dyes. Rudzki and Kleniewska (71) point out that some authorities (e.g., Paschoud) include the parabens (esters of parahydroxybenzene acid) in the "para" group, whereas others do not. In their study, Rudzki and Kleniewska found that of 144 para-phenylenediamine-sensitive patients, 20 were also allergic to parabens, and that of 63 benzocaine-sensitive individuals, 20 were allergic to the parabens.

Aldrete and Johnson (72) studied a patient who illustrated a cross-reaction between PABA esters and paraben.

As far as the parabens are concerned, in his material Fisher has not noted cross-reactions of parahydroxybenzoic acid esters with the other "para" compounds or with benzoic acid itself. However, Fowler (unpublished observation) has seen several cases with positive patch tests to parabens, PABA, and paraphenylenediamine that appeared to be true cross-reactions.

The concept that parabens are not as significant as formaldehyde-releasing preservatives is confirmed by several prevalence studies. The NACDG in 1985 reported on 713 patients with presumed reactions to cosmetic or skin care products. There were 19 reactions to parabens, ranking third on the list of preservatives behind quaternium-15 and imidazolidinyl urea. In comparison, 161 reactions to fragrances were seen (73). In 34 patients with eyelid dermatitis, Nethercott et al. (74) found no reactions to parabens. Menné and Hjorth (75) found about 1% of 8,020 patients tested between 1971 and 1986 were positive to parabens (see Table 17.7).

It has been reported that parabens are enzymatically hydrolyzed to parahydroxybenzoic acid (PHBA) in the skin (76). Because PHBA is apparently a very minimal sensitizer, this transformation may account for the relatively low level of paraben allergy.

Paraben Allergy in Unna Boots

In further support of the concept that paraben allergy is most common when exposure occurs on damaged skin, one report from Cleveland found three cases of paraben allergy from Unna boots used to treat stasis ulcers (77).

Systemic Allergic Contact Dermatitis to Parabens

Veien and colleagues (78) challenged 14 paraben-sensitive patients with 160 mg each of methyl- and propylparaben

TABLE 17.7. *Preservatives Listed by Frequency of Use*

Rank	Preservative	Class	1977	1980	1984	1987	Proj[a]
1	Methylparaben	Paraben ester	5,693	6,785	7,694	7,306	Stable
2	Propylparaben	Paraben ester	5,329	6,174	6,796	6,030	Stable
3	Imidazolindinyl urea	Formaldehyde donor	1,254	1,684	2,315	2,499	Increase
4	Butylparaben	Paraben ester	483	668	803	1,074	Stable
5	Quaternium-15	Formaldehyde donor	599	1,001	1,126	673	Decrease
6	BHA	Antioxidant	440	518	704	662	Stable
7	Ethylparaben	Paraben ester	31	159	365	581	Stable
8	MCI (Kathon CG)[b]	Organic component	0	38	222	512	Decrease
9	MI (Kathon CG)[b]	Organic component	0	38	222	512	Decrease
10	Formaldehyde	Formaldehyde donor	888	874	711	472	Decrease
12	DMDM hydantoin	Formaldehyde donor	15	79	195	318	Increase
13	BNPD (bronopol)[c]	Formaldehyde donor	366	566	429	317	Decrease
20	Diazolidinyl urea	Formaldehyde donor	0	0	53	130	Increase
29	BND (bronidox L)[d]	Formaldehyde donor	0	12	17	44	Stable
44	Paraformaldehyde	Formaldehyde donor	13	20	23	22	Stable
50	MDM hydantoin	Formaldehyde donor	8	15	18	16	Stable

[a]Projected trend in use, in the opinion of the investigator, based in part on usage over the past 15 years. Adapted from reference 76.
[b]Rohm & Haas, Philadelphia, PA.
[c]The Boots Co, Ltd, Nottingham, England.
[d]Henkel Inc, Teaneck, NJ.
Note: As reported to the FDA, in accordance with the code of Federal Regulation, part 720. Adapted from reference 76.

and a placebo control. None reacted to placebo. Two of the 14 reacted with a recurrence of vesicular hand eczema to the parabens, and 1 flared at the patch test site. The authors state that parabens may be found in some systemic medications, as well as in mayonnaise and other condiments, preserved fish and vegetables, fruit and vegetable juices, candies, and cakes.

"Immediate" Urticarial Reactions to the Parabens

Henry et al. (79) reported cases of contact urticaria from parabens in cosmetics. The contact urticaria developed in a patient after topical application of several paraben-containing compounds. Positive results of an open patch test and a passive transfer (Prausnitz-Küstner reaction) test demonstrated an immunologic mechanism for the patient's skin reaction.

Nagel et al. (80) stated that a hydrocortisone preparation containing methylparaben and propylparaben provoked bronchospasm and pruritus when given intravenously to an asthmatic patient, whereas another hydrocortisone preparation without a paraben preservative did not. Direct and transfer (Prausnitz-Küstner) skin tests for immediate hypersensitivity to parabens were positive. Parabens, employed frequently as bacteriostatic agents, are capable of producing immunologically mediated, immediate systemic hypersensitivity reactions.

> **"Immediate" urticarial reactions to the parabens are rare and do not appear to be related to the delayed eczematous reactions.**

Methylchloroisothiazolinone/Methylisothiazolinone (MCI/MI)

MCI/MI (trade names Kathon CG and Euxyl K100, among others) is a preservative first marketed in 1980. Over the past decade its use has increased significantly. Along with this increasing usage has come increasing controversy surrounding the safety of the substance (81).

However, there is no controversy as to its effectiveness as a preservative. It has a broad spectrum of activity against fungi and gram-positive, and gram-negative bacteria. As such, it is comparable to both FRPs and non-formaldehyde-releasing preservatives. The commercial product Kathon CG is a mixture of MCI and MI in a 3:1 ratio. Other related isothiazolinone biocides are also available under trade names such as Kathon WT, Kathon 893, and Proxel GXL. These others, along with Kathon CG, are used as biocides in a variety of industrial products and systems, such as metalworking fluids, water-cooling towers, and latex emulsions.

The controversy over this preservative began when reports from several European centers identified it as a common allergen, with prevalence of positive reactions as high as 8% to 8.5% (82,83). Other centers reported lower rates, as did the NACDG (84). Governmental regulations in some instances limited the use of MCI/MI. In Japan, for example, it may be used in "rinse off" products only at a concentration of 15 ppm or less. Fransway (81) estimated that over 80 research articles were written in a 7-year period regarding the pros and cons of MCI/MI (see Table 17.8).

Guinea pig maximization testing revealed MCI/MI to be a strong sensitizer (85). In addition, primary sensitization by patch testing with MCI/MI 300 ppm aqueous occurred in

TABLE 17.8. *MCI/MI Allergy Prevalences: 1985–1998[a]*

Country	Test conditions	Year(s)	Tested	No. positive	% Positive	Comment
Netherlands	NS	1985	501	7	1.4	Compared to 2% formaldehyde allergy
Sweden	100–150 ppm	1984–1985	658	4	0.6	Most cases occupational, 2+ reaction strength required
Italy	100 ppm	1985–1987	620	52	8.3	All relevant, all PUT (+), all from leave-on product(s)
Denmark	100 ppm	1985–1988	1,396	18	1.3	25% relevant
Netherlands	100 ppm	1986–1987	3,114	155	5.0	70% relevant
Multiple	100 ppm	1984–1986	14,694	165	1.1	Multicenter prevalence range: 0.4%–2.6%
Portugal	NS	1984–1989	4,171	7	0.2	
Switzerland	15 ppm	1984–1986	625	11	1.8	High prevalence at low test concentration
Switzerland	100 ppm	1986–1987	1,320	47	3.6	Multicenter prevalence range: 0.7%–7.5%
North America	100 ppm	1984–1985	495	13	2.6	50% relevant
North America	100 ppm	1985–1987	1,152	20	1.7	
North America	100 ppm	1996–1998	4,083	119	2.9	21st most common allergen
Spain	200 ppm	1989	626	22	3.5	30% relevant
France	100 ppm	1986–1988	540	6	1.1	5/6 relevant
Austria	1.35 ppm	1985–1989	6,202	12	0.2	Claim erroneous test concentration supplied (1.35 ppm)
Austria	100 ppm	1990	400	28	7.0	None reacted at 1.35 ppm
Czechoslovakia	100 ppm	1988–1989	718	6	0.8	All PUT (+)
North America	100 ppm	1988–1989	949	18	1.9	50% PUT (+)
Multiple	100 ppm	1988–1989	4,173	141	3.0	Multicenter prevalence range: 0.4–11.1% "Important new allergen"
France	100 ppm	1987–1989	977	35	3.6	Recommended removal from both rinse-off, leave-on product

[a]PUT, provocative use test
NS, not specified
Adapted from reference 76.

0.8% of 976 patients, a very high rate (86). These data establish the fact that MCI/MI has a high allergenic potential. This may not translate directly into a clinical danger, however. If the levels of MCI/MI are kept to below the recommended maximum (15 ppm), sensitization and even elicitation of ACD in those with positive patch tests is limited. Only 5 of 10 patients with a positive patch test to MCI/MI 100 ppm aqueous reacted to repeated application of a lotion containing 15 ppm MCI/MI (87).

A Danish study confirmed the usefulness of testing MCI/MI at 100 ppm (0.01%) in water (88).

There are several reasons for the international variations in patch test reactions. The preservative was not released in the United States until after several years of use in Europe. European countries do not require ingredient labeling, and there may be less strict quality controls among smaller manufacturers. Apparently some cosmetics and skin care products contained levels of MCI/MI well over the 15 ppm limit. Also, some centers tested with concentrations as high as 200 to 300 ppm, which may have generated false-positive readings, as well as active sensitization. In the United States, where testing has been done at 100 ppm, prevalence rates have been stable at about 2% to 3% positive. Presum-

ably, American manufacturers benefited from the European knowledge and limited the concentration of MCI/MI in products to recommended ranges. The Cosmetic Ingredient Review panel has recommended a maximum level of 15 ppm in rinse-off products, such as soaps and shampoos, and 7.5 ppm in leave-on products.

Occupational exposure to MCI/MI can cause a caustic burn upon direct exposure to the undiluted product. Fowler (unpublished observation) has seen several patients with allergy to MCI/MI after accidental exposure to the chemical in industrial spills. Similar cases have been reported elsewhere (89,90). Gruvberger and Bruze (91,92) have reported that both sodium bisulfite and glutathione can inactivate MCI/MI rapidly. These agents, therefore, could be useful in preventing irritant contact dermatitis and allergic contact dermatitis after an industrial spill.

A report from Sweden found a high rate of allergy to MCI/MI in workers making paints and glues. Allergy was more common to MCI/MI than to formaldehyde or acrylates in the products (36). Metalworkers are also at risk for allergy to MCI/MI (93).

In summary, several statements can be made regarding MCI/MI at this time:

1. In the United States, the prevalence of allergy to MCI/MI is less than allergy to formaldehyde and most FRPs but somewhat greater than to parabens.
2. The high rate of allergy in some countries is probably due to excessive usage concentrations of MCI/MI in cosmetics and skin care products.
3. Patch testing with 100 ppm aqueous is adequate and should be included on routine screening series.
4. Concentrations of MCI/MI of 15 ppm in rinse-off products and 7.5 ppm in leave-on preparations are apparently unlikely to produce excessive sensitization.

Methyldibromoglutaronitrile/Phenoxyethanol

Marketed under the trade name Euxyl K400, this preservative system is a 1:4 mix of the above chemicals. Methyldibromoglutaronitrile (MDGN) is also known as dibromodicyanobutane (94,95). Use of Euxyl K400 in personal care products began in Europe in the mid-1980s and recently has been allowed in the United States. Phenoxyethanol (PE) had been used previously alone in cosmetics. MDGN also had been available as a biocide in latex paints, adhesives, and metalworking fluids. Euxyl K400 is effective at low concentration against both bacteria and fungi (81). The manufacturer (Schulke & Mayr, Hamburg, Germany) recommends a use concentration between 0.05% and 0.02%, depending on the product to be preserved (94).

Despite the finding that neither component of Euxyl K400 was capable of sensitizing guinea pigs in the guinea pig maximization test, multiple case reports of allergy to Euxyl K400 have been published. Only two cases could be found at this writing of allergy to phenoxyethanol (96,97). A number of cases of allergy to MDGN have been reported, however. DeGroot et al. (98) found six cases caused by moist toilet paper. Tosti et al. (97) reported 24 of 2,057 (1.2%) patients reacted to Euxyl K400 (2% pet). In some of these cases, patch tests were positive at very low dilutions, such as 0.001%. This is below the product concentration recommended.

The NACDG has been testing routinely with MDGN/PE since 1994. For the period 1994 to 1996, 2.0% of 3,074 patients were positive to MDGN/PE (1% pet), and none were positive to PE alone (1% pet) (1). Subsequently, from 1996 to 1998 MDGN/PE (at 2.5% pet) was positive in 7.6% of 4,054 patients, whereas MDGN/PE (at 1% pet) was positive in only 2.7% (2). This brings up the concern about patch testing concentrations.

Jackson and Fowler (99) found a positive allergic reaction to 19 of 163 (11.7%) patients tested with 2.5% MDGN/PE (this is equal to 0.5% MDGN). Another 23 patients had mild irritant patch test reactions. Of the 19 with presumed true allergen positives, 7 of 8 with definite relevance were negative to MDGN/PE 1% pet. This suggests that the optimum patch test concentration for MDGN/PE is closer to 2.5% (or 0.5% for plain MDGN). Tosti et al. (100)

and deGroot et al. (101) also feel the higher concentration is more useful.

It should be noted that Euxyl K100 is an isothiazolinone chemically unrelated to Euxyl K400.

> **Euxyl K400 is a preservative system composed of 80% phenoxyethanol and 20% methyldibromoglutaronitrile. Sensitization is usually to the latter compound. Euxyl K100 is chemically unrelated to Euxyl K400.**

Iodopropynyl Butyl Carbamate

The preservative iodopropynyl butyl carbamate (IPBC) is an off-white, crystalline powder of molecular weight 281 and CAS # 55406-53-6 (102). It is moderately water soluble and highly soluble in acetone and benzyl alcohol. It was approved for use in the United States by the Cosmetic Ingredient Review at levels up to 0.1% in topical products in 1996. At that time, 122 products reported to the FDA, mostly shampoos and hair care products, contained it (102). It is also used in paints, wallpapers, metalworking fluids, wood preservatives, and canvas as a biocide. It is particularly active against fungi, but also works against *Staph aureus* and various gram-negative bacilli.

The NACDG began testing with IPBC (0.1% pet) in 1998, and results are not yet available. In Denmark, testing was started in 1996, with 3 of 311 consecutive patients positive (103). Two major questions regarding this potential allergen are unanswered: (a) What is the optimum patch test concentration and (b) Does cross-reactivity occur that can be detected with the carbamate mix?

ALLERGY TO OTHER PRESERVATIVES AND ANTIOXIDANTS

Parachlorometaxylenol (PCMX) and Parachlorometacresol (PCMC)

PCMX, also known as chloroxylenol, is a halogenated phenol used as an additive (preservative) and as an active agent (disinfectant). PCMC, or chlorocresol, is identical to PCMX except for the absence of a methyl group on the basic benzene ring. It is used more commonly in industrial products, such as paints and cutting oils, and less so in topical products than PCMX (81). Both are soluble in oil and water and have activity against both gram-positive and gram-negative bacteria. PCMX may be less initiating than PCMC.

Both of these agents occasionally cause ACD. The two major sources of exposure seem to be occupational products, especially hand cleaners and metalworking fluids, and medical topical products, such as electrode pastes and topical medicaments (104–107). PCMX is the active agent in carbolated Vaseline. Storrs (108) reported seven cases of ACD from electrocardiograph paste or carbolated petrolatum more than 20 years ago. Industrial and medical hand soaps often contain one or the other agent (109). Fowler (110) reported two cases related to medical and industrial hand cleaners.

Cross-reaction between the two agents is common but not absolute. Burry (106) reported ACD in 13 patients related to use of corticosteroid creams. All reacted to PCMX, and eight also reacted to PCMC. Currently, both PCMX and PCMC are tested at 1% pet. Most authors in large studies have reported prevalence rates of positive patch tests in the neighborhood of 1%. PCMX appears to react somewhat more often than PCMC.

A severe hand and foot dermatitis was traced to PCMC in sorbolene cream used by an Australian mechanic as a "barrier cream" (111).

Chloracetamide

Chloracetamide (CAA) is a water-soluble preservative useful especially against yeasts and fungi. In addition, in occasional reports of allergy from cosmetic products, CAA has caused allergy to paints, shoes, adhesives, and cutting oils (81). One report from Australia caused axillary dermatitis from a deodorant (112).

Possibly because of the fairly low frequency of use in cosmetics, prevalence rates of CAA allergy are low. The NACDG found 1 positive of 648 patients tested in 1984 and 1985 (113). In Belgium, 1 of 156 patients thought to be allergic to cosmetics was positive, whereas 0.3% of more than 5,000 total patients reacted (114). Fransway (81) reported a similar frequency. Currently, testing is performed with chloracetamide 0.2% pet. A report from the Swiss Contact Dermatitis Research Group found allergy to CAA in 1.5% of 2,295 patients (8).

Vitamin E (Alpha-Tocopherol)

Vitamin E, used as an antioxidant in foods, is used for the same purpose in some skin care products. In addition, it has become a popular agent used as a marketing device to appeal to consumers wanting to use "natural" products. Although there are occasional reports of vitamin E allergy, they are rare. The NACDG found that 2 of 626 patients suspected of cosmetic allergy reacted to vitamin E but more recently dropped vitamin E from the screening tray due to a lack of response (113).

DeGroot et al. (115) found four cases of allergy to tocopheryl acetate (10% pet). The products involved were a face cream, a cream to treat striae distensae, and a product for cellulitis. These four patients were seen in several practices over a 5-year period, suggesting a low incidence of allergy.

Triclosan

Used as an antibacterial agent and preservative, especially in shampoos, soaps, and deodorants, triclosan is also known as Irgasan DP-300. It has some effectiveness against fungi and bacteria but is not active against *Pseudomonas*. In addition to skin care products, triclosan may be incorporated in footwear to retard odors (81).

Apparently triclosan does not cross-react with the photosensitizing halogenated salicylanilides. Allergy to Triclosan is unusual. Prevalence rates of less than 0.5% are commonly reported (81). In the late 1990s, several new skin lotions, soaps, and even a toothpaste (Colgate-Total, Colgate Palmolive) containing triclosan were marketed in the United States (116).

At one time, a few feminine hygiene sprays contained triclosan.

Thimerosal

This organic mercurial is used as an antiseptic (Merthiolate) and as a preservative, principally in eye medications and cosmetics, contact lens solutions, and injectables such as vaccines.

Frequent positive patch tests are seen to thimerosal 0.1% pet. The most recent NACDG data gives a 10.9% prevalence rate in more than 4,000 patients, with an equal distribution between men and women. Other studies have ranged from a low of 1% to 6% in the Netherlands to a high of 9.5% in Japan, with most reports in the 4% to 5% range (81).

Origin of Thimerosal Sensitivity: Vaccinations

Although many positive, morphologically allergic reactions to thimerosal are seen on patch testing, only one-half or less are deemed relevant when this is specifically evaluated. What, then, is the source of sensitization?

The answer to this question, confirmed by several epidemiologic studies, is that injected vaccinations and allergy immunotherapy lead to frequent development of thimerosal allergy (117,118). Thimerosal is often the preservative used in vaccines and "allergy shots." One study that serves as an example of the evidence implicating vaccination as a source of thimerosal allergy was published by Osawa et al. (119). No reactions were seen in infants who were not yet vaccinated, whereas 25% of 32 persons age 5 to 19 years had positive reactions. Furthermore, over half of a group of guinea pigs given a DPT vaccine containing 0.01% thimerosal became sensitized to thimerosal. Tosti et al. (120) documented that patients who had undergone desensitization injections for allergies had a greater rate of thimerosal sensitivity than other patch test clinic patients. As a natural follow-up to these findings, the question of direct reactions to thimerosal in injections has been studied.

Reactions to Thimerosal in Injectables

Forstrom et al. (118) found that 13 of 45 thimerosal-allergic patients had a local reaction to a subcutaneous injection of thimerosal. One patient developed a generalized dermatitis. Other studies, however, have shown a much lower rate of actual reactions to vaccine injections. For example, Cox and Forsythe (121) found 4 vaccination reactions in 31 individuals allergic to thimerosal but did not prove thimerosal to be the allergen by intracutaneous testing. Other agents, such as aluminum and neomycin, may also cause localized or generalized reactions to injections.

The conclusion is that, although thimerosal in injectables can cause local or systemic reactions, significant occurrences are uncommon.

Life-Threatening Reaction to Thimerosal

Maibach (122) reported a patient who had a marked reaction to thimerosal, after treating his slight sore throat with a thimerosal first-aid spray. The next day, because of continued discomfort, he repeated its use. Laryngeal obstruction followed within hours. Emergency tracheostomy produced prompt improvement. Patch testing revealed an extreme spreading reaction to thimerosal. It was believed that acute laryngeal obstruction developed as a delayed hypersensitivity reaction to this first-aid spray.

The Nature of Thimerosal Allergy

Thimerosal is composed of a thiosalicylate and an organic mercurial. It was once thought that the thiosalicylate fraction is responsible for most of the cases of thimerosal allergy (123). Many years ago a Japanese report showed that almost all 23 tested patients were allergic to the thiosalicylate. More recent studies, however, have suggested about 20% of thimerosal-allergic patients react to thiosalicylate (81).

Patients sensitive to thimerosal (Merthiolate) can be divided into three groups: (a) positive to thimerosal, but negative to other mercurials and to thiosalicylic acid; (b) positive to thimerosal and to some other mercurials, but negative to thiosalicylic acid; and (c) positive to thimerosal and to thiosalicylic acid, but negative to other mercurials.

Allergy to Thimerosal and Photosensitivity to Piroxicam

Piroxicam (Feldane) is a nonsteroidal anti-inflammatory agent that can cause photosensitivity (124). Of 16 patients with a positive thimerosal patch test, 8 had a positive photopatch test to piroxicam (125). The same authors studied 19 thimerosal patients (126). None gave positive regular tests to piroxicam. However, 11 were positive on photopatch testing to 1% piroxicam. Of these, 8 were tested to thiosalicylic acid, 0.1%, and all were positive. All who were piroxicam negative were also thiosalicylic acid nega-

tive. Cirne DeCastro et al. (126) further found that patch tests with a mix of piroxicam and L-cysteine, which was irradiated with UVA in vitro, gave positive results in only the piroxicam-photosensitive patients. This implies that piroxicam must combine with cutaneous amino acids to create a photosensitizing product.

Thimerosal as an Allergen in Eye Preparations

There are numerous reports of allergic contact sensitization to thimerosal (Merthiolate) in various eye preparations and contact lens solutions. The allergic reaction may produce conjunctivitis alone, or a combination of conjunctivitis and eyelid dermatitis. In one instance a sensitized person had a dermatitis of the hands without conjunctivitis.

Fregert and Hjorth (127) stated that allergic reactions to eyedrops often produce both conjunctivitis and eyelid dermatitis, whereas van Ketel and Melzer-van Riemsduk (128) pointed out that thimerosal, present as a preservative in many soft lens solutions, produced allergic conjunctivitis, but no eyelid dermatitis, in three of their patients. Pedersen (129) also described conjunctivitis without eyelid dermatitis.

Sertoli et al. (130) reported that a patient who had allergic thimerosal sensitization developed an allergic contact dermatitis on the fingers and palms; however, when this same solution was applied to the eyes, it did not produce conjunctivitis or eyelid dermatitis. The patient, a 20-year-old woman, had two small patches of dyshidrosiform vesicles. She had worn soft contact lenses for 1 month before the eruption began. When not worn, the lenses were kept in a lens container with a preserving liquid. They were taken out for use individually with the tip of the left index finger, put onto the right palm, and there washed with a liquid using the tip of the left index finger before being put into the eyes.

Rietschel and Wilson (131) reported that soft contact lenses cleaned and stored in thimerosal-containing solutions may produce an ocular inflammatory process and, if untreated, corneal neovascularization. They examined 38 patients who were using soft contact lenses and found that 31 had positive ocular provocation test results to a thimerosal-preserved, artificial tears solution. Delayed hypersensitivity to thimerosal was demonstrated by positive patch tests in 27 patients. Avoidance of thimerosal and the use of unit-dose sterile saline solutions has resulted in complete resolution of ocular symptoms.

Contact urticaria from thimerosal may also cause ocular reaction and contact lens intolerance (132).

Benzalkonium Chloride (BAC)

Benzalkonium chloride (BAC), a mixture of alkyl dimethyl benzyl ammonium chlorides, is a quaternary ammonium cationic detergent. It is used widely as a preoperative skin disinfectant, for disinfection of surgical instruments, and in the treatment of burns, ulcers, wounds, and infected dermatoses. It is also present in some cosmetics, deodorants, mouthwashes, dentrifices, lozenges, and ophthalmic preparations. It is used industrially in the fabrication of textiles and dyes and in metallurgy and agriculture. BAC inhibits a wide variety of bacteria but not *Pseudomonas*. It is less active against fungi (81). BAC is a notorious irritant on patch testing. Therefore, positive reactions must be evaluated critically for relevance. The use or ROAT test is especially valuable with this allergen.

Benzalkonium chloride, present in disinfectants such as Zephiran Chloride, has produced allergic contact dermatitis in medical personnel from exposure to instruments soaked in it and from its use in the treatment of ulcers, burns, and cutaneous infections (133,134). In addition to ACD, irritant dermatitis from BAC may occur.

A bizarre ichthyosis type of dermatitis was reported in Japan to be caused by an ointment containing alkyl benzyl trimethyl-ammonium chloride (135), which differs from BAC only by an additional methyl group. Pandos et al. (136) reported an instance of combined cutaneous and mucous membrane allergic contact reaction from BAC that complicated a tracheostomy procedure.

Benzalkonium chloride (Zephiran Chloride), a widely used antiseptic and preservative, is a rare sensitizer.

Theodore and Schlossman (137) stated that BAC in ophthalmic preparations may produce allergic reactions, but they did not cite specific cases with confirming patch test proof. Fisher and Stillman (138) reported that one of the authors (M. A. Stillman) developed a conjunctivitis from acquired hypersensitivity to BAC in an ophthalmic medicament, which was then made worse when an unsuspecting ophthalmologist prescribed another preparation containing BAC. Allergy to BAC has been seen from plaster of paris and where it was used as a denaturent for ethanol (139,140).

Benzethonium Chloride

This quaternary ammonium compound, which may show cross-reactions with benzalkonium chloride, is also a rare sensitizer (141). Its presence in a roll-on deodorant has produced an allergic axillary dermatitis (142).

Sorbic Acid

Sorbic acid (SA) is known chemically as 2,4-hexadienoic acid and 2-propenyl-acrylic acid. It is a naturally occurring plant substance obtained from the berries of the mountain ash, *Sorbus aucuparia,* L. *rosaceae,* in which it is present as the lactone (parasorbic acid). It is present in cranberries, strawberries, and currants and is used as a preservative in many foods. For commercial purposes, SA may be made synthetically by the condensation of crotonaldehyde with malonic acid.

Sorbic acid is a white, practically odorless, crystalline powder with a faintly acid taste. Potassium sorbate (popularly used salt form) is also a white, almost odorless powder.

SA 0.2% is considered an antimicrobial agent of choice for topically applied vehicles and cosmetics containing fatty acids and polyoxyethylene esters. The sensitizing index of this preservative appears to be low—estimated at 0.3% by Hjorth and Trolle-Lassen (143) and 0.6% by Klaschka and Beiersdorff (144). It appears to compare favorably with the parabens from the standpoint of allergenicity.

SA is soluble in water, alcohol, and propylene glycol. It is an excellent fungistatic agent but has little antibacterial activity. It acts by inhibition of microbial enzyme systems. In addition to use in topical products and foodstuffs, SA may be used in oral medications.

Sorbic Acid—a Rare Cause of Allergic Contact Dermatitis

Fisher et al. (69) found one patient who had allergic hypersensitivity to sorbic acid among 100 patients who were suspected of having allergic reactions to preservatives in topical agents. Klaschka and Beiersdorff (144) reported that in 3 of 735 eczematous patients, sensitization to sorbic acid due to the use of external medicaments could be demonstrated.

Simpson (145) described a British patient with sorbic acid sensitivity from Cortacream paste bandage, which contains sorbic acid as a preservative. This bandage, used in a patient who had stasis eczema, produced a disseminated eruption, and a strongly positive patch test reaction to sorbic acid was obtained.

Saihan and Harman (146) described a patient who acquired an allergic contact dermatitis superimposed upon psoriasis from the presence of sorbic acid in Unguentum Merck. Brown (147) reported that a 75-year-old woman who had a long history of varicose eczema experienced a generalized spread of eczema due to sorbic acid in Unguentum Merck. Gorannson and Liden (148) also reported allergy to sorbic acid in Unguentum Merck.

Sorbic acid is a rare cause of the delayed type of eczematous contact dermatitis.

In the United States, SA has shown a patch test prevalence rate of less than 1%. At the Mayo Clinic, 0.9% of 3,759 patients reacted to SA (2% pet) (81,149). The rate has been constant, with a report of 0.8% in 1985 and 0.7% in 1993 (unpublished observation) by the NACDG. Slightly higher rates have been reported in Europe. The NACDG has not tested with SA in its screening series since 1994.

In Denmark, 10 of 718 (1.4%) patients reacted to SA. Six of these were apparently sensitized through the use of a moisturizing cream (Decubal), which contains 0.15% SA (150). None of these patients were known to react to SA in food, by history, although oral provocation tests were not conducted.

The Use of Sorbic Acid in Foods

Sodium and potassium sorbate are recognized as safe for use in foods under regulations of the Food and Drug Administration. At low concentrations these food additives are effective preservatives for the control of mold and yeast in cheese products, baked goods, fruit juices, fresh fruits and vegetables, wines, soft drinks, pickles, sauerkraut, and certain meat and fish products.

In three patients with known sorbic acid sensitivity who were fed foods known to contain sorbic acid and potassium sorbate for 3 weeks, no flare of dermatitis or patch test sites resulted. Klaschka and Beiersdorff (144) noted that in patients who were allergic to sorbic acid, no reaction could be released orally. Fisher observed one patient who had a 4+ patch test reaction to sorbic acid and who had no flare-up after ingestion of berries. Dillon (151) pronounced that sorbic acid was not a "harmful" food additive. In a report from France, however a patient was definitely reactive to SA present in foods (152). The dermatitis was on the buttocks and perineal area, reminiscent of the "baboon syndrome." Other ingested allergens, such as nickel and propylene glycol, however, have been found to be able to cause systemic ACD. It would seem prudent, therefore, that SA-sensitive patients at least consider the possibility that oral intake might produce dermatitis.

Effect of Sorbic Acid on the Buccal Mucosa

Clemmensen and Schiødt (153) concluded that "[o]ur findings are in accordance with the clinical impression that sorbic acid in the relevant concentrations, when used as a preservative, is not urticariogenic or otherwise harmful to the oral mucosa."

Sorbic Acid—a Common Cause of Nonspecific Erythema and Nonimmunologic Contact Urticaria

In 1958, Fryklof (154) reported an experiment with ointments and creams in which sorbic acid, used as a preservative, was applied to 20 patients in his laboratory. In half of the patients, the application of these products to the face caused a more or less obvious erythema and slight itching, sometimes even slight edema. The reaction appeared 5 to 15 minutes after the application and disappeared completely 1 to 2 hours later.

Hjorth and Trolle-Lassen (143) tested sorbic acid in various bases and reported that in 18 of 26 persons, ointments containing sorbic acid provoked an erythema persisting after 30 minutes. In a control experiment performed simultaneously on the same patients, benzoic acid in identical concentrations and vehicles provoked the same type of response. This was not the case with ointments containing methylparaben.

In 50 consecutive patients that Fisher studied, he found that in more than half of them, a brisk erythema could be produced on the forearms with 5% sorbic acid in petrolatum within a half hour. In most instances, the erythema was not accompanied by any burning sensation or itching. A stinging sensation, however, developed in a certain group of persons who had "status cosmeticus."

Rietschel (155) reported on a patient who had contact urticaria from cassia oil and sorbic acid limited to the face.

Sorbic acid is one of a group of substances that can produce an immediate nonspecific erythema in most individuals (156). Other topical agents that may produce immediate nonspecific erythema include benzoic acid, sodium benzoate, balsam of Peru, cinnamic aldehyde, cinnamic alcohol, and ethyl vanillin.

> **Sorbic acid, like benzoic acid and sodium benzoate, produces an immediate nonspecific erythema and sometimes urticaria in many individuals.**

Fisher has observed this type of nonspecific sorbic acid erythema in infants and in the anogenital area from the use of Diaprene baby wash cloths impregnated with a cleansing solution containing water, SD alcohol-40, propylene glycol, lanolin, sodium nonoxynol-9-phosphate, sorbic acid, citric acid, disodium phosphate, oleth-20, and fragrance.

Potassium Sorbate and Sorbic Acid

Potassium sorbate, because of its high water solubility, is often used to incorporate sorbic acid. The potassium salt of sorbic acid is a weaker preservative than sorbic acid. Like sorbic acid, potassium sorbate is used as a mold and yeast inhibitor, particularly when greater solubility in water is desirable. It should be noted that, depending on the pH, most potassium sorbate–containing products have a certain amount of sorbic acid (see Table 17.9).

Patch tests may be performed with 5% potassium sorbate. No mention is made, however, in the literature of patch tests with potassium sorbate for patients who have sorbic acid hypersensitivity. Sorbic acid hypersensitivity is probably accompanied by hypersensitivity to the potassium salt.

Fisher observed one sorbic acid patient who acquired an allergic reaction to Clinique's Blended Face Powder, which contains potassium sorbate as a preservative. This appears

TABLE 17.9. *Relation of pH to Sorbic Acid/Sorbate Concentrations*

pH	Sorbic acid (%)	Potassium sorbate (%)
4	86	14
5	37	63
6	6	94
7	0.6	99.4
9	0	100

to be the first instance of a patient who had sorbic acid hypersensitivity who acquired an allergic contact dermatitis from exposure to potassium sorbate in a topically applied agent.

Incidentally, polysorbate 60, an emulsifying agent, is not related to potassium sorbate.

> **Sorbic acid and potassium sorbate cross-react to each other but not to polysorbate, which is chemically unrelated.**

Benzyl Alcohol

Benzyl alcohol is used as a preservative instead of thimerosal or phenol in allergenic extracts and injectable biologicals. It is also used occasionally in topical products and ophthalmologic preparations. Other terms for benzyl alcohol include benzene methanol, phenyl methanol, and phenyl carbanol. It has good activity against gram-positive bacteria but is relatively inactive against gram-negative fungi. Like the parabens, benzyl alcohol is deactivated by nonionic surfactants. It appears that the frequency of positive patch tests to benzyl alcohol is less than 1% (81).

Benzyl alcohol is unique in that it is not only a preservative but also a local anesthetic and fragrance. It is used extensively in perfumes and has also been used increasingly in hair dyes, primarily in connection with direct acid dyes rather than the oxidation colors. Benzyl alcohol, soluble only up to about 5% in aqueous systems, tends to adhere to keratin surfaces from such solutions as a result of solubility partition ratios. The use of benzyl alcohol results in deeper shades in dye concentrations at no extra cost (an important commercial feature).

Benzyl alcohol is present as a preservative in Aquatain hydrophilic base, now used in Aristocort and Cyclocort Creams. In Canada, Aquatain is used as a cosmetic, moisturizing cream.

> **Benzyl alcohol, a rare sensitizer, is a preservative and an anesthetic and is used in acid hair dyes to produce deeper shades. Benzyl alcohol may show cross-reactions with balsam of Peru.**

An allergic reaction to benzyl alcohol has been reported by Schultheiss (157) in a patient working with beverages. The patient, however, had been sensitized in childhood to balsam of Peru. Cross-sensitization to benzyl alcohol has been reported in subjects sensitized to balsam of Peru. Lagerholm (158) reported hypersensitivity to a benzyl alcohol preservative in the injectable variety of vitamin B_{12}. No mention is made of any patch tests to benzyl alcohol in this case. Benzyl alcohol was the cause of long-standing vulvar dermatitis due to its presence in various topical agents (159). Indeed, in none of the reported cases of benzyl alcohol sensitivity and dermatitis were scratch and intracutaneous tests compared with patch tests.

Fisher (70) reported two patients who had eczematous contact dermatitis owing to benzyl alcohol, the one from perfume and the other from aftershave lotion. Neither patient, who both had strongly positive patch test reactions to benzyl alcohol, showed positive reactions to scratch and intradermal testing.

> **Patients who had a delayed 48-hour patch test reaction to benzyl alcohol had a negative reaction to scratch and intracutaneous testing, making it likely that benzyl alcohol–sensitive patients will tolerate injections of medications containing benzyl alcohol as a preservative.**

Captan (*N*-Trichloromethylthio-4-Cyclohexene-1,2-Dicarboximide)

Captan (short for mercaptan), which is used primarily as a fungicide, may also be found as a bacteriostat in cosmetic formulations, particularly for the hair (e.g., Selsun and Selsun Blue). In barber shops and beauty salons, it may be employed in Dangard.

This fungicide is used extensively on fruit, vegetables, and plants of all types. Its sensitizing potential was assessed in 205 human subjects by Marzulli and Maibach (160). They sensitized nine (4.4%) human subjects using a concentration of 1%, both for induction and for challenge. Captan 1% in petrolatum was tested on 509 patients by members of the International Contact Dermatitis Research Group. Sixteen (3%) of these patients reacted, but in none was it considered to be clinically relevant, and the reactions were thought to be mild, irritant responses.

After 3 weeks' exposure to captan, a fruit farmer developed dermatitis of his hands and face. Patch tests with captan 1% in Vaseline and with the related chemical phaltan 1% in petrolatum were both positive (161).

Epstein (162) reported an instance of photoallergic contact dermatitis owing to Dangard. The allergic nature of the dermatitis was documented by the eczematous response to a photopatch test and its histologic examination. Dangard is a trade name for the antimicrobial-antiseborrheic ingredient used in QED Hair Groom and QED Shampoo, which are sold exclusively by barbers. Dangard is a recrystallized form of *N*-trichloromethyl-mercapto-4-cyclohexene-1,2-dicarboximide. Another trade name for captan is Vancide 89 RE, which is used in cosmetic and pharmaceutical preparations.

In 1992, captan was deleted from the study series of the NACDG due to an inability to find relevance in most positive reactions. Although it may be useful to retain this allergen for use in agricultural or hairdresser trays, the frequent rate of apparent false positivity makes captan unsuitable for use on a screening series.

> **Captan, used as a fungicide in agriculture and as a preservative in Selsun, is present in Dangard (Vancide) and in QED shampoos used exclusively by barbers.**

Zinc Pyrithione

Muston et al. (163) stated that zinc pyrithione (ZPT) has bactericidal and fungicidal properties and is of value in the treatment of dandruff. It is known under the proprietary names Vancide ZP, Zincon (United States), and Zinc Omadine (United Kingdom) and is an ingredient of various shampoos and other hair care products.

Procter and Gamble stated that shampoos containing ZPT have been popular in the United States since 1963 and in the United Kingdom since 1968. The company estimates that well over 100 million people have been exposed to ZPT shampoos in the two countries. Despite this finding, however, only a few cases of sensitivity have been reported (163).

Pereira et al. (164) reported ACD from ZPT in a shampoo. They were able to identify seven cases from the literature. Nielsen and Menné (165) reported allergy to ZPT in a shampoo that triggered an eruption of pustular psoriasis.

> **Zinc pyrithione may cross-react with piperazine, which is a diethylamine and which in turn may cross-react with ethylenediamine dermatitis.**

Zinc pyrithione is a rare sensitizer that may cross-react with piperazine and ethylenediamine hydrochloride derivatives (see Chapter 14).

Chlorhexidine

Chlorhexidine is used as a disinfectant and bacteriocide in cleansing products, especially those used in health care facilities. As such, it may be considered an "active" agent (see Chapter 12). It also may be used occasionally as a preservative in topical products. In addition to ACD, anaphylactic reactions have been reported from topical contact with chlorhexidine (166).

Benzophenones

At least a dozen different benzophenones exist with widely different uses. Benzophenones are often incorporated in textiles and plastics to impart protection from and colorfastness to ultraviolet radiation. They are put into transparent shades to protect window displays, plastic lens filters for color photography, aerosol sprays to protect color prints, and many polystyrene, acrylic, and rubber products to prevent darkening and loss of strength. They are often included in paints, varnishes, and fluorescent lacquers to inhibit degradation of colors. Of particular interest is their use in cosmetics, such as hair sprays, hair dyes, perfumes, shampoos, and detergent bars.

Reaction to Benzophenones in Sunscreens

Benzophenones, especially oxybenzone (BZP-3), have become the most common photoallergens in sunscreen products. They may also cause "regular" ACD (see Chapter 23). Benzophenone-2 caused ACD in a perfume (167).

> **Benzophenones in a sunscreen may produce immediate urticarial reactions, as well as delayed eczematous responses and photoallergy.**

ANTIOXIDANTS IN TOPICAL PRODUCTS

Antioxidants in topical products protect from oxidation of lipid components, which leads to a rancid odor. These agents are also useful in the protection of fatty foods, such as mayonnaise, oils, and lard. Also, some foods and topical products may discolor on exposure to oxygen. The darkening of fruits and vegetables, for example, is known as "enzymatic browning." A common example of this is the darkening of sliced apples after several minutes of exposure to the air. Antioxidants retard this oxidation-based discoloration. Generally, the antioxidants are lipid-soluble phenolic substances (81,168).

Butylated Hydroxyanisole, Butylated Hydroxytoluene, and Tertiary Butylhydroquinone (BHA, BHT, TBHQ)

BHA and BHT are two of the most commonly used antioxidants in both foods and topical preparations. Other names for these agents are butyl methoxyphenol and dibutyl paracresol, respectively. BHA and BHT are also used in the production of petroleum-based products such as plastic, rubber, and fuels, as well as in animal feeds.

In addition to their antioxidant properties, BHA and BHT have some antibacterial effects, particularly against *Corynebacterium* sp. BHA may have a somewhat broader spectrum of action and also is used in topical products somewhat more frequently than BHT (81).

In general, the prevalence of reactions to BHA or BHT is low. Degreef (169) in 1975 and Fisher (168) in 1976 mention cases of allergy to antioxidants. Meneghini et al. (170) noted only one reaction in 360 patients tested for both BHA and BHT (5% pet). Fransway (81) reported positive rates of 0.7% and 0.5%, respectively, in more than 900 patients. Prevalence of positivity in NACDG studies to BHA was only 0.2% of 4,096 patients (2). The currently used test concentration is 2% pet. Most but not all who react to BHT are also allergic to BHA.

White et al. (171) specifically looked at reactions to BHA and tertiary butylhydroquinone in 1,096 patients with facial eczema. Seven patients (0.7%) were positive to BHA. All five of the patients tested to TBHQ (a related antioxidant) were also positive.

In Denmark, 1,336 patients were tested with BHT, with no positive reactions (172). A computerized database of consumer and industrial products indicated BHT was present in 31 Danish toiletry items out of 440 products overall, mostly coatings, resins, and adhesives.

Norhydroguaiaretic Acid (NDGA)

This agent is not used extensively in the United States. In the 1970s, six patients in Europe were reported allergic to NDGA. Three had been sensitized by one brand of skin cream (173).

Gallate Esters

These agents have little, if any, preservative action in the sense of being antimicrobial. Propyl gallate is the subject of most ACD reports and is used most frequently. Octyl and dodecyl (lauryl) gallate are also used. Various case reports of ACD to gallate in topical products have been reported (81,174–178). Causative agents include antibiotic creams, lipsticks, moisturizers, topical corticosteroids, and eye cosmetics. Propyl gallate was a cause of hand dermatitis in a baker who contacted it in cake icings (J Mark Jackson MD, unpublished observation, 1999). Heine (179) noted six cases from patients using the same body lotion.

Using guinea pig maximization testing, all of eight gallates tested were at least moderate sensitizers. Dodecyl gallate was the strongest (180). In general, those with a longer side chain showed the strongest sensitizing capacity.

The hypothesis that allergenicity of propyl gallate is enhanced by attachment to liposomes has been presented (181). Liposomes, phospholipid spheres, are now becoming popular in moisturizers and are marketed as enhancing smoothing and antiwrinkle capability. Marston (181) noted

a dramatic increase of ACD to propyl gallate with positive patch tests in 13 of 245 women (5.3%) and no men. In 10 of these women, liposomal moisturizers containing propyl gallate were wholly or partly responsible. In 4 of the 10, propyl gallate was the only allergen.

Perhaps the manufacturers of these "night creams" and "antiwrinkle" creams have inadvertently discovered a method to increase contact allergy instead of decreasing the effects of sun and aging.

> **Propyl gallate is a moderate sensitizer in animals but is rarely reported as a cause of ACD in humans. Use of liposome-containing skin creams may unleash a rise in propyl gallate allergy.**

ALLERGY TO OTHER ADDITIVES IN TOPICAL PRODUCTS

PVP/Hexadecene Copolymer

Polyvinylpyrrolidone (PVP)/hexadecene copolymer has been reported to cause allergy in two cases from a bath oil and a cosmetic product (182,183).

Ethylenediamine Tetra-Acetate (EDTA)

Marketed as the calcium disodium salt of ethylenediamine tetra-acetic acid and as Edathamil calcium, calcium edetate, Versene, Sequestrene, and Nullapon, EDTA is well known as a chelating agent with a strong affinity for metals such as calcium, lead, and magnesium. It is classed as a sequestering agent and can bind metallic ions.

EDTA prevents discoloration due to traces of metals in antibiotics, antihistaminics, and local anesthetics. It prevents oxidation by trace metals in cosmetic creams and lotions and is used as a stabilizer in solutions of ascorbic acid, hydrogen peroxide, formaldehyde, folic acid, and hyaluronidase. It is also used systemically for the treatment of lead poisoning. In ophthalmic solutions, it enhances the antibacterial activity of benzalkonium chloride, chlorobutanol, and thimerosal by disrupting the lipid-protein complexes of cell walls. In addition, EDTA has limited antibacterial properties of its own, especially against gram-negative organisms.

A sequestering agent, such as EDTA, is used frequently as a clarifying agent, because it prevents the formation of calcium, magnesium, and iron soaps, which may cause turbidity.

EDTA has rarely caused contact allergy. Raymond and Cross (184) reported it in 1969. A case report of allergy to EDTA in an injected local anesthetic suggests testing with

EDTA 1% pet (185). The patient had facial erythema and edema after a dental injection. Cross-reaction with ethylenediamine did not occur.

One well-documented case report of allergy to EDTA occurred in a leg ulcer patient who was positive to EDTA 1% aq and pet, but not to ethylenediamine (186).

Relation of EDTA to Ethylenediamine HCl

Raymond and Cross (184) stated that two of their patients showed cross-reactions. Eriksen (187) reported patients with cross-reactions, as did Penvy and Shaefer (188). Epstein (189) and Fisher (190), however, could not show any cross-reactions.

Dr. C. V. Denehl of Union Carbide (personal communication) wrote: "We have made a few observations in past years that may offer an explanation for your observation on the lack of cross-sensitization between ethylenediamine hydrochloride and ethylenediamine tetra-acetate. We know that the sensitizing properties of ethylenediamine are reduced each time one of the hydrogens of the amine is replaced, thus:

The fact that the NH_2 group is the active sensitizing part of a compound is supported by the fact that most amines have some sensitizing properties and the property becomes less as hydrogens are substituted."

With these facts in mind it becomes reasonable to conclude that the tetra-acetate that binds each of the hydrogens attached to the nitrogen destroys the sensitizing properties of ethylenediamine. For several years, the NACDG included EDTA in the North American screening tray. There was not a single positive reaction in hundreds of patients who were tested. Furthermore, Fisher (190) tested 100 patients with ethylenediamine hydrochloride sensitivity to EDTA, and in no instance was any cross-reaction evident. Likewise, Balato et al. (191) found no reactions to EDTA in 32 ethylenediamine-allergic patients. We no longer routinely test with EDTA because it is our conviction that EDTA is a minimal sensitizer.

EDTA apparently does not cross-react with ethylenediamine hydrochloride.

Surfactants

Sodium laurel sulfate (SLS) has been long used as a surfactant in skin care preparations. In the last decade, nonionic surfactants have become popular substitutes for SLS. These agents, such as cocamedopropyl betaine (CB), seem to be less irritating than SLS. They are most often used in shampoos and soapless cleansers.

Sodium Laurel Sulfate (SLS)

The Nature of SLS

Sodium laurel sulfate has the following chemical formula: $CH_3(CH_2)_{10}CH_2OSO_3Na$. SLS is an anionic surface active agent used as an emulsifier in many pharmaceutical vehicles, cosmetics, foaming dentifrices, and even foods (192).

SLS as an Irritant

SLS is well known as a standard skin irritant. Its action on surface tension is the cause of its irritancy, and its great capacity for penetration makes it useful to enhance penetration of other substances in patch tests and in animal assay (193).

Recognizing this ability of SLS to damage the epidermal barrier, Kligman (194) proposed the "provocative patch test" for allergic contact patch testing. Dahl and Trancik (195) reported that irritant reactions were induced on the forearms of ten normal subjects with 19% aqueous SLS under patch test occlusion for 24 hours.

In general, irritant patch test responses tend to diminish after the patch is removed, whereas allergic responses often increase in size and intensity. Dahl and Trancik, however, found that as far as SLS is concerned, the inflammatory response may initially accelerate after patch test removal and remain intense for at least 48 hours. Thus, fading of irritant reactions by 48 and 72 hours may not reliably distinguish irritant from allergic patch test reactions. This does not refute the usefulness of a delayed (96-hour) reading, because the irritant inflammation from SLS had decreased significantly by this time, whereas an allergic reaction would usually not be significantly decreased at the end of 96 hours.

In general, then, patch test responses can show significant improvement within 1 to 2 days, and when this occurs, the clinician is usually observing an irritant response. An allergic reaction with the same intensity is likely to persist during this same period. Rapid fading of mild reactions is, however, quite typical of irritant responses.

Bergstresser and Eagelstein (196) showed that hydrophilic ointment and a similar vehicle containing 1% SLS invariably produce contact irritant dermatitis when they are occluded 16 hours a day for more than 3 days and that SLS is the provocative irritant agent. Previous experimental work on SLS suggested that denaturation of epidermal proteins and subsequent loss of the epidermal barrier are likely mechanisms.

These investigators concluded that less irritating emulsifiers, or concentrations of SLS less than 1%, should be used in topical products, especially those that might be used under occlusion.

Krook (197) reported that a 74-year-old man who had stasis dermatitis had an allergic reaction to Ficortril, a Swedish hydrocortisone ointment containing 0.9% SLS. Krook deplored the fact that an ointment used for the treatment of eczema should contain an irritant, such as SLS, in such high concentration, and surmises that the irritating effect of SLS in the vehicle had promoted the sensitization to hydrocortisone.

SLS as a Comedogenic Agent

Fulton et al. (198) reported that the need for a comedogenic-free cosmetic for acne patients led to a study using the rabbit's ear as a model. They found that hydrophilic ointment USP was comedogenic due to the detergent, 1% SLS, in the formula. They declared that SLS was a comedogenic as certain modifications of lanolin and such emulsifiers as butyl stearate and isopropyl myristate, which had proved to be potent acnegens.

SLS as "A Contact Allergen"

Kligman (194) stated that no sensitization to SLS was seen in the 100 cases in which SLS was used in "provocative" or "prophetic" patch test procedures.

Sams and Smith (199) presumed a specific contact sensitization to SLS when used as an emulsifier in a hydrocortisone cream.

Prater et al. (200), using a "lymphocyte transformation test" in 10 of 12 patients who had an eczematous reaction to an SLS wetting test, found an increased incorporation of H-thymidine and claimed that these results are an almost certain sign of sensitization. Patch tests with SLS 0.1% aqueous solution were positive in 2 of 12 subjects with a positive eczematous reaction.

Foussereau et al. (201) reported that in a series of 20 patients treated by "maximization" with a preparation combining hair dyes with SLS, one case of "allergy" to SLS was observed.

> **Sodium lauryl sulfate is a skin irritant and comedogenic agent but is not usually a sensitizer.**

Cocamidopropyl Betaine

Cocamidopropyl betaine (CAPB) is a surfactant used in shampoos and cosmetics. Since its introduction in the 1970s, it has increasingly replaced sodium lauryl sulfate and other anionic surfactants because of its lower irritancy potential. In 1993, the estimated annual worldwide usage of CAPB was 120 million pounds. In addition to shampoos for humans, CAPB may be used in bath gels, body washes, liquid detergents, and pet shampoos. CAPB is valued as a viscosity builder and foam booster. It is formed by linking different fatty acids (variable length) with aminopropyl betaine. Coconut oil forms the source of the commercial

product and therefore may contribute contaminants such as free fatty acids and sterols (202).

According to the Cosmetic Ingredient Review, in 1994, 605 of 9,707 (6.23%) of personal care products voluntarily reported to the FDA contained CAPB. This product list includes hair shampoo and other hair care products, bath products, and other skin care products (202).

The majority of cases of ACD to CB have been caused by shampoos (203–205). Sites of dermatitis are usually the scalp and face. In addition, hand dermatitis was caused by CB in three hairdressers reported by Korting et al. (205) and in one health care worker by Fowler (206). Other allergens were also positive in all three including nickel and glyceryl thioglycolate. Patch tests to CB were negative or equivocal at 48 hours but became positive on the delayed reading.

> **Hairdressers with hand eczema and patients with face or scalp dermatitis should be tested with CAPB.**

Patch testing with CB should be preformed at a concentration of 1% aqueous. Because the substance is a surfactant, mild false-positive irritant reactions are not unusual. Therefore, caution is advised in interpreting patch test readings, and clinical correlation is essential to determine relevance. Out of 12 patients with positive patch tests to CB seen in a 15-month period, we were able to document relevance in 6 by examining shampoo ingredient labeling. In a follow-up study, Fowler et al. (207) could reproduce dermatitis under controlled conditions in a use test study in seven of ten patients positive to CAPB on patch testing. These patients reacted to shampoo and/or bath products with CAPB but not to products lacking CAPB but otherwise identical.

Six of the subjects also reacted to amidoamine (0.1% aq) on patch testing. Amidoamine is a contaminant found in the manufacture of CAPB, at levels of 3,000 to 30,000 ppm. Specially prepared CAPB that was free of amidoamine caused minimal reactivity, suggesting the true allergen may be amidoamine in most cases.

European investigators have suggested that another contaminant, dimethylaminopropylamine, may be an allergen as well (208).

> **Cocamidopropyl betaine, a surfactant, accounts for occasional cases of ACD from shampoos and toiletries. Patch testing can give irritant false-positive results, so clinical correlation is necessary to determine relevance.**

Cocamide DEA/Lauramide DEA

These nonionic surfactants are also known as coconut diethanolamide and lauicacid diethanolamide. DeGroot et al. (209) reported a case of allergy to this in shampoos. Fowler (210) reported three cases of allergy to cocamide DEA (0.5% pet). Other allergens were typically present, but none were allergic to CAPB. In two cases exposure was expected but unproven, due to lack of cooperation from the employer, to be from hydraulic lubricating oils in a mechanic.

Possible exposure sources include personal care products, lubricating oils, and plastics manufacturing where cocamide DEA may be used in lubricants.

Another related surfactant, undecylenamide DEA (UDEA), was shown to cause ACD in one patient. A liquid soap was the source of exposure (211).

Oleamidopropyl and Stearamidopropyl Dimethylamine

Oleamidopropyl dimethylamine (OPD) is a surfactant and emulsifier that has been the cause of occasional reports of allergy. Cosmetics, baby lotions, and body lotions have been held responsible for ACD to OPD (212). However, some older data may need to be revised, as it has been shown that OPD has a propensity to produce irritant patch test reactions (213). It is now recommended that patch testing be done with 0.1% aq OPD. Even this may irritate, however. Many cross-reactions to related amide-amine-type surfactants have been noted (214). Again, irritant reactions are difficult to separate from allergy with these substances.

The related chemical stearamidoethyl diethylamine was held responsible for four cases of ACD, three from a skin lotion and one from a deodorant (215). Testing was done at 0.4% aq. All four were believed to be relevant.

Nonoxynol-9

This is a nonionic surfactant used in spermicides, disinfectants, cleansers, and cosmetics. Fisher (216) reported ACD of the penis from nonoxynol-9 in a condom. Dooms-Goosens et al. (217) found 12 cases of ACD to nonoxynol-9 from various topical antiseptics.

Dihydroxyacetone

This is the principal active agent of self-tanning lotions. The coloration is formed in the superficial epidermal keratin layer. Morren et al. (218) reported two cases of ACD due to the dihydroxyacetone acetone in sunless tanning lotions, confirmed by patch testing with the lotion, as well as dihydroxyacetone 10% (aq).

Hexamidine Isethionate

This agent has been rarely noted to produce ACD. It is occasionally used as an antiseptic and preservative. Patch testing with 0.15% (pet) is recommended (219).

ALLERGY TO VEHICLES IN TOPICAL PRODUCTS

Propylene Glycol

The Nature and Uses of Propylene Glycol

Propylene glycol is a dihydric alcohol, $CH_3CHOHCH_2OH$, that is an odorless, viscous liquid, readily miscible with water, acetone, chloroform, and essential oils. It is stable under ordinary conditions. Propylene glycol is very hygroscopic, with an isotonic concentration of 2% in water.

Propylene glycol is used widely as a vehicle for topical therapeutics, cosmetics, and various hand and body lotions. In recent years, new vehicles based on fatty alcohols and propylene glycol have been developed for corticosteroids. In certain preparations, the amount of propylene glycol may be as high as 70%. Moreover, propylene glycol has been used as the only base for some antiperspirants. It is particularly useful because it has some antimicrobial properties and enhances penetration of topical pharmacologic agents. Above a 25% concentration, propylene glycol is somewhat antibacterial and antifungal and may be considered as a "preservative" in topical medications.

Antimicrobial activity has been shown against *Escherichia coli, Pseudomonas,* and other bacteria, as well as *Candida albicans, Bityrosporum orbiculare,* and some dermatophyte fungi. *In vitro* a 30% concentration has been shown to kill *Candida, E. coli,* and *S. aureus* after 20 hours of exposure. Tinea versicolor and seborrheic dermatitis are both somewhat responsive to treatment with high concentrations of propylene glycol (81).

Fulton et al. (220) have found that propylene glycol does not produce follicular hyperkeratosis and is therefore noncomedogenic. The United States Pharmacopeia has no pH specifications for propylene glycol (221).

Industrial uses of propylene glycol include its use in automotive brake fluid and antifreeze formulations, in alkyd resin manufacture, as a plasticizer for some resin systems, and as a humectant for tobacco formulations.

Propylene glycol is used widely in the food-chemical industry as a solvent, humectant, inhibitor of fermentation, preservative (particularly against molds), softening agent, lubricant for food machinery, and heat-transfer fluid for the processing of foods. It is an excellent solvent for food colors and flavoring agents and is added to foods to obtain desirable aesthetic properties (222).

Propylene glycol, a solvent, humectant, and preservative, is used widely in topical medications, foods, and industry.

Review of the Literature Pertaining to Propylene Glycol Reactions

Warshaw and Herrmann (223), almost 50 years ago, subjected 84 persons to simultaneous testing with several samples of propylene glycol from different sources. These authors concluded that it was often difficult to decide whether a positive reaction to propylene glycol was due to specific sensitization or to irritation. They described one of the patients who had a positive patch test reaction to propylene glycol who acquired cheilitis upon use of a lipstick containing this chemical.

Meneghini et al. (170) performed patch tests with 20% propylene glycol in petrolatum in a series of 50 "healthy" persons. They found that this concentration and vehicle were "nonirritating."

Goldsmith (224) stated that undiluted propylene glycol, especially under occlusion, can be a skin irritant. Fifty percent and 10% aqueous solutions of propylene glycol may also be primary irritants in some patients. Atopics and patients who have eczematous dermatitis may be more sensitive to the irritant effects of propylene glycol than normal people or patients who have other diseases; thus, drugs containing propylene glycol must be used cautiously in these patients. Irritant reactions to propylene glycol are more frequent in winter, and it is speculated that the degree of epidermal hydration may affect the irritant response to propylene glycol.

Trancik and Maibach (225) conducted irritation and sensitization patch test studies using propylene glycol in an attempt to ascertain the nature of the cutaneous response to this common excipient. A total of 10 and 203 subjects completed standard irritation and sensitization protocols, respectively. A provocative use test was conducted on subjects reacting to propylene glycol. Results indicated that propylene glycol is at least a minimal irritant. Fleeting evidence suggestive of sensitization was observed during patch testing but was not substantiated upon provocative use testing.

Hannuksela et al. (226) stated that reactions to propylene glycol were considered to be truly allergic in four patients. These authors stated that evaluating patch test responses is especially difficult when the patient has hyperirritable skin. Their patient had a 3+ reaction to undiluted propylene glycol and a 1+ reaction to 10% propylene glycol.

Braun (227) judged that approximately 3 of 78 patients were sensitive to propylene glycol on the basis of positive reactions to 10% propylene glycol solution. Cross-reactions between propylene glycol and polyethylene glycol were not observed in this group.

The NACDG reported a rate of positive patch tests to propylene glycol 10% pet of 1% to 2% through the 1980s and early 1990s. Several European studies have shown similar results (81). As is true of many allergens, higher concentrations of propylene glycol used for patch testing produce larger numbers of positive results. At concentrations above 10% irritant reactions are more likely and may be misinterpreted as allergic reactions by less experienced testers. In contrast, testing at less than 10% will probably miss some cases of true positive reactions. Currently, the NACDG tests with 30% propylene glycol in water with few irritant results.

Claverie et al. (228) described three patients with allergy to propylene glycol in Zovirax cream. Patch tests were negative with propylene glycol 5% but positive at 10% or 20% only.

> **Patch testing with 10% propylene glycol may give occasional transient irritant responses but probably will miss a few true positives. The NACDG now tests with 30%.**

Illustrative Case of Propylene Glycol Allergy

A 29-year-old nursing mother of a 4-month-old baby had had vulvitis since the birth of her child, for which she had been treated by her gynecologist with Mycolog cream, Lotrimin solution, Neo-Synalar cream, and Kenalog lotion. With the exception of Lotrimin solution, which was ineffective, all of these medications not only afforded no relief but also resulted in more marked vulvitis.

With the approval of the gynecologist and pediatrician, the patient was given systemic corticosteroids and instructed to apply Xylocaine ointment for the marked pruritus. To their astonishment, the vulvitis became worse.

Preliminary patch tests revealed strongly positive results to Mycolog cream, ethylenediamine hydrochloride, Neo-Synalar cream, neomycin, Xylocaine ointment, and Kenalog lotion. Patch tests to Lotrimin solution gave negative results. Further testing with the vehicle screening tray showed a strongly positive patch test reaction to 10% propylene glycol. To rule out an irritant reaction, the patient was tested with 5% and 2% propylene glycol. She showed strongly positive reactions to both 5% and 2% propylene glycol. Thus, this patient was allergic to three individual sensitizers in Mycolog cream—ethylenediamine hydrochloride, neomycin, and propylene glycol.

After delving further into the patient's history, it was revealed that during the middle of her pregnancy she had applied Triple Lanolin Cocoa Cream (which contains propylene glycol) to "prevent" formation of abdominal striae. Not only did striae form, but also severe abdominal dermatitis was produced.

It should be noted that all of the medications, with the exception of Lotrimin solution, contained propylene glycol.

This patient also found that eating foods containing propylene glycol produced systemic contact dermatitis with flares of her healed dermatitis and flares of her previous patch test sites of propylene glycol (see Chapter 34).

Propylene Glycol Dermatitis from Corticosteroid Creams and Gels

Oleffe et al. (229) found that propylene glycol was a sensitizer in corticosteroid cream. Shore and Shelley (230) described contact dermatitis from stearyl alcohol and propylene glycol in fluocinonide cream in a patient who developed "intolerance" to the cream and showed positive patch test reactions to the two agents.

Fowler (231) found that propylene glycol was present in 48 of 82 various corticosteroid creams, gels, ointments, and lotions sold in the United States in 1993. The data is similar today. Because propylene glycol is used so widely in topical corticosteroids, it should be suspected anytime a patient complains of "worsening" after use of such a product. Of course, other excipients and the steroid itself may cause allergy. The clinical picture may be confusing because the benefits of the steroid will moderate somewhat the allergic symptoms.

Propylene Glycol Dermatitis from Deodorants

Agren-Jonsson and Magnusson (232) studied 14 patients who had axillary dermatitis due to an antiperspirant and who had positive patch test reactions to the product. The sensitizer could be demonstrated in 12 cases. Of these, 11 patients had positive reactions to propantheline bromide, three to trichlorocarbanilide, and one to propylene glycol.

Propylene glycol is commonly found in newer clear gel deodorants. In addition to fragrances and preservatives, it should be considered in all cases of presumed deodorant allergy.

Propylene Glycol Dermatitis from Otic Preparations

Five patients in whom a superimposed allergic contact dermatitis developed used corticosteroid preparations in the treatment of otitis externa. It should be noted that those otic preparations, which contain benzocaine and neomycin, are not recommended for the treatment of external ear canal dermatoses, because they act as potent sensitizers in patients who have inflamed ear canals. (Note: The use of a carbol-fuchsin paint [diluted 1:6 with water] may be effective when all else fails in the treatment of otitis externa.)

Propylene Glycol Dermatitis from K-Y Jelly

Propylene glycol was formerly an ingredient of K-Y Jelly that caused occasional allergic reactions (222); it is no longer present in that product (see Table 17.10).

TABLE 17.10. *Lubricants Free of Propylene Glycol*

K-Y Jelly (Johnson & Johnson)
Surgilube (Fougera)
Maxilube Personal Lubricant (Mission)

Propylene Glycol Dermatitis from ECG and TENS Gels

Cases of allergy to propylene glycol in conductive gels used in electrocardiography monitoring and transcutaneous electrical nerve stimulator (TENS) units have been reported (233,234) (see Chapter 20).

Propylene glycol dermatitis can occur from many topical medications, electrocardiogram pastes, and many household products.

"Systemic" Contact Dermatitis Due to Injectable Valium in a Propylene Glycol–Sensitive Individual

A patient who received an injection of Valium preoperatively acquired an eczematous reaction at the sites where she had previously had an allergic contact dermatitis from the application of a steroid gel containing propylene glycol. It had previously been ascertained that she was allergic to propylene glycol in the gel. Propylene glycol was an ingredient in the medication at a concentration of 40%.

Propylene Glycol Intoxication in an Infant

A premature infant became comatose after treatment for burns with dressings containing propylene glycol. Urine levels of propylene glycol were high. Complete recovery ensued after topical treatment was stopped (235).

1,3 Butylene Glycol

Among the qualities associated with butylene glycol (BG) are the following: (a) It is the humectant most resistant to high humidity; (b) it is particularly valuable in hair sprays and setting lotions; (c) it has a marked ability to retard loss of aromas; (d) it preserves cosmetics against spoilage by microorganisms; and (e) it is a superior solvent for benzoates (236; M.V. Shelanski, personal communication).

Several chemists that Fisher consulted stated that from a theoretical chemical viewpoint, they believed that BG would cross-react with propylene glycol. Clinically, however, they believed that testing BG only with propylene glycol–sensitive persons would prove or disprove this "theoretical" viewpoint.

It is claimed that 1,3 BG is as efficient a humectant and preservative potentiator as is propylene glycol. In two patients with propylene glycol sensitivity, Fisher found patch test reactions to 1,3 butylene glycol gave negative results.

A report from Japan identified BG as an allergen in one patient who used multiple cosmetic creams (237). She was not allergic to propylene glycol.

Hexylene Glycol

This glycol is less hygroscopic than propylene glycol or butylene glycol. However, a 10% hexylene glycol (HG) solution showed antibacterial and antiCandidal effects *in vitro* equal to a 30% solution of propylene glycol or butylene glycol (238).

HG is used at concentrations of 0.1% to 25% in skin care products, soaps, hair care products, and eye cosmetics. In a patch test study comparing HG and propylene glycol, 2.8% of over 800 patients tested with 30% or 50% HG in water developed erythema and edema (+ or ++ reactions) (239). However, only 3 of 22 were still positive to patch tests at 1% or 2% HG aq, and they did not react to a use test of a solution of 30% HG. Only one patient with a positive patch test to HG could be identified as definitely clinically relevant. Propylene glycol was shown to have a greater effect on transepidermal water loss than HG in both atopic and nonatopic individuals. The authors concluded that hexylene glycol is an irritant in high concentration, but less so than propylene glycol, and that HG is a rare cause of contact allergy.

Polyethylene Glycol

Polyethylene glycol, $HO (CH_2CH_2)_x OH$, is a mixture of glycols. The lower molecular weights from 200 to 700 are liquids, whereas the higher weights of 1,000 to 6,000 are solids. Polyethylene glycols (PEGs) of varying molecular weights are used extensively as vehicles in topical medicaments, suppositories, shampoos, detergents, hair dressings, insect repellents, cosmetics, toothpastes, and contraceptives (240,241).

In industry the PEGs are used as solvents for nitrocellulose, as plasticizers for glue and casein, and as wetting agents in epoxy hardeners.

PEG ointment (USP) is made up of solid PEG 4000 (USP) and liquid PEG 300. Carbowax is a solid waxy PEG. Carbowax 1500 is a synthetic soft wax, used as a softener and lubricant sizing agent for textiles. Carbowax 4000, a hard, translucent solid, is a binder for pigments and a lubricant in sizing.

Patch Testing with PEG

Maibach (242) stressed that the PEGs of varying molecular weights are used extensively as vehicles in topical medicaments but are not listed as sensitizers in standard reference books. In an experimental study, Marzulli and Maibach (243) used as a screen an experimental bar soap for allergic contact sensitization. The soap was tested at 3% in water with the challenge concentration reduced to 1%. One subject (of 200) had a strong spreading reaction at the final elicitation. This was repeated three times at biweekly intervals with similar results. Breakdown testing of the soap components revealed a strong reaction only to 3% PEG 300 in petrolatum. This was repeated with a similar result. Additional challenges with 3% PEG 100, 1000, 4000, and 6000 were all positive. The same subject also reacted to these at 1% in petrolatum. The subject next received liberal use-type applications twice a day for 7 days of 3% PEG in petrolatum to his cheek and forearm. No dermatitis developed. This patient was apparently not sensitive enough to develop dermatitis in an open use test to 3% PEG 300.

Braun (244) studied 40 patients who showed a delayed allergic contact sensitivity to a medication containing nitrofural, which is a Furacin-like product. In 3 of 40 cases, the active ingredient nitrofural was not the cause of the dermatitis, but the solvent PEG 300 proved to be the culprit. Routine tests in 92 dermatologic patients who had contact allergies gave 4% positive reactions with PEG 300. Group sensitization in the PEG series appeared to occur only with polymers of the same molecular weights. Thus, of 12 subjects sensitized with PEG 300, 5 also reacted to PEG 400 and only 1 of them to PEG 1500 and 6000 as well. No group allergy could be demonstrated between propylene glycol and the PEG derivatives.

Four patients studied by Fisher (241) showed allergic reactions to these liquid PEGs in topical medications. Two had immediate urticarial reactions to PEG 400. Two other patients had delayed allergic eczematous reactions—one to PEG 200 and one to PEG 300. Cross-reactions occurred between PEG 200, 300, and 400, but not between these liquid polyethylenes and the higher molecular weight solid polyethylenes from 1000 to 6000. Two of the patients exhibited an urticarial reaction due to the presence of PEG 400 in the antifungal agents Lotrimin and Tinactin Solutions. The other two patients reacted with a delayed eczematous reaction to PEG 200 and PEG 300 in an ear solution and a topical liquid anesthetic.

In a study from India, Bajaj et al. (245) found 8 of 180 patients with suspected allergy to medicaments reacted to various PEGs. Concentration of the test substances was not given. Four patients reacted only to PEG 400, three to PEG 400 plus either PEG 1500 or 3000, and one to PEG 1500, 3000, and 6000. Relevance was not determined.

In contrast, the NACDG found no reactions to PEG 400 (as is) in 148 subjects tested. Perhaps the difference in sensitization reflects different patterns of medicament usage in India as compared to the United States. The NACDG no longer recommends testing routinely with PEG, but it still may be useful in suspected cases of cosmetic allergy.

The low molecular PEGs from 200 to 400 may cause allergic contact urticaria and eczema. The higher molecular weight PEGs are rare sensitizers.

Glycerin

Glycerin—a Nonirritating, Rare Sensitizer

Among the qualities associated with glycerin are the following: (a) it is a basic readily available raw material of the cosmetic industry; (b) it is stable, nontoxic, nonirritating, and nonallergic; (c) it has good water absorption; (d) it is an effective humectant or hygroscopic agent; (e) it is an effective plasticizer; (f) it is an excellent lubricant; and (g) it imparts "smoothness" to cosmetics.

Allergic reactions to glycerin are rare, and we have not as yet encountered any such reactions. Hannuksela and Forstrom (246) described one patient who was allergic to glycerol (glycerin). This particular patient, on the staff of the allergy laboratory of the dermatologic clinic in Helsinki, noticed eczema on both hands. According to her own observations, a mixture of glycerol (1 part) and 70% ethanol (9 parts) applied on the hands after washing them with soap and water was the apparent cause of her eczema. Glycerol tested at 10%, 5%, and 1% in water and the glycerol-ethanol mixture already mentioned gave 3+ reactions at 48- and 72-hour readings. The reactions were considered to be allergic. The patient stopped using the glycerol-ethanol mixture, and the eczema disappeared within a couple of days.

Glycerin versus Propylene Glycol

Generally, it is agreed that glycerin is much less active than propylene glycol in producing primary irritant and allergic reactions. It is claimed, however, that glycerin is a less desirable solvent than propylene glycol. Also, propylene glycol is said to have better permeation through the stratum corneum, probably because it has different solvent properties (i.e., propylene glycol is more lipid soluble than glycerin). Because of these superior solubility properties, propylene glycol has replaced glycerin in many pharmaceutical and cosmetic preparations. In addition, propylene glycol is less expensive.

Both glycerin and propylene glycol are biodegradable under dilute conditions. Glycerin, however, exhibits antimicrobial properties as a concentrated solution. Thus, glycerin at sufficient concentrations can provide a preservative function in products. Whether or not a product containing glycerin needs a preservative depends on various factors, such as the level of glycerin, other components, and the available water. For example, a dilute solution of glycerin, which contains 10% ethanol, does not need any special preservative because the ethanol will suffice as the preservative. Overall, concentrated glycerin provides a hostile environment for microorganisms and usually does not need a preservative.

> **Glycerin, a rare sensitizer, has many of the qualities of propylene glycol, for which it may sometimes be substituted.**

Petrolatum

Petrolatum is considered one of the most inert of all topical agents. Nevertheless, there are several case reports of petrolatum allergy. Dooms-Goossens and DeGreef commented in three such cases, and Maibach (248) published the first such case in 1978. Grin and Maibach (249) recently reported a patient with both delayed and immediate allergy to petrolatum. On patch testing, all sites of petrolatum allergens were positive at both day 2 and day 4 with urticarial and eczematous patterns. An open test on the forearms produced urticaria at 30 minutes (249).

Emulsifiers

Emulsifiers are common constituents of skin care products, cosmetics, and topical medications. These agents enhance the miscibility of aqueous and fatty components. Generally they are rare sensitizers but mild irritants, especially if applied to damaged skin. Also, irritant patch tests may occur, so delayed readings and clinical correlation are advisable (see Table 17.11).

Triethanolamine

Triethanolamine, also known as trolamine or TEA, a mixture of three alkanolamines, is employed frequently as an excipient in hand and body lotions, shaving creams, soaps, shampoos, bath powders, and occasionally pharmaceutical preparations. An excipient is presumably an "inert" substance that gives a topical agent proper consistency through its action as a dispersant or detergent.

Castelain (250) reported allergic contact dermatitis due to sensitization to triethanolamine. Suurmond (251) showed cross-reactions between triethanolamine and other tertiary amines, such as Phenergan (promethazine). Schwartz (252) cautioned: "These chemicals are combined in the form of an innocuous substance, triethanolamine stearate. On the other hand, in some instances the combined irritant action of chemicals in a cosmetic may be greater than the irritant action of the individual substances."

TEA may be a more common sensitizer in industrial products than in cosmetic agents. A case of allergy to TEA, along with mono- and diethanolamine, in a metal worker has been reported (253). Fowler (unpublished observation) has seen several such cases. A fluorescent marking pen used in patch testing caused allergy from TEA in one patient (254).

TEA-stearate in a sunscreen has caused ACD (255).

> **Triethanolamine is a rare sensitizer that may be a mild irritant.**

TABLE 17.11. *Common Emulsifiers with Selected Patch Test Results*

Emulsifier	Other names	Hannuksela et al. (377) N = 1,200		Tosti et al. (381) N = 739	
		% Pos.	P.T. Conc.	% Pos.	P.T. Conc.
Cetyl alcohol			NT	NT	
Stearyl alcohol			NT	NT	
Cetosteryl alcohol	Lanette O		NT	0.8%	20 pet
Myristyl alcohol			NT	NT	
Stearic acid			NT	NT	
Glyceryl stearate		0	20 pet	NT	
Isopropyl palmitate			NT	NT	
Isopropyl myristate			NT	NT	
Sorbitan sesquioleate	Arlacel 83	0.5%	20 pet	0.9%	20 pet
Polyoxyedilene	Polysorbate 40				
Sorbitan monopalmitate	Tween 40	0.2%	5 pet	0.7%	10 pet
Polyoxyethylene	Polysorbate 80				
Sorbitan monooleate	Tween 80	0.2%	5 pet	0.5%	10 pet
Sorbitan stearate	Span 60	0.4%	5 pet	NT	
Sorbitan oleate	Span 80	0.4%	5 pet	NT	
Triethanolamine		0.4%	5 pet	2.7%	2.5 pet

P.T. = patch test; NT = not tested; Pos. = positive; pet = petrolatum.

Cetyl, Stearyl, and Myristyl Alcohols

The first two alcohols have the formula $CH_3 (CH_2)_{14} CH_2OH$ and $CH_3 (CH_2)_{16} CH_2OH$, respectively. They are often used together under the name cetostearyl alcohol (CSA) as an emulsifier and stabilizer. As such, they may be considered preservatives. Only rare cases of allergy to either or both agents occur. Usually there is a predisposing factor that enhances the patient's sensitivity. For example, De-Berker et al. (256) reported a patient allergic to stearyl alcohol in 5-fluorouracil cream. The irritant effect of the 5-FU probably predisposed to ACD development. Likewise, cases of allergy in leg ulcer patients have been reported (257).

A British study found that of 11 patients previously positive to CSA, only 2 reacted on later testing (258). None reacted to CSA-containing creams in a repeated open application (ROAT) test. The reasons for this apparent "loss of reactivity" are unclear.

Closely related to cetyl and stearyl alcohols, myristyl alcohol has the formula $CH_3(CH_2)_{12} CH_2OH$. It is also known as tetradecanol. There are occasional case reports of allergy to this agent, which may be found in some cosmetics and moisturizing creams (259).

Stearic Acid Glyceryl Stearate

Stearic acid is closely related to stearyl alcohol, containing an extra oxygen atom in place of two hydrogen atoms. Glyceryl stearate is a larger molecule formed by the attachment of glycerin to stearic acid. Both of these agents have been shown to be rare contact sensitizers, although they are used fairly widely in skin care products (260). About 15% of 19,000 cosmetic formulas contained one or the other, according to FDA data in 1984. Cross-reaction between stearic acid, stearyl alcohol, and glyceryl stearate has been

studied, but due to the similarities in chemical structure, these might be expected. Hayakawa (261) studied one patient who had a recurrent cheilitis due to lipsticks. She reacted positively to glyceryl stearate, glyceryl disostearate and tri-isostearate, diisostearyl malate, and stearyl alcohol. Testing to stearic acid was negative.

Oleyl Alcohol

This fatty alcohol has been reported to cause allergy from lipstick and other skin care products. Cross-reactions with castor oil has been observed (262).

Isopropyl Myristate

This emulsifier is a very rare cause of contact allergy (263).

Propolis (Bee Glue) and Beeswax

Propolis (bee glue) is a dark yellow-brown adhesive resin that bees mix with wax to form a cementing substance in their hives. The purified wax from the honeycomb, beeswax, is used widely in cosmetics. Beeswax may be used as cera alba (bleached) or as cera flava (unbleached).

Propolis (Bee Glue)

Propolis (bee glue), derived mainly from poplar and other tree resins, contains, among other things, well-known sensitizers such as cinnamic acid and vanillin and may cross-react with balsam of Peru. Allergic contact dermatitis from propolis is an occupational hazard for beekeepers (264,265). In rare instances a beekeeper may be allergic to beeswax.

Propolis is sold in many health food stores in many forms to be ingested as a cure-all for many diseases, and as a topical agent in the form of various ointments, powders, and cosmetic creams. Solid propolis, which can be chewed, may produce a perioral dermatitis and stomatitis. Thus, Wanscher (266) described two patients who had contact dermatitis from chewing so-called natural propolis products, which are sold without prescription as tablets or as solid propolis in large or small chunks.

Petersen (267) predicted that with the increasing employment of propolis for self-medication, an increasing number of allergic contact eczema to this preparation must be anticipated.

> **Propolis (bee glue), which may cross-react with balsam of Peru, may produce allergic contact dermatitis not only in beekeepers but also in the general population, owing to increasing self-medication with this product.**

Hausen et al. (268) extensively studied various constituents of propolis and found that several caffeates and benzyl isoferulate are strong sensitizers in guinea pigs. A number of these substances are also found in balsam of Peru. From 1988 to 1990, 10 of 137 (0.9%) men and 28 of 2,036 (1.4%) women reacted to propolis on patch testing. One report from Prague, where apparently propolis is used commonly, reported allergy in 25 of 605 patients (4.1%). Thirteen of these also reacted to balsam of Peru (269).

Beeswax

Beeswax is secreted by bees. Camasara (270) reported a woman who was employed in molding art objects from beeswax and who developed chronic palmar dermatitis. A strongly positive patch test to natural beeswax was obtained.

A beekeeper described by Rothenborg (265) reacted to raw, unpurified beeswax but not to purified beeswax. The raw wax was considered contaminated by poplar tree resins to which the was sensitive.

> **Beeswax, which is secreted by bees and is used widely in cosmetics, is a rare sensitizer unless contaminated with propolis (bee glue).**

Honey is a saccharin substance deposited in the honeycomb by the honeybee. It is used as an excipient, as a flavor in gargles and cough medicine, and as a food.

Lanolin

Lanolin (wool fat, wool grease, wool wax, wool alcohol, and adeps lanae anhydrous) and its various esters, fatty acids, and aliphatic alcohols are used in many topical medicaments and cosmetics.

Lanolin is a natural product obtained from the fleece of sheep, and its constituents vary from time to time and place to place.

Composition

Lanolin contains sterols, fatty alcohols, and fatty acids. The lanolin sterols (lanolin alcohols or wood alcohols) include principally cholesterol, lanosterol, and agnesterol and are built from one or more benzene rings.

Commercially, these wool alcohols are called Cerolan, Type HO, Hartolan, Golden Dawn, and Nimco. Cholesterol is the major ingredient of lanolin alcohol, and commercial lanolin products list the cholesterol content. Further studies are required to establish whether these lanolin alcohols are the sole or main sensitizers in lanolin (271).

The fatty alcohols are long-chained and include the closely related stearyl and cetyl alcohols. The fatty acids, the other ingredients of lanolin, have not been found to be sensitizers.

Modifications

Acetylated lanolin (Modulan), according to Cronin (271), is less of a sensitizer than plain lanolin. *Dewaxed lanolin* (Lantrol), formed by a solvent crystallization process, is also claimed to cause less sensitization than lanolin.

Another modification is *hydrogenated lanolin.* Vollum (272) reported that it is used frequently in the pharmaceutical and cosmetic industry because it is colorless, odorless, free from tackiness, and more hydrophilic than lanolin.

Hydrogenation is carried out by heating lanolin with a catalyst to 330°C at a pressure of 180 atmospheres. The absorption of hydrogen is complete within a half hour, and the resulting hydrogenated lanolin contains dihydrocholesterol, other hydrogenated steroids, and some saturated alcohol. It was hoped originally that hydrogenated lanolin, or a modification, could be used in cases of lanolin sensitivity, but some patients show a marked sensitivity to hydrogenated lanolin and not to the plain lanolin. Dermatitis owing to hydrogenated lanolin may be missed if patients are patch tested with wool alcohols for plain lanolin and not the hydrogenated variety.

A "purified" anhydrous lanolin product gave a positive patch test in only 1 of 33 subjects previously positive to lanolin (273). Presumably, the removal of fatty alcohols rendered the "purified" product less allergenic.

Patch Tests for Lanolin Sensitivity

Many investigators routinely test with 30% wool alcohol in petrolatum, but because it may not be the sensitizing substance in lanolin, patch testing should be performed with lanolin. Thune's (274) investigation indicates that the addition of salicylic acid to lanolin or Eucerin may cause false-positive reactions. Patch tests for wool fat sensitivity should be performed with lanolin without the addition of salicylic acid.

Newcomb (275) emphasizes that lanolin is a complex natural material, which is never completely identified because of the wide variations in purity. The development of new derivatives and further purification may contribute to lowering the incidence of skin reactions to this emollient (276).

Oleffe et al. (277) emphasized that lanolin is a complex mixture of esters and polyesters of 33 alcohols with high molecular weights and 36 fatty acids. They made the following points: (a) The response of tested patients varies greatly; thus, a patient may react to one brand of lanolin and not to another. (b) The lanolin alcohols are plainly responsible for allergy to lanolin. (c) The Trolab wool alcohol test is reliable for detecting lanolin allergy. (d) A positive reaction to wool alcohols should prompt the dermatoallergist to test the patient with the lanolin preparation he or she actually will use. (e) The hydrogenated lanolin that was tested had a very slight allergic capacity, whereas in Japan, hydrogenated lanolin appears to be a strong sensitizer.

The exact allergenic fraction awaits clarification. It is still unknown whether or not lanolin-sensitive patients can tolerate modified or purified lanolin and its derivatives.

Most recent NACDG data show that positive lanolin patch test rates are in the range of 3.3% (2).

The results of Giorgini et al. (278) confirm the sensitizing action of lanolin alcohols and the fact that acetylation, ethylenation, and transesterification eliminate the allergenic activity of lanolin.

> **Chemical treatments to reduce the allergenicity of the lanolin alcohols may reduce the usefulness of lanolin as an excipient.**

Sensitizing Potential of Lanolin

The incidence of lanolin sensitivity is a controversial subject. Kligman (279) concludes that "[l]anolin is an extremely weak sensitizer. Its reputation as an allergen has been vastly inflated by reports emanating from European clinics where patients with chronic eczema have been treated with lanolin-based medicaments for many years."

There is general agreement, however, that lanolin frequently produces allergic contact dermatitis when applied to stasis eczemas and ulcers.

> **Lanolin sensitivity is very low in noneczematous skin, moderate in atopic and other eczematous dermatoses, and high in stasis eczema and ulcers.**

Breit and Bandmann (280) found that 13.2% of 326 cases of leg eczema were sensitive to wool alcohols. Of the 43 Eucerin-positive patients of Bandmann and Reichenberger (281), about 70% had stasis eczemas. Thus, stasis dermatitis patients are at unusually high risk.

Lanolin allergy is rare in patients who have chronic skin diseases that are not of the eczematous type (e.g., psoriasis, lichen planus, and bullous diseases).

Cronin et al. (282) showed that the proportion of atopic patients reacting to wool alcohols was comparable to that of other eczematous patients, except those patients who had stasis eczema.

Lanolin derivatives Amerchol L101 and Amerchol CAB are composed of lanolin alcohols and as such may cause allergic sensitization. They are useful in cosmetic products as emulsifiers and emollients. A study by Bojs et al. (283) showed an identical reaction pattern to Amerchol CAB and Amerchol L101 in lanolin-sensitive patients. Amerchol CAB was present in a corticosteroid ointment made in Denmark.

Matthies and Dockx (284) found a great discrepancy in the frequency of positive reactions to lanolin as opposed to Amerchol L101 (wool wax alcohols obtained from hydrolysis of wool fat). Twelve of 323 patients reacted to both lanolin 30% and Amerchol L101 100%, but 32 more reacted to the Amerchol L101 alone. The concern is that some of these may have been irritant reactions. Even so, Amerchol L101 may be a more reliable patch test agent than "standard" wool wax alcohol.

> **Amerchol L101 and Amerchol CAB should be avoided by lanolin-allergic persons.**

Castor Oil

Castor oil is commonly used in lipsticks because of its superior emollient characteristics. Sporadic case reports of allergy to it have implicated ricinoleic acid as the causative agent. Other than one report of allergy to a makeup remover (285), lipsticks have been the source of exposure. An individual who reacts to "all" lipsticks should be tested with castor oil (as is) (286–289).

CUTANEOUS REACTIONS TO COSMETICS

Allergic Reactions to Cosmetics

Allergy to cosmetics constitutes a significant portion of the cases of contact dermatitis seen by dermatologists in the United States (289). In a 64-month study, 11 dermatologists belonging to the NACDG patch tested 13,216 patients; 713 (5.4%) were identified as having reactions caused by cosmetics (73). It is notable that these contact dermatitis experts and their patients did not initially suspect a cosmetic in half the cases later proven to evoke reactions to cosmetics. Patients who experience reactions to newly purchased cosmetics seldom consult a physician and merely discard or discontinue using the suspected item. These circumstances hinder our ability to learn the true incidence of reactions to cosmetics and their ingredients. Nevertheless, this study provides data to alert physicians to suspect cosmetic contact reactions and notes likely offenders. Fifty percent of the reactions occurred on the face, and 79% were in females.

Fragrances and preservatives constituted the majority of reactions, followed by "active ingredients" such as hair coloring or permanent wave chemicals, sunscreens, and nail care products.

A similar study from the Netherlands identified 119 patients with contact allergy to cosmetic products (290). In this study, hair cosmetics, except shampoo and conditioners, were not included in the evaluation. Again, the majority of reactions were due to preservatives (32%) and fragrances (27%).

The majority of cosmetic reactions are not due to allergy, however, but are results of irritation of sensitive skin or urticaria, either immunologic or nonimmunologic (see Table 17.12).

The cosmetics industry has established an expert panel to review the toxicology of the more than 4,000 ingredients used in cosmetics. The deliberations of this Cosmetic Ingredient Review (CIR) Panel should provide additional information about the reactivity of these chemicals. This information should aid responsible manufacturers in formulating safer cosmetics. The reports of the CIR are published periodically in the *Journal of the American College of Toxicology*. Experience in toxicologic testing of cosmetics leads us to question if any truly nonreactive ingredients exist.

Methods of Testing

Closed patch testing can be used safely with many cosmetic preparations in the same way that prepared allergens are tested. When using whole products, however, both false-negative and false-positive reactions may sometimes occur.

TABLE 17.12. *Cosmetic Categories Reported Frequently by Consumers as Causing Adverse Reactions*

Bath soaps and detergents	Mainly irritation
Deodorants (underarm) and antiperspirants	Usually irritation; occasional allergic contact dermatitis
Eye shadow	Mainly irritation
Hair dyes	Allergic contact dermatitis
Mascara	Mainly irritation
Moisturizers	Irritation and allergic contact dermatitis
Permanent waves	Irritation and allergic contact dermatitis
Shampoos	Mainly irritation

False-Negative Reactions

The concentration of an allergen in a cosmetic product may be great enough to produce dermatitis after repeated application on sensitive skin but may be too low to produce a positive patch test on the back. This is especially true of fragrances and preservatives. A negative reaction to a cosmetic, therefore, does not rule out allergy to a component of the product.

False-Positive Reactions

Some cosmetic products are inherently irritating on a closed patch. Cleansing products, hair perms, and artificial nail products are particularly problematic. Volatile solvents, such as are present in some mascaras, may also irritate and therefore should be allowed to evaporate for 10 to 15 minutes before the patch is applied. However, a positive reaction to a nonirritating product such as a makeup or skin lotion virtually confirms contact allergy.

Recommendations for Cosmetic Testing

Table 17.13 gives guidelines for cosmetic product testing. As a general rule, "leave on" products such as moisturizers and makeup are safe for closed patch testing, whereas "rinse off" products may frequently irritate.

Open testing can be done to irritating substances but is much less reliable than properly performed closed patch testing. Often cosmetic manufacturers will supply patch test kits on request with a breakdown of the ingredients in a suspected product. The patch tester should request that materials be provided at proper patch test concentration, not at product use concentrations, to avoid erroneous results. Usually, the proper patch test concentration is higher, but sometimes, in the case of a surfactant or detergent, for example, it may be lower than in the actual product (291).

Immediate testing for contact urticaria may be helpful if clinically indicated and/or regular patch testing is unrevealing. The allergen or product is applied to the volar forearm for about 15 minutes. Readings are taken at intervals over the next 2 hours. Very rarely a "delayed" contact urticaria may occur at a later time (see Table 17.14).

The provocative use test (PUT) or ROAT may identify a reaction if patch testing is equivocal. The suspected product is rubbed into the antecubital skin twice daily for 4 or 5 days. An absence of erythema, pruritus, or other reaction usually confirms lack of allergy.

Finally, a PUT or ROAT may need to be performed on the face or other affected areas. Occasionally, a positive, reproducible reaction will occur only under such testing, especially in the case of contact urticaria.

Photoallergy must also be considered in facial dermatitis in the absence of other positive findings (see Chapter 23).

TABLE 17.13. *Patch Testing Cosmetic Products*

Product	Conc.	Vehicle	Comments
Baby products			
Baby shampoo	1[a]	Aq	Test individual ingredients; detergents may require open test and provocative use tests for confirmation
Baby lotion	as is[b]		
Baby oil	as is		
Baby powder	as is		
Baby cream	as is[b]		
Bath preparation			
Bath oil			
Nonfoaming	as is[b]		Nonfoaming—emulsifiers may irritate.[a]
Foaming			Foaming—treat as detergent; perform open tests and provocative use test[b]
Bubble bath	1[a]	Aq	Test individual ingredients.
Bath capsule			If it contains detergent, dilute 1:100[a]
Other bath preparations			If primarily fragrance, patch test 10% in petrolatum closed and photopatch test. If positive, verify with controls
Eye makeup			
Eyebrow pencil	as is[b]		If positive, verify with controls
Eyeliner	as is[b]		Usually not irritant; if suspected check with open and provocative use test
Eye shadow cream	as is[b]		Rare, irritant reactions. Repeat weak positives with open and provocative use tests
Eye shadow powder	as is		
Eye lotion	as is		
Eye makeup remover	as is[b]		Occasional irritant reaction may contain amphoteric surfactant. Check with open and provocative use tests
Mascara	as is[b]	Dry	Dry 20 minutes to remove volatile solvents. Open and provocative use tests may clarify type of reaction
Fragrance preparations			
Cologne and toilet water	as is	Dry	Dry for 5 minutes. Photopatch test also
Perfume	as is	Dry	Dry for 5 minutes. Photopatch test also
Powder	as is		
Sachet	as is[b]		Photopatch test also
Hair preparations (noncoloring)			
Conditioners	as is[b]		Quaternary ammonium compounds may be irritating under occlusion[c]
Aerosol spray	as is	Dry	
Straightener			Never test except with diluted ingredients
Permanent wave			Never test except with diluted ingredients.
Rinse	2	Aq	
Shampoo	1[a]	Aq	Doubtful value. Test ingredients
Tonic	as is[b]	Dry	Test open and photopatch test. Patch test ingredients. May contain preservatives and fragrance allergens
Hair coloring preparations			
Hair dyes	2	Aq	Prefer: 5 drops dye + 5 drops oxidizer test open and read in 24 hours. Test 1% paraphenylenediamine in petrolatum closed. If negative, test other ingredients
Hair tint			See above: hair dyes
Hair rinse (coloring)			Open test read in 24 hours
Shampoo (coloring)	1[a]	Aq	Irritant due to detergent. If semipermanent dye, test open antecubital area
Bleach			Ammonium persulfate 1 to 2.5% in petrolatum test open (see contact urticaria and text on bleaching)
Makeup preparation			
Blushers	as is		
Face powder	as is		
Foundation	as is[b]		
Leg and body paint	as is		May be an irritant
Lipstick	as is		Phototest also
Makeup base	as is[b]		
Rouge	as is		

(continued)

TABLE 17.13. (Continued)

Product	Conc.	Vehicle	Comments
Manicuring preparations			
Basecoat/undercoat	as is[b]	Dry	May test open
Cuticle softener			Do not patch test as is. Test diluted ingredients only
Nail cream	as is[b]		
Nail extender			Patch test ingredients only
Nail polish and enamel	as is	Dry	May test open
Nail polish remover			Do not patch test as is. Test diluted ingredients only
Oral hygiene			
Dentifrice liquid, paste, powder	2[a]	Aq	Detergents may require open and provocative use tests. If positive, verify with controls
Personal cleanliness			
Bath soaps	1[a]	Aq	Alternatively 5% aq open. Both of doubtful value
Detergents			
Deodorant (underarm)	as is[b]		May be mild irritant. Repeat weak positives open inside forearm twice daily for 1 week. Test diluted ingredients also
Antiperspirants			Test ingredients
Douches			
Feminine deodorant sprays	as is[b]		Usually irritant reactions from being applied too close
Shaving preparations			
Aftershave lotion	as is	Dry	Photopatch test. Provocative use test in small area on beard region
Beard softener			
Men's talc	as is		
Preshave lotion			
Shaving cream aerosol brushless lather	2[a]	Aq	
Shaving soap	1[a]	Aq	
Skin care preparations			
Cleansing lotion, or pads	as is[b]		Likely to be weak irritants
Depilatory			Test diluted ingredients only
Face, body, or hand cream or lotion	as is		
Foot powder or spray			
Hormone cream or lotion	as is		
Moisturizing cream or lotion	as is		
Night cream or lotion	as is[b]		May be weak irritant
Skin lightener			Test ingredients only
Skin freshener	20	Aq	May be irritant. Provocative use test if in doubt
Suntan and sunscreen preparations			
Sunscreen gel, cream or lotion	as is[b]		Photopatch test also
Indoor tanning preparations	as is[b]		

[a]Detergents require provocative use tests.
[b]This category may rarely produce irritancy with occlusive patch test.
[c]Contact manufacturer requesting irritancy controls.

Fisher has suggested an elimination routine that may be helpful in the diagnosis of reactions to cosmetics. All cosmetics are stopped except lipstick, which is allowed if the lips are problem-free. Unscented shampoo and unscented soap are used to cleanse the scalp and the skin. All cosmetics and cosmetic applicators are brought in for the physician to examine and patch test. When the dermatitis has cleared, a program of beginning systematically to use each cosmetic one at a time is initiated. If a reaction recurs, the cosmetic begun most recently is eliminated. The program is begun again, and the suspected cosmetic is used last.

Maibach and Engasser (292) find that a personal, positive approach to the problem produces more compliance.

We emphasize that patients may usually use as much of the following items as they need: (a) lipstick (as in the Fisher regimen), (b) eye makeup of all types (except when the upper lid is involved), (c) all loose powders, (d) glycerin and rose water (stronger rose water NF is prepared by distilling the petals of *Rosa centifolia* L. [fam. Rosacea] with water and separating the volatile oil from the water portion of the distillate. Stronger rose water, diluted with equal parts of purified water, is designated as Rose Water), and (e) cleansing with water.

An "elimination" routine in which individual cosmetics are added gradually may be helpful in diagnosing an irritant or sensitizing cosmetic.

TABLE 17.14. *Test Procedure for Evaluation of Immediate-Type Reactions in Recommended Order*

1. Open application
   Nonaffected normal skin
     Negative
       ↓
   Slightly affected (or previously affected) skin
     Negative
       ↓
2. Occlusive application
   (infrequently needed)
   Nonaffected normal skin
     Negative
       ↓
   Slightly affected (or previously affected) skin
     Negative
       ↓
3. Invasive (inhalant, prick, scratch, or intradermal injection)[a]

IF POSITIVE = DIAGNOSIS OF CONTACT URTICARIA

[a]When invasive methods are employed (especially scratch and inhalant testing), adequate controls are required.

Adapted from Krogh, G von, Maibach, HI. The contact urticaria syndrome—1982. *Semin Dermatol* 1982;1:59. (297)

Ingredient Labeling

The diagnosis and treatment of reactions to cosmetics has been facilitated by the FDA's regulation requiring the ingredient labeling of all retailed cosmetics (293). The ingredients are listed in order of descending concentration. Because of the complexity of the composition of fragrances and trade secrecy concerns, their compositions are not given but are listed simply as "fragrance." This regulation, besides identifying ingredients, is helpful to dermatologists because it mandated a uniform nomenclature for cosmetic ingredients. The *CTFA Ingredient Dictionary,* published by the Cosmetic, Toiletrys, and Fragrance Association, is the source for the official names (294). This dictionary provides a brief description of the chemical, alternative names, and names of suppliers.

Unfortunately, as of this writing, ingredient labeling outside the United States is often not required. The allergic patient is therefore at a major disadvantage.

When the clinical history, appearance of the reaction, or patch test results lead the clinician to conclude that a cosmetic has caused an adverse reaction, it is important to obtain the ingredients for patch testing. The Cosmetic, Toiletry, and Fragrance Association publishes a pamphlet called *Cosmetic Industry on Call.* This pamphlet lists the names of members of the industry (with addresses and telephone numbers) who are willing to answer questions about their products. Physicians can write to or telephone these persons requesting ingredients for patch testing. The letters should request specifically the materials needed. In addition, request any information the manufacturer may have about patch test concentrations. Keep a record of all correspondence, because the patch test materials will arrive frequently without identifying the patient a long time after the request was made. Of course, if the patient does or does not prove to have a reaction due to the cosmetics, the manufacturer should be notified of your results.

On occasion "fractionated" samples will be sent for patch testing. Because irritant concentrations of ingredients may be present in these samples, they are often not suitable to use for closed patch testing. Some manufacturers will supply individual ingredients in the concentration that they appear in the product, as noted earlier. These are often unsatisfactory for patch testing because the nonstandardized concentrations may be too low to provoke an allergic response or may be high enough to elicit irritation under occlusion. See Appendix A in this chapter for sources of information on the cosmetic industry.

Types of Reactions

Reactions to cosmetics can have a varied appearance; this variety of presentation can challenge the clinician's ability to make the correct diagnosis.

Subjective Irritation

When the application of a cosmetic causes burning, stinging, or itching without detectable visible or microscopic changes, this is designated as subjective irritation. This reaction is common in certain susceptible individuals occurring usually on the face. Some of the ingredients that cause this reaction are not generally considered irritants and will not cause abnormal responses in nonsusceptible individuals (295). The burning or stinging lasts usually less than 10 minutes. The clinician is dependent on the patient's subjective responses to the use of a product to identify this type of reaction. This is probably the most common cause of dissatisfaction with cosmetics and skin care products.

Objective Irritation

Predictive testing in human beings and rabbits can reliably detect strong or moderate irritants as ingredients in cosmetics or the products themselves (296). This allows manufacturers to test thoroughly to eliminate these potential hazards before marketing a cosmetic. Mild irritants, however, are more difficult to detect. Because the stratum corneum of the facial skin is penetrated easily, more irritant reactions occur there. Many supposedly nonirritating moisturizers or emollient creams contain surfactants and emulsifiers that may be mild irritants. These cosmetics are applied frequently to facial or inflamed skin, resulting in irritant reactions. In use testing, reproducing an irritant reaction is difficult because penetrability of the stratum corneum varies with environmental conditions such as humidity and temperature. If testing is negative on the back or forearm, provocative use testing may be carried out at the original site of the reactions. This diagnosis rests on the exclusion of contact allergy with patch testing and known exposure to potential irritants.

Examples of irritants in topical products include propylene glycol, PABA, SLS, other surfactants, alpha-hydroxy acids, and retinoids.

Contact Urticaria

A contact urticarial reaction is a wheal-and-flare response to a topically applied chemical that may be immunologic or nonimmunologic. In practice, patients may present with varied complaints: itching, burning, stinging, chronic dermatitis, generalized urticaria, or systemic anaphylactoid reactions. A careful history alerts a physician to perform the tests that are necessary to observe short-term reactions. A flow sheet designed by von Krogh and Maibach (297) can be used to approach testing in suspected cases (see Table 17.14). The details of testing can be studied in this review. The testing should be carried out where emergency resuscitation facilities are available, because anaphylactic reactions have rarely been reported even when chemicals have been applied to intact skin in sensitive individuals.

The cosmetic ingredients and products, cited in Table 17.15, have been implicated in the contact urticarial syndrome.

> **Many cosmetic ingredients can produce contact urticaria, which can be immunologic, nonimmunologic, or of an uncertain mechanism.**

Allergic Contact Dermatitis

Although ACD is the most frequently diagnosed reaction to cosmetics, it is suspected initially in less than half the proven cases. A battery of screening allergens, cosmetic ingredients, and sometimes the cosmetics themselves should be used for testing.

Pigmentation

Hyperpigmentation of the face caused by contact dermatitis to ingredients in cosmetics occurs more frequently in dark complexioned individuals (298). An epidemic of facial pigmentation reported in Japanese women was attributed to "coal tar" dyes (principally Sudan I, a contaminant of D&C Red No. 31) (299,300). The following fragrance ingredients have also been implicated: benzyl salicylate, ylang-ylang oil, cananga oil, jasmin absolute, hydroxycitronellal, methoxycitronellal, sandalwood oil, benzyl alcohol, cinnamic alcohol, lavender oil, geraniol, and geranium oil (301). Histologic examination shows hydropic degeneration of the basal layer and pigment incontinence. There may

TABLE 17.15. *Some Cosmetics and Ingredients That Have Been Reported to Cause Contact Urticaria*

Type of Reaction	Chemical	Product
Nonimmunologic	Acetic acid	
	Alcohols	
	Balsam of Peru	Perfumes
	Benzoic acid	
	Cinnamic acid	
	Cinnamic aldehyde	
	Formaldehyde[a]	
	Sodium benzoate	
	Sorbic acid	Shampoo
Immunologic	Acrylic monomer	
	Alcohols	
	Ammonia	
	Benzoic acid	
	Benzophenone	
	Diethyltoluamide	
	Formaldehyde[b]	
	Henna	
	Menthol	
	Parabens	
	Polyethylene glycol (PEG-8)	
	Polysorbate 60	
	Salicylic acid	
	Sodium sulfide	
Uncertain	Ammonium persulfate	Hair bleaches
	Paraphenylene-diamine	Hair dyes
		Hair spray
		Nail polish
		Rouge
		Toothpaste

[a]Multiple applications may be required for testing.
[b]Single application for testing. Adapted from Krogh, G von, Maibach, HI. The contact urticaria syndrome—1982. *Semin Dermatol* 1982;1:59 (297).

be little other evidence of inflammation. Mathias (302) reported pigmented cosmetic contact dermatitis due to contact allergy to chromium hydroxide used as a dye in toilet soap, and Maibach (248) reported hyperpigmentation in a black man sensitive to petrolatum. These cases are instructive because they alert the dermatologist to search scrupulously for a causative agent; its elimination results frequently in gradual fading of the pigment. Patients require constant encouragement during this slow depigmentation phase; otherwise, they doubt the accuracy of the diagnosis.

Ironically, hydroquinone, used as a bleaching agent, has caused postinflammatory hyperpigmentation. In 1975, Findlay et al. (303) from South Africa reported a long-term complication of the use of hydroquinone—deposits of ochronotic pigment in the skin, along with colloid milia. Black patients had no chemical evidence of alkaptonuria. The melanocyte, despite intense hydroquinone use, escaped destruction, and the site of the injury shifted to the dermis and the fibroblast. Polymeric pigment adhered to thickened, abnormal collagen bundles. Since then, reports of exogenous ochronosis have come from other areas, including the

United States. A biopsy must be performed to establish this diagnosis.

In addition, a few cases of persistent hypopigmentation have incriminated topical hydroquinone (304).

Cinnamic aldehyde, which was present in a toothpaste, caused perioral leukoderma (305).

> **Dihydroxyacetone, present in "tanning lotions," stains the skin but does not affect the melanocyte.**

Paronychia, Onycholysis, Nail Destruction, and Nail Discoloration

The physician should obtain a detailed description of the nail-grooming habits in patients who have paronychia, onycholysis, nail destruction, or nail discoloration because any of these problems may be caused by nail cosmetic usage. Nail discoloration has been reported with the use of hydroquinone bleaching creams and hair dyes containing henna (306). Permanent paresthesia and nail loss following usage of acrylic nails has been reported. Fungal infection with dermatophytes or *Candida* and trauma must also be among the considerations in the diagnoses of nail problems.

Hair Breakage

Permanents and hair straighteners are intended to break the disulfide bonds that give hair keratin its strength. Improper usage or incomplete neutralization of these cosmetics causes hair breakage. Hair that has been damaged by previous applications of permanent waves, straighteners, oxidation-type dyes, bleaches, or excessive exposure to sunlight and chlorine is more susceptible to this damage. The dermatologist should always take a complete history in these cases, including a detailed account of the use of drugs, to detect any causes of telogen or anagen effluvium. Careful examination of the hair shafts is essential to detect any preexisting abnormalities.

Acneiform Reactions

Acne and folliculitis can be precipitated or aggravated by cosmetic usage. Since 1972, when Kligman and Mills (307) proposed the rabbit's ear model to test cosmetics and their ingredients for comedogenicity, screening programs have been conducted.

Classes of ingredients, such as isopropyl myristate and its analogues, lanolin and its derivatives, detergents, and D&C red dyes, have been incriminated by the rabbit's ear test (308). In addition, oils such as mineral oil and petrolatum in topical products may cause occlusive folliculitis and formation of comedones. Bronaugh and Maibach (295) reported that results of the rabbit's ear test correlate well with pustule formation noted in use tests of cosmetics performed on women's faces. They noted instances of skin and hair cosmetics that produce papulopustules after 3 to 7 days of use that are strongly positive in the rabbit's ear model.

> **Cosmetics that produce papulopustules and/or comedones can be detected by the rabbit's ear test.**

Frank (309) accurately pointed out inconsistencies in the results reported from the rabbit's ear test. Many questions remain unanswered: Does the mere presence of a comedogenic ingredient in a cosmetic incriminate the product? Are the effects of multiple, comedogenic ingredients cumulative?

From a practical standpoint even cosmetics touted as noncomedogenic may cause acneiform lesions in some patients. Usually "water-based" or "oil-free" cosmetics will be less likely to do so than those containing oils. Although allergen avoidance is fairly easy by reading labels, acnegenicity in a given individual may have to be determined through the "trial and error" method.

COSMETICS AND TOILETRIES: REACTIONS AND PATCH TESTING

Baby Products

These products are marketed primarily for use on the skin and scalps of infants. Some experimental data suggest that infants are less easily sensitized than adults. Epstein (310) reported that 44% of infants younger than 1 year of age could be sensitized to pentadecyl catechol, but that 87% of children older than 3 years of age were sensitized in the same experiment. In clinical practice, ACD is diagnosed relatively infrequently in young children (311). Patch test results in children mirror frequency of positive reactions in adults, with allergens such as nickel and rubber chemicals often found. Because the diaper area is a frequent site of irritant contact dermatitis, careful attention should be paid to the products used in this area. Often, baby products are fragranced. Baby oil, talc, and cornstarch have simple compositions with little sensitizing potential beside the fragrances. Baby lotions or creams may contain fragrance, preservatives, lanolin, or propylene glycol, which are sensitizers (289). Propylene glycol, present in these lotions and the moistened towelettes marketed for cleansing the diaper area, may be an irritant on sensitive skin. In the treatment of infants with diaper rash, it is important to examine the ingredients of the cosmetics used on the diaper area and to consider in particular their irritant potential.

> **Infantile "diaper dermatitis" may be due to baby skin products containing fragrances, preservatives, lanolins, or propylene glycol.**

Bath Preparations

Adverse reactions to bubble bath reported to the FDA include skin eruptions, irritation of the genitourinary tract, eye irritation, and respiratory disorders (312–314). The genitourinary tract reactions in children have been the most serious; some children have been subjected to extensive urologic work-ups before the cause was established. The skin eruptions are assumed usually to be irritant reactions due to the detergent content of this product. In 1971, the FDA contacted bubble-bath manufacturers and requested that they lower the alkylaryl-sulfonate content below 10%, preferably to between 2% and 5% (Federal Register 42:5368–5370, 1977).

Cocamidopropyl betaine is now present in many bath preparations. Although less irritating than previous surfactants, it may still cause some irritation and allergy. Physicians should warn parents not to allow children to use a bubble bath unsupervised or not to take prolonged bubble baths. Because of their detergent content, these cosmetics may cause or aggravate dryness and inflammation of the skin and are especially unsuitable for atopics.

Eye Makeup Preparations

Mascara, eyeliner, eye shadow, and eyebrow pencil or powders are the most commonly used eye-area makeups. Soft pencils used for shadowing and lining have become popular in recent years, and false eyelashes have become less fashionable. Usually, these cosmetics are unfragranced but do contain one or more preservatives. The parabens are found in almost all eye shadows. Fortunately, these agents are relatively rare sensitizers and may even be tolerated on noninflamed skin in those who are allergic to them (see "The Paraben Paradox" above). Other preservatives, however, may be present and may be more likely causes of allergy. Often overlooked as causes of ACD of the eyelids are the metals nickel, cobalt, and chromate. Nickel is not intentionally present in eye cosmetics but has been found as a contaminant. Both cobalt and chromate may be present in coloring agents.

Metals in Eye Shadows

Sainia et al. (315) tested 88 colors of 25 brands of eye shadow for levels of cobalt, nickel, chromate, lead, and arsenic. Lead and arsenic values were below toxic levels. Over 10 ppm of cobalt was found in 21 (24%) samples, of nickel in 37 (42%) samples, and of chromium in 33 (37%) samples. The highest levels of nickel and cobalt were 41 and 49 ppm, respectively. Chromium levels in three samples were very high, with over 2,000 ppm. This is particularly significant, because usually nickel and cobalt are not listed on ingredient labeling, These levels are significant enough to cause reactivity in some sensitive persons.

Most cases of eyelid dermatitis, in the absence of obvious photosensitivity or primary ophthalmologic disease, can be traced to contact dermatitis, seborrheic dermatitis, or atopic dermatitis. Only rarely is contact urticaria or collagen vascular disease the cause. All but ACD and contact urticaria can usually be diagnosed by history and other physical or laboratory findings.

Because the eyelid skin is thin and sensitive, eyelid ACD may be caused not only by directly applied agents but also by allergens transferred by touch and even airborne contact allergens. In addition to cosmetics, allergens in contact lens solutions or eye medications may directly contact the eyelids. Toluene sulfonamide formaldehyde resin in nail polish is a classic cause of eyelid allergy. Acrylates in artificial nails can cause eyelid dermatitis. Rubber in makeup sponges and eyelash curlers may affect the eyelids. Eyelid dermatitis from chromate in airborne cement dust or from allergens in wood dust may occur. Nethercott et al. (316) reported on 79 cases of eyelid dermatitis, mostly in women. Forty-six percent had ACD, 15% had ICD, and 23% were atopics. Formaldehyde, formaldehyde-releasing preservatives, fragrances, nickel, and neomycin were among the most commonly positive allergens.

More recently gold has been shown to be a not uncommon cause of eyelid dermatitis. Ingredients of shampoos and other hair care products must also be suspected in cases of eyelid dermatitis. Cocamidopropyl betaine and methyldibromoglutaronitrile are two "newer" shampoo components that may cause eyelid ACD.

> **In addition to the ingredients found in eye cosmetics, eyelid dermatitis may be caused by "ectopic" exposures to allergens such as gold, shampoo ingredients, and nail cosmetics.**

Although eye cosmetics may be used "as is" for patch testing, the allergen concentration is often too low to give a positive result. Mascaras may cause an irritant reaction on patch testing unless volatile hydrocarbons are allowed to evaporate for 20 minutes or so before applying the patch (317).

When allergic, seborrheic, and atopic forms of dermatitis are not found, cumulative irritant dermatitis may be present. Dryness, friction, and irritant ingredients of topicals may all contribute to this. Each of these factors must be corrected if treatment is to be successful.

Other than the metals mentioned above, coloring agents are rare sensitizers. In the United States, the pigments used in eye-area cosmetics are restricted. No coal-tar derivatives may be incorporated; only purified natural colors or inorganic pigment or lakes of low allergic potential are used.

Eye infections, of either the cornea or the lids, may be due to abrasions from mascara wands when the mascara is not properly preserved (318). Patients should be urged to use eye cosmetics hygienically and advised not to use eye cosmetics inside the lash line.

Hair Preparations (Noncoloring)

Permanents

Permanent waves are cosmetics that alter the disulfide bonds of hair keratin so that hair fiber configuration can be changed. The disulfide bonds of cystine are broken in the first step when the waving solution is applied to the hair wound around mandrels. In the second step, with neutralization, new disulfide bonds are formed by locking in the curl configuration of the hair.

The waving solutions contain reducing agents that can cause irritant reactions when allowed to run incautiously on the skin surrounding the scalp. Irritant reactions range from erythema to bullous dermatitis. Hair breakage and loss may result when permanent waves are used improperly—in too concentrated a form, for too long a time, or on hair previously damaged by dyes, straighteners, or permanent waves. Old-fashioned hot waves occasionally caused chemical burns, which scarred the scalp, producing permanent alopecia, but modern permanents can cause breakage, which results in temporary loss.

> **Improper use of permanent waves may produce irritant scalp reactions with temporary hair loss.**

Currently, the majority of salon perms use glyceryl thioglycolate (GTG). These are called "acid" or "heat" perms. GTG has become a major allergen in hairdressers and somewhat less so in their clients. Two factors regarding GTG have been elucidated and doubtless contribute to the chronicity of hand eczema in hairdressers (319,320).

GTG persists on permed hair for weeks or months. Hairdressers cutting hair that has been permed previously may still react to the GTG. GTG penetrates intact rubber gloves. The only glove shown to be protective against GTG is a plastic laminate glove (4H glove). Avoidance of this allergen therefore is difficult if not impossible for some hairdressers and may lead to a change in career.

The older type of "cold waves" used for home permanents and salon permanents contain thioglycolic acid combined with ammonia or another alkali to raise the pH. The concentration of the thioglycolic acid and alkali can be varied to change the products' speed of action or to suit the type of hair to be waved (i.e., hard to wave, normal, or easy to wave). The neutralizer contains hydrogen peroxide or sodium bromate. These permanents rarely cause allergic reactions. If a truly allergic reaction is suspected, all the ingredients of the permanent (gums, fragrance, etc.) must be tested as well as the ingredients of the other products used at the same time, such as shampoos, conditioners, and hair sprays. Ammonium thioglycolate can be patch tested as 1% to 2.5% in petrolatum (321). Allergy to these permanents is often assumed but rarely, if ever, proven.

Cross-reactions between GTG and ammonium thioglycolate rarely occur.

Another type of permanent used primarily at home is the sulfite wave. Although the sulfite wave produces less strong curls and is slower, the odor is more pleasant. Neutralization is done usually with bromates. Occasional allergic reactions are seen with these permanents. Use 1% sodium bisulfite in water to patch test (322).

Straighteners

Madame C. J. Walker, in 1901, developed a process to straighten black hair using a heated comb with petrolatum or a mixture of petrolatum, oils, and waxes. The petrolatum or "pressing" oils act as a heat-modifying conductor, which reduces friction when the comb travels down the hair fibers. Mechanical and heat damage can cause hair breakage. Over the years, the heated oils can injure the hair follicles, leading to scarring alopecia ("hot-comb alopecia").

Chemical straighteners containing sodium hydroxide, or "lye," cleave the disulfide bonds of keratin thoroughly and straighten hair permanently (323). Experience and caution in applying these straighteners are important to avoid hair breakage and chemical burns. Similar products that contain guanidine carbonate mixed with calcium hydroxide are reputed to be milder. It is necessary to straighten new growth every few months. Care is taken not to "double process" the distal hair, which is already straightened. Some manufacturers advise against using permanent hair colors that require peroxide on chemically straightened hair to avoid damage.

Sulfite straighteners, chemically similar to sulfite permanents, are best suited for relaxing curly white hair.

"Soft curls" have become a fashionable way of styling the hair of some persons with curly hair (324). Ammonium thioglycolate and a bromate or peroxide neutralizer are used to achieve restructuring of the hair.

Follow-up care is elaborate and includes successive applications of products called moisturizers, curl activators, and oil sheens that saturate the hair and scalp. A plastic cap is worn to bed each night. These cosmetics may contain oils, quaternium compounds, glycerin, propylene glycol, and collagen, as well as fragrance and preservatives.

Shampoos

When shampoos are used, they generally have a short contact time with the scalp and are diluted and rinsed off quickly. (Some residues, inadequately quantitated, remain.) These factors reduce their sensitizing potential. Consumers' complaints are commonly directed at their eye stinging and irritating qualities. The importance of eye safety testing for these products became apparent 25 years ago when shampoos based on blends of cationic and non-ionic detergents caused blindness in some users (325).

Shampoos today generally are detergent-based, with a few containing small amounts of soap for conditioning. Anionic detergents and amphoteric detergents are occasional sensitizers (326,327). The nonionic surfactant cocamidopropyl betaine, discussed earlier in this chapter, may cause hand dermatitis in hairdressers and facial dermatitis in users. Fatty acid amides used in shampoos as thickeners and foam stabilizers have caused allergic contact dermatitis in other products (328,329). In recent years, the fragrance content of shampoos has been increased and used for marketing. Individual ingredient patch testing is necessary to incriminate allergens in shampoos because testing with the actual product will usually cause an irritant reaction.

Hair Coloring Preparations

Millions of persons color their hair using five different types of dyes.

Type 1—Permanent hair dyes are mixtures of colorless, aromatic compounds that act as primary intermediates and couplers. The primary intermediates, principally *p*-phenylenediamine (PPDA), toluene-2,5-diamine (*p*-toluenediamine), and *p*-aminophenol, are oxidized by hydrogen peroxide in the presence of ammonia, polymerize, and combine with couplers to form a variety of colors that blend to give the desired shade. These reactions take place inside the hair shaft, accounting for the fastness of these dyes. Permanent dyes are the most popular in the United States because of the variety of natural colors they can achieve.

Type 2—Semipermanent hair dyes contain low molecular weight nitrophenylenediamine and anthroquinone dyes, which penetrate the hair cortex to some extent. Their color lasts through approximately five shampoos.

Type 3—Temporary rinses are mixtures of mild, organic acids and certified dyes that coat the hair shaft. These rub and shampoo off easily.

Type 4—Vegetable dyes in the United States contain henna, which only colors hair red.

Type 5—Metallic dyes contain lead acetate and sulfur. When they are combed through the hair daily, they deposit insoluble lead oxides and sulfides that impart colors that range from yellow-brown to dark gray.

The vast majority of cases of allergy to hair dyes are caused by PPDA. Cross-reaction may occur to other related amines found in the permanent and semipermanent dyes. Independent sensitization to toluene-2,5-diamine or 2-nitro-*p*-phenylenediamine dyes or resorcinol occurs rarely, but positive patch tests to toluene-2,5-diamine or 2-nitro-*p*-phenylenediamine dyes result generally from cross-sensitization to PPDA (321).

Types 1 and 2 contain coal-tar hair dyes; in the United States, they must bear a label warning about adverse reactions. Instructions for open patch testing are given. The law requires that patch testing be performed before each application of dye; in practice, this is seldom carried out in homes or salons. Coal-tar dyes are added occasionally to temporary rinses. These rinses must also bear a warning label and patch test instructions.

A persistent and significant number of reactions to hair dyes are seen by dermatologists each year. Their severity ranges from mild erythema at the hairline or ears to swelling of the eyelids and face, accompanied by an acute vesicular eruption in the scalp that requires prompt medical attention.

One percent PPDA in petrolatum is used in the standard closed patch test. The most recent NACDG data show a positive patch test rate of 6.8%, with almost all being relevant (1). Broeckx (330) in Belgium reported similar results with 7.2% of more than 5,000 patients reactive to PPDA. Orthonitro PPD and paratoluenediamine were positive in 1.8% and 1.6%, respectively. The products of the oxidation of PPDA are not allergenic. Reiss and Fisher (331) studied the allergenicity of dyed hair. Twenty patients sensitive to PPDA were tested to freshly dyed hair in closed patch tests, and all were negative. The findings of this study are important particularly to hairdressers, sensitive to PPDA, who must work with dyed hair all day. Occasional case reports have appeared that suggested contact reactions occurred to another person's dyed hair (332–335). We assume that the dyeing process must not have been carried out properly and that the unoxidized products remained on the hair.

Patients sensitive to PPDA should be warned about possible cross-reactions with local anesthetics (procaine and benzocaine), sulfonamides, and para-aminobenzoic acid sunscreens. Also, some persons allergic to PPDA may react to disperse or "azo" textile dyes. It is estimated that 25% of patients who are PPDA-sensitive will react to semipermanent hair dyes. Patients who wish to try these as a substitute should do an open patch test with the dye first.

Several patients have been reported who experienced immediate hypersensitivity reactions to PPDA, and this spectrum of reactions to hair dyes should now be considered as a diagnostic possibility in appropriate patients (336). Some patients complain of scalp irritation after dyeing their hair, but we are unaware of published data that study the potential of these dyes for irritation. Some hair dye reactions occur most prominently in light-exposed areas, but the phototoxic and photoallergic potential of coal-tar dyes has not been investigated.

Henna has not been reported to cause allergic contact dermatitis when used as a hair dye, but cases have been reported from coloring the skin with henna (337,338). Cronin (339) described a hairdresser who noted wheezing and coryza when she handled henna; this patient had a positive prick test to henna.

A single case of contact dermatitis due to lead acetate in the metallic dyes has been reported (340).

When hair is bleached, ammonium persulfate, a booster, is added to hydrogen peroxide to obtain the lightest shades.

Ammonium persulfate has several industrial uses as well, and it is known to cause irritant reactions and ACD occasionally (341). One percent aqueous solution of ammonium persulfate can be used in closed patch tests. In addition, observation for immediate reactions should be made at the time of patch testing.

Ammonium persulfate can cause immediate hypersensitivity reactions, including urticaria, facial edema, asthma, and syncope. These reactions are histamine mediated, but at present it is not clear whether or not immunologic mechanisms are involved (342).

Methods of testing for immediate hypersensitivity include rubbing a saturated solution of ammonium persulfate on intact skin, scratch tests or intracutaneous tests using 1% aqueous solution of ammonium persulfate, and inhalation of 0.1 mg of ammonium persulfate powder. All of these methods carry a risk of systemic reactions and, if deemed necessary, should be performed only when emergency treatment for anaphylaxis is available.

Hairdressers should be instructed that clients who develop hives, generalized itching, facial swelling, or asthma when the hair is bleached should not have the process repeated using persulfate. Clients experiencing such reactions should receive immediate medical attention.

Facial Makeup Preparations

Eleven percent of the reactions to cosmetics in an NACDG study in 1985 were to this group of products, which includes lipstick, rouge, makeup bases, and facial powders (73).

Before 1960, allergic reactions to lipsticks were common. Most were caused by D&C Red No. 21 (eosin), an indelible dye used in long-lasting deeply colored lipsticks. The sensitizer in eosin proved to be a contaminant; improved methods of purification have reduced its sensitizing potential. Because eosin is strongly bound to keratin, patch tests are performed with 50% eosin in petrolatum.

> **Various red D&C dyes, including eosin (D&C Red No. 21), are rare lipstick sensitizers.**

Other dyes occasionally have been reported as sensitizers. Cronin (321) reporting on the experience at St. John's Hospital from 1955 to 1976, noted reactions to D&C Red No. 36, No. 31, No. 19, and No. 17 (D&C Red No. 17 is not permitted in lipstick in the United States), and D&C Yellow No. 11. The latter is a potent sensitizer, seldom used in lipsticks but reported as a sensitizing agent in eye cream and rouge as well as lipstick (343). D&C Yellow No. 10, produced by the sulfonation of D&C Yellow No. 11, is not a potent sensitizer (344,345). Other sensitizers have been reported in lipsticks—castor oil acting as a pigment solvent (287), antioxidants propyl gallate and monotertiary-butylhydroquinone (346,347), sunscreens phenyl salicylate,

benzophenone 3, and amyldimethyl aminobenzoic acid (348,349), lanolin (350), and fragrance. Para-tertiary-butylphenol in lipstick caused cheilitis in a patient and depigmentation at the patch test site (351).

Although reactions to lipstick are uncommon, dermatologists should consider this diagnosis even when the eruption has spread beyond the lips, because the sensitizing chemical may be present in cosmetics other than the lipstick. Do not neglect to test each lipstick and lip balm that the patient uses closed as well as performing photopatch tests, because some of the dyes used may be photoallergens.

Rouge or "blush" is manufactured in various forms—powder, cream, liquid, stick, or gel. It is designed to highlight the cheeks with color. The composition is not unique: Powders are similar to face powder, and creams and liquids are similar to foundation. To achieve bright shades, organic colors are added to rouges as they are to lipsticks. D&C Yellow No. 11 caused allergic reactions to rouges as well as lipsticks (343). Some women may use lipstick to color their cheeks in place of rouge, or rouge may be used all over the face to achieve a healthy "glow." These practices need to be taken into account when evaluating patterns of contact dermatitis on the face. Powder blush is less likely to cause allergy than liquid or cream blush probably because it contains fewer preservatives and other sensitizing ingredients. It may also be better for those patients prone to acne.

Facial makeups or foundations are applied to the skin to give an appearance of uniform color and texture and to disguise blemishes or imperfections. Produced in a variety of forms—emulsions of water and oil, oil-free lotions, anhydrous sticks, poured powders, and pancake makeups—the amount of coverage given is determined by the titanium dioxide (TiO_2) content. Because TiO_2 reflects light, some ordinary makeups achieve sun protection factor (SPF) values of 2 or even 4 (352). In recent years, sunscreening agents have been added to some foundations to increase these SPF values. These products with sunscreens may be marketed as "antiaging." PABA derivatives, fragrances, emulsifiers, preservatives, propylene glycol, and lanolin are chemicals with significant sensitizing potential used in makeups. Synthetic esters, such as isopropyl myristate and lanolin derivatives added to these makeups, have been implicated as causes of acne by the rabbit's ear test (307).

In 1975, Calnan (353) described a woman who had a positive patch test to her foundation on two occasions, and her facial eruption flared when she used this foundation. Results were negative, however, when the ingredients of this foundation were used in patch tests. Calnan raised the intriguing possibility of compound allergy—the allergen is produced by a combination of more than one ingredient.

The pattern of dermatitis seen with allergy to facial makeups may be surprisingly irregular, with skipped areas of normal skin interspersed with areas of dermatitis. This raises another interesting question about the existence of resident clones of antigen-presenting cells or T lymphocytes that remain in one area of skin only.

Nail Cosmetics

In the past, adverse reactions have been reported to numerous nail cosmetics, which have been removed subsequently from the market. Nail hardeners containing formaldehyde are in this category (354). In the United States, this type of hardener is permitted for use only on the free edge of the nail when the skin is protected from contact with the hardener. Some manufacturers sell products called "hardeners," but they have merely increased the resin content of ordinary nail enamel.

Nail enamels including base coats and top coats have a similar composition.

1. Film former—nitrocellulose
2. Resins—tosylamide formaldehyde resin, alkyd resins, acrylates, vinyls, or polyesters
3. Plasticizers—camphor, dibutyl phthalate, dioctyl phthalate, and tricresyl phosphate
4. Solvents—alcohol, toluene, ethyl acetate, and butyl acetate
5. Colorants
6. Pearlizers—guanine and bismuth oxychloride

The concentration of each of these chemicals depends on the quality to be achieved in the final product. The base coat will have increased amounts of resin to improve adhesion to the nail plate, but the top coat has increased nitrocellulose and plasticizers to enhance gloss and abrasion resistance.

Patients allergic to nail polish often develop dermatitis at sites distant from the fingers, commonly eyelids, around the mouth and chin, sides of the neck, on the genitalia, and rarely a generalized eruption. Tosylamide formaldehyde resin (TSFR) is responsible for almost all the allergic reactions. In the NACDG study, this resin was the seventh most common ingredient causing allergic contact dermatitis in patients with a cosmetic allergy (73). In a study from the Netherlands, it accounted for 10% of reactions in 119 cosmetic allergy patients, ranking behind only preservatives, fragrances, and emulsifiers (290). A small amount (0.1% to 0.5%) of free formaldehyde is in the resin, but most who react to TSFR are not also allergic to formaldehyde. Patch testing is performed with the resin at 10% pet (321). "Hypoallergenic" brands of nail polish, which substitute alkyd or other resins, are available for those allergic to TSFR. The durability and abrasion resistance of these other resins is said to be inferior to toluene sulfonamide formaldehyde resin (355). Although onycholysis has been attributed to reactions to toluene sulfonamide formaldehyde resin, no published data firmly support this (356).

Fowler has seen one case of allergy to butyl acetate. The patient was unable to find any brand of nail polish she could tolerate. Dermatitis occurred not only on the face but also on the paronychial areas.

Liden et al. (357) show how serious the consequences of ACD to nail polish may be. In a 2-year period, 18 women with nail polish allergy were seen. Eight women had taken 1 or more months of sick leave for a presumed occupational problem before diagnosis. Four were hospitalized, and two lost their jobs.

Yellow discoloration of the nail plate, darkest at the distal end, occurs commonly in women who wear colored nail polish. Samman (306) reproduced this staining with the following colors: D&C Red No. 7, D&C Red No. 34, D&C Red No. 6, and FD&C Yellow No. 5 lake. This discoloration will fade over time only if use of nail polish is discontinued.

Nail enamel removers are mixtures of solvents such as acetone and amyl, butyl, or ethyl acetate to which fatty materials and fragrance may be added (358).

Cuticle removers contain alkaline chemicals, frequently sodium or potassium hydroxide, to break the disulfide bonds of keratin. Many women use these cosmetics weekly without difficulty. They should not be left on for prolonged periods or be used by people who are susceptible to paronychia. Cuticle removers are irritants that should not be used for closed patch testing.

Artificial Nails

"Sculptured nails" have become more popular in recent years because they build an attractive artificial nail on the nail plate. Women who could not grow nails previously can now have the appearance of long nails.

Sculptured nails are applied by a manicurist, or kits may be purchased for home use. The kits consist of a powdered methacrylate polymer, with benzoyl peroxide as an initiator, and a liquid methacrylate ester or mixture of these esters. Polymerization begins when the liquid and the powder are mixed and painted on the nail, which is surrounded by a template that protects the surrounding skin and allows the formation of an artificial extension.

Unfortunately, irritant and allergic reactions to the liquid monomers, as well as secondary infections, may be painful and long-lasting. Paronychia, onycholysis, onychia, and dermatitis of the finger and distant sites may occur. As early as 1957, Fisher et al. (359) reported allergic sensitization to the methyl methacrylate monomers in sculptured nails. In 1974, the FDA banned the use of methyl methacrylate in these cosmetics (360). Analysis of 31 products, however, sold between 1975 and 1981 revealed this monomer was present in nine of them (361). At present, sensitization has also been reported to other monomers, and cross-reactions between acrylate monomers is common (362,363).

Patch testing is essential to determine if an observed reaction is due to acrylate allergy or whether an irritant reaction or allergy to some other component is occurring. A variety of acrylates may be found in artificial nail products (see Table 17.16). A screening series for patch testing is suggested in Table 17.17. If results are negative, the manufacturers of a product used may be able to supply the names of acrylates present. Closed patch testing with acrylic nail products should not be attempted due to the potential for ir-

TABLE 17.16. *Methacrylic Acid Esters Used in Sculptured Nails[a]*

Butyl methacrylate monomer
Diethylene glycol dimethacrylate monomer
Ethylene dimethacrylate
Ethyleneglycol dimethacrylate
Ethoxyethyl methacrylate
Ethyl methacrylate monomer
Isobutyl methacrylate monomer
Methacrylic acid monomer
Tetrahydrofurfuryl methacrylate monomer
Triethylene glycol dimethacrylate
Trimethylopropane trimethacrylate monomer

[a]Modified from Fisher, 1980 (359) and Fuller, 1982 (361).

ritation and active sensitization. However, an open test or use test may be attempted.

Other sensitizers may be present in artificial nail preparations. Benzoyl peroxide is used as a catalyst and hydroquinone as an inhibitor of polymerization. Both of these are occasional allergens. Two rare but very serious reactions to acrylates in artificial nails are the development of paresthesias and nail loss. Fisher (364) reported a case of acrylate allergy that resulted in nail loss. After 16 years there was no regrowth. Parasthesia has been caused by acrylate glues not only from nail preparations but also in dentists and orthopedists using acrylate tissue glues (365). Parasthesias may occur with or without allergic sensitization (366).

Photobonding of acrylate nail extenders using UV light is a newer method of application. Reactions to this process occur just as with non-UV required products.

Cyanoacrylate, or "Krazy Glue," initially thought to be nonsensitizing, has now been shown to be able to sensitize and cause paronychia, onychia, and ACD (367,368).

Preformed plastic nails may be designed to cover the nail plate or extended tips. Their prolonged use causes mechanical damage to the nail, and those covering the entire nail plate may cause injury by occlusion (369). Sensitization to *p*-tertiary butylphenol formaldehyde resin in the nail adhesive and tricresyl ethyl phthalate of the artificial nail has been reported (370).

> **The methacrylic acid esters used in artificial "sculptured" nails may produce severe allergic reactions with resulting onychia and paronychia.**

TABLE 17.17. *Suggested Screening Tray for Artificial Nail Allergy*

Methyl methacrylate 2%
Ethyl acrylate 0.1%
Butyl acrylate 0.1%
Triethyleneglycol dimethacrylate 2%
Bis (hydroxymethacrylpropoxy) phenyl propane 2%
Ethyleneglycol dimethacrylate 2%
Trimethylol propane triacrylate 0.1%

Oral Hygiene Products

See Chapter 36.

Personal Cleanliness Products

The action of bacteria upon sterile apocrine secretions produces a characteristic odor. Work done by Labows et al. (371) incriminated lipophilic diptheroids as the organisms that produce unique axillary odors. Simple deodorants reduce the number of bacteria in the axilla.

Although deodorants are considered cosmetics, antiperspirants are regulated as over-the-counter (OTC) drugs as well as cosmetics. Many of these products have been reformulated over the years in response to health concerns. Hexachlorophene was banned because of its neurotoxicity and halogenated salicylanilides because of their photoallergic nature. Chlorofluorocarbon propellants were removed from aerosols because of their proposed role in depleting the stratosphere of ozone. The chlorofluorocarbons have been replaced by hydrocarbon propellants—isobutane, butane, and propane—which are flammable. The FDA OTC Antiperspirant Review Panel recommended the removal of zirconium-containing chemicals from aerosol antiperspirants because of the potential for formation of granulomata in the lung and skin.

The OTC Review Panel published a list of aluminum and aluminum-zirconium chemicals permitted in antiperspirants (Federal Register vol. 43, Oct. 10, 1978:46694–46732). Irritant reactions to aluminum salts in antiperspirants are common because of the environmental heat, moisture, and friction and the inflammation caused by shaving in the axilla. Occasional allergic dermatitis to aluminum in antiperspirants has been reported. Allergic reactions are usually due to the other chemicals in the antiperspirants, most frequently the fragrance ingredients.

Feminine hygiene sprays are primarily fragrance products that cause irritant reactions when sprayed at too close a range. Allergy from fragrances, preservatives, and antimicrobials may occur.

Shaving Preparations

Preshave toiletries may contain soaps or detergents in their lather. Reactions to aftershaves and colognes, however, account for most of the contact dermatitis that men experience from shaving cosmetics. The reactions, due to fragrance, may or may not be triggered by light (372). Because these toiletries are applied directly to freshly shaved skin, penetration of the fragrance is enhanced.

> **A soapless cleanser such as CAM Lotion or Cetaphil Lotion may be used instead of shaving cream in sensitive subjects.**

In the past, musk ambrette has been reported as a notable photoallergen in aftershaves (373,374). See Chapter 21 for instructions for patch testing fragrance ingredients. When performing a provocative use test with an aftershave, it is preferable to apply the product repeatedly on a quarter-sized area of the skin that is shaved rather than using the antecubital fossa.

> **Fragrances in aftershave lotions are the most common shaving preparation allergens, some of which are photosensitizers, musk ambrette in particular.**

Skin Care Preparations

This category of cosmetics accounted for 28% of all the cosmetic-related contact dermatitis reported by the NACDG (73). Many of these cosmetic products are creams that contain preservatives, emulsifiers, and lanolin, which are responsible for a significant number of adverse reactions.

From 1987 to 1990, the FDA received 12.44 complaints per million units sold of skin moisturizers (375). Because most adverse reactions are not reported to either the FDA or the manufacturers, this number grossly underrepresents the true frequency of such reactions.

Preservatives

Preservatives as a group are the most common cause of cosmetic reactions, followed by fragrances. The formaldehyde-releasing preservatives as a group, especially quaternium-15, are the most frequent preservative allergens. Methylchloroisothiazolinone/methylisothiazolinone and methyldibromoglutaronitrile are fairly common preservative allergens. Parabens, given their frequency of use, are relatively uncommon sensitizers.

Emulsifiers or Surfactants

Creams and lotions require the presence of an emulsifier to allow the combination of water and oil. Emulsifiers may act as mild irritants, especially if applied to slightly damaged skin. It has been hypothesized that increased epidermal cell renewal or "plumping" of the skin may be due to mild, irritant effects of nonionic surfactants (376).

Hannuksela et al. (377) patch tested over 1,200 eczematous patients with common emulsifiers, with results shown in Table 17.11.

> **Emulsifiers are rare sensitizers: Some give irritant reactions with a closed patch test. Provocative use tests should be used to confirm patch test reactions.**

Depilatories

Most depilatories today contain mercaptans such as calcium thioglycolate 2.5% to 4.0% in conjunction with an alkali to bring the pH to between 10 and 12.5 (358). The keratin of the cortex is more vulnerable before it emerges from the follicle, and depilatories attack it there, leaving a soft rather than sharp end. For this reason, the use of depilatories in place of shaving can prevent pseudofolliculitis barbae in some black men. Irritant dermatitis from the keratolytic action on skin is common. Powdered facial depilatories, produced for beard removal, contain barium or strontium sulfide because these chemicals are quicker acting. Unfortunately, these chemicals cause more irritation and produce an unpleasant odor (378). To use the less malodorous thioglycolate depilatories for coarser beard removal, hair accelerators such as thiourea, melamine, and sodium metasilicate are added. Depilatories cannot be patch tested directly, and these thioglycolates are seldom sensitizers.

Epilating Waxes

Epilating waxes are usually warmed to soften, and they harden and enmesh the hair after application. When the wax is pulled off, the hair is removed by the root. Some modified waxes do not have to be warmed and can be applied with a backing material. These cosmetics may contain beeswax, rosin (colophony), fragrance, or rarely benzocaine as potential sensitizers (358). The problems usually seen with these epilating cosmetics are due to mechanical irritation.

> **Depilatories usually contain thioglycolates that are common irritants but rare sensitizers. Epilating waxes often cause mechanical irritation. Those waxes containing rosin, fragrances, or benzocaine may cause allergic reactions.**

Skin Lighteners

All skin lighteners sold in the United States without a prescription contain hydroquinone (1.5% to 2.0%) as the bleaching agent, which inhibits the production of melanin. The adverse reactions attributed to hydroquinone are discussed earlier in this chapter under the section "Pigmentation." Allergic reactions to hydroquinone are infrequent. For patch testing, use 1% hydroquinone in petrolatum.

Cosmetic Intolerance Syndrome

Dermatologists treating reactions to cosmetics will be confronted occasionally by patients who complain bitterly of facial burning and discomfort. This group seriously challenges our diagnostic skills as well as our ability to be em-

TABLE 17.18. *The Face Intolerant to Cosmetics and Skin Care Agents: A Profile of Intolerant Skin Syndrome*

Exogenous	
Subjective irritation	Common but difficult for patients to figure out
Objective irritation	Common but often difficult morphology to observe on face
Allergic contact dermatitis	
Photoallergic contact dermatitis	Less common; discerned retrospectively by testing
Contact urticaria	
Endogenous	
Seborrheic dermatitis	Common; a small percentage of patients have an atypical morphology
Rosacea diathesis	
Atopic dermatitis	May be only residual of childhood atopic dermatitis
Status eczematous[a]	Some patients may have no other definable endogenous or exogenous factors
(Status cosmeticus) Dysmorphobia[a]	Rare diagnosis made by exclusion

[a]These patients are the most difficult to treat successfully.

TABLE 17.19. *Management of Patients Who Are Intolerant to Cosmetic Usage*

1. Examine every cosmetic and skin care agent
2. Patch and photopatch test to rule out occult allergic and photoallergic contact dermatitis, or contact urticaria
3. Limit skin care to:
   a. Water washing without soap or detergent
   b. Lip cosmetics—ad libitum
   c. Eye cosmetics—ad libitum—if the eyelids are not symptomatic
   d. Face powder—ad libitum
   e. Glycerin and rose water as moisturizer only if needed
   f. 6 to 12 months of avoidance of other skin care agents and cosmetics
4. Watch for and test, if necessary, depression and other neuropsychiatric aspects

There is a group of patients who experience continuous facial burning without objective signs whom Cotterill (380) describes as having dermatologic nondisease. Many of these patients have a disturbed body image, dysmorphobia, and complain of physical defects without objective evidence. Frequently these patients are depressed, and in Cotterill's group of 28 patients, several were suicidal. They demand time-consuming care. It is often difficult for these depressed patients to seek the skilled psychiatric care they require.

> **The cosmetic intolerance syndrome is not a single entity, but rather a symptom complex due to multiple factors, both exogenous and endogenous.**

pathetic when the severity of patients' symptoms does not match objective signs of disease (see Table 17.18). These patients may have not only subjective symptoms, but also objective inflammation. Fisher (379) coined the term "status cosmeticus" for the condition in which a patient is no longer able to tolerate the use of any cosmetic. Indeed, some of these patients seem to experience irritation (subjective and/or objective) from cosmetics, but during the evolution of this disorder, they become intolerant of many if not all topical agents. Some patients have occult allergic contact dermatitis, allergic photocontact dermatitis, or contact urticarial reactions, and the causal agents are documented by careful clinical review and patch testing.

Others who have a seborrheic/rosacea diathesis with or without inflammation seem to have flared this condition by abandoning the use of soap and water and by overusing cleansing creams and emollients. Both of these conditions may be accompanied by facial erythema or scaling. Some patients require anti-inflammatory therapy, as do a few atopic patients who develop this state.

Prolonged use of the proposed elimination program seems to aid some women who, after 6 to 12 months or more, are able to gradually return to the use of other cosmetics (see Table 17.19). Additions to their regimens of skin care should be made one at a time—no more frequently than every 2 weeks. The final program should be simple and limited in the number and frequency of cosmetics used.

REFERENCES

1. Marks JG, Belsito DV, DeLeo VA, et al. North American Contact Dermatitis Group patch test results for the detection of delayed-type hypersensitivity to topical allergens. *J Amer Acad Dermatol* 1998; 38:911–918.
2. Marks, JG, Belsito DV, DeLeo et al. North American Contact Dermatitis Group patch test results, 1996–1998. *Arch Dermatol* 2000; 136:272–273.
3. Ebner H, Kraft D. Formaldehyde induced anaphylaxis after dental treatment? *Contact Dermatitis* 1991;24:307.
4. Fisher AA. Formaldehyde: some recent experiences. *Cutis* 1976;17: 665.
5. Tegner E, Fregert S. Contamination of cosmetics with formaldehyde from tubes. *Cont Derm Newsletter* 1973;13:353.
6. Agner T, Flyvholm MA, Menne T. Formaldehyde allergy: a follow-up study. *Amer J Contact Dermatitis* 1999;10:12–17.
7. Nethercott JR, et al. Patch testing with a routine screening tray in North America, 1985 through 1989: 1. Frequency of response. *Am J Cont Derm* 1991;2:122.
8. Perrenoud D, Bircher A, Hunziker T, et al. Frequency of sensitization to 13 common preservatives in Switzerland; Swiss Contact Dermatitis Research Group. *Contact Dermatitis* 1994;30:276–279.
9. Fransway AF, Schmitz NA. The problem of preservation in the 1990s: 2. Formaldehyde and formaldehyde-releasing biocides: incidences of cross-reactivity and the significance of the positive response to formaldehyde. *Am J Cont Derm* 1991;2:78.

10. Parker LU, Taylor JS. A 5-year study of contact allergy to quaternium-15. *Am J Cont Derm* 1991;2:231.
11. Jordan WP. Human studies that determine the sensitizing potential of haptens: experimental allergic contact dermatitis. *Dermatol Clin* 1984;2:533.
12. Stephens TJ, Drake KD, Drotman RB. Experimental delayed contact sensitization to diazolidinyl urea (Germall II) in guinea pigs. *Contact Dermatitis* 1987;16:164.
13. Berke PA, Rosen WE. Germall, a new family of antimicrobial preservatives for cosmetics. *Am Perfum Cosmet* 1970;85:55.
14. Rosen WE, Berke PA. Modern concepts of cosmetic preservation. *J Soc Cosmet Chem* 1973;24:663.
15. Rosen WE, Berke PA, Matzin T, et al. Preservation of cosmetic lotions with imidazolidinyl urea plus parabens. *J Soc Cosmet Chem* 1977;28:83.
16. Ford GP, Beck MH. Reactions to quaternium 15, Bronopol, and Germall 115 in a standard series. *Cont Derm* 1986;14:271.
17. Ziegler V, Ziegler B, Kipping D. Dose-response sensitization experiments with imidazolidinyl urea. *Contact Dermatitis* 1988;19:236.
18. Andersen KE, et al. Guinea pig maximization tests with formaldehyde releasers: results from two laboratories. *Contact Dermatitis* 1984;10:257.
19. Fisher AA. Dermatitis due to formaldehyde-releasing agents in cosmetics and medicaments. *Cutis* 1978;22:655.
20. Fisher AA. Allergic contact dermatitis from Germall 115, a new cosmetic preservative. *Contact Dermatitis* 1975;1:126.
21. Peters MS, Connolly SM, Schroeter AL. Bronopol allergic contact dermatitis. *Contact Dermatitis* 1983;9:397.
22. Croshaw B, Groves MJ, Lessel B. Some properties of bronopol, a new antimicrobial agent active against *Pseudomonas aeruginosa*. *Pharm Pharmacol* (Suppl) 1964;16:127T.
23. Stretton RJ, Manson TW. Some aspects of the mode of action of the antibacterial compound bronopol (2-bromo-2-nitropropane-1 3-diol). *J Appl Bacteriol* 1973;36:61.
24. Marples RR, Kligman AM. Methods for evaluating topical antibacterial agents on human skin. *Antimicrob Agents Chemother* 1974;5:323.
25. Croshaw B. Preservatives for cosmetics and toiletries. *J Soc Cosmet Chem* 1977;28:3.
26. Preservative properties of bronopol. *Cosmet Toiletr* 1977;92:87.
27. Ardo Y. Bronopol as a preservative in milk samples. *Milchwissenschaft* 1979;34:14.
28. Woolford MK, Wilkins RJ. The evaluation of formaldehyde bronopol, tylosin and pimaricin as additives in simulated silage. *J Sci Food Agric* 1975;26:869.
29. Storrs FJ, Bell DE. Allergic contact dermatitis to 2-bromo-2-nitropane-1,3-diol in a hydrophilic ointment. *J Am Acad Dermatol* 1983;8:157.
30. Rosen M. Glydant and MDMH as cosmetic preservatives. In Kabara JJ, ed. *Cosmetic and drug preservation: principles and practice,* Vol 1. New York: Dekker, 1984.
31. DeGroot AC, et al. Patch test reactivity to DMDM hydantoin: relationship to formaldehyde allergy. *Contact Dermatitis* 1988;18:197.
32. DeGroot AC, et al. Contact allergy to preservatives-II. *Contact Dermatitis* 1986;15:218.
33. Bandmann HJ, Breit R, Mutzeck E. Allergic contact dermatitis from formaldehyde in a brewer. *Contact Dermatitis Newsletter* 1974;15:452.
34. Wilkinson DS. Formalin sensitivity in mushroom farming. *Contact Dermatitis Newsletter* 1970;7:162.
35. Fisher AA. *Contact dermatitis.* 3rd ed. Philadelphia: Lea & Febiger, 1986.
36. Gruvberger B, Bruze M, Almgren G. Occupational dermatoses in a plant producing binders for paints and glues. *Contact Dermatitis* 1998;38:71–77.
37. Sanchez I, Rodriguez F, Quinones D, et al. Occupational dermatitis due to formaldehyde in newspaper. *Contact Dermatitis* 1997;37:131–132.
38. Meding B, Ahman M, Karlberg AT. Skin symptoms and contact allergy in woodwork teachers. *Contact Dermatitis* 1996;34:185–190.
39. Cooke MA, Wilkinson JF. Formalin sensitivity in gum arabic. *Contact Dermatitis Newsletter* 1973;13:379.
40. Fabry H. Formaldehyde sensitivity. *Contact Dermatitis Newsletter* 1969;5:56.
41. Fregert S, Dahlquist I, Gruvberger B. A simple method for the detection of formaldehyde. *Contact Dermatitis* 1984;10:132.
42. Gryllaki-Berger M, et al. A comparative study of formaldehyde detection using chromotropic acid, acetylacetone and HPLC in cosmetics and household cleaning products. *Contact Dermatitis* 1992;27:149.
43. Flyvholm M-A, Menné T. Allergic contact dermatitis from formaldehyde (a case study focusing on sources of formaldehyde exposure). *Contact Dermatitis* 1992;27:27.
44. Cronin E. Formaldehyde is a significant allergen in women with hand eczema. *Contact Dermatitis* 1991;25:276.
45. Logan WS, Perry HO. Case dermatitis due to formaldehyde sensitivity. *Arch Dermatol* 1972;106:717.
46. Fabry H. Formaldehyde sensitivity—two interesting cases. *Contact Dermatitis Newsletter* 1968;3:51.
47. Sneddon IB. Formalin dermatitis in a renal dialysis unit. *Contact Dermatitis Newsletter* 1968;3:47.
48. Abdel-Aziz AHM, Hodgson C. Formalin dermatitis in a renal dialysis unit. *Contact Dermatitis Newsletter* 1974;15:441.
49. Hendrick DJ, Lane DJ. Occupational formalin asthma. *Br J Industr Med* 1977;34:11.
50. Fisher AA, Kanof NB, Biondi EM. Free formaldehyde in textiles and paper. *Arch Dermatol* 1962;86:753.
51. Fregert S. Allergic contact dermatitis from formaldehyde in paper. *Contact Dermatitis Newsletter* 1974;15:459.
52. Fregert S. Contamination of chemico-technical preparations with formaldehyde from packages. *Contact Dermatitis* 1977;3:109.
53. Simpson J. Formalin sensitivity—offset printing machines. *Contact Dermatitis Newsletter* 1969;6:133.
54. Black H. Contact dermatitis from formaldehyde in newsprint. *Contact Dermatitis Newsletter* 1971;10:162.
55. Thomsen HF. Hidden sources of formaldehyde. *Contact Dermatitis Newsletter* 1973;13:380.
56. Fisher AA. Dermatitis due to the presence of formaldehyde in certain sodium lauryl sulfate (SLS) solutions. *Cutis* 1981;27:360.
57. Trattner A, Johansen JD, Menné T. Formaldehyde concentration in diagnostic patch testing: comparison of 1% with 2%. *Contact Dermatitis* 1998;38:71–77.
58. Lorenzetti OJ, Weet TC. Topical parabens: benefits and risks. *Dermatologica* 1977;154:244.
59. Rosen WE, Berke PA. Modern concepts of cosmetic preservation. *J Soc Cosmet Chem* 1973;24:663.
60. Schnuch A, Geier J, Uter W, Frosch PJ. Patch testing with preservatives, antimicrobials and industrial biocides: results from a multicentre study. *Br J Dermatol* 1998;138:467–476.
61. Fisher AA. The paraben paradox. *Cutis* 1973;1:830.
62. Schorr WF. Paraben allergy—a cause of intractable dermatitis. *JAMA* 1968;204:859.
63. Hjorth N. *p*-Hydroxybenzoic acid esters (paraben esters, nipagin esters). *Acta Derm Venereol* (Stockh.) 1961;41:97.
64. Schamberg IL. Allergic contact dermatitis to methyl and propyl paraben. *Arch Dermatol* 1967;95:626.
65. Evans S. Epidermal sensitivity to lanolin and parabens—occurrence in pharmaceutical and cosmetic products. *Br J Dermatol* 1970;82:625.
66. Simpson JR. Dermatitis due to parabens in cosmetic creams. *Contact Dermatitis* 1978;5:311.
67. Brauer EW. Parabens in cosmetic creams. *Contact Dermatitis* 1979;5:265.
68. Marzulli FN, Maibach HI. Status of topical parabens: skin hypersensitivity. *Int J Dermatol* 1974;13:3197.
69. Fisher AA, Pascher F, Kanof NB. Allergic contact dermatitis due to ingredients of vehicles. *Arch Dermatol* 1971;104:286.
70. Fisher AA. Allergic paraben and benzyl alcohol hypersensitivity relationship of the delayed and immediate varieties. *Contact Dermatitis* 1975;1:281.
71. Rudzki E, Kleniewska D. Cross reactions between parabens and the para group. *Br J Dermatol* 1970;83:543.
72. Aldrete JA, Johnson PA. Allergy to local anesthetics. *JAMA* 1969;207:356.
73. Adams RM, Maibach HI. A five-year study of cosmetic reactions. *J Am Acad Dermatol* 1985;13:1062.
74. Nethercott JR, Nield G, Holness DL. A review of 79 cases of eyelid dermatitis. *J Am Acad Dermatol* 1989;21:223.

75. Menné T, Hjorth N. Routine patch testing with paraben esters. *Contact Dermatitis* 1988;19:189.

76. Hansen J, et al. Paraben contact allergy: patch testing and *in vitro* absorption/metabolism. *Am J Contact Dermatitis* 1993;4:78.

77. Praditsuwan P, Taylor JS, Rownigk HH Jr. Allergy to Unna boots in four patients. *J Amer Acad Dermatol* 1995;33:906–908.

78. Veien NK, Hattel T, Laurberg G. Oral challenge with parabens in paraben-sensitive patients. *Contact Dermatitis* 1996;34:433.

79. Henry JC, Tschen EH, Becker LE. Contact urticaria to parabens. *Arch Dermatol* 1979;115:1231.

80. Nagel JE, Fuscaldo JT, Fireman P. Paraben allergy. *JAMA* 1977;237:1594.

81. Fransway AF. The problem of preservation in the 1990s: 3. Agents with preservation function independent of formaldehyde release. *Am J Contact Dermatitis* 1991;2:145.

82. DeGroot AC. Methylisothiazolinone/methylchloroisothiazolinone (Kathon CG) allergy: an updated review. *Am J Contact Dermatitis* 1990;1:151.

83. Tosti A. Prevalence and sources of Kathon CG sensitization in Italy. *Contact Dermatitis* 1988;18:173.

84. Rietschel RL, et al. Methylchloroisothiazolinone-methylisothiazolinone reactions in patients screened for vehicle and preservative hypersensitivity. *J Am Acad Dermatol* 1990;22:734.

85. Chan PK, et al. Kathon biocide: manifestation of delayed contact dermatitis in guinea pigs is dependent on the concentration formulation and challenge. *J Invest Dermatol* 1983;81:409.

86. Bjorkner B, et al. Contact allergy to the preservative Kathon® CG. *Contact Dermatitis* 1986;14:85.

87. Marks J, et al. Methylchloroisothiazolinone/methylisothiazolinone (Kathon CG) biocide—United States multicenter study of human skin sensitization. *Am J Contact Dermatitis* 1990;1:157.

88. Fewings J, Menne T. The patch test concentration for methylchloroisothiazolinone/methylisothiazolinone. *Contact Dermatitis* 1998;39:320–321.

89. Kanerva L, Tarvainen K, Pinola A, et al. A single accidental exposure may result in a chemical burn, primary sensitization and allergic contact dermatitis. *Contact Dermatitis* 1994;31:229–235.

90. Primka EJ III, Taylor JS. Three cases of contact allergy after chemical burns from methylchloroisothiazolinone/methylisothiazolinone: one with concomitant allergy to methyldibromoglutaronitrile/phenoxyethanol. *Amer J Contact Dermatitis* 1997;8:43–46.

91. Gruvberger B, Bruze M. Can chemical burns and allergic contact dermatitis from higher concentrations of methylchloroisothiazolinone/methylisothiazolinone be prevented? *Am J Contact Dermatits* 1998;9:11–14.

92. Gruvberger B, Bruze M. Can glutathione-containing emollients inactivate methylchloroisothiazolinone/methylisothiazolinone? *Contact Dermatitis* 1998;38:261–265.

93. Madden SD, Thiboutot DM, Marks JG Jr. Occupationally induced allergic contact dermatitis to methylchloroisothiazolinone/methylisothiazolinone among machinists. *J Amer Acad Dermatol* 1994;30:272–274.

94. DeGroot A C, Weyland J W. Contact allergy to methyldibromoglutaronitrile in the cosmetics preservative Euxyl K400. *Am J Contact Dermatitis* 1991;2:31.

95. Torres V, Soares AP. Contact allergy to dibromodicyanobutane in a cosmetic cream. *Contact Dermatitis* 1992;27:114.

96. Lovell CR, White IR, Boyle J. Contact dermatitis from phenoxyethanol in aqueous cream BP. *Contact Dermatitis* 1984;11:187.

97. Tosti A, et al. Euxyl K400: a new sensitizer in cosmetics. *Contact Dermatitis* 1991;25:89.

98. DeGroot AC, et al. Frequency of allergic reactions to methyldibromoglutaronitrile (1,2-dibromo-2,4-dicyanobutane) in the Netherlands. *Contact Dermatitis* 1991;25:270.

99. Jackson JM, Fowler JF. Methyldibromoglutaronitrile (Euxyl K400): a new and important sensitizer in the United States? *J Amer Acad Dermatol* 1998;38:934–937.

100. Tosti A, Vincenzi C, Trevisi P, Guerra L. Euxyl K400: incidence of sensitization, patch test concentration and vehicle. *Contact Dermatitis* 1995;33:193–195.

101. DeGroot AC, van Ginkel JWC, Weijlad JW. Methyldibromoglutaronitrile (Euxyl K400): an important "new" allergen in cosmetics. *J Amer Acad Dermatol* 1996;35:743–747.

102. Bergfeld WF, Belsito DV, Carlton WW, et al. A final report approved by the Expert Panel of the Cosmetic Ingredient Review: iodopropynyl butylcarbamate (IPBC). Washington, DC, 1996.

103. Bryld LE, Agner T, Rastogi SC, Menne T. Iodopropynyl butylcarbamate: a new contact allergen. *Contact Dermatitis* 1997;36:156–158.

104. Oleffe JA, Blondeel A, DeConinck A. Allergy to chlorocresol and propylene glucol in a steroid cream. *Contact Dermatitis* 1979;5:53.

105. Goncalo M, Goncalo S, Moreno A. Immediate and delayed sensitivity to chlorocresol. *Contact Dermatitis* 1987;17:46.

106. Burry JN, et al. Chlorocresol sensitivity. *Contact Dermatitis* 1975;1:41.

107. Adams RM. *P*-chloro-*m*-xylenol in cutting fluids: two cases of allergic contact dermatitis in machinists. *Contact Dermatitis* 1981;7:341.

108. Storrs FJ. Para-chloro-meta-xylenol allergic contact dermatitis in seven individuals. *Contact Dermatitis* 1975;1:211.

109. Libow LF, Ruskowski AM, DeLeo VA. Allergic contact dermatitis from paracloro-meta-xylenol in hurosep soap. *Contact Dermatitis* 1989;20:67.

110. Fowler JF. Para-chloro-meta-xylenol allergy and hand eczema. *Am J Contact Dermatitis* 1993;4:53.

111. Mackenzie-Wood A, Freeman S. Severe allergy to sorbolene cream. *Australas J Dermatol* 1997;38:33–34.

112. Taran J, Delaney T. Contact allergy to chloroacetamide. *Australas J Dermatol* 1997;38:95–96.

113. Storrs FJ, et al. Prevalence and relevance of allergic reactions in patients patch tested in North America—1984 to 1985. *J Am Acad Dermatol* 1989;20:1038.

114. DeGroot AC, et al. Contact allergy to preservatives—II. *Contact Dermatitis* 1986;15:218.

115. DeGroot AC, et al. Allergic contact dermatitis from tocopheryl acetate in cosmetic creams. *Contact Dermatitis* 1991;25:302.

116. Jackson E. Triclosan in leave on products. *Cosmetic Dermatology* 1998;3:23–26.

117. Moller H. Merthiolate allergy: a nationwide iatrogenic sensitization. *Acta Derm Venereol* 1977;57:509.

118. Forstrom L, et al. Merthiolate hypersensitivity and vaccination. *Contact Dermatitis* 1980;6:241.

119. Osawa J, et al. A probable role for vaccines containing thimerosal in thimerosal hypersensitivity. *Contact Dermatitis* 1991;24:178.

120. Tosti A, Guerra L, Bardazzi F. Hyposensitizing therapy with standard antigenic extracts: an important source of thimerosal sensitization. *Contact Dermatitis* 1989;20:173.

121. Cox NH, Forsythe A. Thimerosal allergy and vaccination reactions. *Contact Dermatitis* 1988;18:229.

122. Maibach HI. Acute laryngeal obstruction presumed secondary to thimerosal (Merthiolate) delayed hypersensitivity. *Contact Dermatitis* 1975;1:221.

123. Takino C. Thimerosal contact dermatitis (Japanese). *Jap J Clin Dermatol* 1971;25:1175.

124. Stern RS. Phototoxic reactions to piroxicam and other nonsteroidal anti-inflammatory agents. *N Engl J Med* 1983;309:186.

125. Cirne DeCastro JL, et al. Mechanism of photosensitive reactions induced by piroxicam. *J Am Acad Dermatol* 1989;20:706.

126. Cirne DeCastro JL, et al. Sensitivity to thimerosal and photosensitivity to piroxicam. *Contact Dermatitis* 1991;24:187.

127. Fregert S, Hjorth H. In: Rook AJ, Wilkinson DS, Ebling JFG, eds. *Textbook of dermatology.* Oxford: 1972.

128. Van Ketel WG, Melzer-van Riemsduk FA. Conjunctivitis due to soft lens solutions. *Contact Dermatitis* 1980;6:321.

129. Pedersen, NB. Allergic conjunctivitis from Merthiolate in soft contact lenses. *Contact Dermatitis* 1978;4:165.

130. Sertoli A, et al. Allergic contact dermatitis from thimerosal in a soft contact lens wearer. *Contact Dermatitis* 1980;6:292.

131. Rietschel RL, Wilson LA. Ocular inflammation in patients using soft contact lenses. *Arch Dermatol* 1982;118:147.

132. Podmore P, Storrs FJ. Contact lens intolerance: allergic conjunctivitis? *Contact Dermatitis* 1989;20:98.

133. Afzelius H, Thulin H. Allergic reactions to benzalkonium chloride. *Contact Dermatitis* 1974;5:60.

134. Wahlberg JE. Two cases of hypersensitivity to quaternary ammonium compounds. *Acta Dermatol Venereol* (Stockh.) 1962;42:239.

135. Seiji M, Mizuno F. Unusual cornification in ichthyosis-like dermatitis. *Acta Dermatol* 1970;50:338.

136. Pandos E, Horowitz ID, Wunder G. Contact dermatitis complicating trachcostomy. *Am J Dis Child* 1965;109:90.

137. Theodore FH, Schlossman A. *Ocular allergy.* Baltimore: Williams & Wilkins, 1958.

138. Fisher AA, Stillman MA. Allergic contact sensitivity to benzalkonium chloride (BAK): cutaneous, ophthalmic and general medical implications. *Arch Dermatol* 1972;106:169.

139. Stanford D, Georgouras K. Allergic contact dermatitis from benzalkonium chloride in plaster of Paris. *Contact Dermatitis* 1996;35:371–372.

140. Ortiz-Frutos FJ, Argila D, Rivera R, et al. Allergic contact dermatitis from benzalkonium chloride used as a denaturant of ethanol. *Contact Dermatitis* 1996;35:302.

141. Fisher AA, Stillman MA. Allergic contact sensitivity to benzalkonium chloride. *Arch Dermatol* 1972;106:169.

142. Shmunes E, Levy EJ. Quaternary ammonium compound contact dermatitis from a deodorant. *Arch Dermatol* 1972;105:91.

143. Hjorth N, Trolle-Lassen C. Skin reactions to preservatives in creams with special regard to paraben esters and sorbic acid. *Am Perfumer* 1962;77:43.

144. Klaschka F, Beiersdorff HU. Allergic eczematous reaction from sorbic acid used as a preservative in external medicaments. *Br J Dermatol* 1965;107:185.

145. Simpson JB. Sorbic acid sensitivity from Cortacream bandages. *Contact Dermatitis Newsletter* 1971;10:232.

146. Saihan EM, Harman RM. Contact sensitivity to sorbic acid in "Unguentum Merck." *Br J Dermatol* 1978;99:583.

147. Brown R. Another case of sorbic acid sensitivity. *Contact Dermatitis* 1979;3:268.

148. Gorannson K, Liden S. Contact allergy to sorbic acid and Unguentum Merck. *Contact Dermatitis* 1981;7:277.

149. Sober AJ, Fitzpatrick TB, eds. *Yearbook of dermatology, 1990.* Chicago: Year Book Medical Publishers, 1990.

150. Ramsing DW, Menné T. Contact sensitivity to sorbic acid. *Contact Dermatitis* 1993;28:124.

151. Dillon HL. Sorbic acid: not harmful as food additive. *JAMA* 1975;233:283.

152. Giordano-Labadie F, Pech-Ormieres C, Bazex J. Systemic contact dermatitis from sorbic acid. *Contact Dermatitis* 1996;34:61–62.

153. Clemmensen OJ, Shiødt M. Patch test reaction of the buccal mucosa to sorbic acid. *Contact Dermatitis* 1982;8:341.

154. Fryklof LE. *A note on the irritant properties of sorbic acid in ointments and creams.* Stockholm: Apotekens Kontrollaboratorium, 1958.

155. Rietschel RL. Contact urticaria from synthetic cassia oil and sorbic acid limited to the face. *Contact Dermatitis* 1978;4:347.

156. Lahti A. Skin reactions to some antimicrobial agents. *Contact Dermatitis* 1978;4:302.

157. Schultheiss E. Benzyl alcohol sensitivity. *Dermatolog Wochenschr* 1957;135:629.

158. Lagerholm B, Lodin A, Gentle H. Hypersensitivity to phenylcarbinol preservative in vitamin B_{12} for injection. *Acta Allerg* 1958;12:295.

159. Li M, Gow E. Benzyl alcohol allergy. *Australas J Dermatol.* 1995;36:219–220.

160. Marzulli FN, Maibach HI. Antimicrobials: experimental contact sensitization in man. *J Soc Cosmet Chem* 1973;24:399.

161. Fregert S. Allergic contact dermatitis from the pesticides captan and phaltan. *Contact Dermatitis Newsletter* 1967;2:28.

162. Epstein S. Photoallergic contact dermatitis. *Cutis* 1968;4:856.

163. Muston HL, Messenger AG, Byrne JPH. Contact dermatitis from zinc pyrithione, an antidandruff agent. *Contact Dermatitis* 1979;5:276.

164. Pereira F, Fernandes C, Dias M, Lacerda MH. Allergic contact dermatitis from zinc pyrithione. *Contact Dermatitis* 1995;33:131.

165. Nielsen NH, Menné T. Allergic contact dermatitis caused by zinc pyrithione associated with pustular psoriasis. *Amer J Contact Dermatitis* 1997;8:170–171.

166. Thune P. Two patients with chlorhexidine allergy—anaphylactic reactions and eczema. *Tidsskr Nor Laegeforen* 1998;118:3295–3296.

167. Jacobs MC. Contact allergy to benzophenone-2 in toilet water. *Contact Dermatitis* 1998;39:42.

168. Fisher AA. Reactions to antioxidants in cosmetics and foods. *Cutis* 1976;17:21.

169. Degreef H, Verhoeve L. Contact dermatitis to miconazole nitrate. *Contact Dermatitis* 1975;1:269.

170. Meneghini CL, Rantuccio F, Lomuto M. Additives, vehicles and active drugs of topical medicaments as causes of delayed-type allergic dermatitis. *Dermatologica* 1971;143:137.

171. White IR, Lovell CR, Cronin E. Antioxidants in cosmetics. *Contact Dermatitis* 1984;11:265.

172. Flyvholm M, Menné T. Sensitizing risk of butylated hydroxytoluene based on exposure and effect data. *Contact Dermatitis* 1990;23:341.

173. Roed-Petersen J, Hjorth N. Contact dermatitis from antioxidants: hidden sensitizers in topical medications and foods. *Br J Dermatol* 1976;94:233.

174. DeGroot AC, Gerkens F. Occupational airborne contact dermatitis from octyl gallate. *Contact Dermatitis* 1990;23:184.

175. Bojs G, Nicklasson B, Svensson A. Allergic contact sensitivity to propyl gallate. *Contact Dermatitis* 1987;17:294.

176. Cronin E. Lipstick dermatitis due to propyl gallate. *Contact Dermatitis* 1980;6:213.

177. Raccagni AA, Frattagli M, Baldari U, Righini MG. Lauryl gallate hand dermatitis in a cheese counter assistant. *Contact Dermatitis* 1997;37:182.

178. Hernandez N, Assier -Bonnet H, Terki N, Revuz J. Allergic contact dermatitis from propyl gallate in desonide cream (Locapred). *Contact Dermatitis* 1997;36:111.

179. Heine A. Contact dermatitis from propyl gallate. *Contact Dermatitis* 1988;18:313.

180. Hausen BM, Beyer W. The sensitizing capacity of the antioxidants propyl, octyl and dodecyl gallate and some related gallic acid esters. *Contact Dermatitis* 1992;26:253.

181. Marston S. Propyl gallate on liposomes. *Contact Dermatitis* 1992;27:74.

182. Fowler JF. Allergic contact dermatitis to polyvinylpyrrolidone/hexadecene copolymer. *Amer J Contact Dermatitis* 1995;6:243–244.

183. DeGroot AC, Brunynzeel DP, Bos JD et al. The allergens in cosmetics. *Arch Dermatol* 1988;124:1525–1529.

184. Raymond JZ, Cross PR. EDTA: preservative dermatitis. *Arch Dermatol* 1969;100:436.

185. Bhushan M, Beck MH. Allergic contact dermatitis from disodium ethylenediamie tetra-acetic acid (EDTA) in a local anaesthetic. *Contact Dermatitis* 1998;38:183.

186. DeGroot AC. Contact allergy to EDTA in a topical corticosteroid preparation. *Contact Dermatitis* 1986;15:250.

187. Eriksen KE. Allergy to ethylenediamine. *Arch Dermatol* 1975;111:791.

188. Penvy I, Shaefer J. Ethylenediamine allergy. *Dermatosen* 1980;28:35.

189. Epstein E. Negative patch tests to ethylenediamine tetraacetate in patients allergic to ethylenediamine. *Contact Dermatitis Newsletter* 1974;16:475.

190. Fisher AA. Does ethylenediamine hydrochloride cross-react with ethylenediamine tetraacetate? *Contact Dermatitis* 1975;1:267.

191. Balato N, et al. Ethylenediamine dermatitis. *Contact Dermatitis* 1986;15:263.

192. CTFA *Cosmetic ingredient dictionary.* 3rd ed. Washington, DC: Cosmetic Toiletry and Fragrance Association, 1982.

193. Nilzen A, Wikstrom K. The influence of sodium lauryl sulfate on the sensitization of guinea pigs to chrome and nickel. *Acta Derm Venereol* 1955;35:292.

194. Kligman AM. The SLS provocative patch test in allergic contact sensitization. *J Invest Dermatol* 1966;36:573.

195. Dahl MV, Trancik RJ. Sodium lauryl sulfate irritant patch tests: degree of inflammation at various times. *Contact Dermatitis* 1977;3:263.

196. Bergstresser PR, Eagelstein WH. Irritation by hydrophilic ointment under occlusion. *Arch Dermatol* 1973;108:218.

197. Krook G. Contact dermatitis due to Ficortril (hydrocortisone 1 percent ointment, Pfizer). *Contact Dermatitis Newsletter* 1974;15:460.

198. Fulton JE, Bradley S, Aqundex A, et al. Non-comedogenic cosmetics. *Cutis* 1976;17:344.

199. Sams WM, Smith G. Contact dermatitis due to hydrocortisone ointment: report of a case of sensitivity to emulsifying agents in a hydrophilic ointment base. *JAMA* 1957;164:1212.

200. Prater E, Goring HD, Schubert H. Sodium lauryl sulphate—a contact allergen. *Contact Dermatitis* 1978;4:242.

201. Foussereau J, Petitjean J, Lants JP. Sodium lauryl sulphate. *Contact Dermatitis Newsletter* 1974;15:460.

202. Expert Panel of the American College of Toxicology. Final report on the safety assessment of cocamidopropyl betaine. *J Am Coll Toxicol* 1991;10:33.

203. VanHoute N, Dooms-Goossens A. Shampoo dermatitis due to cocobetaine and sodium lauryl ether sulphate. *Contact Dermatitis* 1983;9:169.

204. Andersen KE, Roed-Petersen J, Kamp P. Contact allergy related to TEA-PEG-3 cocamide sulfate and cocamidopropyl betaine in a shampoo. *Contact Dermatitis* 1984;11:192.

205. Korting HC, et al. Allergic contact dermatitis to cocamidopropyl betaine in shampoo. *J Am Acad Dermatol* 1992;27:1013.

206. Fowler JF. Cocamidopropyl betaine: the significance of positive patch tests in 12 patients. *Cutis* 1993;52:281–284.

207. Fowler JF, Fowler LM, Hunter JE. Allergy to cocamidopropyl betaine may be due to amidoamine: a patch test and product use test study. *Contact Dermatitis* 1997;37:276–281.

208. Angelini G, Rigano L, Foti C, et al. 3-dimethylaminopropylamine: a key substance in contact allergy to cocamidopropyl betaine? *Contact Dermatitis* 1995;32:96–99.

209. DeGroot AC, et al. Contact allergy to cocamide DEA and lauramide DEA in shampoos. *Contact Dermatitis* 1987;16:117.

210. Fowler J. Allergy to Cocamide DEA. *Am J Contact Dermatitis* 1998;9:40–41.

211. Christersson S, Wrangsjo K. Contact allergy to undecylenamide diethanolamide in a liquid soap. *Contact Dermatitis* 1992;27:191.

212. DeGroot AC, Liem DH. Contact allergy to oleamidopropyl dimethylamine. *Contact Dermatitis* 1984;11:298.

213. Bruynzeel DP, Niklasson B. The patch test dilution of oleamidopropyl dimethylamine. *Contact Dermatitis* 1992;27:190.

214. DeGroot AC, et al. Cross-reaction pattern of the cationic emulsifier oleamidopropyl dimethylamine. *Contact Dermatitis* 1988;19:284.

215. Taylor JS, Jordan WP, Maibach HI. Allergic contact dermatitis from stearamidoethyl diethylamine phosphate: a cosmetic emulsifier. *Contact Dermatitis* 1984;10:74.

216. Fisher AA. Allergic contact dermatitis to nonoxynol-9 in a condom. *Cutis* 1994;53:110–111.

217. Dooms-Goossens A, Deveylder H, D-Alam H, et al. Sensitivity to nonoxynols as a cause of intolerance to antiseptic preparations. *J Am Acad Dermatol* 1989;21:723–727.

218. Morren M. Contact allergy to dihydroxyacetone. *Contact Dermatitis* 1991;25:326.

219. Dooms-Goosens A, et al. Hexamidine isethionate: a sensitizer in topical pharmaceutical products and cosmetics. *Contact Dermatitis* 1989;21:270.

220. Fulton JE Jr, Bradley S, Agundez A, et al. Non-comedogenic cosmetics. *Cutis* 1976;17:344.

221. Fisher AA. Reactions to popular cosmetic humectants: 3. Glycerin, propylene glycol, and butylene glycol. *Cutis* 1980;26:243.

222. Fisher AA. Propylene glycol dermatitis. *Cutis* 1978;21:166.

223. Warshaw TG, Herrmann F. Studies of skin reaction of propylene glycol. *J Invest Dermatol* 1952;19:423.

224. Goldsmith LA. Propylene glycol. *Int J Dermatol* 1978;17:703.

225. Trancik RG, Maibach HI. Propylene glycol: irritation or sensitization? *Contact Dermatitis* 1982;8:185.

226. Hannuksela M, Pirila V, Salo OP. Skin reactions to propylene glycol. *Contact Dermatitis* 1975;1:112.

227. Braun W. Contact allergies against polyethylene glycols. *Z Hautkr Geschlechtskr* 1969;44:385.

228. Claverie F, et al. Eczema de contact au propylene glycol. *Ann Dermatol-Venereol* 1997;124:315–317.

229. Oleffe JA, Blondell A, de Connick A. Allergy to chlorocresol and propylene glycol in a steroid cream. *Contact Dermatitis* 1979;5:53.

230. Shore RN, Shelley WB. Contact dermatitis from stearyl alcohol and propylene glycol in fluocinonide cream. *Arch Dermatol* 1974;109:397.

231. Fowler JF. Contact allergy to propylene glycol in topical corticosteroids. *Am J Contact Dermatitis* 1993;4:37.

232. Agren-Jonsson S, Magnusson B. Sensitization to propantheline bromide, trichlorocarbanilide and propylene glycol in an antiperspirant. *Contact Dermatitis* 1976;2:79.

233. Lewes, D. Electrode jelly in electrocardiography. *Br Heart J* 1965;27:105.

234. Fisher AA. Dermatologic hazards of electrocardiography. *Cutis* 1977;20:686.

235. Peleg O, Bar-Oz B, Arad I. Coma in a premature infant associated with the transdermal absorption of propylene glycol. *Acta Paedatr* 1998;87:1195–1196.

236. Hibbot HW, Monks J. Butylene glycol. *J Soc Cosmet Chem* 1961;12:2.

237. Sugiura M, Hayakawa R. Contact dermatitis due to 1,3-butylene glycol. *Contact Dermatitis* 1997;37:90.

238. Kinnunen T, Koskela M. Antibacterial and antifungal properties of propylene glycol, hexylene glycol, and 1,3-butylene glycol *in vitro*. *Acta Dermatol* 1991;71:148.

239. Kinnunen T, Hannuksela M. Skin reactions to hexylene glycol. *Contact Dermatitis* 1989;21:154.

240. Fisher AA. Contact urticaria due to polyethylene glycol. *Cutis* 1977;19:409.

241. Fisher AA. Immediate and delayed allergic contact reactions to polyethylene glycol. *Contact Dermatitis* 1978;4:135.

242. Maibach HI. Polyethylene glycol: allergic contact dermatitis potential. *Contact Dermatitis* 1975;1:247.

243. Marzulli F, Maibach H. Use of graded concentration in studying skin sensitizers: experimental contact sensitization in man. *Food Cosmetic Toxicol* 1974;12:219.

244. Braun W. Contact allergies to polyethylene glycols. *Z Haut-Geschlechtskrankheiten* 1969;44:385.

245. Bajaj AK. Contact sensitivity of polyethylene glycols. *Contact Dermatitis* 1990;22:291.

246. Hannuksela M, Forstrom L. Contact hypersensitivity to glycerol. *Contact Dermatitis* 1976;2:291.1992;27:1013.

247. Dooms-Goossens A, DeGreef H. Sensitization to yellow petrolatum used as a vehicle for patch testing. *Contact Dermatitis* 1980;6:146–148.

248. Maibach H. Chronic dermatitis and hyperpigmentation from petrolatum. *Contact Dermatitis* 1978;4:62–64.

249. Grin R, Maibach H. Long lasting contact urticaria from petrolatum mimicking dermatitis. *Contact Dermatitis* 1999;40:110.

250. Castelain P. Generalized diffuse eczema due to sensitization to triethanolamine. *Bull Soc Franc Derm Syph* 1967;74:562.

251. Suurmond D. Patch test reactions to Phenergan cream: promethazine and triethanolamine. *Dermatologica* 1966;133:503.

252. Schwartz L. *Sensitivity testing in cosmetics: science and technology.* New York: Interscience Publishers, 1967.

253. Blum A, Lischka G. Allergic contact dermatitis from mono-, di- and triethanolamine. *Contact Dermatitis* 1997;36:166.

254. Hamilton TK, Zug KA. Triethanolamine allergy inadvertently discovered from a fluorescent marking pen. *Amer J Contact Dermatology* 1996;7:164–165.

255. Edwards EK Jr, Edwards EK. Allergic reaction to triethanolamine stearate in a sunscreen. *Cutis* 1983;31:195–196.

256. DeBerker D. Contact sensitivity to the stearyl alcohol in Efudex cream. *Contact Dermatitis* 1992;26:138.

257. Martinez-Falero AA, et al. Allergic contact dermatitis from flucortin butyl. *Contact Dermatitis* 1990;22:241.

258. von-der-Werth JM, English JS, Dalziel KL. Loss of patch test positivity to cetylstearyl alcohol. *Contact Dermatitis* 1998;38:109–110.

259. DeGroot AC, et al. Cosmetic allergy from myristyl alcohol. *Contact Dermatitis* 1988;19:76.

260. DeGroot AC, et al. Cosmetic allergy from stearic acid and glyceryl stearate. *Contact Dermatitis* 1988;19:77.

261. Hayakawa R. Lipstick dermatitis due to C18 aliphatic compounds. *Contact Dermatitis* 1987;16:215.

262. Tan BB, Noble AL, Roberts ME, et al. Allergic contact dermatitis from oleyl alcohol in lipstick cross-reacting with ricinoleic acid in castor oil and lanolin. *Contact Dermatitis* 1997;37:41–42,

263. Calnan CD. Contact dermatitis from drugs: symposium on drug sensitization. *Proc R Soc Med* 1962;55:39.

264. Bunney, MH. Contact dermatitis in beekeepers due to propolis (bee glue). *Br J Dermatol* 1968;80:17.

265. Rothenborg HW. Occupational dermatitis in a beekeeper due to poplar resins in beeswax. *Arch Dermatol* 1967;95:381.

266. Wanscher B. Contact dermatitis from propolis. *Br J Dermatol* 1976;94:451.

267. Petersen HO. Allergy to propolis (bee glue) in patients with eczema. *Ugeskr Laeg* 1977;139:2331.

268. Hausen BM, et al. Propolis allergy (IV). *Contact Dermatitis* 1992;26:34.

269. Machackova J. The incidence of allergy to propolis in 605 consecu-

tive patients patch tested in Prague. *Contact Dermatitis* 1988;18:210–212.

270. Camasara G. Occupational dermatitis from beeswax. *Contact Dermatitis* 1975;1:124.

271. Cronin E. Lanolin dermatitis. *Br J Dermatol* 1966;78:617.

272. Vollum DI. Sensitivity to hydrogenated lanolin. *Arch Dermatol* 1969;100:774.

273. Edman B, Moller H. Testing a purified lanolin preparation by a randomized procedure. *Contact Dermatitis* 1989;20:287.

274. Thune P. Allergy to wool fat: the addition of salicylic acid for patch test purposes. *Acta Derm Venereol* (Stockh.) 1969;49:282.

275. Newcomb, EA. Lanolin allergy. *J Soc Cosmet Chem* 1966;17:149.

276. Peter C, Schropl F, Franzwa H. Experimental investigation regarding allergenic effects of wool wax alcohols. *Hautarzt* 1969;20:450.

277. Oleffe JD, Blondeel A, Boschmans L. Patch testing with lanolin. *Contact Dermatitis* 1978;4:233.

278. Giorgini S, Melli MC, Sertoli A. Comments on the allergenic activity of lanolin. *Contact Dermatitis* 1983;9:425.

279. Kligman AM. Lanolin allergy: crisis or comedy. *Contact Dermatitis* 1983;9:99.

280. Breit R, Bandmann H-J. Dermatitis from lanolin. *Br J Dermatol* 1973;88:414.

281. Bandmann H-J, Reichenberger M. Beobachtungen und Untersuchungen zur Frage der durch Eucerin Bedingten seltenen Allergies. *Hautarzt* 1957;8:11.

282. Cronin E, et al. Contact dermatitis in the atopic. *Acta Derm Venereol* (Stockh.) 1970;50:183.

283. Bojs G, Bruze M, Svensson A. Contact allergy to the lanolin derivative amerchol CAB. *Am J Contact Dermatitis* 1992;3:83.

284. Matthies L, Dockx P. Discrepancy in patch test results with wool wax alcohols and Amerchol L-101. *Contact Dermatitis* 1997;36:150–151.

285. Brandle I. Allergy to castor oil. *Contact Dermatitis* 1983;9:424.

286. Fisher AA. Allergic cheilitis due to castor oil in lipsticks. *Cutis* 1991;47:389.

287. Andersen KE, Nielsen R. Lipstick dermatitis related to castor oil. *Contact Dermatitis* 1984;11:253.

288. Sai S. Lipstick dermatitis caused by ricinoleic acid. *Contact Dermatitis* 1983;9:524.

289. Eiermann HJ, Larsen W, Maibach HI, Taylor JS. Prospective study of cosmetic reactions: 1977–1980. *J Am Acad Dermatol* 1982;6:909.

290. de Groot A, et al. The allergens in cosmetics. *Arch Dermatol* 1988;124:1525.

291. Osolo G, ed. *Remington's pharmaceutical sciences.* 16th ed. Easton, PA: Mack Publishing Co, 1980.

292. Maibach H, Engasser P. In *Fisher's contact dermatitis,* 4th ed. 1995.

293. Food, drug, and cosmetic products warning statements. *Fed Register* 1975;40:8912.

294. Estrin NF, Crosley PA, Haynes CR. *CTFA dictionary.* 3rd ed. Washington, DC: Cosmetic, Toiletry, and Fragrance Association, 1982.

295. Frosch PJ, Kligman AM. A method for appraising the stinging capacity of topically applied substances. *J Soc Cosmet Chem* 1977;28:197.

296. Bronaugh RL, Maibach HI. Primary irritant, allergic contact, phototoxic, and photoallergic reactions to cosmetics and tests to identify problem products. In: Frost P, Horwitz SN, eds. *Principles of cosmetics for the dermatologist.* St Louis: Mosby, 1982.

297. Krogh G von, Maibach HI. The contact urticaria syndrome—1982. *Semin Dermatol* 1982;1:59.

298. Rorsman H. Riehl's melanosis. *Int J Dermatol* 1982;21:75.

299. Sugai T, Takahashi Y, Takagi T. Pigmented cosmetic dermatitis and coal tar dyes. *Contact Dermatitis* 1977;3:249.

300. Kozuka T, Tashiro M, Sano S, et al. Pigmented contact dermatitis from azo dyes: 1. Cross-sensitivity in humans. *Contact Dermatitis* 1980;6:330.

301. Nakayama H, Harada R, Toda M. Pigmented cosmetic dermatitis. *Int J Dermatol* 1976;15:673.

302. Mathias CG. Pigmented cosmetic dermatitis from contact allergy to a toilet soap containing chromium. *Contact Dermatitis* 1982;8:29.

303. Findlay GH, Morrison JGL, Simson IW. Exogenous ochronosis and pigmented colloid millium from hydroquinone bleaching creams. *Br J Dermatol* 1975;93:612.

304. Fisher AA. Hydroquinone uses and abnormal reactions. *Cutis* 1983;31:240.

305. Mathias CG, Maibach HI, Conant MA. Perioral leukoderma simulating vitiligo from use of a toothpaste containing cinnamic aldehyde. *Arch Dermatol* 1980;116:1172.

306. Samman PD. Nail disorders caused by external influences. *J Soc Cosmet Chem* 1977;28:351.

307. Kligman AM, Mills OH. Acne cosmetica. *Arch Dermatol* 1972;106:843.

308. Fulton JE, Pay SR, Fulton JE, III. Comedogenicity of current therapeutic products, cosmetics and ingredients in the rabbit ear. *J Am Acad Dermatol* 1984;10:96.

309. Frank SB. Is the rabbit ear model, in its present state, prophetic of acnegenicity? *J Am Acad Dermatol* 1982;6:373.

310. Epstein WL. Contact-type delayed hypersensitivity in infants and children: Induction of rhus sensitivity. *Pediatrics* 1961;27:51.

311. Hjorth N. Contact dermatitis in children. *Acta Derm Venereol* (Stockh.) 1981;95:36.

312. Marshall S. The effect of bubble bath on the urinary tract. *J Urol* 1965;93:112.

313. Bass HN. Bubble bath as an irritant to the urinary tract of children. *Clin Pediatr* (Phila.) 1966;7:174.

314. Roberts HJ. Bubble bath cystitis and cosmetic vulvitis neglected hazards. *J Fla Med Assoc* 1973;60:31.

315. Sainia E, Jolanki R, Hakalde, Kanerva L. Metals and arsenic in eye shadows. *Contact Dermatitis* 2000;42:5–10.

316. Nethercott J, et al. A review of 79 cases of eyelid dermatitis. *J Am Acad Dermatol* 1989;21:223.

317. Epstein E. Misleading mascara patch tests. *Arch Dermatol* 1965;91:615.

318. Wilson LA, Ahearn DG. Pseudomonas-induced ulcers associated with contaminated eye mascaras. *Am J Ophthalmol* 1977;84:112.

319. Warshawshki L, Mitchell JC, Storrs FJ. Allergic contact dermatitis from glyceryl monothioglycolate in hair dressers. *Contact Dermatitis* 1981;7:351.

320. Rapaport M. Irritant contact dermatitis to glyceryl monothioglycolate. *J Am Acad Dermatol* 1983;9:739.

321. Cronin E. *Contact dermatitis.* New York: Churchill Livingstone, 1980.

322. Schorr WF. Multiple injuries from permanents: cosmetic symposium. *Am Acad Dermatol,* Dec. 3, 1983.

323. Harris RT. Hair relaxing. *Cosmet Toiletr* 1979;94:51.

324. Brooks G, Lewis A. Treatment regimens for styled black hair. *Cosmet Toiletr* 1983;98:59.

325. Henkin H. Technical history of shampoos. *Cosmet Toiletr* 1981;96:39.

326. Sylvest B, Hjorth N, Magnusson B. Lauryl ether sulfate dermatitis in Denmark. *Contact Dermatitis* 1975;1:359.

327. Haute N Van, Dooms-Goossens A. A shampoo dermatitis due to cocobetaine and sodium lauryl ether sulphate. *Contact Dermatitis* 1983;9:169.

328. Hindson C, Lawlor F. Coconut diethanolamide in a hydraulic mining oil. *Contact Dermatitis* 1983;9:168.

329. Nurse DS. Sensitivity to coconut diethanolamide. *Contact Dermatitis* 1980;6:502.

330. Broeckx W. Cosmetic intolerance. *Contact Dermatitis* 1987;16:189.

331. Reiss F, Fisher AA. Is hair dyed with para-phenylenediamine allergenic? *Arch Dermatol* 1974;109:221.

332. Foussereau J, Reuter G, Petitjean J. Is hair dyed with PPD-like dyes allergenic? *Contact Dermatitis* 1980;6:143.

333. Hindson C. *O-nitro-paraphenylenediamine* in hair dye—an unusual dental hazard. *Contact Dermatitis* 1975;1:333.

334. Cronin E. Dermatitis from wife's dyed hair. *Contact Dermatitis Newsletter* 1973;13:363.

335. Warin AP. Contact dermatitis to partner's hair dye. *Clin Exp Dermatol* 1976;1:283.

336. Engasser PG, Maibach HI. Cosmetics and dermatology: hair dye toxicology. In: Rook AJ, Maibach HI, eds. *Recent advances in dermatology,* vol. 6. New York: Churchill Livingstone, 1985.

337. Pasricha, JS, Gupta R, Panjwani S. Contact dermatitis to henna (Lawsonia). *Contact Dermatitis* 1980;6:288.

338. Garcia-Ortiz J, et al. Contact allergy to henna. *Int Arch Allergy Immunol* 1997;114:298–299.

339. Cronin E. Immediate-type hypersensitivity to henna. *Contact Dermatitis* 1979;5:198.

340. Edwards EK, Jr, Edwards EK. Allergic contact dermatitis to lead acetate in a hair dye. *Cutis* 1982;30:629.

341. White IR, Catchpole HE, Rycroft RJG. Rashes among persulfate workers. *Contact Dermatitis* 1982;8:168.

342. Fisher AA, Dooms-Goossens A. Persulfate hair bleach reactions. *Arch Dermatol* 1976;112:1407.

343. Calnan CD. Quinazoline yellow dermatitis D&C Yellow 11 in eye cream. *Contact Dermatitis* 1981;7:271.

344. Sato Y, Kutsuna H, Kobayashi T, Mitsui T. D&C nos. 10 and 11: chemical composition analysis and delayed contact hypersensitivity testing in the guinea pig. *Contact Dermatitis* 1984;10:30.

345. Weaver JE. Disparate skin allergenicity of 2 quinoline dyes. *Contact Dermatitis* 1983;9:526.

346. Cronin E. Lipstick dermatitis due to propyl gallate. *Contact Dermatitis* 1980;6:213.

347. Joost T van, Liem DH, Stolz E. Allergic contact dermatitis to monotertiary-butylhydroquinone in lip gloss. *Contact Dermatitis* 1984;10:189.

348. Calnan CD, Cronin E, Rycroft RJG. Allergy to phenyl salicylate. *Contact Dermatitis* 1981;7:208.

349. Calnan CD. Amyldimethyl aminobenzoic acid causing lipstick dermatitis. *Contact Dermatitis* 1980;6:233.

350. Schorr WF. Lip gloss and gloss-type cosmetics. *Contact Dermatitis Newsletter* 1973;14:408.

351. Angelini E, et al. Allergic contact dermatitis of the lip margins from para-tertiary-butylphenol in a lip liner. *Contact Dermatitis* 1993;28:146.

352. Lanzet M. Modern formulations of coloring agents: facial and eye. In: Frost P, Horwitz SN, eds. *Principles of cosmetics for the dermatologist.* St Louis: Mosby, 1982.

353. Calnan CD. Compound allergy to a cosmetic. *Contact Dermatitis* 1975;1:123.

354. Mitchell JC. Non-inflammatory onycholysis from formaldehyde-containing nail hardener. *Contact Dermatitis* 1981;7:173.

355. Schlossman ML. Nail-enamel resins. *Cosmet Technol* 1979;1:53.

356. Paltzik RL, Enscoe I. Onycholysis secondary to toluene sulfonamide formal dehyde resin used in a nail hardener mimicking onychomycosis. *Cutis* 1980;25:647.

357. Liden C, et al. Nail varnish allergy with farreaching consequences. *Br J Dermatol* 1993;128:57.

358. Wilkinson JB, Moore RJ. *Harry's cosmeticology.* New York: Chemical Publishing, 1982.

359. Fisher AA, Franks A, Glick H. Allergic sensitization to acrylic nails. *J Allergy* 1957;28:84.

360. Food and Drug Administration seizure actions. *FDA Consumer* 1974;8:37.

361. Fuller M. Analysis of paint-on artificial nails. *J Soc Cosmet Chem* 1982;33:51.

362. Marks JG, Bishop ME, Willis, WP. Allergic contact dermatitis to sculptured nails. *Arch Dermatol* 1979;115:100.

363. Fisher AA. Cross reactions between methyl methacrylate monomer and acrylic monomers presently used in acrylic nail preparations. *Contact Dermatitis* 1980;6:345.

364. Fisher A. Permanent loss of fingernails due to allergic reaction to an acrylic nail preparation: a sixteen year follow-up study. *Cutis* 1989;43:404.

365. Fisher A. Paresthesia of the fingers accompanying dermatitis due to methyl methacrylate bone cement. *Contact Dermatitis* 1979;5:56.

366. Baran R, Schibli H. Permanent paresthesia to sculptured nails. *Derm Clin* 1990;8:139.

367. Pigatto P, et al. Unusual sensitization to cyanoacrylate ester. *Contact Dermatitis* 1986;14:193.

368. Belsito D. Contact dermatitis to ethyl cyanoacrylate containing glue. *Contact Dermatitis* 1987;17:234.

369. Baran R. Pathology induced by the application of cosmetics to the nail. In: Frost P, Horwitz SN, eds. *Principles of cosmetics for the dermatologist.* St Louis: Mosby, 1982.

370. Burrows D, Rycroft, RJG. Contact dermatitis from PTBP resin and tricresyl ethyl phthalate in a plastic nail adhesive. *Contact Dermatitis* 1981;7:336.

371. Labows JN, McGinley KJ, Kligman AM. Axillary odor: current status. In: Frost P, Horwitz SN, eds. *Principles of cosmetics for the dermatologist.* St Louis: Mosby, 1982.

372. deGroot AC, Liem DH. Facial psoriasis caused by contact allergy to linalool and hydroxycitronellal in an after-shave. *Contact Dermatitis* 1983;9:230.

373. Raugi GJ, Stoors FJ, Larsen WG. Photoallergic contact dermatitis to men's perfumes. *Contact Dermatitis* 1979;5:251.

374. Giovinazzo VJ, Haber LC, Bickers DR, et al. Photoallergic contact dermatitis to musk ambrette. *Arch Dermatol* 1981;117:344.

375. Jackson E. Moisturizers: what's in them? How do they work? *Am J Contact Dermatitis* 1992;3:162.

376. Pugliese PT. Cell renewal—an overview. *Cosmet Toiletr* 1983;98:61.

377. Hannuksela M, Kousa M, Pirila V. Contact sensitivity to emulsifiers. *Contact Dermatitis* 1976;2:201.

378. Rieger MM. Depilatories: 1979 update. *Cosmet Toiletr* 1979;94:71.

379. Fisher AA. Current contact news (cosmetic actions and reactions: therapeutic, irritant, and allergic). *Cutis* 1980;26:22.

380. Cotterill JG. Dermatological nondisease: a common and potentially fatal disturbance of body image. *Br J Dermatol* 1981;104:611.

381. Tosti A. Prevalence and sources of sensitization to emulsifiers: a clinical study. *Contact Dermatitis* 1990;23:68–72.

APPENDIX A

Cosmetic Industry on Call (contact persons in the cosmetic industry) 8th edition, 1999. Editors: Anita S. Curry and G.N. McEwen, Jr. Ph.D., CTFA.

CTFA International Cosmetic Ingredient Dictionary, 8th edition. Editors: Norman F. Estrin, Ph.D., Patricia A. Crosley, and Charles R. Haynes.

CTFA Cosmetic Ingredient Handbook, 2nd edition.

Additional information available from:

The Cosmetic, Toiletry, and Fragrance Association

1101 17th Street N.W., Suite 300

Washington, D.C. 20036

Telephone: 202–331–1770

Fax: 202–331–1969

Website: http://www.ctfa.org

Complete listing of CTFA publications and/or ordering available from:

CTFA Publication Orders

P.O. Box 75319

Baltimore, MD 21275

Telephone: 301–953–2614

Fax: 301–206–9789

CHAPTER 18

Hand Dermatitis Due to Contactants: Special Considerations

There are several varieties of allergic contact dermatitis (ACD) of the hands. Table 18.1 lists these varieties together with the type of skin testing that may help determine the etiology of the different kinds of hand dermatitis owing to various contactants.

IRRITANT CONTACT DERMATITIS

Irritant contact dermatitis (ICD) due to a nonspecific reaction can occur in all individuals, provided the irritants are in contact with the skin for a sufficient length of time and are in sufficiently high concentrations. This dermatitis is usually characterized by dryness, some fissuring, and thickening of the skin. ICD differs from allergic dermatitis in that vesicles are usually rare. Defatting, degreasing agents, such as detergents and solvents, are the main causes of "gradual" irritant dermatitis. Strong acids and alkalis may produce an acute "severe" irritant dermatitis. In general, irritants damage the skin by direct, cytotoxic action. The diagnosis of irritant dermatitis is one of exclusion, because "proof" cannot be obtained by "skin tests."

One form of ICD was formerly called "housewife's eczema" or "dishpan hands." Medical and dental workers, food preparation and service workers, janitors, housekeepers, and anyone who frequently washes his or her hands or is exposed to cleaners may develop this type of eczema. Patch tests, however, may reveal a superimposed allergic dermatitis. The trapping of soaps and detergents under a ring often initiates an irritant hand dermatitis. It has been estimated that 65% of atopic individuals who do wet work in hospitals develop dermatitis of the hands (1).

Patch Test Reactivity in Hand Eczema Patients

Bjornberg (2) analyzed the skin reactions to 11 primary irritants in patients who had eczema and in normal persons. It has been assumed generally that an irritant reaction ob-served after a 24-hour patch test subsides rapidly. This assumption, which has been used to differentiate allergic from irritant patch test reactions, has often been incorrect. Severe irritant patch test reactions in particular often increase over the first 72 hours (3).

The average concentration of an irritant causing a faint erythema can be taken as a measure of the skin irritancy of a compound. Only 0.2% of croton oil in petrolatum was necessary to evoke this erythema, whereas 0.9% of sodium lauryl sulfate and the surprisingly high figure of 17.5% of potassium soap were necessary. No marked difference was present between patients and controls. Many authors have described the irritant reaction as an "all or none" response, but phenol was the only substance that conformed to this pattern. With all other substances, the intensity of reaction increased in proportion to concentration and exposure time. All age groups react similarly to sodium lauryl sulfate.

The increased skin susceptibility to irritants in remote body regions was an important finding in patients who had hand eczema. This is the first proof of the validity of the commonly used term "status eczematicus" and must be taken into account in establishing the concentration of substances used for patch testing and in assessing the reaction to substances that are at the same time allergens and irritants. This increased reactivity may cause nonspecific patch test reactions, may add to the risk of accidental patch test sensitization, and may cause unexpected side effects from therapeutic agents.

Patients who had healed (in contrast to active) hand eczema showed a normal reactivity to most irritants, but both groups gave stronger reactions to soap, sodium lauryl sulfate, and benzalkonium chloride than did the controls.

Agner (4) used various objective determinations of patch test reactions to sodium lauryl sulfate, including measurements on an evaporimeter, an ultrasound A-scan, a laser-Doppler flowmeter, and a chromameter. He verified the fact that patch test results in hand eczema patients differ from those of controls only when the hand eczema is active.

TABLE 18.1. *Hand Eczema-Skin Test Correlations*

Type	Test
Irritant	No specific test
Allergic	
Contact (delayed)	Patch test
Contact (systemic)	Patch test
Contact (immediate)	Immediate patch, prick, scratch test
Endogenous	No specific tests

> **Patients who have acute hand dermatitis show increased irritability of the skin in sites other than the hands.**

ALLERGIC CONTACT DERMATITIS OF THE HANDS

It is often impossible to distinguish between irritant and allergic contact dermatitis of the hands without performing patch tests. Patch testing is the only scientific "proof" that a contactant is a dermatitis-producing allergen in a particular case. It has been found valuable to patch test patients who have a chronic hand dermatitis with the "standard" patch test series. Jordan (5) reported 220 cases of hand eczema that were evaluated for uncomplicated allergic contact dermatitis. In 12% of the 220 patients, the diagnosis was established with the aid of a standard screening tray. Another 5% of the cases were diagnosed as a result of testing with additional allergens. The hand eczema in these patients (17%) changed dramatically as a result of allergic contact investigation. Wilkinson et al. (6,7) agree that patch testing is of great value in the management of hand dermatitis.

> **Patch testing is essential to distinguish allergic from irritant hand dermatitis.**

EPIDEMIOLOGY OF HAND ECZEMA

Several studies of large groups of individuals have been conducted to analyze the prevalence of hand eczema.

Lantinga et al. (8) studied over 1,900 people in the city of Vlagtweddle in the Netherlands twice over a 3-year period. At the last point in the study, 10% of women and 4.5% of men, age 30 to 60, had hand eczema of some type. ICD alone accounted for about half the cases. ACD alone accounted for 15%, with the remainder being a combination of these or other diagnoses such as atopic or nummular dermatitis. Of 141 patients patch tested, 20% tested positive for nickel (26% women, 7% men). Other allergens were not particularly remarkable.

At about the same time, Kavli and Førde (9) studied hand eczema in northern Norway. This was done by questionnaire, not by patient examination. Five percent of men and 13% of women claimed they had had hand eczema over the preceding 12 months. Of the total sample of 14,667, 49 men (0.7%) and 105 women (1.4%) had taken sick leave for hand eczema during the preceding 3 years.

In a more recent work, Meding and Swanbeck (10) studied hand eczema in Goteborg, Sweden. Twenty thousand persons age 20 to 65 were surveyed by mail, resulting in examination of 1,238 persons with confirmed hand eczema. The 1-year period prevalence was 11.8%. Patch testing of 1,071 patients with 26 standard allergens showed that 15% were allergic to nickel. Other frequent allergens were cobalt (6.7%), fragrance mix (5.8%), balsam of Peru (4.9%), and rosin (3.2%).

Two-thirds of the 1,238 had sought medical help, and 21% had taken sick leave because of eczema. Those with ACD had more serious consequences than those with other forms of eczema (11).

Rystedt (12–14) has extensively studied hand eczema in atopics. She found that those with childhood atopic dermatitis of either moderate or severe degree (44% and 55%, respectively) developed hand eczema even without irritant work exposure, whereas 68% to 81% who worked as housecleaners, nurses, food handlers, or hairdressers developed hand eczema. Those atopics who changed jobs because of hand eczema were less likely to see improvement than nonatopics. Atopics were also less likely to have ACD than nonatopics (22% vs 45%). Although women, those with a family history of atopic dermatitis, and those with respiratory atopy were somewhat more likely to have hand eczema, these factors are of much less significance than a personal history of atopic dermatitis.

ROLE OF CERTAIN ALLERGENS IN THE STANDARD PATCH TEST SERIES IN HAND DERMATITIS

Allergic reactions to nickel, dichromate, ethylenediamine hydrochloride, rubber compounds, paraphenylenediamine, and topical preservatives play a significant role in the production and maintenance of hand dermatitis.

Nickel

As a rule, dermatitis to nickel-plated objects is not confined to the hands, because other sites also are usually exposed to nickel-containing jewelry, clips, and zippers. External hand dermatitis occurs principally as a reaction to handles, knobs, pencils, scissors, surgical instruments, knitting needles, thimbles, and coins. Traces of nickel in detergents are probably not significant in the United States, although in some countries the nickel content may be high enough to cause dermatitis.

Clemensen et al. (15) studied the nickel content of water specimens from consecutive stages during the cleaning process in a Danish hospital. Statistically significant increases of the nickel concentrations were found from step to step of the cleaning, eventually exceeding the theoretical sensitizing safety limit. The dimethylglyoxime test indicates the presence of nickel.

Among hospital cleaners, rubber gloves are used widely. An investigation has shown that nickel penetrates rubber but not vinyl (16).

> **Nickel compounds can penetrate rubber but not vinyl gloves.**

Pompholyx of the Hands Due to "Ingestion" of Nickel (Positive Patch Test)

Allergic contact eczema and hand pompholyx may flare following ingestion of nickel in patients sensitized to this metal, according to several investigators (17–20). It has been reported that the oral administration of nickel in a double-blind test provoked an aggravation of hand eczema in 9 of 12 patients, and in 7 of the patients this was accompanied by secondary eruptions, including outbreaks of earlier, healed eczema.

Nickel excretion in urine in four female patients sensitive to nickel with an intermittent dyshidrotic eruption was measured with flameless atomic absorption. Excretion of nickel increased in association with outbreaks of vesicles. The results would support the idea that the chronic hand condition was maintained by ingestion of nickel in food.

> **Those patients able to reduce nickel intake by at least one-half have a chance of improving nickel hand eczema.**

Christensen (21), after studying female patients who had nickel allergy and hand eczema and who were reinvestigated 6 years after the primary investigation, found that 30% of the patients had healed. Patients who had the pompholyx-type eczema had the worst prognosis. Because the control of pompholyx in nickel-sensitive individuals with diet is difficult, a chelating agent such as disulfiram (Antabuse) has been employed.

Thus, Christensen and Kristensen (22) reported 11 patients who had nickel allergy and hand eczema of the pompholyx type who were treated with disulfiram (Antabuse) at 200 mg daily for 8 weeks. Two patients healed, and eight patients improved considerably. Mild relapses were observed in all patients within 2 to 16 weeks after discontinuation of treatment.

Fowler (23) showed that of nine patients with nickel allergy and hand eczema, eight improved while taking disulfiram 250 mg daily, and none improved and five worsened on placebo. The study was a double-blind, placebo-controlled-crossover evaluation. Some patients were maintained on periodic doses of disulfiram after the study period with continued good results.

Patients receiving disulfiram (Antabuse) must avoid drinking alcohol, and their liver enzymes should be monitored during such therapy. Before using disulfiram, a preliminary patch test with the "thiram mix" should be done to rule out sensitivity to this compound (24).

> **Dietary control of pompholyx with nickel sensitivity is difficult. Antabuse therapy to chelate nickel cannot be used in thiram-rubber-sensitive individuals.**

Potassium Dichromate

Aside from many industrial exposures, particularly cement, individuals sensitized to potassium dichromate may acquire dermatitis of the hands from leather gloves, shoes, and other leather objects. In addition, matches, bleaches, antirust compounds, varnishes, yellow paints, spackling compounds, and certain glues that contain dichromates may cause dermatitis of the hands in sensitized individuals (see Chapter 35).

Role of Dichromate Sensitivity in "Housewife's Eczema"

From Israel, Spain, and Yugoslavia have come reports that the dichromates play an important role in the production of "housewife's eczema" (25–28). In the United States, chromates have not been implicated in "housewife's eczema." Spot tests for chromates may be positive in American soaps and detergents, but the quantity is apparently not sufficient to produce dermatitis. Chromates are part of the earth's crust, and traces of chromates are present in practically all raw materials. Phosphate-containing soaps and detergents have a higher concentration of chromates than do those that are free of this chemical.

In Fisher's series of 50 women who had severe "housewife's eczema," only one showed a positive reaction to potassium dichromate.

Pompholyx from Chromate Ingestion

Cronin (29) reported that the experimental ingestion of 10 drops of a 0.001% solution of $K_2CR_2O_7$ equaling about 0.5 mg $K_2CR_2O_7$ daily for several days can produce vesicular eruption of the palms and flares of dermatitis in chromate-sensitive individuals. Schleif (30) also found that the ingestion of chromates can produce pompholyx-like eruptions and flares of chromate dermatitis in chromate-sensitive individuals. These authors speculated that chromium may be released by cooking acid or salty food in stainless-steel cooking utensils.

Kaaber and Veien (31) also reported that the dermatitis of 11 of 31 patients who had chronic chromate dermatitis was aggravated following the ingestion of an amount of chromate comparable to that found in a normal daily food intake, and that those patients who had pompholyx were the ones most affected by ingestion of chromates.

As Burrows (32) pointed out, however, most chromium is changed in the acid medium of the stomach to trivalent chrome, which is not absorbed. Also, in view of the small quantity of chromium that exists in the diet, apart from the avoidance of cloves, thyme, and pepper, it would be difficult to reduce intake much further. Dermatitis of the hands in professional gamblers and card players may be caused by exposure to chromium salts used for dying green felt or baize, which covers gambling tables (33).

> Reports from abroad implicate chromates in soaps and detergents as significant in the production of housewife's eczema and chromates in food in pompholyx. In the United States, chromates are not yet similarly implicated.

Prognosis of Hand Dermatitis Due to Chromates

Several investigators state that the prognosis is poor for workers who have hand dermatitis owing to exposure to chromates. The term "chrome cripples" has been applied to such workers (34,35).

Fregert (36), however, was more optimistic. He stated that cement chromium hand eczema is often chronic but not as severe as nickel hand eczema, although the change of work does not guarantee healing of the eczema. Fregert advised that chrome-sensitive men should work as carefully as possible and should avoid other chromium sources (e.g., matches). Many people are able to continue their jobs for years with proper topical treatment.

Prevention and Management of Cement Chromate Hand Dermatitis

Because one cannot depend on "hardening" or hyposensitization to occur, early diagnosis of chromate dermatitis and avoidance of chromates is imperative if prolonged disability is to be avoided. Once acquired, chromate dermatitis has a great tendency to become chronic.

The following prophylactic measures have been advocated: (a) Replace the chromates in circulatory water cooling systems with tannins and benzoates. (b) Reduce the sensitizing water-soluble chromates in portland cement by the addition of 0.2% ferrous sulfate. (c) Replace zinc chromate and lead chromate in primer paints and in rust-preventing agents used on iron sheets with molybdates. (d) Use only disposable towels; hand towels used by workers in the chromate industry, even after washing, contain enough chromate to give a positive "spot test" for chromium.

> The addition of ferrous sulfate to cement reduces the sensitizing chromates in cement.

Ethylenediamine Hydrochloride

A positive patch test to ethylenediamine hydrochloride in a patient who had hand dermatitis probably means that the patient was sensitized to this compound through the use of Mycolog Cream (Squibb) or generics. Such patients may need to avoid hydroxyzine and aminophylline. Mycolog II Cream is free of ethylenediamine (see Chapter 17). In addition, it must be remembered that certain epoxy amine hardeners cross-react with ethylenediamine hydrochloride. Such patients must also be patch tested with epoxy amine hardeners, particularly if they have handled epoxy resins.

Rudzki and Krajewska (37) reported that a consecutive series of 1,544 patients and 137 patients in occupational contact with epoxy resins were tested with ethylenediamine or triethylenetetramine; some were tested with diethylenetriamine. Guinea pigs sensitized to triethylenetetramine were tested with ethylenediamine and diethylenetriamine. The results showed that cross-reactions may occur between triethylenetetramine and ethylenediamine, although most patients were sensitized to only one of the compounds.

Rubber

Mercaptobenzothiazole and thiram (tetramethylthiuram disulfide) are the most common causes of allergic rubber dermatitis in the general population. Rubber finger cots, rubber gloves, rubber bands, rubber hoses, tubing, adhesive tape, and adhesive bandages cause allergic rubber dermatitis of the hands, which may also complicate other types of hand dermatoses.

Patients who have hand dermatitis often become sensitized to rubber gloves used to "protect" their hands. Dermatitis owing to rubber gloves should be suspected when a hand dermatitis stops abruptly at the wrists. Patch tests may be performed with a half-inch square cut from the rubber gloves, and those tests may be supplemented by testing with mercaptobenzothiazole and thiram.

> **Mercaptobenzothiazole and the thirams are the most common causes of allergic rubber dermatitis. Dermatitis of the hands from rubber gloves owing to thiram sensitivity will flare if disulfiram is given.**

Rubber may cause allergic contact dermatitis even when completely "cured." It appears that not all antioxidants and accelerators take part in the final crystallization of rubber and are released imperceptibly over many years. Release is enhanced by sweating and heat; this provides the opportunity for sensitization and may even cause occupational depigmentation.

More recently, rubber gloves have been found to cause urticaria, eczema, and even anaphylaxis due to allergy to natural latex proteins. Health care workers are at risk for these reactions. Testing for rubber accelerators is negative. Patch, prick, or scratch tests with latex rubber glove extracts are positive within 10 to 30 minutes (see Chapter 31).

Paraphenylenediamine

Dermatitis of the hands owing to allergic sensitization to paraphenylenediamine (PPDA) occurs mainly in hairdressers and furriers. Hair dyeing, however, may be done occasionally at home by nonprofessionals who may develop allergic contact dermatitis of the hands from the procedure. If the patient has a positive patch test reaction to PPDA and apparently has not handled the dye, patch tests should be performed with other "para-amino" compounds such as benzocaine, procaine, and para-aminobenzoic acid, with which PPDA may cross-react.

In addition, PPDA-sensitive individuals who handle certified azo dyes incorporated into foods, drugs, and cosmetics should be tested with such dyes, as cross-reactions may rarely occur. Allergic dermatitis of the hands from ballpoint pens containing azo dyes may occur in patients sensitized to PPDA.

> **Hairdressers and furriers frequently acquire hand dermatitis from sensitization to PPDA, which may cross-react with azo dyes, benzocaine, and PABA esters.**

Topical Preservatives

Hand eczema, whether it begins as ICD, ACD, or endogenous dermatitis, may become worse because of allergy to preservatives or other agents in topical medicaments and skin care products. The formaldehyde releasers, such as quaternium-15, imidazolidinyl urea, and diazolidynyl urea, are particularly common as causes of ACD. Other preservatives, fragrances, and vehicles may also be a problem in selected individuals. Any time a hand eczema seems to spread or worsen after using a topical product, all of the ingredients in that product must be held suspect as allergens until proven otherwise.

DERMATITIS OF THE HANDS DUE TO CONTACT WITH FOODS

Homemakers, chefs, bakers, and others who handle food may acquire contact dermatitis of the hands (38–40). Such contact dermatitis is of five varieties: (a) an irritant dermatitis, (b) a "delayed" allergic eczematous contact dermatitis, (c) an immediate urticarial type of dermatitis, (d) an immediate vesicular eruption, and (e) a phototoxic dermatitis.

Irritant Contact Dermatitis

The juices of many foods can produce a nonspecific irritant dermatitis of the hands that may be similar to dermatitis from any "wet" work. This type of irritant hand dermatitis is often accompanied by paronychia, particularly of the monilial variety. Irritant dermatitis owing to food is characterized usually by edema, erythema, and fissuring rather than vesiculation and severe pruritus, such as occurs in allergic contact dermatitis. At times, only patch tests will distinguish between the irritant and allergic dermatitis of the hands owing to food. Two recognized irritant hand dermatitides are due to corn and pineapple. Corn dermatitis (corn itch or corn poisoning) is an irritant, occupational eruption of the hands similar to the contact dermatitis seen in other vegetable processing and in wet work in food plants. Excoriations and secondary infections often complicate the dermatitis (41). Pineapple dermatitis is due to pineapple juice, which contains bromelain, a proteolytic enzyme that can readily produce an irritant dermatitis (42).

> **Irritant hand dermatitis can be caused by handling wet foods, fruit juices, corn, and pineapple.**

Allergic Eczematous Contact Dermatitis from Foods

In sensitized individuals, contact with certain foods may produce a classic "delayed" allergic contact dermatitis with a positive patch test reaction. This type of reaction is seen most often with the oleoresins of fruits and vegetables or with spices such as cinnamon. Orange and lemon peel contain oil of limonene and other sensitizing terpenes that may cross-react with turpentine. Limonene is found not only in lemons and oranges, but also in dill, caraway oil, and celery

TABLE 18.2. *Vegetables: "Delayed" Eczematous Dermatitis*

Positive Patch Test

Artichoke	Cucumber
Asparagus	Endive
Carrot	Garlic
Celery	Horseradish
Chicory	Leek
Chives	Lettuce
Corn	Onion

seed oil. In addition, the peel of lime may produce not only allergic contact dermatitis but also photodermatitis.

Patch tests for citrus peel contact sensitivity may be done with either 1% oil of limonene in alcohol or orange, lemon, and lime peel, as is. Should positive reactions be obtained, the test should be performed on three normal controls, because occasionally the oil of these citrus peels may be irritants. In addition, the peel of limes should be tested by both closed and open methods with exposure to sunlight, because certain limes are photosensitizers.

The mango can produce allergic contact dermatitis owing to the oleoresin present in the mango tree sap or the skin of the fruit, which cross-reacts with poison ivy oleoresin.

Limonene is a sensitizing terpene in lemons, oranges, and dill and in oils of caraway and celery. Mango cross-reacts with poison ivy. Limes may be photosensitizers.

Allergic eczematous contact dermatitis from vegetables (see Table 18.2) may be due to the essential oils of edible vegetables including carrots, parsnips, parsley, and celery. Pinene, terpineol, and eucalyptol are probably the actual sensitizers. In addition, onions and garlic may cause a contact dermatitis that may show cross-reactions with tulips and hyacinths.

If prepared oleoresins of vegetables are not available, patch tests may be performed with the fresh vegetables and the results compared with three controls.

Celery, parsnips, and parsley may produce a phototoxic reaction in the presence of moisture and sunlight. Patch tests with celery, parsnip, and parsley should be performed with the vegetable moistened with water and exposed to sunlight or artificial ultraviolet radiation to "prove" phytophoto dermatitis.

Mustard oil (allyl isothiocyanate) is an irritant and a sensitizing chemical found in horseradish, cabbage, broccoli, and brussels sprouts (43).

Celery, parsnips, and parsley are photosensitizing vegetables that may cause phytophoto dermatitis.

TABLE 18.3. *Spices: "Delayed" Eczematous Dermatitis*

Positive Patch Test

Capsicum	Laurel
Cayenne pepper	Mace
Cinnamon	Nutmeg
Cloves	Vanilla

Allergic dermatitis owing to spices (see Table 18.3) occurs in the United States, principally from five spices: capsicum, cinnamon, cloves, nutmeg, and vanilla (44). Blends of mace and nutmeg are used extensively for flavoring foods. Bakers in particular may acquire allergic dermatitis of the hands from handling these spices. Oil of cloves is rich in eugenol, which may be a sensitizer, and is used widely as an ingredient in perfumes, soaps, toothpastes, and mouthwashes.

Dermatitis due to vanilla occurs in individuals employed in the cultivation, trade, or industrial use of vanilla. Vanillism, an allergic contact dermatitis acquired by workers who handle the vanilla plant, produces marked edema and erythema. Rhinitis, asthma, and vertigo may accompany the eruption.

Spencer and Fowler (45) reported a case of hand eczema in a Girl Scout cookie maker due to vanilla.

Nethercott and Holness (40) studied 20 bakers and food service workers in Toronto. Half were felt to have ICD and half ACD. Rubber allergens and fragrance/flavorings such as cinnamic aldehyde and balsam of Peru were most common. Contact urticaria due to shellfish was present in one patient.

Food flavors and spices may produce allergic contact dermatitis in bakers, food handlers, and homemakers.

Sinha et al. (46) studied 53 patients who had a fissured contact dermatitis on the fingertips and who showed positive patch tests to several vegetables, the most common being garlic, onion, tomato, and carrot, in that order of frequency. Of several preparations (made from garlic, onion, tomato, and carrot), the juices used as such gave the maximum number of positive patch test reactions.

Immediate Contact Urticaria of the Hands from Foods

Foods that can cause contact urticaria with resulting hand dermatitis are listed in Table 18.4 (47–52) (see also Chapter 34). Sensitivity to potatoes may be so severe that a wheal may form merely by rubbing the unabraded skin with a raw potato. More often, a strongly positive scratch test reaction to the raw potato consisting of a large wheal and flare is obtained. No reaction occurs in controls. Scratch tests with cooked potatoes usually produce negative results. Potato

TABLE 18.4. *Foods Producing Immediate Urticaria*

Seafood	Fruits
Codfish	Apples
Lobster	Kiwi fruit
Prawns	Peaches
Shrimp	Strawberry
Vegetables	Miscellaneous foods
Bean	Beer
Carrot	Cheese
Lettuce	Egg
Onion	Flour
Parsley	Milk
Parsnip	Mayonnaise (sorbic acid)
Potato	
Rice	
Tomato	
Meat	
Beef	
Calves' liver	
Lamb	
Pork	
Turkey meat	
Turkey skin	

TABLE 18.5. *Foods Causing Immediate Vesicular Eruptions When Applied to Damaged Skin*

Chicory	Lettuce
Endive	Tomato

tomato, and onion revealed positive reactions in patients who had various disorders. These patients had itching and tingling sensations with or without edema of the lips, mouth, and tongue after eating raw fruits and vegetables. In addition, laryngeal and abdominal disturbances, rhinitis, and hand dermatitis were recorded.

Allergic contact urticaria may be caused by many foods. A scratch test on normal skin or on eczematous skin is usually required to produce the urticarial reaction.

---

sensitivity can cause "housewife's" hand eczema and can be classified as an "occupational" allergy.

Sensitized patients also may show positive scratch test results to uncooked fish, shellfish, shrimp, and cheese. Allergic hand dermatitis of the "immediate" variety can be produced by handling these foods, probably because of some proteinaceous substance, particularly in those persons with damaged skin due to an irritant or an allergic contact dermatitis from other causes.

It should be stressed that in these cases of "immediate" food contact dermatitis, the patch tests are negative and therefore scratch tests may be necessary to prove the cause of this variety of contact food dermatitis.

Maibach (51) stressed that the handling of certain foods can produce a burning and stinging sensation in the chronically eczematous skin but not in otherwise normal skin and that tests on intact skin may be negative. Scratch tests with certain foods produced positive results only on intact skin. Intradermal tests with commercial antigens were negative.

When performing scratch tests with whole foods, at least three control subjects also should be tested. A positive reaction in the patient that is not duplicated in the controls makes it likely that the reaction is allergic. At present, it appears that patients who have allergic contact hand dermatitis owing to food handling can eat such foods without experiencing a flare of the dermatitis. It is most likely that either cooking the foods or the action of digestive juices renders the foods hypoallergenic for these patients.

At present, it is not clear whether the food antigens that allergists use in testing for allergic rhinitis, asthma, and gastrointestinal allergy are also the antigens responsible for the immediate allergic contact dermatitis of the hand from handling certain foods (51). Hannuksela and Lahti (52) found that scratch tests with apple, carrot, parsnip, parsley, potato,

Immediate Vesicular Hand Dermatitis

Lettuce, endive, and tomatoes may produce immediate, vesicular, and intensively pruritic eruptions within a few minutes of contact with these vegetables in previously sensitized skin (see Table 18.5). Sometimes a combined urticarial and vesicular eruption arises as a reaction to these vegetables (53). A prerequisite, then, for the appearance of the immediate, vesicular reaction observed in some cases seems to be that the allergen may come into contact with previously damaged skin, even if the skin appears normal to the naked eye.

Parsnip, parsley, and limes are capable of producing phototoxic reactions. They can be tested with ultraviolet light or sunlight (54).

Lettuce, endive, tomatoes, and chicory can produce "immediate" vesicular hand dermatitis.

DERMATITIS OF THE HANDS DUE TO FOOD ADDITIVES

Table 18.6 lists the preservatives added to foods, and Table 18.7 lists miscellaneous food additives and their uses (see also Chapter 30). Other food additives, aside from the

TABLE 18.6. *Preservatives Added to Foods*

Benzoic acid	Polysorbate
Calcium propionate	Quaiac gum
Citric acid	Sodium benzoate
Monoglycerol citrate	Sodium bisulfite
Parabens	Sorbic acid

TABLE 18.7. *Miscellaneous Food Additives and Their Uses*

Additive	Use
Calcium disodium EDTA	Stabilizer—chelating agent
Chlorophyll	Color for pastry
Dyes, certified	Coloring agents
Gum arabic (acacia)	Cream and cheese additive
Karaya	Pastry filler
Lanolin	Chewing gum additive
Propylene glycol aginate	Filler—many salad dressings
Sodium silicon aluminate	Lump preventor in cake mix
Tragacanth	Vegetable gum filler

preservatives, include antioxidants, dyes, flavoring agents, "spoilage retarders," "dough conditioners," "flavor protectors," and "cloudiness preventatives." Some of these chemicals, which may produce contact dermatitis of the hands in certain sensitized individuals, particularly homemakers, food handlers, bakers, and cooks, are often the same agents that have proved to be sensitizers in topical medications and cosmetics (55,56).

Antioxidants in Foods

One of the most common types of food spoilage is an undesirable change in color or flavor caused by oxygen in the air. Thus, sliced, fresh apples and peaches turn brown when exposed to air for any length of time, and foods such as mayonnaise and lard turn rancid and become inedible if kept unprotected too long. Both of these conditions are caused by oxidation and can be retarded by using antioxidants.

The darkening of some fruits and vegetables is a type of oxidation known as "enzymatic browning." If foods containing certain enzymes are cut or bruised or are overmature and exposed to air, the tissues darken and turn brown. Apples, apricots, bananas, cherries, peaches, pears, and potatoes contain such enzymes. Antioxidants prevent or delay this enzymatic browning. Table 18.8 lists the antioxidants that are used in foods.

Oxidation can also cause the rancid taste and odor that sometimes develop in fats, oil, mayonnaise, and lard. Accordingly, processed foods that contain these fatty materials

TABLE 18.8. *Antioxidant Food Additives*

Ammonium persulfate (flour color improver—some European countries)
Benzoyl peroxide (flour color "improver")
Butylated hydroxyanisole
Butylated hydroxytoluene
Dodecyl gallate
Gum benzoin
Lauryl and propyl gallate
Sodium bisulfite
Vitamin E (tocopherols)

must be protected from possible oxidation in order to maintain their best flavor during storage.

> A host of food additives, including preservatives, antioxidants, waxes, gums, and dyes, may produce hand dermatitis.

At present, such antioxidants as butylated hydroxyanisole (BHA) and butylated hydroxytoluene (BHT) are largely replacing gum benzoin. These antioxidants, which may also be present in cosmetics, may be tested 2% in petrolatum.

Butylated Hydroxyanisole

This antioxidant is used in many products, including beverages, chewing gum, ice cream, candy, baked goods, gelatin, desserts, soup bases, potatoes, glacéed fruits, potato flakes, sweet potato flakes, dry breakfast cereals, dry yeast, dry mixes for desserts and beverages, lard, shortening, and unsmoked dry sausage, and in emulsions for stabilizers for shortenings. Roed-Petersen and Hjorth (57) reported that in two patients who had allergic dermatitis owing to BHA or BHT, acute flares of vesicular dermatitis on the fingers appeared after the experimental oral administration of these antioxidants.

Butylated Hydroxytoluene

This antioxidant has uses similar to those of BHA.

Sodium Bisulfite in Salads

Epstein (58) described hand eczema in a salad maker owing to "Veg-White," an antioxidant used to prevent discoloration of fruit and vegetables used in salads. The specific sensitizer in this preparation was sodium bisulfite. Patch tests can be performed with a 10% aqueous solution of sodium bisulfite. Sulfites in foods can also cause immediate anaphylactic reactions in very sensitive individuals.

Lauryl Gallate

Brun (59) reported contact dermatitis in a baker from lauryl gallate added to margarine as an antioxidant.

Propyl Gallate

Liden (60) reported a patient who had allergic hypersensitivity from this preservative in Alphosyl and pointed out that bakers are also exposed to this antioxidant, which is chemically closely related to the parabens.

Potassium and Ammonium Persulfate

These have been used as boosters with hydrogen peroxide to produce "platinum bleached" hair. When they have been used in the past in certain European countries as flour "improvers" to render flour whiter, they have caused dermatitis of the hands in bakers (61).

Benzoyl Peroxide

This is used as an antiacne agent and for the treatment of stasis ulcers. It is also used occasionally as a "flour improver" and can cause hand dermatitis in bakers (62).

Waxes and Gums Added to Foods

These agents include some known skin sensitizers, namely, guaiac, guar, karaya, acacia (gum arabic), tragacanth, benzoin spermaceti, carnauba, and beeswax (the last four being used for glazing confectionery). Acacia (gum arabic) is permitted in chocolate drinks, creams, French dressing, malt liquors, milk, mustard, pickles, cheese, ice cream, and sherbet. Guaiac gum is used as a preservative for fats and oils, and guar gum is used in milk products. Guar gum is also used as a stabilizer; as a thickening and film-forming agent for cheese, salad dressings, ice cream, and soups; and as a binding and disintegrating agent in tablet formulations, suspensions, emulsions, lotions, creams, and toothpastes. Some of these waxes and gums cross-react with balsam of Peru.

Colors Added to Foods

Several "natural" approved colors can be added to foods. In addition, ten synthetic organic dyes are permitted. Citrus Red 2 and Sunset Yellow have formulas that indicate possible cross-reactions with paraphenylenediamine and sulfanilamide.

Spices and Flavoring Agents

Many spices and flavoring agents have been implicated in the production of contact dermatitis owing to foods. These flavoring agents include oil of almond, anise seed, bergamot, capsicum, chamomile, caraway, cinnamon, clove, coconut, ginger, laurel, mace, menthol, minonene, mustard, nutmeg, palm, peppermint, and sesame (63,64).

Potato Chip Dermatitis

Inman (65) traced three cases of contact dermatitis occurring in a potato chip factory that were due, respectively, to cheese powder, wheat filler, and onion powder.

TABLE 18.9. *Metals in Foods**

Aluminum
Chromium
Cobalt
Nickel (may also be added to hydrogenated fats)

*Ethylenediamine tetra-acetate is often added to chelate these metals.

Metals in Foods

Most foods contain traces of various metals, including nickel and chromium. Ethylenediamine tetra-acetate (EDTA) is added to many foods to chelate such metals. It must be emphasized that EDTA is not a sensitizer and does not cross-react with ethylenediamine hydrochloride, which is a notorious sensitizer.

It is interesting to note that the addition of nickel is permitted as a catalyst for hydrogenated fats and that aluminum sulfate may be added to canned fish, pickles, relishes, and starch. Table 18.9 lists metals that may be present in food.

> **EDTA, which is added to many foods to chelate metallic traces, is not a sensitizer and does not cross-react with ethylenediamine hydrochloride.**

Sulfates in Foods

Sodium lauryl sulfate is permitted in egg whites. Sodium sulfate can be added to biscuits, and sodium thiosulfate can be added to table salt (see Table 18.10).

"HOUSEWIFE'S ECZEMA"

"Housewife's eczema" is probably the most common type of contact dermatitis of the hands encountered in clinical practice. This type of eruption occurs principally on the fingers and the webs and dorsa of the hands of women who do house and laundry work that entails more or less regular exposure to soaps, detergents, and other household cleansers. "Housewife's eczema," however, may affect not only homemakers but also those whose profession or other activities involve excessive exposure to soaps and detergents. Included in this group are surgeons, medical personnel, dentists, bartenders, dishwashers, kitchen workers, canners, and individuals employed in those occupations necessitating frequent washing and immersion of the hands in various

TABLE 18.10. *Sulfates in Foods*

Sodium bisulfite (biscuits)
Sodium lauryl sulfate (egg white)
Sodium thiosulfate (table salt)

detergent solutions. The eruption of "housewife's eczema" begins usually with mild dryness, redness, and scaling. As the condition becomes more severe under continued exposure to soap and water, fissuring, crusting, and eventually chronic eczema are produced (66,67).

Hand eczema often begins in cold weather with "chapping" of the hands. A young mother's hands remain frequently in fairly good condition until 3 to 6 months after childbirth. At this time, the increased exposure of the hands to soaps and water in the bathing and care of the infant causes a "breakdown" of the skin. Such eczema may be intensified by any one of many common household irritants such as bleaches, waxes, polishes, and turpentine. The patient not infrequently excoriates the itchy skin, causing secondary infection and lichenifications. Atopic individuals are particularly prone to develop "housewife's eczema" (68,69).

"Housewife's eczema" is an irritant dermatitis that may occur in any individual who is exposed frequently to soaps, detergents, and antiseptics.

Hand Eczema Patterns

Cronin (70) performed an exhaustive study of hand eczema patterns in 263 women. She found that 44% had primary palmar involvement, 15% dorsal, 19% fingers only, and 22% generalized hand eczema. Of those with palmar involvement, only 42% had ICD, whereas 75% of dorsal eczema patients had significant contact with irritants. Those with dorsal or finger involvement were more often atopic than those with palmar predominance. Nickel was the most significant allergen, with about 30% of the women positive. Fragrances and rubber allergens were also common.

ROLE OF RINGS IN HAND DERMATITIS

Allergic reactions to nickel-plated rings may occur in nickel-sensitive individuals. Gold and palladium occasionally cause allergy. Platinum and silver almost never cause ACD. The dermatitis under a ring may be produced in several ways:

1. Soaps, detergents, waxes, polishes, or even cosmetic creams may accumulate under the ring and may cause a primary, irritant type of dermatitis. Therefore, whenever possible, rings should be removed when washing the hands with soaps or exposing them to detergents. Rings must be cleaned at regular intervals to remove such accumulated material.

2. Certain rings, especially alloys of copper and silver, can corrode readily on the skin and form a primary irritant in the presence of an adequate concentration of salt.

3. Industrial smog contains fumes thick with sulfides from the burning of low-grade, sulfur-laden coal and fuel oil, or other corrosive metals such as phosphates. These air pollutants can attack gold alloys directly, even when jewelry is not being worn. When a tarnished ring slips back on the finger, or a bracelet onto the arm, the thin film of tarnish rubs off in a black smudge and may irritate the skin.

4. Simon and Harly (71) reported that radiodermatitis of the fingers is produced by gold rings contaminated with gold seeds containing decayed radon. Leone (72) found that a radioactive gold ring made from improperly salvaged gold radon seeds caused a long-standing radiodermatitis.

Thus, hand eczema begins frequently under a ring. In many instances, when a dermatitis begins on a left fourth finger, the patient changes the ring to the right side and so produces a dermatitis on both hands. If a dermatitis owing to rings is not treated properly, the eruption may spread from the finger onto the hand and to other fingers. The irritated skin produced by a recurring ring dermatitis is subject to secondary infection and sensitization to other chemicals (73).

Removal of a Ring from a Swollen Finger

It is not uncommon for a finger to become swollen suddenly from a contusion, an edematous dermatosis, or some other transient cause.

Leider (74) has described in detail how to remove a ring from a swollen finger without injuring the ring. The procedure is as follows: Lubricate the finger with an oil or petrolatum. Take a longish piece of soft string of moderate caliber and good strength and start winding it from the beginning of the first interphalangeal joint up to the ring, being careful to make every turn comfortably snug and touching close to the preceding one. Such winding progressively reduces the bulk of the tissue and drives edema toward, under, and beyond the ring. When the ring is reached by as many successive turns as it takes to encase completely the swollen digit to that point, feed the advancing end of the string under the ring and beyond it with a slender blunt instrument, such as one prong of a tweezer. This can always be done; there is always enough space to accommodate the girth of a string of loose enough and compressible enough cotton. When the maneuver is accomplished to the point at which the ring is caught by the string (now passed under and beyond it and made taut), start to unwind the turns of the string off the finger gently and slowly, all the while keeping the string taut and almost perpendicular to the finger.

In most cases, the ring will move forward gradually with every unwind, as it is caught by the string which is always behind it. As soon as the second interphalangeal joint is passed, the job is largely done and the ring readily slips off the rest of the finger to the great relief of the patient and the operator. This procedure works almost every time, in all but the most severely swollen fingers. In average cases, the amount of discomfort is moderate and is almost always endurable.

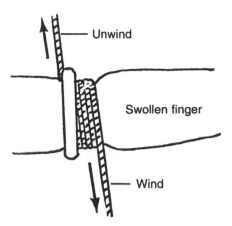

FIG. 18.1. Removal of ring from swollen finger. From Exner FB. *JAMA* 1969;210:558.

> **Hand eczema often begins under a ring, which traps and concentrates irritants.**

Several precautions must be observed: (a) If the finger is swollen from pyogenic infection, has a cut, or is badly abraded, the procedures should not be done. (b) If the unwinding is done roughly or too rapidly, the skin may be too severely crushed, lacerated, or abraded by the moving ring and string as it is unwound. Some slight damage may be done to the epidermis even when this procedure is done gently and slowly, but it is of no great consequence. Such skinning heals readily. (c) If the ring has an impediment such as an expander or a massive setting in the form of a large, bezeled stone or other raised, broad ornament in its position on the dorsal surface of the finger, the string must be depressed parallel to the finger every time the setting is reached and until it is passed each time. The maneuver is gratifyingly successful if it is done skillfully. The string removes the ring as it unwinds, and the patient's praises ring in the operator's ear.

Exner (75) has also removed rings successfully from swollen fingers. Figure 18.1 illustrates the method of removal.

DIFFERENTIAL DIAGNOSIS OF CONTACT DERMATITIS OF THE HANDS

Dermatitides of the hands from entirely different causes may resemble each other so closely that the cause of the dermatitis can often be discerned only after prolonged observation and special diagnostic tests. Thus, allergic and irritant contact dermatitis of the hands may be difficult to distinguish from atopic eczema, tinea infections, psoriasis, nummular eczema, a blistering eruption called pompholyx (dyshidrotic eczema), or a pustular eruption called pustular bacterid or pustular psoriasis (see Table 18.11).

The original condition of the hand dermatitis often becomes changed radically by secondary infection or by a superimposed contact dermatitis resulting from reactions to topical medications and irritating soaps and detergents.

A listing by the physician of all previously used medications, hand creams, and lotions is necessary to evaluate the role of these preparations in alleviating or exacerbating the dermatitis. A detailed history of contactants encountered not only in the workplace but also in various hobbies is important.

Examination of the Patient

Always examine the patient's feet. The patient often protests such a procedure, saying, "I don't have anything on my feet." The physician who believes such a statement is often misled, because the patient may not realize that thickening and yellowish discoloration of the toenails or slight scaling of the soles may mean that he or she has psoriasis or a fungus infection that also affects the hands. Scaling between the toes may indicate an active fungal infection that can cause tiny blisters on the palms, which, in turn, can become "eczematized" and can result in a full-blown hand dermatitis.

> **No study of hand dermatitis is complete unless the feet are also examined.**

TABLE 18.11. *Differential Diagnosis of Contact Dermatitis of Hands*

Dermatophytosis
  KOH, culture
  Examine finger—toenails, soles, and interweb areas
  Rule out dermatophytid of hands (trichophyton test)
Psoriasis
  Examine nails, elbows, knees, scalp, and intergluteal area
Pustular psoriasis
  In psoriatic, discrete pustules in normal or in eczematized skin
Dyshidrosis
Discrete vesicles on sides of fingers, palms, and soles
Atopic dermatitis
  History of asthma, allergic rhinitis, infantile eczema, or presence of eczema—popliteal, antecubital, dorsal aspect of toes and nuchal areas
Pustular bacterid
  Leukocytosis 12,000–19,000 may respond to oral antibiotics focus of infection
Nummular eczema
  Discrete discoid (coin-shaped) lesions on back of hand
Chronic acral dermatitis[79]
  A pruritic, papulovesicular, and keratotic dermatitis of the hands, feet, and extremities had marked elevated serum IgE levels up to 100,000 ng/mL

Examine the soles and heels for blisters or pustules. The presence of a vesicular or pustular eruption on the feet often means that the eruption of the hands is not a "simple" contact dermatitis. Thus, many patients are being treated for contact dermatitis from external or occupational causes when, in reality, they have pompholyx, pustular bacterid, pustular psoriasis, or nummular eczema, which are of endogenic origin (76,77).

Examine the patient's knees, elbows, scalp, and intergluteal area for the dry, scaly evidence of psoriasis. Particularly in dentists and surgeons, psoriasis frequently may localize on the hands because of trauma and may be mistaken for an occupational contact dermatitis (Koebner's phenomenon).

Find out if the patient is atopic. Does the patient have asthma or allergic rhinitis? Does he or she remember having eczema as a child? Examine the antecubital and popliteal areas and the back of the neck for evidence of atopic eczema. Atopic eczema of the hands is often localized on the dorsal surfaces of the joints. Irritants and housework often cause the dermatitis to localize on the hands in an individual who has an atopic constitution.

Examine the dorsal aspect of the extremities for the coin-shaped lesions of nummular eczema, particularly if the hand dermatitis is predominantly on the dorsal aspect. Nummular eczema of unknown origin is often confused with contact dermatitis.

Chronic paronychia, particularly of the monilial variety, is usually evidence that the hands are wet much of the time. Paronychia may be due occasionally to wax, hair, bristles, threads, and scales that enter the paronychial tissues as foreign bodies.

Abnormalities of the nails should be noted, particularly for evidence of fungal infections and psoriasis. The role of such dermatoses in hand dermatitis must be evaluated. Subungual hemorrhages may be caused by excessive exposure to a combination of water, detergents, and trauma, as in the case of professional dishwashers.

Study the distribution of the eruption. A recurrent, pruritic, vesicular eruption on the palms and sides of the fingers that is symmetrical and bilateral will more probably be pompholyx (dyshidrotic eczema) than will one caused by external contactants. The cause of pompholyx is unknown, but in some nickel-sensitive individuals the ingestion of nickel in foods has been implicated as a cause of the eruption. Rarely, penicillin will produce a symmetrical, vesicular eruption of the hands resembling pompholyx.

Examine the eruption for discrete pustules of varying sizes. In the absence of any crusting or itching, such an eruption will most probably be a so-called pustular psoriasis or bacterid rather than an instance of infected contact dermatitis. The etiology of such eruptions is obscure. Some cases respond to antibiotic therapy and removal of foci of infection or to intralesional injection of corticosteroids.

Keratoderma climactericum is a disorder of the palms and soles occurring in menopausal women. The disorder is characterized by discrete oval patches of mild keratoderma. The lesions progress slowly to reach a size and shape that remain almost unchanged in appearance for a long time. The hyperkeratosis is generally quite mild. Vesiculation is not a feature. Both palms and soles may be involved, but usually only the palms are affected. The lesions improve ultimately but are generally unresponsive to therapy.

These dermatoses, which must be distinguished from contact dermatitis, are often complicated by a superimposed, irritant contact dermatitis resulting from the use of soaps, detergents, or chemicals encountered in various occupations. A superimposed allergic contact dermatitis resulting from the use of topical medications or occupational sensitizers is not uncommon. It is, therefore, necessary to find out what medication the patient has used in the past that seemed to make the hand dermatitis worse. In addition, find out the patient's occupation and whether he or she is handling irritants or allergens. The role of irritants is obtained by taking a careful history. The role of allergens is proved by patch tests.

Hand dermatitis often becomes secondarily infected. Sensitization to bacteria may produce an infectious, eczematoid dermatitis with dissemination to the forearms and more distant areas.

Chronic Acral Dermatitis with High IgE

Some patients who have a pruritic, papulovesicular dermatitis of the hands, feet, and extremities have sharply elevated IgE serum levels of up to 100,000 ng/mL. There is no personal or family history of atopic disease. A variety of immunologic, physiologic, and pharmacologic studies of the skin have normal results. The course of this unique dermatitis is chronic, lasting many years, and it is resistant to all treatments except the administration of systemic corticosteroid drugs. Winkelmann and Gleich (78) have labeled this condition "chronic acral dermatitis."

ROLE OF SOAPS AND DETERGENTS IN HAND DERMATITIS

The role of soaps and detergents in hand eczema is controversial. Wechsler (67) suggested that the term "detergent hands" is a misnomer because of the limited role of soaps and detergents as irritants. Indeed, Suskind (79) found that immersion of hands in solutions of soaps or synthetic detergents in the concentrations recommended by the suppliers actually improves hand dermatitis.

Kligman and Wooding (80) pointed out that hand eczema in homemakers was once attributed to soap, but since World War II, synthetic detergents have been incriminated. Their introduction, however, has not led to any notable increase in "housewife's eczema," and widespread use of dishwashers and washing machines over the last ten years has not led to any conspicuous decline.

All investigative methods distinguish between detergents causing a low and high degree of irritancy. The results, however, show unexplained discrepancies, which suggest that detergents are by no means homogeneous and that the damage may be produced by different mechanisms.

Wood and Bettley (81), who studied the denaturing action of detergents upon keratin and irritancy in human skin, also found considerable differences among detergents. Glickman and Silvers (82) found that 82% of patients who have hand eczema have a history of atopy.

Although it is not certain that soaps and detergents play a major role in hand eczema, contact with them should be minimized, especially in atopic persons.

The incidence of "housewife's eczema," "dishpan hands," and "detergent hands" is low compared to the number of people exposed. Cleaning personnel, launderers, dishwashers, and others who earn their living by having their hands immersed in solutions of these detergents, however, do frequently develop dermatitis. In many instances, the inflamed skin does not tolerate soap and detergents well, and contact with these compounds should be avoided, at least until the acute phase has subsided.

Under appropriate circumstances, excessive exposure to water, soap, and detergents leads to changes in the skin. The amount of damage depends on traumatic and environmental influences, such as cold weather, low humidity, impairment in alkali neutralization capacity, emotional stress, hyperhidrosis, exposure to other contactants (e.g., vegetables, fruits, meat juices, and other foods), and contact with cleansing and polishing products containing bleaches, abrasives, alkalis, and solvents.

Soaps and detergents probably damage skin by the following mechanisms:

1. Alkali-induced damage of the keratin layer of the epidermis that increases the permeability of the horny layer
2. Irritative effects of certain fatty acids
3. Removal of lipids and the protective mantle of the skin and prevention of reestablishment of the mantle and its normal acidity
4. Alteration of the buffering capacity of the skin
5. Removal of amino acids with damage to the water-holding capacity of the horny layer; this is particularly likely with synthetic detergents

Often irritation by soaps and detergents is heightened by concentration of the detergent solution on the skin, such as when cleansers become trapped under rings or when, during dishwashing, dishes are held tightly for a period of time in the detergent-moistened hand. Soaps for fine fabrics are probably the least irritating of the detergent cleansers.

Builders

Practically all laundry soaps contain additives, such as sodium carbonate, sodium phosphate, ash, borax, or sodium silicate, that may irritate but not sensitize.

Abrasive Agents

Many powdered, industrial hand cleansers have ingredients to increase the mechanical, cleansing action. The inorganic scrubbers include pumice, talc, sand, and borax; the organic agents include ground nut shells, cornmeal, and wood flours. These agents are effective in removing heavy oil, greases, tar, and other stubborn dirt from the hands, but the inorganic variety is particularly rough on the skin.

Patch Testing with Soaps and Detergents

Patch testing with soaps and detergents is performed usually with a 1% to 2% aqueous solution. The test site occasionally becomes slightly red, desquamates, wrinkles, or appears glazed. These reactions are not indicative of allergic sensitization but are merely owing to the irritant effect of soap or detergent solutions under the covered patch. Patch test reactions with these agents should always be checked on at least three control subjects.

The irritant reactions under a covered patch may interfere with the interpretation of allergic reactions. Whenever possible, therefore, patch tests should be performed with the suspected ingredients. Occasionally, however, photosensitivity reactions owing to antiseptics in soaps are clear, even when the testing is done with soap solutions.

The alkalis and fatty acids of soaps are rare sensitizers. Any white, unscented soap that is free of antiseptics, other medication, or lanolin is hypoallergenic, and patch testing except for investigative purposes is usually unrewarding. Similarly, the synthetic detergents without additives are rarely sensitizing and do not usually yield patch test results of clinical significance.

Numerous methods have been devised for testing new soaps and detergents before they are introduced for general use. Such testing may be of value in detecting unusual, irritant qualities of new products.

The following additives to soaps may be allergens:

1. Lanolin
2. Perfumes
3. Rosin
4. Antiseptics
5. Deodorants
6. Vitamin E
7. Antiperspirants
8. Turpentine (special industry soap)
9. Dyes
10. Surfactants and emulsifiers (rarely)

Rosin (Colophony)

Yellow (soft) laundry bars owe their properties to the presence of rosin, which is the solid resin residue remaining after the distillation of spirits of turpentine derived from the crude oleoresin of certain species of pine. Rosin consists of a mixture of complex abietic acids and esters. It makes laundry bars more soluble and hastens sudsing in cool water. Some toilet soaps also contain a small percentage of this agent.

Perfumes

It should be noted that some soaps, which are labeled "contains no perfume," may contain small amounts of "masking" perfumes to disguise the odor of certain fats. The concentration of such perfumes is not usually a hazard for perfume-sensitive patients.

Some soaps labeled "contains no perfume" or "unscented" may contain a fragrance to "mask" the odor of fatty ingredients.

Enzymes in Detergents

Currently 70% to 75% of laundry detergents sold in the United States contain enzymes. Depending on the brand and type, these products contain as much as 0.1% active enzymes, which are prepared by fermentation with the widely distributed nonpathogenic soil organism *Bacillus subtilis*.

The Food and Drug Administration made public a study in which the average enzyme detergent laundry product in normal use by consumers did not produce more primary irritation of the skin than did similar products containing no enzymes (83). Ducksbury and Dave (84), however, reported that 12 women in the home-help service in Nottingham developed an irritant dermatitis after using enzyme detergents. A survey based on a questionnaire showed an incidence of 5% among people using these products. Onychia may result from their use.

Allergic Reactions to Enzyme Detergents

Exposure to the concentrated enzyme in industry has caused dermatitis, allergic rhinitis, and asthma (85).

Belin et al. (86) stated that sensitization to enzyme detergents can also occur in consumers of enzyme-containing detergents and in every situation in which these enzymes are dust particles. These investigators obtained positive scratch tests in sensitized patients.

Patch test can be done with a 0.25% aqueous solution of the commercial product. The "pure subtilisms" can be patch tested with a 0.1% solution in water.

Enzymes in detergents may rarely cause irritation and sensitization.

BARRIER CREAMS FOR PREVENTION OF HAND ECZEMA

In general, barrier creams have not been proven to be helpful in combating hand eczema. Perhaps this is because the very factors that aggravate hand eczema (friction, solvent and detergent exposure, wet work, etc.) also serve to remove the barrier cream from the skin.

In a study of four "barrier creams," Loden (87) found that three had no effect on absorption of formaldehyde, whereas the other reduced absorption by about 40% only. None had any blocking effect on the solvent benzene.

Some barrier creams may in fact aggravate skin irritation. Frosch et al. (88,89) found that two barrier creams actually increased irritancy from sodium hydroxide in guinea pigs. One other cream did, however, suppress irritation from sodium lauryl sulfate and toluene. These guinea pig studies, of course, cannot duplicate the aggravating factors of actual job performance, so results in actual use would likely be much poorer.

Boman and Mellstrom (90) also found that several barrier creams were of no use in blocking organic solvent absorption in guinea pigs.

The exception to this may be in the use of a barrier cream for prevention of urushiol dermatitis from poison ivy, oak, and sumac. Epstein (91) showed that an organoclay compound may be helpful, and Orchard et al. (92) also found a linoleic acid containing preparation was efficacious. Smith (93), however, found no benefit from a popularly marketed poison ivy shielding preparation.

ROLE OF GLOVES IN THE MANAGEMENT OF HAND DERMATITIS

There are several types of gloves available for hand protection. Those used most commonly are either natural latex rubber or synthetic rubber. Vinyl gloves are available for both home and occupational use. The 4-H glove is a polyethylene laminate glove with good barrier properties for organic chemicals and others. A new plastic polymer glove, Tactyl-1, is available for medical use. It contains no latex or rubber accelerators.

Latex rubber gloves are most commonly used in health care settings because they are inexpensive and easily distensible, allowing for maximum comfort. However, individuals may become sensitive to latex or to the various additives used in glove manufacture, especially when gloves are worn over already dermatitic skin. Vinyl gloves are available for both home and medical use. Vinyl gloves are by nature hypoallergenic, because no rubber accelerators or latex are present. However, vinyl gloves do not fit closely and, therefore, are not good in settings where fine touch is important. This is not so much of a problem for household use. One benefit of vinyl gloves is that they are somewhat more protective than latex gloves for certain allergens, including nickel. Vinyl gloves are more subject to developing microcracks from stretching and, therefore, after being worn for a period of time may decrease in their protective abilities, not only against chemicals but also against microbial agents.

Problem of Protecting the Hands of Orthopedic Surgeons from Acrylic Bone Cement

Acrylic bone cement is a mixture of polymethyl methacrylate and methyl methacrylate (acrylic monomer). It is used for fixation of prostheses to bone in surgical procedures on the hip joint. The brochure describing the bone cement contains the following statement: "The liquid component (methyl methacrylate monomer) is a powerful, lipid solvent. It should not be allowed to come into direct contact with sensitive tissues or be absorbed by the body. Also, it should not be permitted to come in contact with rubber, including rubber gloves."

Ironically, a surgeon can in no way prevent the cement from coming into contact with rubber gloves, because rubber gloves are the only type used regularly in the operating room. The manufacturer of the bone cement recommends: "The surgeon should wear two pairs of rubber gloves when handling the cement directly and discard these for a fresh pair immediately after he [or she] has finished putting the cement in place." This method is thought to provide sufficient protection for an operator unless he or she is sensitive to the methyl methacrylate monomer. In that case, the stratagem may not work.

> **Orthopedic acrylic bone cement is a powerful solvent that penetrates latex gloves. Finger paresthesia may accompany bone cement dermatitis.**

There are many reports of allergic contact dermatitis from acrylic bone cement, which readily penetrates rubber gloves (94–97).

Some surgeons who have become sensitized to bone cement sometimes allow an assistant to perform that part of the operation requiring the handling of bone cement; the sensitized surgeon then completes the operation.

A unique feature of allergic contact dermatitis caused by acrylic monomer is that it is accompanied by a distressing paresthesia of the fingertips in the form of a burning and tingling sensation and a slight numbness. The paresthesia may persist for several weeks after the dermatitis has subsided. The prolonged paresthesia accompanying sensitization to acrylic monomer may occur because the acrylic monomer is a powerful solvent that readily penetrates dam-

aged skin and thus produces an inflammation of the nerve endings in the fingers.

The only currently available glove protective against acrylates is the 4-H plastic polymer glove (Safety 4 Company, Lyngby, Denmark). This glove is thin but has no elasticity and so does not fit snugly against the fingers. A rubber glove, however, can be worn over the 4-H glove to increase fine touch (98).

Nickel

Moursiden and Faber (99) showed that positive patch tests to nickel sulfate (2.5%) could be obtained even when the allergen was separated from nickel-sensitive skin by a segment of rubber glove material. Similar tests, using polyvinyl chloride material instead of rubber, proved negative.

Wall (16) reported that during an investigation of an outbreak of nickel dermatitis in an electrode factory, it was found that the inside lining of the fingertips of the rubber gloves used by the operators was dimethylglyoxime positive, proving that the nickel penetrated rubber gloves.

> **Vinyl gloves give better protection than latex rubber gloves against nitrogen mustard, nickel, hair dyes, and poison ivy.**

Hair Dyes

Moursiden and Faber (99) described a case of allergic, occupational dermatitis in a hairdresser who was sensitive to toluenediamine and aminoazobenzene, which progressed in spite of careful use of rubber gloves. These authors felt that vinyl gloves offer more protection than the rubber variety against hair dyes and most other allergens.

The 4-H glove is also useful in protecting hairdressers from dye and perm chemicals, probably to a greater degree than vinyl gloves (100).

Soaps and Detergents

Homemakers and others who are exposed to soaps and detergents often acquire a dermatitis from the rubber gloves that they use to protect their hands (101). Vinyl gloves adequately protect the hands from soaps and detergents without causing rubber dermatitis.

Nitrogen Mustard

Thomsen and Mikkelsen (102) reported that patients who have early stages of mycosis fungoides are often treated with topical nitrogen mustard (HN_2). HN_2, however, is a potent sensitizer, and 13 of 23 patients who had mycosis fungoides were sensitized.

The only glove that protected the patients against penetration of HN_2 was the one made of polyvinyl chloride. Rubber gloves did not give protection, and a polyethylene glove also permitted penetration of HN_2.

Solvents

Sansone and Tewari (103) have shown that various solvents penetrate most types of gloves. Polyvinyl chloride provided the least protection, and neoprene and nitriles were the most effective.

A study by the National Institute for Occupational Safety and Health revealed that most of the gloves that were tested did not give any protection at all (104). In many cases, they were worse than not wearing anything at all. The study tested the permeation rates of various gloves when immersed in 1,2-dichloroethane, 1,1,1-trichloroethane, 1,1,2-trichloroethane, and a polychlorinated, biphenyl mixture. The glove and garment materials tested included butyl rubber, neoprene rubber latex, nitril rubber latex, polyethylene (medium-density), surgical rubber latex, DuPont's Teflon and Viton, and butylcoated nylon. Normalized times for breakthrough ranged widely, with Viton in all cases resisting permeation the longest.

Viton is a fluorinated elastomer (made by DuPont) that the Norton Company (Charleston Safety Products Division, Charleston, SC) makes into an unsupported, liquid-proof glove.

Surgical Glove Dermatitis

Many surgeons become sensitized to the accelerators or antioxidants used in surgical rubber gloves. In a study of 11 surgeons who acquired an allergic contact dermatitis of their hands from surgical gloves, patch testing revealed that 7 had positive patch tests to mercaptobenzothiazole, a common cause of allergic rubber dermatitis. The other four were allergic to various other rubber chemicals. Such surgeons must use "hypoallergenic" rubber gloves free of mercaptobenzothiazole and other rubber sensitizers in order to avoid hand dermatitis.

Blue nitrite gloves, made of acrylic nitrite and butadiene, have no latex and generally low levels of accelerators.

The Tactyl-1 glove (Smartpractice Co., Phoenix, AZ) is an excellent glove for those with either latex or accelerator allergy but is expensive compared to standard latex gloves (105).

Mechanical Factors

Gloves provide the most effective protection when they can be used, but there are many jobs in the engineering industry in which gloves are dangerously liable to get caught in the moving parts of the machine or in which the components being handled are so small that the wearing of gloves is impossible.

Often, however, patients in certain occupations, such as hairdressing, claim they are unable to do their work properly when they are wearing gloves. When it is pointed out that surgeons must wear gloves when they have to do microsurgery or other delicate operations, such patients sometimes consent to wear gloves.

> It should be pointed out to workers who claim that they cannot wear gloves because their work is "too delicate" that surgeons wear gloves when they do fine heart, brain, and microsurgery.

REFERENCES

1. Lammintausta K, Kalimo K. Atopy and hand dermatitis in hospital wet work. *Contact Dermatitis* 1981;7:301.
2. Bjornberg A. *Skin reactions to primary irritants in patients with hand eczema.* Goteborg, Sweden: Oscar Isacson, 1968.
3. Coenraads PJ, Bleumink E, Nater JP. Susceptibility to primary irritants: age dependence and relation to contact allergic reactions. *Contact Dermatitis* 1975;1:377.
4. Agner T. Skin susceptibility in uninvolved skin of hand eczema patients and healthy controls. *Br J Dermatol* 1991;125:140.
5. Jordan WP. Allergic contact dermatitis in hand eczema. *Arch Dermatol* 1974;110:567.
6. Wilkinson DS. Contact dermatitis of the hands. *Trans St Johns Hosp Dermatol Soc* 1972;58:163.
7. Wilkinson DS, Bandmann HJ, Calnan CD, et al. The role of contact allergy in hand eczema. *Trans St Johns Hosp Dermatol Soc* 1970;56:19.
8. Lantinga H, Nater JP, Coenraads PJ. Prevalence, incidence and course of eczema on the hands and forearms in a sample of the general population. *Contact Dermatitis* 1984;10:135.
9. Kavli G, Førde OH. Hand dermatoses in Tromsø. *Contact Dermatitis* 1984;10:174.
10. Meding B, Swanbeck G. Occupational hand eczema in an industrial city. *Contact Dermatitis* 1990;22:13.
11. Meding B, Swanbeck G. Consequences of having hand eczema. *Contact Dermatitis* 1991;23:6.
12. Rystedt I. Work related hand eczema in atopics. *Contact Dermatitis* 1985;12:164.
13. Rystedt I. Factors influencing the occurrence of hand eczema in adults with a history of atopic dermatitis in childhood. *Contact Dermatitis* 1985;12:185.
14. Rystedt I. Atopic background in patients with occupational hand eczema. *Contact Dermatitis* 1985;12:247.
15. Clemensen OJ, Menne T, Kaaber K, Solgaard P. Exposure of nickel and the relevance of nickel sensitivity among hospital cleaners. *Contact Dermatitis* 1981;7:14.
16. Wall LM. Nickel penetration through rubber gloves. *Contact Dermatitis* 1980;6:461.
17. Fisher AA. Possible role of diet in pompholyx and nickel dermatitis—a critical survey. *Cutis* 1978;22:412.
18. Christensen OB, Moler H. External and internal exposure to the antigen in the hand eczema of nickel allergy. *Contact Dermatitis* 1975;1:136.
19. Menné T, Thorboe A. Nickel dermatitis—nickel excretion. *Contact Dermatitis* 1976;2:353.
20. Hjorth N. Nickel vasculitis. *Contact Dermatitis* 1976;2:356.
21. Christensen OB. Prognosis in nickel allergy and hand eczema. *Contact Dermatitis* 1982;8:7.
22. Christensen OB, Kristensen M. Treatment with disulfiram in chronic nickel hand dermatitis. *Contact Dermatitis* 1982;8:59.
23. Fowler JF. Disulfiram is effective for nickel allergic hand eczema. *Am J Contact Dermatitis* 1992;3:175.

24. Christensen JD. Disulfiram treatment of three patients with nickel dermatitis. *Contact Dermatitis* 1982;8:105.

25. Feuerman EJ. Contact dermatitis in housewives. *Br J Dermatol* 1979;82:205.

26. Wahba A, et al. Housewives' chrome sensitivity in Israel. *Contact Dermatitis* 1979;5:101.

27. Garcia-Perez A, Martin-Pascual A, Sanchez-Misiega A. Chrome content in bleaches and detergents: its relationship to hand dermatitis in women. *Acta Derm Venereol* (Stockh) 1973;53:353.

28. Perisic S, Jovovic D. Allergic contact sensitivity to chromates in housewives. *Dermatovenerol Jugoslav* 1977;4:15.

29. Cronin E. Contact dermatitis XVII: reactions to contact allergens given orally or systemically. *Br J Dermatol* 1972;86:104.

30. Schleif P. Provokation des Chromatekzems zu Testzwecken durch interne chromzufuhr. *Hautarzt* 1968;19:209.

31. Kaaber K, Veien NK. Chromate ingestion in chronic chromate dermatitis. *Contact Dermatitis* 1978;4:119.

32. Burrows D. Chromium and the skin. *Br J Dermatol* 1978;99:587.

33. Fisher AA. "Blackjack disease" and other chromate puzzles. *Cutis* 1976;18:21.

34. Burry JN, Kirk J. Environmental dermatitis: chrome cripples. *Med J Aust* 1975;2:720.

35. Briet R, Turk RMB. The medical and social fate of the dichromate allergic patient. *Br J Dermatol* 1976;94:349.

36. Fregert S. Chromium valencies and cement dermatitis. *Br J Dermatol* 1981;105:7.

37. Rudzki E, Krajewska D. Cross-reactions between ethylenediamine, diethylenetriamine and triethylenetetramine. *Contact Dermatitis* 1976;2:311.

38. Hjorth N. Battery for testing of chefs and other kitchen workers. *Contact Dermatitis* 1975;1:63.

39. Fisher AA. Allergic eczematous contact dermatitis due to foods. *Cutis* 1975;16:603.

40. Nethercott JR, Holness DL. Occupational dermatitis in food handlers and bakers. *J Am Acad Dermatol* 1989;21:485.

41. Seligman EJ, Key MM. Corn dermatitis. *Arch Dermatol* 1968; 97:664.

42. Polunin I. Pineapple dermatoses. *Br J Dermatol* 1951;63:441.

43. Mitchell JC, Jordan WP. Allergic contact dermatitis from radish. *Raphanus sativus. Br J Dermatol* 1974;91:183.

44. Fisher AA. Dermatitis due to cinnamon and cinnamic aldehyde. *Cutis* 1975;16:383.

45. Spencer LV, Fowler JF. "Thin mint" cookie dermatitis. *Contact Dermatitis* 1988;18:185.

46. Sinha SM, Pasricha JS, Sharma RC, Kandhari KC. Vegetable responsible for contact dermatitis of the hands. *Arch Dermatol* 1977;113: 776.

47. Rostenberg A, Jr. Contact urticaria from food. *Arch Dermatol* 1970; 101:491.

48. Fisher AA. Allergic "protein" contact dermatitis due to foods. *Cutis* 1975;16:793.

49. Fisher AA, Stengel F. Allergic occupational hand dermatitis to calves' liver: an urticarial "immediate" type hypersensitivity. *Cutis* 1977;19:561.

50. Hjorth N. Occupational dermatitis in the catering industry. *Br J Dermatol* 1981;105:37.

51. Maibach H. Immediate hypersensitivity in hand dermatitis. *Arch Dermatol* 1976;112:1289.

52. Hannuksela M, Lahti A. Immediate reactions to fruits and vegetables. *Contact Dermatitis* 1977;3:79.

53. Krook G. Occupational dermatitis from *Lactuca sativa* (lettuce) and *Cichorium* (endive). *Contact Dermatitis* 1977;3:27.

54. Sommer RG, Jillson OF. Phytophotodermatitis (solar dermatitis from plants) gas plant and wild parsnip. *N Engl J Med* 1967;276:1484.

55. Fisher AA. Contact dermatitis due to food additives. *Cutis* 1975; 16:961.

56. Mitchell JC. The skin and food additives. (letter to the editor) *Arch Dermatol* 1971;104:329.

57. Roed-Petersen H, Hjorth N. Contact dermatitis from antioxidants. *Br J Dermatol* 1976;94:233.

58. Epstein E. Sodium bisulfite. *Contact Dermatitis Newsletter* 1970; 7:115.

59. Brun R. Eczema de contact à un antioxydant de la margarine (gallate) et changement de métier. *Dermatologica* 1970;140:390.

60. Liden S. *Alphosyl sensitivity*. International Symposium on Contact Dermatitis. Gentofte, Denmark, 1974.

61. Fisher AA. Persulfate hair bleach reactions. *Arch Dermatol* 1976; 112:1407.

62. Fisher AA. Hand dermatitis—a "baker's dozen." *Cutis* 1982;29:214.

63. Fisher AA. Contact dermatitis due to cinnamon and cinnamic aldehyde. *Cutis* 1975;16:383.

64. Neering H, van Ketel WG. *Allergy from spices used in Indonesian cooking*. International Symposium on Contact Dermatitis. Gentofte, Denmark, 1974.

65. Inman PM. Dermatitis in a crisp factory. *Acta Derm Venereol* (Stockh) 1965;45:295.

66. Glickman FS, Silvers SH. Hand eczema and atopy in housewives. *Arch Dermatol* 1967;95:487.

67. Wechsler AL. Soaps, detergents and hand eruptions. *Cutis* 1970; 6:525.

68. Blohm SG, Lodin A. Eczema of the hands in women: "housewives' eczema." *Acta Derm Venereol* (Stockh) 1968;48:7.

69. Calnan CD, et al. Hand dermatitis in housewives. *Br J Dermatol* 1970;82:543.

70. Cronin E. Clinical patterns of hand eczema in women. *Contact Dermatitis* 1985;13:153.

71. Simon W, Harly J. Skin reactions from gold jewelry contaminated with radon deposit. *JAMA* 1967;200:254.

72. Leone RA. Radiodermatitis caused by a radioactive gold ring. *JAMA* 1968;206:2113.

73. Gaul EG. Ring dermatitis. *Arch Dermatol Syphilol* 1958;77:526.

74. Leider M. Removal of ring from a swollen finger without injuring the ring. *J Dermatol Surg Oncol* 1980;6:298.

75. Exner FB. Removal of ring from swollen finger. *JAMA* 1969; 210:558.

76. Epstein E. Therapy of recalcitrant hand dermatitis. *Cutis* 1975; 15:347.

77. Osmet LS. Recurrent and recalcitrant vesiculopustular eruptions of the hands. *Cutis* 1973;11:601.

78. Winkelmann RK, Gleich GJ. Chronic acral dermatitis. *JAMA* 1973; 225:378.

79. Suskind RR. Cutaneous effects of soaps and synthetic detergents. *JAMA* 1957;163:943.

80. Kligman AM, Wooding WM. A method for the measurement and evaluation of irritants on human skin. *J Invest Dermatol* 1967;49:78.

81. Wood DC, Bettley L. The effect of various detergents on human epidermis. *Br J Dermatol* 1971;84:320.

82. Glickman FS, Silvers SH. Hand eczema and atopy in housewives. *Arch Dermatol* 1967;95:487.

83. National Academy of Sciences. *Enzyme-containing laundering compounds and consumer health*. Washington, DC, 1971:15, 23.

84. Ducksbury CFL, Dave VK. Contact dermatitis in home help following the use of enzyme detergents. *Br Med J* 1970;1:537.

85. Weill H, Waddell LC, Ziskind M. A study of workers exposed to detergent enzymes. *JAMA* 1971;217:425.

86. Belin L, Falsen E, Hoborn J, Andre J. Enzyme sensitization in consumers of enzyme-containing washing powders. *Lancet* 1970;2: 1153.

87. Loden M. The effect of four barrier creams on the absorption of water, benzene and formaldehyde into excised human skin. *Contact Dermatitis* 1986;14:292–296.

88. Frosch PJ, et al. Efficacy of skin barrier creams (I). The repetitive irritation test (RIT) in the guinea pig. *Contact Dermatitis* 1993;28:94.

89. Frosch PJ, et al. Efficacy of skin barrier creams (II). Ineffectiveness of a popular "skin protector" against various irritants in the repetitive irritation test in the guinea pig. *Contact Dermatitis* 1993;29:74.

90. Boman A, Mellstrom G. Percutaneous absorption of 3 organic solvents in the guinea pig (III): effect of barrier creams. *Contact Dermatitis* 1989;21:134.

91. Epstein WL. Topical prevention of poison ivy/oak dermatitis. *Arch Dermatol* 1989;125:499.

92. Orchard S, Fellman JA, Storrs FJ. Poison ivy/oak dermatitis: use of polyamine salts of a linoleic acid dimer for topical prophylaxis. *Arch Dermatol* 1986;122:783.

93. Smith WB. Lack of efficacy of a barrier cream in preventing Rhus dermatitis. *Arch Dermatol* 1993;129:787.

94. Fisher AA. "Hypoallergenic" surgical gloves and gloves for special situations. *Cutis* 1975;15:797.

95. Pegum JS, Medhurst EA. Contact dermatitis from penetration of rubber gloves by acrylic monomer. *Br Med J* 1971;2:141.

96. Fisher AA. Contact dermatitis in surgeons. *J Dermatol Surg Oncol* 1975;1:63.

97. Fries IB, Fisher AA, Salvati EA. Contact dermatitis in surgeons from methylmethacrylate bone cement. *J Bone Joint Surg Am* 1975; 57:547.

98. Tobler M, Freiburghaus AV. A glove with exceptional protective features minimizes the risks of working with hazardous chemicals. *Contact Dermatitis* 1992;26:299.

99. Moursiden HT, Faber O. Penetration of protective gloves by allergens and irritants. *Trans St John's Hosp Dermatol Soc* 1973;9:230.

100. McClain TC, Storrs FJ. Protective effect of both a barrier cream and a polyethylene laminate glove against epoxy resin, glyceryl monothioglycolate, frullania, and tansy. *Am J Contact Dermatitis* 1992;3:201.

101. Epstein E. Therapy of recalcitrant hand dermatitis. *Cutis* 1975; 15:346.

102. Thomsen K, Mikkelsen HI. Protective capacity of gloves used for handling nitrogen mustard. *Contact Dermatitis* 1975;1:268.

103. Sansone EB, Tewari YB. The permeability of laboratory gloves to selected solvents. *Am Hygiene Assoc J* 1978;39:169.

104. Protective gear flunks permeation tests (Editorial). *Chemical Week* 1981 Feb 25:20.

105. Lahti A, et al. Patch tests with Tactylon™ in patients with contact allergy to rubber. *Contact Dermatitis* 1992;27:188.

CHAPTER 19

Textile and Shoe Dermatitis

TEXTILE DERMATITIS

Untreated natural and synthetic fabrics and fibers used in the manufacture of clothing cause almost no skin problems. A collection of chemicals and dyes added to these fibers during their manufacture and assembly into garments, however, can cause irritant and allergic dermatitis, as well as petechial and urticarial skin eruptions, in both industrial workers and consumers.

Skin problems from clothing may be attributed to permanent press finishes, dyes, rubber, metals, and glues. Miscellaneous agents such as biocides, spot removers, fire retardants, and smoothers are occasionally causative.

Clinical Picture of Clothing Dermatitis

The distribution of the eruption generally conforms to a pattern that coincides with the places on the skin where the garment fits most snugly. Variation in styling of men's and women's clothing explains some differences in distribution. Men would more likely have a neck dermatitis from a stiffened dress shirt collar, for example. Dermatitis on the anterior and posterior axillary folds from dress or shirt fabrics is typical for women. Pants are worn by both sexes, and a dermatitis on the inner and anterior thighs, as well as on the popliteal fossae, would make them suspect. Any location where the clothing is held more tightly against the skin is a likely spot for textile dermatitis to occur.

Allergy to finishes on bed linens or furniture fabrics may produce a worsening of dermatitis on the back, posterior legs, or other locations of prominent contact. Warmth and moisture, such as from perspiration, tend to increase the appearance of textile allergic contact dermatitis (ACD). Because of wearing heavier clothing, textile dermatitis is worse in the winter in some persons. Sparing of parts of the skin protected by underclothing is a distinctive feature of fabric finish and dye-related ACD, but spreading into these areas may occur. Cross-reaction with formaldehyde-based preservatives may complicate the picture by causing dermatitis on the face and hands (1).

Allergy to rubber additives or latex protein may produce dermatitis around the waist and brassiere straps at sites of elastic contact. Belt buckles and metal buttons produce dermatitis at expected contact sites.

In general, dermatitis from dyes tends to be acute and rapid in onset (2). Durable-press finishes based on formaldehyde resins more commonly produce a smoldering chronic dermatitis. Generalized erythroderma may also result from formaldehyde allergy. Older patients may have a more widespread eruption than younger individuals (3). Purpuric dermatitis is characteristic of an allergy to a rubber antiozonant, N-isopropyl-N-phenyl-paraphenylenediamine (IPPD) (4).

Irritant (ICD) and allergic types of contact dermatitis are the most important cutaneous conditions arising from clothing and other fabrics. In addition, tight clothing may produce follicular irritation with resulting miliaria or folliculitis. Ramam, et al. (5) from India have reported cases of "frictional sweat dermatitis" occurring in hot summer months limited to areas of tight clothing. Clinical features include mild stinging or burning and a glazed, wrinkled skin surface with sharp margins. Recovery is spontaneous. In evaluating possible clothing-related dermatitis, it should be remembered that clothing may trap and hold allergens from the environment or workplace. This can be seen in individuals exposed to airborne dusts or oils, for example. Also, laundry products that are retained in clothing after washing may cause ICD or ACD, although the true occurrence of this is unknown. Fragrances in laundry products are often thought by patients to be a problem, but documentation is difficult.

Fibers Used in Clothing

Natural fibers used in clothing are cellulose (cotton and linen) or protein (wool and silk) in origin. Synthetic fibers can be made from cellulose (rayon) and from proteins such as casein, soybeans, and ground nuts. Azlon, as these reconstituted animal and plant protein fibers are called, is largely obsolete now (6).

Noncellulose-based synthetic fibers are derived largely from petroleum (polyesters and acrylics), although some of

Portions of this chapter are revisions of material written for the 3rd and 4th editions by Frances J. Storrs, M.D. Her contribution is greatly appreciated.

them, such as nylon, can be manufactured from coal tars or even from oat hulls and corncobs (6).

Elastic fibers are made from either natural rubber or synthetic "snap-back" fibers known as elastomers (spandex). Synthetic elastomers are polyurethanes. Fibers used in some drapery materials and in some industrial cloths can be made of spun glass (fiberglass). Metal fibers used in clothing usually consist of aluminum filaments covered with plastics (6).

The fibers used in clothing are made by many different companies. The mode of manufacture of these fibers, as well as an extensive list of their generic and trade names and manufacturers, can be found in a comprehensive text such as Moncrieff's (6). A condensed description of fibers used in clothing is found in Table 19.1.

In 1939, the Wool Products Labeling Act required that all fabrics, except those used in carpets and rugs, indicate on their label the presence of any amount of wool. In 1960, the United States Textile Fiber Products Identification Act extended the Wool Products Labeling Act and directed that all fabrics should be labeled generically according to their fiber content (7). Any fiber present in a concentration greater than 5% must be so designated on the garment label by its percentage in the fabric.

Garments are often made from yarns that are formed by combining natural and synthetic fibers into "blends." These blends, as well as the 100% synthetic and natural fibers that are their parents, have innumerable brand names and manufacturers. Fortunately, the Textile Identification Act not only requires generic names but also allows the use of brand names. Thus, the few brand names in Table 19.1 should be more than sufficient to allow an interested physician to analyze a garment label and make some predictions about the finishing processes that may have been used on any one garment (see Tables 19.2–19.3).

Dermatitis from Natural Fibers

Cotton

Cotton is made from untreated cotton cellulose. Pure cotton has not been reported to cause allergic contact dermatitis.

TABLE 19.1. *Fibers Used in Clothing*

Type	Generic name	Trade name	Raw materials
Natural fibers			
Cotton	Cotton		Cellulose
Linen	Linen		Cellulose
Silk	Silk		Protein
Wool	Wool		Protein
Synthetic fibers			
A. From natural polymers			
Cellulose (1900s)			Wood cellulose
Viscose rayon	Rayon	Topel, Corval, and Coloray	
Cellulose acetate	Acetate	Celanese	
Cellulose triacetate	Triacetate	Celanese	
Animal protein (obsolete)	Artificial wool	Lanital, Merinova, and Fibrolene	Casein in milk
Plant protein (obsolete)	Artificial wool	Ardil, Vicara	Peanut protein Maize protein
B. From synthetic polymers			
Condensation polymers			
Polymides (1930s)	Nylon	Perlon, Antron, and Quiana	Petroleum or oat hulls and corncobs
Polyesters (1950s)	Polyester	Dacron, Terylene	Petroleum
Polyureas (1950s) (obsolete)	Polyurea	Urylon	Rice bran oil
Polyamide aramid		Nomex	
Vinyl-type addition polymers (1950s) (polyacrylonitriles)			
Vinyl chloride	Modacrylic (35%–85% Acrylonitrile)	Dynel	Petroleum
Vinyl cyanide	Acrylic (85% acrylonitrile)	Orlon, Acrilan, and Creslan	Petroleum
Elastomers			
Polyurethanes	Spandex	Lycra, Vyrene	Petroleum
Vinylidene chloride	Saran	Velon, Permalon	Petroleum
Polyvinyl alcohol	Vinylon		Petroleum and coke
Metallic			
Aluminum plus cellulose acetate-butyrate		Lurex, Metlon	Aluminum and cellulose
Aluminum plus polyester		Lurex M M	Aluminum and petroleum

A comprehensive listing and description of fibers used in clothing is found in Ref. 7. Prepared by Frances Storrs MD for the 3rd edition

TABLE 19.2. *Durable-Press Finishing*

Unlikely to be finished	Likely to be finished
100% Cotton denim (e.g., Levi Strauss & Co.'s 501 Shrink-to-Fit Button Blue Jeans)	Rayon
	Any cotton, rayon, or wool blend
100% silk	Corduroy
100% linen that wrinkles	Wrinkle-resistant linen
100% wool[a]	"Shrink-proof" woolens
100% polyester	Any wash-and-wear or wrinkle-resistant 100% cotton
100% nylon	Any synthetic polymer blended with a natural fiber or polymer
100% ultrasuede[b]	

[a]Isolated reports of treatment with formaldehyde resins.
[b]Ultrasuede is a nonwoven polyester held together with a urethane binder and treated with a silicon fluorocarbon finish. No durable press finishes are used (MD Hurwitz, personal communication, 1984).

One can presume that any cotton fiber that claims crease resistance is treated with a durable-press finish, as are virtually all cotton synthetic fiber blends (see section on durable-press finishes). It is impossible to identify with absolute certainty whether a 100% cotton fabric is finish free. Price is not a determinant, although easily wrinkled or shrinkable cottons are less likely to have been treated (Table 19.3).

Genetically enhanced cotton that is less prone to wrinkling is now available, although it does not hold its stiffness as well as fabrics treated with formaldehyde resins.

Cotton "breathes" but does not dissipate perspiration as well as either silk or nylon (8).

> **Clothing made from untreated, finish-free cotton fibers is hypoallergenic.**

Chemical and mechanical processes that may be applied to cotton include:

1. Sanforizing. This is a controlled-shrinkage process. The yarns are rearranged mechanically and are shortened by the amount they would be if they were laundered. No chemicals are used, and no skin hazard exists. Linen is also rarely sanforized.

2. Mercerization. In this finishing process, the cotton is impregnated with a cold, strong (about 25%) sodium hydroxide solution (caustic soda). The process increases the penetrability of finishing resins and dyes and, when done under tension, enhances the fabric's luster. The sodium hydroxide is removed so that no hazard exists to the wearer. Only cotton is mercerized.

3. Sizing. Starch, glues, vegetable gums, rosins, or shellac may be applied to the cotton to impart a stiff, polished, or glazed surface. Organdy, piqué, sheeting, and mosquito netting may be sized. The Levi Strauss 501 "shrink to fit" original blue jeans are finished only with cornstarch, which may reach 10% of the weight of the new garment (SM Rajan, Levi Strauss & Co., personal communication, 1984). The starch may be an irritant in the new, unwashed garment. Traces of glues and rosins in sized cotton cloth may produce dermatitis in sensitized individuals (9). Sizing processes may be used on many fabrics other than cottons.

Linen

This fiber is made from the inner bark of the flax plant. It is treated occasionally with durable-press finishes to combat its tendency to wrinkle. In its unfinished state, it should not cause allergic reactions.

Wool

The warmth, softness, extensibility, ability to felt, and ability to take up a third of its own weight in water without feeling damp are all qualities of wool that have not been duplicated in any synthetic fiber (6). Fibers derived from natural proteins (Table 19.1) approximate the "handle" of wool but fail to reproduce all of its other merits. These synthetic wools are largely obsolete now. Pure woolen garments are not usually treated with durable-press finishes, but some old patents and processes do describe the use of formaldehyde on wool to prevent shrinkage and bacterial degradation (10). Modern wool processing tends to avoid such finishing because it alters the natural handle of wool. Woolen blends may be finished, however.

Allergic dermatitis to natural wool has been very rarely documented (11). Wool is often included in lists of substances that cause contact urticaria and has been documented to do this at least once (1,11–13).

Irritant dermatitis related to wool, particularly in people who have atopic dermatitis, is common (14,15). Atopic dermatitis may be aggravated at sites on the body at which wool touches the skin. Smooth and soft fabrics worn between the atopic skin and wool can minimize this aggravation.

> **Woolen clothing often irritates atopic skin and can cause contact urticaria, but it almost never produces allergic contact dermatitis. Wool finishes may evoke purpuric eruptions.**

During World War II, men wearing woolen khaki shirts developed an unexplained purpuric eruption confined to the shirt area (13). In subsequent investigations, Greenwood (16) inferred that lubricating oils (oleines) containing oleic acid, mineral oils, lanolin, or blended vegetable oils used during the manufacture of woolen fabric may have caused the toxic purpuric eruption as well as a similar eruption that he had seen develop in individuals who used woolen shirts

TABLE 19.3. *Cross-Linking Fabric Finishing Agents (Durable Press)*

Resin type	Abbreviation	Estimated total market share (1990)	Uses and characteristics	Relative formaldehyde release
Polycondensation polymers (1930s) Urea formaldehyde (dimethylol urea)	DMU	6%	Cotton pile fabrics, velvet, corduroy coatings, old-fashioned women's dress goods, flannelettes, upholstery, viscous rayon, used with some water repellents Imparts crease and shrink resistance to cotton and rayon; not chlorine resistant; increases wash fastness, but washes out faster than others; inexpensive	High
Melamine	MF	20%	"Heavy fabrics," "stiff" finishes, draperies, coatings, some collars, some water- and oil-repellent and flame-retardant finishes; effective on synthetic and natural fibers Used with many other finishes to improve durability to washing and dry cleaning	High
Linear reactants Dimethylol carbamates (1960s)	DMC	3%	Less than 2% of clothing; some on sheeting, pillow cases, cotton-polyester blends, fabric liners and draperies, white shirts Soft finish, excellent chlorine resistance; not very light fast and incompatible with some dyes; more expensive	Medium
Cyclic ureas (1960s) N-methylol propylene urea derivatives: (dimethylolpropylene urea) (dimethylolethylene urea) Dimethylol dihydroxyethylene urea (1960s)	DMPU DMEU DMDHEU	3% 16%	Colored cotton textiles and white goods, shirts, some upholstery; more popular in France, Italy, and Spain; little or no use in United States Soft finish, excellent chlorine resistance; used in paper and red wine DMDHEU and its derivatives are used on 80%–90% of U.S. apparel fabric blends; "wash and wear," colored, and white fabrics and shirtings; not used on 100% pure synthetic fabrics; also used on draperies and sheeting; chlorine resistant, stiffer than carbamates, some paper use; relatively inexpensive	Medium Low
DMDHEU blended or reacted with glycols		34%	Performance similar to DMDHEU but slightly slower curing	Very low
Dimethoxymethyl dihydroxyethylene urea (1980s) (methylated DMDHEU)	DMDHEU	10%	As etherified glyoxal reactant; similar uses and characteristics as DMDHEU with lower formaldehyde release, more expensive than DMDHEU	Low
Uron formaldehyde (1950s) N,N'-bis-(methoxymethyl) uron	UF	1%	Soft, white fabrics, used on collar linings in past; durable finishes, some drapery, and upholstery use Not as chlorine resistant as others; little use in United States, but may be added to MF or mixed with other finishing agents	High
N,N'-dimethyl-4,5 dihydroxyethylene	DHDMI or DMcDHEU	1%	Children's apparel at present in United States. May be used in Japan on polyester/cotton blends or on Marks & Spencer fabrics in England; expensive; not as effective as DMDHEU or its derivatives for shrinkage control or durable-press appearance	None

This table was adapted with permission from Frances Storrs MD in Fisher AA, ed. *Contact dermatitis.* 3rd ed. Philadelphia: Lea & Febiger, 1986:288. We also acknowledge the generous assistance of members of the textile industry, especially J. C. Winchester, American Cynamid Co., Manager, Charlotte Laboratory, Charlotte, NC; M. D. Hurwitz, Professor, Clothing & Textiles, University of North Carolina, Greensboro, NC; P.S. Pai, Scientific Applications & Innovations Corp. (textile industry consultant), Charlotte, NC; and R. R. Stewart, Procter & Gamble Co. (textile scientist), Cincinnati, OH.

TABLE 19.4. *Organizations and Journals Serving the Textile Industry*

Organization or publisher	Journal
American Association of Textile Chemists & Colorists P.O. Box 12215 Research Triangle Park, NC 27709 919-549-8141	*TCC and ADR (monthly) Colour Index* (mult. vols.) and *Buyer's Guide* (every July)
McGraw Hill Publishing Co. 4170 Ashford-Dunwoody Road Suite 520 Atlanta, GA 30319 Headquarters' New York 212-512-2000	*Textile World*
Textile Research Institute P.O. Box 625 Princeton, NJ 08540 609-924-3150	*Textile Research Journal*
Institute of Textile Technology 2551 Ivy Road Charlottesville, VA 22903-4614 804-296–5511	*Textile Technology Digest* (Also available on CD-ROM through ITT's Roger Milliken Library and Information Services)

and underwear. Hellier (17), in 1960, and Romaguera et al. (18), in 1981 suggested the possibility that purpuric eruptions associated with wool could be related to allergy from a urea or melamine-formaldehyde resin finish. The sedatives Sedormid and Carbromal, both of which are capable of producing purpuric dermatitis, are also urea compounds (16,17).

Chromium can be used as a mordant in wool-dyeing processes. Allergic dermatitis attributed to chrome has occurred in a woolen blanket factory (19) and in association with the wearing of green, woolen military textiles (20). A woolen dye used in knitting wool explained one case of allergic dermatitis (1).

Silk

Silk is the least extensively used natural fiber (6). Silk, like other fabrics, may be sold under several names, including crepe, satin, chiffon, taffeta, and jersey.

Contact urticaria caused by silk has been reported (21). In a case from Japan, with allergy to silk undergarments, scratch tests were positive to sericin 5% aq, raw silk, and silkworm cocoon. Lymphocyte stimulation tests to sericin was positive (22). Allergic reactions to silk are rare, however, and the nature of the allergen is disputed (23). The silk fiber, the gum or glue (sericin) in raw silk, and the silkworm protein are the antigen candidates. Silk used as a filter for biological products may cause anaphylaxis (24).

Silk is a rare sensitizer.

Dermatitis from Synthetic Fibers (Rayon, Nylon, Polyester, and Acrylics)

Today, synthetic materials are used in greater quantity in clothing manufacture than natural fibers.

Until 1971, nylon led the synthetic fiber market, but since then the polyesters and polyacrylonitrites have surpassed nylon (6). Nylon, Dacron, and Orlon have been the backbone of the synthetic fiber industry for 50 years (6). One would think that as oil reserves decrease, more cellulose-based fibers would be made. The textile industry has become energy efficient, however, and it is estimated that, as of 1983, a pound of polyester can be made from 12 cents' worth of oil (MD Hurwitz, personal communication, November 1983). Rayon constitutes about 17% of synthetic fibers, however, but this percentage is unlikely to increase by much (6).

Nylon clothing dermatitis is usually a miliaria-like eruption because nylon absorbs sweat poorly.

Despite the prevalence of synthetic fibers, allergic reactions to untreated synthetic fibers are rare. Allergic contact dermatitis to virgin nylon has been reliably reported once in the United States and twice in Europe (25,26). One case of allergy to nylon-6 from Japan gave a positive patch test to the nylon monomer epsilon-aminocaproic acid (3% pet) (27). A similar case has been reported from Spain. A textile factory worker was allergic to epsilon-caprolactin (5% pet) used in the synthesis of nylon-6 (28).

Nylon is not very absorbent, and thus a freely perspiring individual may complain of pruritus and dermatitis from the maceration and irritation of unabsorbed sweat when he or she wears nylon garments. Pure rayons and polyester are not known as allergens, but one report has been made of an allergy related to an acrylonitrile used in a finger splint (29). Five workers in a factory producing acrylonitrile (CH_2CHCN) for use in synthetic fibers developed ACD. All gave 3+ reactions to acrylonitrile 0.1% pet. The guinea pig maximization test (GPMT) showed that acrylonitrile has strong allergenic potential (30).

The vinylidene chloride polymers (saran) are used occasionally in belts, suspenders, and raincoats. Dermatitis has been reported in association with Saran Wrap (31). Other vinyl plastics such as polyvinyl chloride may find occasional use in swimwear or as identification armbands. Unexplained irritant dermatitis was reported in seven children wearing such armbands (32). Plasticizers added to the vinyl chlorides (dibutyltin maleate, dibutyl sebacate, dibutyl phthalate, dioctyl phthalate, and epoxy resins) are usually the explanation for both irritant and allergic reactions attributed to the plastic fabrics (33,34).

Contact Urticaria from Nylon

A 21-year-old woman reported urticaria with pruritius within 15 minutes of putting on nylon panties or stockings. Immediate patch tests was repeatedly positive to dye free nylon (35).

Dermatitis from Rubber and Elastomers in Clothing

Pure spandex fibers have not been proven to cause dermatitis. In the past, spandex fibers were treated with mercaptobenzothiazole (MBT). Allergy to this accelerator explained some ACD associated with elastic undergarments (1,36). More recently, a benzotriazole chemical (Tinuvin P) used in spandex in underwear caused one case of ACD (personal communication, FJ Storrs, MD, 1984). Spandex is lighter and whiter than rubber, and its advantages suit its use in underclothes and swimsuits. It is an excellent rubber substitute for people who are sensitive to rubber additives. Antioxidants such as butylated hydroxytoluene also may be used on spandex to prevent deterioration. Clothing containing rubber that has been treated with antioxidants and accelerators, especially thiurams and MBT, can cause dermatitis in sensitized people.

There are several rarer explanations for rubber-related clothing contact dermatitis. IPPD (also called 4-isopropyl-aminodiphenylamine or isopropylphenyl *p*-phenylenediamine [PPD]) is an antiozonant and antioxidant used in the rubber industry. Santoflex IP, Flexzone 3C, and Permanax IPPD are several of the trade names for IPPD. Allergy to IPPD explained a purpuric eczematous dermatitis in 23 patients caused by the elastic in their undergarments (37). IPPD can cross-react with PPD, and patch test reactions to both of these chemicals can be petechial or purpuric (4,38). IPPD imparts a black or gray color to rubber treated with it,

although this color can be masked by weaving the elastic fibers into other material (38). Fisher (39) has noted reactions to IPPD used in a rubber diving suit, in elasticized shorts, and in a rubberized leg support bandage. IPPD can also cross-react with some azo dyes used in textiles.

Thioureas are used increasingly in the production of neoprene rubber and in elastic in underwear (see Chapter 31).

Elasticized clothing may also cause skin eruptions as a consequence of mechanical pressure. Pressure urticaria, acneiform eruptions, exaggeration of preexisting dermatoses, and nondescript erythematous changes may develop at skin sites at which the clothing fits too snugly (40).

Underclothing made of spandex usually avoids allergic contact dermatitis in individuals sensitive to rubber accelerators and antioxidants. Pure cotton French-cut boxer shorts, which button and contain no elastic, are sold by retail stores and in catalogs.

> **Rubber antioxidants, accelerators, and chlorine bleaches produce rubberized clothing dermatitis.**

M. Bourlas and W. P. Jordan of the Medical College of Virginia in Richmond, Virginia (personal communication, 1984) have developed a test that can be helpful in identifying thirams and carbamates in rubber materials.

Office Analysis for Thirams and Carbamates

1. Reagent A is for thirams. Weigh 0.1 g cuprous acetate into a 250-ml volumetric and fill with acetic acid. Stir solution until all of the cuprous acetate has dissolved.

2. Reagent B is for carbamates. A portion of the cuprous acetate solution is diluted in a 3:1 ratio, 3 parts water to 1 part cuprous-acetate solution. This reagent is for all carbamates. Reagent B is made by the dilution of Reagent A.

Procedure for Thirams

1. Acetone is the extracting solvent for samples suspected of containing thirams. Extract approximately 1-g sample of test material in acetone for 2 to 3 minutes (shaking gently). Use from 1 to 3 ml of acetone. Transfer all the acetone to another tube.

2. If over 1 ml of acetone is transferred, let the acetone evaporate until approximately 1 ml remains.

3. Add approximately an equal volume of Reagent A and observe the color change over the next 5 minutes. The "Windex" blue color changes to a mint green, then to a dark green.

Procedure for Carbamates

1. Methylisobutylketone is the extracting solvent for samples suspected of containing carbamates (dithio-).

2. Extract as for thiram instruction.

3. No color is negative, and a positive test is indicated by a change from olive to brown.

Bleached Rubber Syndrome

Jordan and Bourlas (41) reported allergic contact dermatitis to underwear elastic that resulted only when the undergarment was bleached. The rubber accelerator, zinc dibenzyldithio-carbamate, present in the elastic, formed eight reaction products in the presence of sodium hypochlorite (bleach). One of these reaction products, *N,N*-dibenzylcarbamyl chloride, was the sensitizer. Sensitized individuals who wore unbleached underwear avoided the dermatitis.

Fiberglass Dermatitis

Glass can be spun into a fiber and woven into a fabric. It has not been used in garments, however. Glass cloth is used as a fireproof material in curtains, lampshades, furniture covers, and awnings. It has some use in construction as well as for wrapping wires and in insulation.

Fiberglass is an irritant. It has caused a pseudoclothing dermatitis when fabrics made of fiberglass were washed in an automatic washing machine with a family's clothes (42,43). The glass fibers can become embedded in the nonglass garments and subsequently cause a papular, pruritic dermatitis that can resemble scabies. This dermatitis is most likely to be caused by large glass fibers. Small fibers may contact the skin and cause no difficulty (43). When the lesions are biopsied, glass particles may be seen in foreign body granulomas (44). Others have noted that fiberglass particles can induce a spongiotic dermatitis that is patch test negative (45). This observation raises the question of the role that microtrauma can play in inducing eczematous dermatitis seen without allergy (46). It is possible to see the fiberglass fragments in a potassium hydroxide preparation taken from scrapings of the involved skin (47).

> **Biopsies of fiberglass dermatitis may reveal glass particles in a granulomatous reaction or spongiosis mimicking an allergic reaction.**

Although the glass itself does not cause allergic dermatitis, it can be finished with formaldehyde resins like other synthetic fibers. An allergic reaction to such a finish used on fiberglass wool has been noted (44,46).

Fisher (48) has reviewed the similarities and differences between rockwool (mineral wool) dermatitis and fiberglass dermatitis. Rockwool, also known as mineral cotton, silicate cotton, and slag wool, is used for heat and sound insulation. The irritant dermatitis that it causes can be indistinguishable from fiberglass dermatitis.

Dermatitis from Chemical Additives to Clothing

Commercial interest in the modification of cellulosic fabrics by treatment with formaldehyde was first aroused in 1906 when Eschalier took out British and French patents based on the observation that the wet strength of regenerated cellulose or rayon fibers could be improved by an acid formaldehyde treatment (10). This observation was not extensively used until the 1930s, when *N*-methylol (formaldehyde) compounds derived from urea and melamine formaldehyde polycondensation products were polymerized within the interstices of cellulose fibers. The desired property of wrinkle resistance was offset by a tendency of the resins to absorb chlorine from bleaches. The resultant chloramides produced yellowing, breakdown with heat (ironing), and eventual weakening of the fabric. An undesirable amount of formaldehyde was released from the resins during manufacture, storage, and wear (10,49).

In the 1950s and 1960s, escalation in the development of synthetic fibers (Table 19.1) and then mixing (blending) with cellulose (cotton and rayon) was accompanied by the introduction of the cyclic ethylene and propylene urea compounds (Table 19.3). These resins represented an improvement over the condensation resins in that they combine directly with the cellulose fiber. They release less formaldehyde, and they are more wash and chlorine fast. Etherified glyoxal reactant modifications of these cyclic ureas (Table 19.3) are used today and have further decreased formaldehyde release from fabric-finishing resins.

In 1960, it was estimated that 3 billion yards per year of cotton alone was treated with *N*-methylol finishing agents (49). Of the 7.5 billion pounds of formaldehyde consumed in the United States each year, 1% to 2% is used in the textile industry (50). Approximately 140,000 tons of *N*-methylol compounds were produced for use on American fabrics each year.

Alteration in the handle of cellulose (cotton, rayon) or cellulose synthetic fiber blends is the result of the development of covalent cross-linkages that develop between the cellulose and the *N*-methylol (formaldehyde) finishing compounds. Synthetic fibers that are 100% noncellulose do not require finishing with *N*-methylol-containing resins. The resins are incapable of chemically cross-linking 100% synthetic fibers; thus, the resin is left on the surface of the fabric, where its chance of causing allergy or irritation is greater. Only stiff 100% noncellulose synthetics (occasionally nylon) would be expected to be finished with formaldehyde resin. Wool can be treated with *N*-methylol resin to prevent shrinkage. Because the treatment alters the desired natural handle of wool, it is seldom done. Silk is not treated, because the process can actually injure the fibers (6).

The reaction of *N*-methylol finishing agents with cellulose is an acid-catalyzed (e.g., zinc nitrate, magnesium chloride, or alkanolamine hydrochloride) reversible reaction (49).

The reaction is driven by heat during curing. If some acid catalyst remains in the fabric and if no washing or formaldehyde scavenging is done after curing, then hydrolysis can occur under warm, humid conditions. The finishing reaction is reversed and formaldehyde is released. An even more important reason for formaldehyde release from fabric is the failure of some resin to fully cross-link.

During degradation of the resin with use, the amides can react with chlorine in laundry bleaches and can form chloramides. Urea formaldehyde resins do this more than the cyclic ureas.

The textile industry strives continuously to develop finishing agents and a technology that will decrease the amount of formaldehyde releasable from fabrics. The impetus for these efforts has been evidence collected by and for government agencies concerning formaldehyde's potential for carcinogenicity (50,51).

By 1981, the textile industry was able to claim that levels of formaldehyde release had decreased to the point that 100 to 200 ppm rather than 200 ppm was the rule (52). This would provide a level of 0.1 ppm in the air of a textile factory, which is well within NIOSH's (National Institute of Occupational Safety & Health) recommended level of 1 ppm (50). Most of this decrease is probably due to preparation of purer resins and use of less of them. Additionally, the use of methylated dimethylol dihydroxyethylene urea (DMDHEU) (see Table 19.3) eliminates or decreases the NCH_2OH groups in the finish and, thus, the main source of formaldehyde release (52).

An especially hopeful part of this story is the development by the manufacturer BASF of a textile finishing agent for cellulosics (U.S. Patent No. 4,295,846) that does not release formaldehyde at all (Table 19.3) (53). This compound is expensive. The compound is a cyclic urea and consists of N,N'-dimethyl derivatives of 4,5-dihydroxyethylene ureas.

Formaldehyde resins may cause permanent-press finish clothing dermatitis. Most persons are also allergic to formaldehyde itself.

On October 1, 1975, the Japanese Department of Health and Welfare restricted the content of formaldehyde in underclothes to less than 75 ppm for adults and to less than 15 ppm for babies (54). Before the restriction, some Japanese textiles contained more than 10,000 ppm formaldehyde. Formaldehyde and formaldehyde donor release are also restricted in Japanese cosmetics. It is interesting that, in the face of these restrictions, the incidence of patch test positivity to formaldehyde in Japan went from 5.7% in 1974 to 1.9% in 1977 in one series and from 5.4% in 1976 to 1.9% in 1979 in another series (54,55).

The textile resins now in use in the United States are described in detail in Table 19.3. Since 1961, DMDHEU (U.S. Patent No. 2,764,573 1956), which is often blended with glycols, has been the most widely used durable-press finish for apparel in the United States and Britain (1,56). However, Hatch and Maibach (57) stated that the use of this

agent and other high formaldehyde resins is decreasing. They further stated that although U.S. manufacturers are using newer low or no formaldehyde finishes, the amount of clothing made overseas and being imported to the United States is increasing. They reported the introduction in the 1980s of DHDMI-dihydroxydimethyl-imidazolidinone and other agents that apparently do not release free formaldehyde.

In addition to the categories of commonly used compounds described in Table 19.3, the following chemicals (resins or reactants) may also find an occasional place in developing a durable-press finish for textiles (wrinkle, crease, and shrink resistance) (58): polymeric acetates, silicone polymers, triazones, methylol dimenthylhydantoin, epoxide resins, chloro-alkyl cross-linkers, chloromethyl ethers of polyhydric alcohols, divinyl sulfone derivatives, tris (beta sulfato-ethyl) sulfonium salt, formaldehyde, and glyoxal. The organizations and publishing firms listed in Table 19.4 can provide more current information.

Marcussen (59) in Denmark, saw 26 patients with formaldehyde textile allergy between 1934 and 1958. He tested formaldehyde at a concentration of 4%, which may have produced some false-positive irritant reactions. In Norway, Hovding (60) found free formaldehyde between 5,000 and 12,000 ppm in 227 of the 256 rayon and cotton samples he analyzed in 1959. Hovding (61) reported 45 patients whom he saw between 1953 and 1958 among 2,110 routinely patch-tested patients who were formaldehyde sensitive and who had a dermatitis in a clothing distribution.

Cronin (62), in England, saw 30 patients who had a textile dermatitis not caused by dyes between 1953 and 1961. She saw an additional 33 patients from 1970 to 1976 (1). One patient in the first and four in the second group were resin positive and formaldehyde negative. All of the remaining patients were formaldehyde positive. Patch tests to pieces of suspect clothing were often negative, but these same pieces of clothing gave positive chemical reactions for formalin (62). In 1964, Berrens et al. (63) also noted that patients in the Netherlands who were sensitive to formaldehyde (even to concentrations as low as 0.3% to 0.03%) would not react to pieces of suspect clothing, even when it was shown to contain formaldehyde. Avoidance of the formaldehyde-containing clothing, however, resulted in resolution of their dermatitis.

Fisher et al. (64), in 1962, also could not make formaldehyde-positive patients in the United States react to pieces of fabric known to contain formaldehyde. The U.S. patients did not have dermatitis in a clothing pattern, and these authors concluded that American fabrics contained too little formaldehyde release to cause dermatitis. Fisher's patients were chosen, however, for their formaldehyde sensitivity rather than for their clothing distribution.

In 1964, Malten (65) in the Netherlands tested 66 patients who had a suspect textile-finish hypersensitivity dermatitis. Of these 66 patients, 27 reacted to at least one of the 37 substances that were being used in textile finishing. Only seven of the patients reacted to formaldehyde. In addition to Malten's patients and Cronin's (62) aforementioned patient, Fregert and Tegner (66) reported a patient who had a positive reaction to a finishing resin (DMDHEU) and who was negative to formaldehyde.

A most interesting group of formaldehyde-negative, resin-finish-positive patients appeared in Canada in 1973 (67,68). These 11 patients developed an extensive pruritic, follicular eczema after sleeping in colored Wabasso polyester/cotton bedsheets. None of the 11 patients were positive to formaldehyde, nor were 39 additional patients reported from London in 1976 after similar offending sheets were distributed in England (69). Six of the Canadian patients had positive patch tests to white pieces of their own sheets (67). Five of the six reacted to the raw permapress resin (*N,N*-dimethylol-4-methoxy-5,5-dimethyl propylene urea) (68).

> **Patients may be allergic to a formaldehyde resin clothing fabric finish and not to formaldehyde itself.**

Very little textile-related dermatitis has been reported from the United States until recently. Epstein and Maibach (70) identified three patients positive to formaldehyde who had a clothing-pattern dermatitis among 156 patients tested between 1963 and 1965. O'Quinn and Kennedy (71) described three additional patients in 1964 who reacted to formaldehyde and to pieces of textile that contained formaldehyde. Fisher et al. (64) believed that the few U.S. cases could be explained by the fact that after-washing was more common in the finishing process in the United States than it was in Europe.

A dramatic change in this trend was reported by Fowler et al. (2). In a period of 28 months, 17 cases of formaldehyde resin allergy were diagnosed from among 1,022 patients tested in Louisville, Kentucky, and New York City. Clinical data are given in Table 19.5. Five had occupationally related disease. The others tended to be older and to have widespread dermatitis. Only 12 reacted to formaldehyde (1% aq). Twelve also reacted to formaldehyde-related preservatives. Ethylene urea melamine formaldehyde resin (Fixopret AC) (10% pet) was the best screening agent, with

---

TABLE 19.5. *Clinical Patterns of Textile Resin ACD*

Patients tend to be older, with no gender predilection
Face, hand, feet usually spared unless allergic also to formaldehyde-releasing preservatives (FRPs)
Frequent reaction to FRPs (especially quaternium-15)
About 30% negative to formaldehyde alone
Areas of tight clothing (e.g., waist, shoulders, thighs) usually the worst
May go misdiagnosed as scabies, neurodermatitis, etc., for months or years
Itching generally severe

---

14 positives (82%). The authors theorized that a trend toward using imported textiles, even if the finished garment is made in the United States, may account for this upsurge in cases. Alternatively, cases of generalized dermatitis may have previously gone unrecognized as being caused by textile resins. A lack of suspicion of textile allergy may lead to inappropriate withholding of patch testing. Even if patch testing is done, some patients who are formaldehyde negative may be missed on limited screening.

Sherertz (72) reported that 10 of 11 patients with clothing allergy to formaldehyde compounds reacted to urea formaldehyde resin, but only 8 reacted to formaldehyde 1% aq.

In addition to dermatitis, formaldehyde can cause urticaria (73). One case of severe contact urticaria associated with formaldehyde used in leather dresses has been reported from Finland (74).

Consequences of Durable-Press Allergic Contact Dermatitis

If a person is sensitized to *N*-methylol fabric finishing compound and not to formaldehyde itself, simple avoidance of the guilty fabrics should bring relief (65,67–69). When formaldehyde allergy is at the root of the problem, however, the consequences can be more far-reaching. Formaldehyde-sensitive people, for example, can react to a whole series of formaldehyde donors that are used as biocides both in cosmetics and in industry (75–77).

In 1977 and 1979, Raugi and Storrs identified 18 patients who were allergic to quaternium-15 (Q-15, a formaldehyde donor) (S Raugi and FJ Storrs, unpublished results of a presentation to the International Contact Dermatitis Congress, March 29, 1980). Seventeen of these patients were allergic to formaldehyde. Eleven of the 18 patients had positive patch test reactions to melamine formaldehyde (MF), six to dimethylolpropylene urea (DMPU), five to dimethylol carbamates (DMC), and one to DMDHEU. Seven of the 18 patients had a clothing pattern distribution to their dermatitis. They also had relevant clinical dermatitis to Q-15, which preserved cosmetics that they were using.

The decrease in the incidence of formaldehyde allergy in Japan coincident with restrictions on its use has been noted. The North American Contact Dermatitis Group (NACDG) has noted an increase in formaldehyde allergy from 3.4% in 1972 to 1974 to 6.7% in 1980 and 1991 to 9.3 % in 1998 (78,79). Most of this increase was attributed to formaldehyde releasers in cosmetics. A review of the incidence of positive reactors to various allergens around the world gives formaldehyde ratings from 1.3% (Spain) to 7.0% (Japan in 1976) (78). Most Western countries show reaction rates of between 4% and 5% for formaldehyde (78,80,81).

Jordan et al. (82) identified patients who gave allergic responses to aqueous formaldehyde patch tests in concentrations as low as 30 ppm (0.003%). One of their patients could predictably identify (by the development of itching without an observable skin reaction) solutions sprayed into his axilla containing 30 ppm of formaldehyde. No lower concentrations were tested, but Jordan has theorized that sensitive formaldehyde-allergic people might itch without urtication or eczematization from even lower concentrations (WP Jordan, personal communication, 1984).

How does all of this relate to durable-press-type dermatitis? We occasionally encounter patients who insist that they cannot tolerate synthetic blended fabrics on their skin. Fisher (83) encountered four such men whom he labeled as having the "pants paresthesia syndrome." Unsolved suspect fabric dermatitis patients riddle our practices and the dermatologic literature (84,85).

> **Some patients complain of burning, itching, and paresthesia when wearing synthetic fabrics. They present no dermatitis or patch test reaction.**

If one has a clear understanding of how fabrics are processed, it is possible to construct sensible management plans for these patients whose complaints are real but whose difficulty cannot always be proven with a positive patch test, because of the vicissitudes of that diagnostic method.

Patch Testing for Durable-Press Allergy

Although formaldehyde identifies about 70% of people who are allergic to fabric-finishing *N*-methylol resins, it is obvious from the foregoing discussion that some people will be missed if the resins are not tested as well. The fabric is often negative on testing, but it should be included anyway for possible confirmation and to exclude a dye allergy (1). Soaking the fabric in water for 10 minutes before it is applied may produce more positive reactions. Additionally, extraction techniques using solvents such as acetone, methyl ethyl ketone, ethyl alcohol, and pentoxol have been useful in extracting allergens from fabrics when water soaking alone gave negative results (86). Fisher (12) found that butyrolactone may be substituted for any of these solvents.

Patch testing with the substances identified in Table 19.6 detects most allergic contact dermatitis caused by durable-press finishes. Positive reactions are often negative at 48 hours and may not develop until the fifth or seventh day (77,87). Currently, the NACDG uses ethyleneurea melamine formaldehyde resin 5% pet as a screening agent for textile allergy. Scheman et al. (88) recommend dimethyloldihydroxy ethylene urea, however.

In most centers formaldehyde is tested at 1% aq. Fowler has seen cases not infrequently of negative reactions to 1% but definite, relevant positives to 2% aq. Therefore, if formaldehyde allergy is strongly suspected, testing should be done with both 1% and 2% concentrations. Conversely,

TABLE 19.6. *Patch Testing for Textile Resin Allergy*

Formaldehyde[a]	1% or 2% aq
Urea formaldehyde resin	10% pet
Ethyleneurea melamineformaldehyde resin[a]	5% pet
Tetramethylol acetylenediurea formaldehyde resin	5% pet
Dimethylol dihydroxyethylene urea formaldehyde resin	5% aq
Dimethylolpropylene urea formaldehyde resin	5% pet

[a]Best two for screening.

the physician must remember that 2% and occasionally 1% formaldehyde may give a mild irritant reaction. This usually appears as a "glazed" appearance at the site with very mild erythema but without induration or papules. This irritant reaction is not indicative of allergy.

Methods for Detecting Formaldehyde in Textiles

Various methods have been used in the past to determine free formaldehyde release from fabrics. Since 1960, the American Association of Textile Chemists and Colorists' (AATCC) method 112 has been the most popular (52). AATCC-112 measures the formaldehyde released as a vapor from a fabric stored over water for 20 hours at 49°C. Because old methods may have measured formaldehyde release differently, one must compare older reports or ones using non-AATCC-112 methods qualitatively rather than quantitatively.

Such analyses done in 1960 showed 3,900 to 6,200 ppm of formaldehyde released from various resin-treated fabrics. This could be reduced to 1,500 to 3,500 ppm by an afterwash (49). Schorr et al. (89) looked at 112 randomly selected American fabrics in 1974. The treating resin used was not determined, but in general the authors verified that finished cellulose and blends could release up to 3,600 ppm of formaldehyde by the chromotropic acid method. One hundred percent synthetics released 1 to 2 ppm of formaldehyde, which could well have been from biocides in the softeners used on their surfaces.

In yet another refinement, some finishers are employing a fog chamber technique that sprays formaldehyde acceptors or binders ("cappers" or "scavengers") such as ethyleneurea, oxazolidinone, pyrrolidone, propyleneurea, urea, or carbohydrazide onto the fabric immediately after the resin treatment (53,56,90). Using such a scheme, formaldehyde release with the AATCC-112 method is between 0 and 30 ppm (53). The fog method is valuable in that formaldehyde has been shown to migrate into untreated fabrics that are stored with treated fabrics (52). Lowering the formaldehyde-releasing ability of treated fabrics greatly reduces formaldehyde migration.

It can be useful to determine that formaldehyde is in fact present in a substance or fabric. This is of special value when a patient is patch test positive to formaldehyde but negative to the fabric. Such detection methods have shown, for example, that formaldehyde can be present as an occult ingredient in corticosteroid creams or even in cream bases packaged in containers coated by a formaldehyde-containing resin (90,91). Small amounts of formaldehyde present in creams or fabrics may thus play little role in initiating a formaldehyde allergy, but they could contribute to the maintenance of a dermatitis in a previously sensitized person.

Methods that have been used to detect the presence of formaldehyde in fabrics and various cosmetic preparations rely largely on the detection of reducing substances and are not absolutely specific for formaldehyde. The most specific method for formaldehyde is the chromotropic acid test developed by E. Eegriwe in 1937 and modified for textile use by Hovding (10,60). Dahlquist et al. (92) felt that this office procedure modification is not completely specific for formaldehyde. Dahlquist et al. (90) saw false-negative reactions to it. The test detects formaldehyde in a 1:100 solution (60).

> **Several chemical tests are available to determine the presence of formaldehyde in fabrics.**

Chromotropic Acid (4,5-Dihydroxy-2,7-Naphthalenedisulfonic Acid) Methods

1. Bring a 1-cm square sample of fabric to boil in 5 ml of distilled water in a test tube.
2. Let stand for 5 minutes.
3. Add 1 drop of the cooled supernatant to 2 ml of 72% (concentrated) sulfuric acid that contains a few crystals of chromotropic acid.
4. Heat the mixture gently over a flame. An intense red-purple to violet color indicates a positive test (1,10, 60,62,93).

Clinitest Reagent Tablets

1. Soak a small piece (1 sq cm) of suspect fabric in 5 ml of water for 24 hours.
2. Add 1 ml of the supernatant to 1 Clinitest tablet.
3. Any color change in the direction of orange (as diagrammed on the Clinitest container) indicates the presence of formaldehyde.

Miles Laboratory does not recommend this particular adaptation of the Clinitest tablet. However, in a 1980 personal communication, the company verfiied that its data would indicate that using the Clinitest tablet with 1 ml of solution will detect 0.025% formalin in saline.

Numerous other qualitative tests are used to detect formaldehyde (10). When these tests are applied to textiles, controls should always be run, because their results are less predictable than are those with the chromotropic acid and Schiff's aldehyde tests. Another test for formaldehyde, the acetylacetone test, is given in Chapter 17.

Management of Clothing Dermatitis Associated with Permanent-Press Finishes Likely to Release Formaldehyde

These patients are some of the most miserable contact allergy sufferers because of the ubiquitous exposure to the allergens. Often systemic corticosteroids are required for temporary palliation. Even after good efforts at allergen avoidance, some individuals may require several months to completely clear. Counseling and encouragement are especially critical at this stage. Other systemic therapy such as PUVA or immunosuppressive agents may be necessary in some cases of formaldehyde dermatitis.

Table 19.7 lists several instructions for formaldehyde- or textile resin–allergic patients.

Wearing an undergarment made of cotton or silk may allow formaldehyde and formaldehyde-resin-sensitive people to wear treated clothing temporarily. Fowler found silk to be better for this purpose. Cool weather also allows sensitive people to wear treated clothing that they cannot tolerate when they are sweating in hot weather.

Dermatitis from Textile Additives Other Than Durable-Press Finishes

Numerous chemicals other than cross-linking durable-press finishes are applied to textiles to alter the fabrics' "hand" and to impart special characteristics. These include softeners, weighters, acrylic and vinyl hand modifiers, water repellents, biocides, antistats, soil retardants, mothproofers, antislip finishes, and fire retardants. Once clothing is manufactured, it may be treated with spot removers and dry-cleaning agents.

TABLE 19.7. *Instructions for Formaldehyde Resin Patients*

1. Avoid permanent-press, wrinkle-resistant clothing and bed linens as much as possible. If necessary to wear such garments, wear only cool, loose-fitting items for short time periods. Perspiration and heat make the problem worse.
2. Wash *all* new textile products, permanent-press or not, at least twice before using.
3. Soft, easily wrinkled fabrics are safest. Avoid heavy, stiff fabrics.
4. Most blended fabrics (e.g., polyester-cotton) are likely to be treated with resins and should generally be avoided.
5. Silk, linen, wool, denim, and pure nylon are unlikely to be treated and are almost always safe.
6. Rayon blends, corduroy, and "shrink-proof" wool should be avoided.
7. Cotton that is mercerized or sanforized is safe because these finishes do not use formaldehyde.

Descriptions of compounds used for these purposes can be found in the December 1973 issue of *Textile World* and in the American Association of Textile Chemists and Colorists's annual *Buyer's Guide* (58,94) (Table 19.4).

Foussereau et al. (95) found that allergy to alpha-phenylindole explained a dermatitis to American oilcloth in 11 of 18 patients whom they studied. Twenty patients reacted to the entire cloth. This report highlights the fact that although they are most unusual, chemicals other than formaldehyde-releasing fabric finishes are used on fabrics and should, on occasion, be considered when evaluating a baffling case of clothing-related dermatitis.

Softeners

Anionic, cationic, and nonionic softeners are used to modify fabric stiffness. Sulfated natural oils and fatty esters (anionic); fatty acid–diethanolamine condensates, quaternary ammonium salts, and cetyl trimethyl bromide (cationic); ethylene oxide condensates (poly-oxyethylene derivatives); and oleic-acid alcohols and esters (nonionic) all exemplify such softeners. Occasionally, these softeners are preserved with formaldehyde or formaldehyde-releasing preservatives, at very low concentration, probably too low to cause dermatitis. The softener is added to a finishing bath, and modern fabric finishing does not employ afterwashes. Nonetheless, any un-cross-linked formaldehyde preservative remaining in the cloth would be eliminated in the first home wash.

Fabric softeners can also be added to apparel in the home. This is often done during a rinse cycle or in the dryer. Nonwoven fabric strips are impregnated with softening agents and perfume and are added to the dryer tub. Dialkyl-dimethyl ammonium methyl sulfate (DADMAMS), also used in liquid fabric softeners, and a fatty acid ester of a polyhydric alcohol are two softeners that have been added to a popular sheet softener that can be included in home dryers (96). Some dermatologists believe that such heavily scented softening sheets have caused a follicular dermatitis in their patients. Such an association has not been proved, however, as either an irritant or an allergic event.

> **Many textile additives are rare sensitizers. These additives include softeners, weighters, water repellents, biocides, antistatic agents, lubricants, mothproofers, and antislip finishes.**

Weighters

Stannous chloride, sodium, magnesium, calcium, and barium sulfate may all be added to backfill and weight cotton, silk, and polyesters. Knit goods are sold by the pound rather than the yard, which explains the value of these weighters.

Acrylic and Vinyl Hand Alteres and Latices

Polyvinyl acetate and alcohol are used occasionally to finish silk and some synthetics. Polyvinyl chloride is a coating medium for some upholstery and acrylic polymers, and it can modify the hand of textiles. Lattices, based on natural and synthetic rubbers, are used as backing compounds. Butadiene-styrene, polychloroprene, polyisobutylene, and butadiene-acrylonitrile are examples of compounds used for lattices.

Water Repellents

Paraffin wax and aluminum or zirconium salt emulsions are used as water repellents. Fluorocarbon combined with stearomidomethyl pyridinium chloride, melamine, stearamide, and organosilicon compounds are also used. Melamine and urea formaldehyde resins in combination with any of the aforementioned substances can also increase water repellency.

Isophoronediamine (IPDA), used as an epoxy resin hardener, caused occupational ACD in a worker using it to manufacture water-resistant fabric (97). The cloth was intended for use in hospital garments and drapes where blood and water resistance was needed.

Biocides

Biocides are used to inhibit mildew growth and thus prevent the rotting of fabrics likely to be used outside. Tributyl tin, copper-8-quinolate, zinc naphthenate, organomercury compounds, quaternary ammonium compounds, phenols and chlorophenols, zinc dimethyl dithiocarbamate, zinc-2-mercaptobenzothiazole, and even neomycin have all been used as biocides on textiles in the United States. Fregert (98) listed additional textile antimicrobial agents that include carbanilides and salicylanilides in addition to those mentioned above. In the United States, the Environmental Protection Agency closely regulates the use of organomercury compounds.

Fabrics used by the military and canvas fabrics likely to be used for outdoor recreational use may well contain biocides. Molin and Wahlberg (99) reported 70 soldiers who developed an irritant dermatitis on their feet when tribrityltin oxide was used in excess to disinfect their socks. Fisher (personal communication, 1984) reported an allergic contact dermatitis to Triclosan (Irgasan DP 300) used as a fungicide in "Odor Eater" socks by Burlington. Chloracetamide has caused foot dermatitis from its use as an antimicrobial agent in shoe insoles.

Spin Finishes

Biocides can also be used in spin finishes, which are complex aqueous emulsions of oils, waxes, surfactants, and biocides used on synthetic fibers to reduce friction and static. Savage (100) suggested but did not prove that methylol chloracetamide (Grotan HD) caused an allergic hand dermatitis in seven nylon yarn workers who used a nylon spin finish. Burrows and Campbell (101) felt that the ten dermatitis patients whom they saw who developed problems after polyester spin finish exposure had an irritant rather than an allergic contact dermatitis. Their patients' patch test reactions were equivocal. Methylene bisthiocyanate, mixed halogenated amides, N-methylolchloraretamide, and dimethoxane were the biocides used in the spin finishes that they studied. An isothiazolone biocide (Kathon 930) caused hand dermatitis in eight textile workers. The substance was used in a finishing rinse. Interestingly, the patients did not cross-react to Kathon CG (102). In most instances, biocides are added to fabric-finishing compounds in concentrations so low that even patients who are sensitive to a particular chemical have no problem with fabrics so treated (103).

An English textile worker developed ACD from the biocide N,N'-methylene bis-5-methyloxazolidine, used in a nylon spin finish. Testing was positive at 1% aq. This is a formaldehyde-releaser also known as Grotan OX. This patient was not allergic to formaldehyde (28).

Antistatic Agents

Polyethylene glycol and ethylene oxide condensates, as well as polyethylene glycolacrylic esters and iodides, provide antistatic properties in textiles.

Lubricants

Polyalkylene glycol, castor oil, and polyethylene glycols are all used as lubricants on fabric surfaces. Gaul (104) suggested that stearyl and cetyl alcohols, which can be textile lubricants, may have caused an urticaria-like dermatitis in a woman who was working with a green tenting canvas.

Mothproofers

The clothes moth, *Tineola bisselliella,* causes significant damage to clothing. Naphthalene, paradichlorobenzene, and silicofluorides are used as nondurable mothproofers in the United States. Phenyl sulfonic acid derivatives, such as 2,2'-dihydroxy-3,5,3''-tetrachlorotriphenyl methane-2 sulfonic acid, have more durable mothproofing qualities.

Antislip Finishes

Rosin emulsions, colloidal silica, and alumina are nondurable finishes, whereas thermosetting resins, resin-rosin combinations, protein-rosin mixtures, and lattices give more durable antislip finishes.

Soil Retardants and Stain Repellents

Antistatic compounds help reduce soiling. Colloidal alumina, titanium alkylates, methyl and ethyl silica, and fatty alcohol–ethylene oxide condensates also assist in the removal of stains. One patient has been described who had an apparent allergic reaction to Scotchgard, which contained a fluorocarbon, acrylates, and rubber materials. The sensitizer was not identified (105).

Antipill Finish

The tendency of some fabric to produce tiny balls on the surface with friction or wear is called "pilling." An antipill finish, Evafanol-AS-1, containing 1,6-diisocyanatohexane, caused dermatitis in 11 workers at two factories making dresses. This constituted 10% of the workforce. Testing was done at 1% aq strength. Another name for this agent is hexamethylene diisocyanate (106).

Miscellaneous Sources of Potential Allergy and Irritation in Clothing

Detergents

Patients frequently complain that a laundry detergent has caused skin irritation. Often the first thing that is changed in the household when someone develops a dermatitis is the laundry detergent. True rates of allergic or irritant reactions, however, have never been studied and would be very difficult to document. A report from Great Britain discussed 98 patients with a facial rash that occurred while staying at a holiday resort (107). The "attack rate" was 7.0 to 14.2 per 1,000 visitors, depending on the site of the accommodations. Replacement of washed bed linens with new ones resulted in total clearing with no new cases. The author concluded that the "rash" was due to irritation from detergent retained in poorly rinsed linens. Rothenborg and Hjorth (108) found that three-fourths of their perfume-sensitive patients reacted to benzyl salicylate, which is a common detergent perfume ingredient. These patients usually had extremity dermatitis. Enzymes derived from *Bacillus subtilis* are used in detergents. Although they cause irritant dermatitis and respiratory problems in manufacturers, neither irritant nor allergic reactions attributed to the wearing of clothing washed in these products has been proved with certainty (109,110).

Metals

There is probably too little nickel or chrome in detergents produced in the United States to perpetuate a clothing-distributed dermatitis in a nickel- or chrome-sensitive person (1,111). On the other hand, nickel-containing buttons, buckles, snaps, and so on, have become a common cause of dermatitis. Aluminum-containing fibers have caused no known difficulty.

Epoxies

Taylor et al. (112) described three boys who developed an allergic contact dermatitis on their knees that was caused by an epoxy resin (Epon 825) used as a knee-patch adhesive constituent. Epoxies are seldom if ever used now as part of the durable-press finishing of fabrics, although they had some use in the past. Fowler has seen cases of epoxy allergy in workers handling canvas tent fabric, with documentation of the presence of epoxy resin in the fabric.

Textile Allergens

Soni and Sherertz (113) evaluated 72 textile workers over a 5-year period with possible occupational contact dermatitis. Almost three-fourths had work-related ICD, ACD, or a combination, with 38% felt to be ICD. Frictional irritation was prominent. Allergens included textile dyes in 12 cases, formaldehyde finishes in 11, and rubber allergens in 10. The hands were the primary site of involvement, with hand dermatitis found in 82% of those with work-related dermatitis.

Thiourea derivatives have caused allergy in workers handling diazo paper used for patterns (114).

Flame Retardants

Some fabrics such as brushed nylon and wool have an innate flame resistance (6). Polyvinyl chloride fiber and to some extent the modacrylics are flameproof as well (6). Glass and carbon fibers also resist fire but are inherently unsuitable for apparel. An emulsion of polyvinyl chloride with added polyvinyl alcohol can be spun into a blend known as Polychial or Cordelan. It is a Japanese fiber that is flameproof and soft to handle (6). The extent of its use in the United States is unknown. Melamineformaldehyde resins also enhance the flame resistance of polyester blends (see Table 19.8).

Nomex is a synthetic polyamide aramid made by DuPont. Nomex 111A is a blend of Nomex, Kevlar, and carbon core nylon with inherent flame resistance. It is said to be unaffected by most bleaches, solvents, and acids. Vinex is another inherently flame-resistant fabric made of Vinal (a polyvinylalcohol-treated polymer) and polynosic (115).

Flame-retardant chemicals are used in textiles, carpets, home furnishings, plastics, paints, adhesives, and construction materials. In 1977, an estimated 310 million to 360 million pounds of all types of flame-retardant chemicals was used (116,117). Most of this was aluminum oxide used on carpets. Only 3 million to 4 million pounds was used for textiles. Those flame retardants added to textiles can account for 10% to 20% of the weight of the fabric (117). A flame retardant composed of 23-bromocresylglycidyl ether caused severe ACD in a worker after an accidental exposure. It is uncertain whether this is used on textiles (118).

Over 150 flame retardants are available for textile use. Nondurable chemicals are inorganic, water-soluble salts and are not used on clothing. Durable flame retardants used on wearing apparel resist laundering and dry cleaning (116).

Durable flame-retardant chemicals contain phosphorus, nitrogen, chlorine, or bromine. Flame retardants decrease flammability by favoring charring as well as by facilitating the snuffing of a flame in their volatile phase. The major textile flame-retardant chemicals are described in Table 19.8 (116,119).

Many of the flame-retardant chemicals were introduced to meet various federal flammability requirements, beginning with the Flammable Fabrics Act of 1953 (amended in 1967). Some children's sleepwear flammability standards were modified in 1977 in such a way that it was no longer necessary for manufacturers to use a group of chemicals that had been identified as potentially hazardous toxins and carcinogens (M Neilly, Consumer Product Safety Commission, personal communication, 1984) (120). In 1984, most children's sleepwear was made from synthetic fibers that rely on their inherent flame-retardant qualities to meet federal flammability standards. In late 1982 and 1983, some American flannel that was sold for children's sleepwear was again treated with Tetrakis compounds (West Tex, personal communication, 1984) (Table 19.8).

In 1977, the use of TRIS (Tris [2,3-dibromopropyl] phosphate) was banned after it was found to be a bacterial mutagen and an animal carcinogen in rats and mice (116,117,121,122). This ban was overturned subsequently, but its use has been reduced nonetheless.

In 1983, the polybrominated biphenyls were also identified as animal carcinogens, and their use was discontinued as well (123). Subsequently, Tris (1,3-dichloroisopropyl) phosphate (Fyrol FR-2) and the cyclic phosphonate esters (Antiblaze 19) were withdrawn by the industry (116).

The present situation with regard to flame-retardant use in synthetic fabrics is unclear. Toxicologic data and especially carcinogenesis studies are deficient or absent from the literature for most chemicals, and thus manufacturers are hesitant to use expensive and potentially hazardous substances on clothing for daily human use. Those chemicals that have not been withdrawn still find use in plastics and in some specialized industrial or military clothing (Table 19.8) (116).

Most children's sleepwear no longer contains specific chemicals but relies on synthetic fibers (i.e., polyesters), which are inherently flame-resistant.

TABLE 19.8. *Major Flame-Retardant Chemicals Used on Textiles*

Common or trade name	Chemical name	Withdrawn by industry	Textile use	Comment
Tris	Tris (2,3-dibromopropyl)	Yes	Polyester and acetates	Contact sensitization reported; animal carcinogen
Fyrol FR-2	Tris (1,3-dichloroisopropyl)	Yes	Polyester	May be used on polyurethane foams; chromosome aberrations reported
Caliban FR-2 P-53 (DBDPO) Caliban F/R P-44 (DBDPO and antimony trioxide)	Decabromodiphenyl oxide (DBDPO)	No	Polyester	Usually used in combinations with antimony trioxide (caliban F/R P-44). Second most often used flame retardant in United States. Some hepatotoxicity, and some use in plastics
Antiblaxe 19	Cyclic phosphate esters	Yes	Polyester	Used in plastics; toxicology incomplete
Fryol CEF	Tris (2-chloroethyl)	No (seldom used)	Polyesters and acetates	Carcinogenesis is questioned
Fryol 76	Condensate of bis (betachloroethyl) phosphate and alkyl phosphonate	No (seldom used)	Cotton and rayon	May be mutagenic
Pyrovatex CP	N-methylol dimethylphosphonopropionamide	No (seldom used)	Cotton and rayon	Formaldehyde releaser; toxicity studies are in complete and indecisive; reacts with cellulose
Tetrakis (hydroxymethyl) THCPL	Tetrakis (hydroxymethyl) phosphonium chloride	No (popular)	Cotton and rayon	Finished fabric may have up to 500 ppm of formaldehyde on surface
Tetrakis (hydroxymethyl) phosphonium sulfate (THPCS) THPCL or THPCS	Tetrakis (hydroxymethyl) phosphonium sulfate			Cross-links with itself within cellulose and removed with difficulty. THPCL and THPCS used interchangeably. Proban form usually used. Toxicity data incomplete.
plus urea and ammonia = proban				Some use in children's sleepwear. Most frequently used flame retardant in United States

This table was prepared with help from the flame-retardant industry and with special reference to Refs. 116 and 119. It was prepared by Frances Storrs MD for the 3rd edition.

Although TRIS-treated fabrics are presumably no longer used in the United States, it was estimated that prior to 1977 almost 10 million pounds of TRIS was used annually in a variety of products (116). Despite its wide use, only one possible instance of allergic contact dermatitis caused by its presence in protective industrial clothing has been described (124). A second patient who had a positive patch test reaction to TRIS (5% pet) was probably actually sensitized to a related phosphate ester present in her spectacle frames (124). Andersen (124) observed a 46-year-old woman with spectacle frame dermatitis. She had positive patch test results to the dyed plastic frame but not to the sidebars. Supplementary patch tests showed positive reactions to tricresyl phosphate, phenolformaldehyde resin, and a phosphate ester used in Firemaster flame-retardant compounds from Michigan Chemical Corporation consisting of halogenated phosphate esters. Liquid Firemaster caused delayed hypersensitivity maximization test results in human subjects and is classified as a weak to mild sensitizer. Sensitized persons could have reactions to fabrics containing this flame retardant. TRIS is capable of sensitizing humans, and people so sensitized react positively to patch tests with TRIS-treated fabrics (125).

Another flame retardant that has been indicted as a relevant contact allergen is Proban, a polymer produced by cross-linking the condensate of tetrakis (hydroxymethyl) phosphonium chloride (THPCL) and urea with ammonia followed by oxidation (126). Proban-induced dermatitis and urticaria were suspected by Martin-Scott (126) in two children who gave positive patch test reactions to Proban-treated fabric. They were not tested to Proban itself.

The International Contact Dermatitis Research Group included Firemaster LVT 23P in 5% pet in its standard series of patch tests for a limited period of time to determine the incidence of sensitization against Firemaster. Of 1,103 individuals tested, 2 showed a positive response (Maibach H, personal communication, 1986).

Belsito (127) reported 12 patients with ACD from diammonium hydrogen phosphate (DAP) used as a flame retardant in hospital surgical caps. The 100% rayon caps apparently had excessive levels of DAP. Patch testing was done with DAP (0.5% aq).

If the tetrakis phosphonium compounds are applied to cotton or rayon fabrics in their hydroxide form, they react within cellulose to form firm covalent cross-links with themselves. Commercial THPCL has been reported to contain free formaldehyde, and formaldehyde can be recovered from extracts of fabrics that have been cross-linked with THPCL (116,117). One of Martin-Scott's (126) two fabric-positive patients were also formaldehyde patch test positive.

Manufacturers of flame-retardant fabrics indicate that free formaldehyde may be found on the surface of such textiles in concentrations of up to 500 ppm. This is especially true of tetrakis compounds but may occur with other treated fabrics as well (Table 19.8). This formaldehyde is not cross-linked within the cellulosics, and the flame-retardant industry feels that it washes out readily. Information from Westex Inc. indicates that its flame-resistant fabric treatments, Indurn and Proban FR, contain formaldehyde, usually at levels below 0.05% (128).

In 1993, according to Dr. Bernard Miller (personal communication, Textile Research Institute), the textile industry was not actively researching flame retardants because phosphorous-containing compounds had proved satisfactory.

Dry-Cleaning Preparations

The chemicals used in dry cleaning are irritants but are probably only rare allergens. Perchloroethylene (tetrachloroethylene) is used for most closed-machine dry cleaning (1). Vail (129) reported a metalworker who had a 48-hour positive patch test reaction to 1% perchloroethylene in olive oil. Six cases of textile dermatitis were reported in a semiconductor manufacturing facility. The problem was traced to high residual levels of perchloroethylene in dry-cleaned uniform coats. The dermatitis produced was probably irritant rather than allergic contact (130). Other commonly used dry-cleaning compounds include trifluorotrichloroethane (Arklone and Valclene) and trichloroethylene (Trilene). Chloroform, acetone, alcohol, benzene, naphtha, turpentine, carbon tetrachloride, gasoline, kerosene, and ether may also find limited use (12). Their inherent toxicity and flammability make them less valuable. All of these dry-cleaning compounds are irritating and volatile. If garments are properly aired before being worn, they should cause no difficulty.

A Japanese report described three patients with bullous dermatitis, presumed to be irritant, from dry-cleaned clothing. The cleaning agent not perchloroethylene but rather was a "petrolatum solvent" composed of paraffins or paraffin plus naphtens (131).

Garments are "retexed" occasionally in a dry-cleaning establishment. The waxes (paraffin or carnauba), silicones, and rarely lanolin and polyterpene and coumarine-indene resins are used for this purpose (1).

> **Dry-cleaning preparations are usually irritant solvents that are rare sensitizers.**

Spot Removers

Powerful skin irritants such as hydrofluoric acid, glacial acetic acid, carbolic acid, nitrobenzene, and strong alkalis can also find occasional use as spot removers. Van Ketel (132) described two women employees in the clothing industry who developed hand dermatitis while working with stain removers containing hydrazine. They both had positive patch test reactions to hydrazine sulfate 1% in H_2O. They were of special interest in that they showed cross-reactivity to other hydrazine derivatives such as apresoline, phenylhydrazine-HCl, and isoniazid.

Hydrazine "spot" removers may be sensitizers that cross-react with apresoline and isoniazid.

Dyes

Natural fibers have been dyed by people for thousands of years. Natural indigo was known in several parts of the world by 2000 B.C. (133). Billions of yards of natural and synthetic fibers have been colored with a vast array of dyes. Considering the daily exposure to vast numbers of dyes, there are relatively few reports of dye allergy.

As more synthetic fibers were developed in the 1930s and 1950s (Table 19.1), dye technology became more complex in an effort to meet new fiber requirements. Nylon stockings were introduced into the United States in 1939, and shortly thereafter contact dermatitis caused by nylon stocking dyes was reported. Although this problem is much less prevalent now, even at its height, its incidence was estimated to be no more than one case of dermatitis for every 13,309,000 pairs of nylon stockings sold (134).

Textile dye chemistry classification is extraordinarily complex. One must have some familiarity with this nomenclature and with standard sources of dye information in order to approach the rare problem of dye-contact dermatitis at all. Even when a dye can be implicated causally in any one case of allergic contact dermatitis, the already frustrated dermatologist is further dismayed to learn that a garment's final color may be determined by a dye constructed from a whole array of different colored dyes (135). Only the most dogged of investigators is able to trace one dye to one garment. Advising our dye-sensitive patients may seem futile. Despite this seemingly bleak picture, some practical generalizations can be made if we examine how modern fabrics are colored.

"Chemical" Classification

Foussereau et al. (136) break the dyes used for coloring oils, greases, waxes, paints, plastics, soaps, solvents, and textiles into the following chemical groups:

- nitroso compounds
- nitro compounds
- azoic dyes (40% of all textile dyes are azo dyes with the chromophore wQN;wRN. Cross-reactivity with paraphenylenediamine is common)
- insoluble azoics (combination of a diazo compound or diazonium salt with a coupling component inside the fiber)
- stilbene derivatives (optical brighteners used in detergents and on fabrics are usually stilbenes)
- anthraquinone dyes (used in many different textile dye classes such as pigments, acids, mordants, disperse, vats, and reactives)
- indigoids (usually vat dyes)

- diphenylmethane derivatives
- triphenylmethane derivatives
- xanthene dyes
- acridines
- cyanines
- thiazole derivatives
- indamines and indophenols
- azines (cationic dyes that are among the oldest synthetic dyes; azine derivatives can be used for dyeing in gray and black on cellulosics, furs, and hair)
- oxazines
- thiazines
- sulfur dyes (some use for dyeing work clothes, especially black)
- amino and hydro xyketones
- phthalocyanines
- quinolines

Tracing an allergy to any one of these chemical groups may be most difficult in that coupling agents or precursors may be the actual culprit, particularly in the textile industry. Clothing allergy, however, is usually caused by the final reaction product. The chemical textile classes most likely to cause allergic contact dermatitis include azoics, anthraquinones, indigoids, insoluble azoics, stilbenes, and triphenylmethanes.

Azo dyes, which comprise 40% of all textile dyes, may cross-react with paraphenylenediamine and are among the most common causes of allergic textile dye dermatitis.

The work by Cywie et al. (137) describes allergic contact dermatitis in the textile industry from a chemical viewpoint. Of the 62 dyes described in this report, 41 are of the azo type. Dyes were found to be the main cause of allergic dermatitis associated with textiles. Another excellent review was published by Hatch and Maibach (138) in 1995.

Some three thousand chemicals are now used in the textile industry; of these, 1,200 are dyes or pigments (135). Most of the dyes now available that can be used for coloring textiles are compiled in the *Colour Index,* which is a seven-volume encyclopedic reference work published jointly by the American Association of Textile Chemists and Colorists (AATCC) (Table 19.4) and the British Society of Dyers and Colourists (139). It lists over three thousand dyes and pigments manufactured for use in textiles, paints, paper, foods, and leather, together with their published chemical formulas, if available. Unfortunately, not all textile dyes are listed in the *Colour Index.*

The *Colour Index* (C.I.) describes dyes according to their chemical class. It assigns them a generic name and number (refers to their textile use) (see the following) and a specific C.I. number (refers to their chemical constitution).

Chemical formulas, uses, dyeing methods, fastness properties, and a verbal description of the dye's actual color are available in the *Colour Index.*

For example, by consulting the *Colour Index,* one learns that there are many "Acid Blues." One of them, Acid Blue 40 (generic name and number), has a chemical constitution number of 62125. (The generic numbers are short and the chemical constitution numbers long.) Acid Blue 40 is an anthraquinone. Using the *Colour Index,* you could examine its structure; learn its chemical name (1-amino-4-bromo-2 anthraquinonesulfonic acid); discover its chemical properties and its use for dyeing cellulose, acetates, nylon, and silk; and determine that it is really more green than blue.

The AATCC also publishes the *Buyer's Guide* (94). This publication arranges the 1,700 dyes available in the United States to color paper, leather, foods, and textiles according to their trade names, as well as their *Colour Index* generic names. C.I. chemical constitution numbers are often available as well. One dye may have 1 to 30 trade names, depending on the number of manufacturers who provide it. Needless to say, this further confuses an already confusing situation when C.I. Direct Red 111 (no chemical constitution number) is sold only as Pyrazol Fast Brown, whereas Direct Blue 86 (C.I. 74180) can be sold by 26 different trade names, including Carta Turquoise and Solophenyl Turquoise Blue GL Supra. Fortunately, the names, addresses, and phone numbers of the participating U.S. firms are also provided in the *Buyer's Guide.* We have often found that a phone call to a manufacturer may provide helpful background information.

Textile Use Classification

Dye chemists and dyers often prefer to classify dyes according to the procedures involved in applying dyes to the textile materials rather than by their chemical constitution. One "use" category may comprise several different chemical classes.

The classes of dyes used by the *Buyer's Guide* include (94):

acid dyes
azoic compositions
azoic coupling components
azoic diazo components
basic dyes
direct dyes
disperse dyes
fluorescent brightening agents
leuco sulfur dyes
mordant dyes
pigments
reactive dyes
solvent dyes
sulfur dyes
vat dyes

> **Vat dyes are water soluble and hypoallergenic and are used frequently on cellulose (cotton). Disperse dyes are water insoluble and may include azo and anthraquinones, which are suspended by dispersing agents to synthetic fabrics.**

Wick, in Foussereau et al. (136), and Jenkins (133) classified dyes by their textile use in a different manner. They combined their analyses and classifications with Moncrieff's (6) review for some general comments concerning problems that can be associated with the use of dyes on textiles (see below).

Anionic Dyes

Acid Dyes. These are used to dye wool, silk, and polyamides; they are not very color fast. Some are used as food dyes. Acid dyes accounted for 9% of total textile dyes in 1975. They also are used in home dyeing.

A sulfonic acid salt is present somewhere in the dye. The chromophore (color-imparting group) can come from the azoic, anthraquinone, triphenylmethane, azine, or xanthene chemical classes. The group includes metal colorings (metallic complexes with acid dyes).

Mordant Dyes. These are used on animal fibers. The dye is complexed with a metal, usually chromium or aluminum, and sometimes nickel, cobalt, or manganese. The Clean Water Act of 1956 minimized the use of chrome mordants. Mordant dyes totaled only 0.34% of the synthetic dye market in 1974.

Direct Dyes. Used on cotton, cellulosics, wool, leather, and paper; also used for home dyeing. These dyes are not light fast. Direct dyes may be treated with copper, chrome, or formaldehyde to improve fastness.

Many direct dyes are based on benzidine and benzidine derivatives and as such are potential carcinogens. All brown, green, and probably black dyes used for home dyeing in 1975 contained suspect benzidine dyes.

Basic (Cationic) Dyes

These are used in dyed fur, wool, silk, cotton cellulosics, and polyacrylonitriles; home dyeing; and some food dyes. They come from diphenylmethane, triphenylmethane, xanthene, acridine, azine, oxazine, and thiazine chemical classes. Some azo and anthraquinone dyes are also used (some as medications, e.g., gentian violet). Fluorescent textile dyes are in this group.

Sulfur Dyes

These are used for cotton. Only four sulfur dyes were listed in the 1983 *Buyer's Guide.* They are often used for black colors and work clothes.

Vat Dyes

Used for cellulosics and some wool, so named because of original storage in wooden vats. Vat dyes are applied in a colorless reduced "leuco" form. In the fiber, dye is oxidized to its colored form. Chromophore is a quinoid system from anthraquinones or indigoid chemicals. Vat Blue 1 (C.I. 73000) ("Indigo") is used to color Levi Strauss's 501 "Shrink to Fit" blue jeans. It also is used in surgical sutures as D&C Blue No. 6 and in a sulfonated form in foods and drugs as FD&C Blue No. 2 (Buffalo Color Corporation, 1980, and Levi Strauss & Co., 1983, personal communications).

Reactive Dyes

These are used for cellulose, wool, and polyamides. Covalent bonds are formed between hydroxy groups of cellulose and amino groups of wool and polyamides; they are very color fast. Reactive dyes include azo, anthraquinone, and phthalocyanine chemical classes. They are used for some home batik and tie-dyeing. They can be respiratory irritants.

Pigments. These differ from dyes in that they have no fiber affinity. They are used in textile printing. Pigment is held to fabric with a resin binder (e.g., albumin, casein, glue, methacrylate, phenol and urea formaldehyde, polyvinyl condensates, and styrenemaleic acid resins).

These comprise azoics, phthalocyanins, anthraquinones, indigoids, and triphenylmethane chemical classes. In 1969, 75% of 2 billion yards of printed textiles in the United States used pigment printing.

Dyes Synthesized in the Fiber

Insoluble Azoics. Cellulosics and polyesters can be dyed; they are used extensively in underdeveloped countries. They make bad greens.

A coupling component (e.g., Naphthol AS [3,hydroxide-2, naph-thanilide] [C.I. 37505]) plus a diazonium salt or diazo compound form dye in the fiber. Coupling agents have caused pigmented contact dermatitis (140).

Oxidation Colors (Oxidation Base Dyes). These are used to dye fur, hair, and some cotton. Aromatic amines, diamines, and aminophenols oxidized with hydrogen peroxide are used to color the fiber's interior.

Aniline black has been used since 1863 for umbrella fabric. Paraphenylenediamine and derivatives are incorporated in permanent hair coloring. Compounds are being studied today for carcinogenicity.

Phthalogens. Phthalocyanin dyes

Disperse Dyes (Plastosoluble Dyes)

These are used to dye synthetics, especially polyesters; also used on triacetate polyamides and polyacrylonitriles, in printing, and on plastics. Disperse dyes present as colloidal dispersions; the dye dissolves into the fabric. They come from azoic anthraquinone and nitroarylamine chemical classes. This dye class is the principal source of allergic contact dermatitis.

In general, the following textile dye types are most likely to be used on these fabrics:

1. polyamides—acid dyes, metallic, or disperse dyes
2. polyacrylonitrites—cationic or disperse dyes
3. polyesters—disperse dyes
4. cellulosics—direct basic, vat, reactive, and sulfur dyes
5. uniform and canvas tenting in cellulosic fibers—vat dyes
6. work clothes—sulfur dyes
7. furs—oxidation colors and some basic dyes
8. home dyeing for cellulosics and synthetics—direct, acid, basic, and some reactive dyes

Oxidation base dyes used in dyeing furs seldom, if ever, cause dermatitis because they are fully oxidized. In hair dyeing, these dyes are more of a problem. Unfortunately, many individual dye formulas and compositions of dyes remain trade secrets. Additionally, it is known that dyes and dye precursors may be toxic and on occasion carcinogenic. This is especially true of benzidine and its derivatives, which are used in direct dyes.

Allergic Contact Dermatitis from Textile Dyes in Clothing: Clinical Presentation

Dermatitis caused by fabric dyes can be, but is not always, quite acute (1,2). Half of Cronin's (1) series of 21 women patients had their symptoms for less than 3 months, and only 3 were troubled for more than a year before they sought help. Many patients diagnose themselves in that the distribution of the dermatitis tends to mirror the responsible garment. In women, sparing of skin protected by underclothing is characteristic unless, of course, the guilty dye is in the underwear. Involvement of the axillary borders and sparing of the vault is also typical of shirt or dress dye difficulty. Men and women who have trouser dye dermatitis initially develop problems on their anterior thighs. The posterior thighs and popliteal fossae can be involved as well.

Disperse Dyes

Cronin (1) in 1968 and Hatch and Maibach (141,138) in 1985 and in 1995 reviewed textile dye allergy. Aniline black and red were each reported before 1900 to cause a case of ACD, but most cases appeared after the 1930s. It is difficult to tell from these reports which textile classes were incriminated.

> **Dress or shirt dye dermatitis affects the axillary borders, sparing the vault. Trouser dye dermatitis appears initially on the anterior thighs.**

Historical Data on Dye Allergy

Since the late 1960s, and especially with the advent of the more recent editions of the *Colour Index* (139), reporting of allergy to individual dyes is much more accurate. Cronin's (1) experiences with clothing dermatitis owing to dyes between 1970 and 1976 are documented in her textbook. It is clear from these reviews that almost all of the sensitizing dyes belong to the disperse group and that the azo and anthraquinone dyes in this group sensitize more often. Although disperse dyes were developed for use on synthetic fibers, it is difficult to make them fast to the fiber, which may well relate to their tendency to sensitize.

Among Cronin's (3) 16 original patients, a disperse dye was identified as the sensitizer in 14. Four patients were allergic only to anthraquinone dyes, three only to azo dyes, two to both anthraquinone dyes and azo dyes, and three to dyes of different groups. Cronin also had three patients who had reactions to Disperse Black 1 or 2, which is noteworthy in that sensitivity to black dye is rare. Positive cross-reactions to paraphenylenediamine (PPDA) were found in 85% of Cronin's azo dye–positive patients, whereas such cross-reactivity was all but nonexistent in the other groups. Other authors agree that PPDA alone is not a good screen for dye allergy. Seidenari et al. (142) found only 20 PPDA reactors in 100 patients. Many of his patients were allergic to azo dyes, which theoretically may cross-react with PPDA but apparently did not do so clinically. These findings highlight the inadvisability of relying on a paraphenylenediamine patch test reaction to flag clothing dye contact dermatitis. Cronin's initial series also made it clear that the color of the culprit dye often bears no relationship to the color of the offending garment. Thus, a purple suit caused a dermatitis from a disperse yellow dye used as one component of the final purple color.

Cronin (1) also described 21 women and 26 men who had one or more relevant positive reactions to one of a series of routinely tested clothing dyes. Disperse Blue 124 (azo dye) was the most frequent sensitizer among the women and Disperse Orange 76 (azo dye) among the men.

In 1972, Sim-Davies (143) reported 15 men, age 21 to 73, who were all allergic to disperse dyes used in coloring trousers or pajamas made of 100% polyester or Terylene (polyethylene) and polyester wool fabric blends. All of the men were patch test positive to pieces of the guilty fabric. Several men reacted to dyes in more than one chemical class. None of the patients reacted to formaldehyde. Disperse Yellow 39, a methine dye not listed in either the *Colour Index* (Table 19.9) or the *Buyer's Guide*, was the most common sensitizer (6 of 15 patients).

Calnan (144) reported a woman who became allergic to Disperse Yellow 64 (C.I. 47023), which was used to color a green blouse. The dye was a quinoline derivative.

TABLE 19.9. *Some Clothing and Nylon Stocking Dyes Known to Be Potentially Allergenic*

Textile class (generic number)	Color index (C.I.) number	Color index chemical class
Disperse Yellow 1	10345	Nitro
Disperse Yellow 3*	11855	Azo
Disperse Yellow 4	12770	Azo
Disperse Yellow 9*	10375	Nitro
Disperse Yellow 39	—	Indol indigo
Disperse Yellow 49	—	Methine
Disperse Yellow 54	—	Quinoline
Disperse Yellow 64	47023	Quinoline
Disperse Orange 1*	11080	Azo
Disperse Orange 3*	11005	Azo
Disperse Orange 13*	—	—
Disperse Orange 76	—	Monoazo
Disperse Red 1*	11110	Monoazo
Disperse Red 11	62015	Aq
Disperse Red 15	60710	Aq
Disperse Red 17*	11210	Monoazo
Disperse Red 55	—	Aq
Disperse Blue 1	64500	Aq
Disperse Blue 3*	61505	Aq
Disperse Blue 7*	62500	Aq
Disperse Blue 26	63305	Aq
Disperse Blue 35*	—	Aq
Disperse Blue 85*	11370	Azo
Disperse Blue 106*	—	Azo
Disperse Blue 124*	—	Monoazo
Disperse Black 1	11365	Azo
Disperse Black 2	11255	Azo
Disperse Brown 1*	—	—
Acid Black 48	65005	Aq
Acid Yellow 23	19140	Azo
Acid Yellow 159	—	Disazo
Acid Yellow 198	—	Disazo
Acid Red 151	26900	Disazo
Acid Blue 40	62125	Aq
Acid Violet 17	42650	—
Basic Red 46*	—	—
Vat Green 1	59825	Aq
Wool Red B	—	—
Solvent Yellow 1	11000	Azo
Foron Blue	—	Aq
Black Base 1	—	—
Acid Yellow 61	18968	Azo
Acid Red 118	—	Azo
Direct Orange 34	40215	Azo
Acid Red 359	—	Azo
Reactive Red 238	—	—
Reactive Violet 5	—	—
Reactive Blue 122	—	—
Reactive Black 5	20505	—
Reactive Yellow 17	18852	—

This table was prepared with help from E. Cronin and members of the dye industry (1).

Aq, anthraquinone

*Available from Chemotechnique (Malmo, Sweden).

Some dyes do not have assigned *Color Index* numbers.

Modern Dye Allergy Data

Pratt and Taraska (145) reported a "mini-epidemic" of textile dye allergy in Canada. They tested a total of 788 patients over 2½ years, including 271 patients tested with a textile allergen series because of suspected clothing dermatitis. Forty patients reacted to one or more dyes. Disperse Blue 106 and 124 were the most common allergens, with reactions to 53 and 32 patients, respectively. Disperse Red 17 and Red 1 were positive in 10 and 9 patients, respectively. Only 20% were positive to PPDA. Nine of 11 tested patients reacted to blue/black polyester or acetate garment liners.

A report from Israel found that 22 of 55 (40%) patients tested with the same textile series reacted to dyes. The researchers found Disperse Blue 124, Blue 85, Red 17, and Blue 106 most common (146). The editors of the *American Journal of Contact Dermatitis* called Disperse Blue dyes the "allergens of the year" in 2000 (147).

Seidenari et al. (148) studied cross-reactivity in 236 patients with reactions to at least 1 azo textile dye. Of these, 107 reacted to Disperse Orange 3, 104 to Disperse Blue 124, 76 to para-aminoazobenzene (PAAB), 67 to Disperse Red 1, and 43 to Disperse Yellow 3. Those reacting to Disperse Orange 3 and PAAB reacted to PPDA about 66% to 75% of the time, but in less than one-third of the time with the other allergens.

Interesting case reports of dye allergy include one patient with hand and textile dermatitis allergic to multiple disperse dyes (149). The hand dermatitis was due to handling dyed maggots while fishing. In another case, Disperse Blue 85 caused allergy to a knee brace (150). Thioureas are more frequent causes of neoprene knee brace allergy.

Of the 100 patients with dye allergy described by Seidenari et al. (142), the top five sensitizers were all disperse dyes of the azo category listed in Table 19.10. As can be seen from the table, different authors have tested different dye series, so comparison is sometimes difficult. In addition, the prevailing climate, both fashion-wise and meteorological, varies from country to country, possibly allowing for discrepancies in sensitization. It should be noted that the patients of Thierback et al. (151) were chosen for dye testing because of a positive reaction to *p*-aminoazobenzene as a screen.

Screening for Textile Dye Allergy

No one substance is suitable as a screen for textile (mostly disperse) dye allergy. Para-aminoazobenzene, also called Solvent Yellow 1 or Anidine Yellow (C.I. 11000), is probably a candidate but still was positive in only 27% in one study. PPDA reacts in about one-fifth to one-third of patients. Occasional reactions are seen to the "black-rubber mix" of substituted PPDA derivatives. Disperse Blue 106 or 124 would be the single most common screening dye allergen (147).

An Italian group employed a textile-dye mix in retesting 67 patients with known disperse dye allergy. The mix consisted of Disperse Yellow 3, Red 1, and Orange 3, each at 0.25%, and Blue 124 at 0.1% in pet. Sixty of the 67 reacted to the mix (152).

Vat Dyes

Vat dyes rarely cause dermatitis. In fact, Levi Strauss's 501 "Shrink to Fit" jeans, which are dyed with Vat Blue 1 (C.I. 73000), can be a reliable and safe trouser substitute for disperse dye–sensitive people.

Foussereau et al. (136) described a group of cases of allergic contact dermatitis among workers in a factory in which Vat Red 1 (C.I. 73360) was synthesized. A complicated and common green anthraquinone dye, Vat Green 1 (C.I. 59825) was reported by Wilson and Cronin (153) to explain five cases of dermatitis from blue uniforms in nurses. Each nurse was patch test positive to both a piece of her uniform and the dye, 1% in soft paraffin.

> **Blue jeans dyed with a vat blue dye may be used for disperse dye–sensitive individuals.**

Reactive Dyes

Manzini et al. (154) in Italy studied allergy to reactive dyes. These are used on natural fibers cotton, silk, and wool. Eighteen of 1,813 (0.99%) consecutive patients reacted to one or more of 12 dyes tested. Reactive Red 238 (Red Cibacron CR) and Reactive Violet 5 (Violet Remizal 5R)

TABLE 19.10. *Prevalence of Textile Dye Allergy in Selected Studies*

Dye	Author		
	Seidenari (142)	Cronin (1)	Thierback et al. (151)
Disperse Blue 124	36/100 (36%)	—	—
Disperse Red 1	29 (29%)	17/27 (62%)	2/32 (6%)
Disperse Orange 3	28 (28%)	—	24/32 (75%)
Disperse Yellow 3	24 (24%)	27/31 (87%)	3/32 (9%)
Disperse Red 17	20 (20%)	—	3/32 (9%)

gave eight and five positives, respectively. Other reactors included Reactive Blue 122, Reactive Black 5, and Reactive Yellow 17. Testing concentration was at 5% pet. Of the 18 patients, 1 had occupational exposure and 6 were felt to have relevant exposure to these dyes in clothing. Two reacted to disperse dyes. In a separate article, the authors tested 312 patients to five or more reactive dyes, with no positive results (155).

Insoluble Azoics

Dermatitis associated with both the diazonium salts and the coupling agents used to form these dyes within a fabric have been described. The final reaction product would cause clothing allergy, if it exists, whereas the reaction components have caused the problems that have occurred within the textile industry.

Malten (156) described diazonium salt allergy (diazotized ice red color TR) among workers in a Dutch cotton printing mill. Foussereau et al. (136) described the chemistry of this problem in some detail. Ancona-Alayon et al. (140) studied 24 Mexican workers who developed allergic contact dermatitis and 32 who developed hyperpigmentation while working with the coupling agent Naphthol AS (3,hydroxide-2,naphthanilide), coupling component 2 (C.I. 37505), which was being used with an azo dye in a textile mill. The allergic patients had positive reactions to Naphthol AS 5% in water. Kiec-Swierczynska (157) described similar textile workers in Poland who developed hyperpigmentation or allergic dermatitis and who had positive patch test reactions to both "Texas" textiles and to 1% aq Naphthol AS used in the dyes.

A Danish report, using Naphthol AS (1% pet) in a general screening series, detected six cases of allergy (158). One of these was work related, and the rest were clinically typical of textile allergy.

Aniline Dyes

In India, the tie-and-dye industry involves much manual labor and handling of dyestuffs. Mathur et al. (159) found that 20% of 250 workers developed a severe dermatitis. Fourteen of 26 that were patch tested were positive. Red RC salt (C.I. 37120) (0.2% aq) was positive in all 14. Other common reactors were Orange GC (C.I. 37005) in seven and Bordeaux GP (C.I. 37135) in three.

Miscellaneous Dyes

Although basic (cationic) dyes have rarely been implicated in clothing allergy, they have caused allergic dermatitis when used in medicaments (gentian violet, brilliant green, and malachite green), especially on the legs (160). Scheman (161) found a patient allergic to Basic Red 46 in a flame-retardant Nomex fabric.

Acid dyes have also been indicted several times in cases of textile dermatitis. Cronin (1,3) identified Acid Violet 17 (C.I. 42650) as a cause of underwear dermatitis and Acid Black 48 (C.I. 65005) in an instance of clothing dermatitis in a man. We have seen that Acid Red 151 (C.I. 26900) can be associated with a nylon stocking allergy, and Pedersen (162) reported Acid Red 85 (C.I. 22245) as an explanation for a hand dermatitis in a dyehouse worker.

In an Italian study (163), five nondisperse azo dyes were tested in 1,814 patients. Sixteen reactions (0.88%) were noted to Direct Orange 34 (8), Acid Yellow 61 (5), Acid Red 359 (2), and Acid Red 118 (1). These dyes are used mostly on wool, cotton, silk, and polyamide fabrics. In nine cases the allergy appeared relevant to clothing use, and in two there was also occupational exposure. Five of eight reactive to Direct Orange 34 also reacted to PPDA and/or disperse dyes. All dyes were tested at 5% pet.

When leather is used as clothing, dyes incorporated into it can cause problems. Disperse Black 1 and Bismark Brown in a leather watch strap and orthodichlorobenzene in a belt resulted in dermatitis (164,165).

Dermatitis associated with mordant dyes has been described in the section on wool above.

A report from Italy in 1991 implicated several "new" dyes as occasional allergens (166). Unfortunately, dye type and C.I. numbers were not given. Brilliant green (2% pet), said to be used on wool, and Supramine Red (2% pet) for wool and polyamide were each positive in 2 of 569 patch test clinic patients. Supramine Yellow and Red, Turquoise Reactive (cotton), and Neutrichrome Red (wool and polyamide) each reacted once.

Phosgene (2,5-dichlorophenyl) hydrazone from yellow sweaters caused ACD in 12 men in Japan. The chemical was formed by the action of bleach on Pigment Yellow 16 in the garments (167).

Phototoxic Textile Dermatitis

The phototoxic potential of Disperse Blue 35, an anthraquinone-based dye, was elaborately studied by Gardiner et al. (168). They studied 16 employees in a dye-manufacturing factory in which over 130 workers had been seen over a 10-year period for acute redness and swelling of their light-exposed skin. Visible light in the 400-to-700-nm region caused phototoxic skin reactions with the whole dye in individuals whether they had been exposed to the dye in their work or not, verifying a phototoxic as opposed to a photoallergic explanation for the workers' complaints.

Hjorth and Moller (169) described two women who developed phototoxic textile dermatitis and hyperpigmentation on skin covered by bikini bathing suits. Disperse Blue 35 was not absolutely proved to cause this problem, but an extract of the bathing suit dye contained two fractions also found in Disperse Blue 35.

Allergic Dermatitis and Respiratory Disease

Estlander (170) reported five persons who were occupationally sensitized to reactive dyes. Two had only skin disease, but three also had respiratory symptoms. None were atopic. All reacted on patch testing and the latter three also on scratch testing. Involved dyes were in both the azo and anthraquinone families. None of the patients cross-reacted to PPDA or disperse dyes.

Nylon Stocking Dermatitis

Nylon hosiery was introduced in the United States in 1939 and was first made in Britain in 1947 (134,171). By 1940, dermatitis caused either by nylon stocking dyes or finishes was being reported in the United States (172,173). By 1956, nylon stocking dye dermatitis was being described in Britain (174). Although dermatitis associated with dyes used on nylon hosiery has always been infrequent, when one considers the millions of pairs of stockings sold each year, it is even less common now. Technological advances in the dye industry have corrected dye leaching by increasing fastness of the dye to the fiber, and this has helped minimize allergic reactions (134).

In 1947, Dobkevitch and Baer (175) studied 13 patients who had nylon stocking dermatitis caused by azo dyes used in stockings. None of the patients reacted to anthraquinone dyes used in the hosiery. All of them reacted to a piece of the suspected hosiery, to paraphenylenediamine, and to one or more of the suspect azo dyes. These authors felt that the frequency of cross-reactivity between the azo dyes and paraphenylenediamine could be explained by Mayer's hypothesis that they share a common transformation to quinonediimine by cells of the skin.

When Calnan and Wilson (174) described six women who had nylon stocking dermatitis in 1956, all British hosiery manufacturers were using azo dyes. The patients reacted to pieces of stocking and to one or more dyes. Only one patient had a paraphenylenediamine reaction. None of the patients reacted to melamine or urea formaldehyde resins, which at that time were used to provide an antisnag finish.

In the 1940s an emulsion of an acid ester gum was used in hosiery as a finish and caused an epidemic of dermatitis (173). These resins are not used on modern nylon stockings because they provide an intolerable "hand" to the fabric. Hosiery produced today is occasionally finished with a latex polymer or lubricant (e.g., lanolin based) (MD Hurwitz, personal communication, 1984). Calnan and Wilson's patients had no further difficulty when they wore nylons dyed with anthraquinone dyes (Kayser Bondor brand).

Fourteen patients in Finland became allergic to a brown stocking dye mixture (Synten Brown), which consisted of nitro- and aminodiazobenzene and aminoanthraquinone dyes (176). Nine of these patients reacted to aminoazoben-

zene (C.I. 11000), nine to Disperse Orange 3 (C.I. 11005), and four to Disperse Yellow 3 (C.I. 11855). Three of these patients had previously worked with textiles and had hand eczemas. Efforts to flare six of these patients with peroral azo food dyes (tartrazine and amaranth) failed.

In the United States, most black or even navy nylon stockings are not dyed with disperse dyes (Ciba-Geigy Verona Dyestuffs, Division of Mobay Chemical Corporation and Kayser-Roth Hosiery, personal communication, 1984). Furthermore, metallized dyes that utilize nickel or cobalt are used on more expensive dark hosiery. These dyes facilitate an unusually firm binding of the metallic-dye complex to the nylon fiber, providing great color fastness.

Men's nylon socks have been described as sources of allergic contact dermatitis in France, in Britain, and many years ago in the United States (1,134,177). This is a rare event today, inasmuch as men's socks produced today in the United States are dyed usually with acid dyes, because they are more wash-fast. Such a comment is obviously a generalization, and it must be remembered that socks (not women's nylon stockings), like all fabrics, are often blended. In this instance, the textile dye types used on different fabrics, as already described, must be borne in mind. Men's half hose, for example, are often a blend of 75% acrylic and 25% nylon or 70% cotton and 30% nylon. Pure wool or cotton men's or children's socks would most likely not contain disperse dyes.

The following list of dyes contains those that are currently being used most often in the United States to dye nylon stockings (Ciba-Geigy Verona Dyestuffs, Division of Mobay Chemical Corporation and Kayser-Roth Hosiery, personal communication, 1984): C.I. Disperse Yellow 3; C.I. Disperse Red 1; C.I. Disperse Red 55; C.I. Disperse Blue 3; C.I. Disperse Blue 7; C.I. Acid Yellow 159; C.I. Acid Yellow 198; C.I. Acid Red 151; C.I. Acid Blue 40. Acid Yellow 159, Acid Red 151, and Acid Blue 40 are often used together. Acid Yellow 198 is commonly used as well, as are all of the disperse dyes listed.

As already noted, men's socks are usually acid dyed, but if they are blended with nonnylon fabrics, these generalizations can only be applied to the nylon fiber dye. Socks and anklets made of 100% cotton are usually vat dyed (nine out of ten times), although they are colored occasionally with direct dyes or reactive dyes or after-treated with premetallized dyes (copper and cobalt).

Optical Whiteners

"Whiter than white" fabrics are created by the application of colorless dyes, which absorb incidental and invisible ultraviolet light and reflect it as visible bluish light. The resultant reflected light tends to mask off-whites or yellowish tinges and produces radiant whites (6).

The dyes are applied directly to textile fibers, plastics, and papers and can be incorporated into detergents. They tend to concentrate in textile fibers with increasing numbers of washes.

Calnan (178) reviewed some of the real and potential hazards associated with optical whiteners which are also known as optical bleachers, brighteners, blankophores, and fluorescent whitening agents (FWAs) or brightening agents. The *Buyer's Guide* lists 25 "fluorescent brightening agents" available in the United States (94).

Optical whiteners can belong to the acid, basic, or disperse group of textile dyes. They come from six different chemical classes: stilbenes, coumarins, diphenylpyrazolines, naphthalamides, arylazolyl-stilbenes, and combined triazoles and imidazolones. Half of the 35,000 tons of whiteners produced each year are used in detergents, and these are mostly of the stilbene or pyrazoline chemical types (178). Whiteners are not used in cosmetics, toothpastes, toiletries, or food, although they may be used in food packaging. No teratogenic potential appears to be associated with whiteners, although there is suggested but unsubstantiated evidence that they may participate in phototoxic reactions and facilitate cutaneous carcinogenesis. At least one case of suspect phototoxicity has been attributed to an optical whitener.

> At present, dermatitis owing to "optical whiteners" in textiles or detergents is not being encountered. In the past, they produced phototoxic and hyperpigmented dermatitis.

Contact allergic dermatitis has been reported from Denmark and Spain. In 1971, Osmundsen and Alani (179) described 167 patients in Copenhagen who developed a reticulate, occasionally hyperpigmented, long-lasting dermatitis in a clothing distribution. These patients washed their clothing in a detergent that contained 0.02% to 0.2% Tinopal CH 3566 (CPY) as an optical whitener. This compound was a mixture of 1-(3-chlorphenyl)-3-phenyl pyrazoline and 1-(3-chlorphenyl)-3-(4-chlorphenyl)-pyrazoline. All of the affected patients had positive patch tests with the brightener at 0.1% to 1% in petrolatum. Half of the patients who were patch tested to "nylon" pieces washed in the suspect detergent had positive reactions, and 16 of 88 patients tested to benzyl salicylate reacted positively. Benzyl salicylate is a common perfume ingredient in detergents, and this may have represented a cosensitization (108). A special feature of the Danish subjects who had dermatitis was the development of hyperpigmentation in a clothing distribution in nine of them without obvious antecedent dermatitis (175). This pigmentation was reproduced on patch testing. Tinopal CH 3566 (CPY) was shown to be a strong sensitizer in a guinea pig maximization test: CPY was never used in the United States and was withdrawn in Denmark.

The 103 Spanish patients were also associated with CPY and had clinical features like the Danish patients

(180). The Spanish study also had 12 patients who were stilbene sensitive.

Manufacturers of optical whiteners have tried to screen these agents for their sensitizing potential. One such study examined 31 agents and found three sensitizers (181). Two of these chemicals were pyrazolines (one was CPY and the other 1-phenyl-2-(naphtho(2,1-d)oxazol-2-yl) ethylene). This compound was positive in some of Osmundsen's (182) CPY-positive patients.

No recent patients who have textile-distributed dermatitis attributed to optical whiteners have been described in the United States or Europe. The Danish and Spanish epidemics of subtle, long-lasting, elusive dermatitis are, however, a fine example of the value of alertness in examining the sensitizing potential of clothing and its numerous and almost countless additives.

Management of Allergic Contact Dermatitis Caused by Dyes

Fabric that is 100% polyester is most likely to be tolerated by a patient who is allergic to a durable-press finish and is least likely to be tolerated by a person who is allergic to a disperse dye. Because most dye-related clothing dermatitis is caused by disperse dyes, fabrics that usually avoid these dyes should be selected for wear. These would include 100% cellulosics (cotton and rayon) and natural fibers such as linen, silk, and wool. In the past, fabrics that "leached" color most often caused contact allergic dermatitis (134). This problem seldom occurs today but should, however, be watched for. Unfortunately, no guidelines to color avoidance based on the color of the allergenic dye can be given, because a fabric's color is often formed from a collection of dyes (Table 19.11). On the other hand, the number of available dyes and the colors that can be made from them are so endless that often a problem can be traced to a single item of clothing. Discarding the offending item usually solves the problem.

The 501 "Shrink to Fit" button-style blue jeans manufactured by Levi Strauss and Co. can help the durable-press or dye-sensitive patient. These trousers are finished with cornstarch (up to 10% of the garment's new weight) and may have small quantities of polyvinyl alcohol and some softeners and lubricants added. The jeans are dyed with Vat Blue 1 (C.I. 73000), which is certified for use in foods and drugs and is used in some surgical sutures. No case of allergic reaction to it is recorded, despite the fact that it and its close

TABLE 19.11. *Textiles Suggested for Disperse Dye Allergic Patients*

Wear cellulose-based and natural fibers: cotton, rayon, linen, silk, and wool
Wear loose-fitting garments
Wear cotton or silk undergarments
"Pigment dyed" clothing is usually safe
Wash new clothing once or twice before wearing

relatives have been used for several thousand years (120). Levi's 501s are as close to being a truly "hypoallergenic" garment as one could hope to find.

For durable-press-sensitive individuals, 100% polyester garments are recommended. The 501 "Shrink to Fit" button-style blue jeans (Levi Strauss) can be used for durable-press-sensitive or dye-sensitive patients.

Patch Testing in Clothing Dermatitis

A list of allergens that can be used to evaluate a suspect case of clothing dermatitis can be constructed. A collection such as that presented in Table 19.12 should be helpful. It should be remembered, however, that neither formaldehyde nor paraphenylenediamine is an absolute indicator of fabric finish or dye allergy. Often the specific finishes and dyes must be tested individually.

Patch testing with a piece of the suspect fabric is most useful for a dye allergy, in which case it is usually positive. It is of least help for durable-press finishes, in which it is often negative. Aids for extracting finishes have already been mentioned. Dyes can be better extracted by steaming or heating the suspect fabric in hot ethanol (183). We usually simply soak the fabric in water for 10 minutes before applying it. On occasion, more positive reactions are seen with a piece of suspect fabric if it is left in place for longer than 48 hours (e.g., 96 to 120 hours).

Dermatitis from Contaminated Clothing

Poison ivy oleoresin may cling to clothing and retain its dermatitis-producing potential for several days. Residual

---

TABLE 19.12. *Patch Testing for Textile Dermatitis*

I. Most standard screening trays contain
  "Black rubber mix"—dyes and rubber accessories
  Chromate—leather
  Epoxy—adhesives, labels
  Formaldehyde—permanent press
  Lanolin—finishes
  MBT, thiuram, carbamate—rubber, adhesives
  Nickel—metal accessories
  PTBFR—adhesive
  PPDA—some azo dyes
II. Formaldehyde resins: see Table 19.6
III. Dyes: see Table 19.8
IV. Others
  p-aminozobenzene (0.25% pet)—dye marker
  Perchloroethylene (25% olive oil)—dry cleaning
  Triclosan (0.5% pet)—fungicide
  Naphthol AS (5% aq)—dye coupler
V. Piece of suspect clothing: Soak in water for 15 minutes for formaldehyde resins or warmed ethanol for 60 minutes for dyes. Leave on 48 hours. If no reaction, leave another 24 to 48 hours (see text).

MBT, mercaptobenzothiazole
PPDA, paraphenylenediamine
PTBFR, paratertiary butylphenol formaldehyde resin

---

detergents, especially enzyme detergents, can also produce dermatitis.

In India, allergic dermatitis (*dhobi* itch) may be produced by laundry markings made with the oleoresin of the India marking nut tree.

Hosiery can be contaminated by chemicals and dyes leached out of shoes. Hosiery dermatitis may, therefore, actually be due to the chemicals in shoes.

Clothes may be contaminated by oil, grease, cements, insect sprays, and other agents that are handled in work or hobbies.

When fiberglass curtains are washed with clothes, broken particles of fiberglass may be transferred to the clothing. Entire families may suffer from a petechial or scabies type of eruption owing to such contamination.

Dermatitis Due to Mechanical Pressure of Clothing

Stretch garment dermatitis is a syndrome caused by pressure or tension on the skin from the wearing of tight-fitting stretch garments, such as bras, girdles, and socks. The condition is not due to chemical sensitization but is mechanical.

Two principal forms of stretch garment dermatitis are: (a) a nondescript, erythematous and eczematous eruption, usually nonexudative, confined to the area covered by the garment and most severe where it binds most closely; and (b) an exaggeration of an already existing dermatosis in the areas covered by the garment.

Stretch garment dermatitis is an etiologic rather than a morphologic entity and is undoubtedly a variant of Koebner's isomorphic phenomenon. Similar outbreaks of dermatitis may result from wearing garments that are not made of stretch material but are so tight-fitting that they produce friction and pressure (e.g., narrow-cut, short-rise trousers).

Systemic urticaria may also be exacerbated by pressure in areas of tight clothing.

Blousing Garter Dermatitis

This is a syndrome of pigmentation of the ankles and dorsa of the feet in soldiers who wear either blousing garters or bootlaces around their legs to keep fatigues neatly in place. The resultant mild edema and subsequent deposition of hemosiderin and melanin resemble changes of the lower extremities in patients with stasis dermatitis secondary to varicose veins. If the constriction is prolonged, one would assume hemosiderin deposits would occur, as in the pigmented purpuric eruptions. The cutaneous changes occur distal to the site of constriction.

Parasites and Clothing

Parasites may contaminate clothing and produce dermatitis. Arthropods, such as lice and scabies mites, may infest clothing. The body louse, *Pediculus humanus* var. *corporis*, is rarely seen on the patient's skin, because it lays its eggs in and infests the seams of undergarments. It leaves the underclothing only to feed. The dermatitis produced by these blood-sucking lice is most marked in areas that are in most intimate contact with the clothing, such as the upper portion of the back and buttocks. The scabies mite and the louse are most likely to infest hairy or woolen garments.

Bees and Clothing

White or light-colored clothing with a smooth, hard finish is less likely to incite bees to sting than are dark, rough, or wooly materials. Leather, possibly because of its odor, seems to be an attractant.

Clothing Accessory Dermatitis

The many accessories used on clothing, particularly nickel-plated or rubber objects, may produce sharply localized areas of dermatitis. Nickel-plated zippers, clips, buckles, and pins, therefore, may produce dermatitis in nickel-sensitive individuals. Rubber shoulder pads, dress shields, collars, and the rubber portion of girdles and bras can produce dermatitis in sensitized individuals. Other accessories such as studs and buttons, dyed dress labels, clothing marked with inks, and articles carried in pockets may produce dermatitis.

Some garments contain inlaid patches of different colors and materials, such as gloves with leather inlays and socks with stripes of different colors, which may produce circumscribed areas of dermatitis.

Factors Affecting Clothing Dermatitis

Friction, heat, humidity, and particularly excessive perspiration play important roles in the production of clothing dermatitis. Tight-fitting clothing can produce dermatitis, which may not recur when the patient wears a larger garment or loses weight. The patient may acquire dermatitis from a particular article in the summer, but not in cooler weather or in drier climates. Hyperhidrosis, particularly when clothing is nonabsorbent, readily produces miliaria. The change of pH in sweat when evaporation is hindered may be a factor in producing dermatitis. Sweat also leaches dyes and finishes from clothing, which may produce dermatitis in sensitized patients. Control of excessive perspiration enables some patients to wear clothing that would otherwise produce dermatitis.

General Measures for Management of Clothing Dermatitis

When clothing is suspected of producing or aggravating an existing dermatitis, the following procedures should be employed.

Washing of Clothes

Whenever washable garments are suspected of causing dermatitis, such clothes, particularly socks, stockings, shirts, and undergarments, should be washed to remove irritants and sensitizers before being worn again. All undergarments should be carefully washed and rinsed to remove all detergents, sebum, and sweat.

Handling of Dry-Cleaned Clothes

Clothing that has been dry cleaned should be removed from the plastic bag and thoroughly aired before being worn to allow complete evaporation of solvents and irritants used in the dry-cleaning process.

Control of Hyperhidrosis

Attempts to control hyperhidrosis with antiperspirants may aid in the prevention of clothing dermatitis.

Use of Protective Garments

When sleeveless dresses are not feasible, white nylon, cotton, or silk slips with sleeves may protect hypersensitive skin from irritation of rough woolen and tweed dresses. Similarly, a white cotton or silk undershirt may protect the skin from contact with irritating garments. Scarves are useful to protect the neck from the friction of furs and of collars of coats or blouses. Fowler feels that silk is more protective than cotton.

Use of Protective Skin Products

Some individuals have found that spraying the axillae and other skin folds with a topical aerosol spray, such as Decadron (Merck, Sharp & Dohme), may help prevent clothing dermatitis, because the product forms a protective film of isopropyl myristate and corticosteroid.

Spray-on Shield (Kleinert) and Serene (Sheffield) are commercially available sprays containing silicones in solution to act as barriers and protect clothing from perspiration, thereby preventing the leaching of dyes and finishes.

Ivy Block lotion (Enviroderm Inc., Louisville, KY) has been shown to block poison ivy allergy, It is uncertain whether it will block other allergens, but could be tried in areas of clothing dermatitis if allergen avoidance is impossible. Pro-Q foam (Ferndale Labs, Ferndale, MI) is promoted as a skin protectant that has been shown to block irritant effects of sodium lauryl sulfate (184). It may be useful also in clearing dermatitis in intertrigenous areas where sweat and maceration are complicating factors.

Management of Dermatitis from Linings

Dermatitis may occur from the presence of dyes or of formaldehyde used to make linings perspiration-fast. This may sometimes be successfully managed by removing the lining, thoroughly washing and rinsing it, then replacing it. Dermatitis from inexpensive lining material may be due to the presence of dyes that are not light-fast, because these compounds tend to bleed more readily than do dyes used on fabrics exposed to light. Replacement with a lining material of better quality, particularly of a light hue, may enable individuals to wear dresses and coats that previously produced dermatitis.

SHOE CONTACT DERMATITIS

The extraordinary thing about shoe dermatitis is its relative rarity. The hot, humid environment within a shoe, combined with hundreds of chemicals, creates an ideal situation for the development of allergic or irritant contact dermatitis.

Freeman (185) studied 55 patients with shoe dermatitis and was able to follow up with 48 at a later time. Most patients had hyperhidrosis and 43% were atopic. Allergens were rubber (43.1%), chromate (23.6%), p-tert-butylphenol formaldehyde resin (PTBFR) (20.0%), rosin (9.0%), and PPDA (3.6%). Positive reactions to shoe pieces with negative reactions to individual chemicals occurred in 14.5%. At mean follow-up of almost 3 years, 87.5% were clear or better (over half clear), 10% the same, and one patient worse.

In 1969, Epstein (186) had 74 suspected cases of shoe allergy in his busy dermatologic practice. Jordan (187) estimated that he saw one new patient with dermatitis related to shoes every 6 weeks in 1972. From 1977 to 1980, Lynde et al. (188), in Vancouver, Canada, suspected shoe dermatitis enough to apply a shoewear screening tray to 119 of 2,910 patients with eczema whom they patch tested in that period (prevalence of 4.1%). In Italy, Angelini et al. (189) estimated a shoe contact dermatitis prevalence of 6.3% among patients who had dermatitis whom they evaluated for 4½ years up to 1980.

In order to evaluate a patient who has a shoe allergy and to assist that patient in finding shoes that he or she can wear without difficulty, it is important that the physician know how shoes are constructed as well as which chemicals used in shoe manufacture are most likely to cause problems. This is easier said than done.

TABLE 19.13. *Vegetable (Tree) Tannins That May Be Used on Leather* (see page 309)

Common name	Botanical name	Comment
Quebracho	*Schinopsis balansae* and *Schinopsis lorentzii*	Greatest world use; comes from Argentina and Paraguay
Wattle (also called mimosa)	*Acacia pycnantha* and *Acacia molissima*	Second greatest world use; comes from Australia, Brazil, and East Africa
Chestnut	*Castanea sativa*	U.S. use; comes from France and Italy
Mangrove	*Rhizophora muscronata*	No U.S. use; comes from France and Italy
Chestnut oak	Family fagaceae	U.S. use
Hemlock	*Tsuga canadiensis*	Little U.S. use
Turkish oak (also called valonia)	*Quercus aegilops*	U.S. use
Sumac	*Rhus coriaria*	U.S. use; comes from Sicily
Myrabolan (also called Myrobalan)	*Terminalia chebula*	No U.S. use; used in India; boiled water treatment
Douglas fir	*Pseudotsuga meniessi* or *pseudotsuga taxiboles*	Little U.S. use
Myrtan	*Eucalyptus redunca*	No U.S. use; comes from Australia
Gambier	*Terra japonica*	Little U.S. use; comes from Malaysia
Cutch	*Acacia catechu*	Little U.S. use; comes from Malaysia and India
Tara	*Caesalpinia spinosa*	Some U.S. use; comes from Peru, Chile, and Ecuador
Red oak	*Quercus rubra* and *Quercus pedunculata*	U.S. use; from U.S. and Yugoslavia; white oak in Yugoslavia
Lignon sulfonate	Sulfite cellulose	Pulp mill by-product (spruce and birch); some U.S. use; also in linoleum glues and in well drilling

The exact composition of these extracts is often unknown. This highlights the imprecision that can be implicit in patch testing with vegetable tannins.

For patch testing, the powder is applied "as is" or 1% in water or in petrolatum.

References (192, 195, 211, 215) were used to compile this list, as was the expert advice of Anthony Pilar of A.J. & J.O. Pilar, Inc., Pilar River Plate Corp., manufacturers of tanning extracts and materials in Newark, NJ. Table prepared by Frances Storrs MD for the 3rd edition.

TABLE 19.14. *Patch-Test Allergens for Shoe Dermatitis*

From standard tray	
Formaldehyde—tanning agent	
PTBFR—adhesive	
Chromate—tanning agent	
Thiuram, carba mix, MBT, MBT mix, black rubber mix, adhesives	
Colophony—adhesives	
PPDA—dye	
Others	
Para-aminoazobenzene	0.25% pet—dye
Thimerosal	0.1% pet—biocide
Chloracetamide	0.2% pet—biocide
Phenylmercuric nitrate	0.01% aq—biocide
Hydroquinone	1% pet—rubber
Mixed thiourea	1% pet—rubber, adhesive
p-tert-butylphenol (PTBP)	2% pet—adhesive, plastic

Gaul and Underwood (190) noted that their efforts to learn about shoe adhesives were met by a "decided reluctance [of the manufacturing companies] to divulge their ingredients." Hack (191) contacted manufacturers who allegedly made "hypoallergenic" shoes and found that his inquiries "elicited amazed replies in some cases and amazing replies in others." It must be remembered that a modern shoe is so complex that the final assembler may not be aware of all of the chemicals that have been used to prepare each of the shoe's parts, because they may have come from all over the world to finally come together in a finished piece of footwear.

Shoes are being constructed of new materials (e.g., plastics) and glued together with different adhesives. Although groups of chemicals can be collected that are useful for the diagnosis of the cause of shoe allergy (Table 19.14), it has long been the experience of dermatologists who make such investigations that they often fail to find a precise explanation for their patients' obvious shoe dermatitis. Epstein (186) estimated a 20% false-negative shoe test reaction in patients with shoe allergy. Dahl (192) suspected shoe allergy in 59 patients but confirmed specific relevant allergens in only 33 patients, although shoes were positive in 42 patients. Angelini et al. (189) found positive patch tests in only 108 of 165 patients who had clinically suspect shoe allergies, and in many instances these were to medicaments. Only 32 of the 119 suspect patients of Lynde et al. (188) had possibly relevant positive reactions to their shoewear screening tray. Dooms-Goosens in Belgium (personal communication, 1984) echoes the frustration of dermatologists around the world in noting that "we do find a lot of positive tests to the patient's own material, particularly some kind of 'foamy rubber material' present in shoes. We feel that this extra shoe series is not that interesting and that we are certainly missing allergens."

> **Most shoes sold in the United States, particularly women's shoes, are manufactured in other countries.**

In Spain, Grimalt and Romaguera (193) collected 45 unexplained patients who had shoe dermatitis. They were able to explain all but 17 of them by testing with neoprene and polyurethane resins and their constituents (see the following section on adhesives). This fresh approach to a formidable problem has highlighted the need for a reexamination of the composition of the modern shoe.

Constituents of rubber, adhesives, and leather are the most common causes of shoe allergic contact dermatitis. Substances in natural and synthetic fabrics, as well as biocides or dyes added to the finished or refinished shoe, are also suspect but seldom reported. It must be remembered that what is common in one country (e.g., rubber in North America) may be rare in another (e.g., chrome and dyes in Italy) (188,189).

Clinical Picture

The pattern of dermatitis on the foot of a person allergic to a shoewear constituent mimics the location of the offending chemical in the shoe. The patterns of foot dermatitis also reflect the changing vogue in shoe manufacture. Thus, when rubber was being added to the thermoplastic inner box toes of oxfords, shoe dermatitis classically began on the dorsal surfaces of the toes, especially the big toe (190,194,195). Although rubber box toes are no longer used in shoe manufacture, dorsal toe allergic shoe dermatitis is still reported and may well relate to the rubber that covers the outer toe surface of some tennis shoes (196).

When antioxidants used in adhesives caused difficulty, the dermatitis would localize on the entire dorsal surface of the foot where the shoe lining, which was glued down with the suspect glue, lay against the skin (197). "Epidemics" of shoe dermatitis attributed to chromates and vegetable tannins used in leather have also been characterized by dorsal foot involvement (195,198,199). As chrome was fixed more securely to leather, as antioxidants and accelerators were used less in rubber cements, and as rubber itself was used more in the inner, mid-, and outer soles of shoes, the pattern of involvement shifted to the soles of the feet (186,195). Both patterns are seen today, particularly as new synthetic materials are being used in the inner soles and in the adhesives used to secure the various layers of the shoe (200).

The most typical sole involvement spares the instep and the toes' flexural creases. When the instep only is involved with small vesicles or pustules, a shoe dermatitis is unlikely (1). The anterior portion of the sole may be involved exclusively. The dermatitis may be patchy, and amazingly it has often been reported as beginning or even remaining unilateral (186,189). Symmetry is more common, however, as is a history of increased sweating.

Leukoderma may be seen as a late sequela of some phenols used in rubber. Bajaj et al. (201) described 19 cases of depigmentation of the feet, some of which were felt to be due to hydroquinones and/or phenols. In six, dermatitis preceded the depigmentation but patch tests were negative. Even petechial and purpuric eruptions can occur when problems are traced to black rubber boots (4).

> **Shoe dermatitis may involve the dorsal aspect or volar aspect of the feet, usually sparing the instep and flexural creases of the toes. Usually symmetrical, it may remain patchy and even unilateral.**

Once the dermatitis has become established, it may spread to areas that are not in direct contact with offending shoe parts, and the diagnosis may be obscured. Although the toe web spaces are usually spared in both dorsal and ventral surface disease, they may become involved as the dermatitis spreads and necessitate a consideration of coexistent tinea pedis. Such a situation is rare, however (186). Secondary bacterial or fungal infection is more common and may bring a patient with a persistent shoe dermatitis to the doctor.

A secondary vesicular dermatitis on the hands is not uncommon in shoe dermatitis. This "id" reaction or autosensitization was well studied by Gaul and Underwood (190), who observed hand involvement in over half of their 140 patients. The pattern of hand dermatitis tended to mimic the foot's distribution. Hand involvement was most likely when the shoe dermatitis began on the soles and disappeared when the guilty shoes were discarded. Calnan and Sarkany (198), Epstein (186), and Fisher (202) have all reported similar "id"-like reactions with shoe dermatitis. In addition to these hand eruptions, a generalized dermatitis that begins as a shoe allergy has also been described (190). Storrs has seen this happen with mercaptobenzothiazole allergy from a rubber insole (FJ Storrs, MD, personal communication, 1996).

> **Shoe dermatitis is often secondarily infected and may produce eczematous "id" reactions on the hands owing to autosensitization.**

People of all ages may develop shoe allergy. Virtually all reports have included children in the first decade of life, as well as adults in their 60s (186,190,191). Over half of Adam's patients were under 20 years old, and most of Gaul and Underwood's (190) patients were 40 years old or under. Weston et al. (196) studied three children age 1 or under among their nine children who were under 6 years of age

and who had proven relevant shoe allergens. One Italian study of 17 children with foot dermatitis found nine positive patch tests. Two reacted to chromate, two to dodecyl mercaptan in rubber, and six to thimerosal (203). Those with only thimerosal allergy did improve after avoiding certain leather shoes, suggesting the allergen may have been present in the leather.

In a British study, 15 of 29 children and 26 of 57 adults with foot dermatitis had relevant allergies (204). Rubber allergens predominated in both groups, with only one child and three adults allergic to chromate in leather. Somewhat less commonly seen in both groups were allergies to fragrances, preservatives, and topical medication. Similarly, in a small French study all 8 children seen with footwear allergy reacted to various rubber allergens (205).

Differential Diagnosis

The differential diagnosis of shoe allergy includes a mechanical irritant dermatitis, juvenile plantar dermatosis (JPD), atopic dermatitis, tinea pedis, endogenous dermatitis, pustular psoriasis, or even lichen planus.

Ill-fitting shoes and anatomic foot deformities may cause excessive friction and wearing away of protective linings and may thus allow more intimate contact of shoe sensitizers with the skin. New shoes or orthopedic shoes can correct this problem (202). Shoes soaked by perspiration may overdry and become brittle. Ridges may form in the shoes' linings that irritate the skin of the feet. Slow drying of the shoe on wooden shoe trees helps alleviate this problem (206).

Atopic dermatitis may be a special differential diagnostic problem in that irritation can precipitate an attack of dermatitis. An atopic individual often develops dorsal toe dermatitis when wearing an ill-fitting or an old and cracked shoe. Epstein (186) noted that 12 of his 43 patients had a personal or family history of atopy, whereas Gaul and Underwood (190) stated categorically that 90% of their patients were not atopic. As noted previously, almost half of Freeman's (185) 55 patients were atopics.

> **Juvenile plantar dermatosis and the "sweaty sock syndrome" may mimic shoe dermatitis.**

JPD is now an established entity (207). Although its distribution, with instep sparing, can be exactly that of a shoe dermatitis, the absence of vesicles or signs of a more acute dermatitis is a distinguishing feature. The clinical pattern in most cases consists of chronic, scaling, mildly erythematous dermatitis most prominent on the anterior feet. As of 1982, 42% of the 269 reported patients had a personal or family history of atopy (207). Some authors have reported some histologic features of JPD suggesting chronic eczema; thus, these patients have often been patch tested. Ten percent of Mackie's (207) own series of patients had positive patch tests to shoewear constituents, but changes of footwear did not always resolve the dermatitis. Romaguera et al. (208) found relevant shoe allergens in 4 of 15 children whom they initially diagnosed as having JPD. Weston et al. (196) found no positive relevant allergens in any of the 15 children they saw with plantar involvement and called them JPD by default. Steck (209) would agree with the conclusion of Weston et al. He would not diagnose a child as having JPD if he had positive relevant patch tests. Steck felt that JPD is related to the special conditions that are produced by occlusive modern footwear. A sweaty foot that spends most of its time in a "sports shoe" made of occlusive synthetic materials and then dries rapidly when uncovered (especially in winter, when the humidity is low) is bound to develop the "wet and dry foot syndrome," which is Steck's term for JPD.

Other considerations in the differential diagnosis of shoe allergy can be distinguished by appropriate tests (KOH, biopsy, or clinical history).

Leather

Tanning agents and dyes are most likely to explain shoe allergy caused by leather. Reviews of shoe dermatitis have noted that early reports of allergy in the 1930s and 1940s were concerned mostly with leather and dyes. By the 1950s and 1960s, leather had slipped to second place behind rubber constituents in the United States and England (1). In the United States, there are regional differences, as Storrs (personal communication, 2000) in Oregon frequently sees shoe allergy due to leather but Fowler rarely sees it. In Italy, leather allergy was still more common than rubber allergy (189).

Chrome Tanning

Chromium allergy is detected by patch testing with potassium dichromate 0.25% (pet) in the United States and 0.5% pet in some other countries. Although trivalent chrome salts, such as chromic acid, chromic sulfate, and chrome trichloride, are the usual tanning agents, patch testing with trivalent chrome salts is much less reliable than using the hexavent potassium dichromate.

Most shoe leather allergy nowadays is explained by chrome allergy (189). This has not always been the case. In 1959 in Britain, Calnan and Sarkany (198) found that 62% of their 102 patients who had shoe dermatitis reacted to leather, but only 9 of these leather-sensitive patients reacted to chromate. Twelve of these chrome-negative patients were shown subsequently to react to East Indian vegetable-tanned leather (195). In Canada, only 3 of the 32 patients of Lynde et al. (188) who had positive reactions to shoewear reacted to chromate, whereas 49 (30%) of the patients of Angelini et al. (189) had positive and probably relevant reactions in Italy. It is likely that better fixation of chrome to leather, coupled with the cooler climate of North America, explains the decreasing prevalence of chrome allergy. It is known, for example, that individuals sensitized to chrome from other sources can wear chrome-tanned shoes without difficulty (1). Fisher (202) found that only 18 of 68 (26%) dichromate-sensitized persons had shoe dermatitis.

Patch testing with 0.25% potassium dichromate is used to detect shoe dermatitis due to chrome-tanned leather.

In "ideal" circumstances, leather shoe dermatitis caused by chromates can reach epidemic proportions. Scutt (199) saw 86 cases in 3½ years among sailors in the British navy who were assigned to the Far East. These "foreign service invalids" wore unlined chrome-tanned sandals next to their skin. The severe and chronic foot eczema that they developed resulted in "invaliding" to a temperate climate (Britain) at no small cost to the British taxpayer. Once shoe chrome dermatitis develops, it can become chronic, although like other shoe allergies, it may minimize with time (210).

Vegetable Tanning

Vegetable tanning has been done for thousands of years. Very little American leather is vegetable tanned except by special order. British authors have long suspected and documented that vegetable-tanned leather was responsible for many of their unexplained shoe leather–positive patients (195,198). The precise sensitizer was never identified, however. Calnan and Cronin (211) did find one patient in 1978 who reacted to a leather watch strap and to myrabolam extract powder and quebracho extract powder, as well as to potassium dichromate. Lewis (212), however, reported a remarkable case of a man who appeared to have an authentic allergic contact dermatitis to "tannic acid," which he was using as a wet compress. He was patch test positive to tannic acid 0.25% aq.

The tannins are a mixture of naturally occurring compounds that are able to transform skin into leather (tanning). The resulting product is resistant to hydrolytic enzymes. The composition of the various tannins and tannic acids depends on their derivation. Hausen (213) summarized what is known of wood-derived tannins.

The most famous group of patients felt to be allergic to vegetable tannins are those first reported by Lynch (214). Patients developed a vigorous dermatitis under the sandal straps of their Indian leather sandals. Subsequently, reports of this problem came from around the United States and Denmark (215–217). Sumac sap was indicted as the allergen, but patients known to be allergic to poison ivy did not react to the leather (215,216); nor was it possible to extract a catechol-like substance from the Indian sandal leather (217). In fact, Spoor (217) hypothesized that an oil added to the leather as a softening agent and not a vegetable tannin was the actual sensitizer. Some of his patients developed both a generalized and a foot dermatitis.

Because the sensitizers in vegetable tannins remain a mystery, and because the possibility of their involvement in shoe leather allergy is bound to be discussed in the future, a list of vegetable tannins that may be used on leather is presented in Table 19.13.

The reason that so little vegetable tanning is done in the United States is that it is very time consuming. Chrome tanning requires 6 to 14 hours, whereas vegetable tanning can take up to 6 months (206). Vegetable-tanned leathers are more expensive and more easily scuffed. In at least one instance, the leather lining of an American-made shoe was traced to an English supplier who, in turn, acquired the leather from India, where trees such as mimosa were used for leather tanning (216). It should be remembered that, on occasion, leather is both chrome and vegetable tanned.

Military hat bands, peaks of hats, rifle scabbards, pistol holsters, and some belts are leather tanned. Leather prepared from oxen and steers goes into soles, and leather from calves and sheep goes into hat bands and "sweats" (the inner band of a hat) (AJ Pilar, supplier of tanning materials, Newark, NJ, personal communication, 1984). The Ellithorp Tanning Co. (Gloversville, NY) has done vegetable tanning of hat bands and hat peaks for the past 40 years. Vegetable-tanned upper shoe leathers are manufactured by A.F. Gallum & Sons (Milwaukee, WI). A company with great expertise in the matter of leather tanning of all sorts is A. J. & J. O. Pilar (Newark, NJ). Usually only black and brown leathers are available in vegetable tanning (206). Because chrome is used in some brownish dyes, black leather may be "safer" for chrome-allergic people. Synthetic shoe fabrics should be used if other colors are desired.

In Oregon, a stiff leather suitable for saddles, horse collars, heavy straps, boots, prostheses, purses, and wallets is prepared by the Muir and McDonald tannery by a process that this unique firm has used for 120 years. Over a 4-month period, leather is treated with extracts of Douglas fir and hemlock bark; quebracho is added for color. After tanning, the leather is treated with tallow and neat's-foot oil (a pale yellow liquid obtained from the feet of cattle) (Muir & McDonald Tannery, Dallas, OR). On the West Coast, companies such as the Westcoast Shoe Company (Scappoose, OR) make heavy work boots such as logging boots from Muir and McDonald's vegetable-tanned leathers. The leather that is usually used is both vegetable (wattle) and chrome tanned.

Table 19.15 lists other sources of shoes made of exclusively vegetable-tanned leathers for chrome-sensitive people. Unusual sources of vegetable-tanned leathers on the East Coast of the United States may be obtained by contacting the Tanners Council of America (2501 M Street NW, Washington, DC 20036).

TABLE 19.15. *Specialty Shoe Information*

Sandals
  Happy Feet Plastic sandals and open-toe shoes: no rubber, leather, or adhesives. Made of Maclon; for a custom fit, boil for 3 min, place foot in thick sock, step in shoe, and material will mold to foot impression.
  Happy Feet
  P.O. Box 1417
  Corona, CA 91718
  800-COMFORT www.happyfeetintl.com

Plastic (PVC) work boots
  LaCrosse Footwear
  1319 St. Andrews Street
  LaCrosse, WI 54603
  800-451-1806

Custom-made shoes
  P.W. Minor & Son, Inc.
  3 Treadeasy Avenue
  P.O. Box 678
  Batavia, NY 14020
  716-343-1500

Loveless Orthopedics custom-made hypoallergenic boots, women's and men's dress shoes
  2434 SW 29th Street
  Oklahoma City, OK
  405-631-9731
  www.lovelessboots.com

Westcoast Shoe Company can make vegetable-tanned shoes and shoes without rubber cement
  P.O. Box 607
  52828 Northwest Shoe Factory Lane
  Scappoose, OR 97056
  800-326-2711

Sporting shoes
  Nike Air Mariah is supposed to be free of rubber in the shoe but may have rubber glues. Removal of the insole and adding an Aliplast insole may be helpful.
  Puma tennis shoes are usually OK.

Aliplast insoles Will usually block most rubber chemicals from getting to the foot
  Alimed Inc. Aliplast insoles Women's order # 6232; men's order # 6235
  297 High Street
  Dedham, MA 02026-9135
  800-665-2000

Formaldehyde and Glutaraldehyde

Formaldehyde may be used in leather tanning and in leather finishing after dyeing (10,206). It is used principally in the production of white leathers or in leathers designed to have a high degree of water resistance (10). The formaldehyde is believed to react firmly with leather collagen and to be released with great difficulty. Formaldehyde is also employed occasionally as a pretanning agent for heavy leathers that are to be subjected to vegetable tanning. Some synthetic tanning agents (Syntans) utilize water-soluble phenol formaldehyde condensation products containing sulfonic acid groups (10).

Although formaldehyde patch test reactions are seen in patients who have shoe dermatitis, their relevance is suspected but is seldom fully explained (186,188,192). Hack (206) saw a formaldehyde-allergic woman whose shoe dermatitis coincided perfectly with the skin covered by the white leather of her pumps.

> **Formaldehyde and glutaraldehyde used as leather-tanning agents rarely produce allergic contact shoe dermatitis.**

Glutaraldehyde has been used widely to tan upper-shoe leather (218). It is often used to retan chrome-tanned leather. It finds occasional use, as well, in preparing leather for vegetable tanning. It provides great water resistance and reduces shrinkage. For these reasons, glutaraldehyde is used in shoes likely to get wet, such as medical personnel's shoes.

Jordan et al. (218) noted that no primary sensitization from glutaraldehyde in shoe leather has been shown. Although glutaraldehyde is thought to be irreversibly bound to leather, the researchers were able to obtain positive patch test reactions to glutaraldehyde-tanned leather in five patients who had been sensitized to glutaraldehyde in disinfectants. None of these patients had a shoe dermatitis. It is doubtful that glutaraldehyde in leather causes much sensitization.

Dyes

Dyes used to color leather are most unusual causes of leather dermatitis. Cronin (1) reported no cases of shoe dermatitis owing to a dye at St. John's Hospital in London. Fisher (202) had seen no problems from the manufacturer's original shoe dye. However, he had seen problems from shoes that were redyed. He noted that leather dyes are usually azo-aniline group dyes that fix firmly to the leather. Redyed shoes do not fix these dyes as firmly (12). Most shoe dyes are unknown or are trade secrets, but several are listed in Table 19.14 as possible shoe allergens. Para-aminoazobenzene accounted for 5 of 35 reactions in foot dermatitis patients in one Indian study (159).

> **Shoe dye dermatitis is rare, even when the shoes have been redyed.**

Dahl (192) did not list which dyes his five dye-allergic patients, who had shoe dermatitis, reacted to. Some of Dahl's patients also reacted to paraphenylenediamine, which is not uncommon in azo-dye allergy. A proven case of ACD caused by Acid Yellow 36 (C.I. 13065), which was used to dye the inners and stiffeners of an industrial leather protective shoe, was reported by Ancona et al. (219).

Angelini et al. (189) found that 24.8% of their patients with shoe dermatitis reacted to paraphenylenediamine. Paraphenylenediamine is not used to dye shoe leather, and the researchers felt that patients' reactions represented cross-reactions with some rubber additives (see the following section), or with dyes used in fabric or plastic shoes or in stockings. They did not mention any specific guilty dyes. Allergic reactions attributed to dyes used to color leather used as clothing have already been discussed (164,165). Dyes are also used in plastic materials in shoes but have not yet been indicted in a case of shoe dermatitis.

Shoe polishes are also rarely or never the cause of allergic dermatitis (12). Gaul and Underwood (190) listed irritant and questionably allergic reactions to some shoe polishes but did not describe them in any detail.

Rubber

Although shoes produced today favor synthetic materials, rubber allergy is still a common manifestation of shoe contact dermatitis in North America and England (1). The rubber accelerator mercaptobenzothiazole (MBT) leads the list of culprits. The thiurams have also been responsible for some problems, and on rare occasions the accelerator diphenylguanidine (DPG) and other carbamates have caused difficulty as well (194). The antioxidant IPPD has been a problem in rubber boots (4). In the past, monobenzyl ether of hydroquinone (MBH) and 4,4-dioxydiphenyl also caused problems, but this is not as common today (194,197,220). MBH was responsible for three positive reactions in the series of shoe dermatitis patients of Lynde et al. (188). Other rubber allergens with the potential to cause shoe dermatitis are the thioureas and dodecyl mercaptan.

Rubber may be used on the outer sole of shoes, and in the case of some sports shoes it may wrap over the outer upper toe of the shoe. It may also be used as a component of the shoe's midsole. Insoles may still be made of real "foam" or latex-based rubber, but these insoles are made more and more from polyurethanes or leather. At one time, rubber (thermoplastic) box toes were the most common cause of shoe contact dermatitis in the United States (194,202), but they are now essentially obsolete. Modern firm toes, such as the box toe of an oxford, are likely to be made of celastic, which is a cotton flannel impregnated with a cellulose nitrate resin (202). Box toes are even more likely to be made of new synthetic thermoplastic resins such as polystyrenes or fabrics impregnated with polyamide resin systems (D Holmberg, AE Jonas, personal communication, 1984).

No matter where the rubber is in the shoe, it is important to remember that when the shoe becomes wet after being worn, the suspect chemicals can migrate to distant parts of the shoe. Cronin (195), for example, has emphasized the importance of patch testing individuals with shoe dermatitis on their soles to pieces of the outer sole of their shoes. Marcussen (221) showed that MBT can diffuse out of rubber. A piece of canvas became reactive in an MBT-allergic person if it sat for 24 hours in a solution with a piece of rubber that contained MBT. Both deVries (194) and Gaul (220) provide lists of the numerous rubber chemicals likely to be found in shoes, although some may no longer be used.

Mercaptobenzothiazole and Tetramethylthiuram

Cronin (195) noted a trend in favor of rubber allergy and away from leather allergy between 1960 and 1965 at St. John's Hospital in London. Among 100 patients who had positive reactions to rubber in their shoes between 1953 and 1965, Cronin found only two patients who reacted to rubber from their shoes and who were negative to MBT or tetramethylthiuram disulfide (TMTD). Of these 100 patients, 45% were MBT positive, 12% were TMTD positive, and 37% reacted to both MBT and TMTD.

MBT has been identified as the most frequent rubber allergen as well as the most frequent shoe allergen in other series as well (187,188,193,196). MBT accounted for 20% and TMTD for 11% of positive reactions among the shoe-sensitive patients of Lynde et al. (188). Together, they were the most common positives. In a general population of 4,190 eczema patients tested by this same group in Vancouver, between 1972 and 1981, MBT was positive in 3.2% of the patients and the thiuram mix in 5.4% (78). In some countries, rubber allergy is still a less common cause of shoe dermatitis than leather.

Disulfiram (tetraethylthiuram disulfide, Antabuse) is used in the treatment of alcohol abuse. At least one patient with TMT-based rubber allergy from footwear has developed a generalized (systemic) dermatitis after using disulfiram (222).

N-Isopropyl-N-Phenyl-Paraphenylenediamine

N-isopropyl-N-phenyl-p-phenylenediamine (also called isopropylphenyl-p-phenylenediamine or 4-isopropylamino diphenylamine, or IPPD) has caused allergic contact dermatitis in rubber boot wearers (4). One epidemic of 109 patients in Prague is summarized by Cronin (1). Of special interest is the purpuric nature of the eczema that can be reproduced on patch testing (4). IPPD allergy has also been indicted as an explanation for shoe contact dermatitis from Maleki shoes in Iran. The soles of these shoes are made from recycled rubber tires (223).

> Isopropyl-p-phenylenediamine, a rubber antioxidant that can produce a purpuric shoe dermatitis, does not necessarily cross-react with paraphenylenediamine hair dye.

Not all rubber boot allergies are caused by IPPD. In Newfoundland, none of the 30 patients sensitive to rubber boots were found to react to paraphenylenediamine (PPD) (224). IPPD itself was not tested and often does not cross-react with PPD (4). The Newfoundland patients were interesting, nonetheless, in that although some of them reacted to MBT, they also reacted to chemicals used in rubber that are only rarely reported as sensitizers in footwear, such as zinc diethyldithiocarbamate, diphenylguanidine, and trimethylquinoline (224). All of these patients reacted to a piece of boot rubber, but only 13 of them had positive reactions to specific chemicals.

> Reactions to rubber allergens occur in varying numbers, depending on the locations of shoe manufacture and patient exposure. For those that do react to rubber, MBT is the most common allergen, followed by thiurams.

Plastic Allergens in Shoes

Synthetic materials are used commonly in shoe manufacture. Problems with these synthetic materials have mostly to do with adhesives. Some of the same chemicals used in adhesives, however, are also used in solid shoe materials. Roberts and Hanifin (225) reported allergy to ethylbutyl thiourea used as an accelerator in a polychloroprene (neoprene) adhesive used in running shoes. They noted, however, that thioureas may find their way into other neoprene products, such as orthopedic supports and sporting goods.

Polyurethanes are also used in both solid shoe materials and adhesives. Polyurethanes are polyaddition products resulting from the reaction between diisocyanates (Desmodur and Bayer Firm) and polyhydroxy compounds (polyalcohols, polyesters, e.g., Desmophenes and Bayer) with free OH groups (136). Grimalt and Romaguera (193) reported allergy to the polyurethane constituents Desmocoll 400, Desmodur R, and Desmodur RF in 13 patients who had shoe dermatitis in Spain. They also identified 15 patients who were allergic to dodecyl mercaptan, which is used to arrest polymerization in some neoprenes. The Spanish authors confirmed the presence of dodecyl mercaptan in DuPont's Neoprene ACM resin, which is used as glue in the Spanish shoe industry. Such arresters can also be found, however, in solid neoprenes (193).

> The adhesives used in synthetic materials, which may replace leather and rubber in shoes, are the main sensitizers in such shoes.

An understanding of potential allergens used in plastic shoe materials is just developing. Cronin (1), for example, described several patients who were sensitized to polyvinyl chloride (PVC) shoe linings, but the allergen was not identified. Neither Foussereau et al. (136) nor Adams (226) mentions polyurethanes as potential allergens in shoemakers, despite excellent discussions of their chemistry. Bisphenol A, an epoxy resin component, has caused shoe dermatitis from plastic shoes in India (227).

In 1971, Fregert (228) presented a list of such chemicals that could be used in both rubber and plastics such as polythene, polypropylene (neoprene), polyisobutylene, polystyrene, polyamides, pentaplast, polyoxypropylene, PVC, polyolefins, polyformaldehyde, and polyurethane. Many are still used today. Although not all of these chemicals are known as sensitizers, their names are worth bearing in mind as we begin to understand the role that plastic materials may play in shoe contact dermatitis.

In the past, an occlusive plastic shoe made in Japan caused an irritant sort of dermatitis that came to be known as the "Japanese hot foot" (229,230). The dermatitis, which replicated the ripple sole, was attributed to occlusion. The trends in plastic footwear will, in all likelihood, produce similar sorts of hot-foot dermatitis.

Chemicals Used in Both Rubber and Plastics

Phenyl α-naphthylamine
Phenyl β-naphthylamine
p-hydroxyphenyl β-naphthylamine
Aldol α-naphthylamine
N-isopropyl-N'-phenyl-p-phenylenediamine
N,N'-diphenyl-p-phenylenediamine
N,N'-di-β-naphthyl-p-phenylenediamine
Mercaptobenzimidazole
2,6-di-tert-butyl-4-methylphenol
2,6-di(methyl-3-tert-butyl-2-hydroxyphenyl)monosulfide
Bis(5-methyl-3-tert-butyl-2-hydroxyphenyl)monosulfide
2,5-di-tert-butylhydroquinone
2,5-di-tert-amylhydroquinone
Tri(p-nonylphenyl)phosphite
Adhesives

Shoe cements came into use in 1910 (190). Most shoe adhesives were rubber based for many years. In the 1950s and 1960s, neoprene- and urethane-based adhesives became more popular.

Rubber Adhesives and Rosin

The first reports of shoe dermatitis attributed to rubber adhesives were vague. Gaul and Underwood (190) and Fisher (202) noted that their patients who reacted to shoe adhesives or rubber parts were often also allergic to adhesive tape ("plaster"). Although they suspected the same chemicals were used in both the glue and the adhesive tape, the precise chemicals were not named. Fisher, Shatin, and

Reisch all felt that rubber cements were only rarely the cause of shoe allergy.

> **The increased use of occlusive plastic shoes can produce "Japanese hot foot" dermatitis that replicates the ripple sole.**

In 1952, Blank and Miller (197) were actually provided with the chemical ingredients contained in some rubber-based adhesives used for shoe linings. Ten of the 21 patients they tested reacted to the antioxidant MBH. Some of the patients also reacted to MBTs and thiurams. Most of the patients had positive reactions to the cloth linings with the attached rubber adhesive. Patients who wore shoes prepared with glues containing MBH or MBT produced acute dermatitis.

In 1966, Cronin (195) stated that "latex glues are used to stick the inner parts of shoes, but these glues do not contain MBT or tetramethylthiuram disulfide and we have not found a patient with shoe dermatitis caused by latex glues." In her 1980 textbook, however, Cronin (1) stated that thiurams and MBT were used to formulate some latex glues used for shoe linings. She relied on the work of Jordan (187) and Dahl (192), who assumed, but did not verify, that some of their MBT- and TMTD-positive patients were troubled by the presence of these chemicals in latex adhesives.

Modern rubber cements are used usually for sole attaching or for sticking layers below the insole. They help decrease the squeak of leather shoes. They are not as permanent as neoprene or urethane glues and need not be, especially if the sole is sewn. Most of them rely on rosin esters that are present as tackifiers, for example, glyceryl ester of rosin or various esterified wood rosins (usually pine derivatives).

Neoprene Adhesives and Paratertiary Butylphenol Formaldehyde Resin (PTBFR)

Neoprene glues are usually used for the sole attachment but may find use anywhere below the shoe insole (200).

Occasionally, tetramethylthiuram disulfide is added to neoprene glues to control polymerization (226). Such a chemical is known as a "short stop" in the industry. Dodecyl mercaptan (or mercapthane), also used to arrest polymerization in neoprene adhesives (e.g., Neoprene ACM by DuPont), has caused allergic reactions (193). Allergy to ethyl butyl thiourea, used as an accelerator in a neoprene adhesive, has already been mentioned (225).

In general, neoprene cements consist of the following (231):

1. the synthetic rubber neoprene
2. a phenolformaldehyde resin (usually paratertiary butylphenol formaldehyde resin (PTBFR))

3. a catalyst (usually proprietary and unknown)
4. zinc and magnesium oxide, toluene, ethyl acetate, and benzene

PTBFR is added to neoprene to provide stability and durability.

The first cases of allergy to PTBFR in neoprene shoe adhesives were reported by Malten (231) in 1958. None of his ten patients, who were shoemakers, reacted to neoprene AC, but all of them reacted to PTBFR and to PTBP itself. Two patients also reacted to formaldehyde, but it was uncertain whether this was related to formaldehyde's presence in the resin or to a fungicide in the shoe.

By the mid- to late 1960s, patients with shoe allergy attributed to PTBFR were being reported (232). These later PTBFR-positive patients were not always positive to PTBP, which suggested that less free PTBP was present in the newer glues. Although sensitization can occur to either PTBP or PTBFR alone, group sensitization reactions between the two can also occur (232).

The bulky polycondensation plastics such as PTBFR do not themselves often cause primary sensitization, and they may have low-molecular-weight reactive end groups present even at the stage of use (231). Because of this, several authors have suggested that a more simple molecule may be the actual sensitizer in such resin allergies. Schubert and Agatha (233) proposed 2-hydroxy-methyl-4-*tert*-butylphenol (*ortho*-methylol-PTBP) as the actual allergen in PTBFR allergy. Rycroft (234) suggested 2-monomethylol phenol (tested 10% in petrolatum) as the sensitizing molecule in phenol formaldehyde resin allergy. He stressed the importance of testing with a patient's exact resin, because the screening phenol formaldehyde resin may be negative. Malten et al. (200) tested five PTBFR-allergic patients to the molecules just mentioned (1% in pet) but were unable to get uniformly positive reactions. As a result, they concluded that the real causative allergen in PTBFR sensitivity has yet to be revealed. They did emphasize, however, that shoe patch testing series that screen with PTBP alone and leave out PTBFR or the patient's own resin are likely to exclude many shoe adhesive–allergic patients.

PTBFR allergy can explain 10% to 20% of patients allergic to footwear. Four of deVries's (194) allergic patients, 4 of Jordan's (187) 25 patients, and 8 of Dahl's (192) 42 patients were allergic to phenolic resins.

Formaldehyde allergy in association with PTBP/PTBFR allergy is rare, and its relevance is often found outside of the shoe (136,231). Nine of the 108 shoe-allergic patients of Angelini et al. (189) reacted to PTBFR, but none of these 9 patients were sensitive to formaldehyde.

> **Paratertiary butylphenol formaldehyde resin (PTBFR) in neoprene shoe adhesives is a common cause of allergic shoe dermatitis.**

In a study from the Netherlands, 30 of 1,966 (1.5%) patients patch tested reacted to PTBP/PTBFR (235). Of these, six had shoe dermatitis and five were allergic to watchbands. Similarly, 1.6% of over 5,000 North American patients reacted to (1% pet). A clinical correlation was not made in this study.

In 1976, Foussereau et al. (236) collected 106 cases of PTBFR allergy. Thirty-one (29%) of the patients had footwear allergies, and the remaining cases were occupational. Union Carbide's CKR 1634 and CKR 1734 have been blamed for most cases of PTBFR-neoprene adhesive allergy. Foussereau et al. (136,236) provided complete lists of PTBFR-containing neoprene adhesives known to be sensitizing. PTBP/PTBFR-allergic people tend to cross-react to many neoprene adhesives (230). Although some of these resins are known to have a "high" formaldehyde content (e.g., Superbeckacit 1050, Varcum 875, and Varcum 921), Foussereau et al. (236) affirmed that formaldehyde plays only a minor role in PTBFR allergies.

PTBFR adhesives find use in clothing items such as belts, watch straps, and hats. They are used widely in automobile upholstery and for hobby purposes (1,236). Individuals have been reported in whom allergic dermatitis was caused by PTBFR present in their amputation prostheses (237).

> **PTBFR may be an allergen in seating upholstery, belts, purses, orthopedic prostheses, and other leather and vinyl goods.**

Urethane Adhesives

Although urethanes are commonly used as shoe adhesives, allergy caused by them is all but unreported. The nature of polyurethanes and the presence of allergy to their isocyanate component in six shoe-allergic patients has already been alluded to (193,226). It is unclear whether these patients reacted to urethane adhesives or to solid urethane materials such as might be used in the foamy insole material. Textbooks that describe allergy to diisocyanates and to amine catalysts or hardeners used in making polyurethanes do not mention shoemakers or shoe wearers as being troubled by these substances (1,136,226). Tertiary amines such as triethylenediamine, cyclic amines such as diaminodiphenylmethane, plasticizers such as dibutyl tin or tin dilaurate, and the various diisocyanates themselves should all be kept in mind as we attempt to solve mysterious cases of shoe dermatitis associated with modern synthetic shoes that we cannot explain with standard shoe allergens.

Urethanes find wide use as adhesives because of their lightness and durability. Many of them require little curing, and the final product is all but free of extra hardener or isocyanate, which helps explain the lack of allergy attributed to them thus far in shoes.

Patch Testing to Shoes

Patch testing with a standard screening series including chromate, rubber allergens, and PTBFR will detect up to 80% of foot dermatitis caused by shoe allergy. Adding the special "shoe" allergens listed in Table 19.14 will increase that yield. However, as the previous pages have documented, about 10% to 20% of patients with reactions to shoe pieces do not react to these allergens. It is often helpful to patch test directly with pieces of the suspect shoe. Because different parts of the shoe (uppers, lowers, soles, insoles, etc.) contain different allergens, one should attempt to obtain pieces of suspect shoe from an area in contact with the affected skin location. The piece should be thin to avoid pressure effects. Use of an adhesive bandage or plain Scanpor tape is recommended because the Finn chamber causes potential pressure effects as well. The sample can be collected with a biopsy punch, curette, or scissors. It should be remembered that allergens in shoes may migrate under the moist conditions of chronic wearing. An insole, for example, may contain chemicals originally found in the outer sole.

It is difficult in patch testing to replicate the conditions of shoe wearing. For this reason, Jordan (187) has suggested soaking shoe-piece patches in water for 15 minutes before testing. Each piece should be soaked in a different container to avoid contamination. It may be helpful to leave the pieces of shoe in place for 4 or 5 days rather than for the traditional 48 hours.

When a patch test to a piece of shoe is positive but standard allergens are negative, there may be two explanations. Most likely, the allergen is an unusual chemical added to some shoe component such as a biocide in leather or other rarely used additive. However, positive patch tests to shoe pieces have at times been due to uptake by the shoe material of patient applied agents. For example, Storrs (238) has reported a case of allergy to topical steroids that had been absorbed into the shoe material. The patient had not bought any new shoes for several years and was, therefore, reexposing himself to the offending allergens accidentally by wearing his old, "contaminated" shoes.

Guin has described patients who developed positive patch tests to scrapings of scales taken from their foot eruption (J Guin, personal communication, 1984). This observation is fascinating, because it suggests an antigen reservoir in the stratum corneum that may help us understand the chronic dermatitis that plagues some patients.

An equally interesting observation is that two patients with MBT allergy from their shoes gave positive reactions to pieces of white socks that had been soaked in dilute solutions of MBT (0.1% to 1%) for 24 hours and then washed and boiled. Rietschel (239) suggested that shoe allergens may concentrate in stockings and play an additional role in chronicity.

> **Patch testing for shoe dermatitis should include thin shoe samples (7 to 10 mm) soaked in water for 15 minutes and left on for 4 to 5 days.**

Stocking dermatitis may well masquerade as shoe dermatitis; thus, patch testing to stockings themselves or to the stocking dyes listed in Table 19.9 will occasionally verify a patient with shoewear dermatitis.

If a rare problem to a vegetable tannin is suspected, it will be profitable to collect some of the vegetable tannins listed in Table 19.13 and test to them.

Management of Shoe Dermatitis

Once the source of allergy in a shoe is identified, a patient can be guided to a shoe least likely to cause further problems. Because so many American shoes are imported, such guidance is not always easy. The patient can, however, be told what materials to avoid or seek (240).

While the physician sorts out the shoe allergens, or if a trial away from potentially allergenic shoes seems warranted, wooden or plastic shoes may be used as temporary substitutes. Injection-molded 100% plastic shoes are now made by over 20 companies; most of them are made of polyvinylchloride or polyurethanes and should be relatively nonallergenic (J Nielsen, Imperial Adhesives and Chemicals, Cincinnati, OH, and P Brown, Walk In Shoes, Schuylkill, PA, personal communications, 1984). Plastic or wooden shoes should not be purchased with glued insoles. Table 19.15 lists shoe manufacturers for these and other special situations.

For Rubber Allergy

Wear all leather shoes such as sewn leather moccasins with no insole and no attached outer sole. Injection-molded 100% plastic shoes with no insole should be fine. Some tennis shoes are rubber free. These shoes are made of polyolefins, urethanes, and ethylene vinyl acetate. Check the shoe's label for materials. Replace insoles with those listed in Table 19.15. Wooden shoes are also good substitutes.

For Leather Allergy

Wear all-plastic or all-fabric shoes. Remove leather insoles because these may be chrome tanned. Wooden clogs with appropriately tanned leather can help.

For PTBFR Adhesive Allergy

It may be necessary to contact individual manufacturers. One hundred percent leather, plastic (if not neoprene), or wooden shoes should help. Urethane-glued shoes are desired.

Consulting the companies listed in Table 19.15 or the organizations in Table 19.16 can give increased refinement to these general recommendations. In addition, many cities have local manufacturers of special orthopedic or corrective shoes (these can be found in the Yellow Pages). Occasionally, these small companies will take enough interest to provide specially made products to avoid specific allergens. The cost for this may be prohibitive, however.

General Treatment of Shoe Dermatitis

When shoe allergens are not identified but shoe allergy is suspected, a patient should wear wooden or plastic shoes until his or her feet are clear. Superimposed fungal infections or allergy to stockings and medicaments must be excluded. Topical therapy with wet dressings and corticosteroids, as well as the occasional use of systemic corticosteroids, will assist in resolving acute eruptions. Despite these topical measures and even with shoe substitution, chronic foot dermatitis may be a problem. Minimizing shoe friction, using lubricants and occasionally topical corticosteroids, and discarding stockings worn in the guilty shoes will all assist in hastening the resolution of a chronic shoe dermatitis.

Treatment of Hyperhidrosis

People who have hyperhidrosis are especially prone to the development of shoe dermatitis. On occasion, controlling hyperhidrosis will allow a patient with a minimal problem to wear guilty shoes for short periods of time.

TABLE 19.16. *Help with Unusual Shoe Problems*

Shoewear organizations	Glue manufacturers
Footwear Industries of America 3700 Market Street Suite 303 Philadelphia, PA 19104	Imperial Adhesives and Chemicals 6315 Wiehe Road Cincinnati, OH 45237
Prescription Footwear Association 200 Madison Avenue Suite 1409 New York, NY 10016	
United Shoe Machinery (USM Corp.) Bostik Division Middleton, MA 01949	

Zeasorb powder (Stiefel) dusted into shoes and hosiery may lessen perspiration. Drysol (Person & Covey), which is 20% aluminum chloride in ethyl alcohol, can also be used to treat hyperhidrosis. Fluffy tannic acid powders dusted into shoes and stockings and onto the feet will help minimize sweating. Such a powder is manufactured by the Mallinckrodt Co. Tannic acid powder purchased from Aldrich Chemicals or J. T. Baker Co. can be made up with equal parts of bentonite and talc and dispensed in a sifter box for treating hyperhidrosis (12).

The Drionic device (General Medical Corp.) is an iontophoretic device that passes a slight electric current through the skin. Repeated treatments inactivate eccrine sweat glands for periods of up to several weeks. Intradermal injection of botulinum toxin can control hyperhidrosis for up to 6 months.

Tea foot baths are another way to help decrease foot sweating. They also assist in calming an acute dermatitis, but have the side effect of staining the feet and toenails.

Instructions for Tea Foot Baths

1. Boil four to six tea bags in 1 quart of water for 10 minutes.
2. Place in basin and add enough cold water to make lukewarm.
3. Soak feet for 30 minutes before retiring or twice daily if time permits.
4. After 1 to 2 weeks, frequency of treatments can usually be reduced.

Formaldehyde and glutaraldehyde soaks have in the past been used to treat hyperhidrosis. Because of their allergenic potential, however, this cannot be recommended.

It is possible that the patient has a unique allergy to an unusual dye, fungicide, vegetable tannin, or adhesive ingredient that is present in only one pair of shoes. After the dermatitis has been cleared with medical measures and the patient has worn one pair of all-leather, all-wood, or all-plastic shoes (depending on the physician's suspicions), the suspect shoes can be slowly reintroduced. This should be done one pair at a time and no more often than weekly. Such a procedure can be used to apprehend the shoes in question.

REFERENCES

1. Cronin E. Studies in contact dermatitis XVIII: dyes in clothing. *Trans St Johns Hosp Dermatol Soc* 1968;54:156.
2. Fowler J, Skinner S, Belsito D. Allergic contact dermatitis from formaldehyde resin in permanent press clothing. *J Am Acad Dermatol* 1992;27:962.
3. Cronin E. Clothing and textiles. In: Ronin E, ed. *Contact dermatitis.* Edinburgh: Churchill Livingstone, 1980:36.
4. Calnan CD, Peachey RDG. Allergic contact purpura. *Clin Allergy* 1971;1:287.
5. Ramam M, Khaitan B, Singh M, Gupta S. Frictional sweat dermatitis. *Contact Dermatitis* 1998;38:49.

6. Moncrieff RW. *Man-made fibers.* Toronto: John Wiley & Sons, 1975;1.
7. Textile Fiber Products Identification Act. Public Law, 85–897, 72 Stat 1717; codified at 15 USC, 70 approved 9/2/58, effective 3/3/60. Enforced through the Federal Trade Commission.
8. Otomasu K, Yamauchi M, Ohwatari N, et al. Analysis of sweat evaporation from clothing materials by the ventilated sweat capsule method. *European J Appl Physiol* 1997;76:1–7.
9. Braitman M. Dermatitis and fabrics. *J Med Soc NJ* 1955;52:757.
10. Walker JF. *Formaldehyde.* American Chemical Society Monograph Series, no. 159. New York: Robert E. Krieger Publishing Co., 1964:1.
11. Lord LW. Cutaneous sensitization to wool. *Arch Dermatol* 1932; 26:707.
12. Fisher AA. *Contact dermatitis.* 2nd ed. Philadelphia: Lea & Febiger, 1973.
13. Davies JH, Barker AN. Textile dermatitis. *Br J Dermatol Syphilol* 1944;56:33.
14. Hill LW. Wool as cause of eczema in children. *N Engl J Med* 1951; 245:407.
15. Osborne ED, Murray PF. Atopic dermatitis: study of its natural course and of wool as dominant allergenic factor. *Arch Dermatol* 1953;68:619.
16. Greenwood K. Dermatitis with capillary fragility. *Arch Dermatol* 1960;81:947.
17. Hellier FF. Dermatitis purpurica nach Kontakt mit Textilgeweben. *Hautarzt* 1960;11:173.
18. Romaguera C, et al. Occupational purpuric textile dermatitis from formaldehyde resins. *Contact Dermatitis* 1981;7:152.
19. Schwartz L, Dunn JE. Dermatitis occurring in a woolen mill. *Ind Med* 1942;11:432.
20. Fregert S, et al. Allergic contact dermatitis from chromate in military textiles. *Contact Dermatitis* 1978;4:223.
21. Rudzki E. Contact urticaria from silk. *Contact Dermatitis* 1977;3:52.
22. Inoue A, Ishido I, Shoji A, Yamada H. Textile dermatitis from silk. *Contact Dermatitis* 1997;37:185.
23. Urbach E, Gottlieb PM. *Allergy.* New York: Grune & Stratton, 1946:245.
24. Brown SE, Coleman M. Severe immediate reactions to biologicals caused by silk allergy. *JAMA* 1957;165:2178.
25. Morris GE. Nylon dermatitis. *N Engl J Med* 1960;263:30.
26. Prassa MN. Bullous dermatitis of feet caused by pure nylon. *Bull Soc Trans Dermatol Syphilol* 1955;62:508.
27. Tanaka M, et al. Contact dermatitis from nylon-6 in Japan. *Contact Dermatitis* 1993;28:250.
28. Batten K, et al. Occupational ACD from *N,N* methylen bis-5-methyloxazolidine in a nylon spin finish. *Contact Dermatitis* 1999;41:165.
29. Balda B. Allergic contact dermatitis due to acrylonitrile. *Contact Dermatitis Newsletter* 1971;9:219.
30. Bakker J, et al. Occupational contact dermatitis due to acrylonitrile. *Contact Dermatitis* 1991;24:50.
31. Osbourn RA. Contact dermatitis caused by Saran Wrap. *JAMA* 1964; 188:1159.
32. Schulsinger C, Mollgaard K. Polyvinyl chloride dermatitis not caused by phthalates. *Contact Dermatitis* 1980;6:477.
33. Fregert S, Rorsman H. Hypersensitivity to epoxy resins used as plasticizers and stabilizers in polyvinyl chloride resins. *Acta Derm Venereol* (Stockh) 1963;43:10.
34. Morris GE. Vinyl plastics: their dermatological and chemical aspects. *AMA Arch Ind Health* 1953;8:535.
35. Dooms-Goossens A, Duron C, Loncke J, et al. Contact urticaria due to nylon. *Contact Dermatitis* 1986;14:63.
36. Porter PS, Sommer RG. Contact dermatitis due to spandex. *Arch Dermatol* 1967;95:43.
37. Batschvarow B, Minkow DM. Dermatitis and purpura from rubber in clothing. *Trans St Johns Hosp Dermatol Soc* 1968;54:178.
38. Shmunes E. Purpuric allergic contact dermatitis to paraphenylenediamine. *Contact Dermatitis* 1978;4:225.
39. Fisher A. Allergic petechial and purpuric rubber dermatitis: the PPP syndrome. *Cutis* 1974;14:25.
40. Mihan R, Ayres S. Stretch garment dermatitis. *Calif Med* 1968; 108:109.
41. Jordan WP, Bourlas MC. Allergic contact dermatitis to underwear elastic. *Arch Dermatol* 1975;111:593.
42. Abel RR. Fiber glass: washing machine and fiberglass. *Arch Dermatol* 1966;93:78.
43. Heisel EB, Hunt FE. Further studies in cutaneous reactions to glass fibers. *Arch Environ Health* 1968;7:705.
44. Kalimo K, Saarni H, Kytta J. Immediate and delayed type reactions to formaldehyde resin in glass wool. *Contact Dermatitis* 1980;6:496.
45. Cuypers JMC, Hoedemaeker J, Nater JP, deJong MCJM. The histopathology of fiberglass dermatitis in relation to von Hebra's concept of eczema. *Contact Dermatitis* 1975;1:88.
46. Bjornberg A, Lowhagen G. Patch test reactions to rockwool. *Contact Dermatitis* 1975;1:242.
47. Fisher BK, Warkentin JD. Fiberglass dermatitis. *Arch Dermatol* 1969;99:717.
48. Fisher AA. Fiber glass vs mineral wool (rockwool) dermatitis. *Cutis* 1982;29:412.
49. Reid JD, Arceneaux RL, Reinhardt RM, Harris JA. Studies of wrinkle resistance finishes for cotton textiles: release of formaldehyde vapors on storage of wrinkle-resistant cotton fabrics. *Am Dyestuff Reporter* 1960;49:29.
50. *Formaldehyde.* Current Intelligence Bulletin 34, NIOSH, April 15, 1981.
51. *Formaldehyde: an assessment of its health effects.* Prepared for the Consumer Product Safety Commission by the Committee on Toxicology, National Academy of Sciences, Washington, DC, March 1980.
52. Vail SL, Reinhardt RM. What do formaldehyde tests measure? *Text Chem Colorist* 1981;13:13.
53. Peterson H, Pai PS. Reagents for low-formaldehyde finishing of textiles. *Text Res J* 1981;51:282.
54. Sugai T, Yamanoto S. Decrease in the incidence of contact sensitivity to formaldehyde. *Contact Dermatitis* 1980;6:154.
55. Hirano S, Yoshikawa K. Patch testing with European and American standard allergens in Japanese patients. *Contact Dermatitis* 1982; 8:48.
56. Cooke TF, Weigmann L. The chemistry of formaldehyde release from durable-press fabrics. *Text Chem Colorist* 1982;14:25.
57. Hatch K, Maibach H. Textile dermatitis an update I-resins additives and fibers. *Contact Dermatitis* 1995;32:319–326.
58. Guide to textile finishes. *Text World* 1973 Dec.
59. Marcussen PV. Contact dermatitis due to formaldehyde in textiles 1934–1958. *Acta Derm Venereol* (Stockh) 1959;39:348.
60. Hovding G. Free formaldehyde in textiles. *Acta Derm Venereol* (Stockh) 1959;39:357.
61. Hovding G. Contact eczema due to formaldehyde in resin finished textiles. *Acta Derm Venereol* (Stockh) 1961;41:194.
62. Cronin E. Formalin textile dermatitis. *Br J Dermatol* 1963;75:267.
63. Berrens L, Young E, Jansen LH. Free formaldehyde in textiles in relation to formalin contact sensitivity. *Br J Dermatol* 1964;76:110.
64. Fisher AA, Kanof NB, Biondi E. Free formaldehyde in textiles and paper. *Arch Dermatol* 1962;86:97.
65. Malten KE. Textile finish contact hypersensitivity. *Arch Dermatol* 1964;89:102.
66. Fregert S, Tegner E. Non-iron agents. *Contact Dermatitis Newsletter* 1971;9:200.
67. Pannaccio F, Montgomery DC, Adam JE. Follicular contact dermatitis due to coloured permanent-pressed sheets. *Can Med Assoc J* 1973;109:23.
68. Wilkinson RD. Sheet dermatitis. *Can Med Assoc J* 1973;109:14.
69. Rycroft RJG, Cronin E, Calnan CD. Canadian sheet dermatitis. *Br Med J* 1976;2:1175.
70. Epstein E, Maibach HI. Formaldehyde allergy. *Arch Dermatol* 1966; 94:186.
71. O'Quinn SE, Kennedy CB. Contact dermatitis due to formaldehyde in clothing textiles. *JAMA* 1965;194:123.
72. Sherertz E. Clothing dermatitis: practical aspects for the clinician. *Am J Contact Dermatitis* 1992;3:55–64.
73. Schwartz L. Dermatitis from synthetic resins. *J Invest Dermatol* 1945;6:239.
74. Helander I. Contact urticaria from leather containing formaldehyde. *Arch Dermatol* 1977;113:1443.
75. Dahlquist I, Fregert S. Formaldehyde releasers. *Contact Dermatitis* 1978;4:1–13.
76. Dahl M. Formaldehyde sensitivity in patients allergic to formaldehyde-releasing biocides. *Br J Dermatol* 1982;106:119.

77. Robertson MH, Storrs FJ. Allergic contact dermatitis in two machinists. *Arch Dermatol* 1982;118:997.

78. Lynde CW, Warshawski L, Mitchell JC. Screening patch tests in 4190 eczema patients 1972–1981. *Contact Dermatitis* 1982;8:417.

79. Marks J, Belsito D, DeLeo V, Fowler J, et al. North American Contact Dermatitis Group patch-test results, 1996–1998. *Arch Dermatol* 2000;136:272–273.

80. Burry J, Kirk J, Reid JC, Turner T. Environmental dermatitis: changing patterns. *Med J Aust* 1980;1:183.

81. Agathos M. Formaldehyde contact allergy. *Contact Dermatitis* 1982; 8:79.

82. Jordan WP, Sherman WJ, Kins S. Threshold responses in formaldehyde-sensitive subjects. *J Am Acad Dermatol* 1979;1:44.

83. Fisher AA. Contact "pants paresthesia syndrome." *Contact Dermatitis* 1983;9:92.

84. Neilson AW, Reiches AJ. Contact dermatitis due to underwear: observations in fourteen cases with summary of efforts to discover the cause. *Arch Dermatol* 1941;44:218.

85. Barnes R. An unusual "epidemic" in a clothing factory. *Trans Soc Occup Med* 1972;22:137.

86. Fregert S. Extraction of allergens for patch testing. *Acta Derm Venereol* (Stockh) 1964;44:107.

87. Rostenberg A. Dermatitis from formaldehyde resin textiles—discussion. *Arch Dermatol* 1966;94:800.

88. Scheman A, Carroll P, Brown K, Osburn A. Formaldehyde related textile allergy: an update. *Contact Dermatitis* 1998;38:332–336.

89. Schorr WF, Keran E, Plotka E. Formaldehyde allergy. *Arch Dermatol* 1974;110:73.

90. Dahlquist I, Fregert S, Gruvberger B. Detection of formaldehyde in corticoid creams. *Contact Dermatitis* 1980;6:494.

91. Tegner E, Fregert S. Contamination of cosmetics with formaldehyde from tubes. *Contact Dermatitis* Newsletter 1973;13:353.

92. Dahlquist I, Fregert S, Gruvberger B. Reliability of the chromotropic acid method for qualitative formaldehyde determination. *Contact Dermatitis* 1980;6:357.

93. Fenman SE. *Formaldehyde sensitivity and toxicity.* Boca Raton, FL: CRC Press, 1988:105–112.

94. Buyer's guide. *Text Chem Colorist* 1983;15:1.

95. Foussereau PJ, Meynadier J, Reuter G, et al. L'Eczema allergique aux toiles cirées. *Dermatosen Beruf Umwelt* 1980;28:46–50.

96. Weaver JE. Dermatologic testing of household laundry products: a novel fabric softener. *Int J Dermatol* 1976;15:297.

97. Tarvainen K, Jolanki R, Henriks-Eckerman ML, Estlander T. Occupational allergic contact dermatitis from isophoronediamine (IPDA) in operative-clothing manufacture. *Contact Dermatitis* 1998;39:46–47.

98. Fregert S. Antimicrobial agents in textiles. *Contact Dermatitis* Newsletter 1971;9:201.

99. Molin L, Wahlberg JE. Toxic skin reactions caused by tributyltin oxide (TBTD) in socks. *Berufsdermatosen* 1975;23:138.

100. Savage J. Chloracetamide in nylon spin finish. *Contact Dermatitis* 1978;4:179.

101. Burrows D, Campbell HS. Contact dermatitis to polyester spin-finishes. *Contact Dermatitis* 1980;6:362.

102. Kawai K, et al. Occupational contact dermatitis from Kathon 930. *Contact Dermatitis* 1993;28:117.

103. Weaver JE, Maibach HI. Dose response relationships in allergic contact dermatitis: glutaraldehyde-containing liquid fabric softener. *Contact Dermatitis* 1977;3:65.

104. Gaul LE. Dermatitis from cetyl and stearyl alcohols. *Arch Dermatol* 1969;99:593.

105. Eskelson YD, Goodman LS. Contact dermatitis from "Scotchgard," a stain repellent for fabrics. *JAMA* 1963;183:136.

106. Wilkinson S, et al. Allergic contact dermatitis from 1,6-diisocyanatohexane in an anti-pill finish. *Contact Dermatitis* 1991;25:94.

107. Gunnell DJ. Mysterious slapped face rash at holiday centre. *British Medical Journal* 1992;304:477–479

108. Rothenborg HW, Hjorth N. Allergy to perfumes from toilet soaps and detergents in patients with dermatitis. *Arch Dermatol* 1968; 97:417.

109. Carter RO, McMurrain KD. Consumer safety of enzyme detergents. *JAMA* 1970;211:2017.

110. Bolam RM. Severe dermatitis and "biological" detergents (Letter). *Br Med J* 1970;1:818.

111. Cronin E. Contact dermatitis XIII: the significance of nickel sensitivity in women. *Br J Dermatol* 1974;84:96.

112. Taylor JS, Bergfeld WF, Guin JD. Contact dermatitis to knee patch adhesive in boy's jeans: a non-occupational cause of epoxy resin sensitivity. *Cleve Clin Q* 1983;50:123.

113. Soni BP, Sherertz EF. Contact dermatitis in the textile industry: a - review of 72 patients. *Amer J Contact Dermatitis* 1996;7:226–230.

114. Dooms-Goosens A, Boyden B, Ceuterick A, Degruf H. Dimethyl-thiourea, an unexpected hazard for textile workers. *Contact Dermatitis* 1979;5:367.

115. Baltinger, W. *Westex Inc. technical bulletin.* Chicago, 1997.

116. Ulsamer AG, Osterberg RE, McLaughlin J. Flame-retardant chemicals in textiles. *Clin Toxicol* 1980;17:101.

117. Blum A, Ames BN. Flame-retardant additives as possible cancer hazards. *Science* 1977;195:17.

118. Parlew R, King CM, Evans S. Primary sensitization to a single accidental exposure to a flame retardant and subsequent allergic contact dermatitis. *Contact Dermatitis,* 1995;33:286.

119. Drake GC. Flame retardants for textiles. In: *Kirk-Othmer encyclopedia of chemical technology.* New York: John Wiley and Sons, 1980; 10:420.

120. Standard for Children's Sleepwear. Code of Federal Regulations, Title 16, Chap. 2, Part 16–1J, Sizes 0–6X (1972); Part 16–1G, Sizes 0–14 (1975).

121. Children's wearing apparel containing tris: interpretation as banned hazardous substance. *Federal Register* 1977;42:18850–18854; see also 1977;42:28060–28064; and 1977;42:61621–61622.

122. Bioassay of tris (2,3-dibromopropyl) phosphate for possible carcinogenicity. Carcinogenesis testing program, Division of Cancer Cause and Prevention. National Cancer Institute, DHEW Pub. NIH No. 78–1326, 1978, National Toxicology Program Technical Report No. 76, Order No. P-B 280271 from National Technical Information Service, Springfield, VA.

123. Carcinogenesis studies of polybrominated biphenyl mixture (Firemaster FF-1) in F344/N rats and B6C3F, mice. NIH Pub. No. 83–1800, National Toxicology Program Technical Report No. 244, 1983.

124. Andersen KE. Sensitivity to a flame retardant, tris (2,3-dibromopropyl) phosphate (Firemaster LVT 23 P). *Contact Dermatitis* 1977; 3:297.

125. Morrow RW, Hornberger CS, Kligman AM, Maibach HI. Tris (2,3-dibromopropyl) phosphate: human contact sensitization. *Am Ind Hyg Assoc J* 1076;37:192.

126. Martin-Scott I. Contact textile dermatitis. *Br J Dermatol* 1966;78:632.

127. Belsito D. Contact dermatitis from diammonium hydrogen phosphate in surgical garb (Abstract). *Contact Dermatitis* 1990;23:267.

128. Material safety data sheet. Chicago: Westex Inc., 1992.

129. Vail JT. False negative reaction to patch testing with volatile compounds. *Arch Dermatol* 1974;110:130.

130. Redmond S, Schappert K. Occupational dermatitis associated with garments. *J Occup Med* 1987;29:243.

131. Aoki T, Kageyama R. Three cases of dry cleaning dermatitis. *Nippon-Hifuka-Gakkai-Zasshi* 1989;99:1035–1038.

132. Van Ketel WG. Contact dermatitis from a hydrazine-derivative in a stain remover; cross sensitization to apresoline and isoniazid. *Acta Derm Venereol* (Stockh) 1964;44:49.

133. Jenkins CL. Textile dyes are potential hazards. *J Environ Health* 1978;40:279.

134. Fleming AJ. The provocative test for assaying the dermatitis hazards of dyes and finishes used on nylon. *J Invest Dermatol* 1948;10:281.

135. Fregert S, Trulsson L. Difficulties in tracing sensitizing textile dyes. *Contact Dermatitis* 1978;4:174.

136. Foussereau J, Benezra C, Maibach H. *Occupational contact dermatitis: clinical and chemical aspects.* 1st ed. Philadelphia: WB Saunders, 1982:1.

137. Cywie PL, Herve-Bazin B, Foussereau J, et al. Les eczemas allergiques professionnels dans l'industrie textile. Rapport No. 244/R1, ISSN 0397 4529. Vancoevre, France: Institut National de Recherche et Sécurité, Centre de Recherche, March 1977.

138. Hatch KL, Maibach HI. Textile dye dermatitis. *J Amer Acad Dermatology* 1995;32:631–639.

139. *Colour index.* 3rd ed. Vol. 5, *Commercial names and index.* American Association of Textile Chemists and Colorists of the Society of Dyers and Colorists, 1971–1982.

140. Ancona-Alayon A, et al. Occupational pigmented contact dermatitis from Naphthol AS. *Contact Dermatitis* 1976;2:129.
141. Hatch K, Maibach H. Textile fiber dermatitis. *Contact Dermatitis* 1985;12:1–11.
142. Seidenari S, et al. Contact sensitization to textile dyes: description of 100 subjects. *Contact Dermatitis* 1991;24:253.
143. Sim-Davies D. Studies in contact dermatitis XXIV: dyes in trousers. *Trans St Johns Hosp Dermatol Soc* 1972;58:251.
144. Calnan C D. Textile dye disperse yellow 64. *Contact Dermatitis* 1977;3:209.
145. Pratt M, Taraska V. Disperse Blue Dyes 106 and 124 are common causes of textile dermatitis and should serve as screening allergens for this condition. *Amer J Contact Dermatitis* 2000;1:30–41.
146. Lazarov A, Trattner A, David M, Ingber A. Textile dermatitis in Israel: a retrospective study. *Amer J Contact Dermatitis* 2000;1: 26–29.
147. Storrs, F J. Disperse Blue Dyes. *Amer J Contact Dermatitis* 2000; 1:1–2.
148. Seidenari S, Mantovani L, Manzini B M, Pignatti M. Cross-sensitizations between azo dyes and para-amino compound: astudy of 236 azo-dye sensitive subjects. *Contact Dermatitis* 1997;36:91–96.
149. Warren L J, Marren P. Textile dermatitis and dyed maggot exposure. *Contact Dermatitis* 1997;36:106.
150. Lazarov A, Ingber A. Textile dermatitis from Disperse Blue 85 in a knee brace. *Contact Dermatitis* 1998;38:357.
151. Thierback M, et al. Sensitization to azo dyes: Negative patch tests to yellow and red azo dyes in printed paper. *Contact Dermatitis* 1992; 27:22.
152. Francalanci S, Angelini G, Balato N, et al. Effectiveness of disperse dyes mix in detection of contact allergy to textile dyes: an Italian multicentre study. *Contact Dermatitis* 1995;33:351.
153. Wilson H T H, Cronin E. Dermatitis from dyed uniform. *Br J Dermatol* 1971;87:67.
154. Manzini B M, Motolese A, Conti A, et al. Sensitization to reactive textile dyes in patients with contact dermatitis. *Contact Dermatitis* 1996;34:419–422.
155. Manzini B M, Donini M, Motolese A, Seidenari S. A study of 5 newly patch tested reactive textile dyes. *Contact Dermatitis* 1996; 35:313.
156. Malten K E. Eczema in a cotton-printing mill (Proceedings of the XI International Congress of Dermatology). *Acta Derm Venereol* (Stockh) 1957;2:353.
157. Kiec-Swierczynska M. Occupational contact dermatitis in the workers employed in production of Texas textiles. *Dermatosen Beruf Umwelt* 1982;39:41.
158. Roed-Petersen J, Batsberg W, Larsen E. Contact dermatitis from naphthol-AS. *Contact Dermatitis* 1990;22:161.
159. Mathur N, Mathur A, Benerjee K. Contact dermatitis in tie and dye industry workers. *Contact Dermatitis* 1985;12:38.
160. Bielicky T, Novak M. Contact-group sensitization to triphenyl-methane dyes: gentian violet, brilliant green and malachite green. *Arch Dermatol* 1969;100:540.
161. Scheman A. Allergic contact dermatitis from Basic Red 46 in a flame-retardant work clothing. *Contact Dermatitis* 1998;38:340.
162. Pedersen N B. Occupational contact dermatitis from C.I. Acid Red 85 (C.I. 22245). *Contact Dermatitis* 1982;8:142.
163. Seidenari S, Manzini B M, Schiavi M E, Motolese A. Prevalence of contact allergy to non-disperse azo dyes for natural fibers: a study in 1814 consecutive patients. *Contact Dermatitis* 1995;33:118–122.
164. Calnan C D, Woods B. Dermatitis from dye in a leather watchstrap. *Contact Dermatitis* 1978;4:179.
165. Wright R C. Dermatitis from orthodichlorobenzene in a leather dye. *Contact Dermatitis* 1979;5:124.
166. Manzini B, et al. Contact sensitization to newly patch-tested non-disperse textile dyes. *Contact Dermatitis* 1991;25:331.
167. Kojima S, et al. Phosgene (chlorophenyl) hydrazones, strong sensitizers found in yellow sweaters bleached with sodium hypochlorite. *Contact Dermatitis* 1990;23:129.
168. Gardiner J S, Dickson A, Macleod T M, Frain-Bell W. The investigation of photocontact dermatitis is a dye manufacturing process. *Br J Dermatol* 1971;85:264.
169. Hjorth N, Moller H. Phototoxic textile dermatitis ("bikini dermatitis"). *Arch Dermatol* 1976;112:1445.
170. Estlander T. Allergic dermatoses and respiratory diseases from reactive dyes. *Contact Dermatitis* 1988;18:290.
171. Cronin E. Studies in contact dermatitis XIX: nylon stocking dyes. *Trans St Johns Hosp Dermatol Soc* 1968;54:165.
172. Fanburg SJ. Dermatitis following the wearing of nylon stockings. *JAMA* 1940;115:354.
173. Schwartz LW, et al. An outbreak of dermatitis from new resin fabric finishes. *JAMA* 1940;115:906.
174. Calnan CD, Wilson HTH. Nylon stocking dermatitis. *Br Med J* 1956;1:147.
175. Dobkevitch S, Baer RL. Eczematous cross-hypersensitivity to azo dyes in nylon stockings and to paraphenylenediamine. *J Invest Dermatol* 1947;9:203.
176. Kousa M, Soini M. Contact allergy to a stocking dye. *Contact Dermatitis* 1980;6:472.
177. Foussereau J, Tanahaski Y, Grosshans E, et al. Allergic eczema from Disperse Yellow 3 in nylon stockings and socks. *Trans St Johns Hosp Dermatol Soc* 1975;58:75.
178. Calnan CD. Hazards of optic bleachers. *Trans St Johns Hosp Dis Skin* 1973;59:275.
179. Osmundsen PE, Alani MD. Contact allergy to an optical whitener, "CPY," in washing powders. *Br J Dermatol* 1971;85:61.
180. Rinol Aguade J, et al. Dermatitis por blanqueradores opticas. *Medicina Cutanea* 1971;5:249.
181. Griffith JF. Fluorescent whitening agents. *Arch Dermatol* 1973; 107:728.
182. Osmundsen PE. Contact dermatitis from an optical whitener in washing powders. *Cutis* 1972;10:59.
183. Wilkinson DS. Contact dermatitis XVIII: ancillary aids in elucidation of causes of contact dermatitis. *Br J Dermatol* 1972;86:445.
184. Patterson S, Williams V, Marks J. Prevention of sodium lauryl sulfate irritant contact dermatitis by Pro-Q aerosol foam skin protectant. *J Am Acad Dermatol* 1999;40:783–785.
185. Freeman S. Shoe dermatitis. *Contact Dermatitis* 1997;36:247–251.
186. Epstein E. Shoe contact dermatitis. *JAMA* 1969;209:1487.
187. Jordan WP. Clothing and shoe dermatitis. *Postgrad Med* 1972;52: 143.
188. Lynde CW, Warshawski L, Mitchell JC. Patch test results with a shoewear screening tray in 119 patients, 1977–80. *Contact Dermatitis* 1982;8:423.
189. Angelini G, Vena GA, Meneghini CL. Shoe contact dermatitis. *Contact Dermatitis* 1980;6:279.
190. Gaul LE, Underwood GB. Primary irritants and sensitizers used in fabrication of footwear. *Arch Dermatol* 1949;60:649.
191. Hack M. The shoe in contact dermatitis. *J Am Podiatr Assoc* 1976; 66:408.
192. Dahl MV. Allergic contact dermatitis from footwear. *Minn Med* 1975;58:871.
193. Grimalt F, Romaguera C. New resin allergens in shoe contact dermatitis. *Contact Dermatitis* 1975;1:169.
194. deVries HR. Allergic dermatitis due to shoes. *Dermatologica* 1964; 128:68.
195. Cronin E. Shoe dermatitis. *Br J Dermatol* 1966;78:52.
196. Weston JA, Hawkins K, Weston WL. Foot dermatitis in children. *Pediatrics* 1983;72:824.
197. Blank IH, Miller OG. A study of rubber adhesives in shoes as the cause of dermatitis of the feet. *JAMA* 1952;149:1371.
198. Calnan CD, Sarkany I. Studies in contact dermatitis IX: shoe dermatitis. *Trans St Johns Hosp Dermatol Soc* 1959;43:8.
199. Scutt RWB. Chrome sensitivity associated with tropical footwear in the royal navy. *Br J Dermatol* 1966;78:337.
200. Malten KE, Rath R, Pastors PHM. p-tert-butylphenol formaldehyde and other causes of shoe dermatitis. *Dermatosen Beruf Umwelt* 1983;31:149.
201. Bajaj A, et al. Footwear depigmentation. *Contact Dermatitis* 1996; 35:117–118
202. Fisher AA. Some practical aspects of the diagnosis and management of shoe dermatitis. *Arch Dermatol* 1959;79:267.
203. Trevisan G, Kokelj F. Allergic contact dermatitis due to shoes in children: a 5-year follow-up. *Contact Dermatitis* 1992;26:45.
204. Cockayne SE, Shah M, Messenger AG, Gawkrodger DJ. Foot dermatitis in children: causative allergens and follow-up. *Contact Dermatitis* 1998;38:203–206.
205. Raoul S, Ducombs G, Leaute-Labreze C, et al. Footwear contact dermatitis in children. *Contact Dermatitis* 1996;35:334–336.
206. Hack M. Chemical and mechanical etiology of shoe dermatitis. *Cutis* 1970;6:529.

207. Mackie RM. Juvenile plantar dermatosis. *Semin Dermatol* 1982; 1:67.
208. Romaguera C, Grimalt F, Ferrando J. Dry feet syndrome or juvenile plantar dermatosis. *Contact Dermatitis* 1982;8:219.
209. Steck WD. Juvenile plantar dermatosis: the "wet and dry foot syndrome." *Cleve Clin Q* 1983;50:145.
210. Farkas J. Chronic shoe dermatitis from chromium tanned leather. *Contact Dermatitis* 1982;8:140.
211. Calnan CD, Cronin E. Vegetable tans in leather. *Contact Dermatitis* 1978;4:295.
212. Lewis GM. Dermatitis venenata due to tannins. *Arch Dermatol* 1944;50:138.
213. Hausen BM. *Woods injurious to human health: a manual.* Berlin: Walter deGruyter, 1981.
214. Lynch PJ. Indian sandal strap dermatitis. *JAMA* 1969;209:1906.
215. Pilgrim RE, Fleagle GS. Indian sandal strap dermatitis. *JAMA* 1970; 211:1378.
216. Minkin W, Cohen HJ, Frank S. Contact dermatitis to East Indian leather. *Arch Dermatol* 1971;103:523.
217. Spoor HJ. Indian leather dermatitis. *Cutis* 1973;11:805.
218. Jordan WP, Dahl MV, Albert HL. Contact dermatitis from glutaraldehyde. *Arch Dermatol* 1972;105:94.
219. Ancona A, Serviere L, Trejo A, Monroy F. Dermatitis from an azo dye in industrial leather protective shoes. *Contact Dermatitis* 1982; 8:220.
220. Gaul LE. Results of patch testing with rubber antioxidants and accelerators. *J Invest Dermatol* 1957;29:105.
221. Marcussen PV. Rubber footwear as a cause of foot eczema. *Acta Derm Venereol* (Stockh) 1943;23:331.
222. Webb PK, Gibbs SC, Mathias CT, et al. Disulfiram hypersensitivity and rubber contact dermatitis. *JAMA* 1979;241:2061.
223. Leppard BJ, Parhizgar B. Contact dermatitis to PPD rubber in Maleki shoes. *Contact Dermatitis* 1977;3:91.
224. Robb JB. Rubber boot dermatitis in Newfoundland: a survey of 30 patients. *Can Med Assoc J* 1969;100:13.
225. Roberts JL, Hanifin JM. Athletic shoe dermatitis: allergy to ethyl butyl thiourea. *JAMA* 1979;241:275.
226. Adams RM. *Occupational skin disease.* San Francisco: Grune & Stratton, 1983.
227. Srinivas C, et al. Footwear dermatitis due to Bisphenol-A. *Contact Dermatitis* 1989;20:150.
228. Fregert S. Chemicals used both in rubber and plastics. *Contact Dermatitis Newsletter* 1971;9:204.
229. Shellow H. Dermatitis from Japanese rubber thong slippers. *Fam Phys* 1961;1:44.
230. Weiner E. Dermatitis of the feet due to wearing of impermeable shoes. *J Am Podiatr Assoc* 1960;50:545.
231. Malten KE. Occupational eczema due to para-tertiary butylphenol in a shoe adhesive. *Dermatologica* 1958;117:103.
232. Malten KE. Contact sensitization caused by *p*-tert-butylphenol and certain phenol-formaldehyde-containing glues. *Dermatologica* 1967;135:54.
233. Schubert H, Agatha G. The allergenic nature of *p*-tert-butylphenol-formaldehyde resin. *Dermatosen Beruf Umwelt* 1979;27:49.
234. Rycroft RG. Contact sensitization to 2-monomethylol phenol in phenol formaldehyde resin as an example of the recognition and prevention of industrial dermatoses. *Clin Exp Dermatol* 1982;7:285.
235. Geldof B, et al. Clinical aspects of para-tertiary butylphenol-formaldehyde resin (PTBP-FR) allergy. *Contact Dermatitis* 1989;21: 312.
236. Foussereau J, Cavelier C, Selig D. Occupational eczema from para-tertiary-butylphenol formaldehyde resins: a review of the sensitizing resins. *Contact Dermatitis* 1976;2:254.
237. Correcher BL, Perez AG. Dermatitis from shoes and an amputation prosthesis due to mercaptobenzothiazole and paratertiary butyl formaldehyde resin. *Contact Dermatitis* 1981;7:275.
238. Storrs FJ. *Shoe dermatitis.* Presented at American Contact Dermatitis Society Meeting, July 1993, New Orleans, LA.
239. Rietschel RL. Role of socks in shoe dermatitis. *Arch Dermatol* 1984;120:398.
240. Mathias CGT, Maibach HI. Polyvinyl chloride work boots in the management of shoe dermatitis in industrial workers. *Contact Dermatitis* 1979;5:249.

CHAPTER 20

Dermatitis from Medical Devices, Implants, and Equipment

REACTION AND DERMATITIS DUE TO METALS USED IN ORTHOPEDIC SURGERY

Common Prosthetic Metals

Vitallium, stainless steel, and titanium are used widely for prosthetic devices. These metals are resistant to corrosion by physiologic fluids and can be left in the body indefinitely (1,2).

Vitallium, a cobalt-based alloy designed for casting, contains about 30% chromium (Cr) and about 5% molybdenum (Mo). Since 1937, vitallium has been used successfully for orthopedic implants. Being a cast alloy, however, vitallium cannot be drawn into suture wire or worked into other complex shapes.

"Stainless steel" is a generic term covering several dozen iron-chromium alloys. Two of these, AISI Type 302 and AISI Type 316 steels, have found uses in orthopedic surgery. Shortly before World War II, however, it was recognized that Type 316 steel (17% Cr, 13% nickel [Ni], 2.5% Mo) was more inert to physiologic fluids than was Type 302 steel. The addition of molybdenum helps to prevent pitting by body chlorides. Widespread use of AISI Type 316 steel came about during World War II. Type 316 steel has some desirable features that vitallium lacks: greater strength, greater fatigue resistance, the ability to be easily worked into useful forms, and relatively low cost (Table 20.1).

Vitallium, titanium, and Type 316L stainless steel are commonly used in orthopedic implants.

Titanium is one of the newer metals to be used in prosthetic applications. Although it lacks the strength of Type 316 stainless steel or vitallium, it is apparently inert to physiologic fluids. In fact, bone has a tendency to grow in contact with titanium and becomes very adherent to it. Titanium has been used successfully in various reconstructions.

In cases of known or strongly suspected allergy to nickel, cobalt, or chromate, titanium prosthesis may be preferable.

Newer Orthopedic Alloys

Nitinol is an alloy composed of about 55% nickel and 45% titanium. It is called a "metal with a memory" because it returns to its initial shape when heated. It may be used in some suture fixation devices and in spinal rods (2). Other titanium alloys containing zirconium and niobium may be stronger than titanium alone.

Titanium alloys can usually be used when cobalt and nickel sensitivity coexist.

REACTIONS TO IMPLANTED METAL PROSTHESES

Orthopedic implants may be either static, such as rods and screws, or dynamic, such as an artificial hip or knee joint. Most joint implants now have a metal-to-plastic interface. In patients who have old metal-to-metal prostheses, elevated concentrations of chromium and cobalt occur in blood and urine as well as in the tissue adjacent to the joint prostheses. In patients with metal-to-plastic prostheses, the metal concentrations in blood and urine are normal, and only slightly elevated in the tissues when compared with controls (3,4).

Nickel is released from stainless steel prostheses by the action of sweat, blood, and physiologic saline solution. In laboratory animals, solubilized nickel is localized in the tissue near the implant (5).

The sensitization potential of implanted metal alloys has been evaluated in retrospective and prospective clinical studies. The significance of these studies is difficult to interpret, because metal allergy is a common phenomenon in the general population.

321

TABLE 20.1. *Common Metals Used in Orthopedic Implants*

Vitallium—cobalt, chromium steel
Type 316L stainless steel
Titanium alloys
Nitinol-nickel titanium alloy

> **Metal-to-metal prostheses are more likely to produce elevated chromium and cobalt in the blood and tissues than the more commonly used metal-to-plastic articulations, which are less likely to produce metal sensitization.**

In retrospective studies concerning patients with metal-to-metal prostheses (cobalt and chromium), a high incidence of metal sensitivity has been found. In 14 patients who had loose prostheses, 9 were sensitive to either cobalt or chromium. Of 24 patients who had normally functioning prostheses, none was metal sensitive (4). Elves et al. (6) studied 50 patients with metal-to-metal prostheses. Of the 50 patients, 23 had a nontraumatic failure of the prosthesis. Fifteen of these were sensitive to metals, 7 were cobalt-sensitive, 3 were sensitive to cobalt and nickel, 2 to nickel, 2 to chromium, and 1 to both nickel and vanadium. In the other 27 patients who had stable prostheses or who had a traumatic failure, only 4 were metal sensitive. Benson et al. (7) found an incidence of 28% metal sensitivity in patients with metal-to-metal prostheses. Among 34 patients with pain and loosening of the prostheses, Munro-Ashman and Miller (8) found 16 patients with metal sensitivity. Thirteen were sensitive to cobalt, 4 to nickel, and 2 to chromium. The results of these studies are similar and, although retrospective, they suggest that at least cobalt sensitization occurs as a consequence of systematic exposure to the metal when released from an implanted metal alloy.

Lodi et al. (9) patch tested 66 patients an average of 8 years after implantation with a large battery of metal allergens. There was one positive test each to nickel, cobalt, and chromate, but seven to vanadium trichloride (5% pet). Many irritant responses were also seen to the vanadium, so the significance of this data is uncertain. There was no comment regarding the type of prothesis—metal to metal or metal to plastic.

In prospective studies concerning similar patients in whom the preoperative status has been evaluated by patch testing, no evidence was found of sensitization to the implanted metal alloys when retested months to years after the operation (10–13). In the retrospective part of the study by Carlsson et al. (10), a statistically significant increase in the number of metal-sensitive patients was found among those with loose prostheses. Among the patients studied prospectively, only a few had complications with pain and loosening of the prostheses. Rooker and Wilkinson (13) studied 69

patients prospectively. Before the operation, six patients were metal sensitive, but only one remained so afterward. The authors suggested that the minimal systemic exposure to the hapten led to immunologic tolerance. The safety of the metal-to-plastic prostheses from the point of sensitization is in agreement with the small amounts of metal released from this type of prosthesis (3,4).

Sensitization from metal prostheses has been reported mostly in patients with loosening of the prostheses. This does not prove that the allergy is the cause of the loosening. The alternative explanation is that the loosening causes the allergy. The present evidence supports the latter hypothesis (14,15).

> **Loosening of a prosthesis is usually not due to allergy to metals in the prosthesis. Loosening, however, may produce metal changes and sensitization.**

Skin symptoms in patients who have undergone implantation of metal prostheses are rare. They occur in two forms: either as a dermatitis localized to the skin that covers the area of the metal prostheses (8,16) or as a generalized dermatitis (17–19). Those who develop rashes from osteosynthesis screws have a more persistent disease, and removal of the screws has been followed by a rapid clearing of the dermatitis (16,17,19,20).

In a literature review, Dujardin et al. (21) found 54 cases of dermatitis due to various implants. None were caused by titanium. The difficulties of making a firm diagnosis without removal of the prothesis are discussed.

Kubba et al. (18) stated:

> Allergic cutaneous complications of orthopedic implants are rare. However, in an implant recipient in whom a cutaneous problem develops, the likelihood of the cutaneous problem being allergic in nature is slightly greater if the implant is of the static type, if there is a history of metal sensitivity, if the cutaneous eruption shows a predilection for the anatomic zone of the implant, and if the eruption is eczematous and has developed late and persisted.

Oleffe and Wilmet (19) described dermatitis from "static" implants (osteosynthetic screws) in nickel-sensitive individuals.

> **Allergic dermatitis due to orthopedic implants is rare. Such dermatitis is more likely if:**
>
> 1. **The implant is of the static type (screws).**
> 2. **A history of metal sensitivity is present.**
> 3. **The eruption is near the implant.**
> 4. **The eruption is eczematous.**
> 5. **The eruption develops late and persists.**

Reaction to Acrylates in Orthopedic Surgery

Occasionally, allergic reactions have been seen to methyl methacrylate in orthopedic bone cements. More often, the surgeon may suffer a hand dermatitis from these agents. Joint loosening apparently occurs rarely, if at all (21).

Role of Preoperative Patch Testing

Menné and Hjorth (22) stated that the limited number of patients who have allergic reactions owing to implanted metal prostheses does not indicate that all patients should be patch tested preoperatively. Carlsson et al. (10) recommended that a patient who had a history of metal allergy should be examined by a dermatologist and should be patch tested. If a metal allergy is found, an implant should be used that does not contain the metal in question. Only long-term prospective studies can determine whether it is necessary to take any precautions at all.

> The need for preoperative patch testing to metals is controversial, but may be important both from a medical and medicolegal standpoint.

Summary

Gawkrodger (20) reviewed the subject and agreed that modern prostheses of the metal to plastic variety rarely cause metal allergy. Occasionally, eczema, either localized or generalized, may be seen with static implants, but even this is rare.

An important concern in the debate about preoperative patch testing is medicolegal liability. If any adverse event occurs in a metal-sensitive patient after implantation of that metal, the surgeon may be held liable, rightly or wrongly. Therefore, even though cutaneous reactions to implanted metals are rare, avoidance of known allergens in the choice of a prosthesis seems advisable until more definitive data are available.

OSTOMY DERMATITIS

Ostomies are artificial openings to the gastrointestinal (GI) or urinary tracts. They are used widely in the treatment of a variety of inflammatory, neoplastic, and posttraumatic processes. The proper care of the operative stoma and of the appliance fitted to it is crucial to proper functioning of the surgical diversion and to the complete rehabilitation of the patient (see Appendix A).

The peristomal skin is prone to irritation and development of allergic contact dermatitis partly because of the continuous exposure to GI or urinary fluids and moisture, and partly because of the occlusion necessary around the stoma to prevent leakage.

Rothstein (23–26) has written extensively on the care and management of the ostomy site. He states that several factors relating to the stomal surgery itself are important in providing an optimum stoma result. These include gentle handling of the skin to avoid scarring and proper anatomic placement of the stomal stump to avoid surface irregularities that allow for leakage. Also, the length of the stump is critical so that excess irritation from friction or secretions will not occur. Depending on the stoma location, discharge may be more fluid or more solid. Obviously, fluid drainage is more likely to cause irritation because of the presence of fecal enzymes and an alkaline pH.

Peristomal Allergic and Irritant Contact Dermatitis

Irritant dermatitis is common and must be expected to occur in almost any ostomy patient occasionally. Chemical irritation may occur from excreted fluids, from solvents, cleansing materials, or disinfectants used when changing the device, or from pressure and friction from the sealing ring and ostomy pouch. Gentle changing of the ostomy pouch, without the use of solvents, if possible, may be necessary if irritation develops. It has been suggested that the use of a karaya ring instead of common adhesive rings may be useful if irritation develops (27,28). The pouch can be held in place with hypoallergenic tape or a belt temporarily.

Karaya is a gum made from the sterculia tree, a polysaccharide of 9,500,000 molecular weight (26). It is available as a powder, which is good for absorbing moisture, a paste, or as an ostomy ring. Rothstein suggests mixing karaya with milk of magnesia or an antacid such as aluminum hydroxide, which may inhibit fecal enzyme activity (24). Burt-McAliley et al. (29), however, prospectively studied 112 patients given either a karaya-based or a pectin-based barrier. They found that irritation was more likely to develop in those using a karaya-based product.

Allergic contact dermatitis (ACD) may be caused by a variety of allergens in the peristomal area. It has been well documented that ACD is more likely to develop in areas where skin breakdown from other causes occurs, and this situation may be present around a stoma. Pruritus and spread of dermatitis around the affected site are typical of ACD.

Table 20.2 lists some of the reported causes of peristomal ACD. Patch testing is essential to determin the allergen(s) responsible. On screening patch test series, the rubber aller-

TABLE 20.2. *Reported Allergens in Stomal Dermatitis*

Adhesive tapes
Balsam of Peru, fragrances
Deodorizers
Mercaptobenzothiazole
Rosin
Rubber
Stomahesive paste

gens, rosin, epoxy resin, neomycin, fragrance, and preservatives are all candidates to cause peristomal ACD. Other potential allergens include topical antibiotics, preservatives, disinfectants, acrylates, and plasticizers.

Urostomy Dermatitis

Urostomies are subject to encrustations. These are verrucose, gray-white excrescences that seem to grow on the stomal mucosa or on improperly cleaned reusable pouches. They are crystallized alkaline salts, mainly amorphous ammonium phosphates. Because of their gritty texture, they may excoriate the skin if they are allowed to seep beneath the pouch. Prolonged exposure of the skin to moisture creates pseudoepitheliomatous hyperplasia—a condition of epidermal thickening characterized histologically by acanthosis and increased mitoses but without atypia (30).

Urostomy crystals and pseudoepitheliomatous hyperplasia respond to vinegar compresses or lavage with a 50% vinegar solution poured into the pouch and allowed to wash over the stoma. This will not work in urostomy pouches with antireflux valves, however. Dietary modifications may help by altering the urine pH. Local application of a silver nitrate stick will flatten excess tissue or heal small erosions.

Mann et al. (31) reported sensitivity to a urostomy pouch plastic (Squibb System Z Urostomy pouch) in a patient with epoxy resin sensitivity. The patient's eczema cleared completely on subsequently changing the system to a Hollister Lo Profile pouch. Van Ketel et al. (32) also reported epoxyresin dermatitis from a Squibb ileostomy bag, which was made of polyvinyl chloride, in which epoxy resin was used as a plasticizer.

Polyvinyl ostomy bags may be plasticized with epoxy resin, which may cause dermatitis in sensitized individuals.

Contact sensitivity has been reported to Hollister adhesive, Stomahesive, and rubber (25,26,33). The bag itself may cause an irritant reaction owing to friction or a prickly, heatlike eruption owing to sweat retention (27).

Deodorant Dermatitis

Davies et al. (34) reported that an ostomy deodorant sensitized two patients and was due to oil of citronella.

Management of Ostomy Dermatitis

Rothstein (25,26) reviewed important considerations in ostomy management. Obviously, avoidance of further irritation and identification of allergens is a critical first step. Temporary ostomy appliances may be tolerated for several days to allow the skin to heal before reapplying permanent

devices. A topical or oral anti-*Candida* agent will reduce yeast infections and colonization. Low- to medium-strength topical corticosteroids may be needed, but care must be taken so as not to allow development of steroid atrophy or secondary infections. Systemic corticosteroids may be needed for a short time for severe cases.

Covering the pouch with a commercial cloth bag or even flannel or gauze may reduce frictional irritation.

Two new "skin protective" products may offer some benefit at reducing irritation or allergen penetration. These include Pro-Q foam (Ponsus Pharma, Stockholm, Sweden) and Ivy Block Lotion (Enviroderm Inc., Louisville, KY). To be effective, such products would need to be applied to the skin before the appliance is seated and also applied under tape and the pouch.

CONTRACEPTIVE DERMATITIS

The most common contraceptives in use at present—the condom, the diaphragm, chemical contraceptives, female pouches, the intrauterine device, and "the Pill"—may all occasionally produce allergic or other reactions (35).

Condoms

Condoms are popularly called "sheaths," "French letters," prophylactics," "rubbers," "skins," or "safes" and are made mostly of rubber. Allergic reactions to condoms may produce itching and edema of the prepuce or distal part of the shaft of the penis, which may initiate an eczematous dermatitis and spread to the entire shaft, the scrotum, and the inguinal and suprapubic areas. The eruption may spread to other areas of the body.

The rubber condom may also produce an acute dermatitis of the vulva and inner thighs in a rubber-sensitive female sexual partner.

Rubber condom dermatitis is usually due to sensitivity to one or more rubber antioxidants or accelerators or to latex itself (36). (Rubber allergy is discussed more specifically in Chapter 31.) Occasionally, a preservative powder which has been dusted onto the condom is the cause of the dermatitis rather than the rubber itself. In one instance, the powder contained 10% monobenzylether of hydroquinone (agerite alba), which is a sensitizer and depigmenting agent.

Patch tests may be performed with the condom suspected of producing the reaction. If a powder or lubricant is present with the condom, tests should also be performed with these substances. Patch tests should also be performed with the usual rubber allergens.

Immediate hypersensitivity (contact urticaria) to latex may cause localized urticaria in either partner. More severe reactions, including anaphylaxis, have occasionally been reported (see Chapter 31).

Some have found by trial and error that only certain brands of rubber condoms produce allergic reactions, but in general, individuals with rubber sensitivity should use non-rubber condoms.

Nonrubber Condoms

Fourex (Schmidt) and Lambskin (Young) condoms, made of processed lamb cecum, are available for individuals who cannot tolerate rubber condoms. Such preparations are popularly called "fishskins." Because these condoms may not be as effective in preventing the spread of sexually transmitted diseases, a rubber condom may be worn over the natural condom if the man is sensitive or under the natural condom if the woman is sensitive to rubber.

Condoms made of synthetic elastomers that do not contain natural latex are available.

Lubricants Used with Condoms

Many condoms are lubricated with aqueous gums containing preservatives. Some of these preservatives, particularly the parabens, have been shown to be sensitizers. Oils and petrolatum should be avoided as lubricants, because they cause rubber to deteriorate.

> **Condom dermatitis due to rubber chemicals is not rare. Condoms of processed lamb cecum may be used in rubber-sensitive individuals. Anaphylaxis from latex in condoms can occur.**

Allergic Contraceptive Dermatitis in Women

Allergic mucosal reactions can occur from chemical contraceptives. Often, in mild cases, the patient complains of pruritus vulvae or a burning vaginal sensation, and little is noted on examination. This may indicate either an irritant dermatitis or mild ACD. In more severe degrees of allergic reactions, redness and edema of the vulva occurs, and the adjacent skin shows an eczematous reaction.

A rubber-sensitive woman can acquire an acute diffuse dermatitis of the vulva and inner thighs from contact with a rubber condom worn by a man.

Chemical Contraceptives

Many chemical contraceptives are available. They consist essentially of a foaming agent or surfactant substance to emulsify the ejaculate and a spermicide to act upon it. They are produced as creams, jellies, pastes, gelatin vagatories, waxy vagatories, and foaming tablets. These chemical contraceptives are all intended for vaginal insertion before coitus.

These preparations contain monophenoxypolyetoxy ethanol derivatives, hexylresorcinol, and chloramine pre-

dominantly. German manufacturers also commonly use quinine and ammonium thiocyanate. Hungarian "state-manufactured" preparations contain cetylpyridium bromide. In Sweden, sodium dioctylsulfosuccinate and sodium lauryl sulfate are combined commonly in a contraceptive cream. In Russia, quinine pessaries are used widely for contraception.

Sensitizers in Vaginal Spermicides

These chemicals include phenylmercuric acetate, oxyquinoline sulfate, quinine hydrochloride, and hexylresorcinol.

Patch tests with chemical contraceptives must be interpreted with care because some contraceptives contain surfactants that may show nonspecific irritant reactions under a closed patch. A positive patch test reaction to a chemical contraceptive should be followed by testing with the individual ingredients of the product.

Sensitivity to quinine hydrochloride may manifest itself as an allergic purpuric dermatitis medicamentosa.

Hindson (37) recommended patch tests shown in Table 20.3 when contraceptive dermatitis is suspected.

Intrauterine Devices (IUDs)

An IUD made of a copper ring and a polyethylene carrier of metallic copper is available. Several cases of dermatitis due to the IUD in copper-sensitive individuals have been reported (38–41).

Lippe Loop (Ortho) is a polyethylene intrauterine device free of copper.

HEMODIALYSIS (RENAL) DERMATITIS

Formaldehyde, epoxy resin, and tetramethylthiuram may produce allergic contact dermatitis in individuals servicing hemodialysis machines or in patients receiving dialysis.

TABLE 20.3. *Contraceptive Dermatitis Patch Test Series*

Substance	Patch test concentration[a]
Chemical contraceptive used	As is
Dipentamethylenethiuram disulfide	1% pet
Hexylresorcinol	1% pet
Oxyquinoline sulfate	1% pet
Phenoxypolyetoxy ethanol	0.5% pet
Phenyl mercuric acetate	0.01% pet
Quinine hydrochloride	1% aq
Rubber condom	As is
Zinc dithiocarbamate	1% pet
Zinc lupetimide	2% pet
Zinc mercaptobenzothiazole	1% pet

[a]aq, aqueous; pet, in petrolatum

Formaldehyde Dermatitis

Sneddon (42) reported that formaldehyde solutions 2% to 4% are used for sterilization in some renal dialysis units and for home kidney machines. In one such unit, 6 of 13 staff members developed dermatitis of the eyelids, face, and hands. Four staff members were sensitive to formaldehyde. The dermatitis ceased when formaldehyde was replaced by another disinfectant. Abdel-Aziz and Hodgson (43) treated a man who used formaldehyde to sterilize a kidney machine and who subsequently developed an extensive eczema on his hands and arms. Patch testing confirmed the patient's sensitivity to formaldehyde. Three cases of formaldehyde dermatitis occurred in the hospital's dialysis unit. An iodophor-sterilizing solution was substituted for formaldehyde for home dialysis.

Hendrick and Lane (44) stated that formaldehyde used to sterilize artificial kidney machines caused asthma and productive coughs among the staff of a hemodialysis unit. Glutaraldehyde may also be used on dialysis equipment and can cause allergic contact dermatitis in staff and patients.

A prospective double-blind study documented that five of ten patients with anaphylactoid symptoms on dialysis reproduced their symptoms when exposed to formaldehyde sterilized equipment but not when the equipment was gas sterilized (45).

Formaldehyde used to sterilize hemodialysis machines has produced dermatitis and asthma in several individuals who sterilize such machines and in patients themselves.

Epoxy Resin Dermatitis

Mork (46) described contact sensitivity from epoxy resin in a hemodialysis set at the site where an adhesive strip containing epoxy resin fixed the needle. Brandao and Pinto (47) studied two patients on hemodialysis for chronic renal insufficiency who developed dermatitis at the site of needle puncture. Patch tests were positive to epoxy resin and to the glue that binds the needle to the plastic butterfly. Filter paper test and thin layer chromatography confirmed that the glue was a low-molecular-weight epoxy resin of the bisphenol A type.

Both patients changed needles and had no more trouble.

Tetramethylthiuram Dermatitis

Another cause of dermatitis in hemodialysis units has been described by Penneys et al. (48). An outbreak of dermatitis among patients in such a unit was traced to various thiuram compounds, probably leaching out of the rubber components of the hemodialysis apparatus.

Pruritus with Excoriations

Many patients in hemodialysis develop severe itching, which induces scratching and excoriations and which may be a type of preuremic pruritus.

DERMATITIS OF AMPUTATION STUMPS

The skin of an amputee who wears a prosthesis is subject to many abuses, even though the devices have improved greatly in recent years. The artificial limb now weighs about 1 lb compared to 10 to 12 lbs a decade ago. Devices for children can be changed every 2 to 3 months to increase the size as the child grows (49).

With the conventional prosthesis for the below-knee amputee, the stump fits into the hollow of the socket and the device is held on with a pelvic band.

Suction suspension is used more frequently. As the amputee places his weight on the prosthesis, air is forced out through the valve in the socket; then, as the amputee shifts his or her weight to the normal leg, the artificial limb is held to the stump by negative pressure. Uneven loading on the socket, which provides for weight bearing, may cause stress on areas of the stump skin. Common disorders are cysts developed under friction and pressure, dermatitis, and edema at the end of the stump.

Therapy by the dermatologist requires close cooperation with the orthopedic surgeon and prosthetist, which will include eliminating all mechanical factors contributing to edema. These factors can include poor fit and alignment and excessive negative pressure in a suction-socket prosthesis.

Suction-Socket Prosthetic Dermatitis

An amputee can expect edema, hyperemia, and pigmentation resulting from capillary hemorrhage, and other relatively innocuous conditions to occur when starting to wear a suction-socket prosthesis. These changes, which usually do not require therapy, are the result of altered conditions forced on the skin and subcutaneous tissues. They can be partially prevented, however, by gradual compression of the stump tissues with an elastic bandage or "shrinker" sock prior to use of the prosthesis.

"Suction socket" dermatitis consisting of edema, erythema, pigmentation, and capillary hemorrhages may be prevented by use of a "shrinker sock" or an elastic bandage prior to use of the prosthesis.

Nonspecific Eczematization of Amputee Skin

Nonspecific eczematization of the stump skin has been seen in several instances. In one case, the amputee presented a weeping, itching, nonhealing plaque of dermatitis over the distal portion of the stump. The lesion, at first dry and scaly, suddenly and without an apparent reason, became moist. It waxed and waned over a period of months to years. In some instances a significant history of recurrent allergic eczema or active eczematous lesions on other portions of the body was found to account for the eruption on the stump. In other instances, the eczema was secondary to edema and congestion of the terminal portion of the stump, so that only with the alleviation of these problems did the condition clear.

> **Nonspecific eczema of the skin of the stump may be due to a nummular eczema or to edema of the stump.**

Epidermal Cysts in Amputees

Allende et al. (50) reported the following:

1. Epidermoid cysts appearing in the stumps of amputees have been studied from clinical, bacteriologic, and histopathologic points of view.

2. These cysts occur as the result of mechanical shearing forces produced by the socket on the skin, which result in invagination and implantation of keratin plugs and epidermal fragments into the dermis. These plugs become separated from the epidermis and are surrounded by a foreign-body reaction; the cyst that forms may become liquefied and rupture to the surface, producing a sinus. This, in turn, leads to secondary bacterial infection of the cyst.

3. All the therapeutic measures attempted thus far, including surgical incision and drainage, excision and grafting, topical therapy, injection of hydrocortisone and triamcinolone, antibiotic therapy, and griseofulvin therapy, have been only palliative.

4. Improvement in prosthetic fit, with reduction of shearing forces, seems to be the most promising approach to the problem.

> **Good prosthetic fit with reduction of "shearing" force is used in the management of epidermal cysts in amputee stumps.**

Verrucose Hyperplasia

External compression combined with adequate control of bacterial infection proved, through trial and error, to be the best method of treatment.

When support of the stump end was provided in the socket by building up a temporary platform with foam rubber, the verrucose condition was reduced. The greater the compression on the distal stump, the more immediate and lasting was the improvement.

Hyperplasia appeared to be secondary to an underlying vascular disorder, poor prosthetic fit and alignment, and possibly bacterial infection. Working with the orthopedic surgeon and the engineering department permits successful treatment. Levy (49) reported a patient with long-standing verrucose hyperplasia and an ulceration who developed a squamous cell carcinoma of the stump.

Role of Hygiene in Prevention of Amputee Dermatitis

Amputees must be instructed carefully in the hygienic care of their stumps. The primary requirement is that the stump should be kept clean. As soon as the socket is removed after each wearing, the stump skin should be washed with warm water and a disinfectant soap. The soap must then be rinsed away with care, and the skin must be dried thoroughly. Washing should not be done in the morning or just before the prosthesis is put on, because damp skin may swell, stick to the socket, and be irritated by rubbing. The socket itself should be cleansed frequently—every day in warm weather—also after the prosthesis is removed and not just before it is put on. It should be washed with warm water and mild soap, then rinsed with clean warm water, and dried thoroughly. The stump sock should be changed daily and washed immediately after removal, before perspiration dries in it, with mild soap and warm water; it also must be rinsed thoroughly.

Des Groseilliers et al. (51) stated that of 50 amputees seen in 1 year, 17 amputees were affected. The most common lesions were due to badly fitting prostheses or to poor hygiene, which caused callus formation or breakdown of the skin with or without ulceration in 12 patients.

Allergic Contact Dermatitis of the Stump

Table 20.4 lists some allergens.

TABLE 20.4. *Causes of Allergic Contact Dermatitis in Amputees*

Ambroid (pressed amber)
Antibacterial agents
Benzoyl peroxide
Chromates (leather)
Cobalt
Epoxy resin
Methyl methacrylates
Nickel
Paraphenylenediamine
p-tert-butylcatechol
p-tert-butylphenol
p-tert-butylphenol-formaldehyde resin
Rubber alergens—MBT, thiuram, or carbamates
Topical medications

MBT, meraptobenzothiazole

1. *Plastic resins.* The sockets of leg prostheses are commonly finished with an inside application of varnish or lacquer and an outside coating of plastics and resins. These complex organic substances are capable of causing contact dermatitis. The epoxy resins, if cured incompletely in their manufacture, may serve as specific allergic sensitizers or may produce primary-irritant dermatitis. These resins are used frequently to improve the appearance of a socket and to render it impervious to external agents (52). Paratertiary butyl catechol and paratertiary butylphenol formaldehyde resin have caused cases of dermatitis in amputees (53,54). Unsaturated polyester resin caused allergy in a child with an arm prosthesis (55).

Moreover, curing agents, known as catalysts or hardeners, are added to solidify the plastic material. These agents are organic amines of various types and, when left in excess by incomplete baking or curing at high temperatures, are able to produce a dermatitis. Benzoyl peroxide, used as a catalyst in plastic manufacture, caused allergy in one case (56). There are at least two reports of allergic contact dermatitis to methyl methacrylate in leg prosthesis wearers. Other acrylates may also be involved (57,58).

2. *Rubber allergens.* Allergy to thiurams and/or mercaptobenzothiazoles can cause ACD when the stump contains a rubber portion or suction device (59).

3. *Topical medications, cleansers, and antibacterial agents.* These agents applied to the stump or the prosthesis may produce allergic contact dermatitis, which may be revealed by patch testing.

In seven patients with amputation stumps of the thighs, allergic contact eczema could be confirmed by positive patch tests by Fisher. Two patients were allergic to hexomedine, an antibacterial that is often used because it penetrates easily into the skin.

Patch tests with a screening tray and with applied medications may uncover the allergen causing allergic contact dermatitis of the stump skin.

Van Ketel (60) reported that the friction and pressure of prostheses, in addition to close and prolonged contact with the skin, are important factors responsible for the skin becoming easily damaged. Trophic changes in the stumps are mainly the result of these factors.

4. *Leather and metals.* Of five patients wearing leather prostheses, one was sensitized to paraphenylenediamine (1% petrolatum [pet]) and other para dyes. Two patients showed positive patch tests to potassium dichromate (0.5% pet). Because most leathers are tanned with chromium compounds, these reactions could be considered relevant. Another patient reacted to paratertiarybutylphenol (5% in acetone) and paratertiarybutylphenol formaldehyde resin (1%

pet). These compounds are probably used in a glue in the manufacture of prostheses. One patient showed a positive patch test to chamois leather, which was used for patch testing. In this prosthesis, pieces of chamois leather were used to protect the skin from pressure.

Manneschi et al. (61) reported two patients allergic to nickel from metal components of arm prostheses. One also reacted to cobalt, paraphenylenediamine, and a formaldehyde resin.

DERMATOLOGIC HAZARDS OF ELECTROCARDIOGRAPHY

Gels and Pastes Used in Electrocardiography

In the very early days of electrocardiography (ECG), a patient's hands and left foot were placed in three large pots of saline solution. In 1910, with the introduction of contact electrodes, this method of partial immersion in saline solution was replaced by bandaging the limbs with saline pads and malleable metal electrodes. The saline-soaked bedclothes of bedridden patients often produced not only maceration of the skin but also short-circuiting of the equipment. In the 1930s, commercial electrode jellies and pastes consisting principally of sodium chloride and an abrasive became available and are now widely used.

Dermatitis Due to Parabens in a "Nonirritating" Jelly (Natrosol) Used for Long-Term Electrocardiographic Monitoring

An 8-year-old boy with mild atopic dermatitis required long-term ECG monitoring. He began to complain of marked itching under the electrodes. Upon examination, the areas where the electrodes had been applied revealed a sharply demarcated erythematous oozing dermatitis. It was learned that electrode jelly (Natrosol) had been used. A positive patch test to this jelly was obtained. The electrode jelly (Natrosol) consisted of hydroxycellulose, polyvinyl pyrrolidone, sodium, potassium, and calcium chlorides in deionized water, and parabens. Patch tests with the various ingredients gave negative results except for the paraben preservatives (62).

Various ECG gels and pastes and metal and rubber electrodes may produce irritant and allergic contact dermatitis (Table 20–5).

Dermatitis Due to FD&C Yellow No. 5 in Camcreme ECG Paste (Cambridge)

A 40-year-old woman acquired dermatitis at sites where Camcreme ECG paste had been applied. Camcreme is an unusually complex mixture containing sodium sulfate, lanosterol, cholesterol, mineral oil, cetyl alcohol, polyethylene glycol 40 (PEG-40), stearate, stearamide, MEA stearate, glyceryl stearate, stearyl sapamine, laureth-4, preservatives

TABLE 20.5. *Etiology of Allergic Contact Dermatitis Associated with Electrocardiography*

Alcohol sponge (isopropyl alcohol)
Gels or pastes
   FD&C Yellow No. 5
   Parabens
   Parachlorometaxylenol
   Pine oil
   Propylene glycol
Nickel-plated electrodes
Rubber strap fasteners (mercaptobenzothiazole)

(propylparaben, methylparaben, phosphoric acid, and ethoxydiglycol), and fragrances, and colored with FD&C Yellow No. 5 and No. 6. The patient showed a positive patch test reaction to the FD&C Yellow No. 5 and to paraphenylenediamine. FD&C Yellow No. 5 is tartrazine, which has been implicated as a cause of chronic urticaria (63).

Dermatitis Due to Propylene Glycol in Spectra 360 Electro Gel (Parka Lab)

A 62-year-old man acquired dermatitis following the use of this ECG gel, which contains propylene glycol, organic "polymers," and cellulose. Patch test results were positive only to 5% aqueous solution of propylene glycol and negative to the other ingredients (64). Many other brands of electrode gels and pads contain propylene glycol.

Allergic Dermatitis Due to Parachlorometaxylenol (PCMX) in Redux ECG Paste

A 70-year-old woman acquired a sharply defined erythematous vesicular dermatitis at the site where Redux ECG paste had been applied. Positive results were obtained with the paste and with the PCMX, which is used widely as a preservative in numerous topical medications and cosmetics. Storrs (65) documented allergic dermatitis due to PCMX in three men and four women whose dermatitis was precipitated by exposure either to Vaseline First Aid Carbolated Petroleum Jelly or to Redux ECG paste.

Dermatitis Due to Pine Oil in ECG Electrode Jelly (Cambridge)

A 57-year-old man proved to be allergic to this ECG jelly and to pine oil, which is one of its ingredients. Although the pine oil is present in only a 1:10,000 concentration, it was apparently sufficient to produce allergic contact dermatitis. In addition, this jelly contains sodium chloride, gum tragacanth, glycerin, sand, and water. Pine oil is also present in various disinfectants and deodorants and certain liquid scrub soaps. Coskey (66) reported a patient with allergic hypersensitivity to this ECG jelly and incriminated the gum tragacanth as the cause of the allergic dermatitis.

Rubber Straps Used to Fasten ECG Electrodes

Two patients were studied who acquired bandlike, erythematous, vesicular dermatitis at the sites of contact with the rubber straps used to fasten the ECG electrodes. Both patients showed a positive reaction to a piece of the rubber strap and to mercaptobenzothiazole. One patient gave a history of shoe dermatitis with previous hypersensitivity to mercaptobenzothiazole (67).

Nickel-Plated ECG Electrodes

A 26-year-old nurse acquired dermatitis at the sites where electrodes had been applied. It was at first suspected that she was allergic to the ECG pastes, but patch testing with the paste, which was performed elsewhere, gave negative results. The history revealed that she could not wear costume jewelry without acquiring dermatitis. A strongly positive patch test reaction to nickel sulfate was obtained, and the metal electrodes gave a strongly positive reaction to dimethylglyoxime, indicating the presence of "available" nickel in the metal electrode.

Alcohol in a Prepackaged Gauze Pad Used as a Substitute for ECG Paste

A 38-year-old man had a sharply localized rectangular patch of vesicular dermatitis corresponding to the sites of the ECG electrodes. In this patient, alcohol-impregnated cotton sponges were used as conductors instead of ECG paste. This patient was found allergic, on patch testing, to the isopropyl alcohol used in the gauze pad and to ethyl alcohol. No systemic reaction, however, was produced from drinking alcoholic beverages (68).

There are several reports in the literature of various types of topically applied alcohol capable of producing allergic contact dermatitis (69). In some of the patients with delayed-type allergic hypersensitivity to alcohol, an eruption may also develop after the ingestion of alcohol.

Comments

Preservatives, especially parabens, PCMX, and propylene glycol; other additives, such as dyes and alcohols; and rubber and metal may all cause ACD from ECG and other cardiac, neurologic, and electromyographic monitoring procedures.

CARDIAC PACEMAKER DERMATITIS

Contact dermatitis due to a cardiac pacemaker may occur over the site of the pacemaker or may be widespread and may resemble a nummular eczema. Table 20.6 lists the reported causes of pacemaker dermatitis; Table 20.7 lists the composition of a popular pacemaker.

TABLE 20.6. *Causes of Pacemaker Dermatitis*

Epoxy resin
Mercury
Nickel
Polychloroparaxylene (parylene)
Potassium dichromate
Tetramethylthiuram
Titanium

Epoxy resin allergy is one of the most common causes of pacemaker dermatitis. Andersen (70) reported that a pacemaker with an epoxy resin coating produced a dermatitis in a patient who later tolerated a pacemaker in a titanium capsule. Romaguera and Grimalt (71) studied a man with a generalized dermatitis due to epoxy resin cement in a pacemaker that was presumably incompletely polymerized after nearly a year.

Raque and Goldschmidt (72) described a patient with circumscribed eczematous dermatitis occurring over the site of a pacemaker within 3 weeks of implantation. Later, widespread nummular eczema developed. The authors discussed whether it was an irritant dermatitis due to a medical-grade silicone elastomer or nummular eczema provoked by an irritant dermatitis. Patch tests in a patient and two control subjects with the uncured silicone adhesive gave positive reactions that were thought to be irritant reactions. The patient's dermatitis was not resolved.

Polychloroparaxylene, also called parylene, is a widely used coating for pacemakers and has been reported to cause allergy in one patient (73). Polyurethane and titanium patch tests were both positive in one patient with pacemaker sensitivity (74).

Pacemakers caused a localized dermatitis over the sites of implant in two patients investigated by Brun and Hunziker (75). Allergy to mercury accounted for the first patient, but sensitization to titanium was considered the most likely cause in the second case, despite negative patch tests to metallic titanium and titanium tetrachloride. These tests were interpreted as false-negative reactions because compounds for patch testing have yet to be determined.

Peters et al. (76) did find a positive patch test to titanium in one patient with pacemaker dermatitis. A granulomatous reaction to a pacemaker with titanium found on electron probe microanalysis but with negative patch tests has been reported. The eruption resolved spontaneously over several years (77). Other reports have implicated metals including

TABLE 20.7. *Composition of a Popular Pacemaker*

Battery:	Lithium
Casing:	Epoxy resin
	Silicone
	Titanium
Insertion tip:	Iridium (10%)
	Platinum (90%)

nickel, chromate, cobalt, and cadmium, as reviewed by Buchet et al. (78). A pompholyx eruption from a nickel-containing pacemaker has been reported (79). Some reports have failed to identify an allergen but suggest allergy because the dermatitis resolved upon removal of the implant.

At the Seventh International Symposium on Contact Dermatitis, held in East Germany in June 1983, Dr. B. Bandemir, of Neubrandenburg, reported:

> A 76-year-old patient, who had a cardiac infarction in 1978, had a pacemaker with a casing of chromium, nickel, and steel implanted into the left thorax. Some weeks later signs of inflammation as well as an eczematous reaction of the skin appeared in the area of the implanted pacemaker. In the area of the hypogastrium as well as the thighs, small papulous and badly itching efflorescences were seen.
>
> Microorganisms could not be found in the bed of the pacemaker case. Patch tests with the standard series were positive to potassium dichromate after 1 day and 2+ positive after 2 and 3 days with a focal reaction in the area of the implanted pacemaker, the hypogastrium, and the thighs as well as itching on the whole integument. Patch tests with epoxy resin and triethanolamine were completely negative.

In December 1981, a subpectoral implantation of an Axios pacemaker with a pure titanium casing was carried out. Since that time, no reactions of the integument have occurred (79).

Dermatitis from Subcutaneous Pressure?

Wilkerson and Jordan (80) studied a man with localized dermatitis that began 2 years after a pacemaker was inserted over the left upper abdomen. Patch tests were negative. When the pacemaker migrated to a different location, the original dermatitis cleared and the new location became dermatitic. Eventually the unit perforated through the skin and had to be replaced. The authors concluded the dermatitis was caused by an isomorphic response to pressure, as no evidence of allergic contact dermatitis was ever detected. However, the possibility must be considered that an allergy to an unidentified allergen was the true cause.

DERMATITIS ASSOCIATED WITH TRANSCUTANEOUS ELECTRICAL NERVE STIMULATION

Transcutaneous electrical nerve stimulation (TENS) is being used increasingly to relieve postoperative pain and chronic pain from such diverse causes as cancer, bursitis, fractures, causalgia, and postherpetic neuralgia.

TENS uses the passage of small electrical currents through the skin, which are presumed to effect "depolarization" of the affected sensory nerve endings and nerves themselves by the conduction of impulses along them, resulting in the inhibition (of awareness or perception) of paresthesias and particularly pain (81).

The "system" generally used in TENS is a battery-operated "pulse generator" that contains the power source and the electronics of the system. The electrical impulses are transmitted through cables attached to electrodes, which in turn are fastened to the skin by straps, adhesive, or tapes. In most systems, an electrolyte gel is interposed between the electrode and the skin.

Electrical Burns from TENS

Skin burns occur if the patient uses excessive stimulation with small-area electrodes (such as ECG electrodes) or if the interface between skin and electrode is dry. Shealy and Maurer (82) stated that the electrode surface area must be greater than 4 cm^2 for a 500 μsec 85 mA pulse, 185 pps stimulus. The heat produced must be less than 250 mcal/cm^2/sec^3 in order to avoid localized burns.

Burton (83) described another type of injury, which he termed "micropunctate burns," due to poor electrical contact between skin and electrode. The explanation is that current flow is not distributed over a wide surface area but is concentrated in small punctate areas (usually hair follicles). Because of the concentration of a large volume of current in small areas, current density is high and skin burns result. These micropunctate skin burns represent true thermal damage to the skin, but Burton felt that they are of little clinical significance in themselves, and, as with allergic reactions, simple discontinuation of use of the electrodes will allow recovery.

> **Electrical burns may occur from TENS if there is excessive electrical stimulation with small electrodes or poor electrical contact between skin and electrode.**

Skin Irritation from TENS

Even with adequately sized electrodes, skin irritation may occur with the prolonged use of TENS, particularly with a high output. It is advisable in instances of prolonged use to periodically move the electrodes to adjacent positions to prevent such irritation. Loeser et al. (84) noted that if the patient did not heed their warnings about changing the stimulation sites and washing the electrode sponges, areas of erythema might occur after 24 to 48 hours of continuous stimulation. This is easily controlled by discontinuation of stimulation at the inflamed sites.

Zugerman (85) and Bolton (86) stated that multiple irritant follicular papules and erosions may be caused by electrochemical reactions at the electrode-tissue interface. For example, carbon-containing silicone rubber or polyolefin plastic electrodes generate acids at the positive electrode and bases at the negative electrode as electrons are respectively accepted and repelled by the electrode surface during direct current stimulation.

These pH changes are most pronounced at sites of high current density and are associated with the formation of punctate erythema degenerating to bullous lesions, if stimulation is prolonged or intense (current density >10 μA/cm^2).

In the laboratory, it was found that by placing a 1- to 2-mm pad of fabric, thoroughly moistened with physiologic saline or weak buffer solution, between the electrode and the skin, these lesions are prevented by distributing the current uniformly over the entire electrode area and by providing a reservoir of liquid or buffer, which dilutes or minimizes the pH changes. This liquid also serves to hydrate the stratum corneum, the principal barrier to the passage of direct current through the skin.

An alternative way to minimize skin damage associated with these electrochemical reactions is to use a bidirectional pulse or alternating pulse train of opposing polarity, so that the electrochemical effects of each pulse or pulse train are canceled by those of the succeeding one. This would achieve the same neural stimulation effect, while minimizing cumulative electrochemical by-products at the electrode-tissue interface.

> **Prevention of irritant effects from TENS can be accomplished by using either physiologic saline or bidirectional alternating pulses.**

Irritant Dermatitis from TENS Gels

Two patients were encountered who acquired an irritant dermatitis from Sanborn "Redux" Gel. Patch test results did not indicate an allergic reaction but did reveal an irritant, follicular reaction. This type of gel is said to contain silicon oxide, which can produce irritation similar to that of "ground glass" on thin, delicate skin. This patient was able to tolerate EC-Z Cream (Grass Instruments) without difficulty. This TENS cream is said to contain sodium and potassium chlorides as the "active" chemicals. The other contents of EC-Z Cream were not disclosed.

> **Silicon oxide gels may produce irritant follicular eruptions.**

Allergic Reactions to TENS Electrodes

Several types of rubber electrodes are in use. Carbon-impregnated silicone electrodes (Medtronic Inc.) are free of mercaptobenzothiazole. As with ECG electrodes, rubber allergens and metals may cause contact allergy. Theoretically, there should be more chance of reactivity to TENS devices because of prolonged contact with the skin.

Allergic Dermatitis from TENS Gels Containing Propylene Glycol

Three patients acquired a contact dermatitis from Spectra 360 Gel (Parker Lab) because of allergic hypersensitivity to the propylene glycol it contains. One of these patients is reported on through the courtesy of Dr. W. Clendenning of the Hitchcock Clinic in Hanover, New Hampshire. One other patient, seen in consultation with Dr. Mary T. Hunsicker of East Stroudsbourg, Pennsylvania, also proved to have propylene glycol hypersensitivity. The third patient was a New York woman who was allergic to propylene glycol in this TENS gel and in certain of her cosmetics.

Zugerman (85) reported a patient who developed allergic contact dermatitis to propylene glycol in a conductive jelly (Neuromod TENS gel). In an attempt to continue therapy, the patient changed to a poorly conductive surgical lubricant jelly, which caused irritation and micropunctate burns. Electrodes not utilizing conductive jelly were applied subsequently with excellent results.

Although contact dermatitis to propylene glycol in conductive jellies used for TENS may be a common phenomenon, it has rarely been reported in the dermatologic literature. Fisher (81) cited three cases of allergic contact dermatitis due to propylene glycol in electrolyte jelly. He also reported a case of allergic contact sensitivity to propylene glycol in a sterile lubricant (K-Y lubricating jelly) used by a patient undergoing TENS who had previously developed contact sensitivity to propylene glycol in a conductive material (87).

> **Propylene glycol in TENS conductive gels may produce allergic reactions.**

Alternatives for Propylene Glycol-Sensitive Individuals

Two of the above patients were able to continue treatment with the use of a special Lectron II Conductivity Gel (Pharmaceutical Innovations), free of propylene glycol. EC-Z Cream is also free of propylene glycol.

A solvent-activated tape electrode, Epiductive Tape (Medtronic Inc.), has been introduced that does not require any gels. The manufacturer claims that Epiductive Tape is superior for sites where application of the usual conductive rubber electrodes would be difficult, because, according to product literature, it conforms "well to body contours—over, under, and around." The Epiductive Tape is activated by acetone, and its electrical resistance is stated to be substantially lower than that of conductive rubber electrodes.

Other alternatives are available for patients allergic to propylene glycol. The first of these uses an interface pad applied in place of conductive jelly between the black rubber electrode and the skin. Generally, karaya gum or a synthetic gum, to which a small quantity of sodium chloride is added, serves to attach the electrodes to the skin and make electrical contact. In addition, the electrode and interface pad have been integrated into a single unit, which is composed of a polysulfonic acid adhesive backing and stainless steel foil electrode surrounded by foam insulation (Medtronic Inc.). The manufacturer claims that this electrode is more pliant and durable than those using karaya gum interface pads.

DERMATITIS FROM ANTABUSE IMPLANTS

Because some alcoholic patients discontinue the use of oral Antabuse, the subcutaneous implantation of disulfiram pellets has been used to overcome the problems of vacillating motivation (88). Lachapelle (89) described two cases of allergic contact dermatitis due to implanted Antabuse pellets. This side effect had never been reported before. He further stated, "It is also interesting to compare the evolution of both patients. Whereas, one of them was able to take oral disulfiram without any further skin reaction, the other patient developed a severe systemic, eczematous, contact-type dermatitis in the 24 hours following the oral absorption of one tablet of disulfiram. This rash was similar to the one described by Fisher (90) for other drugs."

It is known that alcohol can exacerbate lesions of allergic contact dermatitis from Antabuse. The explanation of this interaction is probably quite different from the aldehyde syndrome. Similarly unexplained is the fact that some patients who have been implanted with Antabuse pellets experience itching, burning, and redness at the site of the implantation when they drink alcohol (91).

> **Antabuse implants containing disulfiram pellets for treatment of alcoholism produce dermatitis in certain rubber-sensitive individuals.**

ACUPUNCTURE NEEDLE DERMATITIS

Romaguera and Grimalt (92) reported that a 48-year-old woman presented with a papulovesicular dermatitis of the neck, elbows, and wrists. She had also been suffering from a vesicular eruption on the forearms, upper part of the back, and face for the previous 8 days. All the lesions were accompanied by marked itching. The patient was receiving treatment with acupuncture for cervical arthritis. She denied any previous reaction to nickel exposures.

Patch tests with the metal series showed a positive reaction to nickel sulfate. The rest of the standard allergens were negative.

An acupuncture needle was introduced experimentally into the forearm; after 8 hours, the needle was removed. Around the site of the puncture a vesicular, edematous plaque with pseudopodia and marked itching was seen. With conventional treatment and termination of the acupuncture sessions, all the lesions disappeared in 18 days. The composition of the metal needles is unknown.

These same authors reported contact dermatitis in a nickel-sensitive individual from a permanent acupuncture needle inserted into the helix of the patient's right ear (93). A severe contact dermatitis appeared at this site around and near the acupuncture needle. Composition of the acupuncture needle, which originated in China, was unknown to the authors.

> **Nickel-plated acupuncture needles may produce dermatitis in nickel-sensitive individuals.**

Eun (94) reported that the earliest needles used were fish bones, bamboo splinters, and pointed stones, which were superseded by needles made of such metals as iron and copper. At present, most needles are made of silver, gold, or stainless steel. Most of the Korean acupuncture needles are composed of iron with 13.3% chromium and 6.7% nickel, as stainless steel. The Chinese and French acupuncture needles, however, were found to be different. Data from Lee's analysis are given in Table 20.8.

Eun (94) tested some of the Korean stainless steel needles presently in use. All samples were dimethylglyoxime spot test negative.

Thin, fiber-shaped gold needles, which are inserted into the body until broken into thin segments and retained permanently as part of a special technique, were also found to be negative to the dimethylglyoxime test.

EYEGLASS FRAME DERMATITIS

Most eyeglass frames are made of metal or plastic. Wood and tortoiseshell are now rarely used. Table 20.9 shows possible sensitizers in eyeglass frames.

Cellulose Plastic Frames

Contact dermatitis from cellulose plastics is infrequent and due usually to cellulose acetate or cellulose propionate. The plastic itself is nonallergenic, but some of the additives used in its manufacture can sensitize. Eyeglass frames are the most common cause of dermatitis from cellulose ac-

TABLE 20.9. *Sensitizers in Eyeglass Frames*

Azo dyes
Beeswax-turpentine mixture
Butyl acrylate
Cellulose acetate
Cellulose propionate
Epoxy resin
Ethyl acetate
Ethylene glycol
Ethylene oxide
Nickel, cobalt (metal frames)
p-tert-butylphenol
Phenyl salicylate
Resorcinol monobenzoate
Tricresyl phosphate
Triphenyl phosphate

etate, but it has also been attributed to ballpoint pens, hearing aids, patch test films, and steering wheels (95).

In addition to the plastic base itself, other ingredients of the finished plastic include a plasticizer, a stabilizer, and a coloring agent. The plasticizer, normally an ester, is added to impart softness and ease of handling; it is rarely a sensitizer. The stabilizers, added to prevent depolymerization, may include at least two classes of compounds (i.e., antioxidants and acid acceptors); these may be sensitizers. Coloring agents include either pigments, which are normally inert, or dyes, frequently amino compounds, which can sensitize. Solvents and formaldehyde resins, used in the processing of some plastics, are not usually used here.

The manufacturing process used in these products is known as "injection molding." In this process, the cellulose (obtained usually from nature in the form of wood fibers), after being esterified, is simply mixed with a plasticizer, a stabilizer, and a coloring agent. The entire mass is then heated to increase mixing of the components and decrease viscosity, but no chemical reaction occurs (i.e., these plastics are not "cured"). Hence, the individual components are not bound chemically to one another and remain more or less available to be leached out. As a final step, the hot mixture is injected into molds of desired shape and is allowed to cool.

Weakley (96) and Vail (97) reported instances of allergic contact dermatitis from Cool-Ray sunglass frames made of

TABLE 20.8. *Quantitative Analysis (% Weight) of Various Acupuncture Needle Materials*

	Iron	Chromium	Nickel	Silver	Copper	Tungsten
Korean	+++	13.3%	6.7%			
Chinese (A)	+++	12.5%	8.5%			
Chinese (B)	+++	10.4%	6.6%			
Handle of needle (A)				+++	1.0%	
Handle of needle (B)					+++	
French						+++

+++ = present, majority component of needle.
From: Fisher A. Allergic dermatitis from acupuncture needles. *Cutis* 1986;38:226–228.

cellulose propionate plastic, due probably to an unknown additive.

Tritolyl Phosphate (Tricresyl Phosphate) and Triphenyl Phosphate

Pegum's (98) patient was sensitive to tritolyl phosphate in polyvinyl chloride (PVC), and she also had dermatitis from triphenyl phosphate in her cellulose acetate eyeglass frames. She reacted to triphenyl phosphate (1% in both peanut oil and acetone), tritolyl phosphate (5% in peanut oil), the eyeglass frames, and PVC from various articles.

Andersen of Denmark (Andersen K, personal communication, 1982) observed a 46-year-old woman with eyeglass frame dermatitis. She had positive patch test results to the dyed plastic frame but not to the sidebars. Supplementary patch tests showed positive reactions to tricresyl phosphate, phenolformaldehyde resin, and a phosphate ester used in Firemaster flame-retardant compounds from Michigan Chemical Corporation consisting of halogenated phosphate esters. Liquid Firemaster caused delayed hypersensitivity maximization test results in human subjects and is classified as a weak to mild sensitizer. Sensitized persons could have reactions to fabrics containing this flame retardant.

The International Contact Dermatitis Research Group included Firemaster LVT 23P in 5% pet in their standard series of patch tests for a limited period of time to determine the incidence of sensitization against Firemaster. Of 1,103 individuals tested, 2 showed a positive response (Maibach H, personal communication, 1986).

"Optyl" Epoxy Frames

Fisher (99) reported a patient with epoxy resin sensitivity acquired from wearing eyeglass frames made of Optyl. It was learned that the eyeglass frames came from Hong Kong and were made of Optyl, a plastic material of the epoxy series. This epoxy plastic is covered with a polyurethane lacquer. Herzberg (100) stated: "Optyl is well suited for the manufacture of [eyeglass] frames; neither the epoxy plastic [n]or its polyurethane lacquer appeared to be [a] sensitizer. More than three million spectacle frames made from Optyl have been delivered, but no adverse effect has been complained about with the possible exception of an 80-year-old woman with a polyvalent sensitization."

Positive patch tests were obtained in Fisher's (99) patient to scrapings from the eyeglass frames but not in three controls. Negative tests were obtained with polyurethane resin monomers. In this instance, an apparently "cured" epoxy resin was capable of producing an allergic contact dermatitis in a sensitized individual.

Turpentine

Jordan (101) reported that a man known to be sensitive to turpentine developed eyeglass frame dermatitis. It was traced to a turpentine-beeswax mixture used in the final polishing. Patch testing revealed that the patient was positive to the turpentine-beeswax polish and a piece of buffed plastic but was negative to beeswax and unbuffed plastic.

Plasticizers in cellulose acetate eyeglass frames can produce contact dermatitis.

Ultraviolet Inhibitors or Stabilizers in Eyeglass Frames

Resorcinol Monobenzoate

Resorcinol monobenzoate is a colorless, ultraviolet light absorber that is added to plastics to prevent deterioration by sunlight. It is no longer used in articles such as eyeglass frames, pens, and hearing aids, but is still added to outdoor plastics, including signs and lighting fixtures (95).

This compound was the sensitizer in two cases of dermatitis from sunglasses reported by Jordan and Dahl (95). In patch tests, both patients reacted to resorcinol monobenzoate 1% pet but not to resorcinol. Two of three patients sensitive to resorcinol monobenzoate were patch tested to balsam of Peru, and both had a reaction to it. Calnan (102) also reported allergic contact dermatitis to resorcinol monobenzoate in eyeglass frames.

Phenyl Salicylate

Rycroft (103), at the 1983 International Contact Dermatitis Symposium in East Germany, reported three cases of contact dermatitis behind the ears from wearing the same brand of industrial safety spectacles. In each case a positive patch test was obtained with scrapings of the plastic. In two cases further patch tests with constituents of the plastic formula were carried out. In both cases positive patch tests were obtained with phenyl salicylate. Phenyl salicylate is used as an ultraviolet inhibitor in some cellulose acetate butyrate and cellulose acetate propionate formulas. It has been reported previously as a contact sensitizer from its use as a sunscreen in a lip salve. Positive patch test reactions were also obtained variously in these cases with balsam of Peru, resorcinol monobenzoate, and epoxy resin.

Resorcinol monobenzoate, and more recently phenyl salicylate, added to plastics to prevent deterioration by sunlight, may produce spectacle dermatitis.

Metal Eyeglasses

Jirasek et al. (104) reported that a celluloid eyeglass frame was reinforced with metal struts made of an alloy containing 30% nickel, 1% to 3% manganese, and 65% to 68% copper. As the plastic aged, the nickel was leached out and caused a retroauricular dermatitis. On patch testing, the patient showed reactions to nickel and corroded plastic, but not to the undamaged celluloid or its components.

Nose-Pad Dermatitis

Hambly and Wilkinson (105) studied a woman with dermatitis from the plastic nose pads of her eyeglass frames. In a patch test she reacted to butyl acrylate 1% (olive oil) but not to ethyl or methyl acrylate. An eyeglass manufacturer confirmed that such acrylates might be present in acrylic frames.

Jordan and Dahl (106) found that eyeglass dermatitis limited to the nose occurred in one patient. Patch testing revealed the offending agent to be a common solvent, ethylene glycol monomethyl ether acetate, used to chemically weld the nose pads to the eyeglass frame. The patient also had an unrevealed allergy to ethyl acetate.

> **Nose pads of eyeglasses can produce dermatitis from acrylates or ethylene acetate solvents.**

TRICHLOROETHANE

Fowler (107) reported a case of contact urticaria in a worker polishing and grinding eyeglass lenses due to trichloroethane.

CONTACT LENS REACTIONS

Contact allergy to ophthalmic drugs and contact lens solutions has been reviewed in detail by Herbst and Maibach (108). They give a suggested patch test tray based on their review. Preservatives (e.g., thimerosal) and antibiotics, especially neomycin, were the most frequent allergens. Other active ingredients and excipients were occasional allergens.

Dr. G. Reuter of Strasbourg, France (at the International Contact Dermatitis Symposium in East Germany in 1983) reported two cases of "intolerance" to soft contact lenses. The clinical aspect of both patients was similar. Both patients showed conjunctival erythema and dermatitis of the eyelids. In one case, patch tests showed an "irritant" reaction to the lens itself. In the other, an allergic reaction was obtained to thimerosal in Hydrocare contact lens solution. Tosti and Tosti (109) reported multiple cases of ACD and conjunctivitis to thimerosal in contact lens solutions. Virtually all such solutions now marketed in the United States are free of thimerosal.

Nickel and cobalt were found in a contact lens solution in Spain that caused intense periorbital dermatitis in a metal-sensitive individual (110).

The surfactants cocamidopropyl betaine and disodium cocoamphodipropionate in contact lens solutions have caused allergy (111,112).

Johnson (113) reported keratoconjunctivitis with involvement of the conjunctiva and the cornea from a contact lens, and Spring (114) from Australia reported several patients with an "allergic-like" eruption from wearing soft contact lenses. These authors did not give results of patch tests.

Two workers manufacturing soft, disposable contact lenses became sensitized to 2-hydroxyethyl acrylate and developed hand dermatitis (115).

> **Allergic reactions to contact lens material itself is rare. Thimerosal or benzalkonium chloride are the usual sensitizers in ophthalmic lens solutions.**

HEARING AID DERMATITIS

A 64-year-old patient who had acquired a new hearing aid soon developed a dermatitis of the ear that was in direct contact with the hearing aid. It was ascertained that this hearing aid was composed of a vinyl plastic. The patient was patch tested with various available types of plastics used in hearing aids and was found to have a strongly positive reaction to the vinyl variety but not to silicone, acrylic, and polyethylene. Table 20.10 lists the various plastics that were supplied for testing purposes by Scientific Plastics, Inc., 79 Madison Avenue, New York, NY (116).

A patient described by Guill and Odom (117) developed dermatitis from a new "in the ear" hearing aid made of cold-cured methyl methacrylate, whereas a replacement with a heat-cured aid was comfortable. Upon patch testing, the patient reacted to 10% methyl methacrylate in olive oil and to pieces of a cold-cured plastic but not to the heat-cured one.

Jordan and Dahl's (95) patient developed a dermatitis from a cellulose ester plastic used in a hearing aid. In this patient the specific sensitizer was resorcinol used as an ultraviolet stabilizer in the plastic. Diethyl phthalate has caused allergy from both hearing aids and eyeglass frames (118). Paratertiary butylphenol formaldehyde resin (PTBFR) may be used to bond plastic parts in hearing aids and has been reported to cause allergy (119).

Hearing aids may contain resorcinol monobenzoate as an ultraviolet stabilizer or as an inhibitor and may produce allergic contact dermatitis in balsam of Peru–sensitive individuals (120).

TABLE 20.10. *Popular Hearing Aid Plastics*

Acrylic	Silicone
Cellulose acetate	Vinyl
Polyethylene	

In two separate studies from Scandinavia, methacrylates were found to be comon sensitizers in hearing aids or the molds for them. In the first study, three lab technicians and four patients were allergic to methacrylates (121). In the second, 6 of 22 patients with chronic dermatitis of the ear canal reacted to methylmethacrylate or related acrylates. Ingredients of topical medications also caused allergy in some cases (122).

Because previous allergic reactions have been reported to acrylic and polyethylene plastics used in hearing aids and none have ever been reported from silicone, it was decided to use silicone hearing aid material. The silicone hearing aid was well tolerated.

In addition to ACD, the differential diagnosis of dermatitis in the area of a hearing aid should include seborrhea, irritant contact dermatitis, psoriasis, and yeast and bacterial infection.

Silicone hearing aids are "hypoallergenic."

NASAL CANNULA DERMATITIS

Wright and Fregert (123) reported two patients who each had dermatitis of their upper lips from the use of an oxygen nasal cannula (123). In the first patient, scrapings from the oxygen cannula showed a positive patch test. The manufacturer of the cannula indicated that vanilla and epoxidized soybean oil were added to polyvinyl chloride in the production of the nasal cannula. A second series of patch tests revealed the following results: vanilla 10% (w/v) in acetone, negative; repeat scrapings from suspect nasal cannula, 2+; scrapings from another nasal cannula made from pure polyvinyl chloride, negative; epoxy resin 1% pet, 2+. A cannula made from pure vinyl chloride was prescribed, and the dermatitis resolved.

The second patient was a 54-year-old woman who had been on continuous oxygen therapy for 10 years and during that period of time had used a plastic oxygen cannula. She had experienced no difficulty until 3 weeks prior to being seen in a dermatologic consultation. She had developed some irritation after using a cannula from a different supplier. On physical examination, dermatitis was present on the upper lip and the cheeks in the area of contact with the cannula. Because of the prior experience with the first patient, a patch test to epoxy resin (1% pet) was carried out and showed a 2+ reaction.

Toome (124) reported a similar case also allergic to epoxy resin. A PVC cannula without epoxy resin was obtained from a different manufacturer.

Irritant dermatitis from the drying effects of the oxygen flow is much more common than ACD.

Vinyl nasal cannula dermatitis may be due to epoxy resin.

STETHOSCOPE DERMATITIS

Several nickel-sensitive physicians and nurses acquired a bilateral, bandlike, linear dermatitis at the sides of their necks whereon the nickel-plated, metallic portion of their stethoscopes rested. The situation was corrected when they used stethoscopes made with stainless steel portions. Rubber or plastic components of the stethoscope may also cause allergy in the wearer.

INFUSION PUMPS

Acrylates and epoxy resins in glues in insulin infusion pumps have caused ACD in diabetics (125,126). Van den Hove et al. (126) suggested that a pump called Pureline Basic or Disetronic Plus has no glue and therefore may be safe for use in these cases.

MEDICAL ADHESIVE TAPES

Medical adhesive bandages (tapes) consist of a pressure-sensitive adhesive and a backing, which is a carrier for the adhesive. Depending on its intended use, the bandage's backing may be made of plastic, cloth, paper, or foam. There are two types of medical adhesive tape: older tapes, based on rubber and rosin; and newer, "hypoallergenic" tapes, composed of acrylic resins.

Rubber, Rosin-Based Adhesives

The rubber-based adhesives contain rubbers, tackifiers, plasticizers, antioxidants, and other stabilizers. Tackifiers provide stickiness and are usually resins derived from terpenes, rosin (colophony), and petroleum. Plasticizers soften and facilitate the conformability of the adhesives. Antioxidants provide resistance to oxygen and thermal deterioration. Abietic acid, a major component in rosin, dihydroabietyl alcohol, plasticizers, and antioxidants have all been shown to cause allergic contact dermatitis (127).

Factitial dermatitis was caused by rosin in adhesive tape in a case from Australia (128).

Rubber in Adhesive Tape

Until recently, the adhesive mass in most adhesive tape contained rubber in the form of either natural latex or synthetic elastomers. Most such adhesive tapes also contained zinc oxide and substances derived from coniferous resins, such as turpentine, balsams, and rosin. In addition, antioxidants, to provide resistance to deterioration, and plasticizers, to facilitate spreading of the adhesive mass on cloth, are the ingredients in many adhesive tapes and plasters.

In a European report, diphenylthiourea was found as a cause of allergy to adhesive tape in eight patients (129).

Zinc diethyldithiocarbamate, a rubber accelerator, was reported as a cause of rubber adhesive dermatitis (130,131).

Resins and turpentine added to rubber bases may also produce allergic dermatitis. Murphy et al. (132) identified diamylhydroquinone as the allergen in both Scotch tape and an adhesive tape.

> **Rubber compounds and rosin are sensitizers in adhesive tapes.**

Adhesive Tape Reactions from TENS Units

Seven patients were either allergic to or irritated by the ordinary adhesive used to fasten the electrodes to the skin. These patients were able to use an acrylate type of adhesive such as Dermicel (Johnson & Johnson) and Micropore (3M). One patient was studied who was allergic to these acrylate adhesive tapes and also could not tolerate ordinary adhesive (133). Special straps had to be used in this instance.

Acrylate-Resin-Based Adhesive Tapes

These single-component adhesives were developed to avoid the allergic reactions and instability associated with rubber-based adhesives. These so-called hypoallergenic adhesives are formed by the combination of an acrylic ester monomer with a polar monomer. On occasion, the acrylic ester monomer is replaced with an acrylic monomer combined with another type of monomer, such as vinyl acetate.

Ethylhexyl Acrylate

Jordan (134) reported that during predictive testing he found seven volunteers who reacted to Curad adhesive but not to Dermicel. All reacted to ethylhexyl acrylate and three to *N-tert*-butyl maleamic acid. No cross-reactions were present between the acrylates and the methacrylates.

Heskel et al. (135) stated that the major components of Curad adhesive are 2-ethylhexyl acrylate and alkyl maleamic acid (a polar monomer). The alkyl group in the maleamic acid is derived from tertiary amines whose alkyl groups range from C_8 to C_{16}, with an average of C_{12} (dodecyl maleamic acid). No tackifiers or plasticizers are used. The resultant polymer is polar and of high molecular weight. During the reaction, approximately 98% of the monomers are converted to a polymer. The polymer is washed, dissolved in solvent, coated on a vinyl film, and heated in order to remove solvents and residual monomers, which are capable of producing sensitization.

The tendency of acrylic ester monomers to cause an allergic reaction has been shown to decrease as the size of the acrylic ester group increases. Methacrylates are less allergenic than the corresponding acrylic esters. Jordan (134) found that allergy to acrylates does not necessarily mean allergy to methacrylates. The di- and triacrylate esters are potent allergens, whose frequency of sensitization increases as the number of unsaturated groups in the monomer increases (136–138).

Heskel et al. (135) reported two patients who proved to be allergic to *N*-dodecyl maleamic acid in a polar monomer used in the production of the adhesive in Curad adhesive plastic bandages.

> **Allergic reactions to acrylate-based adhesive tapes are rare. The acrylate polymer or a monomer such as dodecyl maleamic acid may be sensitizers.**

Allergy to PTBFR was found to cause severe dermatitis in four patients. A particular athletic tape containing PTBFR was the culprit, and one patient also reacted to her athletic shoes (139).

Traumatic, Irritant Adhesive Tape Dermatitis

Most skin reactions related to adhesive tape are mechanical. One type of traumatic adhesive tape reaction results from the shearing stresses at the tape-skin interface and is encountered most frequently when tape is applied with tension that exceeds the physiologic tolerance of skin. Narumi (140) showed that adhesive plaster applied with tension can readily produce erythema and even blistering.

The other type of irritant, adhesive tape reaction, involves the mechanical plugging of the follicular and sweat ostia, producing a follicular rash resembling prickly heat. Also, patients with dermatographism commonly develop erythema and even urticaria at sites ot tape removal, such as in patch tests. This reaction to friction and pressure usually resolves spontaneously within several hours.

Traumatic or irritant adhesive tape dermatitis remains localized usually to the site of contact, but the allergic reactions tend to spread.

Band-Aid Patches

Occasionally, the vinyl film backing of Band-Aids may produce an allergic contact dermatitis because of plasticizers and stabilizers in the film.

DUO Brand Surgical Adhesive (Thayer Co.)

This crepe latex rubber compound is free from the usual antioxidants and accelerators used in rubber cements. Many women use this adhesive to apply false eyelashes. No instance of dermatitis has come to our attention from such use. This adhesive may be used on the scalp for toupees and around ileostomy wounds when other rubber cements irritate the skin or cause allergic reactions. Latex-sensitive persons, however, must not use this product.

Self-Adhering Adhesives

Gauztex (General Bandages Inc.), which is made of gum rubber, does not contain any rubber additives, such as accelerators or antioxidants. In addition, its manufacturer makes an oil-resistant tape that does not contain rubber but is made from plasticized styrene. Gauztex contains mercuric chloride as a preservative.

Salicylic Acid Plaster

Rasmussen and Fisher (141) reported two patients who developed an allergic contact dermatitis while applying 40% salicylic acid plaster to their plantar warts. Patch testing identified the allergen as a dehydroabietic acid, a sensitizer in rosin.

Abietic acid, a component of rosin, may produce allergic reactions in salicylic acid plaster.

Reactions to Transdermal Drug Delivery Systems

Transdermal drug delivery system (TDDS), also called transdermal therapeutic system (TTS), provides a low, continuous dosage of a medication. It is especially useful for drugs with a short half-life that could otherwise require frequent oral dosing or in cases where oral absorption may be impaired. Drugs administered by this route include nitroglycerin, estradiol, scopolamine, nicotine, fentanyl, clonidine, and testosterone (142,143). Reaction can occur either to the active drug or to a component of the patch system (Table 20.11). Reactions to the active drug is more common.

In one study, 21 of 320 patients (6.5%) developed cutaneous reactions to a TDS containing glyceryl trinitrate used for angina pectoris. About half of these had to discontinue therapy. More irritant than allergic reactions were observed (144).

The sensitizing capacity of topical antihistamines was illustrated by a report on an experimental triprolidine TDS.

TABLE 20.11. *Patch Test Series for Suspected Allergy to TDDS*

Clonidine	9.% aq
Estrogen	
Scopolamine	1% aq or pet
Nitroglycerin	2% aq
Nicotine	10% aq
Testosterone	
Hydroxypropyl cellulose	70% alc
Ethanol	5% aq
Acrylates	
Placebo patch	As is

aq, aqueous; pet, in petrolatum; alc, alcohol

Five out of six study subjects exposed twice to this patch in clinical testing developed allergy. Because of this, further development of this technique was halted by these investigators (145).

Nonallergic Reactions

Because the patch may be left in place for several days or more, folliculitis and miliaria rubra may develop from occlusion. Irritant contact dermatitis may occur due to the adhesive and frictional effects of the patch. In one case, apparently a burn was caused by microwave radiation from a leaky oven (142).

Allergy to Active Agents

Scopolamine, clonidine, nicotine, and nitroglycerin have all caused allergic contact dermatitis. Patients allergic to scopolamine have not reacted to atropine. Clonidine is a fairly common cause of allergic contact dermatitis in topical form. Some studies suggest up to 50% of patients may develop allergy to it. However, almost all patients who react topically can tolerate oral clonidine (146). Not only nitroglycerin TDS but also nitroglycerin pastes can cause allergic contact dermatitis. Nicotine reacted in several patients in one Swiss study (147).

Allergy to estrogen in an Estraderm TTS50 patch was followed by generalized dermatitis after oral estrogen administration. Patch test was positive to 17-beta-estradiol (148).

Reduction of Allergy in TDS

Silva and Berman (149) suggested that Maalox applied to the skin before applying clonidine patches reduces the appearance of allergic contact dermatitis in sensitized individuals. Jordan (150) reported that scrotal testosterone TDS was tolerated much better than a nonscrotal system, with less allergy and irritation. Coadministration of a topical steroid also reduces sensitization in TDS (151).

Allergy to Other Patch Ingredients

Various components of the patch, although usually inert, may sometimes cause allergic contact dermatitis. Hydroxypropyl cellulose, the major component of the drug reservoir, caused allergic contact dermatitis in one case (152). Ethanol has also caused allergic contact dermatitis in TDDS (153). Several other instances of apparent allergic contact dermatitis to patch components have been reported, although the offending ingredients were not identified (142,143). Methacrylates in the adhesive of patches may cause allergy (154).

Allergic Contact Dermatitis of the Legs Due to Parabens in Medicated Bandage

A woman used a Dome Paste Bandage on a stasis ulcer that produced a severe superimposed contact dermatitis under the entire bandage. This medicated bandage contains zinc oxide, calamine, and gelatin. The unlisted preservative proved to be the parabens. The patient had strongly positive reactions to a piece of the bandage and to the parabens. This patient tolerated a Primer Medicated Bandage containing zinc oxide in an oil base free of preservatives.

Four cases of allergy to preservatives in Unna boots was reported, three to parabens and one to hexachlorophene. Preservative free wraps were tolerated (155).

ELASTIC LEG SUPPORT BANDAGES

Malten (156), who reported allergic contact dermatitis from paraphenylenediamine and related dyes and mercaptobenzothiazole in rubberized leg bandages and support hose, advocated the use of undyed fabrics with known rubber auxiliary substances declared on the label.

Patients with dermatitis from support bandages usually tolerated the Lycra spandex variety.

> **Medicated leg bandages may contain parabens. Elastic bandages and support hose may contain sensitizing dyes and mercaptobenzothiazole.**

JOINT SUPPORT SLEEVES AND CPAP STRAPS

Tight-fitting elastic sleeves are used to support joints such as knees, ankles, and elbows during athletic activities. These are usually made of neoprene rubber, sometimes with a layer of cloth. Components may be glued or stitched together. In Fowler's (157) experience, allergy to these support devices has usually been caused by thioureas used in the rubber itself or possibly in the adhesives. Scalf and Fowler (158) have also reported allergy to the rubber straps holding a mask used with a continuous positive airway pressure device for treating sleep apnea. Thiourea was again the offending agent.

REFERENCES

1. Ludwigson DC. Today's prosthetic metals. *J Metals* 1964;Mar:1.
2. Kasser J, ed. *Orthopedic knowledge update-5.* Rosemont, IL: American Academy of Orthopedic Surgeons, 1996:41–49.
3. Coleman RF, Harrington J, Scales JT. Concentrations of wear products in hair, blood, and urine after total hip replacement. *Br Med J* 1973;2:527.
4. Evans EM, Freeman MAR, Miller AJ, Vernon-Roberts B. Metal sensitivity as a cause of bone necrosis and loosening of the prosthesis in total joint replacement. *J Bone Joint Surg* 1974;56B:626.
5. Samitz MH, Katz SA. Nickel dermatitis hazards from prostheses. *Br J Dermatol* 1975;92:287.
6. Elves MW, Wilson JN, Scales JE, Kemp HBS. Incidence of metal sensitivity in patients with total joint replacements. *Br Med J* 1975;4:376.
7. Benson MK, Goodwin PG, Brostoff J. Metal sensitivity in patients with joint replacement arthroplasties. *Br Med J* 1975;4:374.
8. Munro-Ashman D, Miller AJ. Rejection of metal prosthesis and skin sensitivity to cobalt. *Contact Dermatitis* 1976;2:65.
9. Lodi A, Chiarelli G, Mancini LI, et al. Skin sensitivity to endoprosthetic materials in the recipients of hip prostheses. *Contact Dermatitis* 1995;32:58–59.
10. Carlsson AS, Magnusson B, Mîeller H. Metal sensitivity in patients with metal-to-plastic total hip arthroplasties. *Acta Orthop Scand* 1980;51:57.
11. Deutman R, Mulder TJ, Brian R, Nater JP. Metal sensitivity before and after total hip arthroplasty. *J Bone Joint Surg* 1977;49A:862.
12. Nater JP, Brian RG, Deutman R, Mulder TJ. The development of metal hypersensitivity in patients with metal-to-plastic hip arthroplasties. *Contact Dermatitis* 1976;2:259.
13. Rooker GD, Wilkinson JC. Metal sensitivity in patients undergoing hip replacement. *J Bone Joint Surg* 1980;62B:502.
14. Metal allergy: a false alarm? *Br Med J* 1980;281:1303.
15. Can metal sensitivity loosen joint replacements? *Lancet* 1980;2:1284.
16. Cramers M, Lucht U. Metal sensitivity in patients treated for tibial fractures with plates of stainless steel. *Acta Orthop Scand* 1977;48:245.
17. Barranco VP, Solomon H. Eczematous dermatitis caused by internal exposure to nickel. *South Med J* 1973;55:447.
18. Kubba R, Taylor JS, Marks KE. Cutaneous complications of orthopedic implants. *Arch Dermatol* 1981;117:554.
19. Oleffe J, Wilmet J. Generalized dermatitis from an osteosynthesis screw. *Contact Dermatitis* 1980;6:365.
20. Gawkrodger DJ. Nickel sensitivity and the implantations of orthopedic prostheses. *Contact Dermatitis* 1993;28:257.
21. Dujardin F, Fevrier V, Lecorvaisier C, Joly P. Allergic dermatitis caused by metallic implants in orthopedic surgery. *Rev-Chir-Orthop-Reparatrice-Appar-Mot* 1995;81:473–484.
22. Menne T, Hjorth N. Reactions from systemic exposure to contact allergies. *Semin Dermatol* 1982;1:15.
23. Rothstein MS. Management of peristomal skin: routine care and maintenance. *J Dermatol Allergy* 1982;5:20.
24. Rothstein MS. Ostomy skin care. *Dialog Dermatol* 1982;10:6.
25. Rothstein MS. Management of stomal wounds. *Clin Dermatol* 1994;12:81–88.
26. Rothstein MS. Dermatologic considerations of stoma care. *JAAD* 1986;15:411–432.
27. Fussell K. Common problems of ileostomies and colostomies. *Practitioner* 1976;216:655.
28. Stevenson CJ. Skin problems with surgical stomata. *Contact Dermatitis* 1975;1:243.
29. Burt-McAliley D, Eberhardt D, van Rijswijk L. Clinical study: peristomal skin irritation in colostomy patients. *Ostomy-Wound-Manage* 1994;40:28–30, 32–34, 36–37.
30. Pappas M. Urostomy skin care. *Ostomy Q* 1979;Fall:50.
31. Mann RJ, Stewart E, Peachey RDG. Sensitivity to urostomy pouch plastic. *Contact Dermatitis* 1983;9:80.
32. Van Ketel WG, van de Burg CKH, de Haan P. Sensitization to epoxy resin from an ileostomy bag. *Contact Dermatitis* 1983;9:516.
33. Scalf L, Fowler J. Contact allergy to Stomahesive paste. *J AM Acad Dermatol* 2000 *(in press).*
34. Davies MG, Hodgson GA, Evans E. Contact dermatitis from an ostomy deodorant. *Contact Dermatitis* 1979;5:317.
35. Fisher AA. Allergic reactions to contraceptives. *Cutis* 1974;13:337.
36. Fisher AA. Practical management of allergic contact dermatitis due to rubber in manufactured articles. *Dermatol Digest* 1963;2:23.
37. Hindson TC. Contact dermatitis: contraceptives. *Trans St John's Hosp Dermatol Soc* 1966;52:1.
38. Barranco VP. Eczematous dermatitis caused by internal exposure to copper. *Arch Dermatol* 1972;106:386.
39. Barkoff JR. Urticaria secondary to a copper intrauterine device. *Int J Dermatol* 1979;15:594.
40. Romaguera C, Grimalt F. Contact dermatitis from a copper-containing intrauterine contraceptive device. *Contact Dermatitis* 1981;7:163.

41. Jouppila P, Ninimaki A, Mikkonen M. Copper allergy and copper IUD. *Contraception* 1979;6:631.
42. Sneddon IB. Formalin dermatitis in a renal dialysis unit. *Contact Dermatitis Newsletter* 1968;3:47.
43. Abel-Aziz AHM, Hodgson C. Formalin dermatitis in a renal dialysis unit. *Contact Dermatitis Newsletter* 1974;15:441.
44. Hendrick DJ, Lane DJ. Occupational formalin asthma. *Br J Industr Med* 1977;34:11.
45. Bousquet J, Rivory J, Maurice F, et al. Allergy in chronic hemodialysis: 1. Double-blind intravenous challenge with formaldehyde. *Clin Allergy* 1987;17:499–506.
46. Mork NJ. Contact sensitivity from epoxy resin in a hemodialysis set. *Contact Dermatitis* 1979;5:331.
47. Brandao FM, Pinto J. Allergic contact dermatitis to epoxy resin in hemodialysis needles. *Contact Dermatitis* 1980;6:218.
48. Penneys NS, Edwards LS, Katsikas JL. Allergic contact sensitivity to thiuram compounds in a hemodialysis unit. *Arch Dermatol* 1976;112:811.
49. Levy SW. Disabling skin reactions associated with stump edema. *Int J Dermatol* 1977;16:122.
50. Allende MF, Levy SW, Barnes GH. Epidermoid cysts in amputees. *Acta Dermato-Venereol* 1967;43:56.
51. Des Groseilliers JP, Desjardins JP, Germain JP, Krol AL. Dermatologic problems in amputees. *Can Med Assoc J* 1978;118:535.
52. Requena L, et al. Epoxy dermatitis of an amputation stump. *Contact Dermatitis* 1986;14:320.
53. Freeman S. Contact dermatitis of a limb stump caused byp-tertiary butyl catechol in the artificial limb. *Contact Dermatitis* 1986;14:68–69.
54. Romaguera C, et al. Paratertiary butylphenol formaldehyde resin in prosthesis *Contact Dermatitis* 1985;12:174.
55. MacFarlane A, Curley R, King C. Contact sensitivity to unstaurated polyester resin in a limb prosthesis. *Contact Dermatitis* 1986;15:301–303.
56. Vincenzi C, et al. Allergic contact dermatitis due to benzoyl peroxide in an arm prosthesis. *Contact Dermatitis* 1991;24:66–67.
57. Foussereau J, Cavelier C, Protois JP, et al. Contact dermatitis from methyl methacrylate in an above-knee prosthesis. *Contact Dermatitis* 1989;20:69.
58. Romaguera C, Vilaplana J, Grimalt F, et al. Contact sensitivity to meth (acrylates) in a limb prosthesis. *Contact Dermatitis* 1989;21:125.
59. Baptista A, Barros M, Azenha A. Allergic contact dermatitis on an amputation stump. *Contact Dermatitis* 1992;26:140–141.
60. van Ketel WG. Allergic contact dermatitis of amputation stumps. *Contact Dermatitis* 1977;3:50.
61. Manneschi V, Palmerio B, Pauluzzi P, Patrone P. Contact dermatitis from myoelectric prosthesis. *Contact Dermatitis* 1989;21:116.
62. Fisher AA. Dermatologic hazards of electrocardiography. *Cutis* 1977;20:686.
63. Lockey SD. Drug reactions and sublingual testing with certified food colors. *Ann Allergy* 1973;31:423.
64. Hannuksela M, Pirila V, Salo PO. Skin reaction to propylene glycol. *Contact Dermatitis* 1975;1:112.
65. Storrs FJ. Para-chloro-meta-xylenol allergic contact dermatitis in seven individuals. *Contact Dermatitis* 1975;1:211.
66. Coskey RJ. Contact dermatitis caused by ECG electrode jelly. *Arch Dermatol* 1977;113:839.
67. Fisher AA. Allergen replacements in allergic contact dermatitis. *Int J Dermatol* 1977;16:319.
68. Richardson DR, Caravati CM Jr, Weary PE. Allergic contact dermatitis to "alcohol" swabs. *Cutis* 1969;5:1115.
69. Lewes D. Electrode jelly in electrocardiography. *Br Heart J* 1965;27:105.
70. Andersen KE. Cutaneous reactions to an epoxy-coated pacemaker. *Arch Dermatol* 1979;115;97.
71. Romaguera C, Grimalt F. Pacemaker dermatitis. *Contact Dermatitis* 1981;7:333.
72. Raque C, Goldschmidt H. Dermatitis associated with an implanted cardiac pacemaker. *Arch Dermatol* 1970;102:646.
73. Iguchi N, Kasanuki H, Matsuda N, et al. Contact sensitivity to poly-chloroparaxylene-coated cardiac pacemaker. *Pacing-Clin-Electrophysiol* 1997;20:372–373.
74. Abdallah H, Balsara R, O'Riordan A. Pacemaker contact sensitivity: clinical recognition and management. *Ann Thorac Surg* 1994;57:1017–1018.
75. Brun R, Hunziker N. Pacemaker dermatitis. *Contact Dermatitis* 1980;6:212.
76. Peters MS, Schroeter AL, Van Hale HM, et al. Pacemaker contact sensitivity. *Contact Dermatitis* 1984;11:214.
77. Viraben R, Boulinguez S, Alba C. Granulomatous dermatitis after implantation of a titanium pacemaker. *Contact Dermatitis* 1995;33:437.
78. Buchet S, Blanc D, Humbert P, et al. Pacemaker dermatitis. *Contact Dermatitis* 1992;26:46–47.
79. Landwehr A, van-Ketel W. Pompholyx after implantation of a nickel-containing pacemaker in a nickel-allergic patient. *Contact Dermatitis* 1983;9:147
80. Wilkerson PG, Jordan WP. Pressure dermatitis from an implanted pacemaker. *Dermatol Clin* 1990;8:189.
81. Fisher AA. Dermatitis associated with transcutaneous nerve stimulation for control of pain. *Surg Neurol* 1974;2:45.
82. Shealy CN, Maurer D. Transcutaneous nerve stimulation for control of pain. *Surg Neurol* 1974;2:45.
83. Burton C. Transcutaneous electrical nerve stimulation to relieve pain. *Postgrad Med* 1976;59:105.
84. Loeser JD, Black RG, Christman A. Relief of pain by transcutaneous stimulation. *J Neurosurg* 1975;42:308.
85. Zugerman C. Dermatitis from transcutaneous electric nerve stimulation. *J Am Acad Dermatol* 1982;6:936.
86. Bolton L. Tens electrode irritation [Letter]. *J Am Acad Dermatol* 1983;8:134.
87. Fisher AA, Brancaccio RR. Allergic contact sensitivity to propylene glycol in a lubricant jelly. *Arch Dermatol* 1979;115:1451.
88. Fisher AA. Dermatologic aspects of disulfiram (Antabuse) use. *Cutis* 1982;30:461.
89. Lachapelle JM. Allergic "contact" dermatitis from disulfiram implants. *Contact Dermatitis* 1975;1:218.
90. Fisher AA. Allergic "contact" dermatitis from disulfiram implants. *Contact Dermatitis* 1975;1:218.
91. Swinson RP. Disulfiram implant. *J Alcohol* 1970;5:40.
92. Romaguera C, Grimalt F. Nickel dermatitis from acupuncture needles. *Contact Dermatitis* 1979;5:195.
93. Romaguera C, Grimalt F. Contact dermatitis from a permanent acupuncture needle. *Contact Dermatitis* 1981;7:156.
94. Eun HC. Nickel in acupuncture needles. *Contact Dermatitis* 1981;7:334.
95. Jordan WP, Dahl MV. Contact dermatitis from cellulose ester plastics. *Arch Dermatol* 1972;105:880.
96. Weakley DR. Two cases of contact dermatitis from cheap polaroid sunglasses. *Schoch Letter* 1970;Sep.
97. Vail JT. Allergic contact dermatitis due to eyeglass frames. *Cutis* 1972;9:703.
98. Pegum JS. Contact dermatitis from plastics containing tri-aryl phosphates. *Br J Dermatol* 1966;78:626.
99. Fisher AA. Epoxy resin dermatitis. *Cutis* 1976;17:1027.
100. Herzberg J. Investigations on a new epoxy material, Optyl, used in the manufacture of spectacles. *Berufs-Dermatosen* 1973;21:1.
101. Jordan WP. Turpentine in eyeglasses. *Contact Dermatitis Newslett* 1972;12:309.
102. Calnan CD. Resorcinol monobenzoate. *Contact Dermatitis* 1975;1:59.
103. Sonnex T, Rycroft R. Dermatitis from phenyl salicylate in safety spectacle frames. *Contact Dermatitis* 1986;14:268–270.
104. Jirasek L, Kobikova M, Jiraskova M. Retroauricular eczema caused by the nickel of celluloid-rimmed spectacles. *Cesk Dermatol* 1976;51:369.
105. Hambly EM, Wilkinson DS. Contact dermatitis to butyl acrylate in spectacle frames. *Contact Dermatitis* 1978;4:115.
106. Jordan WP, Dahl MV. Contact dermatitis to a plastic solvent in eyeglasses: cross-sensitivity to ethyl acetate. *Arch Dermatol* 1971;104:524.
107. Fowler J. Contact urticaria to 1,1,1 trichloroethane. *Am J Contact Dermatitis* 1991;2:239–240.
108. Herbst R, Maibach H. Contact dermatitis caused by allergy to ophthalmic drugs and contact lens solutions. *Contact Dermatitis* 1991;25:305–312.
109. Tosti A, Tosti G. Thimerosal: a hidden allergen in ophthamology. *Contact Dermatitis* 1988;18:268–273.

110. Vilaplana J, Romaguera C, Grimalt F. Contact dermatitis from nickel and cobalt in a contact lens cleaning solution. *Contact Dermatitis* 1991;24:232–233.

111. Cameli N, Tosti G, et al. Eyelid dermatitis due to cocamidopropyl betaine in a hard contact lens solution. *Contact Dermatitis* 1991; 25:261.

112. De-Groot A, Weijland J. Contact allergy to disodium cocoamphodipropionate. *Contact Dermatitis* 1996;35:248.

113. Johnson DS. Contact lens reactions. *J Can Ophthalmol* 1973;8:92.

114. Spring TF. Reactions to hydrophilic lens. *Med J Aust* 1974;24: 449.

115. Peters K, Andersen K. Allergic hand dermatitis from 2-hydroxyethyl acrylate in contact lenses. *Contact Dermatitis* 1986;15:188–189.

116. Fisher AA. Allergen replacement (alternatives) in the management of contact dermatitis. *Cutis* 1981;28:368.

117. Guill MA, Odom RB. Hearing aid dermatitis. *Arch Dermatol* 1972; 105:880.

118. Oliwiecki S, Beck M, Chalmers R. Contact dermatitis from spectacle frames and hearing aid containing diethyl phthalate. *Contact Dermatitis* 1991;25:264–265.

119. Matrolonardo M, Loconsole F, Conte A, et al. Allergic contact dermatitis to PTBFR in a hearing aid. *Contact Dermatitis* 1993;28:197.

120. Jordan WP. Resorcinol monobenzoate, balsam of Peru sensitivity. *Arch Dermatol* 1973;108:278.

121. Koefoed-Nielsen B, Pedersen B. Allergy caused by light cured ear moulds. *Scand-Audiol* 1993;22:193–194.

122. Meding B, Ringdahl A. Allergic contact dermatitis from the earmolds of hearing aids. *Ear-Hear* 1992;13:122–124.

123. Wright RC, Fregert S. Allergic contact dermatitis from epoxy resin in nasal cannulae. *Contact Dermatitis* 1983;9:387.

124. Toome BK. Allergic contact dermatitis to a nasal cannula. *Arch Dermatol* 1989;125:571.

125. Boom B, et al. Allergic contact dermatitis to epoxy resin in infusion sets of an insulin pump. *Contact Dermatitis* 1985;12:280.

126. Van den Hove J, et al. Allergic contact dermatitis from acrylates in insulin pump infusion sets. *Contact Dermatitis* 1996;35:108.

127. Cronin E, Calnan CD. Allergy to hydroabietic alcohol in adhesive tape. *Contact Dermatitis* 1978;4:57.

128. Dwyer P, Freeman S. Allergic contact dermatitis to adhesive tape and contrived disease. *Australas J Dermatol* 1997;38:141.

129. Dooms-Goossens A, et al. Contact and photocontact sensitivity problems associated with thiourea and its derivatives. *Br J Dermatol* 1987;116:573–579.

130. Cronin E. Sensitivity to zinc diethyldithiocarbamate. *Contact Dermatitis Newsletter* 1972;13:379.

131. Calnan CD. Diethyldithiocarbamate in adhesive tape. *Contact Dermatitis* 1978;4:61.

132. Murphy JC, Reif AE, January HL. Cutaneous hypersensitivity to adhesive and scotch tapes. *J Invest Dermatol* 1958;31:45.

133. Marron P, DeBerker D, Powell S. Methacrylate sensitivity and transcutaneous electrical nerve stimulation (TENS). *Contact Dermatitis* 1991;25:190.

134. Jordan WP. Cross sensitization patterns in acrylate allergies. *Contact Dermatitis* 1975;1:13.

135. Heskel NS, Samour CM, Storrs FJ. Allergic contact dermatitis from dodecyl maleamic acid in Curad adhesive plastic bandages. *J Am Acad Dermatol* 1982;7:747.

136. Rycroft RJG. Contact dermatitis from acrylic compounds. *Br J Dermatol* 1977;96:685.

137. Nethercott JR. Skin problems associated with multifunctional acrylic monomers in ultraviolet curing inks. *Br J Dermatol* 1978;98: 541.

138. Emmett EA. Contact dermatitis from polyfunctional acrylic monomers. *Contact Dermatitis* 1977;3:245.

139. Shono M, Ezoe K, Kaniwa M, et al. Allergic contact dermatitis from PTBP-FR in athletic tape and leather adhesive. *Contact Dermatitis* 1991;24:281–288.

140. Narumi J. Friction dermatitis due to adhesive plaster. Narumi Dermatology Clinic, Beppu, Japan. *Jpn J Clin Dermatol* 1970;24:1185.

141. Rasmussen JE, Fisher AA. Allergic contact dermatitis to salicylic acid plaster. *Contact Dermatitis* 1976;2:237.

142. Hogan DJ, Maibach HI. Adverse dermatologic reactions to transdermal drug delivery systems. *J Am Acad Dermatol* 1990;22:811.

143. Holdiness MR. A review of contact dermatitis associated with transdermal therapeutic systems. *Contact Dermatitis* 1989;20:3.

144. Kounis N, Zavras G, Papadaki P, et al. Allergic reactions to local glyceryl trinitrate administration. *Br J Clin Pract* 1996;50:437–439.

145. Robinson M, et al. Evaluation of the primary skin irritation and allergic contact sensitization potential of transdermal triprolidine. *Fundam-Appl-Toxicol* 1991;17:103–119.

146. Maibach HI. Oral substitutions in patients sensitized by transdermal clonidine treatment. *Contact Dermatitis* 1985;19:225.

147. Bircher AJ, Howald H, Rufli T. Adverse skin reactions to nicotine in a transdermal therapeutic system. *Contact Dermatitis* 1991;25:230.

148. El-Sayed F, Bayl-Lebey P, Marquery M, et al. Sensibilisation systemique au 17 beta-oestradiol induite par la voie transcutanee. *Ann-Dermatol-Venereol* 1996;123:26–28.

149. Silva SK, Berman B. The effect of topical Maalox on transdermal clonidine induced contact dermatitis. *Am J Contact Dermatitis* 1992; 3:79.

150. Jordan W. Allergy and topical irritation associated with transdermal testosterone administration: a comparison of scrotal and nonscrotal transdermal systems. *Am J Contact Dermatitis* 1997;8:108–113.

151. Amkraut A, Jordan W, Taskovich L. Effect of coadministrations of corticosteroids on the development of contact sensitization. *J Am Acad Dermatol* 1996;35:27–31.

152. Schwarz BK, Clendenning WE. Allergic contact dermatitis from hydroxypropyl cellulose in a transdermal patch. *Contact Dermatitis* 1988;18:106.

153. Pecquet C, et al. Allergic contact dermatitis from ethanol in a transdermal estradiol patch. *Contact Dermatitis* 1992;27:275.

154. Dwyer C, Forsyth A. Allergic contact dermatitis from methacrylates in a nicotine transdermal patch. *Contact Dermatitis* 1994;30:309.

155. Praditsuwan P, Taylor J, Roenigk H. Allergy to Unna boots in four patients. *J Am Acad Dermatol* 1995;33:906–908.

156. Malten KE. Sensitizers in leg bandages. *Contact Dermatitis* 1977;3: 217.

157. Fowler J. Contact allergy to a rubber knee brace. *Am J Contact Dermatitis* 1991;2:211–212.

158. Scalf L, Fowler J. Allergic contact dermatitis caused by dialkyl thioureas in a patient with sleep apnea. *Am J Contact Dermatitis* 1999;10:169–171.

APPENDIX A

Sources of Ostomy Information and Supplies

Bard Consumer Products Division
C.R. Bard Inc. (Health Care Products)
8195 Industrial Boulevard
Covington, GA 30014
800-526-4455

Blanchard Ostomy Products
1510 Raymond Avenue
Glendale, CA 91201

Coloplast Corp.
1955 West Oak Circle
Marietta, GA 30062
800-533-0464

Convatec
P.O. Box 5254
Princeton, NJ 08543
800-422-8811

Cymed
1336A Channing Way
Berkeley, CA 94702
800-582-0707

Dansac AS
DK 3480
Fredenborg, Denmark

Ferndale Laboratories Inc.
780 West Eight Mile Road
Ferndale, MI 48220

Hollister Inc.
2000 Hollister Drive
Libertyville, IL 60048

Incutech Inc.
P.O. Box 1608
Kernersville, NC 27285
800-699-4232

Marlen
5150 Richmond Road
Bedford, OH 44146
216-292-7060

Nu-Hope Laboratories Inc.
P.O. Box 331150
Pacoima, CA 91333
800-899-5017

Ostomy USA
P.O. Box 859
Tallevast, FL 34270-0859
800-846-5994

Spenco Medical Corp.
P.O. Box 2501
Waco, TX 76712
800-877-3626

Torbot Group Inc.
1185 Jefferson Boulevard
P.O. Box 6008
Warwick, RI 02887-6008
800-545-5254

The United Ostomy Association
118 Monmouth
Lakewood, NJ 08701
800-551-7110

VPI
1100 West Morgan
Spencer, IN 47460
812-829-4891

APPENDIX B

Information on TENS Units

EMPI Medical
599 Cardigan Road
St. Paul, MN 55126
800-325-5663

Grass Instrument Division
AstroMed Inc.
600 East Greenwich Avenue
West Warwick, RI 02893
401-828-4000

Parker Laboratories Inc.
286 Eldridge Road
Fairfield, NJ 07004
800-631-8888

Pharmaceutical Innovations Inc.
897 Frelinghuysen Avenue
Newark, NJ 07114
973-242-2900

CHAPTER 21

Fragrance Allergy

Fragrance materials are among the most common causes of allergic contact dermatitis. In addition to ACD, photodermatitis is seen occasionally, as is contact urticaria, irritation, and depigmentation. Fragrances have widespread use and are found not only in hair and skin care products, but also in laundry products, dentifrices, and cleaning products. Usually the source of the fragrance exposure is a skin or hair care product rather than a cologne or perfume itself. Only one-fourth of the patients with a fragrance allergy in a European study reacted to perfume or cologne (1).

Fragrance allergy generally has be recognized only since the 1940s. Bonnevie (2) in 1948 reported that balsam of Peru (BOP) was a common allergen and identified cinnamic aldehyde as an important allergenic constituent. In 1961, Hjorth (3) extensively described BOP allergy, both topically and systemically. Larsen (4) in 1977 developed the fragrance mix and reported on its usefulness as a screening allergen. These pioneers have allowed us to have a much clearer understanding of the diagnosis and prevalence of fragrance allergy.

The approximate concentration of perfume oils used in various products is shown in Table 21.1. More than five thousand fragrance materials are in use today. Fragrance sales are more than $4 billion per year, worldwide. A typical complete perfume may consist of 10 to 300 separate components. Defining the specific offending allergens can, therefore, be difficult. Fortunately, there are often chemical similarities among fragrances that lead to cross-reactions.

PREVALENCE OF FRAGRANCE ALLERGY

Twenty years ago, a prospective cosmetic adverse reaction study showed that fragrances are the leading cause of allergic contact dermatitis due to cosmetics (5). A follow-up study by the same investigators found 713 patients over a 6-year period with cosmetic dermatitis (6). Of 536 positive patch tests, 161 (30%) were to fragrances. Preservatives accounted for 27% of reactions.

The most recent data from the North American Contact Dermatitis Group (NACDG) (1996–1998) indicate that fragrance mix (FM) (8% pet) was positive in 11.7% of 4,095 patients tested, and BOP was positive in 11.8%. This compares with 14.0% and 10.4%, respectively, seen in the period 1994–1996 (7). These patients were all suffering from suspected ACD. Only nickel and neomycin gave more positive reactions in the 1996–1998 data.

DeGroot and Frosch (8) summarized fragrance allergy in Europe. Prevalence rates of about 5% to 11% are reported in various studies, with a European multicenter study reporting 8.3% of 1,072 tested patients positive to the fragrance mix (9).

In the general population, the frequency of fragrance allergy is uncertain. In a study from Denmark, about 1% of unselected subjects were positive to the fragrance mix (10). Guin and Berry (11), however, found that 18% of 90 student nurses were positive to the fragrance mix (16% concentration).

SCREENING FOR FRAGRANCE ALLERGY

Because there are hundreds of individual fragrance chemicals, the use of screening allergens is essential in diagnosing fragrance allergy.

Balsam of Peru

Balsam of Peru (BP) is generally included in standard screening patch test series as an indicator of fragrance sensitivity. A naturally occurring substance obtained from fir trees, BP is composed of many allergens including benzyl acetate, benzyl alcohol, cinnamic acid, cinnamic alcohol, cinnamic aldehyde, eugenol, and isoeugenol.

BP itself is rarely used in fragrances, although distillates are used that may be less allergenic. Some individuals may be sensitized to BP through medicinal exposure. Cross-reactions with benzoin and resorcinol have been reported. BP as a marker substance is positive in about 50% of cases of fragrance allergy.

Fragrance Mix

A second agent used to screen for fragrance allergy is a fragrance mix. Typically, a mixture of eight common individual fragrance allergens, listed in Table 21.2, is used. Cur-

TABLE 21.1. *Approximate Concentrations of Perfumes in Various Products*

Colognes	4.0%
Cosmetics	0.5%
Masking perfumes	0.1% or less
Perfumes	20.0%
Toilet water	5.0%

The current fragrance mix and balsam of Peru detect the vast majority of cases of fragrance allergy. Adding oils of sandalwood, narcissus, and ylang-ylang allows detection of almost 100% of known fragrance allergy.

rently, each allergen is included at a 1% concentration (8% total). This is superior to a 16% mix in terms of reduced irritancy, but may miss some reactions that would be positive at 16%. Santucci et al. (12) found a 3.6% to 5.2% range of positive reactions to fragrance mix depending on concentrations.

An interesting observation by Enders et al. (13) has led to the discovery that sorbitan sesquioleate (SS), an emulsifier, can enhance the diagnostic value of patch testing fragrances. They noted that less than half the patients positive to fragrance mix reacted to any of the agents separately. Subsequently, after finding the presence of SS in the mix, but not the individual allergens, they retested patients after adding SS to each single allergen. Ninety-three percent reacted to one or more allergen and none to SS (20% pet). The authors suggest that adding SS or another emulsifier may enhance patch test diagnostic power (14).

If an irritant reaction from fragrance mix is suspected and it is crucial to rule in or rule out fragrance allergy, then retesting at a later time with the individual components with SS is recommended. If a particular product is suspected as the cause, a request to the manufacturer for patch test materials containing a breakdown of the fragrance components is often helpful. Although fragrance formulas in many products are closely guarded, a coded patch test series may be supplied. Without divulging the whole formula, the manufacturer may disclose only the agents causing positive reactions. The Cosmetics, Toiletry and Fragrance Association (CTFA) and/or the Research Institute for Fragrance Materials (RIFM) can be helpful in supplying information to assist the physician investigating fragrance or other cosmetic problems (see Appendix A).

Testing with BP and fragrance mix will probably detect over 90% of the cases of fragrance allergy. Larsen et al. (15) tested known perfume-sensitive patients and found that over 90% reacted to BOP, FM, or both. Three essential oils, sandalwood, narcissus, and ylang-ylang, detected almost all the remaining few patients who did not react to BOP or FM.

TESTING WITH INDIVIDUAL FRAGRANCE AGENTS AND PATIENT-SUPPLIED MATERIALS

Perfumes and colognes usually can be tested as is, although the patch should be allowed to dry before application to avoid irritation from volatile solvents. Individual fragrance should be tested at concentrations listed in Table 21.3.

The NACDG collected data on frequency of positive patch tests to individual fragrance chemicals before 1991. For the years 1989–1990, 614 patients were tested with these allergens (Table 21.3). Twenty-two percent had one or more reactions. Twelve of these 135 patients (9%) had occupationally related fragrance allergy. Of the 199 total reactions, 162 (81.4%) were considered relevant to a past or current skin problem. The data from a European multicenter study is presented in Table 21.4. Oak moss was the most common individual allergen positive in patients allergic to the FM (9).

Cinnamic Alcohol and Cinnamic Aldehyde

These two commonly used fragrance materials are well-known allergens. Cinnamic aldehyde and alcohol and chemically related components are used primarily as flavoring agents, as well as fragrances. They are used in beverages (cola), vermouths, bitters, chewing gums, mouthwashes, soaps, and toothpaste. Sanitary napkin dermatitis due to cinnamic alcohol has been reported.

Because of its sensitizing capacity, the International Fragrance Research Association (IFRA) recommends that cinnamic alcohol should not be used as a fragrance ingredient at a level of more than 4% in fragrance compounds.

Cinnamic aldehyde has shown stronger sensitization than cinnamic alcohol in guinea pig tests (16). There is some apparent cross-reactivity between the two. The enzyme alcohol dehydrogenase, present in human skin, can convert the alcohol to the aldehyde.

Geraniol

This substance is found in many essential oils, including rose, geraniums, citronella, jasmine, and lavender oils. It is colorless with a scent of roses (8).

TABLE 21.2. *Components of the Fragrance Patch Test Mixture*

An essential oil from a lichen

1. oak moss absolute	2. cinnamic aldehyde	3. cinnamic alcohol	4. alpha-amyl cinnamic alcohol
5. geraniol	6. hydroxycitronellal	7. isoeugenol	8. eugenol

TABLE 21.3. *Positive Patch Tests to Fragrances in 614 Patients*

Allergen (pet)	Positive (%)
Cinnamic alcohol 5%	47 (7.6)
Cinnamic aldehyde 1%	30 (4.9)
Hydroxycitronellal 4%	13 (2.1)
Eugenol 4%	33 (5.4)
Isoeugenol 4%	19 (3.1)
Oak moss %%	11 (1.8)
Benzyl alcohol 5%	8 (1.3)
Geraniol 5%	17 (2.8)
Alpha-amyl cinnamic alcohol 5%	1 (0.2)
Benzyl salicylate 2%	7 (0.2)
Anisyl alcohol 5%	3 (0.5)
Sandalwood oil 2%	10 (1.6)
Coumarin 5%	8 (1.3)
Musk ambrette 5%	3 (0.5)

Source: NACDG. Unpublished data, 1991.

Alpha-Amyl Cinnamic Aldehyde

This is a synthetic fragrance with a jasmine odor. It is a weak sensitizer, as noted in studies where individual fragrance allergens are tested (Tables 21.3 and 21.4).

Hydroxycitronellal

Hydroxycitronellal is a fragrance used widely in floralizing perfume materials. It may also be found as a fragrance in antiseptics and insecticides. This widely used fragrance material is synthetic and is not found in nature.

Isoeugenol and Eugenol

Eugenol is a component of essential oils obtained from spices, including cloves and cinnamon leaf, with an odor and taste of cloves. Positive patch tests to eugenol and isoeugenol, respectively, were found in 1.4% and 2.4% of 1,016 patients reported by the NACDG. Of the patients reactive to either substance, 13% reacted to both, indicating a low degree of cross-reactivity. The chemical structure of these substances is very similar (Table 21.2). Eugenol is found in mouthwashes, toothpaste, dental cements and

TABLE 21.4. *Fragrance Mixture Results*

1995	Tested	Positive	%
Fragrance mix	1,072	89	8.3
Oak moss		24	2.24
Isoeugenol		20	1.86
Eugenol		13	1.21
Cinnamic aldehyde		10	0.93
Geraniol		8	0.75
Hydroxycitronella		8	0.75
Cinnamic alcohol		6	0.56
Alpha-amyl cinnamic aldehyde		5	0.47
Sorbitan sesquioleate		5	0.47

Source: Adapted from Frosch et al. 1995.

packing agents, antiseptics, and inhalants, as well as in fragrance mixtures. Eugenol has been shown to have the ability to "quench" nonimmunologic contact urticaria when applied before urticants such as sorbic acid and cinnamic aldehyde (17). Unfortunately, it does not inhibit allergic contact dermatitis in the same situations (18).

Isoeugenol has a weaker odor than eugenol and may be found in ylang-ylang and nutmeg oil. In 1998, the IFRA suggested reducing the limit of 0.2% in consumer products to 0.02%. White et al. (19) reported that isoeugenol acetate (1.2% ethanol), a possible replacement for isoeugenol, gave positive patch tests in most isoeugenol sensitive patients.

Oak Moss Absolute

Oak moss absolute is a natural product derived from a tree lichen, *Evernia prunastri*. Atranorin, a potent sensitizer, is present in oak moss, which is made from tree moss (20). Other allergens include evernic acid and fumarproto-cetaric acid. Consort contact dermatitis has been reported in a woman due to exposure to her husband's aftershave lotion, which contained oak moss (21,22). Oak moss absolute is a commonly used fragrance material in aftershave lotions.

Benzyl Alcohol

Benzyl alcohol is a fragrance ingredient that is also used as a preservative and antiseptic topically and as a preservative in injectable medications (see Table 21.5). Allergy to benzyl alcohol as a fragrance ingredient has been reported (23). However, allergy from other exposure sources, such as preservatives and solvents, is also common. Shaw (24) gives an excellent review of the topic.

TABLE 21.5. *Some Topical Products and Injectable Medications Containing Benzyl Alcohol*

Topical	Injectables
Aristocort A Cream	Intron A
Cyclocort Cream/Ointment	Kenalog
Lotrisone Cream	Depo-Medrol
Lotrimin Lotion	
Loprox Cream/Lotion	
Naftin Cream	
Mycelex-7 Vaginal Cream	
Theraplex Lotion	
Zostrix Cream	
Itch-X Gel	
Rhuligel	
Capitrol Shampoo	
Theraplex-T Shampoo	
Ivy Block Lotion	
Photoplex Sunscreens	
Zonalon	
Zilactin	
Aldara	

Musk Ambrette and Musk Moskene

Musk ambrette is a synthetic chemical that has been used widely for the last 60 years (25). Its use in fragrances, soaps, detergents, creams, lotions, and dentifrices in the United States amounts to about 100,000 lb per year. This nitro-musk compound is used as a fixative in perfume formulations in concentrations from 1% to as high as 15%. In 1978, Larsen (26) reported the first case of photoallergic contact dermatitis to musk ambrette. The patient used a well-known aftershave lotion and broke out with a severe dermatitis on the sun-exposed areas of the face and neck.

Since that time, numerous reports of photosensitivity to musk ambrette have been made (27). In addition, musk ambrette can cause nonphotoallergic contact dermatitis. Harber sensitized guinea pigs to musk ambrette, whereas Kligman was not able to sensitize humans (27). Until now, almost all clinical cases have been male patients. It is apparent that putting aftershave lotion on a recently shaved face and going outdoors is analogous to a continuous photomaximization test. Musk ambrette should be a component of any photo patch testing series.

In addition to photoallergy, an apparent case of airborne ACD of the face with hyperpigmentation has been reported. Chronic burning of incense for several years was the source of exposure (28).

A case of ACD to musk moskene, a related perfume, has been reported from contact in facial cosmetics (29). Testing at 5% pet was negative in controls. Musk moskene is reported to cause less photosensitivity and allergy than musk ambrette.

The IFRA recommends that musk ambrette should not be used as a fragrance ingredient at a level of more than 4% in fragrance compounds. It recommends further that musk ambrette should not be used at a level of more than 0.5% in fragrance compounds intended for use in aftershave products.

> **Musk ambrette and methylcoumarin are photosensitizing fragrances.**

6-Methylcoumarin

The synthetic compound 6-methylcoumarin is a related structurally to the furocoumarins. In 1980, an epidemic of photodermatitis occurred in people using a popular sunscreen with an increased level of 6-methylcoumarin (30). The reaction occurred primarily in women and developed within several hours after they applied suntan lotion and went into the sun. The U.S. Food and Drug Administration (FDA) received many consumer complaints, and it initiated a shelf recall of all those suntan products containing this ingredient (31). Subsequent phototesting suggested that 6-methylcoumarin is indeed a potent photosensitizer, at least under the conditions of this particular application (32).

The IFRA recommends that 6-methylcoumarin and also 7-methylcoumarin should not be used as a fragrance ingredient.

Versalide (AETT)

Versalide (AETT) is a tetralin musk formerly used widely as a musk fixative in many cosmetics, including soaps, colognes, and antiperspirants. It found wide use as a masking agent in nonscented antiperspirants. In 1979, Avon toxicologists discovered that during routine dermal tests with rats exposed to perfume oil, the skin and internal organs of the rats developed a blue color. The central nervous system was among those organs showing the most intense coloration. The pathologic change found in the nervous tissue was demyelinization of nerve tracts (33). This neurotoxic effect was reported to the RIFM, and the two fragrance companies that made versalide stopped supplying this compound for use in consumer products. The FDA took no action because the compound was no longer available for human use. The IFRA recommends that versalide should not be used in any fragrance compounds.

Tea-Tree Oil

The extracts of the Melaleuca plant, tea-tree oil, is promoted as being useful for a wide spectrum of skin disorders, and therefore is found in assorted topical products (34). Allergy in patients was reported by Rubel et al. (35). Extensive patch testing with tea-tree oil components documented allergy to these sesquiterpenoid fractions. Another report implicated a monoterpene, O-limonene, as responsible for tea-tree oil allergy in six cases (36). Cross-reactivity with balsam of Peru on patch testing appears to be common.

Fowler noted frequent cross-reactivity between tea-tree oil and BOP and FM (Fowler J, personal communication, 2000).

Rose Oil

Scheinman (37) reported 9 of 299 (3%) consecutive patients positive to rose oil (2% pet). In an Indonesian study, 7 of 32 patients positive to FM also reacted to rose extract (38).

Further study of rose oil/extract would seem to be in order.

UNSCENTED COSMETICS AND MASKING FRAGRANCES

Some cosmetics and skin care products are labeled "unscented" but actually contain a low concentration of a "masking fragrance." The masking fragrance is intended to cover the fatty odor of soap or the "medicinal" smell of some chemicals without giving a recognizable aroma of its own. Ethylene brassylate (Musk T) is often used for this purpose. It is uncertain how often this fragrance cross-reacts with other fragrances, but if a patient wishes to completely avoid fragrance exposure, this substance should be looked for in ingredient lists. Generally, products labeled "fragrance-free" have no fragrance chemicals, including a masking fragrance. Therefore, the fragrance-sensitive consumer should look for this designation rather than the label "unscented."

> **Some cosmetics labeled "unscented" contain a "masking" fragrance in a very low concentration. The term "fragrance-free" usually is more reliable than "unscented."**

FRAGRANCES MASQUERADING AS "BOTANICAL" OR "HERBAL" INGREDIENTS

In recent years some personal care products such as skin lotions and soaps have been marketed as being "unscented" or "fragrance-free," yet they contain herbal ingredients or oils from botanicals. Technically, although they import a fragrance, they are classified as "moisturizers" rather than fragrances. Unwitting consumers may be duped by marketing claims stating that a product contains only "natural" ingredients and may not realize that these herbal and botanical extracts can cause allergy in fragrance-sensitive persons (37,39).

Both Scheinman (39) and Nakayama et al. (40) reported cases of allergic contact dermatitis from "hidden" fragrances in soaps and other toiletries. Offending allergens included rose oil, vanilla, and sweet almond oil.

Fragrance-allergic patients should be counseled to read ingredient labels and avoid products containing covert fragrance allergens such as "herbal," "natural," or "botanical" extracts. As Fisher is fond of saying, the notorious sensitizer poison ivy is a natural substance.

CONTACT URTICARIA

Contact urticaria may be allergic or nonallergic (41). BP and some of its derivatives can cause nonallergic urticaria. The chief agent responsible for this is cinnamic aldehyde, although cinnamic acid, benzoic acid, and benzaldehyde are also active. The mechanism of action is probably a non-allergic histamine-liberating effect that may be more than a purely cutaneous phenomenon, because some individuals suffering from chronic respiratory allergies precipitate symptoms of their condition on exposure to certain fragrance materials. Fowler has observed immediate, presumably nonimmunologic contact urticaria at patch test sites of cinnamic aldehyde and BOP. Cancian et al (42) reported generalized urticaria with foci at patch sites of FM and BOP that resolved after 6 hours. Terpinyl acetate used in a spray starch has been reported to cause contact urticaria (43).

Further discussion of contact urticaria is found in Chapter 6.

"PREDICTIVE TESTING" FOR FRAGRANCE SENSITIZATION

Klejak (44) correlated the quantitative aspects of fragrance sensitivity in the guinea pig. Using the open epicutaneous method, Klejak presented the dose of a fragrance required to induce and elicit sensitization. In humans, most fragrance allergy potential is documented with the maximization method. False-negative assays, however, occur with this method (45).

Malten et al. (46) reported on 22 fragrance substances included by the RIFM in human maximization testing. Some agents showing a high rate of sensitization, such as diethylmaleate, are listed as prohibited in Table 21.6. However, several agents, including eugenol, hydroxycitronellal, and cinnamic alcohol, that showed a very low sensitization potential were proven to give positive patch tests in certain ACD patients.

The fragrance industry is trying constantly to eliminate those fragrance materials that cause adverse reactions. The IFRA recommends chemicals not to be used at all as well as those with limits and concentrations (consult Table 22.6). If the fragrance industry follows these recommendations, the

TABLE 21.6. *Suggested Restrictions in Ingredient Usage*

Excluded	Limit on concentration on product use*	Use with quenching agent(s)
AETT (acetyl ethyltetramethyltetralin	5-acetyl-1,1,2,3,3,6-hexamenthyl indan	Carvone oxide
Acetyl isovaleryl	Allyl heptine carbonate	
Allanroot oil (elocampane oil)	Amyl cyclopentenone	Cinnamic aldehyde
Allylisothiocyanate		
Anisylidene acetone	Angelica root	Cinnamic aldehyde methyl anthranilate Schiff base
	cis- and *trans-* asarone	
Benzylidene acetone	Bergamot oil	Citral
p-tert-butylphenol	Bitter orange oil expressed	
Chenopodium oil	*p-tert*-butyl-dihydrocinamaldehyde	
Cinnamylidene acetone		

continued

TABLE 21.6. *Suggested Restrictions in Ingredient Usage (Continued)*

Excluded	Limit on concentration on product use*	Use with quenching agent(s)
Colophony	Cassia oil	Phenylacetaldehyde
Costus root oil, absolute and concrete		
3,7-dimethyl-2-octen-1-ol (6,7-dihydrogeraniol)		
Diethyl maleate	Cinnamic alcohol	
Dihydrocoumarin	Cinnamon bark oil, Ceylon	
2,4-dihydroxy-3-methyl-benzaldehyde	Citrus oils and other furocoumarins containing essential oils	
4,6-dimethyl-8-t-butyl coumarin	Coatus root, essential oil, absolute and concrete	
Dimethylictraconate	Cumin oil	
Diphenylamine	Cyclamen alcohol	
Esters of 2-octynoic acid, except methyl and allyl heptine carbonate	Grapefruit oil expressed	
Esters of 2-nonynoic acid, except methyl octine carbonate	*trans*-2-hexenal	
	α-hexylidene cyclopentanone	
	Hydroxycitronella	
	Isocyclogeraniol	
	Isoeugenol	
Ethyl acrylate	Lemon oil, cold pressed	
Ethylene glycol monoeathyl ether and its acetate	Lime oil, expressed	
Etylene glycol monomethyl ether and its acetate	Marigold oil and absolute (tagetes oil and absolute)	
Fig leaf absolute	Menthadienyl formate	
Furfurylideneacetone	Methoxy dicyclopentadiene carboxaldehyde	
	2-methoxy-4-methylphenol	
trans-2-heptenal	Methyl heptadienone	
Hexahydrocoumarin		
trans-2-hexenal diethyl acetal		
trans-2-hexenal dimethyl acetal		
Hydroabietyl alcohol		
Hydroquinone monoethylether		
Hydroquinone monomethylether		
6-isopropyl-2-decalol	Methyl heptine carbonate	
Massoia bark oil	*p*-methylhydrocinnamic aldehyde	
Massoia lactone		
Melissa oil		
Methyl methacrylate		
7-methoxycoumarin	Methyl *N*-methyl anthranilate	
	3-methyl-2(3)-nonenenitrile	
	Methyl octine carbonate	
	Oak moss extracts	
	1-octen-2-yl acetate	
N-methyl anisylidene acetone	Opoponax	
6-methylcoumarin	Perilla aldehyde	
	Balsam of Peru	
7-methylcoumarin		
4-methyl-7-ethoxy coumarin	Propylidene phthalide	
Methylcrotonate	Rue oil	
Musk ambrette		
Nitrobenzene	Safrole, isosafrole, dihdyrosafrole	
	Styrax	
	Tree moss extracts	
	1-(trimethylcyclohexenyl/cyclohexadienyl)-2-butenn-1-ones (Rose ketones)	
Pentylidene cyclohexanone	Verbena absolute	
Phenylacetone (methyl benzyl ketone)		
Phenylbenzoate		
Pseudoionones		
Pseudomethylionone		
Thea sinensis absolute		
Verbena oil		

*These items are restricted to various maximum concentrations in the final product. Based on IFRA guidelines, 1999.

incidence of fragrance sensitivity, including photosensitivity, may decrease.

THE FUTURE

We will not learn about new fragrance allergens unless we look for them by testing all cosmetic and toiletry cases and by determining the offending allergens. This is done most easily by testing the actual product as is, except when it is irritating, as with shampoos and cleansers. If testing of the final formulation is positive, all the components, including the fragrance, should be obtained and should be tested separately. Most major cosmetic and toiletry manufacturers will assist by sending patch test materials when requested. If the fragrance component is positive, further breakdown of the fragrance to its individual components should be done to discover new fragrance allergens. (See Table 21.7 for an example of the component breakdown of one product (Mycolog Cream) (47).)

> **Many fragrance allergies are occult; thus, we should look for fragrance allergy in any nonhealing, recurrent, or chronic dermatitis.**

TABLE 21.7. *Ingredients of Mycolog Cream Perfume: An Example of the Complexity of Perfume Formulations*

Acetophenone extra
Alpha-amyl cinnamic alcohol
Anisyl alcohol
Benzyl acetate extra
Benzyl alcohol
Brazilian bois de rose oil
Cinnamic alcohol
Citral pure
Citronellal extra
Coumarin in benzyl alcohol
Gardinol
Geranium boubon
Hydroxycitronellal
Lavadin
Lime distilled
Linalyl acetate
Linalyl formate
Lovage extra, oil
Mousse d'abre absolute (oak moss absolute)
Musk T special
Orange sweet California
Orange terpenes
Patchouli oil
Petitgrain cordillera
Resinoid labdanum in benzyl benzoate
Sandalwood
Terpineol prime
Terpinyl acetate

See Ref. 47.

PREVENTION

The avoidance of fragranced cosmetics and toiletries is fairly straightforward if patients read labels. More cosmetic lines are developing fragrance-free cosmetics, allowing for a wider choice of products by consumers. However, no commercial sources of perfumes and colognes with fragrance ingredients on the labels are available. Some companies will answer whether a specific product does or does not have a given fragrance component.

> **Because cosmetic labeling does not include fragrance component labeling, use tests may be done with the cosmetics and perfumes.**

Those individuals with fragrance allergy are suggested to avoid fragrances entirely. Patients also must be cautioned against using products with "natural" extracts of botanicals and herbs. Those who will not or cannot do this may perform a use or ROAT test (repeated open application test). Application of a product such as a lotion or perfume to the antecubital space twice daily for 5 days is recommended. A lack of response suggests that the product contains little or no fragrance chemical in question.

REFERENCES

1. DeGroot AC, Bruynzeel DP, Bos J, et al. The allergens in cosmetics. *Arch Dermatol* 1988;124:1525.
2. Bonnevie P. Some experiences of war-time dermatoses. *Acta Derm Venereol* (Stockh) 1948;28:231–237.
3. Hjorth N. Eczematous allergy to balsams, allied perfumes and flavoring agents with special reference to balsam of Peru. *Acta Derm Venereol* (Stockh) 1961;41(Suppl 46):1–216.
4. Larsen W. Perfume dermatitis. *Arch Dermatol* 1977;113:623–626.
5. Eiermann HJ, Larsen WG, Maibach HI, Taylor JS. Prospective study of cosmetic reactions, 1977–80. *J Am Acad Dermatol* 1982;6:909.
6. Adams RM, Maibach HI. A five-year study of cosmetic reactions. *J Am Acad Dermatol* 1985;13:1062.
7. Marks J, Belsito D, DeLeo V. North American Contact Dermatitis Group patch test results, 1996–1998. *Arch Dermatol* 2000;136:576–578.
8. DeGroot A, Frosch P. Adverse reactions to fragrances. *Contact Dermatitis* 1997;36:57–86.
9. Frosch P, Pilz B, Andersen K, et al. Patch testing with fragrances: results of a multicenter study of the EECDRG with 48 frequently used constituents of perfumes. *Contact Dermatitis* 1995;33:333–342.
10. Nielsen N, Menne T. Allergic contact sensitization in an unselected Danish population. *Acta Derm Venereol* (Stockh) 1992;72:456–460.
11. Guin J, Berry V. Perfume sensitivity in adult females. *J Am Acad Dermatol* 1984;11:1168–1174.
12. Santucci B, et al. Contact dermatitis to fragrances. *Contact Dermatitis* 1987;16;93.
13. Enders F, Przybilla B, Ring J. Patch testing with fragrance mix at 16% and 8%, and its individual constituents. *Contact Dermatitis* 1989;20:348.
14. Enders F, Przybilla B, Ring J. Patch testing with fragrance-mix and its constituents: discrepancies are largely due to the presence or absence of Sorbitan sequioleate. *Contact Dermatitis* 1991;24:238.
15. Larsen W, Kakayama H, Fischer T, et al. Fragrance contact dermatitis—a worldwide multicenter investigation. *Am J Contact Dermatitis* 1996;7:77–83.

16. Basketter DA. Skin sensitization to cinnamic alcohol: the role of skin metabolism. *Acta Derm Venereol* (Stockh) 1992;72:264.
17. Safford RJ, et al. Immediate contact reactions to chemicals in the fragrance mix and a study of the quenching action of eugenol. *Br J Dermatol* 1990;123:595.
18. Basketter DA, Allenby CF. Studies of the quenching phenomenon in delayed contact hypersensitivity reactions. *Contact Dermatitis* 1991;25:160.
19. White I, Johansen D, Arnau E, et al. Isoeugenol is an important contact allergen: can it be safely replaced with isoeugenol acetate? *Contact Dermatitis* 1999;41:272–275.
20. Thune P, et al. Perfume allergy due to oak moss and other lichens. *Contact Dermatitis* 1982;8:396.
21. Held JL, Ruszkowski AM, Deleo VA. Consort contact dermatitis due to oak moss. *Arch Dermatol* 1988;124:261.
22. Opdyke DL. Musk ambrette: monographs of fragrance raw materials. *Food Cosmet Toxicol* 1975;13:875.
23. Corazza M, Mantovani L, Maranini C, et al. Allergic contact dermatitis from benzyl alcohol. *Contact Dermatitis* 1996;34:74–75.
24. Shaw D. Allergic contact dermatitis to benzyl alcohol in a hearing aid impression material. *Am J Contact Dermatitis* 1999;10:228–232.
25. Raugi GH, Storrs FJ, Larsen WG. Photoallergic contact dermatitis to men's perfumes. *Contact Dermatitis* 1979;5:251.
26. Larsen WG. Photoallergy to musk ambrette found in an aftershave lotion. Presented at the American Academy of Dermatology Meeting, San Francisco, Dec 1978.
27. Kochever IE, et al. Assay of contact photosensitivity to musk ambrette in guinea pigs. *J Invest Dermatol* 1979;73:144.
28. Hayakawa R, Matsunaga K, Arima Y. Airborne pigmented contact dermatitis due to musk ambrette in incense. *Contact Dermatitis* 1987;16:96.
29. Hayakawa R, Hirose O, Arima Y. Pigmented contact dermatitis due to musk moskene. *J Dermatol* 1991;18:420.
30. Jackson RT, Nesbitt LT, Jr, DeLeo VA. 6-methylcoumarin photocontact dermatitis. *J Am Acad Dermatol* 1980;2:124.
31. Eiermann HJ. Regulatory issues concerning AETT and 6-MC. *Contact Dermatitis* 1980;6:120.
32. Kaidbey KH, Kligman AM. Identification of topical photosensitizing agents in humans. *J Invest Dermatol* 1978;70:149.
33. Spencer PS, et al. Neurotoxic changes in rats exposed to the fragrance compound acetyl ethyl tetramethyl tetralin. *Neurotoxicology* 1979;1:221.
34. Altman P. Australian Tea-Tree oil: a natural antiseptic. *Aust J Biotechnol* 1989;3:247–248.
35. Rubel D, Freeman S, Southwell I. Tea-tree oil allergy: what is the offending agent? *Aust J Dermatol* 1998;39:244–247.
36. Knight T, Hausen B. Melaleuca oil (tea-tree oil) dermatitis. *J Am Acad Dermatol* 1994;30:423–427.
37. Scheinman P. Is it really fragrance free? *Am J Contact Dermatitis* 1997;8:239–242.
38. Roesyanto-Mahadi I, Guersen-Reitsma A, vanJoost T, et al. Sensitization to fragrance materials in Indonesian cosmetics. *Contact Dermatitis* 1990;22: 212–217.
39. Scheinman P. The foul side of fragrance-free products: what every clinician should know about managing patients with fragrance allergy. *J Am Acad Dermatol* 1999;41:1020–1024.
40. Nakayama H, Nogi N, Kashara N, et al. Allergen control, an indispensable treatment for allergic contact dermatitis. *Dermatol Clin* 1990;8:197–204.
41. Von Krogh G, Maibach HI, eds. The contact urticaria syndrome. In: Marzulli FN, Maibach HI, eds. *Dermatotoxicology,* 2nd ed. New York: Hemisphere Publishing, 1983:301.
42. Cancian M, Fortina A, Peserico A. Contact urticaria syndrome from constituents of balsam of Peru and fragrance mix in a patient with chronic urticaria. *Contact Dermatitis* 1999;41:300.
43. McDaniel WR, Marks JG. Contact urticaria due to sensitivity to spray starch. *Arch Dermatol* 1979;115:628.
44. Klejak W. Allergic contact dermatitis in the guinea pig. In: Marzulli FN, Maibach HI, eds. *Dermatotoxicology,* 2nd ed. New York: Hemisphere Publishing, 1983.
45. Marzulli F, Maibach HI. Contact allergy: predictive testing of fragrance ingredients in humans by draizé and maximization methods. *J Environ Pathol Toxicol* 1980;3:235.
46. Malten KE, et al. Reactions in selected patients to 22 fragrance materials. *Contact Dermatitis* 1984;11:1.
47. Larsen WG. Allergic contact dermatitis from the perfume in Mycolog Cream. *Arch Dermatol* 1972;105:896.

APPENDIX A

INFORMATION SOURCES FOR FRAGRANCES

Research Institute for Fragrance Materials (RIFM)
2 University Drive, Suite 406
Hackensack, NJ 07601–6209
Telephone: 201-488-5527
Fax: 201-488-5594

International Fragrance Research Association (IFRA)
Square Marie-Louise
49-B 1000 Brussels, Belgium
Telephone: 32-2-238-99-05
Fax: 32-2-230-02-65
E-mail: ifra@dial.eunet.ch
Web site: http://www.ifraorg.org

Cosmetics, Toiletry, and Fragrance Association (CTFA)
1101 17th Street, N.W. #300
Washington, DC 20036
Telephone: 202-331-1770
Fax: 202-331-1969
Web site: http://www.ctfa.org

To order CTFA publications, write to:
CTFA Publications Orders
P.O. Box 75319
Baltimore, MD 21275
Telephone: 301-953-2614
Fax: 301-206-9789

CHAPTER 22

Allergic Sensitization to Plants[1]

Plant dermatitis may be classified as allergic sensitization, mechanical irritation, chemical irritation, phytophotodermatitis, and pseudophytodermatitis.

The plant substances responsible for dermatitis do not enter directly into the metabolism of the plant and are classified as secondary products. The relative proportion of these secondary products depends on vigor of growth, cultural conditions, and the stage of development of the plant. Thus, the amount of ragweed oleoresin increases tenfold when the plant pollinates and is at the height of growth.

> **Contact with certain *uninjured* plants may produce allergic dermatitis; other plants must be *crushed* to release dermatitis-producing chemicals.**

Another factor that may be clinically significant is the distribution of the dermatitis-producing substances in the plant. For example, primin, the antigenic substance of the primrose, is stored in fragile cells in superficial glandular hairs and is released by casual contact. In contrast, the sensitizing substance in some daisies is stored in resin canals and is released only when the plant is bruised or crushed (1). In some plants, the sensitizers may be in the leaves and stem; in others, they are found, in addition, in the flowers, pollen, and roots.

Pentadecylcatechols in the plant oleoresin, consisting of 1,2-dihydroxy benzenes (catechols) with a 15-atom side chain in the third position, are the sensitizers in the *Toxicodendron* plants. These pentadecylcatechols may show cross-reactivity with other phenolic compounds, such as resorcinol, hexylresorcinol, and hydroquinones, but not with phenol.

A 1:10 dilution of the oleoresin in acetone usually equals a 1:1,000 dilution of pentadecylcatechols in antigenicity. Patch testing, except for investigational purposes, is not advisable.

The oleoresin contains unstable, unsaturated compounds that are probably more potent sensitizers than the stable, unsaturated pentadecylcatechols. Members of the Anacardiaceae plant family include common poison ivy *(T. radicans)*, poison oak *(T. toxicodendron, T. diversiloba)*, poison sumac *(T. vernix)*, mango, lacquer tree, cashew nut, Indian marking nut, and rengas tree (black varnish tree). The ginkgo tree fruit contains related allergenic catechols.

TOXICODENDRON PLANTS

In the United States, the *Toxicodendron* group of plants is responsible probably for more cases of allergic contact dermatitis than are all other provocatives combined.

In the eastern United States, *Toxicodendron* dermatitis occurs usually in the spring and summer, but in the Southwest, where outdoor living is common all year, poison oak dermatitis appears at any time, regardless of the season. Even in the East, poison ivy may be acquired from the roots of the plant throughout the year.

Poison ivy and poison oak are the principal causes of *Toxicodendron* dermatitis in the United States. Poison oak *(T. toxicodendron, T. diversiloba)* is more prominent on the West Coast than elsewhere, but poison ivy *(T. radicans)* occurs throughout the United States. Poison sumac or poison dogwood *(T. vernix)* is found only in woody, swampy areas. Cross-sensitivity between the *Toxicodendron* plants exists, and the antigens of all of them are essentially the same. Table 22.1 shows some distinctive characteristics of the various *Toxicodendron* plants.

> **Poison ivy, oak, and sumac contain identical antigens and produce identical eruptions.**

Poison ivy, the most ubiquitous of the *Toxicodendron* group, is a versatile plant that may climb for many feet on a pole, a tree, or a house. On several occasions poison ivy has been discovered being cultivated as an ornamental vine, growing up the side of a house as high as the second story and producing severe, recurrent poison ivy dermatitis on the unsuspecting occupants. The leaflets of the poison ivy

---

[1]This is a revision of a chapter written for the 3rd edition by A. A. Fisher and John C. Mitchell.

TABLE 22.1. *Characteristics of Poisonous Toxicodendron Plants*[a]

Name	Habitat	Identification aids
Poison ivy *(T. radicans)*	United States (except extreme Southwest) and southern Canada	Groups of three leaflets, the margins of each entire, to toothed, to lobed, flat, or wavy. *Leaflets 5 to 15 cm long,* apex pointed. Fruits off-white. Stems with or without aerial rootlets, usually clambering or climbing.
Poison oak *(T. toxicodendron, quercifolia)*	Same as above	Groups of three leaflets, the margins of which are more wavy, more lobed, more "oaklike" than *T. radicans,* and the plant appears more shrublike and less vinelike. *Leaflets 5 to 15 cm long,* more apex pointed than rounded. Conservative botanists consider this a variety or form of poison ivy. Fruits off-white.
Poison oak *(T. diversiloba)*	Generally west of the Cascade and Sierra Nevada mountains, from the Puget Sound to Mexico	Group of three to five leaflets, the margins of each wavy to deeply lobed, more "oaklike" than either of the two above. *Leaflets 3 to 7 cm long,* apex rounded. Fruits off-white. Stems smooth to pubescent, usually stiff and shrublike, less commonly vinelike. This is the poison oak variety found in California.
Poison sumac *(T. vernix)*	Damp, swampy places east of the Rocky Mountains, particularly east of the Mississippi River	Groups of 7 to 13 leaflets, arranged as pairs along central rib, with single leaflet at the end. Fruits white.

[a]In the United States and Canada, any species of Toxicodendron with white fruits should be avoided until positive identification is made. Red-fruited species generally are safe.

and oak plants usually grow in groups of three, giving rise to the warning "Leaves three, leave them be!"

The poison toxicodendron plants are related to the Japanese lacquer and cashew nut trees, the mango, and the marking nut tree of India.

The allergic contact dermatitis whether produced by poison ivy, poison oak, or poison sumac is the same. Furthermore, because the *Toxicodendron* plants belong to the Anacardiaceae family, cross-reactions may occur with the following related plants and substances:

1. A furniture lacquer that may sensitize is obtained from the Japanese lacquer tree.

2. The oil from the shell of the cashew nut contains a potent sensitizer, which is destroyed by heat. Imported Haitian voodoo dolls and swizzle sticks made from cashew nuts may produce a reaction resembling poison ivy dermatitis. Cashew oil may be used in the synthesis of phenol-formaldehyde resins and in mucilages, varnishes, and printer's ink. Components of the oil of cashew nut shells may cross-react with the fruit pulp of the ginkgo tree. The ginkgo fruit pulp may produce an eruption indistinguishable from that of poison ivy dermatitis.

3. The rind of the mango contains a catechol similar to the catechol of the poison ivy group.

4. The marking nut tree of India produces a black, tarry oleoresin used to mark laundry. Because this black ink is a potent sensitizer unaffected by boiling, it can cause repeated attacks of allergic contact dermatitis (dhobi itch) when used to mark clothing. (A *dhobi* is a laundryman.)

Dark-skinned individuals seem less susceptible than others to *Toxicodendron* dermatitis. It has been estimated that at least 70% of the population of the United States would acquire it if exposed casually to the plants. Prolonged exposure would probably sensitize even more of the population. Although elderly individuals are not usually as susceptible to poison ivy as are younger people, Fisher (2) observed poison ivy dermatitis in several individuals who were in their late 70s. Newborn infants can readily be sensitized by a single application of the oleoresin to a localized area, such as a patch test site. More than 50% of infants thus sensitized showed positive patch test reactions 2 to 3 weeks after the initial sensitizing application.

Toxicodendron **dermatitis may occur in persons of all races and ages.**

TABLE 22.2. *Anacardiaceae Plants Related to the Poison Ivy Group*

Common names	Scientific names	Distribution	Modes of contact
Brazilian pepper	*Schinus terebinthifolius*	Brazil, Hawaii, France, Florida	Direct—plant to skin
Cashew nut shell oil		India, Africa, Central America, East Indies	Direct—plant to skin Voodoo dolls, swizzle sticks, resins, mucilages, printer's ink, electric insulation
Cashew oil	*Anacardium occidentale*		
El litre tree	*Lithraea caustica*	Chile	
Ginkgo tree	*Ginkgo biloba*	Southeastern United States, China, Japan, Europe	Oriental lacquerware, stepping in seeds
Indian marking nut dhobi (laundryman) itch	*Semecarpus anacardium*	India, Malaya	Laundry marking ink
Lacquer tree	*Rhus vernicifera*	China, India, Japan	Wood boxes, bracelets, bar rails
Mango	*Mangifera indica*	Hawaii, California, Florida, India, Central America, Mediterranean	Direct—plant to skin
		Florida, India, Central America, Mediterranean	skin
Pepeo tree	*Mauria puberula*	Venezuela	Direct—plant to skin Direct—plant to skin
Rengas tree Black varnish tree	*Anacardium melanorrhoea* melanorrhoea	Malaya	Furniture, wood carvings

Table 22.2 has a list of plants that contain urushiols, which are related to the poison ivy group. Tests for the pyrocatechols in these anacardiaceous plants are presented in Table 22.3.

Goldstein (3) pointed out that rengas trees, which grow primarily in Malayan jungles, furnish lumber resembling mahogany that is used for furniture. Unlike mahogany, however, rengas sap cross-reacts with other urushiol plants and trees. If rengas wood furniture is varnished before it is dried thoroughly, the sap may come through the varnish and cause reactions in those using it.

Indian sandal strap dermatitis may be due to the urushiol-containing sumac used to tan leather in certain Indian villages.

A contact dermatitis can be caused by the oleoresin of the mango tree sap or the skin of the fruit. Ingestion of the fruit may produce anaphylactic reactions.

Japanese Lacquer Tree

Dermatitis from the Japanese lacquer tree is known to be due to urushiol. The lacquer resin of *Melanorrhoea usitata* is used for the same purposes in Thailand. The allergen is closely related to urushiol and is known as thitsiol. In Vietnam, the lacquer contains laccol (4).

TABLE 22.3. *Tests for Pyrocatechols*

Green to black with ferric chloride
Green to brown with alcohol and caustic soda
White with lead acetate

Japanese Wax Trees

In Japan, Australia, and New Zealand, *Rhus succedanea* and *R. vernicifua* are sources of poison ivy. Known collectively as Japanese wax trees, the fat from the berries is used for candles and the resin for lacquer. These ornamental sumacs are valued for their bright red-orange leaves in fall (5).

In South America, the *Lithraea* genus causes allergic contact dermatitis. *Lithraea molleoides, caustica,* and *brasiliensis* are commonly referred to as Aroeira or Aruera, followed by the suffix *brava,* which means "harmful" or "hazardous." These are trees *(L. molleoides)* or shrubs *(L. brasiliensis).* They are members of the Anacardiaceae family and do cross-react with *Toxicodendron.* In a study of 17 *Lithraea*-sensitive patients, all reacted to urushiol. This is not surprising, given that the allergens identified in *Lithraea* include 3-pentadecylcatechol, 3-pentadecenylcatechol, 3-heptadecenylcatechol, and 3-hepta-dec-dienilcatechol (6).

Dermatitis-Producing Factors of the Toxicodendron Plants

The leaves, stems, seeds, flowers, berries, and roots of certain plants contain a milky sap that turns into a black substance resembling varnish on exposure to air. Alcohol and other solvents can be used to extract a crude yellow-brown viscous substance from the sap. The residue remaining after evaporation of the solvents is the antigenic oleoresin. The term "urushiol" is often used for the oleoresins of the

Anacardiaceae plants, including the *Toxicodendron* group. Urushiol is antigenic even after the plant has died.

The dermatitis-producing principle of the oleoresin is related to the presence of pentadecylcatechols (PDCs), which are 1,2-dihydroxy benzenes (catechols) with a 15-atom side chain in the third position. Some investigators, however, suggest that individuals may be sensitive to another component of the oleoresin. Some people with allergic hypersensitivity to PDCs show cross-reactivity to other phenolic compounds, such as resorcinol, hexylresorcinol, and the hydroquinones, but not to phenol.

A 1:10 dilution of the oleoresin in acetone usually equals a 1:1,000 dilution of PDCs in antigenicity. The oleoresin contains unstable, unsaturated compounds, however, which are probably more potent sensitizers than the stable, saturated PDCs.

> **The oleoresin (urushiol) of the sap of the *Toxicodendron* plants contains catechols, which are the sensitizing chemicals.**

Aside from phenolic substances, the oleoresins contain variable mixtures of polymers of unknown chemical composition.

NATURE OF TOXICODENDRON DERMATITIS

The eruption produced by poison ivy is an allergic eczematous contact dermatitis usually characterized by redness, papules, vesicles, and bullae, plus linear streaking. Occasionally, urticaria and eruptions, resembling erythema multiforme, measles, or scarlatina, occur from systemic absorption of the poison ivy antigen.

The dermatitis is produced by exposure to some portion of the bruised plant, allowing the oleoresin to contact the skin. The uninjured plant is innocuous. Pure smoke from burning the poison ivy plant is also harmless provided the particulate matter does not contain the oleoresin. Involvement of the mucous membranes, with stomatitis or proctitis, due to chewing of the leaves or overdosage in oral hyposensitization, is not rare.

The fluid content of vesicles and bullae present in poison ivy dermatitis is not antigenic. Patch tests performed with it give negative reactions.

One can acquire poison ivy dermatitis from oleoresin-contaminated animals, clothing, tools, golf clubs, fishing rods, and baseball bats. Fomites contaminated with the oleoresin in a dry atmosphere may remain antigenic for a long time, whereas a warm, moist climate favors loss of potency. The urushiol of the Japanese lacquer tree *(Toxicodendron verniciflua)* polymerizes to a nonallergenic state over 10 to 20 or more years, but heating accelerates this. The reaction seen from urushiol stored at 20°C for 10 years is equal to that seen with urushiol stored at 110°C for 1 week or 150°C

for 11 hours (7). Washing with soap or detergents renders oleoresin-contaminated clothing and objects harmless. The *Toxicodendron* oleoresin may remain under a person's fingernails unless removed deliberately by thorough cleansing. If not removed, for several days after contact with the plants, the antigen may be spread from the fingers to the covered parts of the body and even to other individuals.

> **Soap and water and organic solvents render *Toxicodendron* oleoresin harmless.**

After first exposure to the oleoresin, sensitization and dermatitis occur after 7 to 10 days. After a previously sensitized person contacts the oleoresin, the eruption appears usually within 2 days, and delay of onset rarely exceeds 10 days. In a few cases, the skin reaction may occur within 8 hours of exposure. Such temporal differences are due probably to the degree of exposure, individual susceptibility, and regional variation in cutaneous reactivity. In some recent experimental work with urushiol antigen, it was observed that most subjects react between day 4 and 5 after exposure to a moderate antigen dose (RLR, personal observation).

Toxicodendron dermatitis begins usually with itching and redness. Streaks of erythema or papules in linear arrangement soon appear. Complications include eosinophilia, kidney damage, urticaria, dyshidrosis, and marked pigmentation or leukoderma. Impetigo and pyoderma are frequent complications.

In the differential diagnosis, it must be remembered that arthropod bites, particularly those due to bedbugs, often cause a linear eruption. In addition, phytophotodermatitis (dermatitis bullosa striata pratensis) due to the psoralen of plants may produce lesions consisting of bullae that are striate or irregularly linear on exposed portions of the body. The lesions develop 12 to 24 hours after plants, such as celery, parsley, gas plants, limes, and figs, have been crushed on the skin and after subsequent exposure to sunlight. The bullae heal, leaving pigmentation that may persist for many months.

Toxicodendron plants are not photosensitizers, and the dermatitis is distinguished by occurring on both covered and uncovered parts of the body and by not requiring sunlight for its development.

> **The linear configuration of poison ivy dermatitis must be differentiated from striate plant photodermatitis.**

Patch Testing for Poison Ivy Sensitivity

The plant oleoresin diluted 1:10 in acetone may be used for patch testing. The pure synthetic antigen, 3-pentadecylcatechol, a stable crystalline material, may also be used in various dilutions, but it is not readily available. There is also some question as to whether it contains all the antigenic materials of the poison ivy oleoresin.

Patch testing reveals that about 50% of the population of the United States has been sensitized to poison ivy. A strong possibility exists that 5% to 10% of nonsensitized individuals may become sensitized by being patch tested with either the synthetic antigen or the natural oleoresin.

The diagnosis of poison ivy dermatitis is usually fairly obvious, and there is not much point in proving the diagnosis by such a procedure. Patch testing with the oleoresin or pentadecylcatechol should be restricted to investigative procedures or to proving hyposensitization by prophylactic treatment.

> **Patch testing with *Toxicodendron* oleoresin should not be done routinely: This is an investigative procedure.**

The only objective proof of successful hyposensitization procedures is a negative or weakly positive patch test reaction to poison ivy in individuals who had previously shown a strongly positive reaction to the oleoresin. The oleoresins may give intense vesicular and even bullous reactions in sensitized individuals.

Urushiol is insoluble in water, as is its component, PDC. This limits some of the *in vitro* investigations that can be carried out. A water-soluble allergen, tetrahydrourushiol glycoside (THUG), gives concordant reactions with urushiol and PDC. Similar intensity of patch test responses was observed with 0.002% urushiol in petrolatum as compared with 0.1% PDC in petrolatum and 0.1% THUG in water (8).

General Prophylaxis of *Toxicodendron* Dermatitis

The best prophylaxis for any type of allergic contact dermatitis is complete avoidance of the allergen. Patients should be taught to recognize and avoid the *Toxicodendron* group. They should carefully observe and search surrounding terrain before choosing a picnic or camping site. When a poison plant is present in the garden or cannot be avoided, its chemical destruction or physical removal is indicated. Farmer's Bulletin No. 2158, *Chemical Control of Brush and Trees* (9), issued by the U.S. Department of Agriculture, should be consulted for information on specific chemicals for destroying poison ivy or poison oak.

> **The best prophylaxis for *Toxicodendron* dermatitis is the avoidance and destruction of the *Toxicodendron* plants; topical prophylaxis is less predictable.**

All individuals exposed to these plants should thoroughly wash the entire body with soap and water. One need not use strong soaps for this purpose. Complete change of clothing is also advisable, and, whenever possible, contaminated clothing should be washed with soap and water.

The poison ivy antigen enters the skin so rapidly that the oil must be totally removed within 10 minutes of exposure. When such early washing is not feasible, however, it is worthwhile for the individual to wash at the first opportunity to remove any oleoresin remaining on the skin and thereby prevent its being transferred to other parts of the body.

Topical prophylaxis of poison ivy/oak has been demonstrated with topical linoleic acid dimer (10).

In a double-blind evaluation of seven different barrier creams, three were deemed significantly more effective in protecting against experimental toxododendron dermatitis. Stokogard, Hollister Moisture Barrier, and Hydropel were helpful, and Stokogard proved most effective, but no product was completely effective (11).

Experimentally induced poison ivy dermatitis was effectively prevented by application of a 5% quaternium-18 bentonite lotion. About 70% of the 144 urushiol-sensitive subjects had total or near total protection (12). The product is sold under the brand name Ivy Block, and the active agent has been renamed bentoquantum.

POISON IVY

Some Unusual Features of the *Toxicodendron* Group

"Leaves three, leave them be!" is the common warning. However, as Gillis (13) stated, "Although typical poison ivy and poison oak normally have but three leaflets, occasionally additional leaflets are formed. Added leaflets are common especially in western poison oak, in which nearly every clone studied can be found to have some leaves with *five or more* leaflets. I have seen one population that consistently produced additional leaflets, ranging even up to seventeen!"

> **Although poison ivy and poison oak usually have three leaves, additional leaves are not uncommon in western poison oak.**

Lack of Protection by Rubber Gloves

The catechols in urushiol are soluble in rubber. Therefore, rubber gloves do not protect the hands from poison ivy. Use heavy-duty vinyl gloves instead.

Black Lacquer Deposits Due to Self-Blackening of Toxicodendron Sap

Guin (14) demonstrated that a black enamel–like deposit is seen frequently on injured areas of *Toxicodendron* plants.

The black deposit can be produced by crushing leaves from the plant onto a sheet of white paper and exposing the paper to the air for a few minutes. When the oleoresin is released by injury to the plant, it darkens and hardens to form a black "lacquer." Mallory et al. (15) reported four patients with clinical *Toxicodendron* dermatitis that presented with dramatic black lacquer–like deposits on several lesions. This black deposit was also observed at sites of injury on poison ivy plants and was reproduced on volunteers by the application of plant sap on the skin. Histologically, the observed material was identified in the stratum corneum.

The Role of Age, Sex, Color of Skin, and Species

Poison ivy does not spare age, sex, color of skin, or race. Poison ivy dermatitis can occur at any age, although infants are apparently not as easily sensitized as adults. After the age of 3, children become highly susceptible, and by 12 years of age nearly all have become sensitized to poison ivy (16).

Of all animals, only humans and a few of the higher primates are sensitive to poison ivy. Even rhesus monkeys may be sensitized only with difficulty, and they lose their sensitivity relatively rapidly. A few instances are on record of deliberately sensitizing dogs once the poison was applied directly to the skin with the hair removed.

> *Toxicodendron* dermatitis affects only humans and some higher primates. Other species do not acquire poison ivy dermatitis.

Urushiol

The oleoresin component of poison ivy contains the pentadecylcatechols that produce dermatitis. These catechols are soluble in rubber and in oil and fat solvents.

Urushiol retains its antigenic potential in the dry state indefinitely. Thus, several 100-year-old herbarium specimens containing urushiol have been known to produce dermatitis in a sensitized individual who has handled them (17).

The reaction of urushiol with the sensitized skin is almost immediate, a complex protein being formed almost at once.

> Urushiol remains antigenic indefinitely in the dry state unless washed off a few minutes after exposure dermatitis occurs in highly sensitive individuals.

It is known that the sap from *Toxicodendron* plants turns black when touched to surfaces other than skin. The juice from the vine made a satisfactory indelible ink, and some Native American tribes even made a black dye from the vines. This use is similar to that of the Japanese lacquer tree, whose sap, when exposed to the air, forms a black varnish. *Semecarpus anacardium,* the usual cause of dhobi mark dermatitis, is used to make laundry marks in India because of similar properties. Contact urticaria from a dhobi mark has been reported (18).

Fisher (19) pointed out that urushiol binds with sensitized skin, forming a catechol-protein complex that is not removed by thorough washing. The black deposits could not be removed with soap and water in volunteers after 4 hours, although no attempt was made to remove the deposit with an organic solvent. The oleoresin-protein complex or the oleoresin itself probably accounts for the yellowish, amorphous material observed in the stratum corneum of biopsies.

> The sap of the poison ivy plant family turns to a black varnish when exposed to dry surfaces and skin.

No amount of washing will remove the already reacted complex of catechol protein. After the dermatitis appears, washing will have no effect. Washing may remove excess ununited urushiol from dry areas of the skin.

Urushiol is nonvolatile and dries quickly on clothing, shoes, and tools, retaining its potency for months or even years on such fomites. Cleaning fluid solvents can effectively remove urushiol from fomites, and for contaminated clothing ordinary laundering is usually effective in removing urushiol.

Epstein et al. (20) reported that 21 adults, highly sensitive to urushiol, ingested up to 300 mg of urushiol over 3 to 6 months. A control group received placebo capsules. The study was done double blind to evaluate changes in patch test reactivity to urushiol, altered reactivity to an unrelated contact sensitizer, side effects, and duration of hyposensitization. A significant number of subjects in the experimental group (15 of 21) became hyposensitized. Such hyposensitization was not seen in the control group (2 of 12), and the difference between groups was significant. No change in reactivity to an unrelated contact sensitizer occurred in subjects hyposensitized to urushiol, suggesting antigen specificity. Retesting up to 3 months after completion of the protocol indicated that subjects remained hyposensitized without a "rebound" effect during that time. Side effects, detected by a questionnaire, were limited to vesicular and urticarial rashes and pruritus ani in 18 of 21 test subjects.

Geography

Poison ivy is most abundant along the sandbars off the coast of New Jersey, New York, through the Carolinas, and along the rocky coast of New England (14). Poison ivy can grow to a rather large size. At least one poison ivy tree is on record from Sanibel Island, Florida, that stands 15 to 20 feet high. Poison ivy vine can grow as high as 30 feet on a telephone pole.

Poison ivy is native to North and South America and eastern Asia. In the lower Mississippi River basin, a form of poison ivy exists that is confined virtually to the cotton-growing areas of rich soils in places such as the Delta region of Arkansas, Louisiana, and Mississippi (21).

In the Edwards Plateau region of Texas and continuing north to the Arbuckle Mountains of Oklahoma, another subspecies of poison ivy is found with sharply pointed lobes on the leaflets. A species of poison ivy, which is common in Mexico in the Sierra Madre Occidental, extends northward into the southeastern corner of Arizona, and to the southern tip of Baja, California (22). Reports of poison ivy dermatitis in Europe and Australia involve introduced plants.

Complications

On rare occasions, patients with poison ivy dermatitis may develop immune complex disease with accumulations of IgG in the kidney and skin associated with the appearance of skin sensitive antibodies to urushiol in serum with resulting nephrosis (23).

Nephrosis is a rare complication of severe poison ivy dermatitis.

Hyperpigmentation is a common complication of poison ivy dermatitis in black skin, but is rare in white skin. Urticaria or erythema multiforme or scarlatiniform eruptions may occur occasionally from systemic absorption of poison ivy antigen.

Oral or injected administration of poison extract can produce an allergic systemic contact dermatitis with a flare of poison ivy dermatitis at previously affected sites.

Differential Diagnosis

Three dermatoses resembling each other clinically and characterized by linear or striate papules and vesicles, and sometimes urticaria, include poison ivy dermatitis, phytophotodermatitis, and Portuguese man-of-war envenomization. Allergic contact dermatitis from scorpion weed, *Phacelia,* in the southwestern United States closely resembles poison ivy/oak dermatitis.

Immunity and Desensitization

The U.S. Food and Drug Administration (FDA) has not approved as yet any desensitizing procedure (24).

At present, there is no FDA-approved desensitization procedure for *Toxicodendron* dermatitis.

Natural Desensitization or Hardening

Immunologists cannot explain why repeated skin exposure to poison oak and poison ivy allergens often reduces patch test reactivity. The phenomenon of "hardening," which occurs presumably with certain industrial chemicals, has been reported in certain settings. Japanese lacquer craftspeople who are new to the job are exposed to 60% to 65% urishiol in raw lacquer. After 1 month on the job, five of eight such individuals became sensitized with patch test verification (25). After 9 to 10 months, seven of eight showed decreased sensitivity, and the one who did not "harden" was suspected to have had antecedent sensitization (25). Another study of the Japanese lacquer industry by questionnaire revealed that 81% of 232 craftspeople developed dermatitis, but only 1.3% did not decrease reactivity, and those with more than 2 hours per day exposure "hardened" better than those with less exposure (26). This usually occurred within 1 month. These observations are similar to those found in the cashew nut shell oil industry, where 9 of 13 workers showed decreased or no reactivity to poison ivy/oak after several months of occupational exposure (27).

Repeated patch tests with urushiol give unpredictable results, sometimes reducing, sometimes heightening responses. Administration of live, attenuated measles virus vaccine to a small group of subjects resulted in a *temporary* reduction of sensitivity to poison ivy most marked between the third and sixth weeks after immunization (28).

Some persons appear to be relatively immune to poison ivy. Probably few persons are potentially totally immune, but rather have a high threshold for sensitization or have never been sensitized.

The "Spread" of Poison Ivy

Poison ivy may be spread in the smoke of burning poison ivy because of tiny droplets of the urushiol present on the particles of dust and ash in the smoke. Smoke that does not contain urushiol is not antigenic. Such "airborne" urushiol, however, may produce severe involvement of the eyelids and conjunctivitis. It must be emphasized that urushiol is not volatile even at the usual temperature of bonfires and therefore cannot be spread from burning poison ivy as a gas.

Urushiol is not volatile and cannot be spread from burning poison ivy as a gas but can be spread if the smoke contains droplets of urushiol in the dust and ash in the smoke.

The "Exotic" Members of the Anacardiaceae Family

Poison ivy closely related to the East Coast variety is found in China and Japan. The lacquer from the lacquer trees of

China and Japan consists of a dried urushiol, and even when dried, the lacquer can still produce dermatitis.

The nuts of the cashew tree contain cardol oil, a urushiol whose sensitizing property is destroyed by roasting. Brake linings, electrical insulations, resins, mucilages, and printer's ink are made from cashew nut shell oil. Swizzle sticks (drink stirrers) and voodoo dolls made from cashew nuts may cause urushiol dermatitis.

The ginkgo fruit pulp contains catechols that may produce cheilitis, stomatitis, proctitis, and pruritus ani when ingested by sensitized individuals (29). The seeds of the ginkgo tree fruit are free of catechols (30).

The catechols of the mango are restricted to the stem or pedicle and the exocarp ("skin") of the fruit (31). Black deposits on the edible mango can also result from contamination by sap from the stem.

Poison Ivy and Brazilian Pepper ("Florida Holly")

Morton (32) reports that the Brazilian pepper tree (*Schinus terebinthifolius,* of the family Anacardiaceae) is closely related to poison ivy and is native to Brazil. It has been commonly cultivated in Florida for more than 50 years as an ornamental, and use of its sprays of showy red fruits for Christmas decoration gave rise to the popular misnomer "Florida holly." Too late, it was found to become a large, spreading tree; aggressive seedlings began springing up near and far. Jungles of *Schinus* have crowded out native vegetation over vast areas of Florida and the Bahamas, as in all the islands of Hawaii.

When in bloom, the tree is a major source of respiratory difficulty and dermatitis. The abundant nectar yields a spicy, commercial honey, and beekeepers are opposed to eradication programs. This plant has produced many cases of severe dermatitis in Florida.

"Florida holly" (Brazilian pepper tree) is a member of the poison plant family.

Hurtado et al. (33) found that the oleoresin of *Mauria puberula,* a poisonous species of the Anacardiaceae that is indigenous to the Venezuelan Andes, can cause both primary irritant dermatitis and allergic contact dermatitis in guinea pigs and humans. Cross-sensitization reactions were found in persons with known allergy to *Toxicodendron* spp. or *Lithraea caustica* and in guinea pigs sensitized to 3-n-pentadecylcatechol. These results suggest that the active principles of *Mauria* are chemically related to, but not identical to, those of *Toxicodendron.*

Eradication of Poison Ivy

The following is reprinted from *Poison Ivy, Poison Oak and Poison Sumac* by Donald M. Crooks and Dayton L. Kling-man, Farmer's Bulletin No. 1972, published by the U.S. Department of Agriculture, U.S. Government Printing Office, Washington, D.C., 1976 (22).

Control by Mechanical Means

Poison ivy and poison oak can be grubbed out by hand quite readily early in spring and late in fall, only if a few plants are involved. Roots are most easily removed when soil is thoroughly wet. Grubbing when soil is dry and hard is almost futile because the roots break off in the ground, leaving large pieces that later sprout vigorously. Grubbing is effective if well done.

Poison-ivy vines climbing on trees should be severed at the base, and as much of the vine as possible should be pulled away from the tree. Often the roots of the tree and weed are so intertwined that grubbing is impossible without injury to the tree. Bury or destroy roots and stems removed in grubbing, because the dry material is almost as poisonous as the fresh.

Smoke from burning poison-ivy plants or contaminated articles may carry the poison in a dispersed form. Take extreme caution to avoid inhalation or contact of smoke with the skin or clothing. (Pure smoke from burning poison ivy plants, since it does not contain any particles of the plant, will not cause any dermatitis.)

Old plants of poison ivy produce an abundance of seeds, and these are freely disseminated, especially by birds. A poison-ivy seedling 2 months old usually has a root that one mowing will not kill. Seedling plants at the end of the first year have well-established underground runners that only grubbing or herbicides will kill. Seedlings are a threat as long as old poison ivy is in the neighborhood.

Plowing is of little value in combating poison ivy and poison oak. Mowing with a scythe or a sickle is not an efficient means of controlling poison ivy and poison oak. It has little effect on the roots unless frequently repeated. Weed burners are also inefficient in controlling poison ivy and poison oak.

Control by Herbicides

Poison ivy and poison oak can be destroyed with herbicides without endangering the operator. One usually may stand at a distance from the plants and apply the herbicide without touching them. Most herbicides are applied as a spray solution by sprayers equipped with nozzles on extensions 2 feet or more in length. The greatest danger of poisoning occurs in careless handling of gloves, shoes, and clothing after work is finished.

The most satisfactory herbicides for control of poison ivy, poison oak, and poison sumac are: 1) amitrole (3-amino-s-triazole); 2) silvex [2-(2,4,5-trichlorophenoxyl) propionic acid]; 3) ammonium sulfamate; and 4) 2,4-D [2, 4(dichlorophenoxy) acetic acid]. These herbicides are sold under their common names and under various trade names.

Any field or garden sprayer, or even a sprinkling can, can be used for applying the spray liquid, but a common compressed-air sprayer holding 2 to 3 gallons is convenient and does not waste the spray.

Use moderate pressure giving relatively large spray droplets, rather than high pressure giving a driving mist, because the object is to wet the leaves of the poison ivy and poison oak and avoid wetting the leaves of desirable plants. High pressures cause formation of many fine droplets that may drift to desirable plants.

Follow the manufacturer's recommendations shown on the container label in preparing the spray solution. Cover all foliage, stems, shoots, and bark of poison plants with herbicide spray. Although best results normally are obtained soon after maximum foliage development in the spring, applications may be made up to 3 weeks before fall frost is normally expected under good growing conditions in humid areas.

Many herbicides used on poison ivy and poison oak will injure most broad-leaved plants. Apply them with caution if the surrounding vegetation is valuable. During the early part of the growing season, the leaves of poisonous plants usually tend to stand conspicuously apart from those of adjacent plants, and they can be treated separately if sprayed with care. Later in the season, the leaves become intermingled, and injury to adjacent species is unavoidable. Chemicals other than oil are not injurious to the thick bark of an old tree, and poison ivy clinging to the trunk safely can be sprayed with them. Cutting the vine at the base of the tree and spraying regrowth, however, may be more practical.

Apply sprays when there is little or no air movement. Early morning or late afternoon, when the air is cool and moist, is usually a favorable time. No method of herbicidal eradication can be depended on to kill all plants in a stand of poison ivy and poison oak with one application. Retreatments made as soon as the new leaves are fully expanded are almost always necessary to destroy plants missed the first time, to treat new growth, and to destroy seedlings. Plants believed dead sometimes revive after many months. An area under treatment must be watched closely for at least a year and retreated where necessary.

Dead foliage and stems remaining after the plants have been killed with herbicides are slightly poisonous. Cut off dead stems and bury or burn them, taking care to keep out of the smoke. (The smoke may carry droplets of the catechols that also may cause the dermatitis.)

Precautions

1. Herbicides used improperly may cause injury to [humans] and animals. Use them only when needed and handle them with care. Follow the directions and heed all precautions on the labels.
2. Keep herbicides in closed, well-labeled containers in a dry place. Store them where they will not contaminate food or feed, and where children and animals cannot reach them.

3. When handling a herbicide, wear clean, dry clothing.
4. Avoid repeated or prolonged contact of herbicides with your skin.
5. Wear protective clothing and equipment if specified on the container label. Avoid prolonged inhalation of herbicide mists.
6. Avoid spilling herbicide concentrate on your skin, and keep it out of your eyes, nose, and mouth. If you spill any on your skin, wash it off immediately with soap and water. If you spill it on your clothing, remove clothing immediately and wash contaminated skin. Launder the clothing before wearing it again.
7. After handling a herbicide, do not eat, drink, or smoke until you have washed your hands and face. Wash any exposed skin immediately after applying a herbicide.
8. Avoid drift of herbicide to nearby crops.
9. To protect water resources, fish, and wildlife, do not contaminate lakes, streams, or ponds with herbicide. Do not clean spraying equipment or dump excess spray material near such water.
10. It is difficult to remove all traces of herbicides from equipment. For this reason, do not use the same equipment for applying herbicides that you use for insecticides and fungicides.
11. Dispose of empty herbicide containers at a sanitary land-fill dump, or crush and bury them at least 18 inches deep in a level, isolated place where they will not contaminate water supplies. If you have a trash-collection service, wrap small containers in heavy layers of newspapers and place them in the trash can.

PLANTS AND SPICES

Most of the dermatitis-producing plants belong to a limited number of families, and many of the plant sensitizers that have been isolated also appear to belong to closely related chemicals, such as catechols and lactones.

Many cases of plant dermatitis are occupational. The *Toxicodendron* group (poison ivy, oak, and sumac) produces many instances of both occupational and nonoccupational dermatitis. In Europe, *Primula obconica* (primrose) is the principal cause of nonoccupational plant dermatitis.

> **In the United States, the poison ivy group produces most cases of both occupational and nonoccupational plant dermatitis, whereas in Europe, *Primula obconica* is the principal cause of plant dermatitis.**

Sex Distribution of Plant Dermatitis

Even among city dwellers, ragweed dermatitis occurs almost exclusively in men. Primula dermatitis occurs principally in women. *Toxicodendron* reactions occur equally in both sexes and at all ages.

Plant Sensitizers

The most recent development in the study of plant dermatitis has been the isolation of specific chemicals that are the sensitizers. It is hoped that these chemicals will become useful in hyposensitizing procedures.

Sesquiterpene Lactones

Mitchell et al. (34,35) showed that such lactones are the allergens responsible for allergic contact dermatitis caused by ragweed *(Ambrosia)*, sneezeweed *(Helenium)*, sagebrush, wormwood and mugwort *(Artemisia)*, boneset *(Eupatorium)*, poverty weed *(Franseria)*, marsh elder *(Iva)*, cocklebur *(Xanthium)*, burdock *(Arctium)*, chamomile *(Anthemis)*, artichoke *(Cynara)*, gaillardia, and chrysanthemum species (tansy, feverfew, and pyrethrum).

The presence of an alpha-methylene group exocyclic to the gamma-lactone appears to be the immunochemical requisite for such dermatitis. For patch test purposes, Mitchell and Dupuis (34) used alantolactone 0.25% in petrolatum.

A major allergen in airborne and occupational contact dermatitis from Compositae is parthenolide, which is the main sesquiterpene lactone in feverfew and tansy, according to Hausen (36). Parthenolide is water soluble. In fact, one-third of the allergen extractable with chloroform can actually be removed with water alone. Parthenolide may make up 0.3% to 1% of tansy and feverfew, respectively, and is found in 12 other Compositae and Magnoliaceae species (36).

Compositae dermatitis presents a pattern on exposed surface mimicking either a photodermatitis or windblown distribution, but when carefully studied, hand eczema was more common than these more widespread patterns (37).

Because more than 1,350 sesquiterpene lactones have been identified so far, no ideal substance has been found for fool-proof patch testing. A 1% costus oil in petrolatum test was used in a study of 740 patients, and 1.5% of patients (13) were found sensitive (37). Nine of the 11 patients had hand eczema. Mixtures of sesquiterpene lactones have been evaluated in an attempt to provide an improved screening tool. About 1.5% of patients undergoing diagnostic patch testing were found to be positive to a 0.1% petrolatum mix of equimolar amounts of alantolactone, costunolide, and dihydrocostus lactone (38). Of the positive reactions, 41% were deemed relevant to the dermatitis evaluation.

A similar study found a Compositae mix to give reactions in 124 of 3,489 patients. About half were sensitive to yarrow, and none were photoaggravated (39). The airborne nature of the clinical presentation was believed to be caused by an increase in allergen concentration as the plants withered.

Lovell and Rowan (40) concluded that shortcomings of any mix attempting to cover so many possible allergens can be anticipated. The commercial sesquiterpene lactone mix failed to detect five of seven patients sensitive to *Tarax-*

acum officinale, a dandelion in the chrysanthemum family. A 3:1 chloroform/methanol extract in petrolatum at 1% concentration was positive from the leaf, flower, and root (40). The possibility of cross-reactions further confuses some of the investigations of plant contact dermatitis. A cross-reaction occurs between marigolds *(Tagetes)* and the Compositae plant *Arnica* and other sesquiterpene-lactone-containing species, even though the genus *Tagetes* is not known to produce sesquiterpene lactone, but rather thiopene compounds (41).

When patients report summer-exacerbated dermatitis, suspect (a) sensitivity to flowers or plants, (b) sensitivity to pollen (especially in atopic individuals or, (c) photosensitivity, but keep in mind that half of patients sensitive to Compositae plant extracts are not photosensitive (42).

> **Sesquiterpene lactones appear to be the specific sensitizers in chrysanthemum, pyrethrum, ragweed, and other weeds.**

Similar lactones have been implicated as the sensitizers in *Frullania,* a genus of liverworts. Like ragweed dermatitis, many cases of Frullania dermatitis occur in males. Mitchell (43) also reported that dermatitis may be due to usnic acid, which is derived from lichens. Such dermatitis occurred only during work in forest areas and was worse during wet weather. These cases may represent multiple sensitization to usnic acid, lichen chemicals, and lactones.

Calnan (44) reported two patients who developed allergic contact dermatitis from incense cedar wood *(Libocedrus decurrens)* used in pencils. The allergen was thymoquinone. Calnan stated that there are at least eight different cedar woods belonging to several species, and that the terms "cedar wood dermatitis" and "cedar poisoning" are inaccurate.

Various other plants, including trees, grasses, flowers, vegetables, fruits, and weeds, as well as airborne pollens, can produce contact dermatitis. The term "phytodermatitis" is usually applied in such cases.

Most cases of plant dermatitis are the result of allergic hypersensitivity, which is dependent on immunologic changes induced by previous contact with the same plant or with a closely related species (45). Certain plants are such potent sensitizers that brief contact is sufficient to produce sensitization in a considerable proportion of those exposed. This is true for poison ivy. Sensitivity may develop within 7 to 10 days of first contact or only after many years of exposure. No plant can be dismissed as a cause of dermatitis solely because the patient has handled it for a long time with impunity (46).

Other plants that are fairly common sensitizers include the following:

Family Compositae. The members of this family that are sensitizers include chrysanthemums and daisies.

Family Ambrosia. These include both giant and dwarf ragweed.

Family Liliaceae. This group consists of the tulip, hyacinth, and asparagus (47).

Family Alleaceae. Garlic and onion.

Family Amaryllidaceae. Includes the daffodil and narcissus.

Family Umbelliferae. Carrots, celery, and wild parsnips are members of this group.

Family Cannabidaceae. Includes hops.

Family Rutaceae. The sensitizers in this family include the orange, lemon, and grapefruit. *Dictamnus albus* (the gas plant fraxinella, burning bush, or dittany) is a photosensitizer.

PLANT SENSITIZERS

The sensitizing substances of many plants are present mainly in the oleoresin fraction. In a few plants, the allergens are water-soluble glucosides or other aqueous fractions (48).

Oleoresin Fraction

This fraction consists of a mixture of substances, including essential oils, terpenes, resins, phenols, and camphors. The potency and amount of oleoresin increase as the growth of the plant becomes more vigorous. The oleoresin may be present throughout the plant and in the pollen. When the pollen is freely airborne, contact dermatitis occurs without touching the plant. In ragweed dermatitis, the contact is usually from such pollen and from small light fragments of dry dead plant material and detached plant hairs that are blown about as a dust.

Essential Oil Fraction

This fraction of oleoresin contains most of the sensitizing substances identified until now. Essential oils ordinarily occur in localized regions of the plant, for example, predominantly in the flowers (lavender), leaves (eucalyptus), bark (cinnamon), wood (sandalwood), and peel (citrus fruits).

An essential oil is a volatile, nongreasy, nonsaponifying oil with a characteristic odor, which is obtained from plants or plant constituents by distillation. Accidental contact with the oleoresin essential oils may occur when the plant is crushed or bruised. More than five hundred compounds have been identified in essential oils. These compounds may be classified into five main groups:

1. phenols and aromatic alcohols and aldehydes
2. terpenes
3. aliphatic and aromatic esters
4. substituted benzene hydrocarbons (including the mustard oils)
5. quinones

> **The term "essential" refers to oils' use in perfume essences.**

Of special interest to the dermatologist are phenols, aromatic alcohols, aldehydes, and terpenes. The phenols include dihydric phenols, plus catechols, resorcinols, and hydroquinones. The catechols and related compounds are the sensitizing substances in the *Toxicodendron* (poison ivy) plants and other members of the Anacardiaceae family, which include the marking nut tree of India, the Japanese lacquer tree, the mango, and the cashew nut (49).

Substituted Catechols

These substances, including eugenol and vanillin, are occasionally sensitizers. Eugenol is used in dentistry and is present in cinnamon oil, oil of cloves, some perfumes and soaps, and bay rum. More complex substituted catechols are now appearing in industry. The *p*-tertiary butyl catechol, for example, is used in duplicating papers, in paint, in rubber manufacture, in the oil industry, and as an oxidation catalyst in the manufacture of polyester and polystyrene resins.

The chemical 2-methoxy-6-*n*-pentyl-*p*-benzoquinone is the major allergen of *Primula* (primrose) (50). Other plants and woods contain allergenic quinones that show cross-sensitivity to primin. This assumption is supported by the finding of a coincidence between positive reaction to *Primula obconica* leaf and Dalbergia wood.

Oranges

This fruit may be treated with ethylene gas and biphenyl, a mold retarder. In addition, the azo dye (Citrus Red No. 2) may be used for the peel of Florida oranges, but not those from California (JC Mitchell, personal communication). This azo dye is a rare sensitizer, which may be tested as 2% in acetone.

The outer layer of orange peel consists of numerous oil-containing cells from which an oil of limonene, other terpenes, linalool, and a resinous residue can be expressed. The natural coloring is mainly hesperidin and carotene. The terpene limonene is probably the principal sensitizer of orange peels.

Patch tests with the orange peel may lead to primary irritant reactions.

> **Florida oranges may be dyed with Citrus Red No. 2, an azo dye.**

Lemons

This fruit may produce dermatitis in sensitized individuals because of lemon oil, which contains terpenes (limonene)

(51). Allergic dermatitis may also occur in carpenters from contact with lemon wood and sawdust. In addition, an irritant dermatitis may occur in waiters and bakers from contact with citric acid, which also has been implicated in the production of aphthous ulcers.

Turpentine

Turpentine is extracted from species of pine. The irritant and sensitizing potentials vary from country to country. An individual who is sensitized may show cross-reaction with balsam of Peru, benzoin, ragweed oil, chrysanthemum, and pyrethrum. The most commonly used products containing turpentine include varnishes, sealing wax, paint thinners, and dry-cleaning materials. Freshly distilled turpentine is less antigenic than turpentine that has been stored and become oxidized. The principal sensitizer in turpentine is a carene; pinene and limonene (dipentene) may be less potent sensitizers (52).

The principal sensitizers in turpentine are the oxidized terpenes that are tested as turpentine peroxides 0.3% in olive oil; occasionally, alpha-pinene (test 15% in olive oil) or dipentene (test 10% in methyl ethyl ketone) may also be sensitizers.

Terpenes

These substances are sensitizing agents in dermatitis caused by citrus fruits, celery, and turpentine (Table 22.4). Terpenes or their derivatives are present in other plants, such as chrysanthemums, and plant products, such as resins and balsams.

In discussing the terpenes, D.S. Wilkinson (personal communication) stated that, in addition to carbohydrates, proteins, and glycerides, plants contain oily substances, which are insoluble in water. Many of these essential oils are terpene, but oils of wintergreen, aniseed, and mustard are not.

The true terpenes (e.g., limonene, pinene, and camphene) are hydrocarbons with the molecular formula $C_{10}H_{16}$; their alcohols, aldehydes, ketones, and other related compounds are equally important and widespread (e.g., menthol and camphor).

The function of terpenes in the life of the plant is not known; they may attract or repel insects or may be waste products of metabolism. Their precursors in nature are also unknown, although two possibilities are leucine and certain carbohydrates.

Camphene is solid, but the other true terpenes are liquids, boiling between 155°C and 185°C. They have strong, not unpleasant smells, and are volatile in steam.

TABLE 22.4. *Sources of Exposure to Turpentine*

Polishes: automobile, metal, porcelain and metal, shoe, stove, silver (dip type), wood and furniture
Preservatives: paintbrush, wood
Repellants: bird
Waxes: general purpose, paste
Fertilizers
Cosmetics: liquid soaps, soap powders, bath oils, emollient creams, hair tonics, hand tonics, hand lotions, lilac and lily of the valley perfumes, talcum powders, and suntan preparations
Cleaners: metal, general-purpose industrial soaps
Insecticides: products with pine oil, tree sprays, dairy stock sprays, and preparations for dog and cat fleas and lice, floral garden pests, grubs, mites, moths, thrips, ticks, flies, and aphids
Mange treatment
Deodorizers: cleanser type
Degreasers
Liquid starch
Paints: including anticorrosion paints
Solvents and thinners: for paints, dry cleaners, and waxes
Varnishes, shellacs, and lacquers
Stains and finishes
Terpineol: solvent for resins
Dutch Drops (Haarlem Oil): proprietary remedy for colds and fever
Any cleaning, cosmetic, or painting product having a pine odor
Shoe polish
Eyeglass frames
Substances that may cross-react with turpentine: ragweed, burwood marsh elder, chrysanthemum, and pyrethrum (found in disinfectants, insecticides, fungicides, soil conditioners, wood preservatives, repellents, dog and cat soaps)

Geraniol, $C_{10}H_{17}OH$, is a straight-chain terpene alcohol. It occurs in many Indian grasses and as a glucoside in Pelargonium odorantissimum.

Citral, $C_9H_{15}CHO$, is the aldehyde of lemon grass oil.

Citronellol, $C_{10}H_{19}OH$, is an alcohol in rose oil and geranium oil. It is also a glandular secretion of the alligator.

Linalool, $C_{10}H_{17}OH$, has many botanical sources (e.g., oil of linaloe).

Monocyclic terpenes. These compounds always have one ring in the molecular structure.

Myrcene, $C_{10}H_{16}$, is an open-chain hydrocarbon with three double bonds and is found in oil of bay and oil of hops.

(+) *Limonene* is found in lemon oil, oil of neroli, dill and bergamot, oil in orange peel, caraway oil, and celery seed oil.

(−) *Limonene* is found in spearmint and pine needles. Dipentene is a form of limonene.

Cineole occurs in wormseed oil, cajeput oil, eucalyptus oil, and rosemary.

Phellandrene occurs in elemi oil, ginger grass oil, oil of cinnamon, and bitter fennel oil.

(−) *Phellandrene* occurs in eucalyptus oils, pimento oils, Canada balsam oil, and Japanese peppermint oil.

(+) *Phellandrene* occurs in fennel oil, and lemon oil.

Carvone, $C_{10}H_{14}O$, is a constituent of dill and caraway oils.

(−) *Menthone,* $C_{10}H_{18}$, which occurs in oil of peppermint, is a liquid.

(−) *Menthol,* $C_{10}H_{19}OH$, occurs in peppermint oils and Japanese mint oil.

Dicyclic terpenes. These compounds, $C_{10}H_{16}$, always have one six-membered ring, a second closed chain, and one olefinic link.

Alpha-pinene is the principal constituent of oil of turpentine, which is obtained from members of the order Coniferae.

(+) *Camphor,* $C_{10}H_{16}O$, occurs in the camphor laurel and in feverfew oil.

Camphene occurs widely in nature, particularly the (−) form, which is found in the oil of *Abies sibirica.*

Borneol, $C_{10}H_{17}OH$, occurs in many oils, such as pine oil. Wilkinson (personal communication) states that the terpene-free diet shown in Table 22.5 may, on occasion, be useful for trial on patients who are allergic to flavors and perfumes.

RESINS AND BALSAMS

Resins and balsams are plant products that may be sensitizers. Balsams are similar to resins but are pathologic secretions after injury to the plant. Resins are acidic substances occurring either as amorphous vitreous solids or as solutions in essential oils. Some are phenolic derivatives, but others are polymerization and oxidation products of terpenes. The residue remaining after distillation of crude oil of turpentine is rosin or colophony, which consists mainly of abietic acid and pimaric acids. Some resins are plant exudations containing mixtures of true gums, oils, and resin.

Balsam of Peru

The term "balsam of Peru," a viscid fluid with an odor recalling cinnamon and vanilla, is a misnomer. Hjorth (53) in his fine monograph, *Eczematous Allergy to Balsams,* points out that the balsam comes almost exclusively from El Salvador. The balsam is not found preformed in the wood of the tree *(Myroxolon balsamum)* from which it is obtained, but it is produced by inflicting wounds on the tree's bark. The balsam then exudes out as a sort of granulation tissue to heal the bark's lesions and is used subsequently in many ways.

Hjorth (53) stated that approximately two-thirds of Peruvian balsam comprise the volatile oil cinnamein, which contains the following chemicals: cinnamic acid, cinnamic aldehyde, cinnamic alcohol, methyl cinnamate, benzyl cinnamate, vanillin, and eugenol.

TABLE 22.5. *Terpene-Free Diet*

No oils of:
Lemon, spearmint, rosemary, cinnamon, bitter fennel, pimento, peppermint, camphor, eucalyptus, orange, caraway, dill, and red palm—or any foods or condiments containing them (e.g., fruit drinks, boiled sweets, flavorings, or colorings)

No red or yellow fruits:
Including apples, apricots, bananas, blackberries, cherries, gooseberries, oranges, pears, peaches, plums, pineapples, prunes, raspberries, and strawberries

Fruits allowed:
Currants, damsons, figs, grapefruit, white grapes, white melon, raisins, sultanas, and nuts

No green, leafy vegetables:
Including asparagus, broccoli, cabbage, brussels sprouts, carrots, French beans, runner beans, cauliflower, endive, leeks, lettuce, mint, parsley, peas, spinach, and tomatoes

Vegetables allowed:
Artichokes, broad beans, butter beans, beetroot, celery, cucumber, horseradish, lentils, marrow, onions, parsnips, split dried peas, potatoes, shallots, rutabaga, and radishes

Foods to avoid:
Liver, kidneys, and heart
Fatty fish (e.g., herring, kippers, salmon, sardines, and oysters)
Dairy products, including milk, butter, margarine, cheese, egg yolks, and cream
Avoid any foods containing them (e.g., cakes, sweets, and puddings)

Foods allowed:
Skimmed milk
Egg white
Vegetable oils
Bacon, pork, beef, mutton, and poultry
White fish
All cereals, including wheat, rye, macaroni, rice, and semolina
Sugars, jams, honey, and syrups
Tea, coffee, rose hip syrup, and ribena
Beers, ciders, wines, and spirits

The remaining one-third consists of polymers of esters of coniferyl alcohol with benzoic acid and cinnamic acid that may prove to be the major allergens of balsam of Peru.

The following food items and other products may contain balsams (NK Veien, personal communication):

Products that contain the peel of citrus fruits (oranges, lemons, grapefruits, bitter oranges, tangerines, and mandarin oranges), e.g., marmalade, juice, and bakery goods.

Flavoring agents, such as those found in Danish pastries and other bakery goods, candy, and chewing gum

Perfumed products, such as perfumed tea and tobacco

Certain cough medicines and lozenges

Eugenol used by dentists

Suppositories containing balsam of Peru

Ice cream

Cola and other spiced soft drinks

Spices such as cinnamon, cloves, vanilla, and curry. These spices are used in such products as ketchup, chili sauce, chutney, spiced herring, pickled vegetables like beets and cucumbers, highly spiced bakery goods, liver paste, vermouth, and various other bitter, spiced drinks.

The following compounds often show cross-reactions with balsam of Peru: cinnamon, clove, orange peel, benzoin, rosin, vanilla, cinnamic aldehyde and alcohol, cinnamates, benzyl benzoate, benzyl salicylate and alcohol, eugenol, and various perfumes (53).

Chrism

Chrism is a consecrated oil used by certain churches in various rites, such as baptism. Such aromatic oil may contain or cross-react with balsam of Peru.

Many patients with allergic perfume sensitivity show strong patch test reactions to balsam of Peru.

> **Allergic reactions to balsam of Peru may signify perfume or flavor cross-reactivity.**

Many topical medications and sunscreens contain balsam of Peru (see Chapter 11).

Allergic Reaction to Certain Flavoring Agents

Cinnamon oil is used for flavoring foods, cakes, toothpaste, chewing gum, tobacco, vermouth, aperitifs, bitters, and beverages of the cola type. Cassia is a Chinese cinnamon. The ingestion of cinnamon oil may produce an eczematous contact–type flare-up in individuals previously sensitized by contact with the oil. Fisher (54) observed a balsam of Peru–sensitive patient, sensitized to a cinnamon in a toothpaste, whose dermatitis flared after drinking vermouth containing cinnamon.

Hjorth (55) reported two children who were sensitive to balsam of Peru and orange peel and whose eczema flared after eating fruits and ices. Hjorth also described a man with a severe hand eczema who was allergic to balsam of Peru and whose eczema flared when he ate a jar of orange marmalade. The patient then avoided perfumes, cola drinks, vermouth, throat tablets, and cinnamon, and his hand eczema cleared up.

Pirila (56) reported that eating vanilla sugar caused a flare of eczema in a patient sensitive to balsam of Peru. Thus, dermatitis due to sensitization to balsam of Peru may flare with ingestion of cinnamon, oranges, and other flavors. A low-balsam diet has produced long-term benefit in 47% of patients, but a positive provocation has not proved to be predictive of those who will derive benefit (57).

> **Sensitization to balsam of Peru may produce dermatitis in dentists, bakers, food handlers, beekeepers, and laboratory technicians; exposure may occur from chrism oil in baptismal rites.**

Resorcinol Monobenzoate, Steering Wheels, and Balsam of Peru

Jordan (58) reported: "Resorcinol monobenzoate (RMB) has . . . been described as a cause of allergic contact dermatitis in seven patients who had been in close contact with cellulose ester plastics." A 69-year-old man with an intractable palm eczema was patch test positive to his car steering wheel, RMB, and balsam of Peru. The plastics manufacturer confirmed the existence of RMB in the steering wheel. Steering wheels made of cellulose ester plastic should not contain RMB after 1971.

Jordan and Dahl (59) also reported that plastic sunglasses, hearing aids, and ballpoint pens contain resorcinol monobenzoate as an ultraviolet stabilizer or inhibitor and may produce allergic contact dermatitis in balsam of Peru–sensitive individuals. Thus, resorcinol monobenzoate allergy should be considered when a candidate for plastic dermatitis reacts to balsam of Peru. To date, six RMB-sensitive patients have reacted to balsam of Peru.

> **Plastics containing resorcin monobenzoate may produce reactions in patients sensitive to balsam of Peru.**

Colophony (Rosin)

The sap tapped from pine trees is referred to as gum rosin, whereas wood rosin refers to rosin extracted from pine stumps or wood. The more liquid tall oil rosin is a by-product of the pulp industry (60). Gum rosin is mostly abietic acid. Modified rosin is usually treated with maleic anhydride or fumeric acid with the subsequent product used as paper size. The modified rosin esters are used as printing ink, varnish, or adhesives. The major allergen in the modified rosin has been reported to be maleopimaric acid (60).

Mitchell and Rook (61) found that the constituents of rosin are about 90% resin acids and 10% neutral matter. Of the resin acids, about 90% are isomeric with abietic acid ($C_{20}H_{30}O_2$); the other 10% is a mixture of dihydroabietic acid ($C_{20}H_{32}O_2$) and dehydroabietic acid ($C_{20}H_{28}O_2$). Malten et al. (62) found that rosin is a mixture of certain resin acids, namely, abietic acid and its isomers; neoabietic acid, palustric acid, pimaric acid, and levopimaric acid.

Ehrin and Karlberg (63) concur that 90% of colophony is resin and found 30% to 50% of the resin to be abietic acid, which, along with dihydroabietic acid, has been linked to allergy. Pimaric acids in colophony appear to be nonallergenic. The importance of colophony as an allergen is its widespread use, with 1.2 million tons produced in 1988. Of this production, 66% was used for paper, adhesives, and printing inks. The rosin content of most paper is 0.1% to 0.2% of the weight, whereas rosin core solder is 15% to 20% rosin, and tall oil is 2% to 20% rosin. Soluble cutting oils tend to be 15% to 20% tall oil or 0.4% to 4.0% rosin (63).

Rosin may be combined with glycerin or alcohol to form emulsions of acid ester gums that may be used as fabric finishers and can produce allergic contact dermatitis when sensitized persons come in contact with the clothing.

Exposure to and Dermatitis from Rosin (Colophony)

There are many opportunities for a person to become exposed to rosin and in some cases sensitized to it. The North American Contact Dermatitis Group lists of over three hundred products that contain rosin (Table 22.6).

Agrup (64) found that dermatitis due to adhesive tape, furniture polish, and sawdust was often caused by sensitivity to rosin. Kirk (65) reported a case of "colophony collar dermatitis," whereas Fregert (66) found that colophony in cutting oil and in soap water used as cutting fluid produced allergic dermatitis in certain workers. Adams (67) reported that rosin could be an industrial cause of contact dermatitis, and Wilkinson and Calnan (68) cited a patient with allergic

TABLE 22.6. *Exposure to Rosin (Colophony)*

Adhesives, adhesive plasters, and tapes
Asphaltic products, emulsions, and foundry supplies
Caulking compounds
Cements (linoleum, rubber, shoe, thermoplastic tile, lens-coating), cement agents
Chewing gum
Cleaners for leather and office machines, and grease remover for clothes
Corrosion inhibitors (automobile cooling systems, brake-shoe lining)
Cosmetics (brilliantine, depilatories of wax, eyeshadow, mascara, rouge, hair pomade, nail varnish)
Disinfectants and insecticides
Fillers (putty, wood dough)
Fireworks
Glues
Grease and lubricant thickener, axle grease, and greases
Insulating tapes (less frequent)
Jointing tapes
Linoleum, floor coverings, and floor tiles: adhesive bedding, cement
Insulations, electrical and thermal
Match tips
Medicaments (human and veterinary)
Modeling clay
Ostomy appliances
Paints: oleoresinous, anticorrosion, antifouling, house paint and enamel, finishes, varnishes (metallic drier, paint drier, emulsifiers)
Paper: Paper can be coated with rosin size. Rosin is added to paper to increase its water resistance, to prevent feathering or spreading of ink. Protective coating for glossy paper, price labels, plastics, and stickers. Rosin is applied as a finishing film to protect print on paper and as a surface coating for price labels. Ink can contain rosin derivatives (ceramic, marking, mimeograph, printing inks). Water-fast colors in artists' pens. Photographic paper. One of the largest single uses of colophony is in the sizing of paper and paperboard. Small quantities of resin acids can be transferred from paper to articles packed in it (e.g., food substances).
Polish (floor, furniture, metal, shoe, car)
Polythene (polyethylene)
Rosins and derivatives: gum rosin, wood rosin, rosin oil, tall oil (rosinol, retinol abitol), and ester gums. Resins (alkyd, synthetic ester, metals, phenolic resin modifier). Epoxy resins
Sawdust and resin of pine and spruce
Sealants and wood swellers
Shoes and clothing
Soaps: Brown soap, clear (transparent) soap, yellow soap, soap water used with cutting oil, yellow (soft) laundry bar soap. Rosin makes laundry bars more soluble and hastens sudsing in cool water
Soldering fluxes and soldering agents
Solvents
Stains
Surface coatings (lager beer casks, rust-proof coatings, coatings for price labels, can labels), polish for roasted coffee beans

continued

TABLE 22.6. *(Continued)*

Tacky substances—to prevent slipping
    Athletic grip aids
    Carpentry nails, rosin applied with tar
    Drive belts and clutches in automobile industry and engineering
    Grafting wax for trees
    Machine belts in industry
    Nonslip applications
    Postage stamp glue
    Powdered rosin as an application to belts on machinery to prevent slipping
    Rosin bag for baseball players
    Sticky flypaper
    Handles for sports (golf club, tennis racket, etc.)
    Rosin applied to bows of stringed musical instruments and to dancers' shoes
    Rosin for wrestlers, gymnasts, ballplayers, and bowlers
    Mixed with rubber (e.g., in car tires). Rubber-compounding aids, reclaiming agents, and emulsifying
        agents in producing synthetic rubber
    Rosin used on floors to prevent slipping
    Rosin is not infrequently used as an adulterant of other resinous products. Traces of turpentine may be
        present in gum rosin. Evidence for cross-sensitivity between colophony (rosin) and balsam of Peru is
        scanty
Tall oils, cutting oils, and core oils
Varnishes: Rosin reacts with maleic anhydride to produce adducts known as maleic resins
    These are used extensively in oil and spirit varnishes and lacquers
Water-proofing agents (cardboard, walls) and oilcloth
Wax: sealing, shoemaker, tree wax, and grafting wax. Wax modification. Car, floor furniture wax and
    polish.
Physiotherapy wax (contaminated)
Zein compositions

reactions to rosin used for a belt-driven machine. Perioral lip lickers–like dermatitis has also been traced to colophony in chewing gum (69).

Relationship of Abietic Acid to Rosin (Colophony)

Abietic acid is a principal sensitizer in rosin. During a 6-month period, Wahlberg (70) found 15 patients who were allergic to rosin; of these 15, 6 were also allergic to abietic acid.

Cronin and Calnan (71) found a patient who was allergic to hydroabietic alcohol (Abitol) in adhesive tape but not to abietic acid or rosin. Dooms-Goossens et al. (72) reported on a woman with mascara dermatitis who was allergic to both dihydroabietyl alcohol (as Abitol is known in Europe), present in mascara, and hypoallergenic adhesive tape containing methyl abietate. Results also indicated that colophony cross-reacted with abietic acid. Because Abitol is produced from abietic acid and other rosin acids, it would be expected that cross-reactions could occur readily between Abitol and abietic acid.

Rapaport (73), reviewing sensitization to Abitol, stated,

> Abitol is a colorless, tacky balsamic resin. It is a high molecuculate primary monohydric alcohol derived from rosin acids that have been hydrogenated to reduce unsaturation. It has a high refractive index, excellent color, low odor, good adhesion, and resistance to oxidation. Typically, Abitol has found wide application with natural and synthetic rubber, nitrocellulose, and other polymers as a plasticizer and with

emulsions, solvents, and hot-melt adhesives as a tackifier. Toxicologic data have shown Abitol to be safe. It was tested many years ago by a modified Schwartz technique and showed little irritation. It was interpreted as a nonsensitizer from data at that time (p. 137).

> **Abietic acid is the principal sensitizer in rosin (colophony).**

Rasmussen and Fisher (74) described salicylic acid plaster dermatitis from rosin. Fisher (75) reported contact dermatitis in a violinist from rosin. Solder flux, newsprint paper, and sandcores have produced rosin dermatitis (76–78).

DERMATITIS DUE TO PLANT OLEORESINS, INCLUDING POLLEN

Dermatitis from plant pollens, particularly that of ragweed, is a fairly common cause of plant dermatitis. The shell of the pollen grain contains the allergen, a resin-like material. Reactions occur mostly in farmers, gardeners, carpenters, salespeople, harvesters, and others who work outdoors and have prolonged contact with pollen-bearing plants.

The typical seasonal appearance is often masked because of the secondary lichenification and infection, which prolong the duration beyond the pollen seasons. In persons who have the dermatitis throughout the year, however, a careful history reveals that exacerbations occur during the pollen seasons. Often such cases masquerade as neurodermatitis.

> Pollens may contain two *distinct* antigens: a protein fraction, causing asthma or rhinitis, and an oleoresin, producing contact dermatitis.

The principal sites of pollen dermatitis are the exposed surfaces, namely, the face, neck, V area of the chest, arms, and legs. This pattern is always suggestive of an airborne dermatitis. Pollen dermatitis is usually subacute, but vesiculation may be found on the areas where pollen grains have adhered. The diffuse and even distribution of the eruption is attributed to the coalescing of minute individual papules produced by the grains of pollen.

Aside from the oleoresin, an aqueous protein fraction in pollen may produce asthma, hay fever, and occasionally atopic dermatitis. Rarely is there both an immediate urticarial sensitivity reaction (due to the protein fraction) and a delayed eczematous sensitivity reaction (due to oleoresin) to the pollen. In some patients, exacerbations of atopic dermatitis in the summer, aside from those due to humidity and sweating, are thought to be caused by inhalation of plant pollens.

Airborne pollen dermatitis with marked involvement of the exposed areas may resemble a photosensitivity dermatitis due to plants, drugs, or topical substances. Lesions on exposed areas due to simple pollen dermatitis, without photosensitivity, are not usually as sharply demarcated from normal skin as in the case of a photosensitizing dermatitis, because the pollen grains often get inside the collar and extend the dermatitis to the upper part of the chest and shoulders. Similarly, pollen grains may get inside trousers and affect the legs and even the inguinal area and genitals. Such involvement under the clothes may help differentiate simple pollen dermatitis from photosensitivity reactions. It must be remembered, however, that certain pollens, particularly ragweed, are photosensitizers as well as causes of dermatitis venenata.

> Ragweed dermatitis may mimic a photodermatitis.

Ragweed Oil Dermatitis

The oleoresin that produces ragweed dermatitis is present in the pollen and the stem and leaf of the plant. Ragweed pollen has two chief components: an inner core containing the water-soluble protein fraction, which may produce allergic rhinitis or asthma, and an outer portion, which is waxy and can produce allergic contact dermatitis in the sen-

sitized individual at the time of ragweed pollination (79). The sesquiterpene lactone parthenin is oil-soluble and has been detected in the waxy coat of the allergenic plant *Parthenium hysterophorus.* Ragweed oil dermatitis and ragweed hay fever are unrelated entities caused by different antigens of the ragweed plant. Most individuals with ragweed oil dermatitis are *not* atopic and do *not* have ragweed rhinitis or asthma.

Sensitized individuals may acquire dermatitis also by contact with the stem or leaves of the ragweed plant in the spring or summer, even before pollination takes place. In most instances, however, ragweed oil dermatitis is due to contact with airborne pollen when the plant is at maximal growth and its oleoresin is most concentrated (80,81).

> Men are much more commonly affected than women in a ratio of about 20:1.

Dermatitis due to airborne pollen is seasonal, lasting initially from August to the first frost. As the patient advances in age and as the seasonal exposures continue, the dermatitis may begin in June and extend to December.

The early, uncomplicated case usually involves the face, particularly the eyelids, the sides of the neck, the sternal area, and the extensor region of the arms. The dermatitis is often sharply limited by a protective undershirt. In chronic cases, it may extend to involve the trunk, groin, and lower extremities and become so widespread that it resembles a generalized erythroderma. Spontaneous remissions of ragweed oil dermatitis are rare, but even the untreated patient may show variations in severity.

The patient who is sensitive to ragweed oil may have associated allergic contact hypersensitivity to pyrethrum, chrysanthemum, and turpentine (81). Synonyms for Compositae dermatitis are shown in Table 22.7. Some of the numerous members of the Compositae family are shown in Table 22.8.

Compositae Family

Sesquiterpene lactones present in the oil-soluble plant oleoresin are responsible for allergic dermatitis caused by these plants. The presence of an alpha-methylene group exocylic

---

TABLE 22.7. *Compositae Dermatitis Synonyms*

Australian bush dermatitis
Chrysanthemum dermatitis
Compositae dermatitis/airborne contact
Parthenium dermatitis
Pollen dermatitis
Ragweed (oil) dermatitis
Sesquiterpene lactone dermatitis
Sesquiterpenoid dermatitis
Weed dermatitis

TABLE 22.8. *Some Plants Known to Contain Sesquiterpene Lactones*

Common name	Genus
Arnica	Arnica
Artichoke, globe	Cynara
Artichoke, wild	Olearia
Bitterweed	Helenium
Boneset	Eupatorium
Broomweed	Amphiachyris
Burdock	Arctium
Burrobrush	Hymenoclea
Capeweed	Cryptostemma
Chamomile, German	Matricaria
Chamomile, Roman	Anthemis
Champaca of perfumery	Michelia[a]
Chicory	Cichorium
Chrysanthemum	Chrysanthemum
Cocklebur	Xanthium
Cosmos	Cosmos
Costus of perfumery	Saussurea
Cottonthistle	Onopordon
Encelia	Encelia
Feverfew	Parthenium
Fireweed	Gaillardia
Fleabane	Erigeron
Guayule	Parthenium
Hempweed	Mikania
Ironweed	Veronia
Laurel oil	Laurus
Leafcup	Polymnia
Lettuce	Lactuca
Liverwort	Frullania
Marguerite	Chrysanthemum
Marigold	Calendula
Marsh elder	Iva
Oxeye	Telekia
Pyrethrum	Chrysanthemum
Ragweed	Ambrosia
Sagebrush	Artemisia
Sneezeweed	Helenium
Sowthistle	Sonchus
Starthistle	Centaurea
Stinkwort	Inula
Sunflower	Helianthus
Tansy	Tanacetum
Tulip tree	Liriodendron[a]
Whitewood of commerce	Liriodendron[a]
Wormwood	Artemisia
Yarrow	Achillea

[a]Not a member of the Compositae family.

to the gamma-lactone appears to be the immunochemical requisite for such dermatitis. A screening test for Compositae with 0.1% sesquiterpene lactone mix has been evaluated against individual Compositae oleoresins. The mix identified only 35% of the cases. The mix is considered an inadequate screening tool based on these results (82).

This family of plants includes ragweed *(Ambrosia)*, sneezeweed and bitterweed *(Helenium)*, sagebrush, wormwood, mugwort *(Artemisia)*, boneset *(Eupatorium)*, poverty weed *(Franseria)*, marsh elder *(Iva)*, cocklebur *(Xanthium)*, burdock *(Arctium)*, chamomile *(Anthemis)*, ar-

tichoke *(Cynara)*, gaillardia, chrysanthemum, tansy *(Tanacetum)*, feverfew *(Chrysanthemum parthenium)*, pyrethrum *(Chrysanthemum species)*, and broomweed *(Amphiachyris dracunculoides)*.

Ragweeds of the plant genus Ambrosia have water-soluble antigens, which release IgE from the basophils and mast cells of the nose, producing hay fever: This is a Type 1 reaction. The same plant, ragweed, may produce contact dermatitis through a Type 4 reaction to one of the several lipid-soluble antigens, among which are the sesquiterpene lactones. Thus, ragweed possesses several different antigens that can cause different types of hypersensitivity responses.

Ragweed and parthenium dermatitis occur almost exclusively in adult men. Children and women seem to be immune. Oral hyposensitization in cases of Compositae allergic contact dermatitis cannot be recommended with complete confidence, but may be somewhat helpful (80). Airborne contact dermatitis from Compositae oleoresin simulating photodermatitis has been reported from the United States, India, Australia, United Kingdom, and most recently from Scandinavian countries (34).

Ragweed dermatitis appears initially in the fall and clears after the first frost, but untreated cases may become perennial. Cross-reactions between Compositae species are often observed, owing to some 3,500 cross-reacting allergenic sesquiterpene lactones distributed in this family.

It was thought originally that Compositae dermatitis was not present in Europe. Hjorth et al. (81), however, reported a series of Danish patients who had been treated for 1 to 50 years for photodermatitis (or in one instance of actinic reticuloid), all of whom turned out to be strongly positive to oleoresin from several Compositae species.

Can Ragweed Dermatitis Be Airborne?

After Fisher studied 18 male New Yorkers who were not farmers and had not been exposed to ragweed plants, he became convinced that ragweed dermatitis can be airborne from pollen containing the oleoresin.

Howell (83) stated, however, that he could not produce dermatitis by blowing ragweed onto the moistened skin of patients with ragweed dermatitis.

Grater (84) stated, "Everyone who has made an allergy extract knows that the pollen contains a considerable amount of oleoresins. In the preparation of extracts for pollens, they are defatted with ether, thus the hyposensitization has none of the active principle causing the dermatitis." (p. 159)

Hjorth et al. (81) stated flatly that wind-borne plant material is responsible for a true airborne contact etiology. Furthermore, Burry et al. (85), in discussing Compositae dermatitis in Australia, suggested that "Australian bush dermatitis" as a suitable name for a chronic dermatitis of exposed areas occurring in men living in the Australian bush. Sensitivity to ragweed revealed by patch testing was common to five patients suffering from the dermatitis, but was thought to be incidental and not clinically relevant. Wind-borne pollens or dust, released during dry, summer conditions by other plants of the Compositae family present in the Australian bush, are suggested as probable causes. The incapacitating chronicity of Australian bush dermatitis indicates that dermatologic, botanical, and chemical research into its origins is desirable.

> **Although it is not unanimous, most investigators have found that ragweed dermatitis is airborne due to floating pollen containing oleoresin.**

Ragweed dermatitis is not often recognized, usually being misdiagnosed as "photodermatitis" from other causes (86,87). Coexistence of ultraviolet light sensitivity and Compositae sensitivity do occur, however (88).

As commercial sesquiterpene lactone patch test mixes have become available, the diagnosis of Compositae dermatitis has been established in 1% to 2% of patients patch tested, with clinical relevance found in about one-half of the positive cases (38). The trend that has evolved is for hand eczema to be as or more prevalent than photodermatitis or airborne dermatitis. At the European Contact Dermatitis Society meeting in Brussels, October 1992, Ross reported 1.8% of 7,420 patients were allergic to sesquiterpene lactones and about one-third showed an airborne pattern, one-third hand eczema, and one-fifth generalized dermatitis. The remainder had facial dermatitis. Only 22% of the sesquiterpene lactone allergic patients were found photosensitive (89). At the same meeting, du Peloux Managé reported 9% of these patients who were photosensitive reacted to ultraviolet B (UVB) only, 82% to ultraviolet A (UVA) and UVB, and 8% were sensitive to UVA, UVB, and visible light (89).

Parthenium Dermatitis Exported to India

Parthenium hysterophorus (feverfew, carrot weed), an American weed introduced accidentally to India by a shipment of American wheat, has produced hundreds of cases of severe contact dermatitis in the Poona area, located on the western coast of India near Bombay. In some cases, the dermatitis progressed to a generalized erythroderma with fatal results. The weed has spread to other parts of India and so devastated the countryside that it has been called the "scourge of India" (90).

Parthenium, a member of the Compositae group of plants, which includes tansy and pyrethrum, cross-reacts with ragweed *(Ambrosia)*. As in ragweed dermatitis, the contact sensitizer parthenolide is an oil-soluble oleoresin present throughout the plant and pollen. Up to one-third of the oil-soluble fraction can be removed with water alone (36). In contrast, ragweed and parthenium allergic rhinitis and asthma are due to water-soluble proteins present only in the pollen. Parthenolide makes up 0.3% to 1% of the plant weight and is found in 12 other Compositae species (36).

The principal source of exposure to parthenium is direct contact with the living plant whose plant hairs (trichomes) contain abundant dermatitis-producing sesquiterpene lactones. The airborne pollen of parthenium, however, also contains the oleoresin, and the resulting contact dermatitis may be entirely "airborne." In addition, the plants crumble during the dry season to a fine dust that is scattered throughout the countryside. This dust is another source of "airborne" contact dermatitis (91). Because spontaneous cures of parthenium and ragweed dermatitis apparently do not occur, hyposensitization procedures are worthwhile, particularly in those patients who cannot avoid exposure to the plants. An allergenic sesquiterpene lactone, parthenin, has been detected in parthenium pollen.

> **Parthenium weed accidentally introduced into India has become the "scourge of India," producing a severe ragweed-like dermatitis in thousands of individuals, particularly males after puberty.**

Features of Parthenium Dermatitis

1. This is the first instance of an "imported" sensitizer causing allergic contact dermatitis in thousands of people.
2. The eruption may become generalized and produce a universal erythroderma that is not amenable to systemic corticosteroids and may be fatal.
3. The only effective treatment presently is to remove the patient from the area in which the weed is growing in India. Because thousands of Indians are affected, such a procedure is not practical.
4. In the southwestern United States, parthenium usually causes only a mild dermatitis, subsiding after the first frost when the plant becomes dormant. Shelmire (92), however, described a patient in Texas with a generalized parthenium dermatitis who showed a positive patch test reaction to a 1:100,000 parthenium extract. The eruption was recurrent from May to December.
5. In India, parthenium is no longer a rural problem. The weed is extraordinarily prolific and aggressive, growing rapidly all over the city in vacant lots and any open space in cities, on roadsides and paths, and even from crevices in the walls of buildings and houses. In Poona, a city with a population of 1.5 million, a bank manager, an urban physician, and other office workers were affected with dermatitis. The plant in pastureland is harmful to cattle, contaminates milk, and interferes with crops and agricultural food production.
6. The principal sensitizing chemical of parthenium is the sesquiterpene lactone, parthenolide. Patch testing has revealed cross-reactions to numerous other plants of the

Compositae group and to their sesquiterpene lactones (36,93).

7. Although Indian authorities claim that no herbicide is effective, Hausen (94) has stated that control of *Parthenium hysterophorus* is possible with Ansar-529, a weed killer containing arsenic.

8. Parthenium dermatitis, like ragweed dermatitis, affects men almost exclusively. The dermatitis is rare in women and does not affect children. About 4% of exposed males acquire parthenium dermatitis.

9. Parthenium dermatitis, like ragweed dermatitis, resembles photodermatitis because skin surfaces not usually covered with clothing are initially involved.

The parthenium oleoresin may contain phototoxic chemicals (95). Mitchell (96), in discussing "dermatitis at a distance," states that it is possible that the airborne pollen of parthenium is capable, on phytochemical grounds, of providing allergens for the production of dermatitis. Recently, allergenic oil-soluble sesquiterpene lactones have been detected in the waxy coat of parthenium pollen.

Dr. A. Lonkar (personal communication) wrote:

The treatment of parthenium dermatitis has been frustrating. The systemic as well as topical steroids are of limited value. Prolonged corticosteroid administration has its own hazards. The clue given by the age of the patients, involvements of only postmenopausal women, although rarely, absence of the disease before puberty and activation or increase due to sunlight stimulated me in trying short courses of antimalarials and female hormones. I use Chlorquin 200 mg tid for about 1 week and then taper it off to suit the need. Ethinyl estradiol 0.05 mg at bedtime for about 3 weeks is given to both adult males and females. This combination does seem to modify the course of the disease. I have not advocated this as a standard treatment in parthenium dermatitis, but I feel that it provides a clue in the pathogenesis of the disease.

The Effect of Pyrethrin Insecticides on Ragweed-Sensitive Individuals

Fisher (97) stated that a sharp distinction must be made between pyrethrum and the commercially refined pyrethrin extracts used in insecticides.

It has been known for a long time that insecticidal pyrethrins present in pyrethrum powder are not the cause of respiratory allergy (98). As far as the dermatitis-producing oleoresin is concerned, Mitchell et al. (99) have shown that the oleoresin fraction of ragweed that produces contact dermatitis is a sesquiterpene lactone and that the dermatitis-producing fraction of pyrethrum is pyrethrosin, a sesquiterpene lactone that is not used for insecticidal properties. Furthermore, Head (100) has shown that pyrethrosin is not present in the commercially refined pyrethrin extracts used as insecticides. Hausen and Schulz (101) confirmed Mitchell's observation that the pyrethrins (i.e., constituents with strong insecticidal activity) play no role in chrysanthemum and pyrethrum dermatitis.

In addition, Fisher (2) completed a study of 50 patients with either ragweed dermatitis or ragweed rhinitis or asthma. Twelve of these patients were men with ragweed dermatitis, with a strongly positive patch test reaction to ragweed oleoresin. Thirty-eight patients had ragweed rhinitis or asthma with positive scratch test reactions to the aqueous ragweed fraction. None of these patients showed any patch or scratch test reaction to RID (Pfizer), a pediculicide that contains purified pyrethrins.

One can, therefore, conclude that pyrethrum-derived pyrethrin insecticides are safe for patients with respiratory allergy or dermatitis due to ragweed.

> **Although pyrethrum may cross-react with ragweed protein and oleoresin, the refined pyrethrins used in insecticides are safe for patients with ragweed rhinitis or asthma or ragweed dermatitis.**

FRULLANIA (LIVERWORTS)

Liverworts of the genus *Frullania* are small, reddish or brownish plants, which frequently grow with mosses and lichens, from which they may be distinguished by their compact ropelike appearance. So-called cedar or hemlock poisoning is a misnomer because the dermatitis is actually caused by liverwort plants growing on the trees and in nearby forests or due to lichens.

Mitchell et al. (102) identified *Frullania* (liverwort) as the causative agent of some cases of so-called cedar wood poisoning in the forests of the Pacific Northwest. They demonstrated positive patch tests in addition to several members of the Compositae family or their oleoresin extracts, and deduced that the sesquiterpene lactones were the chemicals common to Compositae and the unrelated *Frullania*. Some of the patients were said to exhibit evidence of photosensitivity. Comparison of the chemical structures of a series of sesquiterpene lactones indicated that the presence of an exocyclic, carbon-to-carbon double bond (methylene) conjugated with the cyclic carbonyl (lactone) was essential for antigenicity.

Storrs et al. (103) emphasized the unvarying clinical picture of both Compositae and *Frullania* dermatitis, with the exception that the Frullania reactors by contrast flare in the wet winter in the Pacific Northwest. They suggest that the more water-soluble oleoresin sensitizers may even contaminate rainwater, which might explain slight submental-sparing simulating photodermatitis.

Despite initial clinical impressions, phototesting was negative. The authors drew attention to several positive patch tests to balsam of Peru, turpentine, and colophony, which contain terpenes and might be cross-reactive.

Storrs et al. (103) stated that many individuals with allergic hypersensitivity to the d-usnic acid in lichens are also allergic to *Frullania*. This is not a true cross-reaction, because reactions to d-usnic acid probably represent separate sensitization to lichens rather than a true cross-reaction to sesquiterpene lactones. D-usnic acid is not a sesquiterpene lactone, does not occur in *Frullania* or Compositae, and exhibits stereoisomeric specificity in the production of delayed hypersensitivity (only the d- form is active). As a sensitizer, d-usnic acid is not as potent as the sesquiterpenoids. Stereoisomeric specificity was reported for two species of *Frullania*. *F. dilatata* produced the 1 or (-) form of frullanolide, and *F. tamarisci* produced the d- or (+) form. These enantiomers (mirror images) did not cross-react. Routine screening with frullanolide is not recommended, as it may sensitize. It should be used as an "aimed test" when highly likely to be helpful on clinical history (104).

Frullania (liverwort) dermatitis is caused by a lactone similar to ragweed and resembling ragweed dermatitis. Co-reactions with lichens may occur; however, such reactions are not true cross-reactions but represent coincidental sensitization.

Allergic contact dermatitis due to *Frullania* and Compositae responds rapidly to withdrawal of the patient from exposure to the causative antigen. Systemic and topical corticosteroids hasten recovery. The only patients who have not had continued problems are those who have changed occupations or retired. In the case of forest workers, this involves total avoidance of tree bark. Fallers, buckers, log truckers, toppers, hook tenders, choker setters, scalers, and timber cruisers are all susceptible. Switching from one to another of these occupations does not benefit the patient; however, because persons who work with debarked trees (sawyers, graders, and finishers) seem to have no difficulty with *Frullania* sensitivity, transfer to one of these jobs can be a suitable alternative to switching industries completely.

Persons sensitive to *Frullania* must also be cautioned to avoid the particular members of the Compositae family to which patch testing has revealed sensitivities. Thus, transfer of a sensitized logger to a ranching position might result in continued dermatitis from tansy or sagebrush. Conversely, a sagebrush-sensitive rancher might have problems as a logger.

Some French investigators (105) have been able to hyposensitize some of their *Frullania*-sensitive patients using repeated biweekly applications of whole *Frullania*. Theoretically, oral hyposensitization with plant extracts could be achieved in a manner similar to that used for the treatment of ragweed or *Toxicodendron* dermatitis. In Oregon, Storrs et al. (103) attempted this procedure in four patients, using mixtures of Compositae oleoresins prepared according to the patient's specific sensitivity pattern by Hollister-Stier. Two of these treated patients believed that their summer tansy-related dermatitis was "somewhat better" while taking the oleoresin-filled capsules. An explosive flare of dermatitis occurred in one patient each time he began oral hyposensitization. In the fourth patient, the severe dermatitis never cleared sufficiently to allow therapy without fear of worsening the condition. Oral hyposensitization therapy in cases of Frullania and Compositae allergic contact dermatitis cannot yet be recommended with confidence.

DERMATITIS DUE TO LICHENS

Lichens, plants composed of fungi living in symbiosis with algae, have caused allergic contact dermatitis in foresters. The specific sensitizing substance is apparently usnic acid, which accumulates in lichenized fungi. It is chemically related to the furocoumarins, but it is apparently not a photosensitizer.

So-called cedar poisoning or wood cutter's eczema may actually be a contact dermatitis due to lichens. The general population may be exposed by burning lichen-infested logs in fireplaces. Lichen mosses used to simulate trees and shrubs are the source of exposure in model railroad operators and architects. Lichens may also be used in making clothing dyes and funeral wreaths. Litmus is derived from lichen pigment. Ointments containing usnic acid are used for treatment of skin infections, particularly in Scandinavia and Germany. Patch tests may be performed with 1% usnic acid in petrolatum.

Salo et al. (106) reported the frequency and immunologic background of dermatitis occurring in lichen pickers who were studied in a small community in northern Finland. Thirty of 164 lichen pickers had suffered from dermatitis at least on the fingers and the dorsa of their hands, and many of them also had dermatitis on their forearms and faces. Fifteen were subjected to epicutaneous and photoepicutaneous testing with crushed *Cladonia alpestris* (L.) Rab. and some fractions of it. Allergic contact reactions were seen in nine subjects, three of whom also had positive photoepicutaneous test reactions from lichen allergens. No immediate reactions were seen in scratch or scratch chamber tests with crushed *Cladonia alpestris* or with its alcoholic extract.

Lichens cause allergic dermatitis; usnic acid is the specific sensitizer.

PLANT DERMATITIS DUE TO MECHANICAL IRRITATION

Mechanical irritation may be produced by spines, thorns, specialized bristles, and hairs. The large or small wounds produced by such mechanical irritation may be complicated by bacterial or fungal infection, particularly sporotrichosis. Many grasses and cereals, including barley, millet, rice, and bamboo, have sharp trichomes, which may produce urticarial papules in workers handling crops or litter straw. Dogwood has t-shaped hairs, which may produce urticaria when the leaf is rubbed on the skin in the direction of the hairs.

Many European herbs of the borage family are covered with coarse, stiff hairs, which can produce an irritant dermatitis. Certain tropical plants, including palms and cacti, have spicules, which may also produce dermatitis.

The prickly pear cactus has barbs (glochidia), which can enter the skin, producing a dermatitis resembling scabies. Covered parts of the body may be secondarily affected through the transfer of the broken-off barbs from primarily affected sites. In Israel, harvesting the pears of this plant produces an occupational hazard called sabra dermatitis. Mechanical removal of the barbs is difficult. Peeling ointments or salicylic acid plasters may be used to bring about exfoliation of the skin with the embedded barbs.

PRIMARY IRRITANT DERMATITIS DUE TO PLANT CHEMICALS

Chemical irritation may occur from contact with fluids or crystals in specialized hairs or other portions of the plant.

Plants may injure the skin by direct chemical action. No allergic mechanism is involved, and if the degree of exposure is sufficiently great, a reaction is provoked in everyone so exposed. Variation in susceptibility is attributed to anatomic factors, notably, the thickness of the horny layer, and to climatic factors, which favor or impede the penetration of the irritant substances. Primary irritant dermatitis is particularly common in children.

> **Some plants have irritant hairs; others have caustic juices that are powerful primary irritants.**

Aside from irritant hairs, many plants contain chemicals that are strong primary irritants. The buttercup is an important irritant plant. It contains an unsaturated lactone, protoanemonin, formed by the breakdown of a glucoside in injured plants. Children chewing the leaves or stems of the injured plants may acquire blisters on the face and around the lips.

Certain members of the daisy family may also produce an irritant bullous eruption when crushed on the skin.

Cactus-like plants (spurges) of South Africa contain a copious milky latex in their stems, which has strong caustic properties. The manchineel tree of the West Indies and certain vegetables, such as tropical gourds and cucumbers, contain a juice that can irritate the skin.

Plants of the mustard and radish family contain the glucoside sinigrin, which is harmless in the dry state, but is converted into the irritant, volatile oil of mustard in the presence of water.

Pineapple juice contains bromelin, a proteolytic enzyme that can cause a primary irritant dermatitis. The enzyme

TABLE 22.9. *Irritant Dermatitis Due to Plants*

Chemical
1. *Euphorbiaceae*—
   a. *Euphorbia* (spurge)
   b. *Hippomane mancinella* (manchineel tree)
2. *Mucuna pruriens* (cowhage)
   Itch powder
   Proteolytic enzyme
3. Pineapple
   Calcium oxalate and bromelin, a keratolytic enzyme
Mechanical irritant
   a. Opuntia family—prickly pear cactus pines (glochidia), produce foreign body granulomas
Pharmacologic
Nettles (Urticaceae family): 5-hydroxy tryptamine, histamine, acetylcholine

causes separation of the superficial layers of the skin and increases skin and capillary permeability. These effects resemble the mechanical damage produced by needle-shaped calcium oxalate crystals of tulip bulbs. Both the enzyme and the crystals produce itching and increased permeability of capillaries with the formation of wheals, which are suggestive of histamine liberation in the skin.

The tropical plant *Mucuna pruriens* (itch plant) is a member of the bean family. It does not occur in the United States, but it grows wild in all tropical areas. Short, barbed spicules cover its seed pods. The active itch-producing principle of the plant is a proteolytic enzyme named mucunain, which is the principal ingredient of the "itch powder" used by practical jokers.

Sometimes irritant effects give way to more classic delayed reactions. A 9-year-old boy fell into a nettle bush and experienced a 12-hour bout of urticaria, which at 48 hours changed to a vesicular dermatitis (107).

Table 22.9 summarizes plant irritant dermatitis.

Phytophotodermatitis

Photosensitization contact dermatitis due to plants is caused largely, if not entirely, by photosensitizing compounds related to furocoumarin (psoralens). Some other chemical compounds, such as thiophenes, have so far been reported to induce phototoxicity only in microbial systems (108). Phytophotodermatitis can be diagnosed usually by the clinical history and characteristic skin lesions that follow exposure to psoralen-containing plants.

Two requisites for the initiation of phytophotodermatitis are contact with a sensitizing furocoumarin in the juice of the plant and subsequent exposure to ultraviolet radiation of wavelengths greater than 320 nm (usually sunlight). All individuals exposed sufficiently to the plant are susceptible, because a phototoxic and not an allergic mechanism is involved.

Table 22.10 shows the differential diagnosis of an allergic contact plant dermatitis (poison ivy) and one due to

TABLE 22.10. *Clinical Features of Poison Ivy-Oak (Toxicodendron) Dermatitis and of Phytophotodermatitis of Plants with Psoralens*

Disorder	Onset	Mechanism	Symptoms	Course
Poison ivy dermatitis	First exposure can result in sensitization and dermatitis after 5 or more days; on reexposure, dermatitis appears within 48 hours, often within 12 hours	Contact allergic	Itching	Fresh disseminated lesions often appear during 1 week after exposure
Phytophotodermatitis	First exposure can result in redness and blistering of the skin, which appears at about 48 hours; on reexposure, the reaction time is about 48 hours	Phototoxic	Burning pain	Reaction is confined to initial sites of contact

phytophotodermatitis. Table 22.11 lists plants implicated in causing phytophotodermatitis.

Phytophotodermatitis, evoked by exposure to UVA and a psoralen plant, such as the gas plant or a plant product (such as a bergamot orange oil in perfume), is a cutaneous phototoxic reaction. First exposure can result in redness, burning pain, and blistering of the skin that appears at about 48 hours; the reaction is confined to the initial sites of contact. Hyperpigmentation, which can result, even without obvious dermatitis, often persists for months.

> **Phytophotodermatitis produces erythema and vesiculation on first exposure, followed by persistent hyperpigmentation.**

> **Psoralen, as from the Egyptian umbelliferae plant, ammi majus, is used in PUVA therapy.**

TABLE 22.11. *Common Plants Implicated in Causing Phytophotodermatitis*

Common name	Botanical name	Family
Angelica	Angelica archangelica	Umbelliferae
Bergamot	Citrus bergamia	Rutaceae
Bitter orange	Citrus aurantium	Rutaceae
Celery	Apium graveolens	Umbelliferae
Citron	Citrus medica (C. acida)	
Cow parsley	Heracleum sphondylium	Umbelliferae
Cow parsley, wild chervil	Anthriscus sylvestris	Umbelliferae
Dill	Anethum graveolens	Umbelliferae
	Peucedanum oreoselinum	Umbelliferae
Fennel	Foeniculum vulgare	Umbelliferae
Figs	Ficus carica	Moraceae
Gas plant, burning bush	Dictamnus albus (D. fraxinella)	Rutaceae
Giant hogweed	Heracleum mantegazzianum	Umbelliferae
	H. maximum (H. dulce)	Umbelliferae
Lemon	Citrus limon	Rutaceae
Lime	Citrus aurantifolia	Rutaceae
Lovage	Levisticum officinale	Umbelliferae
Masterwort	Peucedanum ostruthium	Umbilliferae
	Ammi majus	Umbelliferae
Parsnip (garden variety)	Pastinaca sativa (P. urens)	Umbelliferae
Parsnip (wild parsnip)	Heracleum giganteum	Umbelliferae
Persian lime	Citrus aurantifolia	Rutaceae
(Tahitian)	"Persian"	Rutaceae
Rue	Ruta graveolens	
Wild carrot, garden carrot	Daucus carota	Umbelliferae

Meadow grass dermatitis (dermatitis bullosa striata pratensis) is a phototoxic eruption produced by contact with wild parsnip and other vegetation and exposure to sunshine. A network of crisscross, striate bullae, resembling poison ivy dermatitis, is produced. The lesions develop 12 to 24 hours after the plants have been crushed on the skin and there has been subsequent exposure to sunlight. If the skin is moist, the photodynamic effect is enhanced. The bullae soon heal, leaving marked pigmentation, which may persist for many months.

Furocoumarins continue to be identified in a variety of plants including lovage, which is an herb that contains 0.64 μg/g of psoralen and caused phytophotodermatitis in a woman harvesting it (109). Celery that has been rendered most resistant to fungal contamination ironically contains psoralens that caused phytophotodermatitis in grocery store clerks (105). Celery normally contains psoralen precursors. Under attack by fungus, celery produces psoralen as a defensive mechanism. Fungus-infected celery (pink rot) causes blisters on the hands of harvesters in sunlight. Botanists have produced strains of celery that contain psoralens and are therefore resistant to pink rot. Psoralen-containing strains of celery produce hyperpigmentation of the forearms of produce workers. Picking the leaves and flowers of *Ruta corsica* can produce phytophotodermatitis (110).

Primula dermatitis is not usually a photodermatitis, but one case has been reported in which 5.9 J of UVA caused a positive patch test to 0.01% primin in petrolatum, whereas the unirradiated test was negative (111) (see also Chapter 23).

PSEUDOPHYTODERMATITIS

Pseudophytodermatitis is an eruption that appears to be due to plants, but in reality is produced by arthropods infesting the plants or by dyes and waxes applied to the skin of citrus fruits and plant insecticides.

Pseudophytodermatitis Due to Mites

Grain Itch Mites

Pediculoides ventricosus, the North American itch mite, feeds on various insect larvae that infest wheat, barley, rye, and other grain straw and beans. The mites attack humans, especially persons sleeping on straw mattresses, and may produce a generalized eruption consisting of petechiae, wheals, vesicles, and pustules.

Farmers, harvesters, chaff cutters, handlers of old hay, strawboard factory workers, millers, bakers, packers, unloaders, and persons working in grain elevators or places where grain and straw are handled may become infested with grain itch mites.

Frequent bathing and change of clothing may prevent infestation when there is massive exposure to the mites. The wearing of clothing impregnated with benzyl benzoate may be effective. Prophylactic use of Kwell or Eurax is beneficial.

Food Mites

Tyroglyphus farinae, the flour mite, may infest not only grain stores, mills, and bakeries, but also food in homes. Contact with the food produces a papular dermatitis.

Tyroglyphus siro, the cheese mite, infests not only cheese but also dried fruit, sugar, roots, bulbs, and copra. Grocer's itch, a pruritic papular eruption, is produced in persons handling these infested plant products. Cheese mites do not suck blood, but their migration under superficial scales of the epidermis produces pruritus and an eruption that is difficult to distinguish from that of allergic contact dermatitis.

Cheese mites have been controlled by painting the cheese with paraffin and by wiping or dipping cheese with mineral oil, cotton seed oil, or glycerin. Good packaging to prevent the mites from obtaining entrance to the food is important for prevention of infestation.

> **Mites and caterpillars on plants may be the causes of "plant dermatitis" known as pseudophytodermatitis.**

Miscellaneous Mites

Barley itch usually occurs in dock workers unloading barley infested with food mites. Baker's itch occurs among workers in granaries, flour mills, and bakeries, particularly in small establishments that do not use mechanical processes and have few sanitary arrangements to destroy mites.

Individuals handling cotton seed in bulk may acquire a mite rash known as cotton seed itch. When the seeds are handled in bags, dermatitis does not occur. The mite in cotton seed is related to *Pediculoides ventricosus*. Bulb mite itch is contracted by individuals who store infested bulbs above their beds on shelves or in attics; these persons, while asleep, are attacked by the mites.

Bakers, workers in sugar refineries or chocolate candy factories, and those who can and pack fruits and syrups may acquire a dermatitis from the sugar mite.

Dried fruits may be infested by the mite *Carpoglyphus passularum*. Sorters, peelers, and packers of infested prunes may acquire a follicular, papular eruption. Women sorting partly damaged dates may also be affected. Dock laborers and workers engaged in shoveling figs for a jam factory have developed dermatitis produced by a fruit mite. A mite found on dried beans can produce dermatitis in workers handling these legumes.

Pseudophytodermatitis Due to Contact with Poison Hairs of Caterpillars

Outdoors, exposure to caterpillars is not uncommon. In the home, caterpillars may crawl into clothes and bedding. Fomites infested with caterpillars may produce dermatitis for long periods, even in cold storage. Caterpillar dermatitis is an occupational disease in plantation workers.

Dead larvae and cocoons of caterpillars as well as debris from infested pine forests can cause dermatitis. Caterpillar dermatitis, therefore, may occur throughout the entire year. The eruption is caused by microscopic hairs containing a toxin that produces lesions in all individuals exposed. An entire community may suffer from urticaria epidemica due to caterpillars.

This type of dermatitis appears usually as a urticarial, papular eruption, but vesiculation and even necrosis may also occur. Nodular conjunctivitis and severe damage to the eyeball are serious complications.

Pseudophytodermatitis Due to Dyes

Certified azo dyes applied to the skin of oranges and grapefruits rarely cause dermatitis.

Pseudophytodermatitis Due to Waxes

Carnauba wax, from the South American palm, is used to wax oranges and is an ingredient of shoe, furniture, and automobile polishes, cosmetic creams, lipsticks, and solid perfumes. J. C. Mitchell has not encountered allergic contact dermatitis from this wax.

Plant Insecticides

Various plant insecticides, including arsenical sprays and malathion, can produce contact dermatitis, which may initially be diagnosed as plant dermatitis.

DERMATITIS DUE TO FLOWERS AND DECORATIVE PLANTS

Many varieties of wild and cultivated flowers may cause dermatitis.

Sensitivity occurring in gardeners and florists is confined usually to the hands, forearms, face, and neck; episodic, acute vesicular reactions occur. Dermatitis in commercial flower growers is a known hazard of the trade. Those affected are often seasonal workers who leave the work when dermatitis appears or carry on despite it and do not come to the attention of dermatologists. The growing of chrysanthemums by commercial growers and hobby gardeners involves close contact by "pinching out" the buds of the plants as they mature. Cutting back and pruning many garden plants (e.g., English and Algerian ivy) involve contact with the sap and risk of contact dermatitis.

Chrysanthemum

Chrysanthemums, asters, and daisies all belong to the same family of plants. Most of these flowers can produce dermatitis under certain conditions. Chrysanthemums are the most common offenders, and the resulting dermatitis appears usually in the late fall and early winter—the blooming season. Because the blooms emit a pollen, the eyelids may be the first areas involved. Many sensitized individuals also have facial involvement. Widespread chrysanthemum dermatitis is not uncommon. The diagnosis may be confirmed by a patch test. Patients who react to one species of chrysanthemum may react to other Compositae plants as well. For example, cross-reactions may also take place with arnica and aster.

Philodendron

This plant is widely used for interior and patio decoration. Contact dermatitis from several species, especially *Philodendron cordatum,* has occurred. Hands and arms are usually involved. Exposure takes place when the patient washes, oils, or plucks the leaves. Because the plant grows indoors, there is no relationship of the dermatitis to a particular season. A patient may have numerous attacks of dermatitis, which are not readily diagnosed. Dieffenbachia, a common house plant related closely to the philodendron, may also cause dermatitis.

Contact dermatitis to philodendron (*Philodendron scandens)* is common in Hawaii. The allergen in philodendron is an alkylresorcinol, which is chemically close to the catachols found in *Toxicodendron.* However, a study of patients sensitive to one or the other of these two plants found cross-activity to be rare (112).

Algerian Ivy

This plant may be used as a ground cover. The history reveals usually that the patient cut the ivy a day or so before the onset of the dermatitis.

English Ivy

A dermatitis may be caused by the leaves, stems, and even the roots of this ornamental plant. The lesion sometimes resembles a *Toxicodendron* eruption.

Oleander

Dermatitis results when crushed leaves of this plant come into contact with the skin of persons who have become sensitized by previous exposure. Often children playing near shrubs are affected. Because oleander is not deciduous, it may produce dermatitis at any time of year. Patch testing confirms the diagnosis.

Castor Bean

Dermatitis may occur at any time of year when there is exposure to the juice of the leaves or stems of the plants or to the beans. Castor oil extractors, fertilizer workers, and farmers may acquire occupational dermatitis from handling the plants or the beans. The beans are poisonous when ingested.

Daffodil/Narcissus

These plants can cause a papular, pruritic eruption with most severe involvement on the face, hands, and forearms. Daffodils and narcissi are members of the Amaryllidaceae family. Those affected are usually engaged in cutting, bunching, or packing daffodils and narcissi. Daffodil pickers characteristically get a papular and excoriated dermatitis on the dorsum of their hands due to the manner in which the flower is harvested. The hand is exposed to the calcium oxalate crystals in the sap, and this produces an irritant contact dermatitis. Paronychia are common in these individuals (113).

Chinese Rice Paper Plant

This popular ornamental shrub may cause severe dermatitis. The toxic substance is present in a heavy yellow pollen produced in the fall and winter. Irritant contact dermatitis can be caused by the trichomes of the Chinese rice paper tree *(Tetrapanax papyriferum)*. This is a member of the Araliaceae family, which contains other plants known for both irritant and allergy, such as *Hedera helix, Fatsia japonica,* and *Schefflera* sp. (114).

Dendropanax

In Japan, the plant commonly known as kakuremino (because it resembles a Japanese straw coat) is *Dendropanax trifidus* Makino. There has been some confusion as to whether this member of the Araliaceae family cross-reacts with the Japanese lacquer tree or *Fatsia japonica*. The allergen has been identified as cis-9,17-octadecadiene-12,14-diyne-1,16-diol. This is an analog of falcarinol. The apparent cross-reactions to urushiol were considered coincidental. Falcarinol is the allergen found in *Hedera helix* and *Schefflera arboricola* (115).

The allergen identified in Dendropanax has been found to be present in 7 times greater concentration than in Fatsia japonica. Two additional allergens have been found in Dendropanax trifidus: 16-hydroxy-cis-9,17-ocadecadiene-12,14-diynoic acid and cis-9,trans-16-octadecadiene-12,14-diynoic acid (116).

Phacelia Crenulata

This plant is known as the desert or false heliotrope. It blooms profusely in March and April in the desert areas of southern Utah, New Mexico, Arizona, southeastern California, and the Baja peninsula. The plant produces an eruption similar to that of poison ivy dermatitis.

Bougainvillea

This popular genus of South American origin is planted both indoors and outdoors. Localized urticaria outbreaks accompanied by some shortness of breath have been reported (117). A scratch chamber test reproduced the urticarial reaction in 20 to 30 minutes (117).

Coleus

Facial dermatitis suspected to be due to airborne contact with dried leaves of coleus has been reported (118). The allergen coleon O tested at 0.01% has been deemed a strong sensitizer (118).

Gardenia Fruit

A folk remedy known as Sokujikoh in Japan was found to contain 16% powdered gardenia fruit (*Gardenia jasminoides,* member of the Rubiaceae family), which was responsible for contact dermatitis (119). Extracts with alcohol of the pericarp and seeds were positive (119).

Centella Asiatica

This plant is known as the Indian penyworts and is an Umbelliferae. A 2% extract of *Centella asiatica* was included in a vasotonic cream that also contained neomycin, lavender, and geraniol, but the plant extract proved to be the allergen (120).

Hydrangea

There are 25 species of hydrangea, and the allergen is found in both leaf and flower (121). Hydrangenol is tested at 0.1% in petrolatum and is extractable with alcohol (122). Hydrangenol is not uniformly found throughout the 25 species (121). Generally, rubber gloves are protective (122).

Dahlia

There are three patterns of dermatitis reported among 20 patients with dahlia dermatitis. Hand dermatitis was seen in 10, hand and face in 7, and an airborne pattern in 4. The exposure was occupational in 87% of these cases (123). A 1:10 ethanol extract can be used for patch testing.

Elecampane

Crude extracts of elecampane (*Inula helenium* L.) are potent sensitizers at 1% concentration. Positive reactions to helenin 0.1% and alantolactone 0.1% were found in these cases (124).

> **Weed dermatitis may be confined to the hands, as in milker's eczema due to weed oleoresin contaminating cows or winter fodder mixed with weeds.**

> **Tulip bulb fingers may be due to trauma or an allergic reaction to a specific lactone; narcissus and hyacinths produce "bulb fingers" mostly due to irritation from calcium oxalate crystals.**

Narcissus and Hyacinths

Dermatitis from these plants may be allergic, but it is usually an irritant reaction to bundles of needle-shaped crystals of calcium oxalate in the outer layers of the bulbs. These do not occur in tulip bulbs. The outer scales of hyacinth bulbs contain about 6% calcium oxalate, and the dust on worktables has a similar concentration. The crystals penetrate the skin and cause a dermatitis resembling fiberglass dermatitis. Itching can be abolished by washing with dilute acetic acid. Hyacinth itch is thus rarely of allergic origin.

Marigold

Three potential sensitizers have been identified in marigolds (*Tagetes* sp.). Tests in guinea pigs have defined the allergenic potential of these compounds as 5-(3-buten-1-ynyl)-2,2′-bithiophene [strong], alpha-terthienyl [less strong], and hydroxytremetone [weak]. Thiophenes abundantly occur in many species of Compositae, and both phototoxic and sensitizing properties have been found (125).

Trachelium

A plant know as *Trachelium caeruleum* grows in the western Mediterranean region and is used in cut flower bouquets. It is a member of the Campanulaceae (bellflower) family and has caused allergic contact dermatitis in a male florist who had previously had contact allergy to chrysanthemum. No cross-reactivity was suspected, as the plants come from different families, and the patient's allergy developed after about 1 year of exposure to *T. caeruleum* (126).

Verbena

Anaphylactic symptoms developed in a teenage boy after contact with *Verbena hybrida.* The incident followed retrieving a ball from a garden. A 62000 Dalton allergen caused specific IgE mediated response. *Verbena elegans* 'Cleopatra' has also produced contact urticaria and delayed hypersensitivity (127).

Gerbera

Contact urticaria, conjunctivitis, and rhinitis would occur in a botanist who studied *Gerbera hybrida,* which is a member of the Asteraceae family (Compositae). Type 1 reactions to this family are rare. Prick tests and RAST were positive. Pollen gave stronger reactions than did petals or leaves (128).

Dittrichia Viscosa

Dittrichia viscosa (L.) Greuter is a member of the Compositae (Asteraceae) family, which grows in Portugal. It contains sesquiterpene lactones rather than alantolactone or isoalantolactone (129).

Miscellaneous Flowers and Shrubs

Less commonly, dermatitis venenata is produced by dichondra, magnolia, tea roses, greasewood, *Wigandia caracasana,* daffodils, poinsettias, *Ficus repens,* century plants, and Australian silk oak trees.

DERMATITIS DUE TO TREES

Colloquial, common, and trade names of commercial woods can be completely misleading; for example, Canadian hemlock is often shipped as Alaska pine. A dictionary of commercial trees lists in several languages the large number of trade names of commercial woods. No reliance can be placed on the trade name of a wood as an indication of the botanical species of the tree from which the wood is derived. Expert identification by a department of botany or by a forest products laboratory is essential for meaningful tests in suspected contact allergy from sawdust (130).

Forest workers who fell trees and cut them up can be irritated or sensitized by the wood itself, but more common is sensitivity to lichens and *Frullania* (a liverwort resembling a moss) that grows on the bark of the trees. Sensitized workers develop, during work with vegetation in forest areas, occupational allergic contact dermatitis of exposed skin surfaces, which resolves on leaving work in the forests.

Dermatitis from the solid wood of finished articles is much less common, but has followed prolonged contact with musical instruments, bracelets, or knife handles made of the strongly allergenic Dalbergia rosewoods. Furniture made of rengas or obeche can also give trouble.

Hausen (131) listed the main sensitizers in woods (see also Table 22.12). Fisher and Bikowski (132) reported allergic contact dermatitis due to a wooden cross made of *Dalbergia nigra.* A search of the available literature revealed

TABLE 22.12. *Concentrations of Essential Contact Allergens of Wood Species for Epicutaneous Tests*

Sensitizer	Timber	Concentration
Anthothecol	*Khaya anthotheca*	1
Chlorophorin	*Chlorophora excelsa*	1–10
Cordiachromes	*Cordia* and *Patagonula* species	0.1
Deoxylapachol	*Tectona grandis; Tabebuia* species	0.01–0.1
R-3,4-dimethoxydalbergione	*Machaerium* species	0.01
S-4,4′-dimethoxydalbergione	*Dalbergia* species	1
S-4′-hydroxy-4-methoxydal	*Dalbergia* species	1
2,6-dimethoxy-1,4-benzoquinone	Various wood species	10
Lapachol	*Tectona grandis; Bignoniaceae* species	1–10
"Macassar quinone"	Oxidation product of Macassar II from *Diospyros celebica*	1
Mansonone A	Mansonia altissima	0.1
Obtusaquinone	*Dalbergia retusa*	1
Oxyayanin A and B	*Distemonanthus benthamianus*	1
Thymoquinone	*Calocedrus decurrens*	0.1

that all previous reports of allergic contact dermatitis due to *Dalbergia nigra* were concerned with occupational exposure to the wood in carpenters, woodworkers, and cabinetmakers. This is apparently the first report of "nonoccupational" dermatitis from *Dalbergia nigra*. It is of interest to note that this wooden cross produced an erythema type of eruption.

Martin et al. (133) reported a case of erythema multiforme–like eruption from Brazilian rosewood in a 35-year-old carpenter who initially developed rhinitis and conjunctivitis, which was succeeded by a generalized erythema multiforme–like eruption. A patch test with the wood dust produced a positive + + + reaction at 48 hours.

Hausen and Rothenborg (134) reported a case of allergic contact dermatitis caused by olive wood jewelry. Chemical analysis revealed that the olive wood contains quinoid compounds similar to sensitizers in teakwood and East Indian rosewood. Exposure to olive wood can take place not only from wood jewelry, but also from napkin rings, knife handles, and musical instruments.

Eucalyptus

IgE-mediated contact urticaria to eucalyptus pollen without any systemic symptom has been reported (135). Eucalyptus oil has been found allergenic also. Tea-tree oil has been used as a topical medicament and produced contact dermatitis, which upon oral ingestion causes a flare of the prior dermatitis and a generalized eruption (136). Tea-tree oil contains 98.5% eucalyptol, which is 1,8-cincole, and cajapulol. This is the primary ingredient in eucalyptus oil, and as little as 3.5 g of ingested eucalyptol can be fatal (136). Tea-tree oil comes from *Melaleuca alternifolia*.

> **Allergic reactions to tropical woods may produce erythema multiforme–like eruptions.**

Trees may contain irritants or sensitizers in the bark, wood, or pollen.

Irritation Dermatitis

Sawdust and fragments of wood produced by machine tools can cause contact dermatitis. The severity depends on whether the cut fragments are hard or soft, dry or moist.

About 120 commercial woods exist that can cause contact dermatitis in sawyers, carpenters, and those who come in contact with sawdust. The hands and face are affected, together with skin folds in which dust accumulates. Involvement of the face, ears, and scalp can resemble seborrheic dermatitis or an airborne photodermatitis. Table 22.13 lists steps for testing with sawdust.

Sensitization Dermatitis to Sawdust

Sensitizing chemicals are more often found among the extractives of the heartwood and therefore affect sawyers, carpenters, joiners, polishers, and finishers exposed to fine dust. The picture is that of an airborne contact dermatitis, beginning on the dorsa of the hands and forearms, eyelids, face, and neck and rapidly involving the genitals through handling in urination. In bald men, the scalp is often affected. If the clothing gives poor protection, fine dust may

TABLE 22.13. *Steps Recommended for Patch Testing Workers Suspected of Allergy to Sawdust*

1. Obtain botanical identification if possible from the wood (not the dust).
2. Place no reliance on trade (lumber) names.
3. Patch test with dry and then with damp sawdust. (Damp sawdust may release formic acid and other irritants.)
4. It is best to patch test with freshly ground sawdust 10% in petrolatum and test controls.
5. Care must be taken not to actively sensitize workers by using allergens in too strong a concentration.

drift inside it and may affect the sweaty area of the axillae, waistband, and groin and sometimes the ankles and dorsa of the feet.

Mild cases have only erythema and slight irritation, but often there is papular or vesicular dermatitis, which may progress to chronic dermatitis, after repeated exposure. Severe fissured lichenification of the palms was described as *mains de crocodile.*

The latent period varies from a week to many years, but is most commonly 10 to 15 days. In successive attacks, the latent period becomes shorter and eczema usually increases in severity, but hardening is not unusual. Cross-reactions to other woods, or other sources of related antigens, are common.

Allergic Dermatitis

In the United States, the native woods that are cutaneous sensitizers include acacia, alder, ash, beech, birch, chestnut, cedar, elm, maple, mesquite, oak, pine, poplar, prune, and spruce. Some patch test concentrations for specific extracts are found in Table 22.12.

The major components of wood, such as cellulose and lignin, are not sensitizers, but the minor components, such as resins, terpenes, oils, phenols, formic acid, and nitrogen-containing substances, may cause allergic contact dermatitis. In addition, certain species of poplar contain a glucoside that may be a primary irritant.

Freshly cut woods are more apt to cause a dermatitis than are older woods, but Rengas wood, used in furniture making, may produce dermatitis only when it is old and begins to disintegrate.

Birch bark contains a fine powder on its inner aspect, which can produce a follicular acneiform eruption by mechanically plugging the follicles of exposed skin.

The bark of aspen trees *(Populus tremula)* was found to contain salicyl alcohol, the source of contact dermatitis in a farmer who developed the dermatitis while pruning using a chain saw (137). Synonyms for salicyl alcohol include 2-hydroxybenzyl alcohol and 2-methylolphenol. Bruze used the latter term in his work with phenol-formaldehyde resins in which cross-reactions occurred between phenol-formaldehyde resins and 2-methylolphenol. Balsam of Peru can also cross-react with this constellation of seemingly diverse allergens.

Tropical Woods

Working with tropical wood may result in inflammations of the oral mucosae and the respiratory system, as well as acute contact dermatitis, especially of the face and extremities. The condition often occurs in persons who are exposed to high concentrations of fine sawdust. Exotic woods seem to be the most sensitizing. Obeche wood may cause contact urticaria. Teak and mansonia contain sensitizing quinones.

> **Some tropical woods contain quinones, which are strong sensitizers.**

Other types of dermatitis that have been mistakenly called wood poisoning include bacterial and fungal infections, seborrheic and atopic dermatitis, and contact dermatitis from common weeds, such as poison oak. In addition, chemicals sprayed onto the wood and agents, such as chloronaphthalenes, impregnated into wood for protection may cause dermatitis.

These woods are used in musical instruments, in boat construction, in furniture, and as handles for kitchen utensils. Cocus wood, known as "green ebony" or "grenadil," is used to make flutes, recorders, and clarinets. Wood shavings can produce positive patch tests, and the allergens Cocus I and II tested at 1% in ethanol. The structure of Cocus II is not fully known, but Cocus I is 7,8-dihydroxy-2,4,5-trimethoxisoflavan (138). Clarinetists and saxophonists may develop cheilitis from cane reeds used in the instruments (139,140). A scratch or prick test is sometimes positive when patch tests are negative (140). A plastic-coated reed (Plasticover, available from Encore Music Co., Woodburn, IN 46797) is a suitable alternative for these patients (140).

Fig and rubber trees, belonging to the *Ficus* genus of plants, contain a milky sap, which is commonly called latex. Fig tree latex may produce both allergic dermatitis and photodermatitis. Rubber latex rarely sensitizes.

Latex from other trees, such as gutta percha, chicle, and balata gum, rarely cause dermatitis.

The fruit of the female ginkgo tree may produce an allergic dermatitis simulating poison ivy dermatitis. Ginkgo fruit and *Toxicodendron* contain related catechols.

Brazilian Box Tree Wood

Sources of dermatitis from this plant include "orange sticks" for manicuring and unvarnished surfaces of organs. Dermatitis appears on hands, fingers, eyelids, and face. Both irritant and allergic reactions to *Aspidosperma* sp. occur (141).

Planthymenia

The Brazilian tree *Plathymenia foliosa,* also known as vinhatico, is a member of the Leguminosae family. A carpenter exposed to the dust of this tree developed a pigmented contact dermatitis. This is not surprising, as the tree is thought to contain psoralens (142).

Tali Wood

The wood of *Erythrophleum guianense* is an irritant to nasal mucosa and can cause bradycardia, vomiting, and vertigo. A patch test to a 10% ethanol extract in petrolatum confirms contact dermatitis. This wood is used for flooring (143).

Australian Blackwood

There are 125 Australian and 3 African species of *Acacia,* and the *A. melanoxylon* R. Br. is known as the Australian blackwood. The sensitizers are 2,6-dimethoxy-1,4-benzoquinone, acamelin, and melacacidin. The latter substance occurs in all species (144).

Apuleia Leiocarpa

Carpenters at times are exposed to exotic woods and can develop airborne contact dermatitis to sawdust from these materials. Such was the case for a 42-year-old man who became allergic to *Apuleia leiocarpa* wood. This tree from Brazil is also known as tatajuba, bagasse, and crebianco giono (145).

Jelutong

Wood from the *Dyera costulata* tree in southeastern Asia is commonly known as jelutong. It is a soft wood used for carving; the sap is used for chewing gum and some medicine. This tree is from the family Apocynaceae. Contact dermatitis was found in 19% of teachers who used the wood in woodworking classes. This finding, plus guinea pig sensitization studies, confirms this material to be a potent sensitizer (146).

Milo Wood

Thespesia populnea is a tree native to Hawaii. The wood is used for carved bowls and artifacts. The tree is commonly known as milo in Hawaii and portia in California. In the Philippines, it is known as banago. The allergen in this wood is mansonone: 7-hydroxy-2,3,5,6-tetrahydro-3,6,9-triimethylnaphtho [1,8 bc] pyran-4,8-dione. It is a moderate sensitizer (147).

Sucupira Wood

Bowdichia nitida of the family Papilionaceae or Fabaceae is known as sucupira wood. Because it is very hard, it is used for railroad ties, stakes, floors, and joists. This wood contains benzoquinone, and cross-reactions with hydroquinone and primula (which contains benzoquinone) have been reported (148).

Iroko

Iroko (*Chlorophora excelsa),* also known as African teak, is a member of the Moraceae family. It was used in building a staircase and ship repair by a man who in that setting developed airborne contact dermatitis. The allergen in this wood is chlorophorin, which is an oxystilbene (149).

Iroko is also known as kambala, rokko, African oak, swamp mahogany, rock elm, West African mulberry, and bush oak. It caused dermatitis in a Swiss carpenter working as a joiner (150).

Obeche Wood

Obeche wood comes from the African whitewood or African maple (*Triplochiton scleroxylon).* It is very resistant to warping and does not get as hot as other woods; therefore, it is used to make sauna benches. In Finland, occupational asthma has frequently been traced to obeche wood. A carpenter who used obeche wood to make organs developed contact urticaria when sitting on obeche wood in saunas and occupational rhinitis. He did not develop contact urticaria from the wood unless moisture was a part of the exposure (151).

Tree Pollens

Contact dermatitis may be caused by ether-soluble portions of tree pollen oleoresin. Like ragweed oil dermatitis, tree pollen oil dermatitis is usually confined to a short season during which the pollen is airborne. The history usually reveals that the skin becomes clear after the pollination has ended and remains clear until the next season. Individuals sensitized to the oil fractions of the pollen, which produce allergic contact dermatitis, may not be sensitized to the aqueous protein fraction, which produces allergic rhinitis and asthma.

Airborne contact urticaria manifested as erythema, edema of the hands and neck, and angioedema of the lips and eyes was found to be due to mulberry (*Morus alba)* pollen rather than mulberry leaves. Prick test to the pollen extract was positive, and specific IgE to the pollen was elevated (152).

Beekeepers can acquire an allergic contact dermatitis from bee glue (propolis) derived mainly from poplar and other tree resins. This glue is also used as a local anesthetic in Russia. In Africa, it is used as a wood and leather varnish and as a base for ointments, cosmetics, and polishes.

A tree surgeon who developed dermatitis while working on poplar trees was found sensitive to a mixture of three caffeic acid pentenyl esters thought to be the major sensitizers in poplar bud resin. The individual also reacted to propolis, balsam of Peru and Tolu, wood tars, eugenol, and isoeugenol (153).

CONTACT DERMATITIS DUE TO VEGETABLES

The essential oils of the edible umbellifers carrots, parsnips, parsley, squash, asparagus, and celery (including celery salt) may cause allergic eczematous dermatitis in sensitized individuals (154). Pinene, terpineol, and cineole are probably the sensitizers. Some members of this family are also photosensitizers. Onions and garlic may cause a contact dermatitis that can cross-react with tulips and hyacinths (155).

Corn dermatitis (corn itch or corn poisoning) is an occupational eruption similar to the contact dermatitis seen in other vegetable processing or wet work with food plants (156). Excoriations often complicate the dermatitis, and occasionally secondary infection occurs. Protective gloves and barrier creams help reduce exposure. In addition, a photosensitizing dermatitis may appear in workers harvesting celery parasitized by fungi (rusts or smuts) (157).

Carrots

Klauder and Kimmich (158) described a patient with a sensitivity to carrots who developed a cheilitis and perioral dermatitis when she ate this vegetable raw or cooked.

If the oleoresin of carrots is not available for testing, patch tests may be performed with the external surface of an unpeeled raw carrot or with the surface of a slice of carrot. The reaction is usually stronger to the slice than to the outside portion. The essential oil of carrot contains pinene, terpineol, cineole, and limonene.

Celery

This plant may cause an ordinary allergic contact reaction and photocontact dermatitis. Cross-reaction may occur with the essential oil of orange, lemon, bergamot, caraway, dill, and balsams.

Wild Parsnips and Parsley

The dermatitis produced by these vegetables is usually due to photosensitization. Moisture is necessary for the reaction. Some individuals acquire the photocontact dermatitis only when they are perspiring profusely or have become wet from water (157).

Exposure to sunlight within 48 hours after the moist contact with the plants is necessary for the phototoxic reaction.

Photo patch tests with parsnip and parsley can be performed with the vegetable moistened with water and exposed to sunlight or artificial ultraviolet radiation.

Both contact urticaria and chronic urticaria have occurred from eating *Eruca sativa,* a popular salad garnish in Italy. A positive reaction was found with RAST and scratch tests but not open application to skin (159).

Squash

Butternut squash caused hand dermatitis in a 30-year-old woman who had no antecedent history of atopic dermatitis. Rechallenge with the plant *(Cucurbita moschata)* reproduced the eczematous reaction. Previous reports of squash dermatitis were due to turban or winter squash *(C. maxima)* (160).

Asparagus

Harvesting and canning of asparagus is associated with allergic contact dermatitis. The frequency of reactions is such that the condition has been called "asparagus scabies." The allergen in asparagus *(Asparagus officinalis)* has been identified as 1,2,3-trithiane-5-carboxylic acid. This is a growth inhibitor, which is present in asparagus mainly in the early part of the season (161).

TULIP BULB DERMATITIS

Alpha-methylene-gamma-butyro-lactone is the chemical cause of tulip dermatitis. This lactone, which is split off the plant glycoside, is most highly concentrated in the bulbs. Less is found in the stems, and the least in the petals. The lactone, found in members of both *Tulipa* and *Alstroemeria,* is known as Tuliposide A.

Patch tests with the pure allergen in dilutions down to 1:600 may give positive reactions in control subjects, whereas patients suffering from "tulip fingers" usually have positive reactions to a concentration of 1:20,000. Because the pure tulip allergen is not available for clinical use, patch tests can be performed with the moist, fleshy outer layers of the bulb, from which the thin outer skin has been removed. Tests in control subjects are required to exclude irritant reactions.

Tulip bulbs may cause a painful, dry, fissured, and hyperkeratotic eczema, at first underneath the free margin of the nails, then extending to the fingertips and periungual region. Dermatitis of the face, the hands and forearms, and the genital region may also occasionally occur.

Sensitivity to other bulbs, such as hyacinth *(Hyacinthus)* and daffodil *(Narcissus)* are important causes of contact dermatitis in the bulb-growing industry.

Alstroemeriaceae (Alstroemeria)

Alstroemeria (Peruvian lily), which can produce allergic contact dermatitis of the hands in floriculturalists, cross-reacts with *Tulipa;* both contain the allergen Tuliposide A. Alstroemeria dermatitis can be confined to the fingertips of workers who string the flowers on garlands (162,163).

Although *Alstroemeria* has gotten a good deal of recent attention as a cause of dermatitis among florists, a study of 164 persons working in floral shops found 46% had a rash at some time. The most commonly suspected plant was daffodil stems followed by primula, Christmas tree, and Cupressus for wreaths (164). Wholesale florists usually are reactive to chrysanthemums, tulips, and alstroemeria (165).

Dry fissured fingertips have been associated with *Alstroemeria,* garlic, tulip bulbs, and the northern India shrub

Tabernaemontana coronaria, a member of the Apocynaceae family (166).

MISCELLANEOUS PLANT FAMILIES THAT PRODUCE DERMATITIS

Alliaceae (Onion Family)

Onion *(Allium cepa)* and garlic *(A. sativum)* can produce irritant and allergic contact dermatitis on cooks' hands. The eruption tends to start on the fingertips and to be unilateral. By patch test, onion and garlic do not always co-react. The allergen may be allyl disulfide.

Capparidaceae (Caper Family) and Cruciferae (Mustard Family)

The mustard family and its tropical counterpart, the caper family, characteristically contain thioglucosides (167,168). These release isothiocyanates, which, by their irritant and vesicant action, provide the counterirritant effect of a traditional mustard plaster. In making the familiar condiment, mustard powder, the ground dry seeds of *Brassica nigra,* is wetted, thus allowing action by the plant enzyme, myrosinase, and release of isothiocyanate from its thioglucoside.

Crushed seeds of mustard have been reported to cause a dermatitis deemed irritant. The dermatitis flared 5 days after oral ingestion of mustard. One month later, patch tests were negative to commercial mustard 1:10, crushed seeds 1:1 in olive oil, and allylisothiocyanate up to 1% in ethanol. At this point, oral ingestion was asymptomatic (169).

Familiar members of these families are *Capparis* (the pickled flower buds form capers), horseradish *(Armoracia),* cress *(Lepidium),* cabbage, brussels sprouts, cauliflower and broccoli *(Brassica* species), and nasturtium *(Tropaeolum);* the pickled seeds of the last can form a poor man's caper.

A compress of leaves and fruit of capers *(Capparis spinosa)* resulted in a dermatitis detected by patch tests to the leaf and fruit as is, mustard oil 1% and 0.1% in petrolatum, allyl isothiocyanate 0.1% and 0.05% in petrolatum, and benzyl isothiocyanate 0.1% in petrolatum. Other isothiocyanate plants were negative (170).

The radish *(Raphanus)* is not only pungent and irritant but also sensitizing, and it is likely that the pronounced irritant effects of isothiocyanates have obscured their allergenic potential.

Allyl and benzyl isothiocyanates present in mustard oils are usually primary irritants that produce vesiculation. Occasionally, however, they may also be sensitizers. These chemicals can be tested at a concentration of 0.05% in petrolatum.

The botanical sources of allyl isothiocyanate and benzyl isothiocyanate are as follows: 1) *Allyl isothiocyanate:* wild garlic, madwort, horseradish, winter cress, mustard greens, black mustard, (root) cabbage, kohlrabi, kale, brussels sprouts, cauliflower, broccoli, sea rocket, shepherd's purse, sea kale, and white wall rocket). *Benzyl isothiocyante:* blister cress, rocket, candytuft, charlock, wild mustard, hedge mustard, penny cress, wild garlic, bitter cress, wart cress, garden cress, cow cress, pepper grass, and mignonette nasturtium of gardens.

Primrose Family

Primin, 2-methoxy-6-*n*-pentyl-*p*-benzoquinone, is the major allergen of primrose dermatitis. A patch test concentration of 0.01% primin in petrolatum was evaluated in 3,075 patients. Of this group, 1.8% were positive, and only two patients were sensitized by the patch test itself. There was an active primin dermatitis present at the time of testing in 41% of those who tested positive (171). Allergy to primin was rarely found in patients under age 35 (171).

Primrose dermatitis is common in Europe. Although the plant is not supposed to grow in the United States, the late Dr. Neils Hjorth in a personal communication stated that he had seen plenty of primrose in California. The allergen content of the plants varies considerably, depending on the season, the number of hours of sunshine, the method of cultivation, and the horticultural variety. Patch testing with the leaf may be unreliable because of these variations, which result in false-negative patch test reactions, especially during winter. Therefore, an extract of *Primula obconica* is preferable for routine patch testing (172,173).

Several other plants and woods containing allergenic quinones show cross-reactivity with primin, particularly rosewood extract (50).

> **The primrose family of plants, originally thought to be unique to Europe, has been found in California.**

Chenopodiaceae (Spinach Family)

Russian thistle *(Salsola kali)* is a widespread weed native to Russia but a common and troublesome pest in arid regions of the United States, where it can cause "tumbleweed dermatitis." The spines of the plant by mechanical injury produce a papular eruption and contact urticaria.

Powell and Smith (174) reported that Russian thistle *(Salsola kali),* the most common plant referred to as "tumbleweed" in the western United States, can cause a dermatitis in persons who come into direct contact with it. Tests were conducted to determine the mechanism of this dermatitis. Mechanical contact with plant branches, as well as scratch, patch, and photopatch tests with Russian thistle extract and scratch tests with 1.5% potassium nitrate, a plant constituent, was used. The tests, along with transparent adhesive tape preparations and a skin biopsy, showed that in nonsensitized persons, dermatitis was due only to mechanical irritation of plant floral bracts. In sensitized individuals, Russian thistle floral bracts pierced the skin and stimulated a urticarial reaction.

Cannabidaceae (Hemp Family)

Hops *(Humulus lupulus)* are used to flavor beer. Hop pickers' dermatitis is an affliction of seasonal workers who pick the female inflorescence (hop cone), which is aromatic with hop oil and sticky with resin containing humulone and lupulone. These chemicals may be the sensitizers. The dermatitis affects the dorsa of hands, forearm flexures, and face. Possibly 1 in 30 pickers are affected, but the incidence is difficult to determine because of the casual workforce. The milder cases may clear or become "hardened," but the more severe ones tend to get worse; some quit the casual work without coming to medical attention.

Tobacco (*Nicotiana Tabacum*)

The green and yellow cured tobacco leaf, but not nicotine or pesticide, caused contact dermatitis in a 40-year-old female seasonal tobacco plantation worker. One percent ether, acetone, and alcohol extracts in petrolatum were all positive (175).

Cactaceae (Cactus Family)

In addition to the obvious and injurious spines of cacti, the hobbyist may encounter tufts of short, fuzzy, barbed bristles, or glochids, five to eight on each of the 25 to 30 areolae per opuntia (cactus) leaf. The glochids have barbs that prevent their ready extraction once in the skin.

The glochids of *Opuntia lingularis* (cholla) cause immediate pain on entering the skin. Erythema and swelling develop in 72 hours and subside after 1 to 3 days, only if the glochids are removed. Retained glochids produce papules and plaques, sometimes like granuloma annulare, with a central punctum and bristle. It may take 3 to 4 months for these changes to resolve once the bristles have been rejected, and during extrusion the epidermis may become warty.

Allergic reactions consisting of flesh-colored, domed papules, 2 to 4 mm in diameter, each with a central black dot, can occur on the limbs, usually in groups of 3 to 6, and last for 2 to 8 months. Skin tests with glochid extracts have given positive responses.

O. ficus indica, prickly pear or sabra of North America, Mexico, and the Mediterranean region, causes dermatitis in workers who pick, distribute, and sell the fruit. Vacationers in the Mediterranean have also been affected. The glochids break off readily, get into the clothes, and cause sabra dermatitis, a pruritic papulovesicular eruption that looks rather like scabies. To remove glochids, depilatory wax or adhesive tape can be applied to the skin and pulled off.

Cactus spines, when embedded in the skin and not readily visible at the surface, can cause deep injuries, such as pseudotumors of bone.

> **Prickly pear or sabra dermatitis, caused by the broken glochids of cacti, may resemble scabies.**

Agave Americana

The century plant derives its name from the legend that it flowers only once every one hundred years. Although this is not true, the *Agave americana* produces contact dermatitis more often than that. It is highly irritating and contains sapogenins, hecogenins, oxalic acid, and calcium oxalate crystals (176).

Araceae (Arum Family)

Plants of the Arum family are grown mainly as houseplants, some as outdoor plants in warm areas for their attractive foliage. The plant tissues contain sharp, stinging calcium oxalate crystals, which are irritant to the lips and tongue. Acute cheilitis, stomatitis, and glossitis can occur in those, usually children, who chew the stems of dieffenbachia and monstera. Some other chemicals besides the crystals, and as yet unidentified, probably play a part.

The common houseplant philodendron is a sensitizer for nursery workers and hobbyists; the allergen is an alkyl-resorcinol similar to those of Proteaceae and with phytochemical affinities to the allergenic catechols of Anacardiaceae. Co-reaction of the genus *Philodendron* and *Toxicodendron*, however, has not been reported. Contact may be accidental during watering the plant or result from plucking or polishing the leaves. Hobbyists are exposed far less than nursery workers, as they water the plant with greater care and handle it less. Dermatitis from *P. scandens* and related species resembles mild poison ivy reactions with streaky, blotchy vesicular erythema on the hands and forearms, less often on the abdomen and lower limbs. The eyelids may be affected alone, or as part of widespread dermatitis.

> **Philodendron dermatitis may resemble that of poison ivy.**

Hammershoy and Verdich (177) reported allergic contact dermatitis due to *P. scadens*. In four patients with dermatitis, allergy to philodendron was found through patch testing with leaves, stems, and ether extracts from eight philodendron species. Although this allergy appears to be rare, it ought to be considered in patients with dermatitis on hands, arms, and face.

Scindapsus aureus is a popular indoor climber in Scandinavia despite its needle-like hairs; biting the stem causes intense irritation, and the plant is also allergenic. Reactions from it as a garden plant are known in Hawaii (178).

> **In Florida, *Scindapsus*, colloquially named hunter's robe and taro vine, is a cause of dermatitis in nursery workers.**

The roots of some Arum contain a starchy material that is edible if boiled or otherwise treated to destroy irritant calcium oxalate crystals. The starch from the tubers of *Arum maculatum* (cuckoo pint, wake robin, and lords-and-ladies) forms arrowroot, which is made into biscuits. In Elizabethan times, the starch of this species used to stiffen ruffs irritated the hands of laundresses. In 1713, Ramazzini, the father of occupational medicine, described gangrene of the genitals of an apothecary who contacted another arum *(A. arisarum)*. Many others, perhaps most of the 2,000 species in the plant family, have irritant properties. The clinical history obtained in cases of dermatitis will suggest immediate irritancy rather than a delayed allergic effect. For example, in Venezuela, laborers cutting *Montrichardia arborescens* with a machete develop erythema instantly on contact with the sap. The erythema fades in 24 to 72 hours.

Araliaceae (Ivy Family)

Hedera (ivy), the best known genus, is popular as a houseplant or as ground cover in the garden. Algerian or Canary Island ivy *(H. canariensis)* causes more dermatitis than English ivy *(H. helix)*, possibly because it grows faster and requires more cutting back. Like poison ivy, the plant parts of ivy must be bruised to release the allergenic sap. The clinical picture of Hedera dermatitis resembles that from poison ivy but tends to be seasonal, corresponding to the time of pruning. Co-reaction with schefflera *(Brassaia)*, a botanically related and popular houseplant, has been reported.

Hydrophyllaceae (Phacelia)

Reynolds et al. (179) stated that dermatitis due to *Phacelia crenulata*, or desert heliotrope, is quite common, with dermatitis frequently seen on the ankles and legs of persons walking in the desert during the spring blooms. Desert heliotrope grows during the spring months throughout the arid southwestern United States (California, Arizona, southern Utah, and southern Nevada) and is commonly found along the sand and gravel of desert highways and roadsides.

The major contact allergen of *P. crenulata* (Hydrophyllaceae) has been identified as geranylhydroquinone. A maximization test of geranylhydroquinone showed this to be a potent sensitizer comparable in degree to poison oak/ivy urushiol. Comparative patch testing on humans with urushiol established that the phacelia allergen does not cross-react with poison oak or ivy.

> **The potent contact allergen of the desert heliotrope is a hydroquinone that does not cross-react with poison ivy.**

Aspidiaceae (Fern Family)

Considering the wide use of ferns as houseplants, dermatitis from them is rare. Leatherleaf fern *(Arachnoides adiantiformis)*, used as a background for floral arrangements, caused dermatitis on the palms and fingers of a florist. An allergen, present only during sporogenesis, has been isolated, but not identified (180). Sporogenesis refers to the time when spore capsules are present on the under surface of the leaves.

Nursery workers are exposed to many plants, but de Cock et al. (181) were able to trace the source of dermatitis in a 23-year-old woman to contact with ferns. The specific plant was *Pteris ensiformis* 'Evergemiensis.' This fern is a member of the Pteridaceae family. Unlike previous fern allergy that required spores to be present, in this case the plant was allergenic without spores.

Euphorbiacae *(Croton, Codiaeum Variegatum)*

There were several reports of allergic contact dermatitis to this plant family. Tafelkruyer and van Ketel (182) described a male flower grower with hyperkeratotic eczema localized to the tips of the thumb and index finger and onycholysis of these nails. The unknown sensitizer seems to be soluble in water but not in alcohol.

Codiaeum is often called croton by growers. The genus *Croton* and the genus *Codiaeum* are members of the large Euphorbiaceae family.

Codiaeum variegatum is not to be confused with *Croton tiglium*, from which croton oil is derived. Croton oil, which is a brownish-yellow oil expressed from the seeds of *Croton tiglium*, is a violent purgative and irritant.

Hausen and Schulz (183) reported that one of the most decorative and popular ornamental potted plants is croton. Eczema of the hands developed in a nursery gardener who handled this plant for a period of 6 months. Patch tests with croton leaves gave positive results. Control test results remained negative. Sensitization experiments in guinea pigs with a methanolic extract of the leaves were successful.

The results of the study indicate that the latex of croton produces no primary irritant reaction and the latex is able to induce contact allergy. Further experiments are being continued in an attempt to isolate irritant and allergenic factors from the latex of various Euphorbiaceae species. Many plants of this family, particularly the genus *Euphorbea*, are irritant, having a milky sap that is injurious to the skin and the eye.

Grass

Allergy to grasses is commonly associated with repiratory allergy, but Wong et al. (184) found that military personnel who complained of grass allergy could have either immediate or delayed hypersensitivity. Of 23 patients, 2 were prick test positive and 3 were patch test positive to grass *(Axonopus compressus)*. The authors pointed out that Bermuda grass *(Cynodon dactylon)* and crab grass *(Digitaria sanguinalis)* have also caused contact dermatitis.

Intolerance of grass was the subject of a study of patients in Singapore (185). Of the 46 patients with this complaint, 11% were confirmed to have a positive patch test to one of five grasses: carpet grass *(Axonopus compressus)*, seashore centipede grass *(Ischaemem muticum)*, lalang *(Imperata cylindrica)*, Guinea grass *(Panicum maximum)*, or elephant grass *(Pennisetum purpureum)*.

Fungicide Dermatitis

The fungicide Plondrel can cause dermatitis that appears to be caused by the plant, because positive patch tests may be obtained with leaves that still contain traces of the fungicide (186).

> **Plant fungicides may cause dermatitis that can be mistaken for dermatitis due to the plants.**

CLINICAL AND BOTANICAL INVESTIGATION

When the dermatologist or the patient suspects that a plant is causing contact dermatitis, samples must be obtained of all the plants to which exposure may have occurred. Flowers and leaves of all the suspected plants should be brought in by the patient and stored temporarily in a refrigerator in the physician's office. The patient should be warned that he or she must be thorough and bring samples of all plants, including those considered "weeds."

The plants selected for the first set of patch tests should be those recognized as causing dermatitis. If these first tests are negative, tests with the remaining plants should be carried out. In some instances, repeated search may be required before the offending plant is detected. An absolute necessity is botanical identification of the plants used for testing. Sources of information are listed in Table 22.14. It is fruitless and misleading to look up the common or colloquial name of the plant in any book. An expert identification of the suspected plants by a plant taxonomist is essential.

Speed is also essential in identifying a suspected plant. Wasted time leads to lack of interest by patient and physi-

TABLE 22.14. *Sources for Botanical Identification of Plants Suspected of Causing Contact Dermatitis*

Botanical gardens
Botanist (plant taxonomist if possible) at national, state, or private herbarium or high school
County agricultural agents and soil conservation agents (U.S. Department of Agriculture)
Department of Botany at a university
Curator of herbarium

cian, and important information may be lost by delay. Each case is a minor or even a major research exercise. The suspected offending plant should promptly be divided into three approximately equal portions. One portion for botanical identification should be dried or stored in the freezer. The second and third portions should be stored in a freezer, one portion for patch test purposes and the other for possible later chemical studies.

An interested patient available for patch testing, the suspected plants reliably identified, and the samples safely frozen in three portions provide the opportunity for a significant and rewarding investigation. Armed with the names of the plants, one can turn to the literature.

Avoidance of Testing Irritant Plants

It is useless to patch test with irritant plants; some plant families, such as the Euphorbiaceae (spurge) family, contain mostly irritant plants. A partial list of irritant plant families appears in Table 22.15.

> **Irritant plants give false-positive patch test reactions and can cause not only irritant dermatitis but also stomatitis when chewed.**

Patch Testing with Plants

The steps to be carried out are summarized in Table 22.16.

There is no point in patch testing with the known irritant plants shown in Table 22.17. If irritancy seems possible, it is necessary to patch test with caution. In all cases, patch

TABLE 22.15. *Botanical Families that Contain Many Irritant Plants[a]*

Family	Genus
Araceae	Dieffenbachia
Capparidaceae (caper)	*Capparis* (Cleopatra's needle)
Cruciferae (mustard)	*Brassica* (mustard)
Euphorbiaceae (spurge)	*Euphorbia* (spurge)
Ranunculaceae (buttercup)	*Ranunculus* (buttercup)
	Clematis (pasqueflower)
	Anemone (windflower)

[a]Plants of the genera noted are often irritant.

TABLE 22.16. *Steps for Preserving Plants for Patch Testing*

Recommended steps for patch testing with a plant:
1. Divide the plant into three parts. Air dry or freeze one part and keep for botanical identification (flowers needed).
   Label, date, source, geographic site obtained.
   Put two parts into freezer:
   a. For patch testing
   b. For making extract dilutions and for chemical studies
2. Patch test with leaf, flowerhead, stalk, and petal.
   Tests in control individuals are essential.

tests to plants in a patient suspected to be allergic should be accompanied by control patch tests in at least 5, preferably 20, volunteer subjects. The literature abounds with invalid reports in which alleged allergenic plants have not received the simple, but crucial, tests for irritancy in controls. No plant can be considered proven allergenic unless tests are negative in a substantial number of controls.

The actual plants to which the patient was exposed should be used for patch testing. Rarely is it possible to use dried herbarium specimens of identified species for this purpose.

> A "positive" plant patch test reaction must be checked on several controls.

To prepare a plant for patch testing, leaves and petals should be lightly crushed, and stalks and thick leaves should be cut into thin slices. Having established the allergenicity of a plant by suitable patch testing and by the use of controls, one can proceed to test more thoroughly with various parts of the plant root, stalk, leaf, flower head, and other parts of the flower. Controls are required for each part tested because the parts of a plant often vary in their chemical composition. Hausen recommends a 60-second dip in either as an all-purpose extraction procedure for plant allergens, notably sesquiterpene lactones from plant hairs.

Several methods of making plant allergens for patch testing have been suggested. The 60- to 90-second dip in diethyl ether provides for an adequate extraction. This is evaporated to dryness and resuspended in either petrolatum or acetone in a concentration of 1% to 10%. Some prefer to

TABLE 22.17. *Irritant Hairy Plants*

Many plants of Borage family, *Borago*, etc.
Cortusa—relative of *Primula*
Begonia rex and hybrids
Sparmannia (indoor linden) (this plant is also allergenic)
Ulmus (elm)
Cornus sanguinea (blood-twig dogwood)—T-shaped hairs
Nettles—*Urtica*

use acetone for the extraction. Alternatively, a 1-hour patch test can be performed (187).

Role of Age of Plants

Often, mature plants are more allergenic than immature plants. With age, secondary products of metabolism accumulate in plants because they have little or no excretory mechanisms. Therefore, mature plants should be used for patch testing. Some provisional evidence suggests that immature plants of *Asparagus* (asparagus) and *Chicorium* (chicory) may be more allergenic than flowering specimens. If this is the case, these plants are exceptions to the rule noted previously. These plants are commonly used for commercial and culinary purposes when in a state of immaturity; therefore, maximum exposure occurs to immature rather than to mature plants. Until this aspect is clarified, it is probably best to use mature plants for patch testing.

Timing and Site of Patch Tests

If plant dermatitis is suspected clinically but no clear lead is provided by the history, it may be useful to limit screening patch testing to plants within these commonly offending families; otherwise, patch tests with innocuous but popular plants may continue to be performed.

One should wait until acute dermatitis has subsided before patch testing, in order to avoid the risk of provoking a focal or disseminated flare. The skin site selected for patch testing should be clear of dermatitis for at least 2 weeks, preferably 1 month, before such testing is carried out—hence the usefulness of freezing plants. The irritant plant *Ranunculus* (buttercup) becomes more irritant after freezing; as the tissues are rewarmed, the cells burst and enzyme action releases an irritant compound, protoanemonin. Dried buttercups are hardly irritant at all, because protoanemonin is converted into an innocuous polymer, anemonin. There is no firm evidence that plant allergens are made innocuous by freezing. False-positive reactions can result from testing during status eczematicus—the so-called angry back. The back is more sensitive than are the extremities. Confusion may occur from discoloration of the skin at the test site by the presence in a plant of a red dye that simulates an erythema. An irritant patch test reaction can never be reliably distinguished from an allergic patch test reaction on morphologic grounds alone.

Patch Testing with Bulbs

The bulbs of the tulip *(Tulipa)*, hyacinth *(Hyacinthus)*, and daffodil *(Narcissus)* are important causes of contact dermatitis in the bulb-growing industry. The problem is well known to the growers, but cases are rarely seen by a dermatologist. For patch testing, the thin dried outer scale of the bulb should be removed. The moist fleshy outer layers of the bulb, which are actually leaves modified to storage, should be used for patch testing. Tests on control subjects are required to exclude irritancy.

Patch Testing with Hairy Plants

Patch testing with hairy plants can produce irritant patch test reactions. Some irritant, hairy plants are listed in Table 22.17. Indoor linden *(Sparmannia)* can produce irritant patch test reactions and is also probably allergenic. Thus, judicious patch testing with the plant and its extracts is required. The T-shaped hairs of blood-twig dogwood *(Cornus sanguinea)* produce urticarial reactions if the leaf is rubbed on the skin in the direction of its long axis. Some other commonly grown hairy plants produce irritant patch test reactions from their leaves (for example, cineraria *(Senecio),* primrose *(Primula sinensis),* and fig *(Ficus macrophylla).*

Photopatch Testing

Phytophotodermatitis is caused by a photochemical reaction mediated by psoralens and possibly by other plant chemicals. No allergic mechanism is implicated, and any individual exposed adequately to the plant juices and then to sunlight will react. Skin tests are meaningless if the suspected plant is known to contain psoralens, but they may be of interest if such information is lacking in the world literature and facilities for photochemical studies are not available. The tests can be carried out on any volunteer to avoid inconveniencing the patient, who is often a child.

Purification and Identification of Plant Allergens

Purification and identification of plant allergens have been accomplished only in a few instances. The method used has been summarized by Benezra (188). To carry an investigation this far is a major research exercise.

Some plants are irritant and allergenic. When such plants are suspect, it is necessary to use plant extracts, diluted to a nonirritant level for patch testing. This complex but not unimportant problem is summarized in Table 22.18.

TABLE 22.18. *Patch Testing with Irritant, Suspected Allergenic Plants*

Patch testing with an irritant but suspected allergenic plant:
1. Make 20% aqueous extract. Allergen of *Allium* (garlic), for example, is water soluble.
2. Use 10% ethanol extract. Most plant allergens are soluble in organic solvents.
3. Patch test the patient and controls.
4. If negative, try 20% or more to find a nonirritant, allergenic concentration. A variety of organic solvents can be tried.

Control Tests

Regarding controls, synthetic primin, the allergenic quinone of *Primula obconica,* provides a useful example. Concentration 1:100 is always irritant; 1:1,000 is often irritant; 1:10,000 produces active sensitization (sensitization by patch testing); 1:50,000 elicits positive reactions only in sensitized individuals. The allergen of *Tulipa* (tulip) (alpha-methylene-γ-butyrolactone) is irritant at a concentration 1:600 but produces positive patch test reactions in sensitized persons 1:20,000. An overriding consideration is that the concentrations should *not* be great enough to cause active sensitization. Twenty-five microliter pipettes may be used for applying the fluid extracts. The test response depends on the amount of allergen deposited per surface area and not on the total dose.

The patch test unit to be used requires consideration. The A1 test patches have a 1-cm circular cellulose disc. Plant chemicals in solution may be retained in the interstices of the cellulose disc. False-negative reactions can be produced. It is preferable to apply the solution to the skin, to await evaporation, then to occlude the site.

DERMATITIS DUE TO SPICES

At least 60 spices, with their essential oils, are in use. Six of these are of particular interest to the dermatologist because they produce allergic contact dermatitis.

In the United States, the five spices that most commonly produce dermatitis are capsicum, cinnamon, cloves, nutmeg, and vanilla. In Europe, laurel is apparently the most common cause.

All these spices can produce flares at the healed sites of allergic contact dermatitis when they are ingested or inhaled. In addition, spices may produce urticaria when ingested with foods or drink or when inhaled.

Spices have been used in perfumes, cosmetics, and topical medications.

Highly seasoned foods were known to cause rosacea, particularly rhinophyma, a fact immortalized in the following poem more than three and a half centuries ago (189):

> Nose, nose, nose, nose!
> And who gave thee this jolly red nose!
> Nutmeg, and ginger, cinnamon and cloves,
> And they gave me this jolly red nose

All the spices contain essential oils, which can irritate the skin in concentrated form. The dust that forms when spices are ground produces an irritant dermatitis mechanically as well as chemically. Many of the essential oils also are sensitizers (190). Spice allergy may be underdiagnosed, because 47% of patients reacting to standard substances like colophony, balsam of Peru, fragrance mix, and/or wood tars also reacted to one or more spices (paprika, cinnamon, laurel, celery seed, nutmeg, coriander, cacao, or garlic) (190). In this study, powdered spices were moistened with a bit of water. Of those reacting to spices, 28% were to nutmeg, 19% to paprika, and 12% to clove (191).

Many spices, particularly mustard and capsicum, can irritate the mucous membranes of the eyes and respiratory passages. The oleoresin of capsicum is such an efficient lacrimator that it is employed in the United States as tear gas (192,193).

Cayenne Pepper (*Capsicum Frutescens*)

This pepper, from which the oleoresin of capsicum is extracted, is distributed worldwide. One patient was recently studied who had an acute eczematous dermatitis on one side of the neck after being playfully sprayed with an aerosol containing the oleoresin of capsicum at a New Year's Eve party. One year before this episode, the patient had a stiff neck and applied Capsolin Rubefacient, which contains oleoresin of capsicum, camphor, oil of turpentine, and oil of cajeput (a pungent oil from an East Indian myrtle tree). Patch tests revealed a maximal reaction to capsicum and negative reactions to the other ingredients.

On two occasions, the dermatitis of the neck flared after the ingestion of pickles that had been flavored with capsicum. Ginger ale and liqueurs flavored with capsicum can produce similar eczematous contact dermatitis in sensitized individuals (194).

The oleoresin of capsicum is a powerful irritant, which may be used as a tear gas.

Cinnamon and Cassia

There has been a confusion between cinnamon and cassia. When we order cinnamon toast, we should, to be correct, ask for cassia toast, because cassia has almost entirely replaced cinnamon as a spice in the United States.

In Great Britain, the word "cinnamon" applies only to *Cinnamomum zeylanicum* and cassia to *C. cassia*. In the United States, the Food, Drug and Cosmetic Act of 1938 officially permitted the word "cinnamon" to be used for both *C. zeylanicum* and *C. cassia,* as well as other species of cassia. The nomenclature in various countries is listed in Table 22.19.

Cinnamon is the bark of the cinnamon or cassia tree. The flavor is derived from oil of cinnamon, which contains cinnamic aldehyde and eugenol. Oil of cinnamon is used mainly for flavoring food, toothpaste, chewing gum, tobacco, aperitifs and bitters, and cola beverages. Because of its sensitizing properties, it is used for perfumes only to a limited extent, and always in low concentrations.

Occupational dermatitis from oil of cinnamon may occur in bakers and candy makers, but cinnamon dermatitis has also been observed among cooks and homemakers (195). Oil of cinnamon has further been reported as the cause of allergic dermatitis from ammoniated toothpaste (196), bubble gum, and lipstick. Sensitization to balsam of Peru may result in a high degree of cross-sensitivity to oil of cinnamon (53). Ingestion of oil of cinnamon may produce an eczematous contact type of flare-up in individuals previously sensitized by contact with the oils (197).

Nutmeg and Mace

The nutmeg tree, *Myristica fragrans,* produces two closely related but separate spices, nutmeg and mace. The terms for nutmeg in different countries are listed in Table 22.19.

The essential oils of nutmeg and mace contain myristicin, which is highly toxic and a powerful narcotic. The fatty oils of nutmeg are used in the manufacture of soap and perfumes and may be the cause of allergic dermatitis. Blends of mace and nutmeg are used extensively for flavoring foods. Bakers may acquire allergic dermatitis from handling these spices. Pure nutmeg oil contains eugenol, isogenol, safrole, myristicin, elemicin, and limonene (198). Nutmeg oil has been found to inhibit prostaglandin synthesis due to its eugenol content (198).

Connecticut is known as the "Nutmeg State." This nickname resulted from the ingenuity of Connecticut Yankee peddlers of the early nineteenth century who were charged with the sale of wooden imitation nutmegs as the genuine article to unsuspecting housewives.

TABLE 22.19. *Cinnamon, Cassia, and Nutmeg Terminology in Various Languages*

	Cinnamon	Cassia	Nutmeg
Spanish	Canela	Canella de la China	Nuez Moscada
French	Cannelle	Cannelle de Cochinchine	Muscade
German	Zimt	Zimtkassie	Muskatnuss
Swedish	Kanel	Kassia	Nuskot
Arabic	Qurfa	Darasini	Babbasa
Dutch	Kaneel	Kassia	Notemuskaat
Italian	Cannella	Cassia	Noce Moscata
Portuguese	Canela	(none known)	Noz-Moscada
Russian	Koritsa	(none known)	Oryekh Muskatny
Japanese	Seitron-Nikkei	Bokei	Nikuzuku
Chinese	Jou-Kuei (or Jou-Kwei)	Kuei (or Kwei)	Jou-Tou-K'ou

When the word "mace" is mentioned in the United States, most dermatologists think of chemical Mace, referring to a tear gas. The term is an acronym derived from the chemicals involved—*M*ethylchloroform chlor*ACE*tophenone (199). Chemical Mace is a potent sensitizer and, of course, is unrelated to mace, the spice.

For patch test purposes, capsicum and mace are tested in a 1% alcoholic solution.

Cloves

The word "clove" *(Syzgium aromaticum)* is derived from the French *clou,* referring to the flower bud of the tree.

Oil of clove is rich in essential oils, particularly eugenol, which are widely used in perfumes, soaps, toothpastes, and mouthwashes.

Eugenol is a pale yellow liquid with a strong smell of carnation used in zinc oxide-eugenol dental cement. It may also be combined with rosin and zinc oxide. It is the essential chemical constituent of clove oil and is also present in cinnamon oil, perfumes, soaps, and bay rum. Individuals sensitized to eugenol should avoid exposure to such products. Eugenol is both a primary irritant and a sensitizer, and for patch testing a 10% solution in olive oil or a 5% solution in petrolatum is used.

Eugenol, one of the main constituents of oil of bay, may show cross-reactions with balsam of Peru. Sometimes oil of cloves and of cinnamon are added to bay rum. Both oils are sensitizers, and cinnamon oil may cross-react with eugenol and balsam of Peru. Eugenol, when used in dental preparations, such as impression pastes, surgical packings, temporary fillings, and cements, may produce stomatitis venenata and allergic eczematous eruptions in dental personnel (200).

Oil of cloves incorporated into a liniment has been reported as a cause of allergic dermatitis (201,202). The mucilage of postage stamps may also contain clove oil, and cause glossitis in persons who lick the stamps. Clove oil may be patch tested with a 1% alcoholic solution.

Individuals sensitized to oil of cloves or eugenol may have to avoid ingestion of foods containing the spice or the essential oil in order to avoid a flare of dermatitis. Indians use cloves to flavor the betel nut; the English use oil of cloves in apple tarts; the French love onion soup with cloves. In the United States, cloves are frequently used with pork.

Vanilla and Vanillin

Vanilla is a flavoring extract made from the pod of the vanilla plant. Vanillin is a crystalline compound, which is the fragrant constituent of vanilla. The vanilla bean is the dried and fermented fruit of an orchid, *Vanilla planifolia.* Vanillin, a benzaldehyde, is formed from glycosides, such as glucovanillyl alcohol and glucoconiferyl alcohol, the latter being converted into glucovanillin, glucose, and vanillin.

Contact dermatitis due to vanilla occurs in individuals used in the cultivation, trade, or industrial use of vanilla. One variety of vanilla dermatitis is a pseudophytodermatitis caused by mites, living on vanilla pods, of the same species as meal mites *(Tyroglyphus farinae),* which produce an eruption of urticarial papules, called vanilla lichen (203), on exposed parts of the body. Vanillism, an allergic contact dermatitis acquired by workers handling the vanilla plant, produces marked edema and erythema. Rhinitis, asthma, and vertigo may accompany the eruption.

Synthetic vanillin can be produced from pine tree sap, eugenol, wood pulp, sugar, and coal tar. The U.S. Food and Drug Administration requires that the term "imitation vanilla" appear on the label if the product contains synthetic ingredients. If the label has the term "vanilla extract," the product must be derived from vanilla beans. Some individuals are sensitized to synthetic vanillin and not to the natural spice, and vice versa (190).

An unusual source of exposure to vanillin is smoking certain types of tobacco. For patch test purposes, a 10% alcoholic extract of vanilla in acetone can be used. Vanillin may be tested 10% in petrolatum.

Laurel

The bay tree, *Laurus nobilis,* also known as sweet bay, is native to the Mediterranean region and Asia Minor. This bay tree is not related to the West Indian bay tree *Pimenta acris,* leaves of which are distilled to produce bay rum.

Laurel oil is used in medicine and in the textile and soap industries. Laurel leaves are used in cooking because of their flavoring and antioxidant properties. They are also used in meat and fish preservation, pickled gherkins, condensed soups, and spiced sauces.

The bactericidal properties of laurel oil have been known for a long time in Germany and made use of in an ointment for abscesses. In France, laurel oil is used in only one Codex listed product (Fioravanti balsam) and in the commercial product Vegebom. Fioravanti spirit, which is also called turpentine spirit mixture, contains 0.4% of *L. nobilis* berries, 20% of larch tree turpentine, and other products. Among the Vegebom preparations, only the ointment, the suppositories, and an adhesive for prosthetic dentistry (Dental Vegebom) include appreciable quantities of laurel oil (1.2% in the ointment).

Laurel oil is often used in the textile industry to improve the luster of felt hats. In the store, the hatband becomes contaminated when the hats are stacked and produces hatband dermatitis in the wearer.

In the United States, dermatitis from laurel is apparently rare. Sensitization to laurel is not uncommon, however, in Europe. Most cases have been observed in Germany, Switzerland, and France (204).

In Germany, sensitization occurs from the use of laurel in the felt industry. In France and Switzerland, the source of exposure is ointments containing the oil of laurel (Vegebom ointment).

Cosmetics and food may also be sources of exposure. It is surprising to learn that in Strasbourg, laurel oil is a more common sensitizer than nickel or mercury.

In the United States, bay leaves are practically never used for medicinal purposes; consequently, sensitization from topical exposure is eliminated. Bay leaves are used to season some dishes, particularly bean soup. Bay leaves are popular in French cuisine for flavoring meats, fish, poultry, vegetables, and stews. It is conceivable that such extensive use may have sensitized some individuals.

Patch tests with laurel oil may be performed with a 2% concentration in petrolatum or with a 5% solution of essential oil in alcohol.

Laurel, rarely implicated in the United States, is a common sensitizer in Germany, Switzerland, and France.

Additional Foods Capable of Producing Contact Dermatitis

A dry, often fissured, fingertip dermatitis is most frequently associated with garlic. Of 155 persons tested to a slice of fresh garlic, 8 reacted (205). Additional patch tests to garlic powder as is, 2% and 5% diallyl disulfide in petrolatum, ethanol (2%), and aqueous (10%) were conducted, and five of five women with an irritant-appearing dermatitis were positive to all of the tests confirming diallyl disulfide as an allergen and the utility of any of the materials for test purposes. Inasmuch as fresh garlic under a Finn chamber patch test unit causes irritant reactions (206), the powder would give more reliable results.

Lettuce

Gosta Krook of Malmo, Sweden (personal communication), reported a gardener with a dermatitis of his hands, face, arms, and legs from contact with lettuce. During the winter, when he did not work with lettuce, he did not develop dermatitis. Positive patch tests were obtained to the lettuce stalk and leaf.

Rinkel and Balyeat (207) also reported a patient with contact dermatitis due to lettuce.

Closson (208) described a patient with oral mucosal edema and swelling of the eustachian tubes due to the ingestion of lettuce.

Two patients with a gardening hobby became sensitized to sesquiterpene lactones in weeds and flowers. Ingestion of lettuce caused a flare of the patients' dermatitis and burning of the mouth. Extracts of lettuce and chicory were positive

at 10% in petroleum, and these are known to be sources of sesquiterpene lactones (209).

Kiwifruit

Cheilitis, pruritus, and burning tongue with accompanying swelling was seen within minutes of eating kiwifruit (*Actinidia chinensis*). The pulp gave a positive scratch test, but application to intact skin was negative (210).

Mushrooms

The mushroom *Agaricus bisporus* caused an occupational hand eczema in a mushroom picker. Patch tests to the cap with spores as well as the stem were positive in the patient and negative in 25 controls (211). The second most commonly produced mushroom in the world is the shiitake (*Lentinus edodes*) (212). The hyphae have been the source of allergic contact dermatitis among growers, and in guinea pig maximization testing, the shiitake mushroom is a moderate sensitizer (213). A dermatitis has been described after ingestion of shiitake mushrooms. Small 1-mm papules widely disseminated occur and may be accompanied by petechia from scratching. The Koebner phenomenon may be seen. One to 2 days after eating half-baked raw shiitake, the trunk exhibits the majority of the rash, followed by the face and head. The duration ranges from 2 to 14 days and averages 8 days. The overall picture suggests a mobilliform pattern not unlike a drug eruption (212). There are no gastrointestinal, central nervous system, or mucosal symptoms. Patch and intracutaneous tests are not helpful, and complete boiling of the mushrooms seems to eliminate the potential for dermatitis (212).

Pleurotus ostreatus is a commercially cultivated mushroom in the order Agaricales and family Tricholomataceae. It can cause contact dermatitis in those who harvest the mushroom. Other mushrooms reported to cause contact dermatitis are *Lentinus edodes, Suillus, Agaricus, Boletus,* and *Ramaria flava* (214).

Mushroom pickers are at risk for occupational contact dermatitis to shiitake mushroom (*Lentinus edodes*), white mushrooms (*Agaricus hortensis*), brown mushrooms (*Agaricus bisporus*), yellow boletus (*Boletus luteus*), finger mushrooms (*Clavaria flava*), orange agaric mushroom (*Lactarius deliciosus*), and *Suillus* and *Pleurotus ostreatus* (215).

Chamomile

Oil of chamomile is found in herbal remedies often used by lactating women for treatment of nipple eczema. A 0.1% in petrolatum concentration is adequate for patch tests purposes. There are both German and Roman sources, and they come from different genera. The German source is *Matricaria recutita* and the Roman source *Chamalmelum nobile*. Both are in the Compositae (Asteraceae) family, and the

Roman product appears more allergenic (216). The ingestion of chamomile tea can exacerbate contact dermatitis from chamomile (216).

MISCELLANEOUS FOOD DERMATITIS

Mango

Contact dermatitis can be caused by the oleoresin of the mango tree sap or the skin of the fruit. Patients who are sensitized to poison ivy may acquire an allergenic cheilitis from eating mango, which contains a catechol related to that of poison ivy.

Dang and Bell (217) reported an anaphylactic reaction to the ingestion of mango.

Litchi

Litchi or lichee or lychee *(Litchi chinensis)* is a fruit that has caused generalized urticaria, angioedema, and bronchospasm after ingestion. Positive prick tests to the mesocarp

TABLE 22.20. *Botanical Glossary*

Common name	Genus, species	Family
Alstroemeria	*Alstroemeria aurantiaca*	Alstromeriaceae
Anemone	*Anemone* sp	Ranunculaceae
Angelica	*Angelica silvestris*	Umbelliferae
Angelica (garden)	*Angelica archangelica*	Umbelliferae
Arnica	*Arnica montana*	Compositae
Asparagus	*Asparagus officinalis*	Liliaceae
Burdock	*Arctium minus*	Compositae
Buttercup	*Ranunculus* sp	Ranunculaceae
Cabbage	*Brassica oleracea*	Cruciferae
Camomile, chamomile	*Matricaria chamomilla*	Compositae
Caper	*Capparis decidua*	Capparidaceae
Carrot	*Daucus carota*	Umbelliferae
Cashew nut tree	*Anacardium occidentale*	Anacardiaceae
Cauliflower	*Brassica oleracea botrytis*	Cruciferae
Celery	*Apium graveolens*	Umbelliferae
Chicory	*Cichorium intybus*	Compositae
Chrysanthemum of florists	*Chrysanthemum hortorum*	Compositae
Clematis	*Clematis* sp	Ranunculaceae
Congress weed	*Parthenium hysterophorus*	Compositae
Costus	*Saussurea lappa*	Compositae
Daffodil	See *Narcissus*	
Dock	*Rumex* sp	Polygonaceae
Endive	*Cichorium endivia*	Compositae
False ragweed	*Franseria* sp	Compositae
Feverfew	*Parthenium hysterophorus*	Compositae
Field chamomile	*Anthemis arvensis*	Compositae
Fig tree	*Ficus carica*	Moraceae
Frullania	*Frullania nisqualensis*	Jubulaceae
Garden cress	*Lepidium sativum*	Cruciferae
Gas plant, fraxinella	*Dictamnus albus*	Rutaceae
Gingko (ginkyo) tree	*Ginkgo biloba*	Ginkyoaceae
Horseradish	*Armoracia rusticana*	Cruciferae
Ivy, Algerian	*Hedera canariensis*	Araliaceae
Ivy, English	*Hedera helix*	Araliaceae
Jonquil	See *Narcissus*	
Laurel oil	*Laurus nobilis*	Lauraceae
Mango	*Mangifera indica*	Anacardiaceae
Maple	*Acer* sp	Aceraceae
Marsh elder	*Iva* sp	Compositae
Milfoil, Yarrow	*Achillea millefolium*	Compositae
Mugwort	*Artemisia* sp	Compositae
Mustard	*Brassica nigra, Sinapsis alba*	Cruciferae
Narcissus	*Narcissus* sp	Amaryllidaceae
Nettle	*Urtica* sp	Urticaceae
Norway spruce	*Picea excelsa*	Pinaceae
Ox-eye daisy	*Chrysanthemum leucanthemum*	Compositae
Parsley	*Petroselinum sativum*	Umbelliferae

Used with permission. Mitchell JC. Plant dermatitis in Vancouver. *Can J Dermatol* 1993;5:389.

and epicarp were obtained in a 34-year-old woman who exhibited these symptoms. Additionally, a positive patch test was found to the epicarp. The patient also reacted to mango, which is in the Anacardiaceae family. Both litchi and mango are in the order Sapindales (218).

Pineapple

Pineapple juice contains bromelin, a proteolytic enzyme that can cause a primary irritant dermatitis (219). The enzyme causes separation of the superficial layers of the skin and increases skin and capillary permeability. These effects resemble the mechanical damage produced by needle-shaped calcium oxalate crystals of tulip bulbs. Both the enzyme and the crystals produce itching and increased permeability of capillaries with the formation of wheals, which are suggestive of histamine liberation in the skin.

Coffee

Lupton (220) described a persistent cheilitis due to coffee. In this instance, the coffee produced a positive patch test reaction on the skin.

Malt Flour

Calnan (221) studied a 19-year-old woman who was working as a research assistant in an experimental test bakery. Once a week she used a malt flour. Patch tests were positive to malt flour on two occasions. Six control subjects were negative.

Calnan stated that cases of dermatitis from grain and flour are difficult to evaluate and quoted personal communications from Solomons, who described reactions to barley and oats, and from Malten, who described reactions to bran, maize, barley, vitamins, and beet pulp.

Hjorth (222) suggested that chefs and kitchen workers with dermatitis should be patch tested not only with the standard patch tests but also with the following foods: garlic, onions (various kinds), chives, leek, carrot, cucumber, horseradish, lemon peel, endive, lettuce, asparagus, and artichoke. Cinnamon might also be added to this list.

BOTANICAL NOMENCLATURE

Common names are used in this chapter, but this usage has limitations, particularly in countries where the common names vary. To assist the reader with the proper scientific names, the glossary developed by John Mitchell is provided in Table 22.20 (223).

REFERENCES

1. Rook A. Plant dermatitis in general practice. *Practitioner* 1962; 188:627.
2. Fisher AA. *Contact dermatitis,* 3rd ed. Philadelphia: Lea & Febiger, 1986.
3. Goldstein N. The ubiquitous urushiols—contact dermatitis from mango, poison ivy, and other "poison" plants. *Cutis* 1968;6:679.
4. Kullavanijaya P, Ophaswongse S. A study of dermatitis in the lacquerware industry. *Contact Dermatitis* 1997;36:244.
5. Rademaker M, Duffill MB. *Toxicodendron succedaneum* (Rhus tree), New Zealand's poison ivy. *Contact Dermatitis* 1995;33:357.
6. Ale SI, Ferreira F, Gonzalez G, Epstein W. Allergic contact dermatitis caused by *Lithraea molleoides* and *Lithraea brasiliensis:* identification and characterization of the responsible allergens. *Am J Contact Dermatitis* 1997;8:144.
7. Kawai K, et al. Heat treatment of Japanese lacquerware renders it hypoallergenic. *Contact Dermatitis* 1992;27:244.
8. Kawai K, et al. Tetrahydrourushiol glycoside, o-mono-glycosylated hydrourushiol, can be used for the investigation of contact allergy as a water-soluble urushiol. *Contact Dermatitis* 1994;31:59.
9. Farmer's Bulletin No. 2158, *Chemical control of brush and trees.* Washington, DC: US Department of Agriculture, US Government Printing Office.
10. Orchard S, Fellman JH, Storrs FJ. Poison ivy/oak dermatitis use of polyamine salts of a linolein acid dimer for topical prophylaxis. *Arch Dermatol* 1986;122:783.
11. Grevelink SA, Olsen EA. Efficacy of barrier creams in suppression of experimentally induced Rhus dermatitis. *Am J Contact Dermatitis* 1991;2:69.
12. Marks JG Jr, Fowler JF Jr, Sheretz EF, Rietschel RL. Prevention of poison ivy and poison oak allergic contact dermatitis by quaternium-18 bentonite. *J Am Acad Dermatol* 1995;33:212.
13. Gillis WT. Poison-ivy and its kin. *Arnoldia* 1975;35:93.
14. Guin JD. The black spot test for recognizing poison ivy and related species. *J Am Acad Dermatol* 1980;2:332.
15. Mallory SB, Miller OF, III, Tyler WB. Toxicodendron radicans dermatitis with black lacquer deposit on the skin. *J Am Acad Dermatol* 1982;6:363.
16. Kligman AM. Poison ivy (*Rhus*) dermatitis. *Arch Dermatol* 1974; 90:535.
17. Gillis WT. Systematics and ecology of poison ivy and the poison oaks (Toxicodendron, Anacardiaceae). *Rhodora* 1971;73:72.
18. Shankar DSK. Contact urticaria induced by *Semecarpus anacardium. Contact Dermatitis* 1992;26:200.
19. Fisher AA. Poison ivy—the poison "Rhus" plants. *Cutis* 1966;2:316.
20. Epstein WL, Byers VS, Frankart W. Induction of antigen specific hyposensitization to poison oak in sensitized adults. *Arch Dermatol* 1982;118:630.
21. Cooley GR. The vegetation of Sanibel Island, Lee County, Florida. *Rhodora* 1955;57:268.
22. Farmer's Bulletin No. 1972, *Poison ivy, poison oak and poison sumac.* Washington, DC: US Department of Agriculture, US Government Printing Office, 1976.
23. Devich KB, et al. Renal lesions accompanying poison oak dermatitis. *Clin Nephrol* 1975;3:106.
24. Block SH. Rhus hyposensitization dermatitis. *JAMA* 1973;224:627.
25. Kawai K, et al. Hyposensitization to urishiol among Japanese lacquer craftsmen: results of patch test on students learning the art of lacquerware. *Contact Dermatitis* 1991;25:290.
26. Kawai K, et al. Hyposensitization to urishiol among Japanese lacquer craftsmen. *Contact Dermatitis* 1991;24:146.
27. Reginella RF, Fairfield JC, Marks JG, Jr. Hyposensitization to poison ivy after working in a cashew nut shell oil processing factory. *Contact Dermatitis* 1989;20:274.
28. Blumhardt R, Pappano JE, Moyer DG. Depression of poison ivy skin tests by measles vaccine. *JAMA* 1968;206:27.
29. Becker LE, Skipworth GB. Ginkgo tree dermatitis, stomatitis and proctitis. *JAMA* 1975;231:1162.
30. Mitchell JC, Rook AJ. Diagnosis of contact dermatitis from plants. *Int J Dermatol* 1977;16:257.
31. Fisher AA. The notorious poison ivy family of Anacardiaceae plants. *Cutis* 1977;20:570.
32. Morton JF. Brazilian pepper—its impact on people, animals and the environment. *Economic Botany* 1978;32:353.
33. Hurtado I, et al. Studies on the skin-sensitizing properties of the "pepeo" tree, *Mauria puberula* (Anacardiaceae). *J Am Acad Dermatol* 1982;7:341.
34. Mitchell JC, Dupuis G. Allergic contact dermatitis from sesquiterpenoids of the Compositae family of plants. *Br J Dermatol* 1971;84:139.

35. Mitchell JC, et al. Allergic contact dermatitis from ragweeds (*Ambrosia* species): the role of sesquiterpene lactones. *Arch Dermatol* 1971;104:73.

36. Hausen BM. A simple method of isolating parthenolide from *Tanacetum* and other sensitizing plants. *Contact Dermatitis* 1991; 24:153.

37. Fitzgerald DA, English JSC. Compositae dermatitis presenting as hand eczema. *Contact Dermatitis* 1992;27:256.

38. Ducombs G, et al. Patch testing with the "sesquiterpene lactone mix": a marker for contact allergy to Compositae and other sesquiterpene-lactone-containing plants. A multicentre study of the EECDRG. *Contact Dermatitis* 1990;22:249.

39. Hausen BM, et al. Peroxyachifolid and other new sensitizing sesquiterpene lactones from yarrow (*Achillae millefolium* L., Compositae). *Contact Dermatitis* 1991;24:274.

40. Lovell CR, Rowan M. Dandelion dermatitis. *Contact Dermatitis* 1991;25:185.

41. Pipker C, et al. Cross-reactivity with *Tagetes* in *Arnica* contact eczema. *Contact Dermatitis* 1992;26:217.

42. Wrangsjo K, Ros AM, Walhlberg JE. Contact allergy to Compositae plants in patients with summer-exacerbated dermatitis. *Contact Dermatitis* 1990;22:148.

43. Mitchell JC. Allergy to *Frullania*. *Arch Dermatol* 1969;100:46.

44. Calnan CD. Dermatitis from cedar wood pencils. *Trans St John Hosp Derm Soc* 1972;58:43.

45. Rook A. Plant dermatitis: the significance of variety-specific sensitization. *Br J Dermatol* 1961;73:283.

46. Curtis GH. Plant dermatitis. *Va Med Monthly* 1960;87:301.

47. Bleumink E, et al. Allergic contact dermatitis to garlic. *Br J Dermatol* 1972;87:6.

48. Cairns RJ. Plant dermatoses. *Trans St John Hosp Derm Soc* 1964; 59:137.

49. Kligman AM. Poison ivy *(Rhus)* dermatitis. *Arch Dermatol* 1958; 77:149.

50. Hjorth N, Fregert S, Schildknecht H. Cross-sensitization between synthetic primin and related quinones. *Acta Derm Venereol* (Stockh) 1969;49:552.

51. Puglisi V. Dermatoses caused by lemons. *Gior Ital Derm e Sif* 1951; 92:239.

52. Pirila V., et al. Chemical nature of eczematogens in oils of turpentine: pattern of sensitivity to different terpenes. *Dermatologica* 1969; 139;183.

53. Hjorth N. *Eczematous allergy to balsams: allied perfumes and flavoring agents.* Copenhagen: Munksgaard, 1961:134.

54. Fisher AA. The clinical significance of patch test reactions to balsam of Peru. *Cutis* 1976;13:910.

55. Hjorth N. Allergy to balsams. *Spectrum* 1971;8:97.

56. Pirila V. Endogenic contact eczema. *Allerg Asthma* 1970;16:1.

57. Veine NK. Systemically induced eczema in adults. *Acta Derma Venereol* [Suppl] 1989;147:9.

58. Jordan WP. Resorcinol monobenzoate, steering wheels, Peruvian balsam. *Arch Dermatol* 1973;108:278.

59. Jordan WP, Dahl MV. Contact dermatitis from cellulose ester plastics. *Arch Dermatol* 1972;105:880.

60. Karlberg A-T, et al. Maleopimaric acid—a potent sensitizer in modified rosin. *Contact Dermatitis* 1990;22:193.

61. Mitchell J, Rook A. *Botanical dermatology.* Vancouver: Greengrass, 1979.

62. Malten KE, Nater JP, van Ketel WG. *Patch testing guidelines.* Amsterdam: Dekker and van de Veg Nijmegen, 1976.

63. Ehrin E, Karlberg AT. Detection of rosin (colophony) components in technical products using an HPLC technique. *Contact Dermatitis* 1990;23:359.

64. Agrup G. Hand eczema and other hand dermatoses in South Sweden. *Acta Derm Venereol* (Stockh) 1969;49:1.

65. Kirk J. Colophony collar dermatitis. *Contact Dermatitis* 1976;2: 294.

66. Fregert S. Colophony in cutting oil and in soap water used as cutting fluid. *Contact Dermatitis* 1979;5:52.

67. Adams RM. *Occupational contact dermatitis.* Philadelphia: JB Lippincott Co, 1969.

68. Wilkinson DS, Calnan CD. Rosin used for belt-drive machine. *Contact Dermatitis* 1975;1:64.

69. Satyawan I, Oranje AP, van Joost T. Perioral dermatitis in a child due to rosin in chewing gum. *Contact Dermatitis* 1990;22:182.

70. Wahlberg JE. Abietic add and colophony. *Contact Dermatitis* 1979; 4:55.

71. Cronin E, Calnan CD. Allergy to hydroabietic alcohol in adhesive tape. *Contact Dermatitis* 1978;4:57.

72. Dooms-Goossens A, Degreef H, Luytens E. Dihydroabietyl alcohol (abitol): a sensitizer in mascara. *Contact Dermatitis* 1979;5:350.

73. Rapaport MJ. Sensitization to Abitol. *Contact Dermatitis* 1980;6: 137.

74. Rasmussen JE, Fisher AA. Allergic contact dermatitis to a salicylic acid plaster. *Contact Dermatitis* 1976;2:237.

75. Fisher AA. Allergic contact termatitis in a violinist: the role of abietic acid sensitizer in rosin (colophony) as the causative agent. *Cutis* 1981;27:466.

76. Widstron L. Contact allergy to colophony in soldering flux. *Contact Dermatitis* 1983;9:205.

77. Bergmark G, Meding B. Allergic contact dermatitis from newsprint paper. *Contact Dermatitis* 1983;9:330.

78. Dahlquist I. Contact allergy to colophony and formaldehyde from sandcores. *Contact Dermatitis* 1981;7:167.

79. Fisher AA. Some plant chemicals that produce allergic reactions. *Cutis* 1977;20:441.

80. Fisher AA. Some immunologic phenomena in treatment of and patch testing for ragweed oil dermatitis. *J Invest Dermatol* 1952;19:271.

81. Hjorth N, Roed-Petersen J, Thomsen K. Airborne contact dermatitis from Compositae oleoresins simulating photodermatitis. *Br J Dermatol* 1976;95:613.

82. Green C, Ferguson J. Sesquiterpene lactone mix is not an adequate screen for Compositae allergy. *Contact Dermatitis* 1994;31:151.

83. Howell JB. Contact dermatitis from weeds: facts and fallacies. *Contact Dermatitis* 1979;4:365.

84. Grater WC. Hypersensitivity dermatitis from American weeds, other than poison ivy. *Ann Allergy* 1975;35:159.

85. Burry NJ, Kuchel R, Reid KJ. Australian bush dermatitis: Compositae dermatitis in South Australia. *Med J Aust* 1973;1:110.

86. Crounse RG. Plant dermatitis due to the Compositae (Asteraceae) family. *J Am Acad Dermatol* 1980;2:417.

87. Arlette J, Mitchell JC. Compositae dermatitis: current aspects. *Contact Dermatitis* 1981;7:129.

88. Frain-Bell W, Johnson BE. Contact allergic sensitivity to plants and the photosensitivity dermatitis and actinic reticuloid syndrome. *Br J Dermatol* 1979;101:503.

89. Rietschel RL. Selected highlights of the European *Contact Dermatitis* Society meeting: Brussels, Belgium, October 8–10, 1992. *Am J Contact Dermatitis* 1993;4:66.

90. Mitchell JC, Calnan CD. Scourge of India: Parthenium dermatitis. *Int J Dermatol* 1978;17:303.

91. Lonkar A, Mitchell JC, Calnan CD. Allergic contact dermatitis from *Parthenium hysterophorus*. *Trans St John Hosp Derm Soc* 1974; 60:43.

92. Shelmire B. Contact dermatitis from vegetation. *South Med J* 1940; 33:338.

93. Rodriguez E, et al. Role of sesquiterpene lactones in contact sensitivity to some North and South American species of feverfew (Parthenium-Compositae). *Contact Dermatitis* 177;3:155.

94. Hausen BM. Allergy to parthenium, occupational and environmental dermatoses. *Dermatosen* 1978;26:115.

95. Fisher AA. Contact dermatitis due to American parthenium weed in India. *Cutis* 1979;23:20.

96. Mitchell JC. Parthenium pollen—parthenium dermatitis. *Contact Dermatitis* 1981;7:212.

97. Fisher AA. Safety of pyrethrin insecticides in ragweed sensitive patients. *Contact Dermatitis* 1978;22:141.

98. Feinberg SM. Pyrethrum sensitization—its importance and relation to pollen allergy. *JAMA* 1934;102:1557.

99. Mitchell JC, Dupuis G, Towers GHN. Allergic contact dermatitis from pyrethrum (*Chrysanthemum* spp). *Br J Dermatol* 1972;86:568.

100. Head SW. The quantitative determination of pyrethrins in gas-liquid chromatography. *Pyrethrum Post* 1966;8:3.

101. Hausen BM, Schulz KH. Experimental studies on the identification of chrysanthemum allergens. *Contact Dermatitis* 1975;4:244.

102. Mitchell JC, Schofield WB, Singh B, Towers GHN. Allergy to *Frullania*: allergic contact dermatitis occurring in forest workers caused by exposure to *Frullania nisquallensis*. *Arch Dermatol* 1969;100:46.

103. Storrs FJ, Mitchell JC, Rasmussen JE. Contact hypersensitivity to liverwort and the Compositae family of plants. *Cutis* 1976;18:681.

104. Tomb RR. Patch testing with *Frullania* during a 10-year period: hazards and complications. *Contact Dermatitis* 1992;26:220.

105. Bancons F. *L'Allergie au frullania: son role dans la "dermite du bois de chene."* Bordeaux, France: Thesis, 1967.

106. Salo H, Hannuksela M, Hausen B. Lichen picker's dermatitis [*Cladonia alpestris* (L.) Rab.]. *Contact Dermatitis* 1981;7:9.

107. Edwards EK Jr, Edwards EK Sr. Immediate and delayed hypersensitivity to the nettle plant. *Contact Dermatitis* 1992;27:264.

108. Camm EL, Gowers GHN, Mitchell JC. Ultraviolet-mediated antibiotic activity of some Compositae species. *Phytochemistry* 1975;14:2007.

109. Ashwood-Smith MJ, et al. Photosensitivity from harvesting lovage (*Levisticum officinale*). *Contact Dermatitis* 1992;26:356.

110. Ena P, Camarda I. Phytophotodermatitis from *Ruta corsica*. *Contact Dermatitis* 1990;22:63.

111. Ingber A. Primula photodermatitis in Israel. *Contact Dermatitis* 1991;25:265.

112. Knight TE, Boll P, Epstein WL, Prasad AK. Resorcinols and catachols: a clinical study of cross-sensitivity. *Am J Contact Dermatitis* 1996;7:138.

113. Julian CG, Bowers PW. The nature and distribution of daffodil pickers' rash. *Contact Dermatitis* 1997;37:259.

114. Giannattasio M, et al. Contact dermatitis from *Tetrapanax papyriferum* trichomes. *Contact Dermatitis* 1996;35:106.

115. Oka K, Saito F, Yasuhara T, Sugimoto A. The major allergen of *Dendropanax trifidus* Makino. *Contact Dermatitis* 1997;36:252.

116. Oka K, Saito F, Yasuhara T, Sugimoto A. The allergens of *Dendropanax trifidus* Makino and *Fatsia japonica* Decne. et Planch. and evaluation of cross-reactions with other plants of the Araliaceae family. *Contact Dermatitis* 1999;40:209.

117. Fisher T. Bougainvillaea contact urticaria. *Contact Dermatitis* 1991;24:376.

118. van Hecke E, et al. Airborne contact dermatitis from coleus in a housewife. *Contact Dermatitis* 1991;25:128.

119. Kubo Y, Nonaka S, Yoshida H. Allergic contact dermatitis from gardenia fruit. *Contact Dermatitis* 1990;22:65.

120. Izu R, et al. Allergic contact dermatitis from cream containing *Centella asiatica* extract. *Contact Dermatitis* 1992;26:192.

121. Kuligowski ME, Chang A, Leemreize JHM. Allergic contact hand dermatitis from hydrangea: report of a 10th case. *Contact Dermatitis* 1992;26:269.

122. Meijer P, Coenraads PJ, Hausen BM. Allergic contact dermatitis from hydrangea [Comments]. *Contact Dermatitis* 1990;23:59.

123. Sharma SC, Kaur S. Contact dermatitis from *Dahlia pinnata*. *Contact Dermatitis* 1990;23:204.

124. Aberer W, Hausen BM. Active sensitization to elecampane by patch testing with a crude plant extract. *Contact Dermatitis* 1990;22:53.

125. Hausen BM, Helmke B. Butenylbithiophene, alpha-terthienyl and hydroxytremetone as contact allergens in cultivars of marigold (*Tagetes* sp.). *Contact Dermatitis* 1995;33:33.

126. van Baar HMJ, van der Valk PGM. Contact allergy due to *Trachelium caeruleum*. *Contact Dermatitis* 1994;31:118.

127. Potter PC, et al. Immediate and delayed contact hypersensitivity to verbena plants. *Contact Dermatitis* 1995;33:343.

128. Estlander T, Kanerva L, Tupasela O, Jolanki R. Occupational contact urticaria and Type 1 sensitization caused by gerbera. *Contact Dermatitis* 1998;38:118.

129. Estrela F, Tapadinhas C, Pereira F. Allergic contact dermatitis from *Dittrichia viscosa* (L.) Greuter. *Contact Dermatitis* 1995;32:108.

130. Woods B, Calnan CD. Toxic woods. *Br J Dermatol* 1976;94(Suppl 13):3.

131. Hausen BM. *Woods injurious to human health.* New York: Walter deGruyter, 1981.

132. Fisher AA, Bikowski J, Jr. Allergic contact dermatitis due to a wooden cross made of Dalbergia Nigra. *Contact Dermatitis* 1081;7:45.

133. Martin P, Bergoend H, Piette F. Erythema multiformelike eruption from Brazilian rosewood. Barcelona: 5th International Symposium on Contact Dermatitis, March 28, 1980.

134. Hausen BM, Rothenborg HW. Allergic contact dermatitis caused by olive wood jewelry. *Arch Dermatol* 1981;11:732.

135. Vidal C, Cabeza N. Contact urticaria due to eucalyptus pollen. *Contact Dermatitis* 1992;26:265.

136. de Groot AC, Weyland JW. Systemic contact dermatitis from tea-tree oil. *Contact Dermatitis* 1992;27:279.

137. Jolanki R, et al. Contact allergy to salicyl alcohol in aspen bark. *Contact Dermatitis* 1997;37:304.

138. Hausen BM, Bruhn G, Koenig WA. New hydroxyisoflavans as contact sensitizers in cocus wood *Brya ebenus* DC (Fabaceae). *Contact Dermatitis* 1991;25:149.

139. van der Wegen-Keijser MH, Bruynzeel DP. Allergy to cane reed in a saxophonist. *Contact Dermatitis* 1991;25:268.

140. McFadden JP, Ingram MJ, Rycroft RJ. Contact allergy to cane reed in a clarinetist. *Contact Dermatitis* 1992;27:117.

141. Jemec GB, Hausen BM. Contact dermatitis from Brazilian box tree wood (*Aspidosperma* sp.) *Contact Dermatitis* 1991;25:58.

142. Pires MC, Manoel Silva dos Reis V, Mitelmann R, Moreira F. Pigmented contact dermatitis due to *Plathymenia foliosa* dust. *Contact Dermatitis* 1999;40:339.

143. Gamboa PM, et al. Allergic contact dermatitis from tali (missanda) wood (*Erythrophleum guianense*). *Contact Dermatitis* 1991;24:309.

144. Hausen BM, Bruhn G, Tilsley DA. Contact allergy to Australian blackwood (*Acacia melanoxylon* R. Br.): isolation and identification of new hydroxyflavan sensitizers. *Contact Dermatitis* 1990;23:33.

145. Dejobert Y, Martin P, Bergoend H. Airborne contact dermatitis from *Apuleia leiocarpa* wood. *Contact Dermatitis* 1995;32:242.

146. Meding B, Karlberg A-T, Ahman M. Wood dust from jelutong (*Dyera costulata*) causes contact dermatitis. *Contact Dermatitis* 1996;34:349.

147. Hausen BM, Knight TE, Milbrodt M. *Thespesia populnea* dermatitis. *Am J Contact Dermatitis* 1997;8:225.

148. Gonçalo S. Allergic contact dermatitis from *Bowdichia nitida* (sucupira) wood. *Contact Dermatitis* 1992;26:205.

149. Stingeni L, Mariotti M, Lisi P. Airborne allergic contact dermatitis from iroko (*Chlorophora excelsa*). *Contact Dermatitis* 1998;38:287.

150. Hinnen U, Willa-Craps C, Elsner P. Allergic contact dermatitis from iroko and pine wood dust. *Contact Dermatitis* 1995;33:428.

151. Kanerva L, Tuppurainen M, Keskinen H. Contact urticaria caused by obeche wood (*Triplochiton scleroxylon*). *Contact Dermatitis* 1998;38:170.

152. Munoz FJ, et al. Airborne contact urticaria due to mulberry (*Morus alba*) pollen. *Contact Dermatitis* 1995;32:61.

153. Oliwiecki S, Beck MH, Hausen BM. Occupational allergic contact dermatitis from caffeates in poplar bud resin in a tree surgeon. *Contact Dermatitis* 1992;27:127.

154. Gougerot H, Carteaud A. *Les dermatoses professionelles.* Paris: Norbert Maloine, 1952.

155. Burks JW. Classic aspects of onion and garlic dermatitis in housewives. *Ann Allerg* 1954;12:592.

156. Seligman EI, Key MM. Corn dermatitis. *Arch Dermatol* 1968;97:664.

157. Somner RG, Jillson OF. Phytophotodermatits (solar dermatitis from plants) gas plant and wild parsnip. *N Engl J Med* 1967;276:1484.

158. Klauder JV, Kimmich J. Sensitization to carrots. *Arch Dermatol* 1956;74:149.

159. Pigatto PD, et al. Ig-E-mediated contact and generalized urticaria from *Eruca sativa*. *Contact Dermatitis* 1991;25:191.

160. Potter TS, Hashimoto K. Butternut squash (*Cucurbita moschata*) dermatitis. *Contact Dermatitis* 1994;30:123.

161. Hausen BM, Wolf C. 1,2,3-trithiane-5-carboxylic acid, a first contact allergen from *Asparagus officinalis* (Liliaceae). *Am J Contact Dermatitis* 1996;7:41.

162. Van Ketel WG, Mijnssen GAWV, Nerring H. Contact eczema from *Alstroemeria*. *Contact Dermatitis* 1975;1:323.

163. Mijnssen GAWV. Pathogenesis and causative agent of "tulip finger." *Br J Dermatol* 1969;81:737.

164. Merrick C, et al. A survey of skin problems in floristry. *Contact Dermatitis* 1991;24:306.

165. Hausen BM, Oestmann G. Untersuchungen über die Häufigkert berufsbedingter allergischer Hauter-Krangen auf einen Blumengrossmarkt. *Dermatosen* 1988;36:117.

166. Bajaj AK, et al. *Tabernaemontana coronaria* causing fingertip dermatitis. *Contact Dermatitis* 1996;35:104.

167. Mitchell JC. Contact dermatitis from plants of the caper family, Capparidaceae—effects on the skin of some plants which yield isothiocyanates. *Br J Dermatol* 1974;91:13.

168. Mitchell JC, Jordan WP. Allergic contact dermatitis from the radish, *Raphanus sativus*. *Br J Dermatol* 1974;91:183.

169. Kohl PK, Frosch PJ. Irritant contact dermatitis induced by a mustard compress. *Contact Dermatitis* 1990;23:189.

170. Angelini G, et al. Allergic contact dermatitis from *Capparis spinosa* L. applied as wet compresses. *Contact Dermatitis* 1991;24:382.

171. Ingber A, Menné T. Primin standard patch testing: 5 years' experience. *Contact Dermatitis* 1990;23:15.

172. Fregert S, Hjorth N, Schultz KH. Patch testing with synthetic primin in persons sensitive to *Primula obconica. Arch Dermatol* 1968;98:144.

173. Agrup G, et al. Routine patch testing with ether extract of *Primula obconica. Br J Dermatol* 1968;80:497.

174. Powell RF, Smith EB. Tumbleweed dermatitis. *Arch Dermatol* 1978;114:751.

175. Gonçalo M, Couto J, Gonçalo S. Allergic contact dermatitis from *Nicotiana tabacum. Contact Dermatitis* 1990;22:188.

176. Brazzelli V, Romano E, Balduzzi A, Borroni G. Acute irritant contact dermatitis from *Agave americana* L. *Contact Dermatitis* 1995;33:60.

177. Hammershoy O, Verdich J. Allergic contact dermatitis from *Philodendron scandens* Koch et Sello subsp. oxycardium (Schott) bunting ("Philodendron scandens cordatum"). *Contact Dermatitis* 1980;6:95.

178. Mitchell JC, Rook A. Scindapsus dermatitis. *Contact Dermatitis* 1976;2:125.

179. Reynolds G, et al. A potent contact allergen of *Phacelia* (Hydrophyllaceae). *Contact Dermatitis* 1980;6:272.

180. Hausen BM, Schulz KH. Occupational allergic contact dermatitis due to leatherleaf fern *Arachnoides adiantiformis* (Forst) Tindale. *Br J Dermatol* 1978;98:325.

181. de Cock PAJJM, Vorwerk H, Bruynzeel DP. Hand dermatitis caused by ferns. *Contact Dermatitis* 1998;39:324.

182. Tafelkruver J, van Ketel WG. Sensitivity to *Codiaeum variegatum. Contact Dermatitis* 1976;2:288.

183. Hausen BM, Schulz KH. Occupational contact dermatitis due to Croton (Codiaeum variegatum [1] A. Juss var. pictum [Lodd] Muell Arg.): sensitization by plants of the Euphorbiaceae. *Contact Dermatitis* 1977;3:289.

184. Wong WK, Ng SK, Goh CL. Grass allergy among national servicemen in Singapore: a preliminary report. *Contact Dermatitis* 1994;30:108.

185. Koh D, et al. Allergic contact dermatitis from grass. *Contact Dermatitis* 1997;37:32.

186. van Ketel WG. Allergic contact dermatitis from a new pesticide. *Contact Dermatitis* 1975;1:297.

187. Guin J. Patch testing to plants: some practical aspects of what has become an esoteric area of contact dermatitis. *Am J Contact Dermatitis* 1995;6:232.

188. Benezra C. Allergänes vegetaux. Mëthodes chimiques d'isolement et d'identification. *Rev Fr Allergol* 1973;13:51.

189. Rosengarten F. *The book of spices.* Wynnewood, PA: Livingston Publishing Co, 1969.

190. Schwartz I, Tulipan L, Birmingham DJ. *Occupational diseases of the skin,* 2nd ed. Philadelphia: Lea & Febiger, 1957.

191. van den Akker TW, Roesyanto-Mahadi ID, van Toorenenbergen AW, van Joot T. Contact allergy to spices. *Contact Dermatitis* 1990;22:267.

192. Fisher AA. Dermatitis due to tear gases (lacrimators). *Derm Int* 1970;9:91.

193. Gleason MN, et al. *Clinical toxicology of commercial products,* 3rd ed. Baltimore: Williams & Wilkins, 1969.

194. Ormsby OS, Montgomery H. *Diseases of the skin,* 8th ed. Philadelphia: Lea & Febiger, 1954.

195. Kern AB. Contact dermatitis from cinnamon. *Arch Dermatol* 1960;87:599.

196. Leifer W. Contact dermatitis due to cinnamon. *Arch Dermatol* 1951;64:52.

197. Fisher AA. Systemic eczematous "contact-type" dermatitis medicamentosa. *Ann Allergy* 1966;24:415.

198. Rasheed A, et al. Eugenol and prostaglandin biosynthesis [Letter]. *N Engl J Med* 1984;310:50.

199. Fisher AA. Mace—modern acronym and an ancient nomenclature [Letter]. *JAMA* 1970;212:320.

200. Goransson L, et al. Some cases of eugenol hypersensitivity. *Derm Venereol Tandlak T* 1967;60:545.

201. Gaul LE. Dermatitis of the hands from oil of cloves. *Skin* 1963;2:413.

202. Gaul LE. Contact dermatitis from synthetic oil of mustard. *Arch Dermatol* 1964;90:158.

203. Matheson R. *Medical entomology,* 2nd ed. Ithaca, NY: Comstock Publishing Co, 1950.

204. Foussercau J, et al. Contact dermatitis from laurel: I. Clinical aspects. *Trans St John Hosp Derm Soc* 1967;53:141.

205. Lembo G, et al. Allergic contact dermatitis due to garlic (*Allium sativum*). *Contact Dermatitis* 1991;25:330.

206. Lee TY, Lam TH. Contact dermatitis due to topical treatment with garlic in Hong Kong. *Contact Dermatitis* 1991;24:193.

207. Rinkel HJ, Balyeat RM. Occupational dermatitis due to lettuce. *JAMA* 1932;98:137.

208. Closson JB. Oral allergy after lettuce ingestion (questions and answers). *JAMA* 1974;230:113.

209. Oliwiecki S, Beck MH, Hausen BM. Compositae dermatitis aggravated by eating lettuce. *Contact Dermatitis* 1991;24:318.

210. Veraldi S, Schianchi-Veraldi R. Contact urticaria from kiwi fruit. *Contact Dermatitis* 1990;22:244.

211. Korstanje MJ, van de Staak WJM. A case of hand dermatitis due to mushrooms. *Contact Dermatitis* 1990;22:115.

212. Nakamura T. Shiitake (*Lentinus edodes*) dermatitis [published erratum appeared in Dermatitis 1992;27:351]. *Contact Dermatitis* 1992;27:65.

213. Ueda A, et al. Allergic contact dermatitis in shiitake (*Lentinus edodes* [Berk] Sing) growers. *Contact Dermatitis* 1992;26:228.

214. Rosina P, Cheiregato C, Schena D. Allergic contact dermatitis from *Pleurotus* mushroom. *Contact Dermatitis* 1995;33:277.

215. Kanerva L, Estlander T, Jolanki R. Airborne occupational allergic contact dermatitis from champignon mushroom. *Am J Contact Dermatitis* 1998;9:190.

216. McGeorge BC, Steele MC. Allergic contact dermatitis of the nipple from Roman chamomile ointment. *Contact Dermatitis* 1991;24:139.

217. Dang RW, Bell DB. Anaphylactic reaction to the ingestion of mango. *Hawaii Med J* 1967;27:149.

218. Giannattasio M, et al. Contact urticaria from litchi fruit (*Litchi chinensis* Sonn.). *Contact Dermatitis* 1995;33:67.

219. Polunin I. Pineapple dermatoses. *Br J Dermatol* 1951;63:441.

220. Lupton ES. Cheilitis due to coffee. *Arch Dermatol* 1961;84:798.

221. Calnan CD. Malt flour dermatitis. *Contact Dermatitis Newsletter* 1973;14390.

222. Hjorth N. Battery for testing of chefs and other kitchen workers. *Contact Dermatitis* 1975;2:63.

223. Mitchell JC. Plant dermatitis in Vancouver. *Can J Dermatol* 1993;5:389.

CHAPTER 23

Photocontact Dermatitis

Dermatologic conditions resulting from exposure to light can occur in several forms and can be caused by both local and systemic processes. The differential diagnosis of a photosensitive eruption includes autoimmune diseases, such as lupus erythematosus, metabolic alterations, such as the porphyrias, photosensitivity caused by internal or external exposure to photoactive agents, and diseases of unknown mechanisms such as polymorphous light eruption and chronic actinic dermatitis. In addition, "regular" contact dermatitis can occur in a photodistribution. For example, allergy to a sunscreen chemical can give this clinical pattern. For the purposes of this text, this chapter will concentrate on reactions to topically encountered agents, realizing that there is often overlap with systemic photosensitivity. The other cutaneous photosensitivity reactions are reviewed in several texts and articles (1–3).

Photocontact dermatitis may be divided into two broad categories, photoallergic and phototoxic dermatitis, depending on whether the reaction is immune mediated or not. It may be difficult clinically to distinguish between the two, and sometimes a chemical can cause both types of reactions. Table 23.1 lists characteristics helpful in separating photoallergic and phototoxic reactions.

In either case, by definition, light energy, along with exposure to the chemical in question, is required to produce a reaction. It should be noted, however, that some chemicals are able to act as regular allergens as well as photoallergens. Although direct sunlight (ultraviolet light) is almost always needed to produce a photoreaction, occasionally artificial light sources may be sufficient (4).

Photocontact dermatitis reached the proportions of a mini-epidemic in the 1960s in the United States, Europe, and Australia. Thousands of individuals developed photosensitivity after exposure to antibacterial agents in soaps and other cleaning products (5,6). Fortunately, the causative agents were recalled by the U.S. Food and Drug Administration and other regulatory agencies, but not before some patients developed chronic photosensitivity.

During the 1980s and 1990s, a shift occurred to new agents causing photodermatitis. Sunscreen agents and fragrances have been responsible for the majority of photoallergic reactions in the last decade (7–9). The plant-derived furocoumarins remain as the most frequent cause of phototoxic reactions. In some countries where topical nonsteroidal anti-inflammatory drugs (NSAIDs) are used, the NSAIDs have caused very frequent phototoxicity and some photoallergy (8).

CLINICAL FEATURES OF PHOTODERMATITIS

Exposed areas, such as the face, the V of the neck, the back of the hands, and the dorsal forearms, are the most frequent sites of contact photodermatitis. Any skin area receiving sufficient light and a photosensitizing chemical, however, may develop a reaction. The scalp and other densely hairy areas, the periorbital areas, and the skin immediately under the chin are rarely involved. When lesions are present on the forearms, the extensor and radial aspects are almost always the most extensively involved. The cubital fossae are frequently spared. Sharply demarcated areas of involvement may appear below the sleeves. Photodermatitis from sunlight exposure, while driving an automobile with a left-hand drive, affects the left side of the face and the uncovered left arm and forearm most severely. Often such a photodermatitis presents in a unilateral pattern.

Phototoxic reactions often resemble sunburn and are limited invariably to areas exposed to light. Many types of reaction patterns, however, can occur. The eruption may be eczematous, bullous, or fissured, may resemble lichen planus, or may mimic lupus erythematosus. Phototoxic dermatitis usually disappears promptly when the photocontactant is avoided. The eruption is rarely persistent. Dermatitis that is limited to, or occurs predominantly on, areas exposed to light should be investigated for the possibility of being a photosensitive reaction. Dermatitis due to airborne contactants can closely simulate photodermatitis.

> **Airborne contact dermatitis may closely mimic photodermatitis. Sparing of the skin folds of the neck, the retroauricular, nasolabial, and submental areas favors a diagnosis of photodermatitis.**

TABLE 23.1. *Characteristics of Contact Photosensitivity: Phototoxic and Photoallergic Reactions*

Characteristics	Reaction	
	Phototoxic	Photoallergic
Incidence	Usually relatively high (theoretically 100%)	Usually low
Clinical manifestations	Usually resemble sunburn	Varied morphology
Possibility of reaction on first exposure	Yes	No
Incubation period after first exposure	No	Yes
Development of persistent light reaction	No	Yes
Possibility of "flares" at distant previously involved sites	No	Yes
Cross-reactions to structurally related agents	No	Frequent
Broadening of cross-reactions following repeated photopatch testing	No	Possible
Concentration of drug necessary for reaction	High	Low
Chemical alteration of photosensitizer	Sometimes	Yes
Covalent binding with carrier protein	No	Yes
Cellular passive transfer abolition with anti-T-cell sera	No	Possible
Lymphocyte stimulation test	No	Possible
Macrophage migration inhibition test	No	Possible

PHOTOTOXIC CONTACT DERMATITIS

Phototoxic contact dermatitis can occur in virtually anyone upon first exposure to the phototoxin and under appropriate conditions, such as sufficient intensity of light (Table 23.2). Phototoxic reactions are not dependent on immunologic mechanisms, and therefore previous sensitization is not required for expression of the condition. Phototoxicity is clinically similar to a severe sunburn, with severe blistering reactions possible.

Each compound causing a photocontact dermatitis will absorb only specific wavelengths of light. Its absorption spectrum is determined by its chemical structure. This spectrum usually closely approximates the wavelengths responsible for the clinical reaction, the so-called action spectrum. Most phototoxic sensitizers have an action spectrum in the ultraviolet band between 280 and 430 nm. Certain dyes, however, such as eosin photosensitize in the visible light region. Window glass, which usually absorbs ultraviolet radiation of wavelengths shorter than 320 nm, will protect patients from those phototoxic reactions that have an action spectrum below 320 nm, but fails to protect against photosensitizers with a higher action spectrum such as tar and the psoralens that produce most cases of phototoxic contact dermatitis (4).

Phytophotodermatitis Due to Furocoumarins in Plants

When a phototoxic chemical is contacted by exposure to a plant, vegetable, or fruit, the resulting photodermatitis is referred to as phytophotodermatitis. Bowers (10) in a fine review of this topic, stated that as early as 1500 B.C. Egyptians used an extract from *Ammi majus* to treat vitiligo. This plant, called false bishop's weed, is a commonly seen member of the Umbelliferae family.

The most common presentation of phytophotodermatitis is linear streaks of pruritic dermatitis on sun-exposed skin surfaces. Depending on the degree of exposure to the offending plant and the level of sun exposure, painful blisters may occur. Marked hyperpigmentation develops after the acute phase heals. This usually resolves slowly after several months without sequelae. Common phototoxic plants are listed in Table 23.3.

Phytophotodermatitis has also been described in individuals exposed to the oil of Persian limes and in carrot processors and celery pickers (Tables 23.3 and 23.4) (11). Such

TABLE 23.2. *Topically Encountered Phototoxic Drugs and Chemicals*

Coal-tar derivatives
  Acridine
  Anthracene
  Phenanthrene
Drugs
  Phenothiazines
  Sulfonamides
Dyes
  Anthraquinone
  Eosin
  Methylene blue
  Rose bengal
Plant derivatives—furocoumarins
  Psoralens
  Dictamnin

TABLE 23.3. *Common Plants in the United States Known to Cause Phytophotodermatitis*

Family	Botanical name	Common name
Compositae	Achillea millefolium	Milfoil, yarrow
	Anthemis cotula	Stinking mayweed
Umbelliferae	Angelica gigas	Angelica
	Ammi majus	False bishop's weed
	Anthriscus sylvestris	Cow parsley, wild chervil
	Apium graveolens dulce	Celery
	Daucus carota	Carrot
	Foeniculum vulgare	Fennel
	Heracleum lanatum	Cow parsnip
	Heracleum mantegazzianum	Giant hogweed, wild parsnip
	Pastinaca sativa	Parsnip
	Petroselinum crispum	Parsley
Papilionaceae	Psoralea corylifolia	Psoralen
Rutaceae	Citrus aurantifolia, begamia	Lime, bergamot lime
	Citrus limon	Lemon
	Citrus sinensis	Orange
	Dictamnus albus	Gas plant, burning bush, fraxinella
	Cneoridium dumosum	Coast spice bush
	Pelea anisata	Mokihana
	Ruta graveolens	Rue
Moraceae	Ficus carica	Fig

Partially adapted from Bowers, Reference 10.

phytophotodermatitis, as well as that which follows contact with plants of other species, is probably caused primarily by furocoumarin compounds, which are present in the plants. These phototoxic substances are lipid-soluble and penetrate into the epidermis with ease.

> **Phytophotodermatitis is a plant-solar dermatitis produced on skin exposed to plant psoralens (furocoumarins) in the presence of sunlight. Such dermatitis is followed by marked hyperpigmentation.**

For phytophotodermatitis to occur, there must be contact with a plant containing the sensitizing furocoumarin with concomitant or subsequent exposure to ultraviolet light in the ultraviolet A (UVA) range (e.g., sunlight). Absorption of psoralens into the skin is enhanced by high humidity (12). The most common phototoxins are activated by UVA radiation (320–400 nm).

Therapeutically, psoralens, purified from plant materials or synthetically produced, have become common agents in the treatment of many cutaneous diseases, most notably psoriasis and vitiligo. Photochemotherapy utilizes either topical or systemic psoralens and ultraviolet radiation in the UVA (320–400 nm) range and is referred to as PUVA (13).

> **A bullous plant photodermatitis is often mistaken for a poison ivy eruption or bullous reactions from blister beetles or insect bites.**

Berloque Dermatitis

Certain clinical manifestations of phytophotodermatitis have been given specific names, such as Berloque dermatitis and meadow grass dermatitis. Berloque dermatitis is produced at sites exposed to a combination of certain perfumes and sunlight. The streaky erythema of the eruption is followed by pigmentation. Oil of bergamot, containing bergapten (5-methoxy-psoralen), is probably the principal cause of photodermatitis produced by perfumes and toilet waters (14,15).

Phytophotodermatitis from Wild or Cultivated Plants

Farmworkers are probably the most likely group to be at risk for phytophotodermatitis. A major outbreak involving 11 people occurred while weeding parsnips by hand on an "organic" farm. Surreptitious use of pesticides was suspected before the true diagnosis was established (16). Lovage and angelica have caused reactions in workers (17,18).

In Hawaii, the Mokihana bush (*Pelea arisata*), which grows in the mountains of Kauai, is a common cause of

TABLE 23.4. *Occupations at Risk for Phytophotodermatitis*

Occupation	Photosensitizer
Bartenders	Persian limes, lemons
Cannery packers	Celery, figs, carrots
Dairy workers	Parsnips
Vegetable harvesters, produce workers	Fennel, parsley, celery, dill, parsnips, carrots

phytophotodermatitis (19); the berries are used to make garlands.

Meadow grass dermatitis (dermatitis bullosa striata pratensis), another example of phytophotodermatitis, is produced by contact of the skin with meadow grass and subsequent exposure to sunlight. The eruption is a phototoxic reaction characterized by bizarre, criss-cross, linear streaks of erythema and vesicles or bullae, which heal with hyperpigmentation. The photosensitizing agent is not grass, but is either the yellow-flowered wild meadow parsnip, which belongs to the carrot family, or a common wild yellow-flowered herb of the rose family. The skin of individuals who sunbathe in meadows may become impregnated with the juices of these weeds or wild flowers containing furocoumarins. Subsequent exposure to sunlight produces the phototoxic dermatitis.

Occasionally, the bites of chiggers or other arthropods infesting grass may produce a pseudo-phytophotodermatitis that may be confused with meadow grass dermatitis. Itching is more intense and pigmentation is less marked in dermatitis produced by arthropods than in meadow grass dermatitis.

The gas plant (Dictamnus alba) has been reported to cause typical phytophotodermatitis in gardeners. In addition to psoralens, it contains an alkaloid, dictamnin, which is also a phototoxin (20).

The coast spice bush or berry rue (Cneoridium dumosum) is a common plant in southern California and Mexico, usually growing in dry areas below 2,500 ft elevation (21). This member of the Rutaceae family is a slender branched evergreen shrub growing 3 to 5 ft tall, with white flowers and red berries. Exposure to this plant during a field trip caused photodermatitis with severe blistering in two naturalists and multiple students. The vesicular dermatitis was experimentally reproduced later in a volunteer, with minimal exposure to the plant (21).

Phototoxic Tar Dermatitis

Coal-tar derivatives are among the most commonly encountered photosensitizers. At least 400 compounds have been isolated from coal tar, many of which are used in diverse industries, including the manufacture of drugs, dyes, perfumes, synthetic resins, explosives, insecticides, and disinfectants. The known active photosensitizers of coal tar are acridine, anthracene, benzpyrene, phenanthrene, and pyridene. Wood tars generally are not photosensitizers and do not contain any of these photosensitizing chemicals. The action spectrum for coal-tar contact photosensitivity is in the 320 to 430 nm range.

Photodermatitis due to tar and pitch may appear as a severe sunburn referred to as "flashes" and "smarts" in workers exposed to tar, pitch, or creosote and sunlight. Actual contact with pitch or creosote is not necessary for the production of a photosensitive reaction, because the volatile fumes emanating from these products when heated can produce a photodermatitis. Moderate to marked pigmentation may occur at the sites of tar photodermatitis. In one series, 70% of white workers exposed to pitch fumes were affected, whereas black workers were not affected (22). The increased pigmentation of the skin of black workers proved to be protective against pitch photosensitivity. Smarting and erythema may continue 1 to 3 days after exposure to pitch fumes. There may be a latent period of 2 weeks or more between the initial exposure to pitch fumes and the appearance of photosensitivity.

The ability of coal-tar derivatives to cause photosensitivity contributes to the treatment of psoriasis using the classic Goeckerman therapy.

Contact with coal tar or with volatile derivatives, such as pitch or creosote, may produce a photocontact dermatitis and "smarting."

PHOTOALLERGIC CONTACT DERMATITIS

Photoallergic contact dermatitis (photo-ACD) is similar to "regular" delayed hypersensitivity in that the pathogenesis is a T-cell-mediated immunologic response. The concentration of the allergen needed to elicit a photoallergic reaction is lower than that needed to produce a phototoxic reaction, and there is no clinical reaction on first exposure. Some photoallergens can also produce "ordinary" ACD in the absence of light (Table 23.5).

Clinical differentiation between photoallergic and phototoxic contact dermatitis may be difficult at times. The criteria in Table 23.1 may be helpful in distinguishing between the two types.

TABLE 23.5. *Topically Encountered Photoallergenic Drugs and Chemicals*

Antifungal agents
Fenticlor
Jadit
Multifungin
Fragrances
Methylcoumarin
Musk ambrette
Halogenated salicylanilides
Bithionol
Dibromosalicylanilide
Tetrachlorosalicylanilide
Tribromosalicylanilide
Trichlorocarbanilide
Phenothiazines
Sulfonamides
Sunscreens
Whiteners
Stilbenes

Photo-ACD to Antiseptics and Disinfectants

The most widespread outbreak of photoallergic reactions to topically encountered agents resulted from the use of soaps and cleansers containing halogenated salicylanilides and related compounds. Although most of these substances are no longer used in consumer products in the United States and in Western Europe, patients are occasionally encountered with "persistent light reactions" initiated by these agents 10 to 15 years ago. They should, therefore, be considered as possible etiologic agents in the differential diagnosis of photosensitivity. These compounds should also be included in the group of antigens used in routine patch testing procedures.

Tetrachlorosalicylanilide (TCSA: Impregon)

In Great Britain, many instances of photodermatitis were reported from exposure to soap containing TCSA (23,24). In a small U.S. market test of a product containing 0.5% tetrachlorosalicylanilide, several instances of photosensitization were reported and verified by patch tests (25). The individuals developed intense itching and erythema in areas exposed to the sun. In some instances, papules and vesicles also appeared. This agent is still available in the United States as a surface disinfectant and mold inhibitor.

> Present statutes do not require that all agents incorporated into a nondrug or cosmetic preparation be identified on the package; some unlisted ingredients may be photosensitizers.

Tribromosalicylanilide (TBS)

This antiseptic was a favorite deodorant agent in many soaps and detergents and produced allergic photocontact dermatitis from its presence in Lifebuoy, Safeguard, and Praise soaps (26).

Dibromsalan (4,5-Dibromosalicylanilide; DBS)

This chemical, which was present in Lifebuoy soap, also caused photoallergic contact dermatitis.

Trichlorocarbanilide (TCC)

This agent, used in the past in Dial, Zest, and Safeguard soaps, is a potent photosensitizer (27).

There are numerous reports in the literature of these halogenated salicylanilides and related chemicals producing photodermatitis (28–31).

Jadit (Chlorosalicylamide)

This antifungal agent with the formula 4-chlorohydroxybenzoic acid-n-butilamide, used in Australia and Europe, can cause a photoallergic reaction that may be persistent. The photosensitizing action is probably related to that of the halogenated salicylanilides (39).

> The halogenated salicylanilides and related chemicals, used as antiseptics in deodorant soaps and cosmetics, were the causative agents in most patients with allergic contact photodermatitis in the 1960s. Fenticlor seems to give frequent positive reactions, but exposure sources are often uncertain.

Phenothiazine and Its Derivatives

Phenothiazine is used as an insecticide and as an anthelmintic in human and veterinary medicine, as well as an antipsychotic agent. It is a parent substance for methylene blue, a dye that is a powerful photosensitizer (40).

Orchard workers using phenothiazine as an insecticide against moths exhibited photosensitivity. Because many individuals were involved, it was presumed that the reaction was one of phototoxicity rather than of photoallergy (40).

Chlorpromazine (Thorazine)

Allergic photocontact dermatitis occurs principally among medical and nursing personnel who contaminate their hands while injecting the drug (41,42). Those receiving the drug systemically may acquire a phototoxic dermatitis.

> Phenothiazine and its derivatives, Thorazine and Phenergan, produce allergic contact dermatitis (without light) and photocontact dermatitis.

Bithionol (Bisphenol, Actamar)

Bithionol, 2-2′-thiobis (4,6-dichlorophenol), is a bacteriostatic agent related to hexachlorophene. It can produce both ordinary and photoallergic dermatitis. Bithionol often shows cross-reactions not only to the hexachlorophene but also to the halogenated salicylanilides (32–36).

Hexachlorophene

This formerly widely used halogenated phenol antiseptic rarely produces ordinary contact allergy. Cross-contact sensitivity and photocontact sensitivity to hexachlorophene have been observed in guinea pigs with primary photosensitivity to tetrachlorosalicylanilide and tribromosalicylanilide (5). It is not certain whether hexachlorophene is a primary photosensitizer, although such photosensitivity has been reported (29).

Cross-Reaction between Bithionol, Hexachlorophene, and the Halogenated Salicylanilides

Cross-reaction may occur with tetrachlorosalicylanilide and tribromosalicylanilide, and bithionol is apparently a primary photosensitizer engendering cross-sensitivity to both. Reactions to hexachlorophene in patients with contact photodermatitis from bithionol not requiring any light represent cross-sensitivity between a photosensitizer and a simple contact allergen.

Fentichlor [bis(2-Hydroxy-5-Chlorophenyl) Sulfide] and Bromosalicylchloranilide (Multifungin, 5-Bromo-4′-Chlorosalicylanilide)

These topical antifungal agents, used in Australia, are photoallergens. Fentichlor, chemically related to bithionol, also cross-reacts with hexachlorophene.

A number of positive patch test reactions are seen to Fentichlor that defy clinical explanation. Multifungin is chemically related to tribromosalicylanilide, with which it cross-reacts (37,38).

Promethazine Hydrochloride (Phenergan)

This antihistamine can also produce phototoxic and photoallergic reactions. In France, where Phenergan Cream was used extensively as a topical antipruritic, many instances of photocontact dermatitis occurred. Photosensitivity seems to be induced primarily by contact with promethazine, whereas systemic administration without topical application does not appear to induce photosensitivity (43,44). Cross-photosensitivity may occur between promethazine and chlorpromazine (45).

Many phenothiazine compounds can also produce ordinary allergic contact sensitization. Cross-reactions between the phenothiazine compounds may include both the photoallergic and the ordinary allergic variety. Sometimes the cross-reactivity extends only to the photoallergic phenomenon (46).

More recently, dioxopromethazine (in Prothanon Gel), used topically for pruritus, has been reported (47). The acute episode was followed by development of persistent light reactivity for over 1½ years. Cross-photoreactivity occurred to promethazine but not to chloropromazine.

Sulfanilamide

This antibacterial agent can apparently produce both phototoxic and photoallergic reactions (48). Phototoxic reactions are also produced by systemic administration of the drug. Window glass usually protects the individual from such phototoxic reactions. However, the topical application of sulfanilamide preparations may engender photoallergic contact sensitivity. Fortunately, topical sulfanilamide preparations are not commonly used at this time. Other topically applied sulfonamide compounds, such as sulfacetamide, sulfathiazole, and sulfadiazine, are apparently not common photosensitizers. Hypoglycemic sulfonamides, such as chloropropamide (Diabinese) and tolbutamide (Orinase), thiazide diuretics, such as chlorothiazide (Diuril) and hydrochlorothiazide (Esidrix, HydroDIURIL, and Oretic), and quinethazone (Hydromox), however, may produce phototoxic and photoallergic reactions when administered systemically (49).

SUNSCREEN AGENTS

Sunscreen agents have become the most common causative substances of photoallergic contact dermatitis in the United States (9,50,51). These chemicals are also able to cause "regular" allergic contact dermatitis without UV light exposure. A list of the most commonly used agents is given in Table 23.6. Many sunscreen lotions contain two or more active ingredients to provide a broader spectrum of photoprotection. In addition, many cosmetic products and moisturizing creams incorporate a sunscreen agent. Although in the past, PABA derivatives were the most common sunscreen allergens, now oxybenzone is the most common (9,51).

TABLE 23.6. *Examples of Sunscreen Agents*

UVA absorbers
Anthranilate derivatives
Camphor derivatives (e.g., Mexoryl SX)
Dibenzoylmethane derivatives (e.g., Eusolex 9020, Parsol 1789)
UVB absorbers
Benzophenones
   Oxybenzone (BZP 3) (e.g., Eusolex 4360, Uvinul M40)
   Sulisobenzone (BZP 4) (e.g., Escalol 577, Uvasorb S5)
   Dioxybenzone (BZP 8)
   Mexenone
   Octocrylene (e.g., Neo Heliopan 0S)
Camphor derivatives
   Methyl benzilidene camphor and others
Cinnamates
   Octylmethoxycinnamate (e.g., Parsol MCX)
   Cinoxate
   Other methoxycinnamates
PABA and derivatives
   PABA (Para-aminobenzoic acid)
   Padimate-A (amyldimethyl PABA)
   Padimate-O (octyldimethyl PABA)
   Glyceryl PABA and others
Salicylates
   Homosalate (homomenthyl salicylate)
   Octylsalicylate
   Other salicylates

Para-Aminobenzoic Acid (PABA) and Its Esters

These chemicals are among the earliest sunscreen agents and are still used. They are primarily effective at blocking UVB light. Some persons report a transient stinging or burning reaction upon application, especially to sensitive skin areas. This is much more common than a true allergy but may lead the patient to believe that he or she is "allergic" to the chemicals. A number of sunscreen lotions are mistakenly marketed as being "hypoallergenic" because they contain no PABA.

DeLeo et al. (9) found 3 of 187 patients with allergic contact dermatitis to PABA or octyldimethyl PABA (PABA-O), 3 with photoallergic contact dermatitis to PABA, and 2 with combined photoallergic contact dermatitis and ACD; almost 4% of the 187 patients tested and 22% of the 37 patients with any positive reaction. The researchers also reported 3 of 11 patients tested with pentil-dimethyl PABA had a reaction of either ACD or photoallergic contact dermatitis, or both (9). Fotiades et al. (52) found no cross-reactivity between PABA and the PABA esters PABA-O and amyl-dimethyl PABA (PABA-A). There were 9 positive patch tests to one of the esters (out of 138 tested) and 3 to PABA (52). In contrast, 54 suspected photosensitive cases were tested by Lenique et al. (53) in France with no reaction to PABA, and only 1 to PABA-O. However, seven were positive to oxybenzone (see below). Berne and Bos (54) found only 2 positives to PABA out of 355 patients (0.6%) tested to PABA (5% alcohol). They did not test with PABA esters. However, in a report from France, photoallergic contact dermatitis to PABA was second only to oxybenzone (51).

> In studies from the 1980s, allergies to PABA and its esters were common. In the 1990s, oxybenzone became the most common sunscreen photoallergen, with far fewer cases of PABA allergy.

Many patients with positive patch tests to PABA may react due to cross-sensitivity between other para-amino substances such as paraphenylenediamine (PPDA) or benzocaine. Theeuwes et al. (55) showed that these reactions may not be clinically relevant. Fifty-four of 74 patients with positive reactions to a sunscreen agent (not photoreaction) had no history of problems from cosmetics or sunscreens. All 54 were positive to either PABA or PABA-O. Also, 46 of 328 patients reactive to PPDA and 51 of 180 benzocaine-allergic patients were positive to PABA or PABA-O.

Oxybenzone

Oxybenzone, also known as benzophenone-3 and Eusolex 4360, is the most frequently used benzophenone in sunscreens. It is also the most common sunscreen agent to cause photoallergic contact dermatitis. Sczurko et al. (51) found 35 cases of photo-ACD to oxybenzone out of 283 patients tested (12.4%). In over one-third, exposure was not from a sunblock product but from a daily moisturizer. In a large Italian study of 1,050 patients, 31 showed reactions to sunscreen agents, with oxybenzone the most common at 10. Overall, oxybenzone was the fourth most common photoallergen after phenothiazines and Fentichlor (56).

Of the 54 patients treated by Lenique et al. (53), 7 (13%) reacted to oxybenzone. There were three cases of pure photoallergic contact dermatitis, two cases of allergic contact dermatitis, and two cases with both. Only two of the seven reacted to other photoallergens (53). Photoallergy to oxybenzone has been reported in a patient with a clinical pattern similar to erythema multiforme (57). Use of sunscreens without oxybenzone is suggested in patients with known or presumed photoallergy.

Other benzophenones, sulisobenzone and mexenone, are rarely used in sunscreens. There are scattered case reports of ACD and photoallergic contact dermatitis and even contact urticaria from these agents (58).

Butylmethoxydibenzoylmethane (Parsol 1789)

This chemical is a newer, particularly effective, UVA blocker currently used in the United States and elsewhere. In some newer studies, this agent has moved into second or third place in frequency of allergy to sunscreens. Schauder and Ippen (59) from Germany reported 15 cases of ACD and 13 cases of photoallergy from 402 patients tested. Because it is one of the better UVA blockers, frequency of use of, and therefore of photoallergy to, this agent will likely increase in the coming years.

Isopropyl Dibenzoylmethane

This agent was withdrawn from the market in 1993 due to frequent reports of photosensitization. It was by far the most common sunscreen photoallergen in one study (59) from the 1980s to early 1990s.

Cinnamates

These are primarily UVB absorbers and are used in many sunscreens. They are poorly soluble in water and therefore are common in "waterproof" sunscreens (58). In one study from Germany, out of 402 patients, there were 7 cases of allergy and 14 cases of photoallergy to either octyl-methoxycinnamate or isoamyl p-methoxycinnamate (59). In a study from France, however, only 3 of 283 reacted to a cinnamate (51), whereas, in a study from Italy, 6 of 1,050 reacted (56). Allergy to these agents is unusual. Probably the most significant feature is their cross-reactivity with fragrances and flavorings, particularly cinnamic aldehyde, alcohol, and cinnamon oil. Avoidance of perfumes and cinnamon-type spices in food may be necessary.

Methyl Benzilidene Camphor

This UVB blocker is apparently a better allergen than a photoallergen. In Germany, there were 32 cases of allergy but only 5 of photoallergy (59). In France, there were three positive patch tests and no positive patch tests (51).

Salicylates

Although they are only weak UVB absorbers, salicylates are popular in sunscreens because of their safety, solubility, and stability. Although not used in routine patch test batteries, apparently contact allergic reactions are very rare (60).

Anthranilates

These are UVA absorbers, which are combined with other agents to provide broad-spectrum photoprotection. Allergy to these agents has not yet been documented.

Physical Sunscreens

These "nonchemical" sun blockers act by physically blocking light rays away from the skin by virtue of their opacity. Titanium dioxide and zinc oxide are most commonly used. Allergy and photoallergy have not been reported. The opaque appearance may be either desirable or objectionable, depending on the individual.

> **Sunscreen agents have become the most common cause of photoallergic contact dermatitis. Oxybenzone and PABA and its esters are the most frequent sensitizers. Physical sunscreens containing titinium dioxide are free of chemical sunscreen agents and can be used if photoallergy to sunscreens is suspected.**

NONSPECIFIC SUNSCREEN REACTIONS

Many "reactions" to sunscreen products are not due to photoallergy. Additives such as fragrances and preservatives are more likely to cause ACD. Even more commonly, transient reactions such as stinging occur, especially with PABA. Other dermatologic entities, such as acne and urticaria, may develop after sunscreen use. An Australian study of 603 adults using a single sunscreen product found that 19% complained of some sort of reaction (61). None of these were due to photoallergy to the active agents. More than 90% were not allergic at all. Atopics were more likely to experience an adverse reaction than others.

Photoallergic Contact Dermatitis from Perfumes

Contact photoallergic reactions to perfumes are due to either of two major components contained in the product: the fragrance per se or the fixative used to hold the fragrance or to enhance its scent.

Fragrances in their natural form are essential oils obtained from plants or flowers. In an attempt to reduce cost, synthetic fragrances have been produced and are widely used. These less expensive agents are organic compounds of the aldehyde, ketone, or alcohol variety.

The fixatives used in perfumes are usually secretions from the sexual scent glands of animals. They can also be synthesized, as exemplified by musk ambrette.

Musk ambrette, a synthetic fragrance fixative, is used in both the food and cosmetic industries. Its potent, floral odor has been considered quite desirable and in the past was present in concentrations as high as 15% in the final perfume product. Raugi and Storrs (62) reported localized photocontact dermatitis to men's aftershave lotions and traced the source to musk ambrette. Musk ambrette, like the halogenated salicylanilides, has also been reported to induce persistent light reaction in several patients (63,64).

6-methylcoumarin, a synthetic organic lactone, is structurally related to the furocoumarins. Unlike the psoralens, however, 6-methylcoumarin was thought after initial testing to be a nonphotoactive substance. Since the early part of the last century it has been used extensively in the United States both in cosmetics and as an artificial flavoring agent in several foods. In the late 1970s, several reports of severe photosensitivity reactions occurring after patients used a suntanning preparation, in which 6-methylcoumarin had been incorporated as a fragrance, were noted in the southern United States (65). Interestingly, in these patients, the clinical reaction had morphologic features both of phototoxicity and of photoallergy. The eruption occurred in some patients without a history of prior exposure to the suntanning product; lesions occurred within a few hours of exposure and were followed by long-lasting pigmentary changes in the skin. This finding suggested phototoxicity. Conversely, the eruption was a papulovesicular one morphologically; it occurred in a relatively small number of users of the product, and the reaction spread to areas not exposed to the product or irradiation. This pattern is associated usually with a photoallergic reaction. Similarly, reactivity could be elicited experimentally in only a small percentage of test subjects, suggestive of photoallergy (66). The photosensitivity could be induced in guinea pigs and is immunologic (67). Confirmation by routine phototesting in humans was unrewarding until it was discovered that to produce positive patch test reactions, the test substance must be applied shortly before irradiation rather than at the routine 24 to 48 hours. When done at the later time, false-negative results were obtained.

Since then, 6-methylcoumarin has been removed from suntanning products. It is believed that 6-methylcoumarin represents a substance of low photosensitizing potential that under most circumstances does not result in photocontact dermatitis unless used in high concentrations with adequate exposure to ultraviolet irradiation.

Miscellaneous Photoallergic Sensitizers

Epstein reported that ragweed pollen (68), benzocaine (69), and Dangard (70) are photosensitizers. Dangard, a chloromercaptodicarboximide, is used by barbers as an antiseborrheic agent. Dangard is also a trade name for Vanicide 89 Re, which is used as an antiseptic in cosmetic and pharmaceutical preparations.

Photoallergy has been reported from Japan to three pesticides, maneb, fenitrothion, and Daconil (tetrachloroisophthalonitrile). Test concentrations were 0.01% aq, 0.01% aq, and 0.002% aq, respectively. The first two were used in rice paddies and the latter in recreational gardening (71,72).

Photosensitivity reactions from blankophores (optical brightening agents) (73), cadmium sulfide (74,75), the yellow pigment in tattoos, fluorouracil and the chromates (76,77), cobalt (78), diphenhydramine (79,80), amantadine, quindoxin, and dibucaine (81–83) have been reported.

> **Photosensitivity reactions have been reported from such diverse substances as benzocaine, ragweed pollen, fluorouracil, blankophores, cobalt, chromates, diphenhydramine, amantadine, and quindoxin.**

PERSISTENT LIGHT REACTIVITY

A small number of individuals who develop a photoallergic contact dermatitis to certain agents will retain a persistent reactivity to light (PLR) long after all exposure to the photosensitizing compound has ceased. This phenomenon was probably first recognized in soldiers photosensitized in North Africa after topical application of sulfanilamide in World War II. Promethazine, chlorpromazine, bithionol, and most notably the halogenated salicylanilides were reported to induce this type of reaction in the 1950s and 1960s (84–87). The perfume component musk ambrette has caused PLR (63,64). Occasionally systemic agents including quinine, NSAIDs, and thiazides may produce a PLR phenomenon (88,89).

Regardless of the particular photosensitizers involved, patients who become affected are for all practical purposes incapacitated, because they cannot tolerate exposure to sunlight. In fact, they may be so exquisitely photosensitive as to react adversely even to light emitted from artificial sources, such as household fluorescent tubes (90). An important and still puzzling feature of the phenomenon is that the action spectrum of the patient's photosensitivity extends beyond those wavelengths that initiated sensitization. Also, people who develop a PLR regularly show an abnormal reaction to UVB. Accordingly, clinical erythema with an eczematous histology occurs with doses in fractional amounts of the normal minimal erythema dose (MED) for UVB. It should be stressed, however, that the histopathol-ogy of this reaction is different from that described for sunburn and that it is an acute eczematous reaction.

In cases of presumed PLR, studies for other photosensitivity diseases, such as lupus erythematosus and porphyria, are negative. The persistent light reactors have no more-than-average incidence of atopy. They do include a preponderance of males in the fifth, sixth, and seventh decades of life.

The mechanism of persistent light reaction remains unclear, but a plausible theory may be that the patient has become autophotosensitized to a carrier protein that absorbs photons in the UVB range, thereby producing erythema and an eczematous response (91). Roelandts (89) suggested that somehow a state of "conditioned hyperirritability" could develop in PLR patients due to endogenous or exogenous influences.

Classification of Persistent Light Reactivity

Persistent photosensitivity reactions that first appear morphologically as edematous or vesicular reactions and later resemble chronic dermatitis can be differentiated according to several criteria. The following discussion outlines a working classification of these types of reactions on the bases of whether photosensitivity is localized or generalized and of the response of the patient to phototests and photopatch tests. This classification is summarized in Table 23.7.

Localized Specific Nonimmunologic Persistence of Photosensitivity

This type of reactivity was first described in Swedish sailors tattooed with cadmium sulfide, a yellow pigment (92). Localized swellings confined solely to the yellow portions of the tattoos occurred whenever the sailors were exposed to sunlight. Studies indicated that the action spectrum of cadmium was in the UVA and visible light ranges. All phototests and photopatch tests on nontattooed sites are normal. This type of phototoxic reactions arises from the local retention of the photosensitizer in macrophages.

Localized Specific Immunologic Persistence of Photosensitivity

This reaction was well described by Burry (93) in 1967. He studied Australian patients with photoallergic contact dermatitis. Several patients had incurred repeated topical exposure to Fentichlor and Multifungin, which are commercially available topical antibiotic preparations containing halogenated salicylanilides or closely related compounds. Burry reported that at such sites as the forearms where a severe, chronic, lichenified photodermatitis occurred, the patients remained photosensitive to UVA light for months with no continued exposure to the halogenated salicylanilides. In contrast, phototests on normal-appearing unin-

TABLE 23.7. *Persistent Light Reaction to Topically Encountered Agents*

Condition	Example	Response					Mechanism	Other features
		Photo Patch +UVA	UVB	UVA	Visible	Heat		
1. Localized specific nonimmunologic persistence of photosensitivity	Cadmium	0	0	+++	+++	0	Tattoo procedures, permanent deposition of phototoxic agents	Has persisted for years in Swedish sailors
2. Localized specific immunologic persistence of photosensitivity	Fentichlor	+++	0	+++	0	0	Retention of photoallergen at site of repetitive photoallergic reactions (light-exposed area)	Classic photoallergic (T-cell) reaction with photoantigen "trapped" in skin; lasts for months to years
3. Classic generalized immunologic "persistent light" reactivity	Halogenated salicylanilides	+++	+++	0	0	0	Autophotosensitization (carrier protein?)	Persists for years
4. Polyvalent light	No known agents	0	+++	+	+++	0	Unknown	Persists for years
5. Chronic actinic dermatosis	Various agents	?	+++	+++	+++	0	Unknown	Related to lymphomas?

0, Normal response
3 +++, abnormal response

volved skin exposed to UVA radiation were negative. Photopatch tests with Fentichlor and Multifungin plus UVA light on these same uninvolved sites, however, were strongly positive. A possible explanation of this phenomenon is that the damaged skin at the previously light-exposed sites retained some of the photosensitizers for more extended periods of time than did normal skin.

Classic Generalized Immunologic Persistent Light Reactivity

These patients fulfilled the criteria described by Jillson and Baughman (85), that is, a lowered MED to UVB and a positive photopatch test reaction to a sensitizer plus UVA. A small subgroup of patients among the classic reactors demonstrates atypical generalized immunologic persistent light reactivity. They differ from the "classic" patients only in that they demonstrate a positive phototest response on normal gluteal skin to UVA radiation alone. The response, however, is weaker than that at the photopatch test site. No satisfactory explanation has been offered for this phenomenon.

Polyvalent Light Sensitivity with Persistent Photosensitivity

This term describes patients who respond initially to both UV and visible light with marked erythema and who subsequently develop pruritic, lichenified plaques. No known phototoxic or photoallergic agent can be identified from the patient's history or by phototesting. Unfortunately, the disability persists for years.

Chronic Actinic Dermatitis (CAD)

CAD encompasses the diagnosis actinic reticuloid as well as other chronic photosensitivity dermatoses for which the cause remains elusive. Most patients are men over the age of 50. The clinical picture is similar to other types of photodermatitis, although generalization to non-sun-exposed areas is common. Often persistence throughout the year is seen, although worsening usually occurs in summer (90). The term "actinic reticuloid," first used by Ive et al. (94), describes a subgroup of photosensitive persons with histologic changes suggestive of lymphoma. Actual progression to malignancy apparently occurs rarely, if at all (95,96).

The majority of patients are abnormally sensitive to both UVA and UVB. Menage et al. (97) reported that 83% of 89 patients had reduced MEDs to both UVA and UVB, 9% to UVB alone, and 8% to UVA, UVB, and visible light. They also found that 36% had a positive patch or photopatch test to sesquiterpene lactone mix (0.1% pet, Hermal, Rheinbeck, Germany). Some patients reacted to other allergens, including colophony, fragrances, and sunscreens. Relevance of reactions was not always clear.

Phototesting and Photopatch Testing

Phototesting and photopatch testing can be performed in the outpatient setting as long as a light source and photoallergens are available. The most important equipment needed to perform photopatch tests is an artificial light source with relatively good spectral irradiance in the UVA range. A combined UVB/PUVA box can be used to deliver the appropriate radiation dosages. Handheld light sources are also available. Selected examples of these light sources are listed in Table 23.8. The light source should be calibrated with a UV photometer to insure that the desired dosage is accurately delivered.

The usual dose of UVA light for phototesting and photopatch testing is 10 joules (J)/cm^2. Occasionally, if extreme UVA photosensitivity is suspected, phototesting can also be performed to 1 and 5 J/cm^2. If 10 J/cm^2 or less causes erythema, the next lower dose is then used for photopatch tests. Regardless of skin color, reaction to 10 J/cm^2 of UVA indicates UVA photosensitivity.

The dosage of UVB light for phototesting is not so clear-cut. The minimal erythema dose (MED) varies normally with the skin color. An MED of 30 mJ/cm^2 may be normal in a fair-skinned person (types I or II) but would be abnormal in a dark-skinned patient. Doses between 5 and 100 mJ/cm^2 of UVB may be given in phototesting, depending on the patient's skin type.

Photopatch testing is conducted with UVA radiation because the vast majority of photo-ACD reactions are due to UVA. The chemicals currently recommended by the North American Contact Dermatitis Group (NACDG) for photopatch testing are listed in Table 23.9. Duplicate sets of patches are prepared and are placed on symmetrical sites of the back, as in ordinary patch-test procedures. One set of the duplicate patches will be irradiated with UVA light, whereas the nonirradiated set serves as a control.

Photopatch testing using patient-supplied or "nonstandard" materials can be performed in the same fashion. Perfumes and sunscreen preparations generally can be tested full strength (as is). Pieces of plants or plant juices can be tested to prove phytophotodermatitis. Because of the likelihood of producing persistent pigmentation, however, testing on a covered area such as the buttock is recommended.

TABLE 23.8. *Light Sources Used in Photopatch Testing*[a]

Light source	Comment
Fluorescent tubes (PUVA box)	Excellent rapid source of UVA; need to carefully cover all of patient except photopatch site
Wood's light (Blak Ray)	Simple, inexpensive
Hot quartz	Simple, inexpensive; needs proper filter

[a]Other light sources, such as ordinary black lights, UVB fluorescent tubes, and cold quartz, are not effective for photopatch testing.

TABLE 23.9. *Suggested Photopatch Test Allergens[a]*

Sunscreen agents
  Octylmethoxycinnamate 7.5% pet
  Para-amino benzoic acid (PABA) 5% pet
  Octyldimethyl PABA (padimate-O) 5% pet
  Oxybenzone (benzophenone-3) 2% pet
  Sulisobenzone (benzophenone-4) 10% pet
  Butyl methoxybibenzoylmethane (parsol 1789) 5% pet
  Octyl salicylate 5% pet
  Homosalate 5% pet
  Menthylanthranilate 5% pet
  2-hydroxy-methoxy methyl benzophenone
  2-phenylbenzimidazol-5-sulfonic acid 2% pet
Antiseptic agents
  Dichlorophene 1% pet
  Hexachloropene 1% pet
  Triclosan 2% pet
  Chlorhexidine diacetate 0.5% aq
  Bithionol 1% pet
  Tribromsalicylanicide 1% pet
Fragrances
  Musk ambrette 1% pet
  Sandalwood oil 2% pet
  Musk ambrette 1% in alcohol
Miscellaneous
  Thiourea 0.1% pet
  Sesquiterpene lactone mix 0.1% pet
  Lichen acid mix 0.3% pet
  Fentichlor 1% pet
  Ketoprofen 5% pet

[a]Based on current guidelines from the North American Contact Dermatitis Group.

After application of the chemicals, the two sets of patches are both covered with light-opaque material, such as aluminum foil or dark-colored nylon cloth. After 24 or 48 hours, both sets of patches are removed and each site is evaluated for any visible reaction. A positive test indicates the presence of either an "ordinary" allergic contact dermatitis or, rarely, a primary irritant reaction to the applied chemical. After the uncovered sites are evaluated, one set is irradiated with 10 J/cm² of UVA, as recommended by the NACDG. The British Photodermatology Group, however, recommends testing with 5 J/cm² (98). After completion of irradiation, the photopatch test sites are covered again with light-opaque material. Forty-eight hours later, 96 hours after initial patch application, a second reading is performed. Some authors suggest a further delayed reading of the irradiated side in another 2 to 4 days.

TABLE 23.10. *Interpretation of Photopatch Tests*

Reading at irradiated site[a]		Reading at non-irradiated site[a]	Interpretation
0		0	Normal
1–3+		0	Contact photoallergy
1–3+	=	1–3+	Contact allergy alone
1–3+	>	1–2+	Contact photoallergy and contact allergy

[a]Evaluations are scored 0 through 3, as described by the North American Contact Dermatitis Group.

If the irradiated site shows a positive reaction and the nonirradiated site shows a negative one, contact photoallergy is present. If both sites show equally positive reactions, then contact allergy is present (Table 23.10).

ALLERGEN CONCENTRATIONS IN PHOTOPATCH TESTING

Hasan and Jansen (99) studied a number of photo allergens in varying concentrations and with varying doses of UVA (99). With PABA, for example, they found allergen concentration to be very important in photocontact reactions, but less so in "regular" ACD. The dosage of UVA did not make much difference, however, so they recommend 5 joules for routine testing. The British Photodermatology Group also recommends 5 joules (98). However, testing with 10 joules may result in a few more positive reactions without any increase risk.

Hazards of Photopatch Testing

It should be emphasized that photopatch testing is not always an innocuous procedure. Some hazards and complications associated with it are outlined in Table 23.11. The patient should be aware that strong reactions characterized by vesiculation may cause discomfort. Photopatch testing should be avoided, if possible, in patients with acute active dermatitis, because false-positive reactions may result from the "hyperirritability" of the skin.

MANAGEMENT OF PHOTOCONTACT SENSITIVITY

Exposure to the photosensitizing agent must be eliminated, and the patient should minimize exposure to sunlight for at least 2 weeks (93). It is advisable to give the patient a list of related drugs or chemicals that produce cross-photosensitivity and that are to be avoided. This list is important, particularly when the salicylanilides and phenothiazines are implicated. When topical therapeutic or cosmetic agents are involved, the patient should be given a list of nonsensitizing substitutes.

Individuals with an acute photosensitivity reaction with severe erythema and edema may obtain relief with ice cold compresses of Burow's solution diluted 1:10. It is often

TABLE 23.11. *Hazards and Complications of Photopatch Testing*

1. Inadvertent sensitization to photopatch test materials
2. Mechanical or radiation injury due to improper use of light sources
3. False-positive and false-negative tests due to selection of inappropriate type or amount of light
4. Discomfort at patch test sites and "flares" at previously involved sites
5. Masked photopatch reaction
6. Persistent hyperpigmentation at test sites

beneficial to superimpose these compresses on a thin layer of petrolatum to prevent excessive drying.

In acute phototoxic reactions (sunburn), aspirin is very helpful if given as soon as possible after the exposure. Two or three tablets every 4 to 6 hours for about 48 hours, if tolerated, is usually sufficient.

In generalized cases, systemic corticosteroid therapy often gives prompt symptomatic relief. The dosage is similar to that for any generalized acute dermatitis.

In chronic cases that are only responsive to systemic corticosteroids, and in which a significant morbidity is present, immunosuppressive agents may be helpful (89). Azathioprine seems to be the most efficacious of these agents.

Although it may seem paradoxical, PUVA therapy has proven helpful, especially in some cases of chronic actinic dermatitis (100). Apparently, clinical improvement is related to inhibition of T cells and Langerhans cells.

Cyclosporine, alone or with PUVA, has been noted to be beneficial in sporadic case reports, as has the anabolic steroid danazol (101,102).

Protection against Light

The avoidance of sunlight must often be extended beyond the period of acute dermatitis because excretion of the photosensitive chemical from the skin may be delayed. In severe cases, confinement of the patient in a darkened room for several days may speed recovery. Window glass does not usually protect against contact phototoxic or contact photoallergic reactions.

Knowledge of the action spectrum of a photosensitizer is often of value, because ordinary window glass (3 mm thick) usually affords protection only against UV radiation less than 320 nm (103).

Patients with a photosensitivity dermatitis may obtain protection by using adequate clothing. Closely woven dark fabrics are best. The weave pattern of the fabric is much more important than the color or fabric type (104). White shirting becomes much more permeable to erythema-producing radiation when it is wet with water or perspiration.

Repeated, short exposures to sun have occasionally helped in desensitizing individuals. Such desensitization is probably nonimmunologic and is due to increased melanin formation and thickening of the horny layer. Dark-skinned individuals are less apt to have photosensitizing reactions than are fair-skinned people. Birmingham et al. (11) noted that the skin of Mexican and black harvesters affords protection against the phototoxic effects of the celery pink rot. Crow et al. (22) noted that dark-skinned workers are protected against photodermatitis from pitch.

Pigmentation of skin, color of clothes, and reflection and scattering of sunlight may affect the intensity of photodermatitis.

Use of Sunscreen Agents

Unfortunately, sunscreens seem to be of only modest benefit in the treatment of photodermatitis, especially the chronic varieties. For those who are allergic to the active sunscreen agents, physical sunscreens such as titanium dioxide and zinc oxide may be useful. However, some of these products produce a visible opaque coating on the skin.

The sunless tanning agents do not offer photoprotection even though the skin darkens slightly with their use.

Birmingham et al. (11) reported that physical sunscreens protect celery harvesters against phototoxic reactions due to pink rot in celery, but chemical sunscreens did not.

Management of Contact Photodermatitis Due to Specific Phototoxins

Tar

Individuals receiving tar therapy in whom a photosensitivity reaction is to be avoided should apply the tar at night only and should remove it carefully in the morning. Patients should be warned that, even though the tars have apparently been completely removed from the skin, avoidance of exposure to strong sunlight for several days is important, because traces of the tar alone may cause phototoxic reactions. Purified or refined tars are less apt to cause photosensitivity reactions. It may be desirable occasionally to substitute wood tars (e.g., pine tar), which are not photosensitizers.

The Phenothiazines

Medical and nursing personnel and those in the pharmaceutical industry who handle Thorazine and certain insecticides should be warned of their photosensitizing capabilities.

REFERENCES

1. Harber LC, Bickers DR. *Photosensitivity diseases: principles of diagnosis and treatment.* Philadelphia: WB Saunders, 1981.
2. Gould J, Mercurio M, Elmets C. Cutaneous photosensitivity diseases induced by exogenous agents. *J Am Acad Dermatol* 1995;33:551–573.
3. Gonzalez E, Gonzalez S. Drug photosensitivity, idiopathic photodermatoses and sunscreens. *J Am Acad Dermatol* 1996;35:871–885.
4. Baer RL, Harber LC. Photosensitivity induced by drugs. *JAMA* 1965;192:989.
5. Harber LC, Targouik SE, Baer RL. Studies on contact photosensitivity to hexachlorophene and trichlorocarbanilide in guinea pigs and man. *J Invest Dermatol* 1986;51:373.
6. Harber LC, Levine GM. Photo sensitivity dermatitis from household products. *GP* 1969;39:95.
7. Menz J, Muller SA, Connolly SM. Photopatch testing: a six-year experience. *J Am Acad Dermatol* 1988;18:1044.
8. Hölzle E, et al. Photopatch testing: the 5-year experience of the German, Austrian, and Swiss Photopatch Test Group. *J Am Acad Dermatol* 1991;25:59.
9. DeLeo V, Suarez S, Maso M. Photoallergic contact dermatitis: results of photopatch testing in New York, 1985–1990. *Arch Dermatol* 1992;128:1513.

10. Bowers A. Phytophotodermatitis. *Amer J Contact Derm* 1999;10: 89–93.

11. Birmingham DJ, et al. Phototoxic bullae among celery harvesters. *Arch Dermatol* 1961;83:73.

12. Pathak MA, Daniels Jr F, Fitzpatrick TB. The presently known distribution of furocoumarins (psoralens) in plants. *J Invest Dermatol* 1962;39:225.

13. Parrish JA, Fitzpatrick TB, Tanenbaum L, Pathak MA. Photochemotherapy of psoriasis with oral methoxsalen and longwave ultraviolet light. *N Engl J Med* 1974;291:1207.

14. Harber LC, et al. Berloque dermatitis. *Arch Dermatol* 1964;90:572.

15. Sams EM. Photodynamic action of lime oil *(Citrus aurantifolia)*. *Arch Dermatol* 1941;44:571.

16. Aberer W. Occupational dermatitis from organically grown parsnip *(Pastinaca sativa L.) Contact Dermatitis* 1992;26:62.

17. Ash-Wood-Smith MF, et al. Photosensitivity from harvesting lovage *(Lesisticum officinale). Contact Dermatitis* 1992;26:356.

18. Hann SK, et al. Angelica-induced phytophotodermatitis. *Photodermatol Photoimmunol Photomed* 1991;8:84.

19. Elpern DJ, Mitchell JC. Phytophotodermatitis from Mokihana fruits *(Pelea anisata* H. Mann, fa. Rutaccae) in Hawaiian lei. *Contact Dermatitis* 1984;10:224.

20. Schempp C, Sonntag C, Schopf E, et al. Dermatitis bullosa striata pretensis durch *Dictamnus albus* L. (Brennender Busch). *Hautarzt* 1996;47:708–710.

21. Tunget C, Turchen S, Manogiuerra A, et al. Sunlight and the plant: a toxic combination. Severe phytophotodermatitis from *Cneoridium dumosum. Cutis* 1994;54:400–402.

22. Crow KD, et al. Photosensitivity due to pitch. *Br J Dermatol* 1961; 73:220.

23. Calnan C, Harman R, Wells G. Photodermatitis from soap. *Br Med J* 1961;2:1266.

24. Wilkinson DS. Photodermatitis due to tetrachlorosalicylanilide. *Br J Dermatol* 1961;73:213.

25. Vinson LK, Flatt RS. Photosensitization by tetrachlorosalicylanilide. *J Invest Dermatol* 1962;38:327.

26. Osmundsen PE. Contact photodermatitis due to tribromosalicylanilide. *Br J Dermatol* 1969;81:929.

27. Auerbach R, Pearlstein HH. Photosensitivity and soap. *NY J Med* 1971;72:747.

28. Harber LC, Harris H, Baer RL. Photoallergic contact dermatitis. *Arch Dermatol* 1966;94:255.

29. Freeman RG, Knox JM. The action spectrum of photocontact dermatitis caused by halogenated salicylanilides and related compounds. *Arch Dermatol* 1968;97:130.

30. Epstein JH, Woepper KD, Maibach HI. Photocontact dermatitis to halogenated salicylanilides and related compounds. *Arch Dermatol* 1968;97:236.

31. Harber LC, Harris H, Baer RL. Structural features of photoallergy to salicylanilides and related compounds. *J Invest Dermatol* 1966; 46:303.

32. Gaul LE. Sensitivity to bithionol. *Arch Dermatol* 1963;87:383.

33. Jillson OF, Baughman RD. Contact photodermatitis from bithionol. *Arch Dermatol* 1963;88:409.

34. Epstein J, Rees W, Baughman RD. Contact photodermatitis from bithionol. *Arch Dermatol* 1964;90:153.

35. O'Quinn SE, Kennedy B, Isbell KH. Contact photodermatitis due to bithionol and related compounds. *JAMA* 1967;199:89.

36. O'Quinn SE. The sun and your skin. *Cutis* 1968;4:585.

37. Burry JM. Photoallergies to Fentichlor and multifungin. *Arch Dermatol* 1967;95:287.

38. Burry JM. Cross sensitivity between Fentichlor and bithionol. *Arch Dermatol* 1968;97:496.

39. Burry JM, Hunter GA. Photocontact dermatitis from jadit. *Br J Dermatol* 1970;82:224.

40. DeEds F, Wilson RH, Thomas JO. Photosensitization by phenothiazine. *JAMA* 1940;114:2095.

41. Cahn MM, Levy EJ. Ultraviolet light factor in chlorpromazine dermatitis. *Arch Dermatol* 1957;75:38.

42. Epstein JH, Brunsting LA. Topical application of chlorpromazine: its effect on the erythema response to ultraviolet light. *J Invest Dermatol* 1958;30:91.

43. Sidi E, Hincky M, Gervais A. Allergic sensitization and photosensitization to Phenergan Cream. *J Invest Dermatol* 1955;24:345.

44. Newill RGD. Photosensitivity caused by promethazine. *Br Med J* 1960;2:359.

45. Epstein S. Allergic photo-contact dermatitis from promethazine (phenergan). *Arch Dermatol* 1960;81:175.

46. Epstein S, Rowe RJ. Photoallergy and photocross sensitivity to phenergan. *J Invest Dermatol* 1957;29:319.

47. Schauder S. Dioxopromethazine induced photoallergic contact dermatitis followed by persistent light reaction. *Amer J Contact Derm* 1998;9:182–187.

48. Epstein S. Photoallergy and primary photosensitivity to sulfanilamide. *J Invest Dermatol* 1939;2:43.

49. Harber LC, Lashinsky AM, Baer RL. Photosensitivity due to chlorothiazide and hydrochlorothiazide. *N Engl J Med* 1959;261: 1378.

50. Journe F, Marguery M, Rakotondrazafy J, et al. Sunscreen sensitization: a 5-year study. *Acta Derm Vener* 1999;79:211–213.

51. Szczurko C, Dompmartin A, Michel M, et al. Photocontact allergy to oxybenzone: ten years of experience. *Photodermatol Photoimmunol Photomed* 1994;10:144–147.

52. Fotiades J, Soter NA, Lim HW. Results of evaluation of 203 patients for photosensitivity in a 7.3 year period. *J Amer Acad Derm* 1995;33:597–602.

53. Lenique P, et al. Contact and photocontact allergy to oxybenzone. *Contact Dermatitis* 1992;26:177.

54. Berne B, Bos A. Seven-year experience of photopatch testing with sunscreen allergen in Sweden. *Contact Dermatitis* 1998;38:1–4.

55. Theeuwes M, Degreef H, Dooms-Goossens A. Para-aminobenzoic acid (PABA) and sunscreen allergy. *Am J Cont Derm* 1992;3:206.

56. Pigatto PD, Legori A, Bigardi AS, et al. Gruppo Italiano ricerca dermatiti da contatto ed ambientali. Italian multicenter study of allergic contact photodermatitis: epidemiological aspects. *Amer J Contact Derm* 1996;7:158–163.

57. Zhang XM, Nakagawa M, Kawai K, et al. Erythema-multiforme-like eruption following photoallergic contact dermatitis from oxybenzone. Contact Dermatitis 1998;38:43–44.

58. Sterling GB. Sunscreens: a review. *Cutis* 1992;50:221.

59. Schauder S, Ippen H. Contact and photocontact sensitivity to sunscreens: review of a 15-year experience and of the literature. *Contact Dermatitis* 1997;37:221–232.

60. Fisher AA. Sunscreen dermatitis: part IV—the salicylates, the anthranilates, and physical agents. *Cutis* 1992;50:397.

61. Foley P, et al. The frequency of reactions to sunscreens: results of a longitudinal population-based study on the regular use of sunscreens in Australia. *Br J Dermatol* 1993;128:512.

62. Raugi GJ, Storrs FJ. Photosensitivity from men's cologne. *Arch Dermatol* 1979;115:106.

63. Giovinazzo VJ, Harber LC, Bickers DR, Armstrong RB. Photoallergic contact dermatitis to musk ambrette: histopathologic features of photobiologic reactions observed in a persistent light reactor. *Arch Dermatol* 1981;7:344.

64. Burry JN. Persistent light reaction associated with sensitivity to musk ambrette. *Contact Dermatitis* 1981;7:46.

65. Jackson RT, Nesbitt Jr LT, De Leo VA. 6-methylcoumarin photocontact dermatitis. *J Am Acad Dermatol* 1980;2:124.

66. Kaidbey KH, Kligman AM. Contact photoallergy to 6-methylcoumarin in proprietary sunscreens. *Arch Dermatol* 1978;114:1709.

67. Harber LC, Armstrong RB, Ichikawa H. Current status of predicting animal models for drug photoallergy and their correlation with drug photoallergy in humans. *J Natl Cancer Inst* 1982;69:237.

68. Epstein S. Role of dermal sensitivity in ragweed contact dermatitis. *Arch Dermatol* 1960;82:48.

69. Epstein S. Photocontact dermatitis from benzocaine. *Arch Dermatol* 1965;92:591.

70. Epstein S. Photoallergic contact dermatitis: report of a case due to Dangard. *Cutis* 1968;4:856.

71. Nakamura M, Arima Y, Nobuhara S, et al. Airborne photocontact dermatitis due to the pesticides maneb and fenitrothion. *Contact Dermatitis* 1999;40:222–223.

72. Matsushita S, Kanekura T, Sarvinatari K, et al. Photoallergic contact dermatitis due to Daconil. *Contact Dermatitis* 1996;35:115.

73. Burckhardt W. Photoallergic eczema due to blankophores (optic brightening agents). *Hautarzt* 1957;8:486.

74. Bjoernber A. Reactions of light in yellow tattoos from cadmium sulfide. *Arch Dermatol* 1963;88:267.

75. Goldstein N. Mercury-cadmium sensitivity in tattoos: a photoallergic reaction in red pigment. *Ann Intern Med* 1967;67:984.

76. Sams WM. Untoward response with topical fluorouracil. *Arch Dermatol* 1968;97:14.

77. Tronnier H. Photosensitivity of eczema patients (with particular reference to chromate eczema). *Arch Klin Exp Derm* 1970;47:494.

78. Romaguera C, Lecha M, Grimalt F, et al. Photocontact dermatitis to cobalt salts. *Contact Dermatitis* 1982;8:383.

79. Yamada S, Tanaka M, Kawahara Y, et al. Photoallergic contact dermatitis due to diphenhydramine hydrochloride. *Contact Dermatitis* 1998;38:282.

80. Horio T. Allergic and photoallergic dermatitis from diphenhydramine. *Arch Dermatol* 1976;112:1124.

81. Urrutia I, Jauregui I, Gamboa P, et al. Photocontact dermatitis from cinchocaine (dibucaine). *Contact Dermatitis* 1997;39:139–140.

82. Zaynoun S, Johnson BE, Frain-Bell W. The investigation of quindoxin photosensitivity. *Contact Dermatitis* 1976;2:343.

83. Frain-Bell W, Gardiner J. Photocontact dermatitis due to quindoxin. *Contact Dermatitis* 1975;1:256.

84. Wilkinson DS. Patch test reactions to certain halogenated salicylanilides. *Br J Dermatol* 1962b;74:302.

85. Jillson OF, Baughman RD. Contact photodermatitis from bithionol. *Arch Dermatol* 1963;88:409.

86. Sidi LE, Hincky M, Gervais A. Allergic sensitization and photosensitization to phenergan cream. *J Invest Dermatol* 1955;24:345.

87. Wiskemann A, Wulf K. Untersuchungen uber den auslosenden spektral Bereich und die direkte licht Pigmentierung bei chronischen und akuten licht Auschlagen. *Arch Klin Exp Derm* 1959;209:443.

88. Guzzo C, Kaidbey K. Persistent light reactivity from systemic quinine. *Photodermatol Photoimmunol Photomed* 1990;7:166.

89. Roelandts R. Chronic actinic dermatitis. *J Am Acad Dermatol* 1993;28:240.

90. Willis I, Kligman AM. The mechanism of the persistent light reactor. *J Invest Dermatol* 1968b;51:385.

91. Katsamura Y, Tanaka J, Ichikawa H, et al. Persistent light reaction: induction in the guinea pig. *J Invest Dermatol* 1986;87:330–333.

92. Bjornberg A. Reactions to light yellow tattoos from cadmium sulfide. *Arch Dermatol* 1963;88:267.

93. Burry JN. Photoallergies to Fentichlor and Multifungin. *Arch Dermatol* 1967;95:287.

94. Ive FA, Magnus LA, Warin RP, et al. Actinic reticuloid: a chronic dermatosis associated with severe photosensitivity and the histological resemblance to lymphoma. *Br J Dermatol* 1969;81:469.

95. Toonstra J, Henquet C, van Weelden H. Actinic reticuloid. *J Am Acad Dermatol* 1989;21:205–214.

96. Bilsland D, Crombie I, Ferguson J. The photosensitivity dermatitis and actinic reticuloid syndrome: no association with lymphoreticular malignancy. *Br J Dermatol* 1994;131:209–214.

97. Menage H, Ross J, Norris P, et al. Contact and photocontact sensitization in chronic actinic dermatitis: sesquiterpene lactone mix is an important allergen. *Br J Dermatol* 1995;132:543–547.

98. British Photodermatology Group. Workshop report: photopatch testing—methods and indications. *Br J Dermatol* 1997;136:371–376.

99. Hasan T, Jansen CT. Photopatch test reactivity: effect of photoallergen concentration and UVA dosaging. *Contact Dermatitis* 1996;34:383–386.

100. Hindson C, et al. PUVA therapy of chronic actinic dermatitis: a 5-year follow-up. *Br J Dermatol* 1990;123:273.

101. Gareazábal J, et al. Successful treatment of musk ketone-induced chronic actinic dermatitis with cyclosporine and PUVA. *J Am Acad Dermatol* 1992;27:838.

102. Humbert P, et al. Chronic actinic dermatitis responding to danazol. *Br J Dermatol* 1991;124:195.

103. Blum HF. Sunburn. In: Hollander A, ed. *Radiation biology,* vol. 2. New York: McGraw-Hill, 1955.

104. Robson J, Diffey B. Textiles and sun protection. *Photodermatol Photoimmunol Photomed* 1990;7:32.

CHAPTER 24

Paresthesia Due to Contactants

The chemicals and fabrics shown in Table 24.1 can produce abnormal sensory symptoms without dermatitis.

PARESTHESIA FROM SYNTHETIC PYRETHROID INSECTICIDES

Knox et al. (1,2), stating that occupational exposure to fenvalerate, a synthetic pyrethroid insecticide, has been reported to cause paresthesia, developed a protocol that involved the topical application of 0.05 ml of field-use diluted technical Pydrin (1:180) or a placebo (ethyl alcohol) to the ear of 36 volunteer subjects. Numbness, itching, burning, tingling, and warmth were the most commonly reported sensations. These sensations usually began after 1 hour, peaked at 3 to 6 hours, and lasted less than 24 hours. For technical Pydrin, the average score of intensity on a scale of 0 (no sensation) to 4 (markedly intense) was 1.40; the score of intensity for the placebo was 0.36. This finding demonstrates that a statistically significant sensation (p = .001) occurred after application of Pydrin.

As field use of fenvalerate has increased in recent years, several reports of cutaneous paresthesias among occupationally exposed individuals have appeared (3). These cutaneous sensations occur topically without erythema, edema, vesiculation, or any other sign of cutaneous irritation.

> **Contact exposure to synthetic pyrethrin insecticide can produce numbness, itching, burning, tingling, and warmth without dermatitis; the effect takes place after 1 hour and may last for 24 hours.**

LeQuesne et al. (3) reported that among 23 workers exposed to synthetic pyrethroids, 19 had experienced one or more episodes of abnormal facial sensation developing between 30 minutes and 3 hours after exposure and persisting for 30 minutes to 8 hours. There were no abnormal neurologic signs, and electrophysiologic studies (of the arms and legs) were normal. The sensations were variously described as "tingling," "burning," "like coming in from the cold," or like "nettle rash," but no study participants complained of loss of sensation; when directly questioned, they said it was quite different from the sensation after administration of a local anesthetic for dental treatment. The subjects were not aware of loss of sensation when they touched the affected area, and the sensation was unaffected by rubbing the skin.

The abnormal sensations were usually distributed symmetrically over the cheeks, particularly under the eyes and sometimes on the nose. In three subjects, unilateral symptoms on the face occurred after an accidental splash or direct contact with a pyrethroid solution. In other instances, subjects said they developed symptoms when working with pyrethroids in the form of a fine powder of one- to four-particle size or dissolved in a volatile solvent, but not when working with pyrethroids in other forms.

A delay characteristically followed exposure to the pyrethroids before the onset of symptoms. The shortest delay was 30 minutes after beginning to work with pyrethroids, and the longest interval before symptoms developed was 3 hours after exposure ceased. The duration of symptoms varied from 30 minutes to 8 hours.

It should be emphasized that the facial dysesthesia is not accompanied by dermatitis. The dictionary definition of "dysesthesia" is impairment of sensation short of anesthesia or a condition in which a disagreeable sensation is produced by ordinary stimuli.

Descriptions of the facial symptoms have varied. A few subjects said the sensation that followed pyrethroid exposure resembled that after direct skin contact with some solvents, for example, dimethylsulfoxide (DMSO). However, DMSO has an immediate effect, and all sensations are rapidly relieved by washing the exposed area of skin. For several reasons it is unlikely that a solvent is responsible for the symptoms described here. Similar symptoms occurred with a variety of solvents and in the absence of a solvent (the only common exposure was a pyrethroid). The delay in onset of symptoms after exposure and their duration are unlike those that follow skin contact with other irritant solutions.

It seems likely that direct skin contact with a pyrethroid is necessary for the development of symptoms. In a few instances, there was a clear history of contact before symp-

TABLE 24.1. *Contactants Producing Paresthesia*

Methyl methacrylate monomer
Pants paresthesia syndrome (from synthetic fabric)
Physical pressure
Solvents: turpentine, benzene, and acetone
Synthetic pyrethroids
Wool in atopics
Acrylonitrile

> **Topical vitamin E oil has been recommended to prevent contact paresthesia from pyrethrin insecticides; topical vitamin E, however, may cause allergic eczematous and urticarial contact dermatitis.**

toms developed, and other workers related the occurrence of symptoms to the degree of exposure. It is noteworthy that one field operator found he was protected from symptoms only when wearing a full head and facial mask with breathing canister. In this group of workers, symptoms occurred only on the face. It may be that, apart from the hands, the face receives the greatest exposure and absorption occurs more easily through the facial skin than through other exposed areas. Thus, the symptoms are most likely to result from transient lowering of the threshold of sensory nerve fibers or sensory nerve endings after exposure of the facial skin to pyrethroids. This is similar to the phenomena described after exposure of animal nerves to pyrethroids.

A field survey by Tucker and Flannigan (4) disclosed that a stinging sensation about the face and arms was reported by workers occupationally exposed to fenvalerate. Direct contact with the liquid was not necessary to induce the paresthesia. It was believed that cutaneous exposure to aerosol or vapor was responsible for several reported cases. Interestingly, a similar sensation was reported by investigators in 1941 after exposure to *Chrysanthemum cineariaefolium* flowers (5). The patient described tingling of his face after entering a room with an open cannister of airdried flowers. To continue his work, he was forced as a prophylactic measure to smear petrolatum over all exposed areas of his body.

Tucker et al. (6) performed pilot studies on various topical agents to assess their ability to prevent dysesthesia accompanying exposure to the synthetic pyrethroid, Pydrin. Six compounds were evaluated for their prophylactic efficacy on four participants on separate occasions. Nature's County Natural Vitamin E Oil (25,000 IU/2.1 fl oz) was the most effective prophylactic agent evaluated, with a prophylactic index (PI) of 97.3%. In contrast, Lilly Zinc Oxide Paste (USP 25%) appeared to be synergistic when applied, resulting in a negative PI index. A cost-effective therapeutic agent would be Arrowhead Mills Brand Corn Oil. Owing to the comedogenic properties of vegetable oils, however, it was not recommended.

Contact dermatitis in response to synthetic pyrethroids is very rare. In a survey of 230 subjects (7), two cases of allergy to fenvalerate were reported, along with one allergic reaction to cypermethrin and two irritant reactions to resmethrin.

THE PANTS PARESTHESIA SYNDROME

Fisher (8) studied four men who complained bitterly of itching, tingling, and formication of the lower extremities, particularly the inner aspects of the thighs, whenever they wore trousers not made exclusively of cotton. Examination of the skin revealed no abnormalities. Two of the patients were examined by neurologists who also found nothing objectively. Patch tests to formaldehyde and various resins and textile finishes were negative. Two of the patients believed that the "weight of the material itself" caused a burning sensation.

> **Some individuals, particularly men, complain of paresthesia when wearing trousers made of synthetic fibers. They tolerate only cotton fabrics. No dermatitis is present.**

Dr. F. Storrs, who interviewed two of the patients, reported to Dr. Fisher (9):

> I don't have any more ideas about those burning and itching male patients of yours than I did last year. I still think that one of the formaldehyde polymers or dyes could be causing the problem. Ask your patients to wear well-washed Levis blue jeans for a month and only Levis blue jeans. If they become substantially better, I think you can, in fact, look to a fabric finish or a dye as the cause of the difficulty. Perhaps they developed contact urticaria. Remember that the Levis must be the so-called "bread and butter Levis" that are found on whole shelves. They cannot be the so-called designer Levis. (p. 482)

Dr. Calnan of London informed Fisher that several patients were "running around" in London frustrated because dermatologists were unable to come up with an answer to this problem.

Dr. Devel of Belgium sent Fisher the following information:

> Referring to your letter on "pants" problem (*Contact Dermatitis* 9:92): I have sent you the following short communication read in the Flemish newspaper *De Standaard* on Saturday 11, March 1983: "My son likes to wear velvet jean trousers, but they cause him skin irritation on the thighs, even if consisting of 85% cotton and only 15% polyester. Frequent washings, water softeners, abstinence of ironing, lining as low as the knees, . . . it doesn't make any difference. Who knows what to do?" (p. 482)

One dermatologist reported that he personally suffers from this pants syndrome.

All the patients mentioned were men. Dr. L. Alston, however, writes as follows:

> Regarding contact "pants paresthesia syndrome," I have had a patient who has driven me nuts for the past year complaining bitterly of discomfort, tingling and funny sensations on her inner thighs. She is a 40-year-old slightly chubby woman who usually wears slacks. She felt the seams of her slacks were causing the problem. She would sew handkerchiefs into her slacks to cover those seams. That helped just a little. For a period of time she had a deep erythema in that region. I did patch test her to dyes, formaldehyde, etc., pieces of fabric from her slacks and could not find anything on patch testing. The rash gradually diminished with a topical steroid. She has switched to wearing dresses. She seems to fit the pattern of your male patients with the burning and itching. I cannot find anything at least in what I have patch tested her to regarding formaldehyde, resins, and textile finishes. She does not wear Levis at all so it really is not a problem with Levis. She usually wears brown, black, or navy polyester slacks. (p. 482)

PARESTHESIA FROM WOOL AND MOHAIR

Wool is the natural, highly crimped fiber from sheep. Minute scales on the fiber allow interlocking to form felt cloth and mill-finished worsteds. These scales may be harsh enough to cause mechanical irritation in many persons.

Friction with woolen garments, particularly in association with sweating and atopic dermatitis, may produce a nonspecific pruritus and burning sensation.

Mohair is the resilient hair fiber obtained from the Angora goat. It provides a crisp, firm, and slightly scratchy feel to fabrics even when used in low percentage blends with other fibers. Its addition to clothing produces itching and discomfort in many persons, but allergic sensitivity has not been reported.

PRESSURE PARESTHESIA

Choy (10) reported as follows:

> A stockbroker appeared at my office with a chief complaint of hypesthesia in a palm-sized area over the left suprapatellar area of several months' duration. Another physician had ordered roentgenograms of the lumbar spine, which were normal. Physical examination showed hypesthesia and obvious hair loss over the involved area.
>
> Careful questioning revealed that the telephone in his office was so placed that reaching for it necessitated turning his body more than 90° to the right. This motion was always accompanied by scraping the anterior surface of his left lower thigh (the affected area) against the kneehole of the desk.
>
> In a follow-up visit, he reported that in discussing his now famous knee with his office colleagues, another stockbroker with the same telephone-desk configuration came forward with an almost identical complaint of hypesthesia in the left suprapatellar area.
>
> Perhaps an appropriate diagnosis in these two cases would be stockbroker's knee. (p. 482)

An orthopedic surgeon reported that the pressure of a wallet in a hip pocket can produce a neuralgia-simulating sciatica.

PARESTHESIA FROM SOLVENTS

Strong solvents, such as turpentine, acetone, and benzene, may produce dryness and fissuring of the skin accompanied by paresthesia of the fingers. Such paresthesias may persist for several weeks after the dermatitis has subsided and the patient no longer has contact with the solvents.

One consultant neurologist stated he had observed similar peripheral neuritis and paresthesia accompanying industrial dermatitis from benzene (Fisher AA, Contact Dermatitis. Lea & Febiger 1986, p. 483).

Acrylonitrile, which is recognized as a skin irritant, was found to produce five cases of allergic contact dermatitis in an occupational setting. One of these was accompanied by paresthesia that had not previously been reported with acrylonitrile (11).

Strong solvents may produce paresthesia that may persist long after any dermatitis has subsided.

LOSS OF TASTE

Contact dermatitis in the form of cheilitis and perioral eczema due to anethole was associated with a loss of taste (12). The sense of taste returned about 2 to 3 weeks after the cheilitis cleared. Anethole is found in oil of anise, star anise, and fennel. It can be found in toothpaste.

METHYL METHACRYLATE MONOMER

Fisher (13) reported that surgeons and dentists who became sensitized to methyl methacrylate monomer in acrylic bone cement may suffer a distressing paresthesia of the fingertips in the form of a burning sensation, tingling, and slight numbness. The paresthesia may persist for several weeks to months after the dermatitis has subsided. Fisher saw this type of paresthesia in two orthopedic surgeons who became sensitized to acrylic monomer. In one, the paresthesia persisted for 3 months after the dermatitis subsided. In the other, the paresthesia persisted for 4 months.

Five dentists who acquired an acrylic monomer dermatitis had persistent dermatitis for 3 to 6 months after the dermatitis subsided. Dermatitis and paresthesia of the fingertips of the first three fingers of both hands were found to be due to a dental acrylate containing 2-hydroxyethyl methacrylate (14). A local effect on peripheral nerves is thought to be responsible for the paresthesia, which can last for up to 6 months after exposure is discontinued.

It should be noted that the acrylic monomer is such a strong solvent that it can readily penetrate rubber gloves.

Some surgeons wear three pairs of gloves during surgery. The acrylic monomer readily penetrates damaged skin, producing an inflammation of the nerve endings in the fingers with resultant persistent peripheral neuritis and paresthesia.

> **Methyl methacrylate monomer can penetrate rubber gloves and produce persistent neuritis in dentists and orthopedic surgeons.**

ADVERSE SUBJECTIVE REACTIONS TO TOPICAL AGENTS

Grove et al. (15) state that certain topical products, especially those applied to the face, can pass all the standard tests yet still be unacceptable because they induce strong, disagreeable sensations (e.g., stinging, burning, or itching). These investigators indicate that these disagreeable sensations occur frequently enough to warrant serious study. This is not an easy task, as the adverse reactions are purely subjective and generally not accompanied by any visual signs by which the degree of response can be graded. Thus, the ear, not the eye, serves as the detector regarding problems of adverse subjective reactions.

> **Many topical agents produce stinging, burning, and other disagreeable sensations without producing dermatitis.**

Testing for "Stinging" Topical Agents

Stinging is a problem that occurs primarily on the face, particularly on the nasolabial folds and cheeks. The extreme sensitivity of this region is a reflection of its microanatomic features, including a more permeable horny layer, a high density of appendages (hair follicles and sweat glands) that serve as diffusional shunts, and an elaborate network of sensory nerves. In humans, every vellous hair is associated with specialized nerve endings that connect to an elaborate dermal nerve network (16). Thus, it is not surprising that the face is so sensitive to touch and pain (see Chapter 5).

Stinging seems to be a variant of pain that develops rapidly and fades quickly any time the appropriate sensory nerves are stimulated. This type of response is usually quite well tolerated. Consumers have come to expect just such a short burst of stinging from alcoholic formulations, for example, aftershave lotions, astringents, and toners. With the intolerable variety of stinging with which we are concerned, the response is not only more intense but somewhat delayed and sustained. Typically, it begins within 1 or 2 minutes after product application and intensifies over the next 5 to 10 minutes. This sharp stinging then fades slowly

over the next 15 to 20 minutes. Despite the fact that this crescendo-type stinging may become so intense that frantic attempts are made to wash off the offending material, visual indications of the adverse response, for example, erythema, are rarely seen.

Frosch and Kligman (17) were prompted to develop a practical test for uncovering new facial products that may have potential to produce stinging. The essential features of this procedure were that the test materials were applied to the nasolabial folds and cheeks of preselected sensitive individuals who were brought to a state of profuse sweating in an environmental chamber. Once again, no strong correlation between irritancy and stinging was observed. For example, strong irritants, such as quaternary ammonium surfactants, undiluted kerosene, and 5% sodium lauryl sulfate, did not produce stinging under these conditions, whereas weak irritants or nonirritants, such as Escalol 506, provoked intense stinging.

> **Escalol 506, the amyl ester of PABA in sunscreens, produces a marked, stinging sensation in some persons.**

Initially, Frosch and Kligman (16,17) thought that most persons who experienced stinging would be light-complexioned persons of Celtic ancestry who were easily sunburned and tanned poorly.

Grove et al. (15) reported that skin type is not a reliable predictor of stinging proclivity. People with a darker complexion can also experience moderate or intense stinging in response to 10% lactic acid applied to the nasolabial folds and cheeks. Persons who experienced such positive reactions judged themselves as having unusually "sensitive" skin and usually reported a variety of past troubles with cosmetics, soaps, and related items. Thus, it is more expedient to prescreen candidates on the basis of a history of problem or sensitive skin than on the basis of a fair or dark complexion.

The actual premarket testing of products for stinging capacity is performed on preselected "stingers" who are brought to a state of profuse sweating in an environmental chamber. Test materials can be classified into one of three categories, based on results obtained with the improved facial sting test. The first class includes materials that exhibit little or no potential for stinging during normal use. The second class includes products that have a slight potential for stinging and that might pose a problem for some sensitive-skinned persons. The third class includes products with a strong potential for stinging; these would be intolerable to sensitive-skinned persons and perhaps other consumers as well. In this manner, problem products can be readily identified, and intolerable stinging induced by facial products need no longer be experienced by today's consumers.

> **A 10% lactic acid solution may be used to detect persons who are "stingers."**

Testing Topical Agents that Cause "Burning"

Using a 20:80 mixture of chloroform:methanol, Frosch and Kligman (16) found that the nasolabial fold is the region most sensitive to both "burning" and "stinging" sensations. Heavy users of cosmetics were most susceptible to the lactic acid "stinging" test and the chloroform:methanol "burning" test.

> **Burning and stinging from cosmetics usually occurs in women who use a great many cosmetics.**

Testing for Itching in Response to Cosmetics

Frosch and Kligman (16) found that fragrances and sunscreen lotions are the major culprits of itching from cosmetics. They used a "histamine itching test" to determine which woman would itch from exposure to topical agents.

Using this test, Fisher (9) found no correlation between the size of the wheal and the sensation of itching. Frosch and Kligman (16) also found no correlation between wheal size and itching. There appears to be no correlation between itching and stinging or burning.

STATUS COSMETICUS (PROBLEM SENSITIVE SKIN)

Frosch and Kligman (17) came to the conclusion that a small but significant number of young women have "problem-sensitive skin." Fisher found that not only young women but also many older women have "problem-sensitive skin," which has long been called "status cosmeticus" (18).

In some patients, the problem-sensitive skin is localized to the eyelids and does not affect the face at all.

> **Status cosmeticus (problem sensitive skin) can affect women at any age and is sometimes confined to the eyelids.**

Fisher (9) observed that many women with status cosmeticus are particularly affected not only by lactic acid but also by sorbic acid, isopropyl myristate, and urea.

REFERENCES

1. Knox JM, Tucker SB. A new cutaneous sensation caused by synthetic pyrethroids. *Clin Res* 1982;30:915A.
2. Knox II JM, Tucker SB, Flannigan SA. Paresthesia from cutaneous exposure to a synthetic pyrethroid insecticide. *Arch Dermatol* 1984; 120:744.
3. LeQuesne PM, Maxwell IC, Butterworth ST. Transient facial sensory symptoms following exposure to synthetic pyrethroids: a clinical and electrophysiological assessment. *Neurotoxicology* 1980;2:1.
4. Tucker SB, Flannigan SA. Cutaneous effects from occupational exposure to fenvalerate. *Arch Toxicol* 1983;54:195.
5. Martin TJ, Hester KHC. Dermatitis caused by insecticidal pyrethrum flowers (*Chrysanthemum cineraiaefolium*). *Br J Dermatol* 1941;53:127.
6. Tucker SB, Flannigan SA, Smolensky MH. Comparison of therapeutic agents for synthetic pyrethroid exposure. *Contact Dermatitis* 1983;9:316.
7. Lisi P. Sensitization risk of pyrethroid insecticides. *Contact Dermatitis* 1992;26:349.
8. Fisher AA. Contact "pants paresthesia syndrome." *Contact Dermatitis* 1983;9:92.
9. Fisher AA. *Contact dermatitis,* 3rd ed. Philadelphia: Lea & Febiger, 1986.
10. Choy DSJ. "Stockbroker's knee." *Arch Dermatol* 1977;113:1300.
11. Bakker JG, Jongen SM, Van Neer FC, Neis JM. Occupational contact dermatitis due to acrylonitrile. *Contact Dermatitis* 1991;24:50.
12. Franks A. Contact allergy to anethole in toothpaste associated with loss of taste. *Contact Dermatitis* 1998;38:354.
13. Fisher AA. Paresthesia on the fingers accompanying dermatitis due to methylmethacrylate bone cement. *Contact Dermatitis* 1979;5:56.
14. Kanerva L, et al. Fingertip paresthesia and occupational allergic contact dermatitis caused by acrylics in a dental nurse. *Contact Dermatitis* 1998;38:114.
15. Grove GL, Soschin D, Kligman AM. Guidelines for performing facial sting tests. In: *Proceedings of the 12th International Congress of the I.F.S.C.C.,* Paris.
16. Frosch P, Kligman AM. A method for appraising the stinging capacity of topically applied substances. *J Soc Cosmet Chem* 1981;28:197.
17. Frosch P, Kligman AM. Recognition of chemically vulnerable and delicate skin. In: Frost P, ed. *Principles of cosmetics for the dermatologist.* St. Louis: Mosby, 1984;287.
18. Fisher AA. Cosmetic actions and reactions: therapeutic, irritant, and allergic. *Cutis* 1980;26:22.

CHAPTER 25

Occupational Dermatitis[1]

Dermatitis is by far the most frequently reported occupational disease, and patch testing with a standard screening series of allergens reveals a substantial number of relevant causes. In addition, of course, special test series may have to be performed on workers exposed to diverse contactants.

> **Dermatitis is the most common industrial disease. Contact allergens play such a significant role in industry that all patients with chronic dermatoses should be patch tested not only with specific industrial contactants but also with the "standard" or "routine" series.**

In industry, as elsewhere, patch testing is indicated only in the diagnosis of allergic eczematous contact dermatitis. Aside from investigative procedures, patch tests are of no value in the primary irritant type of contact dermatitis. The diagnosis of industrial dermatitis depends not only on the patch test results but also on the history, clinical picture, and proved exposure to the suspected contactant (1,2).

The patch test is particularly valuable in ascertaining the cause of outbreaks of isolated cases of allergic contact dermatitis in an industry in which workers are directly or indirectly exposed to many sensitizing chemicals. Although a careful history and personal investigation of the patient's exposure to contactants often reduce the necessity for routine patch tests, such procedures are often necessary to confirm a diagnosis of allergic contact dermatitis.

Most insurance carriers and industrial boards accept a significant patch test reaction as proof of the etiologic basis of an allergic contact dermatitis. A properly performed and correctly interpreted patch test is scientific proof of the relationship of a specific contactant to a particular dermatitis.

Patch testing may also help in differentiating occupational and nonoccupational dermatitis, particularly when a person with contact dermatitis is exposed to sensitizers not only at work but also at play or in pursuit of hobbies. Properly performed patch tests may pinpoint the offending contactant quickly and efficiently, whereas reliance on history and trial and error may prolong the dermatitis while the offending allergen is being pursued.

Many workers have a superimposed allergic contact dermatitis from sensitizing topical medications. Such a complication can be proved only by patch testing.

The factory dispensary or "first aid" room is sometimes the source of a superimposed allergic contact dermatitis, because sensitizing topical medications are often dispensed or used on industrial dermatitis, burns, and other injuries. Table 25.1 lists the sensitizing medications often found in factories as well as nonsensitizing alternatives.

> **Factory dispensaries and "first aid" rooms often provide workers with such sensitizing topical medications as benzocaine, topical antihistamines, neomycin, and other creams that produce superimposed contact dermatitis.**

In an English contact dermatitis clinic, of 1,153 patients evaluated, 17% were diagnosed as having occupational dermatitis. The final diagnosis was irritant contact dermatitis in 53% and allergic contact dermatitis in 47% (3). The most common job associated with occupational dermatitis was metal processing, followed by nursing, catering, hairdressing, cleaning, then shop work.

Occupational dermatitis involves both irritant and allergic contact dermatitis, and when aggregated the individuals who develop occupational contact dermatitis as compared with nonoccupational contact dermatitis are younger, less likely to be atopics, more likely to be male, have hand and arm dermatitis, and show positive patch test responses to metals, rubber compounds, p-phenylenediamine, epoxy, and rosin. However, when the irritant occupational contact dermatitis cases are compared with the allergic occupational contact dermatitis cases, the allergic cases are likely to be female, atopics, and have dermatitis of the hands, arms, and eyelids (4).

A survey of Gothenberg, Sweden, sampled 7.6% of the population by questionnaire, with an 82.9% response rate. At issue were whether the populace experienced hand

---

[1]This chapter is the revision of a chapter written for the third edition by Robert M. Adams.

TABLE 25.1. *Suggested Nonsensitizing Medications for Factory First-Aid Treatment*

Medication	Low sensitizers	Potent sensitizers
Anesthetics	Pramoxine HCl cream or lotion Xylocaine ointment	Topical "caine" anesthetics, especially those containing benzocaine
Antibiotics	Ilotycin ointment	Topical antibiotics containing neomycin
Antifungal agents	Micatin, Lotrimin lotion, Whitfield's ointment	Mycolog cream
Antihistamines	Oral antihistamine to relieve itching	Topical antihistamine-containing creams
Antiseptics	Hydrogen peroxide	Thimerosal (Merthiolate)
	Betadine solution	Nitrofurazone (furacin)
Steroids	Hydrocortisone cream 0.5% to 2.5%	Paraben-containing steroid creams
	Fluorinated corticosteroid creams 0.01% to 0.05%	
Vitamin preparations	Petrolatum	Vitamin E–containing creams

eczema and what role was played by occupation. It was learned that 1,385 respondents had experienced hand eczema in the previous 12 months, and it was the result of occupational exposure in 11.8%. Cleaners had the highest period prevalence (21.3%). Most cases were irritant, and the most common allergen was nickel, followed by cobalt, fragrance mix, balsam of Peru, and colophony. Colophony, an allergen associated with paper products, increased in prevalence with administrative work (5). Holness and Nethercott (6) surveyed 230 workers over a 5-year period and learned that 48% of their occupational cases of dermatitis were allergic and 52% irritant. Persons who did not remember their diagnosis correctly were twice as likely to have active dermatitis and dermatitis that was more severe. The majority of patients did not accurately recall their diagnosis. Wall and Gebauer (7) investigated the outcome of occupational skin disease in 771 patients, more than 60% of whom were followed more than 2 years from the initial diagnosis. Wall and Gebauer found that 50% were still suffering from the original dermatitis. Furthermore, if these patients had changed jobs, many were back in work environments that put them at the same risk as in the first job. More than 10% had persistent postoccupational dermatitis without obvious cause (11.5%) (7).

PATCH TESTING WITH NEW INDUSTRIAL COMPOUNDS

Particular care must be exercised when new manufacturing processes and compounds are introduced. Under such circumstances, the dermatologic hazards of the new procedures and chemicals must be evaluated properly and as fully as possible before a large number of workers are exposed and sensitized.

Animal studies are of value when the chemical is a strong primary irritant. Preliminary human patch tests for primary irritant effects are useful, but they should be done on volunteer or paid subjects rather than on the workers to prevent undue apprehension among them, complaints from labor unions, or legal action.

The application of a new compound every day or two for 2 to 3 weeks may simulate working conditions and may prove of value in determining the irritant properties of the substance.

Whenever new chemicals are tested and the proper concentration for testing has not been established, it is much safer to perform the preliminary patch test by the open method. If the reaction is negative, it is then relatively safe to patch test by the usual covered method.

Solutions of dyes, paints, or liquid resins may be painted on the skin and left uncovered, because they evaporate and adhere to the site. Volatile solvents should be allowed to evaporate before being covered. If it is suspected that the chemical to be tested is a strong sensitizer, it is wise to observe the patient in the office for an hour or so after the patch test has been applied. Such observations may sometimes detect chemicals that are producers of nonimmunologic or immunologic contact urticaria.

RULES FOR TESTING WITH UNLISTED OR UNKNOWN SUBSTANCES

1. Test liquid substances with litmus paper to ascertain whether they are strongly acidic or alkaline. Such substances must be tested carefully and in the proper dilutions to avoid severe irritation or burns.
2. Determine whether the substance to be tested is soluble in water, acetone, or olive oil or can be dispersed in petrolatum. Petrolatum is the preferred dispersing agent because it is suitably occlusive and nonirritating.
3. Always test unknown or unlisted substances at first by the "open" method. Start with a 0.1% concentration. If there is no reaction, test with a 1% concentration. If there is then no reaction, proceed to "closed" patch testing starting with a 0.1% concentration and then to a 1% concentration. Should a positive reaction be obtained, test three controls to rule out an irritant reaction.
4. Test substances stored in rubber-stoppered bottles or containers may be contaminated with rubber chemicals and may thus give false-positive reactions.
5. Observe the patient in the office for 1 hour after the patches are applied. Examine for evidence of contact urticaria.

> **Do not patch test with occupational chemicals until the nature of the substance is known and the proper solvent and concentration for safe testing are obtained.**

INTERPRETATION OF PATCH TEST RESULTS WITH NEW COMPOUNDS

The interpretation of results of patch testing with new compounds is fraught with pitfalls, because it may be difficult to distinguish an allergic from a primary irritant reaction. A neat vesicular eruption consisting of closely set, clear vesicles is probably an allergic response, particularly if the site itches and the reaction persists and spreads.

An erosion or a single bulla covering the entire patch test site and confined almost exactly to the area of application is probably a primary irritant reaction. Less marked primary irritant reactions may consist of minute papules and pustulovesicles irregularly situated at follicular or sweat gland orifices, and follicular crusts and minute superficial etched-out ulcers. Primary irritant reactions tend to disappear rapidly when the covering patch is removed, but allergic reactions often become more intense. Unfortunately, irritant reactions occasionally intensify for 1 to 2 days after a patch test is removed, so that the intensification phenomenon is not an absolute distinguishing feature.

Whenever the results of patch testing with a new compound are doubtful, the chemical should be tested on three normal controls. A primary irritant will usually cause a reaction in one or two of the controls, but an allergen should not cause a reaction in them.

Another type of irritant or false-positive reaction may occur when the skin is hyperirritable or an acute dermatitis is present. In such instances, even testing substances used in nonirritating concentrations may produce reactions that are difficult to distinguish from a true allergic response. In case of doubt, patch tests should be repeated after a week or so when the skin is less irritable or the dermatitis less acute.

PREEMPLOYMENT PATCH TESTING

The routine use of preemployment patch tests should be avoided. Workers who do not have a history of allergic dermatitis or who do not present with a dermatitis that is compatible with an allergic contact dermatitis should not be subjected to preemployment patch test procedures. Although a properly performed patch test does not usually sensitize those who would not in all likelihood have become sensitized by the occupational exposure, workers who react positively may claim that the procedure caused the sensitization.

A contrary view has been presented for people entering the hard metal industrial trades. Prescreening with patch tests showed 28 of 79 male students training for work in the metalworking industry were sensitive to nickel, cobalt, or chromate, leading the authors to conclude that screening was valuable (8).

> **Routine preemployment patch testing should be avoided for medicolegal reasons.**

If the worker gives a history of allergic contact dermatitis or presents with a dermatitis compatible with such a diagnosis, preemployment patch testing may be indicated. Such testing alerts him or her to avoid further exposure, in the new occupation, to a specific chemical to which he or she had become sensitized in the past.

A worker who shows a strongly positive patch test reaction to a chemical must avoid not only that particular chemical but also immunochemically related allergens. For example, individuals who demonstrate allergic hypersensitivity to paraphenylenediamine should also avoid azo and aniline dyes. However, a positive patch test reaction to the dichromates does not preclude exposure to other metals, such as nickel and copper, because cross-reactions between these metals do not usually occur.

It is unfair to exclude a worker from employment merely because he or she has had an allergic contact dermatitis in the past. As a rule, aside from cross-sensitization reactions, allergic contact hypersensitivity is specific and is restricted to one group of chemicals. It would also be unfair to deny employment to an individual because he or she has had an allergic contact dermatitis and has an "immunologic" scar or his or her skin had been damaged in the past.

Although strongly positive patch test reactions usually indicate that the patient will acquire severe contact dermatitis if exposed to the sensitizer, mild positive reactions, such as a 1+ rating, need not necessarily exclude a worker from handling the sensitizing compound.

In many instances in which a highly skilled worker has a minimal dermatitis with a weakly positive patch test reaction to a particular chemical, the dermatitis remains mild despite continued exposure to the allergen. Fisher (9) observed several furriers with mild test reactions to paraphenylenediamine and minimal dermatitis who continued to be exposed to the dye for years without much difficulty. Such instances are not examples of hardening, but of a low-grade sensitization, which may at any time suddenly become more marked. Fisher (9) also observed low-grade sensitizations with minimal dermatitis from dichromates and formaldehyde in patients who continued to be exposed without acquiring disabling eruptions.

Great care must be taken to dilute strong sensitizers so that a strongly positive patch test reaction may be avoided. Such reactions may produce marked itching and discomfort for several weeks and may cause a disgruntled employee to claim that he or she never had any "skin trouble" until the patch test was performed. Medicolegal complications may result from such severe reactions.

USE OF PATCH TESTS TO DETERMINE HARDENING IN INDUSTRY

The term "hardening," as originally introduced by J. Jadassohn, indicated a condition in which an allergic contact dermatitis in sensitized persons disappeared or failed to reappear on repeated exposure to the sensitizing chemical. This concept of a specific hardening has been broadened to include a nonspecific variety.

"Nonspecific hardening" refers to instances in which a patient acquires a dermatitis from a primary irritant, such as fiberglass, and subsequently can handle it without acquiring an eruption. The type of nonspecific hardening is neither proved nor disproved by patch testing.

> **Specific desensitization or "hardening" is the exception rather than the rule.**

Specific hardening may be described as a form of natural hyposensitization in which certain individuals suffering from an allergic dermatitis may become hyposensitized to the allergen in spite of continued exposure. The term "hyposensitization" is preferred to "desensitization," because in many instances the hypersensitivity returns, particularly if there is reexposure after a period of avoidance.

Hardening is said to occur under conditions of diminished but continuous contact with the allergen, and it is more likely to occur if the allergic dermatitis appears after a short exposure than after prolonged contact. It is also claimed that hardening is less likely to occur after a severe dermatitis than after a mild attack. Hardening after allergic sensitization is more likely to occur with certain sensitizing chemicals, for example, tetryl, than with sensitizers such as the dichromates.

It was Fisher's opinion (9) that hardening, or hyposensitization, occurs only in rare instances and may be attributed to better hygiene so that contact with the allergen is avoided. In most instances in which hardening is cited in the literature, the impression is "clinical" only. Scientific proof of specific hardening would be established when the following criteria have been satisfied:

1. The patient has had an allergic contact dermatitis due to a specific chemical that caused a *strongly* positive patch test reaction.
2. The allergic contact dermatitis produced by the chemical clears and remains clear despite exposure to the chemical that caused the positive patch test reaction.
3. The previously strongly positive patch test reaction to the chemical becomes negative or only weakly positive.

Fisher's experience (9) was that hardening, or desensitization, that fulfills these criteria occurs only in rare instances and usually cannot be relied upon in the management of allergic contact dermatitis due to occupational exposures. A recent study of the persistence of allergic eczematous sensitivity to paraphenylenediamine revealed that such hypersensitivity persisted for 10 to 15 years in more than 90% of patients, and strongly positive patch test reactions were obtained in sensitized individuals even when they apparently no longer came in contact with the sensitizer.

More recent reports suggest that some form of hardening may have occurred in Japanese lacquer workers and in cashew nut shell oil dermatitis (10,11). Rietschel et al. (12) tried to induce hardening with an irritant-maleic acid. After 6 weeks of daily exposure in 50 human volunteers, only about 20% demonstrated some diminution of reactivity, and nearly as many developed intense, vesicular dermatitis of sudden onset after 2 to 4 weeks of exposure, indicating the onset of true allergy. None of this latter group could be hardened, and further exposure only exacerbated the dermatitis. The investigators concluded that hardening of any type, specific or nonspecific, was the exception rather than the rule and could not be anticipated as a clinically useful outcome (12).

Workers who acquire an allergic contact dermatitis from a chemical that produces a strongly positive patch test reaction should not be exposed to the sensitizing compound in the hope that hardening, or desensitization, may take place. This expectation is almost never fulfilled.

Attempts at desensitization by exposing the patient's skin to gradually increasing concentrations of the contact allergen also fail. Therapeutic hardening by feeding or injecting graduated amounts of specific contact allergens has been successful only partially with poison ivy and ragweed oleoresins.

Nonspecific hardening does frequently take place with continued use of mild or moderate primary irritants because of gradual thickening and pigmentation of the skin.

> **Desensitization procedures with occupational chemicals usually fail.**

OCCUPATIONAL CONTACT PSORIASIS OF THE HANDS FROM TRAUMA (KOEBNER PHENOMENON)

Pressure and friction from occupational procedures may produce psoriasis of the hands, particularly the palms and volar surface of the fingers. This Koebner phenomenon was seen in a pharmacist (from the pressure of opening and closing containers with child-resistant caps), a surgeon, a dentist (from the pressure of various instruments), a bus driver (from the pressure of the steering wheel), and in an office worker (from pounding a stapler) (13).

Also, fresh lesions of psoriasis that appear after trauma from scratching, abrasions, lacerations, folliculitis, and acne have led many workers to press for compensation in the belief that the disease was caused or activated by their occupation. If a "koebnerized" lesion is followed quickly by a severe flare of the disease, the idea of occupational causation seems even more likely to the worker. Trauma may undoubtedly incite the development of new lesions of psoriasis, but only in persons who already have the disease, if only in latent form. For this reason, careful consideration should be given to the job placement of persons with active psoriasis and even to those with a history of the disease. Thus, Koebner phenomenon is medicolegally important when it follows industrial injuries. Lichen planus may occasionally also produce an industrial Koebner phenomenon.

> **Koebner phenomenon with the production of contact psoriasis is often a source of medicolegal problems in industrial cases.**

OCCUPATIONAL SITE SURVEY: PRINCIPLES AND SIGNIFICANCE

The procedure of occupational site survey includes teamwork between physicians, nurses, industrial hygienists, biostatisticians, and epidemiologists. The personnel involved in data collection should be chosen so as to obtain the most information during a single visit to an industrial plant and to best interpret the data gathered. It is important to make an appointment before visiting an industrial plant and never to visit unannounced.

White and Rycroft (14) discovered, on a visit to an industrial plant in which there had been an outbreak of dermatoses among the employees of a soft lens factory, that the dermatitis was the result of low relative humidity in the ambient atmosphere.

> **Low or high humidity or poor ventilation may produce an industrial dermatitis that can only be diagnosed by a visit to the industrial plant.**

OCCUPATIONAL DERMATITIS THAT IS SELF-INFLICTED

Meneghini and Angelini (15) state that cases of occupational dermatosis of this type fall into two pathogenetic groups: (a) dermatoses produced directly on healthy skin and (b) aggravation of preexisting dermatoses of spontaneous origin.

The malingerer uses various noxious, usually exogenous, agents; mechanical, physical (red-hot metal objects, boiling water, or olive oil), and chemical solutions of strong acids or alkalis, (chromium salts, aqua regia, or other solvents); or substances of vegetables (capsicum and cactus) or animal (cantharides) origin.

Most of the lesions are found mainly at the sites exposed to the possible action of occupational factors. The lesions almost always show regular punched out outlines, are monomorphic, and are surrounded by normal skin.

Fisher (9) saw patients, however, who were accused of being malingerers but who actually had porphyria cutanea tarda with punched out ulcers of the dorsum of the hands on apparently normal skin.

In many cases the morphology of the lesions alone may provide sufficient grounds for the diagnosis of dermatitis artefacta. The diagnosis is also helped by the fact that the malingerer often attempts to reproduce the clinical picture of occupational contact dermatitis on healthy skin and does not realize that this is difficult to do.

Angelini et al. (16) state that some patients produce persistent edema of the hand by the application of a tourniquet or by repeated self-inflicted contusion of the dorsum of the hand, the so-called Secretan's syndrome.

The diagnosis is more difficult when the malingerer seeks to aggravate or perpetuate the preexisting eczematous dermatosis. Continued observation in the hospital may be necessary to solve this diagnostic problem.

> **Self-inflicted lesions often appear on normal skin. Factical-like lesions, however, may appear in patients with porphyria cutanea tarda due to trauma.**

ASSESSMENT OF OCCUPATIONAL CUTANEOUS IMPAIRMENT AND DISABILITY

The evaluation of impairment is usually possible through the exercise of sound clinical judgment and depends on a detailed medical history, a thorough physical examination, and a judicious use of diagnostic procedures. Some articles are recommended in the reference section to help in such an assessment (17–21). The role of a chronic allergic occupational dermatitis in a patient who develops mycosis fungoides is a difficult assessment to make. Able (22) did not find a correlation between specific industrial exposures and the occurrence of mycosis fungoids in a carefully controlled study.

> **The possible role of chronic allergic occupational dermatitis in the production of mycosis fungoides is medicolegally significant.**

A Method of Evaluation for Patients with Occupational Contact Allergy[2]

"Standard" patch test series contain the most frequently encountered allergens found in the home and work environment and are especially valuable for the discovery of sensitivities to cosmetics and medications. For workplace allergens, only the rubber chemicals, epoxy resin, dichromate, rosin, nickel, and p-tert-butylphenol formaldehyde are included on the most frequently employed standard patch test series.

A search for a hidden allergen need not offer formidable difficulties, nor be especially time-consuming, if a program of logical steps is followed.

Occupational History

The cornerstone of the investigation is the occupational history, which must be obtained as soon as possible after the onset of the dermatitis. The dermatitis is often no longer present by the time of the patient's initial visit, especially if the worker is referred for evaluation by an insurance company or by a lawyer. The physician must, therefore, reconstruct the conditions surrounding the onset through detailed questioning, with sufficient time reserved for the interview, usually 30 to 45 minutes.

It is important to learn the area of skin involved at the onset of the dermatitis. This information can often provide a clue to the initial event and to the substances contacted at that time. The next regions involved and any subsequent spreading must be noted. Details of early treatment should be recorded. Improvement away from work and regular recurrence on returning to the same activity is relevant, as this is often the sole criterion required in worker's compensation law to substantiate a work relationship. Other workers may be similarly affected, which may suggest the presence of an unrecognized irritant, improper work practices, or the existence of a newly introduced allergen.

It is common for workers to have fixated on a putative cause that may or may not be correct, and they will want to direct the entire interview toward this substance. It actually saves time to ask patients to put that subject aside and go back to the beginning of their skin problem. Inquire where it occurred, what they did about it first, and what they did next. Reassure patients that you want to be comprehensive and know as much as possible about what they have been going through. This will eliminate a lot of otherwise missed information that is required for compensation forms and depositions. Keep asking "What did you do next, and what did you do after that?" until you come up to the present day.

It is important to document treatment from the plant dispensary, as well as the use of home remedies, barrier creams, special soaps, and whether gloves and other protective clothing have been worn.

Considerable questioning is usually necessary to learn the details of the work performed. Workers who do their jobs automatically, especially when the work is repetitive, often have difficulty explaining what they actually do. In these cases, it is necessary to urge the patient to recite a detailed step-by-step explanation of the exact movements required by the job. The worker should also be asked to describe the materials contacted at work, and from this the physician must estimate to what degree and in what manner they contact the skin.

Information can sometimes be gained from previous occupations and any work-related skin conditions arising from that work. A general medical history is also important, with special emphasis on a personal or family history of atopy. Previous contact dermatitis, especially reactions to cosmetics, topical medications, and jewelry, should be recorded. Also important are hobbies and other recreational activities, as well as the existence of a second job.

Material Safety Data

Material safety data sheets are documents required by the U.S. Labor Code Section 6390, which provide information about particular hazardous substances or mixtures in the work environment. Every employer is required to have available, or have requested from a manufacturer, producer, or any other seller of a hazardous substance, a completed material safety data sheet (MSDS) for each hazardous substance in use at the place of employment, and to make this information available upon the request of an employee, a union representative, or an employee's physician. These documents are supposed to provide pertinent information regarding ingredients, including the chemical names, physical data, fire and explosive information, reactivity data, leak, spill, and clean-up procedures, and special protective and handling information.

Unfortunately, MSDSs frequently contain little or no information of value to dermatologists. On many of them, ingredients are not precisely listed or are not named at all. Often they are recorded only in general terms, such as "amine" or "hydrocarbon." Substances in concentrations of less than 1% are frequently not included.

This situation can create difficulties, as important skin allergens are usually found in this fraction, especially germicidal agents, antioxidants, and fragrance materials. A telephone number at the upper-right-hand corner of the first sheet, however, will lead the physician to a person who can provide the required information. It is important to identify oneself as a physician, to explain that the information is required to study a patient properly, and that the knowledge gained may result in keeping the worker on the job. This approach is usually sufficient to loosen any tight reins on disclosure of any "proprietary" information.

---

[2]This section is by Robert M. Adams, clinical professor of dermatology, Stanford University Medical Center, and author of *Occupational skin disease*. Philadelphia: WB Saunders, 1990.

Sometimes a company may agree to release information only after a secrecy agreement has been signed. Agreeing to this stipulation will usually open up a free-flowing dialogue of vital information.

> **Material safety data sheets are usually of limited value to dermatologists.**

When several ingredients are listed, a dermatologist experienced in contact dermatitis can readily identify those chemicals that are known to cause allergic reactions, as well as those usually associated solely with irritancy.

Industrial Plant Visits

While material safety data sheets, when properly used, are indispensable for learning the chemical hazards of a given workplace, additional information can be obtained from an industrial plant visit, which can be profitable in many ways. Familiarity with work materials, job processes, the industrial plant environment, and the attitudes of workers and management enable physicians to more adequately diagnose and treat occupational skin diseases arising from working conditions in the plant. The physician will also be in a better position to recommend preventive measures and to assist in the placement of workers.

A visit can be arranged by the manager of a small industrial plant, or the safety or personnel departments of larger industrial plants. If the industrial plant has a part-time or full-time physician, arrangement can be made through him or her. Another method is to obtain an appointment through an industrial engineer of the local or state health department. Visits should be made early in the day, at the beginning of the day shift (at 7:00 A.M.), and can usually be completed within an hour or so.

Physical Examination

Although most cases of occupational skin disease involve only the hands and forearms, it is important to examine the entire skin to rule out other diseases or contributory conditions. It should be emphasized it is impossible to differentiate in every case between an allergic and an irritant contact dermatitis from the appearance of the eruption alone. Allergic reactions are often more explosive in onset, with marked vesiculation and itching. They are also often intermittent, appearing 1 or 2 days after contact with the allergen in a previously sensitized individual. However, mild irritant reactions develop more gradually, requiring days or weeks to evolve. In almost every case, however, it is impossible to differentiate between allergic and irritant dermatitis from appearance alone.

Patch Testing

The only certain way to diagnose allergic contact dermatitis in the workplace is through diagnostic patch testing. One is sometimes tempted to test with a product used by the worker without knowledge of its exact contents and potential for irritancy. Even substances that appear fairly innocuous may produce an irritant reaction when tested full strength under an occluded patch test for 48 hours, and the result can easily be interpreted incorrectly as a true allergic response.

When the history, examination, and information from the MSDS cause one to suspect one or more ingredients in a given compound as allergens, the next step is to obtain these chemicals in as pure a state as possible. If they are not present on a standard patch test series, they must be obtained from a chemical company. Catalogs are available on request. A supply company will refuse occasionally to sell a chemical to a private physician, but one can usually avoid this by appeal to higher officials of the company, or by buying the material through a hospital pharmacy or university chemical department. The costs are minor in small amounts, and after preparation any excess of the test materials can be stored for future use.

Appropriate concentrations for patch testing can be found in textbooks on contact dermatitis. A pharmacist can be found to prepare the mixtures, usually in white petrolatum, and the compensation insurance carrier can be billed for the cost, which is usually minor.

Determination of Relevance

When a positive test result is obtained with one or more known ingredients of a substance, the next step is to attempt to reproduce the dermatitis by a "use" test. The material itself, unless irritating, can be applied, in the concentration normally contacted by the patient, to a small area of skin, usually on the inner aspect of the arm just above the elbow, twice daily for 7 days, or until a reaction appears. The physician must recognize nonspecific irritant reactions due to lack of sufficient skin penetration.

Finally, relevance must be confirmed by again questioning the worker regarding the actual way the substance contacted the skin during the work process. It is reasonable that this substance could be responsible for the worker's dermatitis. If this seems to be true, one can be reasonably certain that a given substance containing an allergen to which the worker is found sensitive is indeed the cause of the dermatitis under investigation. At the same time, contributing factors such as nonoccupational activities can be placed in perspective.

A study of this magnitude is important because knowledge of the exact chemical responsible will enable the physician to help the patient avoid future contact with the allergen, either by substitution with unrelated and nonallergenic substances, or by suggesting an appropriate job change. Without this information, the worker is condemned to repeated episodes of dermatitis.

> **The proper application of a "use" test may determine the relevance of a suspected contact allergen in occupational dermatitis.**

RESOURCES FOR INFORMATION OR ASSISTANCE IN OCCUPATIONAL DERMATITIS

The following agencies can help the physician to obtain information concerning occupational exposures and injury:

1. National Institute for Occupational Safety and Health
   Clearinghouse for Occupational Safety and Health Information
   4676 Columbia Parkway
   Cincinnati, OH 45226
2. Consumer Product Safety Hotline
   Injury Information Clearinghouse
   1111 18th Street, N.W.
   Washington, DC 20207
3. Occupational Safety and Health Administration
   Director, Office of Information and Consumer Affairs
   200 Constitution Avenue, N.W.
   Washington, DC 20210
4. Environmental Protection Agency
   Public Information Center
   401 M Street, S.W.
   Washington, DC 20460

Valuable information can also be obtained from the *Dictionary of Occupational Titles,* 4th ed., US Department of Labor, 1977.

Catalogs of Chemical Companies

Eastman Organic Chemicals Catalog
Fischer Scientific Company
JT Baker Company
R & K Laboratory of Rare and Fine Chemicals
Subdivision of ICN Pharmaceuticals, Inc.
121 Express Street
Plainview, NY 11803

Manufacturers of Occupational Protective Materials

Protective Clothing

American Optical Corporation, 14 Mechanic Street, Southbridge, MA 01550
Mine Safety Appliances Co., 400 Penn Center Boulevard, Pittsburgh, PA 15235

Safety Clothing and Equipment Co., Division of Safety First Industries, Inc., 1522 East 69th Street, Cleveland, OH 44103
Uniroyal Protective Clothing, Washington, IN 47501

Protective Sleeves and Aprons

American Optical Corp., 14 Mechanic Street, Southbridge, MA 01550
Mine Safety Appliances Co., Penn Center Boulevard, Pittsburgh, PA 15235
Standard Safety Equipment Co., 431 North Quentin Road, Palatine, IL 60067
Surety Rubber Co., Box 97-G-12, Carrollton, OH 44615
Wheeler Protective Apparel, Inc., 226 West Huron Street, Chicago, IL 60610

Industrial Rubber Gloves and Synthetic Rubber Gloves

Edmont-Wilson, 3167 Walnut Street, Coschocton, OH 43812
Mine Safety Appliance Co., 400 Penn Center Boulevard, Pittsburgh, PA 15235
Pioneer Rubber Co., Tiffin Road, Willard, OH 44890
Surety Rubber Co., Box 97-G-12, Carrollton, OH 44615

Industrial Cleaners

Calgon Corp., Calgon Commercial Division, 7501 Page Street, St. Louis, MO 63133
Dameron Enterprises, Inc., 7635 National Turnpike, Louisville, KY 40214
Milburn Co., 3246 Woodbridge, Detroit, MI 48207
Sugar Beet Products, P.O. Box 1387, Saginaw, MI 48605
West Chemical Products, Inc., 4216 West Street, Long Island City, NY 11101

Waterless Hand Cleaners

Dameron Enterprises, Inc., 7635 National Turnpike, Louisville, KY 40214
Go-Jo Industries, Inc., P.O. Box 991, Akron, OH 44309
Sugar Beet Products, P.O. Box 1387, Saginaw, MI 48605
West Chemical Products, Inc., 4216 West Street, Long Island City, NY 11101

Protective Ointments and Barrier Creams

Amar-Stone Laboratories, Inc., 601 East Kensington Road, Mount Prospect, IL 60056
Ayerst Laboratories, 685 Third Avenue, New York, NY 10017
Calgon Corp., Calgon Commercial Division, 7501 Page Avenue, St. Louis, MO 63133
E. I. Du Pont de Nemours & Co., 1007 Market Street, Wilmington, DE 19898

Milburn Co., 3246 E. Woodbridge, Detroit, MI 48207

Mine Safety Appliances Co., 201 North Braddock Avenue, Pittsburgh, PA 15208

West Chemical Products, Inc., 4216 West Street, Long Island City, NY 11101

Zee Medical Products, 11800 Woodruff Avenue, Downey, GA 90241

LICHENOID ERUPTIONS AND LEUKODERMA IN THE PHOTOGRAPHY INDUSTRY

Photographers may acquire lichen planus–like eruptions from CD2-type color developers. The chemicals involved are derivatives of paraphenylenediamine or aniline. Most reports incriminate Kodak CD2 and Kodak CD3 (23–27).

Roed-Petersen and Menné (28) reported that these color developers are now being used in the processing of high-speed black-and-white film. At present, there are fewer reports of lichen planus–like eruptions as a result of industrial automatization that successfully stopped the previous epidemic of dermatitis. Most film developing is performed at large-scale, fully automated plants. Sporadic skin reactions occur among amateurs, newspaper photographers, and others who develop their own films manually.

> **Lichen planus–like eruptions and contact leukoderma are unusual types of dermatitis that photographers may develop.**

Automated photoprocessing might seem to eliminate contact with color film developer chemicals, but facial dermatitis from airborne contact from this source has occurred (29). Color developers CD2, CD3, and CD4 were the source. Lichenoid changes were not observed in this context.

Another type of unusual reaction that may occur in the photography industry is a contact leukoderma (vitiligo). This type of depigmentation is due to hydroquinone used in the developing process (30–32). This type of eruption also usually occurs mostly in amateurs who develop their own films. Adams (9) saw a high school student who took a course in photography and who developed a leukoderma of the hands.

Goh (33) reported allergic hand eczema due to Colorprint 101ER Developer Replenisher. The dermatitis was accompanied by onycholysis and was traced to hydroxylamine sulfite, which is tested at 2% aqueous concentration.

Photographers are exposed to many irritants and allergens, such as the following:

1. *Developers* (hydroquinone, *p*-amino-phenol, pyrocatechol, pyrogallol, metol, and paraphenylenediamine). These developers are dissolved in irritant alkaline solutions containing sodium sulfate and sodium carbonate or sodium hydroxide.

> **Leukoderma from hydroquinone may occur from the developing process.**

2. *"Stop bath"* (bromoresol purple). The "stop bath" consists of a weak solution of acetic acid. The concentrated acid can cause burns, and inhalation of the vapors can irritate the breathing passages and throat. Potassium chrome alum, sometimes used as a stop hardener, contains chromium and can cause ulcerations, especially in cuts and nasal membranes, and allergies.

3. *Fixers.* The fixer usually contains sodium sulfite, acetic acid, sodium thiosulfate (hypo), boric acid, and potassium alum. Hypo and the mixture of sodium sulfite and acetic acid produce sulfur dioxide, which is highly corrosive to the lungs. Potassium alum, a hardener, is a weak sensitizer and may cause some skin dermatitis.

4. *Bleaches.* Bleaches may contain potassium dichromate, hydrochloric acid, or mercuric chloride.

5. *Reducers.* Reducers may contain potassium ferricyanide.

6. *Toners.* Toners contain both irritants and allergens. Many toners contain highly toxic chemicals. These include selenium, uranium, liver of sulfur (corrosive to skin and breathing passages), gold, platinum (allergies), and oxalic acid (corrosive).

7. *Hardeners and stabilizers.* Hardeners and stabilizers often contain formaldehyde, which is poisonous and is very irritating to the eyes, throat, and breathing passages. They can cause dermatitis, severe allergies, and asthma. Some of the solutions used to clean negatives contain harmful chlorinated hydrocarbons.

8. *Print flattening solutions* (formaldehyde, hydrazine).

9. *Antifoggants* (Benzotriazole). The greatest skin hazard occurs during the preparation and handling of concentrated stock solutions of the various chemicals.

PIGMENTARY AND PURPURIC ERUPTIONS IN THE TEXTILE INDUSTRY

A survey of 72 textile workers found irritant contact dermatitis related to work exposures in 27 (38%) (34). Allergic contact dermatitis was due to occupational contactants in 21 (29%). The most frequent allergens were textile dyes in 12 workers, textile finishes in 11, and rubber-related allergens in 10. The textile finishes were formaldehyde-related permanent press finishes, and no one dye predominated.

Textile workers may acquire purpuric dermatitis presumably from formaldehyde resin and extensive hyperchromatism presumably due to naphthol compounds added to dyes in the process of preliminary dyeing (35,36).

Dooms-Goossens et al. (37) describe contact dermatitis caused by dimethylthiourea, an additive in diazo-sensitized paper used for textile cutting patterns. Table 25.2 shows

TABLE 25.2. *Patch-Test Series for Dermatitis Acquired in the Textile Industry*[a]

Patch test allergens	Patch test concentration
Azo dyes	
C.I. Disperse Black 2	1% pet
C.I. Disperse Yellow 35	1% pet
C.I. Disperse Red 1	1% pet
C.I. Disperse Yellow 3	1% pet
Cresol	2% pet
Dimethylolurea	10% pet
Ethylene glycol	2.5% aq
Ethylene urea	50% aq
Formaldehyde	2% aq
Hydrazine	1% pet
Melamine-formaldehyde resin	10% pet
Paraphenylenediamine	1% pet
Pentachlorophenol	3% pet
Phenylmercuric nitrate	0.05% pet
Potassium dichromate	0.5% pet
Quaternary ammonium salts	0.1% aq
Triethylene-imino-phosphine oxide	1% olive oil
Urea-formaldehyde resin	10% pet

[a]Aq, aqueous; Pet, in petrolatum.

patch test series suitable for dermatitis acquired in the textile industry.

> **Textile industry workers may develop purpuric dermatitis and extensive hyperchromatism.**

OCCUPATIONAL DERMATITIS IN THE PAINTING INDUSTRY

As a consequence of the decreasing use of solvent-based glues and paints and the increasing use of water-based products, manufacturers face problems with preservation.

Merthiolate, phenyl mercuric nitrate, and more recently chloracetamide have been used for this purpose. Chloracetamide has proved to be a common sensitizer in the painting industry (38–40).

Many painters have been exposed to chloracetamide in hanging wallpaper and fiberglass fabrics. Painters are also exposed to glues that may contain chloracetamide. It should be known that chloracetamide is also used as a preservative in cosmetic creams and lotions. The pesticide chlorothalonil has been added to some paints, which has led to facial dermatitis in people inhabiting freshly painted rooms due to the vapor pressure of chlorothalonil (41). In this case, the patch test was positive from 1% down to 0.0001% aqueous solution (0.4 ppm chlorothalonil). This potent sensitizer is used as a wood preservative and a pesticide in floriculture (41). In addition, various acrylates found in paint are shown in Table 25.3. Table 25.4 shows the numerous compounds found in paint (42), and Table 25.5 lists the suggested patch test series for painters.

TABLE 25.3. *Acrylates Found in Paints*[a]

	Patch test concentration
Butyl acrylate	1% pet
Epoxy acrylate	1% pet
Ethyl acrylate	1% pet
2-ethyl-hexylacrylate	1% pet
N-methylolacrylamide	1% pet
Pentaerythritol triacrylate	0.2% pet
Trimethylolpropane triacrylate	1% pet
Tripropylene glycol triacrylate	1% pet

[a]Pet, in petrolatum.

> **The newer water-based paints include merthiolate, phenyl mercuric nitrate, and chloracetamide, which are used as preservatives. These preservatives may produce allergic contact dermatitis; they are also used in cosmetics and topical medications.**

TABLE 25.4. *Miscellaneous Compounds Found in Paints*

Pigments
  Alizarin
  Chromates
  Lithol red
  Nickel dust
  Para-red
  Phthalocyanine blue
  Rhodamine
  Thioflavin
  Toluidine toners
Vehicles (binders)
  Linseed oil (rare)
  Rosin
  Synthetic resins, catalysts, and plasticizers
  Tung oil
Miscellaneous
  Antifoam agents
    Dibutyl phthalate
    Pine oil
  Antioxidants
    Hydroquinone
  Driers
    Cobalt naphthenates
  Paint thinners
    Diptene
    Turpentine
  Plasticizers
    Acrylates
    Dibutyl phthalate
    Polyester resins
    Sulfonamides
  Preservatives
    Chloracetamide
    Chlorothymol
    Mercuric oxide
    Organic mercurials
    Tetramethylthiuram disulfide
    Thimerosal
    Thymol

TABLE 25.5. *Test Tray for Painters[a]*

Allergens	Patch test concentration
Acrylates	1% pet
Betanaphthol (wallpaper adhesive)	10% olive oil
Δ³-Carene-turpentine sensitizer	1% as peroxide in olive oil
Chloracetamide	1% pet
Chloroparanitraniline red	2% pet
Cobalt chloride (dyes and driers)	2% pet
Colophony (rosin)	20% pet
Dipentene	10% MEK (methyl ethyl ketone)
Epoxy resin	1% pet
Epoxy resin hardeners	1% pet
Ethylene glycol	2.5% aq
F4R red	2% pet
Formaldehyde	2% aq
Hansa yellow	2% pet
Hydroquinone	1% pet
Para red	2% pet
Paratoluenesulfonamide	2% pet
Phenylmercuric nitrate (germicidal)	0.5% pet
Polyester resin monomer (polyester paint)	10% pet
Potassium dichromate (green and yellow)	2% pet
Propylene glycol	5% aq
Thimerosal (germicidal)	0.1% pet
Toluidine red (helio red)	2% pet
Tricresyl phosphate	5% pet
Turpentine	20% olive oil

[a]Aq, aqueous; Pet, in petrolatum.

Painters may become sensitized to resin additives. 1,2-benzisothiazolin-3-one (BIT) is a preservative that can be found in paints and combined with ethylenediamine in a product called Proxel XL 2 or Proxel CRL. It has caused contact dermatitis in painters, and sensitization to Kathon CG is commonly seen in these cases (43).

Another paint additive that has caused contact dermatitis is dichlofluanide, a fungicide that is also used in agriculture. Five cases of dichlofluanide allergy from glazing paints were reported by Gruvberger et al. (44). One of these patients developed erythema multiforme–like dermatitis. In guinea pigs, dichlofluanide is a strong sensitizer.

Painters may acquire dermatitis from turpentine and dipentene, which is used as a paint thinner.

PROTECTION FOR ARTISTS AND "DO IT YOURSELF" HOME DECORATORS AND PAINTERS

Dermatitis is one of the biggest dangers of working with art materials. The best way to prevent dermatitis is to prevent hazardous substance contact with the skin, particularly the hands, by wearing plastic or rubber gloves, especially when working with organic solvents, acids, and caustics. There are two basic requirements in choosing the type of glove: first, that the glove should be impervious to the materials being used; and second, that the glove should allow the degree of "feel" required for one's art.

For many purposes, polyvinyl gloves are suitable, such as cheap, disposable "surgeons' gloves" and heavier lined gloves for greater comfort. These polyvinyl gloves protect against most solvents except those containing large amounts of ketones, such as acetone.

Butyl rubber or natural rubber gloves will protect against ketones but not against aromatic solvents (toluol, xylol, and polyester resin) or most chlorinated hydrocarbons, and only provide fair protection against petroleum distillates (naphtha, mineral spirits, and kerosene) and acids. Neoprene rubber gloves have almost the exact opposite characteristics of other rubbers.

For work with acids and caustics, either polyvinyl chloride or neoprene rubber is best. For work with concentrated solutions, the gloves should be the gauntlet type with a cuff to turn back the acid or caustic. If protection from acrylates is required, the 4-H glove is better than rubber and vinyl, which provide no meaningful protection. The 4-H glove has recently been shown to provide protection for up to 1 week in electron microscopists exposed to 1-hexadecene and 2-hydroxyethyl acrylate (45).

If one cannot wear gloves, the use of barrier creams ("invisible gloves") might help by providing an impermeable barrier between the skin and the toxic material. There are different types of barrier creams, some water soluble and others water insoluble, but silicone types are supposed to be best. These barrier creams have to be renewed regularly. After use, the barrier creams are washed off with a mild soap and water. Unfortunately, even barrier creams that test well in the laboratory do not always help in practice. A clinical study of 12 patients showed that with the use of the best laboratory-tested barrier creams, 7 experienced return of dermatitis (46).

In cleaning hands, it is important to wash carefully and frequently with soap and water (especially before eating and smoking). Do not use harsh or abrasive soaps, because these can cause dermatitis themselves and can just increase the problem. With some materials, including paints, ink, and oils, waterless hand cleansers are helpful. These hand cleansers are often available in hardware and art supply stores. Cleansers containing kerosene are not recommended because of their defatting action. One hand cleaner, Centrex Red, has been reported to cause allergic contact dermatitis due to a sulfosuccinate derivative tested at 5% in petrolatum. The substance was sodium ricinoleic monoethanolamido-sulfosuccinate, which was the liquid detergent present at 0.47% in the product (47). After washing with these cleansers, one should also wash with plenty of soap and water. One should then use a hand lotion or cream containing lanolin to replace any skin oils lost.

Detailed information on the subject of art hazards is contained in the following publications: Gail Coningsby Barazani, *Safe Practices in the Arts and Crafts: A Studio*

Guide, available from the College Art Association, 16 East 52nd Street, New York, NY 10022; and Michael McCann, *Artist Beware: The Hazards and Precautions in Working with Art and Craft Materials,* published by Watson-Guptil, New York. For additional information and assistance, artists may consult the *National Poison Control Network,* Pittsburgh, PA, and the *Center for Occupation Hazards and Art Hazards Information Center,* 5 Beekman Street, New York, NY 10038.

OCCUPATIONAL DERMATITIS IN THE PRINTING INDUSTRY

The printing industry (not only newspapers, books, and magazines but also containers) has been almost revolutionized by a new drying method using polyfunctional acrylics (some also with an epoxy), a benzophenone photoactivator, and ultraviolet light. The old methods of solvent drying with all their difficulties can be dispensed with, and the time of cure is only seconds. Most cases of dermatitis have occurred in those persons who make the inks; hardly at all in the users, so far.

Malten et al. (48) state that the manufacture of photopolymer printing plates in general is based on a light-induced curing of synthetic resin applied on a metal or plastic carrier sheet. Ultraviolet light causes a radical donor to decompose into radicals, inducing cross-linking by a hardener between (long) chains bearing reactive sites. The irradiated parts of the plate are thus cured within a few seconds, making these parts resistant to subsequent processing (blowing or dissolving) means to remove the unirradiated parts of the plate.

Modern printing exposes the printer to various acrylate compounds and epoxy resins, as well as phototoxic reactions from isomers of para-aminobenzoic acid.

The composition of the inks varies widely and consists of pigments dispersed in a vehicle that contains various resins, photoinitiators, diluents, hydrogen transfer agents, stabilizers, surfactants, flattening agents, and inhibitors. Allergic sensitization to several polyfunctional acrylic monomers, epoxy acrylate oligomers, and associated isocyanate compounds has recent been reported, as has phototoxicity from exposure to mixed isomers (ortho and para) of amyl dimethylaminobenzoate (48–57).

In printing plants, printers, typesetters, and press operators are exposed to several irritants that include alcohols, alkalis, developers, etching solutions, grease, waxes, inks, resins, soaps, detergents, and solvents. Workers in printing operations may also be exposed to the following contact allergens: potassium dichromate, dyes, formaldehyde, hydro-

TABLE 25.6. *Test Tray for Printers[a]*

Allergens	Patch test concentration
Brown Sudan (naphthylaminoazonaphthol)	2% pet
Chloroparanitraniline red	2% pet
Eosin	50% pet
Epoxy acrylate	1% pet
Ethylene glycol	2.5% aq
Formaldehyde	2% aq
Hexanediol diacrylate	1% pet
Impression plates (acrylics)	as is
Lake Red C	2% pet
Mercaptopropionic acid	1% pet
Methacrylics	5% pet
Other plates (polyurethane)	as is
Para red	2% pet
p-phenylene diamine	1% pet
Pentaerythritol triacrylate	0.2% pet
Polythiol (pentaerythritol + mercaptopropionic acid)	0.1% acetone
Potassium dichromate	0.5% pet
Propylene glycol	2.5% aq
Toluidine red (or helio red)	2% pet
Trimethylol propane triacrylate	1% pet
Turpentine Δ^3-carene (peroxides)	1% pet
UV drying inks	1% pet

[a]Aq, aqueous; Pet, in petrolatum.

quinone, glues, and gums. Table 25.6 is a suggested patch test series for printers.

OCCUPATIONAL DERMATITIS FROM PESTICIDES

Those occupations, most often exposed to various pesticides that are likely to acquire pesticide dermatitis are listed in Table 25.7. A classification of the pesticides and repellents is given in Table 25.8.

Many of these pesticides are dispensed in solvents that are irritating to the skin. The pure active ingredient should be obtained if possible for patch tests. Impurities may cause more trouble than the active pesticides. Thus, Milby and Epstein (58) reported that the allergen in malathion is not the chemical itself but diethyl fumarate, which is present as a contaminant.

Pesticide dermatitis may be due to the pesticide chemical, to solvents, or to impurities.

TABLE 25.7. *Occupational Exposures to Pesticides*

Agricultural workers	Farmers
Cattle breeders	Foresters
Dairy workers	

TABLE 25.8. *A Classification of Pesticides and Repellents*

Acaricides
Animal repellents, including rodenticides
Fungicides
Herbicides
Insecticides and insect repellents

Both at home and abroad numerous reports indicate that pesticides produce many instances of occupational dermatitis (59–66).

Fungicides

Patch-test procedures with various fungicides are listed in Table 25.9. The dithiocarbamates listed in Table 25.10, which are widely used as fungicides, have caused numerous instances of allergic contact dermatitis (65,67–71).

In the midwestern section of the United States, the dithiocarbamate Maneb, used widely to prevent the ginseng weed from producing potato blight, has resulted in many severe cases of allergic contact dermatitis among farmers.

If is of interest to note that the agricultural fungicides thiram and the dithiocarbamates are closely related to

TABLE 25.9. *Patch Testing for Fungicides[a]*

	Patch test concentration
Chloronitrobenzenes	
DNCB	0.1% aq
Pentachloronitrobenzene	1% pet
Dicarboximides	
Captan	1% pet
Difolatan (captafol)	0.1% pet
Phaltan	0.1% pet
Dithiocarbamates (see Table 25.10)	
Mercaptobenzothiazole	1% pet
Mercury compounds	
Phenyl mercuric nitrate	0.01% pet
Nitrophenols	
4,6,-dinitro-o-cresol	0.5% aq
Dinobuton (acrex)	10% pet
Dinocap	0.5% pet
Nitrofen	0.5% pet
Organ-tin compounds (tributyltin oxide)	0.01% aq
Phenols	
Pentachlorophenol	1% aq
p-chloro-o-cresol	0.1% alcohol
Tetrachlorodihydroxydiphenyl	1% aq
Sulfide (vancide bl)	1% aq
O-benzyl-p-chlorophenol (Chlorophene, santophen 1)	1% aq
Phosphothioate	
Plondrel (ditalimfos)	0.01% pet
Quinones	
Chloranil	1% pet
Dichlone	1% pet
Dithianone	1% pet

[a]Aq, aqueous; Pet, in petrolatum.

Antabuse, which causes "flushing" when used in the treatment of alcoholism.

> **Thiram and the dithiocarbamates, agricultural fungicides, are closely related chemically to Antabuse, which is used in the treatment of alcoholism.**

Potato farmers in Ecuador have a high prevalence of dermatitis and frequent exposure to the fungicide Maneb. A comparison of farmworkers with those applying the fungicide found significant differences in dermatitis frequency (72). Conjunctivitis was present in 7% of fungicide applicators but in none of the workers or controls. Dermatitis was present in 68% of the workers, 55% of those applying fungicide, and 31% of controls. These findings are somewhat different from those reported from California, where dermatitis was due to vegetation in about 50% of cases and to pesticides in 20%.

Such dicarboximide fungicides as captan, phtahan, and difoltan can also produce allergic contact dermatitis (73–75). The less widely used fungicides such as phenylmercuric nitrate and the "quinone," dithianone, have caused dermatitis (76,77). Hearn (59) analyzed 250 cases of poisoning due to pesticides that occurred between 1957 and 1971. "Dermatitis" was a feature in 54 cases and chemical burns occurred in 18 cases. Many different chemicals were involved, but the most frequent causes of dermatitis were the organomercurial compounds, paraquat and thiram. The soil fumigant DD-95 is predominantly 1,3-dichloropropene, a severe irritant, but allergy can be distinguished by patch testing at 0.005% in petrolatum, because 0.05% was negative in 20 volunteers (78). Tin compounds such as tributyl tin oxide (hexa-n-butyl distanoxane) is corrosive at 0.1% as a patch test, and clothing contaminated by it should be discarded, as it does not wash out (79). This compound is also found in papermaking, timber preservation, polymerization of silicon, and stabilization of plastic, and is a biocide in paint (79).

Insecticides

Table 25.11 lists the insecticides. Rycroft (80) stated that the organophosphorus compounds were introduced originally as insecticides, but members of the group are now used as fungicides, herbicides, and plant growth regulators. Instances of contact dermatitis may be due to the pure chemical or to impurities in such compounds (58,81,82).

Herbicides

Table 25.12 lists the herbicides in current use. Peachey (83) states that no cases of contact dermatitis due to the herbicides paraquat or diquat have been reported so far, but

TABLE 25.10. *Dithiocarbamates[a]*

Chemical name	Common name	Patch test concentration
Chloro butynyl-chlorophenyl-carbamate	Barban (carbyne)	1% pet
Iron dimethyldithiocarbamate	Ferbam	1% pet
Manganese and zinc ethylene-bis-dithiocarbamate	Mancozeb	1% pet
Manganese ethylene-bis-dithiocarbamate	Maneb	0.5% pet
Methyl-butylcarbamoyl-benzimidazole carbamate	Benomyl (benlate)	0.1% pet
Mixture of polyethylene-bis-thiram sulfides	Carbatene	1% pet
Sodium methyldithiocarbamate	Metam-sodium	1% pet
Tetraethylthiurammonosulfide	Tetmosol	1% pet
Tetramethylthiuram disulfide	Thiram	1% pet
Triscopper dimethyldithiocarbamate-bis-chloride	Cuprobam	1% pet
Zinc dimethyldithiocarbamate	Ziram	1% pet
Zinc ethylene-bis-dithiocarbamate	Zineb (dithane)	1% pet
Zinc propylene-bis-dithiocarbamate	Propineb	1% pet

[a]Pet, in petrolatum

Sharvill (84) described skin ulceration due to contact with paraquat solution, and Samman and Johnston (85) reported softening and discoloration of fingernails due to contact with the concentrated chemical. Spencer (86) reported contact dermatitis due to the herbicide Randox.

Pentachlorophenol, which was used in a Japanese herbicide, caused dermatitis and death (87).

Insect Repellents

The US Department of Agriculture has tested more than 9,000 insect repellents and found that *n,n'*-diethyl-*m*-toluamide (commonly known as deet) is the best all-purpose repellent. Other effective agents include ethyl hexanediol, dimethyl phthalate, dimethyl carbate, and butopyronoxyl (Indalone).

More than 50 repellent preparations are available commercially: Most of them contain either DEET (Off and McKesson Mosquitone) or ethyl hexanediol (6–12 Brand and SkeetoGo). They are available in several forms, including liquid, foam, pressurized spray, stick, cream, and wipe-on tissue. Concentrations of the active ingredient vary with both type of formulation and brand. Preparations in which deet is the only repellent contain from less than 5% (in wipe-on tissues) to more than 40% (in liquids).

Factors Affecting Repellent Action

Some compounds are more effective than others against certain insects; for example, Indalone is better than deet in preventing tick bites. The concentration of the active compound can affect both the range of susceptible effects and the duration of effect.

TABLE 25.11. *Insecticides[a]*

	Patch test concentration
Carbamates (methyl)	1% pet
Cyclodienes	
Aldrin	1% pet
Dieldrin	1% pet
Dazomet (mylone) (hydrolyzes to formalin)	0.25% aq
DDD-dichloro-bis-chlorophenyl	1% acetone
Dichloro-diphenyl-trichloro-ethane (DDT)	1% pet
Lindane	1% pet
Omite	0.05% pet
Organophosphorus compounds	
Malathion	0.5% pet
Naled (dibrominated)	1% pet
Parathion	1% alcohol
Organothiocyanates	
Rodannitrobenzine	1% pet
Inorganic insecticides	
Arsenic	1% pet
Fluorides	1% pet
Botannical insecticides	
Benzyl benzoate	5% pet
Nicotine sulfate	5% aq
Pyrethrum powder	as is
Rotenone	5% in talcum powder

[a]Aq, aqueous; Pet, in petrolatum.
Note: The esters derived from pyrethrum powder are active insecticides as pyrethrens and cinerins. These do not contain sensitizers that cross-react with sesquiterpene lactones, which cause dermatitis from the chrysanthemum plant and ragweed.

TABLE 25.12. *Herbicides in Current Use[a]*

	Patch test concentration
Amides	
Propachlor	1% pet
Randox (A chloracetamine)	0.1% pet
Pentachlorophenol	1% pet
Quaternary salts	
Diquat	0.1% pet
Paraquat	0.1% pet
Triazines	
Atrazine	1% pet
Desmetryne	1% pet
Methotryne	1% pet
Prometryne	1% pet
Simazine	1% pet

[a]Pet, in petrolatum.

Cronce and Alden (88) reported a case of flea collar dermatitis. An insecticide (2,2-dichlorovinyl dimethyl phosphate and related compounds) in antiflea dog collars caused primary irritant contact dermatitis in four patients who handled dogs wearing these collars. The insecticide is a known poison that inhibits cholinesterase, and it is capable of producing primary irritant dermatitis and even chemical burns when it is incorporated into soft, plastic, antiflea dog collars in a 9% to 10% concentration. Fortunately, this insecticide is liberated slowly from the collar under normal circumstances, and the dog's hair helps to prevent dermatitis on its neck.

Shell's No-Pest Strip contained the same insecticide as do flea collars. Deet may produce a bullous reaction resembling a blistering insect eruption (89). In addition, deet may produce contact urticaria (90).

> **The insect repellent diethyl-*m*-toluamide (deet) may produce eczematous, bullous dermatitis and contact urticaria.**

Animal Repellents

The animal repellents are shown in Table 25.13. Warfarin, which is used widely as a rodenticide, causes death by producing hemorrhage in animals.

Antu, also known as Antirax, may be patch tested 2% in petrolatum. Antu, which is a thiourea compound and is also a widely used rat poison, can cause contact dermatitis in humans (91).

The acaricides are listed in Table 25.14. Omite, a sulfite compound, may be tested 0.05% in petrolatum, and even under this dilute concentration may produce irritant reactions (92). Dinobuton (Acrex), a nitrophenol compound, can cause yellow staining of the hair and nails and skin irritation. This compound is closely related to picric acid,

TABLE 25.13. *Animal Repellents[a]*

	Patch test concentration
Birds	
Anthraquinone powder[b]	as is
Dogs and cats	
Citronella oil	1% pet
Diethyl phthalate	2% pet
Eucalyptus oil	1% pet
Nicotine sulfate	5% aq
Oil of lemongrass	1% pet
Pine tar	1% pet
Synthetic oil of mustard	0.1% pet
Rabbits, deer, and meadow mice	
Thiram (used up to 20%)	1% pet
Rodents	
Antu (naphthylthiourea, Antirax)	1% pet
Warfarin	0.05% pet
Squirrels	
Oil of lemongrass	1% pet
Paradichlorobenzene	1% alcohol
Synthetic oil of mustard	0.1% pet

[a]Aq, aqueous; Pet, in petrolatum.
[b]Used on seeds to make them distasteful to birds.

which can cause a similar type of staining. Patch testing may be performed with 10% in petrolatum.

Bird Repellents

Anthraquinone is used to make seeds distasteful to birds and thus acts as a repellent. Because some anthraquinone dyes cross-react with paraphenylenediamine, contact with such seeds in a paraphenylenediamine-sensitive individual could possibly cause an eruption.

Farmers and Agricultural Workers

Not only are such workers exposed to pesticides, but also the average farmer engages in a wide variety of activities, including the rearing and feeding of animals, milking, veterinary care, treatment of soil and crops, harvesting, and maintenance of the farm building and machinery (93). Furthermore, mechanized farming may expose the farmer to dyes in gasoline, rubber tires, various lubrications, and greases. Piglet dealers who sedate pigs going to market with Stresnil, which contains azaperone (4'-fluoro-4-(4-(2-pyridyl)-1-piperazinyl) butyrophenone, may experience

TABLE 25.14. *Acaricides[a]*

	Patch test concentration
Benzyl benzoate	5% pet
Dinobuton (Acrex)	10% pet
Omite (propargite)	1% pet
Sulfur compounds	5% pet

[a]Pet, in petrolatum.

photocontact dermatitis. A 0.4% aqueous concentration plus 10J of UVA light can confirm this allergy (94).

The feed additive olaquindox causes photosensitivity in white pigs that must be kept indoors when fed this substance, and it can cause photoallergic contact dermatitis in pig farmers (95). Olaquindox forms a reactive oxyziridine on light exposure. The closely related quindoxin, which was marketed in the 1970s, was withdrawn due to persistent light reactions.

A group of 15 pig farmers were reported with photodermatitis from olaquindox airborne exposure (96). Prolonged UVA sensitivity accompanied the photoallergic dermatitis in almost all patients and prolonged UVB sensitivity in about half of the cases.

A study of farmers in Finland found that 8.6% had hand eczema (97). Furthermore, 70% of hand dermatitis cases were work related. Cow allergy was the main problem, and this was seen as both immediate sensitivity identified by skin prick test and delayed hypersensitivity to cow dander seen by patch tests.

Between 1990–1994 there were 2759 cases of occupational allergic contact dermatitis in Finland: 30% due to contact urticaria and 70% to allergic contact dermatitis of a delayed type (98). Contact urticaria was found in women more commonly than men by 70% to 30%. The most common causes of contact urticaria as an occupational skin disease were cow dander (44%); natural rubber latex (24%); flour, grains, and feed (11%); foodstuffs (3%); industrial enzymes (2%); and decorative plants (2%).

Aside from the allergens listed in Table 25.15, these workers may be exposed to various plants, woods, lichens, fertilizers, insecticides, and animal feed additives.

Dairy Workers

As with farmers and agricultural workers, dairy workers are exposed to many allergens besides pesticides. Rubber sensitivity is quite common in dairy workers because they are in frequent contact with water, detergents, and hypochlorite chemicals from the rubber (99). Black (100) and Lintum and Nater (101) reported hand eczema in dairy workers due to sensitization to isopropyl-phenyl-paraphenylenediamine in the black rubber hosing of milking machines. Further cases were reported by Nurse (99). Besides contact with hypochlorite solutions and detergents used for sterilizing the milking machinery and rubber hosing, dairy workers also have contact with iodine-containing preparations, which are used for washing the cows' teats before milking and as a teat-dip after milking. Chlorhexidine may also be used in treat care. The animals' fur may also pose a source of dermatitis, as was reported (102) among ewe milkers who work bare-handed. A patch test to ewe's wool was positive, and there was no cross-reaction with wool alcohol (30%) or lanolin (100%).

Suggested patch test allergens for dairy workers are listed in Table 25.16. It should be noted that milk samples may be preserved with dichromates that are sent for laboratory analysis for lipids and proteins. Such dichromates may cause dermatitis in laboratory workers (103).

Cattle Breeders

Cattle breeders may be exposed to insecticides, insect repellents, animal feed additives, and other allergens listed in Table 25.17.

Forest Workers

Although pesticide dermatitis occurs in this group of workers, irritant dermatitis from wet work and plant dermatoses are probably more common.

Contact with the bark of trees in felling or processing the trees also often produces an allergic dermatitis due to a *d*-usnic acid found in the lichens on tree barks. In addition,

TABLE 25.15. *Farmers and Agricultural Workers[a]*

Allergens	Patch test concentration
Antu (thiourea rat poison)	2% pet
p-dimethylaminoazobenzene (gasoline dye)	1% pet
Dithiocarbamates	
Maneb	1% pet
Thiram	1% pet
Zineb	1% pet
Ziram	1% pet
Potassium dichromate (leather gloves)	0.5% pet
Ragweed oleoresin	1% pet
Red Sudan IV (gasoline dye)	2% pet
Rubber chemicals (boots and gloves)	
Miscellaneous	
Animal feed additives (antibiotics and preservatives)	
Fertilizers	
Insecticides	
Lichens	
Mercury (organic and inorganic)	
Plants	
Wood	

[a]Pet, in petrolatum.

TABLE 25.16. *Dairy Workers[a]*

Allergens	Patch test concentration
Benzalkonium chloride (disinfectants)	0.01% aq
Chlorpromazine (medications)	1% pet
Cinnamon oil (medications)	0.5% pet
Coal tar (dust control oils)	5% pet
Cobalt chloride (animal feed additives)	1% pet
Dichlorophene (disinfectants)	1% pet
Neomycin sulfate (feed additives and medications)	20% pet
Rosin (medications)	20% pet
Rubber chemical series (milking machines and rubber gloves)	

[a]Aq, aqueous; Pet, in petrolatum.

TABLE 25.17. *Cattle Breeders*[a]

Allergens	Patch test concentration
3,5-dinitro-o-toluamide	1% pet
Ethoxyquin	0.5% pet (photopatch test)
Furadantin	5% pet
Furazolidone	3% pet
Furfuraldehyde	3% pet
Isopropylparaphenylenediamine (IPPD) (rubber)	0.5% pet
Lauryl gallate	2% pet
Neomycin	20% pet
Nitrofurazone	3% pet
Penicillin	1% pet
Phenothiazine	2.5% pet
Piperazine (diethylenediamine)	5% aq
Quindoxin	0.1% pet (photopatch test)
Rubber chemicals	see standard tray
Spiramycin	10% pet
Tylan (tylosin)	1% pet

[a]Aq, aqueous; Pet, in petrolatum.

sesquiterpenes in liverworts (Frullania), a primitive plant found on the surface of smooth barked trees such as the alder and hemlock, produce many instances of allergic dermatitis that may be confused with a photodermatitis (104). These sesquiterpenes cross-react with chrysanthemum, ragweed, and other members of the Compositae family (105–108). Table 25.18 lists the plant chemicals for patch testing forest workers who have dermatitis.

TABLE 25.18. *Forest Workers*[a]

Allergen	Patch test concentration
Alantolactone	0.1% pet
Δ^3-Carene (turpentine)	1% peroxides in olive oil
Frullania, whole plant (liverwort)	as is
Parmelia (lichen)	as is
Pine bud	as is
Pine sap	10% pet
Poplar resin	10% pet
Plant extracts	Hollister-Stier in alcohol
Chrysanthemum (chrysanthemum)	
Cocklebur (xanthium)	
Feverfew (chrysanthemum parthenium)	
Marsh elder (iva)	
Sagebrush (artemisia)	
Short ragweed (ambrosia)	
Tansy (tanacetum)	
Rosin	20% pet
Usinic acid (sensitizer in lichens)	1% pet
Various sawdusts (moist with water)	as is

[a]Pet, in petrolatum.

Gardeners

An extensive survey of Danish gardeners and greenhouse workers found 17% to have occupational allergic contact dermatitis (109). Plants were the overwhelming source of the dermatitis compared with pesticides and rubber allergens, which were rarely the source. The Compositae plants produced most of the reactions. The 17% prevalence of dermatitis was the same as that found among tulip workers by Bruze in Sweden (110).

Short-lived skin irritation of urticarial-type symptoms is commonly reported among gardeners and greenhouse workers. In a Danish study of such workers, 25% had short-lived symptoms (111). When prick tested for plant sensitivity, 33% of 105 tested workers had a reaction to one or more plants. The most commonly identified reaction was to Christmas cactus (*Schlumbergera* hybrids).

OTHER BIOLOGIC CAUSES OF CONTACT DERMATITIS

Italian cheese (taliggio) is wrapped in rags during its manufacture, which supports the growth of the mite Rhizoglyphus (112). This mite causes rhinitis, asthma, and dermatitis on exposure. This is confirmed by prick tests and tests with other mites that proved negative (112).

Marine organisms cause hand and forearm dermatitis among North Sea fishermen trawling the Dogger Bank. *Alcyonidium gelatinosum* or *hirsutum* causes most of the cases. Other organisms that cause what is referred to as "white seaweed" dermatitis include *Electra pilosa* and *Sertularia argentae,* which cause contact urticaria; *Flustra folicea* (a bryozoan); and *Abieturiasia abretina* and *Hydralmania falcata* (coelenteratis) (113).

A coffee worker developed dermatitis from roasted espresso coffee in powdered form and as a drink. Prior reports have been of dermatitis from green coffee beans (114).

PAPER DERMATITIS

More than 600 products are used in the manufacture of paper from the cellulose fibers of trees (spruce, pine, and hemlock). These products include fillers, preservatives, plasticizers, whitening agents, chelators, adhesives, dispersing agents, corrosion inhibitors, and many other additives such as ammonia, hydrogen sulfide, sulfuric acid, carbon monoxide, sodium hydroxide, and chlorine (115).

The Role of Formaldehyde and Formaldehyde Resins

Formaldehyde and its reactive derivatives are used in the paper industry to improve the wet-strength, water-resistance, shrink-resistance, grease-resistance, and other characteristics of paper and paper products. In addition, formaldehyde serves as a disinfectant and preservative in paper manufacture and in the preparation of finishes, sizing agents, and parchment paper.

Paper towels may contain melamine formaldehyde resin to increase resistance to water, and paper money may contain formaldehyde and its resins to prevent mildew (116). Wrapping paper, inexpensive paper, and newspapers may produce dermatitis from the presence of free formaldehyde (117).

Many types of paper contain formaldehyde or its resin to increase "wet strength" and to prevent mildew.

Glossy table paper contains a formaldehyde resin and free formaldehyde. The shiny, heavy, more expensive table paper is much more likely to contain formaldehyde than the thinner, less expensive, duller, more fragile type of paper. To be on the safe side, formaldehyde-sensitive patients should be protected from table paper with an all-cotton sheet.

The handling of most newspapers, magazines, both hard-cover and paperback books, and glossy paper readily produces dermatitis in formaldehyde-sensitive individuals.

In connection with paper dermatitis, Black (118) reported a formaldehyde-sensitive individual who was allergic to blank newsprint. The estimation of free formaldehyde content of the newsprint showed it to be 0.02%. A similar estimation done on paper towels used in Black's hospital as an "economy" measure was 0.03%.

The formaldehyde-sensitive patient also acquires dermatitis from many types of paper tissues, paper towels, paper plates, and cups, except Marcal products. Although formaldehyde is not present in the actual ingredients of Dixie plates and cups, a minute quantity of formaldehyde is present in the lubricants used to keep the paperboard from wrinkling during its manufacture.

The formaldehyde-sensitive individual cannot tolerate any art paper used for acrylic paint or water colors, except for paper with the Grumbacher label. Incidentally, Boncour acrylic paint is tolerated by formaldehyde-sensitive individuals, but Liquitex is not.

Quaternium Ammonium

Paper strength is increased by the addition of modified cationic starch to the pulp and sizing. The manufacture of this type of starch involves a quaternium ammonium compound known as 2,3-epoxypropyl trimethyl ammonium chloride. This potent sensitizer in guinea pigs sensitized several Finnish workers exposed to this occupationally (119). It is also known as glycidyl trimethyl ammonium chloride. Beyond usage in paper manufacture, this chemical is useful in the production of cellulose textile fibers, hair dye, dispersing and emulsifying agents, surfactants, fabric softeners, and adsorbents for the removal of dyes from wastewater. A patch test concentration of 0.5% in petrolatum was effective in identifying the cases.

Colophony

Hand eczema can occur from handling paper and newsprint (without ink) due to colophony (120). Patch tests with the paper are usually negative. A proper patch test is prepared from an acetone extract of paper at about 10% concentration.

Carbon Paper

Calnan (121) stated that there are only two reports of proven reactions to carbon paper. Hjorth (122) described a man with a positive patch test to one type of carbon paper and to the plasticizer triphenyl phosphate, which was present at a concentration of 30% in the film emulsion. The second report by Calnan and Connor (123) described a man with dermatitis from nigrosine that was present only in a special carbon paper used for computer work.

A carbon paper ink consists basically of three elements: waxes, oils, and colors (Table 25.19). Each of these elements consists of complex mixtures. The oils are nondrying to produce softness and compactness of the ink; the waxes keep the ink hard and dry at room temperature and are a vehicle for the colors. The quality of the paper on which the ink is deposited is also important, because it must be thin and free of pinholes (124).

> **Although carbon paper contains various waxes, oils, and dyes, the only proved allergens have been nigrosine dye and triphenyl phosphate, a cellulose ester plasticizer.**

Carbonless Paper

Calnan (125) describes carbonless paper as pressure-sensitive paper for which either a ballpoint pen or an electric typewriter is the most suitable writing instrument. The principle consists of coating the undersurface of the top or writing sheet of paper with a thin emulsion that contains microcapsules of "ink." The "inks" are "color formers" that are colorless at one pH and colored at another. The pH inside the capsules is acid, and the pH outside the capsules is alkaline.

TABLE 25.19. *Constituents of Carbon Papers*

Oils	Waxes
Mineral and castor oils	Beeswax
Stearic and oleic acids	Cardelilla
Pigments and dyes	Carnauba
Carbon black	Montan
Methyl and crystal violet	Oricony
Miliori blue	Paraffin wax
Nigrosine	
Victoria blue	

The top surface of the second sheet is coated with a material that absorbs the "ink" (color former) when the microcapsules are broken by the pressure of the ballpoint pen. This material is alkaline, and so the color appears.

The color formers are mostly triphenyl methane dyes such as gentian violet and malachite green, which are dissolved in organic solvents inside the microcapsules. The solvents include kerosene diarylethanes, alkyl naphthalenes, cyclohexane, and dibutyl phthalate, which may be diluted with odorless kerosene. Some of these papers contain formaldehyde, others contain ammonia.

Complaints from handling the carbonless copy papers include mild dermatitis and rather severe upper respiratory symptoms. Some individuals complain of an irritating odor emanating from handling the papers (121,125,126).

> **Dermatitis and upper respiratory symptoms from handling carbonless copy paper may be due to the solvents in the paper. Adequate ventilation is often helpful in solving complaints.**

Rycroft and Calnan (127) stated that there have been several instances of irritation of the skin, eyes, and upper respiratory tract in office workers handling carbonless copy paper. Symptoms that these carbonless copy papers produced were dismissed initially by some physicians as psychoneurotic, but their occurrence now in several different groups of employees seems to make it certain that this is a physical phenomenon. The symptoms are suggestive of an airborne irritant, and research into release of chemicals from the complex chemical system incorporated in the paper is needed. It appears at present that the most likely candidates for the cause of these irritant symptoms reside among a range of organic solvents that are an essential component of these systems. The symptoms attributed to NCR paper of skin and mucous membrane irritation, itching, headache, and fatigue have more recently been attributed to "sick building syndrome" (128). The chemicals used to manufacture NCR paper have been virtually dermatitis free even though 1.8×10^6 tons are produced worldwide (128).

Marks (129) reported an allergic reaction to a component of a carbonless paper containing a color former composed of paratoluene sulfinate of Michler's hydrol (PTSMH). Paratoluene sulfinate of Michler's hydrol is a colorless dye salt that forms a colored print on transfer to a suitable receiving paper. The reaction of Michler's hydrol and paratoluene sulfinic acid produces PTSMH. This chemical coating was developed to improve business copy papers.

Copy Paper

Table 25.20 lists the four methods of copying or duplicating.

TABLE 25.20. *Methods of Paper Copying (Duplication)*

Photocopying
Dyeline or diazo method
Thermofax (heat process)
Electrostatic or xerographic procedure

1. *Verifax* (Eastman Kodak) is a photocopying method. Two men were sensitized while employed making the powder for the sensitized emulsion. Both men developed severe and widespread eczema and were sensitized by 4-phenyl catechol, patch tested 0.5% in petrolatum (130).

Jensen and Roed-Petersen (131) described patients who had itchy erythema of the face and headaches from vapor evaporating from wet toners used in photocopy machines, but they were unable to identify the precise chemical. Adequate ventilation solved the problem.

2. *Diazo or dyeline process.* The dyeline or diazo process is a paper copying method. An original pattern is placed on diazo-sensitized paper and is exposed to ultraviolet light. The ultraviolet light decomposes the diazonium salts in the diazo paper, except where they are shielded by the pattern. The paper is then developed with ammonia gas, which causes a change of color in the unexposed portions of the diazo-sensitized paper. Diazonium salts interact with "coupling agents" present in the paper to give a blue, black, or brown copy by the formation of azo dyes (130).

The coupling agents are generally aromatic alcohols such as phenol and resorcinol derivatives. Other components such as stabilizing agents are also present. Zinc chloride and acids such as citric acid inhibit chemical interactions at room temperature, thus preventing premature coupling. Antioxidants, for example, thiourea, prevent yellowing of the white nonimage area. Ammonia is also used in the process. Nickel salts are present in some papers. The allergen in diazo paper is usually *p*-diethylaminobenzene diazonium chloride (diazodiethyl aniline hydrochloride, DDA), which is reduced to an amine that may cross-react with paraphenylenediamine. Cross-reactions do not appear to occur with other azo compounds.

The DDA is not a sensitizer when it is irradiated. Thus, patch tests with the nonirradiated paper are positive in sensitized individuals but are negative with irradiated paper. There are several reports of dermatitis from such diazo papers as Amonax, Ozalid, and Radex papers (130, 132–134).

An irritant dermatitis may occur from the ammonia used in the process. The DDA was tested in a 10% aqueous solution by Mijnssen and Verspyck (132), who found that sensitized patients gave a positive reaction to the nonirradiated paper.

> Nonirradiated diazo paper is a sensitizer, but not when irradiated. An "amine" is produced on reduction of the dye that cross-reacts with para-phenylenediamine (PPDA). Thiourea, to prevent yellowing of the paper, may produce both ordinary and photoallergic contact dermatitis.

Dooms-Goossens et al. (37) reported a textile cutter who had conjunctivitis and an erythematous itching dermatitis of the eyelids, nasal mucous membranes, and the corners of the mouth. Patch testing revealed a strong positive reaction to the textile cutting patterns that she handled, which were duplicated by diazo processing. The contact dermatitis reaction was caused specifically by thiourea (dimethyl-thiourea), an additive in diazo-sensitized paper that prevents discoloration of the paper. Sengel et al. (135) reported a similar case. Van der Leun et al. (136) described a case of photodermatitis from thiourea in copy paper. Thiourea may be tested 5% in aqueous solution.

3. *Thermofax* (heat process). This heat process used in duplication paper produced many instances of allergic sensitization to 4-tertiary butyl catechol, which may cross-react with pentadecylcatechol in poison ivy.

Dermatitis from thermofax paper was reported by Fisher (137) and also by Harman and Sarkany (130). Degos et al. (138) reported dermatitis due to methyl gallate, an antioxidant used in thermofax paper.

Patch tests may be performed with the butyl catechol, 0.5% in petrolatum, and methyl gallate, 2% in petrolatum. The thermofax paper may be tested "as is."

> Dermatitis from thermofax paper may be due to tertiary butyl catechol that can cross-react with the catechol in poison ivy. The antioxidant methyl gallate may also be a sensitizer.

There are several reports of thermofax dermatitis that stops when the subject is no longer in contact with the duplication paper or if the subject uses a different paper. Thermofax paper allergy can be suppressed by using the two new nonsensitizing thermofax papers Jl and Jlo. Cases of allergy to the hypoallergenic thermofax paper have been reported (139–141). Hand dermatitis that improved on job leave and vacation and relapsed on return to work was traced to colophony in telefax paper that contained 1% colophony. Patch testing with this fax paper gave only ± reactivity (142).

4. *The electrostatic or xerographic method.* No instance of contact dermatitis has been reported from this process of duplication.

Typewriting Paper

Wikstrom (143) reported that in dermatitis due to typewriting paper the allergen appeared to occur in the "size" contained in the paper, a gum resin that consisted partly of rosin. Sensitivity to the typewriting paper can be accompanied also by sensitivity to rosin, juniper tar, and styrax. All of these substances contain mixtures of resinous acids, one of which is abietic acid. Allergic reactions to abietic acid were shown in sensitivity to typewriting paper.

> Abietic acid in the rosin in typewriting paper may produce allergic contact dermatitis.

Typewriter Correction Paper

Jordan and Bourlas (144) found that a patient had an allergic reaction from a phenol formaldehyde resin, Arochem 455, tested 1% in alcohol. The resin is used as a binder for the powdery coating on the paper. Patch tests should be done with the powdered side of the paper.

Perfume in Paper

Perfumed facial tissues, toilet paper, and sanitary napkins can produce allergic contact dermatitis, particularly if they contain cinnamic aldehyde or cinnamic alcohol (145–147).

> Cinnamic alcohol and aldehyde in perfumed facial tissue and sanitary napkins can produce allergic contact dermatitis.

Parks (148) believed that perfume in toilet tissue is unlikely to cause sensitivity because of its low concentration and the manufacturing practice of applying it to the inner core of the roll. The perfume is probably there in low concentration, because it has to be carried to the paper by diffusion.

BAKERS' DERMATITIS

In a population-based study of occupational skin disease, bakers had a higher risk of dermatitis (191 per 10,000 employees) compared with confectioners (84 per 10,000) and cooks (34 per 10,000) (149). Irritant contact dermatitis was the most common diagnosis. Occupationally relevant type 1 allergy was found in 36% of bakers, 16% of confectioners, and 9% of cooks.

Many cases of hand dermatitis of bakers are irritant, infectious, or due to infestation: Some cases are atopic in nature or due to dyshidrosis (150).

TABLE 25.21. *Irritants That Bakers May Encounter*

Acetic acid	Fruit juices
Ascorbinic acid (flour improver)	Lactic acid
	Potassium bicarbonate
Bleaching agents	Potassium iodide and
Calcium acetate and sulfate	bromate
Emulsifying agents	Wet dough
Enzymes	Yeast

1. *Irritant dermatitis.* Most instances of hand dermatitis in bakers are due to a nonspecific dermatitis from various irritants, such as the wet, sticky dough, sweetening agents, enzymes, and various flavors. Soaps and detergents used for cleansing the hands are also often the cause of irritant bakers' dermatitis. In such instances, the patch tests are negative. Table 25.21 lists the numerous irritants to which bakers are exposed.

2. *Paronychia.* Monilial and bacterial paronychia occurs frequently in bakers. Painting the paronychial area with a Betadine solution is often effective for both types of paronychia.

3. *Food mite dermatitis.* Food mite dermatitis may be papulofollicular rather than eczematous and most prominent on the dorsal aspect of the hands. Flour mites (Tyroglyphus) may be found in the flour and on the bakers' skin. This type of "bakers' itch" occurs particularly among workers in flour mills and bakeries in small establishments that do not use mechanical processes and have few sanitary arrangements. Pastry bakers are subject to a dermatitis due to the sugar mite (151).

4. *Bakers' "psoriasis."* Bakers with psoriasis may develop a fissured, hyperkeratotic, psoriatic lesion on their palms due to the Koebner's phenomenon from trauma to their hands. Wütrich (152) used the term "bakers' psoriasis" for palmar keratoderma of bakers due to this phenomenon.

Hand dermatitis in bakers may be due to various nonallergic causes, including irritants, parasites, fungi, bacteria, and dyshidrosis.

---

5. *Dyshidrotic eczema.* Several bakers were observed with dyshidrotic eczema of the hands. In two bakers, however, the dyshidrosis continued after they discontinued their jobs as bakers. Young (153) reported that he observed bakers with positive intracutaneous tests to flour extracts and with skin eruptions of atopic dermatitis or dyshidrotic eczema, and that an inhalant allergy to flour may cause eczema of the hands as the only symptom.

6. *Atopic dermatitis.* Hjorth (154) stated that most bakers' dermatitis was associated with an immediate type 1 sensitivity. Herxheimer (155) found that skin sensitivity to pollen and flour often occurred together. Jarvinen et al. (156) found that a disease of the atopic group was established in 25% of bakery employees investigated and that 9% had asthma, 25% had allergic rhinitis, and 5% had atopic eczema. They concluded that an individual with atopy is unsuitable for bakery work.

Bakers may develop asthma, allergic rhinitis, and atopic eczema from flour.

---

7. *Contact urticaria due to flour.* Flour can produce a contact urticaria of the baker's hands that the baker scratches and excoriates. When it can be seen, the hand dermatitis resembles an eczematous dermatitis. A careful history usually reveals that the baker complains of immediate burning and itching when handling flour. The hands soon become red and edematous. Patch tests are negative, but moistened flour on the scratch produces an urticarial wheal in the baker and not in controls. Fisher (157) and Odom and Maibach (158) reviewed this type of urticarial reaction to various food products.

Enzymes are added to flour because most are deficient in amylase. Enzymes such as *Aspergillus orzae* and *Bacillus subtilis* may cause contact urticaria in bakers (159). In bakers, alpha-amylase can cause both immediate and delayed hypersensitivity (160) and has caused contact urticaria and protein contact dermatitis. Kanerva et al. (161) found that differences in allergenicity of alpha-amylase exist depending on whether the enzyme is of bacterial or fungal origin. Their patient was sensitive only to enzyme of fungal origin, which would allow for an allergen substitution of the bacterial alpha-amylase.

In addition to alpha-amylase, other enzymes are used industrially. Skin reactions have been reported to cellulase found in feeds, baking, brewing, detergents, pulp/paper, textile processing; glucoamylase in alcohol production and baking; papain in brewing, contact lens detergents and pharmaceuticals; and xylanase in the pulp/paper industry (162).

8. *Sorbic acid reactions.* This preservative is sometimes added to flour, particularly in the making of rye bread. An eczematous contact dermatitis of the hands from hypersensitivity to sorbic acid with positive patch test reactions to sorbic acid and potassium sorbate can be demonstrated.

In addition, a baker developed an immediate reaction consisting of redness and slight itching of hands where he contacted flour containing sorbic acid. The 48-hour patch test was negative. The baker, however, developed an immediate wheal from the application of 5% sorbic acid in petrolatum (163).

Potassium sorbate, which cross-reacts with sorbic acid, is used as a preservative in meringue.

> Contact urticaria in bakers may occur from flour and also from sorbic acid and enzymes added to flour.

9. *Flour flavors.* Malten (164) reported several bakers with contact dermatitis from flavors in flours and pointed out cinnamon as an occupational hazard of bakers. Table 25.22 lists the various flavors that may be used by bakers.

Five cases of occupational contact dermatitis due to spices were reported in chefs and kitchen or restaurant workers (165). All had hand dermatitis. The incriminated spices were garlic, cinnamon, ginger, allspice, and clove. Patch tests were also positive to foods including tomato, lettuce, and carrot.

10. *Karaya gum.* Karaya gum, a vegetable gum derivative, is used as a pastry filler and as a stabilizer of meringue, which is a frothy pastry topping consisting of beaten egg whites and sugar. Patch testing reveals a positive reaction to karaya gum, which is a rare sensitizer (166). Karaya is also widely used in hair waving lotions, denture adhesive powders, furniture polishes, and as a cement for ileostomy appliances. Karaya may occasionally produce allergic reactions (167).

11. *Ammonium persulfate reactions.* Ammonium persulfate was used previously in certain European countries as a flour "improver" to render the flour white. In Greece, until recently, this chemical was added to flour, but it has never been permitted in flour in the United States.

Ammonium persulfate and benzoyl peroxide are still permitted in flour in the Netherlands and in Great Britain, but although benzoyl peroxide is still widely used, many millers have replaced persulfates with potassium bromate, which is equally efficient and easier to handle. Ammonium persulfate not only may produce an eczematous contact dermatitis, but in certain individuals severe urticaria and anaphylactic shock may occur (168,169).

12. *Benzoyl peroxide.* This antioxidant flour bleaching agent may produce allergic contact dermatitis in sensitized bakers (170).

13. *Antioxidants in flour.* The antioxidants, butylated hydroxyanisole (BHA), butylated hydroxytoluene (BHT), and lauryl and propyl gallate may produce contact dermatitis in bakers (171–173).

14. *Chromates in flour.* There are no reports of dermatitis in bakers from chromium compounds in this country. Heime and Fox (174) in Germany reported, however, that they

TABLE 25.22. *Flavoring Used by Bakers*

Anise	Lemon juice
Cardamom	Lemon oil
Cinnamon	Methyl salicylate
Cloves	Nutmeg
Ginger	Peppermint
Laurel	Vanilla

TABLE 25.23. *Allergens in the Baking Industry*[a]

	Patch test concentration
Alpha-tocopherol (antioxidant for fats)	10% pet
Ammonium persulfate (Europe)	1% aq
Balsam of Peru (cross-reacts with flavors)	25% pet
Beeswax (artificial flowers)	5% pet
Benzoyl peroxide	1% pet
Butylated hydroxyanisole [(BHA) (antioxidants for lards and greases)]	2% pet
Butylated hydroxytoluene (BHT) (antioxidants for lards and greases)	2% pet
Cinnamic aldehyde	1% pet
Cinnamon oil	0.5% pet
Eugenol	5% pet
Food dyes	1% pet
Karaya gum (sterculia gum)	as is
Lauryl gallate (antioxidant in margarines)	5% pet
Limonen, oil of	1% in alcohol
Methyl salicylate (flavorings)	2% in olive oil
p-amino-azo-benzene (indicator for azo dyes)	0.25% pet
Potassium bromate	5% aq
Potassium dichromate	0.25% pet
Sorbic acid (preservative)	5% pet
Vanilla (alcoholic extract)	10% in acetone
Vanillin	10% pet

[a]Aq, aqueous; Pet, in petrolatum.
Note: Flour may be tested as is for delayed hypersensitivity. Urticarial reactions with flour should be tested with moistened flour on a scratch.

studied a baker with eczema of the hands with relapses that obviously occurred because of contact with flour. Patch testing revealed only hypersensitivity to chromate. Four sorts of flour used in Germany were analyzed, and it was found that the chromium content ranged from 0.01 to 0.09 mg/dL in these four flour samples. These authors concluded that even those comparatively low chromium levels were capable of giving rise to eczema in chromate-sensitive individuals.

> A rare cause of bakers' dermatitis in Germany was due to the presence of chromates in flour.

Table 25.23 lists the allergens that bakers may encounter.

DERMATITIS IN HAIRDRESSERS

Hairdressers are exposed to several irritants and allergens (175). In many cases, the hand dermatitis is a combination of an irritant and allergic variety. A hairdresser can acquire a dry irritant dermatitis over the metacarpophalangeal joints while shampooing a client's hair. Some hairdressers de-

TABLE 25.24. *A "Screening" Patch Test Series for Hairdressers*

Bleaching
   Ammonium persulfate 2.0% (Caution: may cause syncope)
Fragrance[a]
   Fragrance mix no. 3 (standard tray)
Hair dyes[b]
   o-nitro-p-phenylenediamine 1%
   p-aminophenol 1%
   p-phenylenediamine 1%
   p-toluylenediamine 1%
   Pyrogallol 1%
   Resorcinol
Metals[a]
   Nickel 5% (standard tray)
Perfumes
   Balsam of Peru 25%
Permanent waving
   Ammonium thioglycolate 2.5%
   Glyceryl monothioglycolate 2.5%
Preservatives
   Formaldehyde 1% aqueous
   Proteins
   Quaternium 15 (Dowicil 200)
Rubber chemicals
   Carbamate mix
   Mercaptobenzothiazole 2%
   Thiram mix

[a]Standard tray.
[b]All these may cross-react with paraphenylenediamine except resorcinol and pyrogallol.
Note: All are tested with petrolatum except formaldehyde (1% aqueous).

velop eczema of the fingers. In those who give up hairdressing, the dermatitis generally improves or heals; in those who continue hairdressing, the dermatitis is likely to persist especially in atopic individuals (176–180).

Irritant hand dermatitis in hairdressers facilitates allergic hypersensitivity to hair dyes, rubber chemicals, nickel, and the allergens to which hairdressers are exposed (Table 25.24).

In a 4-year study of hairdressers, allergic contact dermatitis was more common than irritant contact dermatitis in this occupation (181). The principal allergen was glyceryl thioglycolate. Avoidance of glyceryl thioglycolate proved problematic, as it contaminated the work surfaces of the shop, so that avoidance of permanent wave solution was insufficient for prevention. Other important allergens in this industry were ammonium persulfate and nickel. Also found were the shampoo ingredients cocamidopropyl betaine and sodium coco hydrolyzed animal protein, as well as the hair dye chemicals.

When hairdressers were followed from apprenticeship to a point 8 years into their careers, dermatitis was found to be a problem in 51%, even though they had no dermatitis before entering the profession (182). Of those who gave up practicing hairdressing, only 33% had hand eczema. In this long-term study, no relationship was found between atopy or nickel sensitivity and the development of hand dermatitis, but dry skin was a risk factor.

Dahlquist et al. (183) demonstrated that nickel is released from hair clips and nickel-plated metal by ammonium thioglycolate in permanent wave liquids. This finding might explain to some extent the high frequency of nickel allergy among hairdressers who are exposed to nickel-plated scissors, clips, pins, rollers, rods, and grips. It would, therefore, seem advisable for nickel-sensitive hairdressers to use stainless steel or plastic utensils only.

Hand dermatitis in hairdressers is often a combination of irritant and allergic reactions and is especially severe in atopic and nickel-sensitive individuals.

The introduction of glyceryl thioglycolate as a hairwaving chemical has produced many instances of hand dermatitis in hairdressers (184).

Two unusual cases of contact urticaria in hairdressers to an egg shampoo have been described (185). Both patients had had continuous contact with raw egg in the course of their work; while massaging or packing, egg emulsion was rubbed on their skin.

The first patient, a 24-year-old beautician, first observed the symptoms on her palms after using quail eggs for massage, and later contact with raw hen's egg caused urticaria. After eating egg, she developed urticaria all over the body accompanied by tightness of the chest and angioedema. Epicutaneous testing showed sensitivity to both the white and the yolk of raw egg, with wheals all over the body, and also produced shock. In the case of boiled egg only, the white produced contact urticaria that was not accompanied by general symptoms. In the course of oral exposure only, the yoke of the egg produced disseminated urticaria within 30 minutes that was followed by coughing.

In the other patient, a 31-year-old hairdresser, consumption of egg dishes resulted in local and generalized urticaria. Epicutaneous testing with the white of raw egg gave a positive reaction. Oral testing showed sensitivity to the white of boiled egg, causing continuous urticaria and hard breathing. Raw egg was not tested orally because of the risk of severe symptoms.

Contact urticaria of the hands in beauticians can occur from egg shampoos.

Egg is a complex albumen; thus, isolation of the material responsible for antigenicity is rather problematic and has not yet been solved. Antigenicity is influenced strongly both by pH changes and heat (186).

Lynde and Mitchell (187) reported that over a period of 8 years, 66 hairdresser patients were patch tested to the North American Contact Dermatitis Group screening series, to a hairdressers' screening series, or to both. Paraphenylenediamine (PPD) produced positive reactions in 45% and nickel sulfate in 27% of the patients tested. Apart from the PPD substances and glyceryl thioglycolate, other chemicals tested produced allergic reactions in no more than 4 of 66 (6%) patients.

Paraphenylenediamine, nickel, and glyceryl thioglycolate were the most common causes of allergic contact dermatitis in hairdressers.

Henna

Urticaria of the face, sinusitis, and headache can occur from airborne henna powder in hairdressers who have immediate hypersensitivity to henna. Henna is derived from *Lawsonia inermis,* and the allergen is thought to be 2-hydroxy-1,4-naphtoquinone (lawsone). The case reported by Majoie and Bruynzeel (188) was prick test negative to the lawsone but positive to henna 1% in ethanol and water. They cited other cases in hairdressers with similar symptoms and asthma, some of whom were positive to lawsone and others not. Therefore, another unidentified allergen is likely to also be present in henna.

Hydrogen Peroxide

Two hairdressers who were allergic to multiple salon products were also found to be allergic to hydrogen peroxide used in hair bleaching and coloring operations (189). A 3% aqueous preparation of hydrogen peroxide was used for patch test purposes. The normal use concentration in salon products is 3% to 5%.

Ammonium Persulfate

Ammonium persulfate is used in bleaching procedures in hairdressing salons, and potassium persulfate is used industrially as a bleaching, oxidizing, and antiseptic agent. It is also a polymerization promoter in the processing of textiles and in photography. Sensitization to potassium persulfate was confirmed in a laboratory assistant by 2.5% in petrolatum (190). This patch test concentration was negative in 20 controls. Although the laboratory assistant had never dyed or bleached her hair, she had a positive reaction to ammonium persulfate.

The most common causes of allergic contact dermatitis in hairdressers are paraphenylenediamine, nickel, and glyceryl monothioglycolate.

Protection of the Hands for Hairdressers

Hairdressers should choose vinyl or nitrile gloves instead of the rubber variety, because many hairdressers become sensitized to the rubber gloves. In addition, the hair perming chemical glyceryl thioglycolate passes through rubber gloves more readily than through vinyl gloves. 4-H gloves are more preferable for protection than rubber or vinyl but are hard to work in. Nitrile gloves provide better protection and dexterity.

FORMALDEHYDE AND FORMALDEHYDE-RELEASING MATERIALS

Hand eczema is a persistent occupational and nonoccupational problem. Cronin (191) pointed out the importance of formaldehyde in perpetuating this type of contact dermatitis. Her table on formaldehyde-free products can be of use to individuals with this problem (Table 25.25). Cutting fluids remain a frequent source of formaldehyde-releasing preservatives (191). Prevention of metalworking fluid dermatitis has been reported by applying grapeseed oil, which contains vitamin E (192). The grapeseed oil should be removed with soft paper, then soap and water. Formaldehyde-releasing materials have been linked to hand dermatitis additionally in gum arabic in printing materials, wallpaper adhesives, tape, flame retardants, cleaners, and fabric softeners (191).

ELECTRONICS

Six categories of skin hazards have been identified in the electronics industry (193).

1. *Solder.* Irritant reactions are more common than allergic reactions due to acids and solvents, but rosin-based solder poses a colophony risk that can be direct contact dermatitis, airborne dermatitis, or contact urticaria. Other potential allergens are hydrazine and aminoethyl ethanolamine.

2. Solvents generally are irritants and include isopropanol, *n*-butyl acrylate, freon, xylene, acetone, methanol, petroleum distillates, trichloroethane, methylene chloride, tetrachloroethylene (may cause Stevens-Johnson syndrome), ethylene glycol, and methyl ethyl ketone.

3. Hydrofluoric acid is the most common cause of chemical burns in the semiconductor industry.

4. Epoxy resins are the major allergens in the electronics industry. Also of concern is triglycidyl isocyanurate.

5. Metals of potential concern include ammonium bichromate, adhesion of phosphor in color TV screens, cobalt (magnets), platinum (connectors), and gold.

6. Irritation to cyanoacrylate glue with low relative humidity, which is corrected by greater than 55% relative humidity.

TABLE 25.25. *Products That, as Far as the Manufacturers Know, Do Not Contain Formaldehyde or a Formaldehyde Donor[a]*

Washing-up liquids	
Fairy Liquid (both regular and lemon fresh perfumed)	Procter and Gamble
Sunlight Lemon Liquid	Unilever
Hard surface cleaners	
Impact Bathroom Cleaner	Benckiser
Impact Kitchen Cleaner	Benckiser
Mr. Muscle Kitchen Cleaner	Bristol-Myers Co. Ltd.
Mr. Muscle Bathroom Cleaner	Bristol-Myers Co. Ltd.
Shiny Sinks	Homecare Products
Flash Powder	Procter and Gamble
Flash Liquid	Procter and Gamble
Handy Andy	Unilever
Cooker cleaners	
Mr. Muscle Oven Cleaner	Bristol-Myers Co. Ltd.
Easy-Do Powder Cleanser	Easy-Do Products Ltd.
Hob Brite Cleanser	Homecare Products
Window cleaners	
Mr. Muscle Window Cleaner	Bristol-Myers Co. Ltd.
Windowlene Spray	Reckitt and Colman
Windowlene Plus (trigger pack)	Reckitt and Colman
Silver brass and copper polishers	
Silver Polish	Johnson Wax
Long Term Brass Polish	Johnson Wax
Long Term Copper Polish	Johnson Wax
Bleaches	
Vortex Bleach	Procter and Gamble
Domestos	Unilever
Clothes washing preparations	
Bold 3	Procter and Gamble
Bounce	Procter and Gamble
Ariel	Procter and Gamble
Fairy Snow	Procter and Gamble
Persil	Unilever
Persil Automatic nonbiological	Unilever
Persil Automatic New System	Unilever
Surf	Unilever
Surf Automatic	Unilever
Wisk	Unilever
Breeze Automatic	Unilever
Lux Flakes	Unilever
Fabric softener	
Lenor Concentrate	Procter and Gamble
Dishwasher products	
Finish Dishwasher Powder (standard and lemon)	Benckiser
Finish Concentrated Dishwasher Liquid (standard and lemon)	Benckiser
Finish Compact Dishwasher Detergent	Benckiser
Finish Rinse Agent	Benckiser
Finish Dishwasher Cleaner and Freshner	Benckiser
Sun Machine Dishwashing Liquid	Unilever
Other domestic products	
Vanish Stain Removing Bar and Stain Stick	Benckiser
Vanish Machine Carpet Shampoo with De-foamer	Benckiser
Calgon	Benckiser
Scale Away	Benckiser
Lime Away	Benckiser
Dettol Liquid	Reckitt and Colman
Harpic Dual Action	Reckitt and Colman
Shampoos	
Flex Shampoo	Revlon
Other hair preparations	
Silvikrin Styling Mousse	Beecham Products
Silvikrin Hair Spray	Beecham Products
Flex Conditioner	Revlon

[a]From Cronin E. Formaldehyde is a significant allergen in women with hand eczema. *Contact Dermatitis* 1991;25:276. Used with permission.

CERAMICS

A study of 139 ceramics workers making floor and wall tile found 52 experienced dermatitis, of which 37% were allergic and 63% irritant (194).

In pottery workers, 24 cases of hand dermatitis occurred when a change was made from Portuguese to Indonesian turpentine (195). Oil of turpentine is still used in the pottery industry and to some extent in the perfume industry. The most common turpentine ingredient found to cause reactions was alpha-pinene rather than delta-3-carene, which has been said to be the principal allergen. These cases were in fine china workers, and heavy metals used for ceramic decoration were not a common problem. Reverting to Portuguese oil of turpentine alleviated the epidemic.

CRYSTAL-ARSENIC

In the manufacture of crystal, arsenic is added to facilitate melting of the crystal. A 29-year-old man who mixed and carried powders to make crystal became sensitized to arsenic, which was detected by 1% sodium arsenate aqueous. Avoidance was curative (196).

NITROGLYCERIN

In the explosives industry, contact dermatitis to nitroglycerin has occurred 4 to 24 years after initial exposure, whereas medical use of nitroglycerin topically may cause dermatitis in as little as 3 days (197). The allergens in dynamite or nitroglycerin include dinitrotoluene and ethylene glycol dinitrate, which can be tested at 0.1% to 0.5% in petrolatum. Nitroglycerin itself can be tested at 0.5% to 2.0% in petrolatum.

LABORATORY WORK

Analytic chemicals produce contact dermatitis in chemists and technicians. One such example is the reagent ethyl chloro oximido acetate, which subsequent animal work has established as a strong irritant and strong allergen (198).

CONSTRUCTION

A study of Spanish construction workers found that 65% showed one or more reactions to occupationally relevant allergens (199). Of the 268 such workers, the most common allergen was chromate (42%), followed by cobalt (20%), nickel (10%), and epoxy resin (7.5%). A total of 106 workers were allergic to rubber components, with thiuram mix being the most prevalent rubber allergen. A German study of 205 construction workers found that chromate was the most frequently encountered allergen (32%), followed by cobalt (15%), nickel (8%), thiuram (8%), and p-phenylenediamine (8%) (200).

Several studies have attempted to assess whether addition of ferrous sulfate to cement will actually lower the prevalence of contact dermatitis to chromium (201–203). This addition reduces hexavalent chromate to trivalent chromate, which is less likely to penetrate skin and lead to adverse reactions. Studies from Denmark, Sweden, and Finland all point to favorable results with a reduction of chromium cases of occupational dermatitis to less than one-third of previous levels (201). However, if the cement is stored for more than 6 months, the benefit tends to be lost. The lower levels of chromium dermatitis may be due to factors other than the addition of ferrous sulfate to cement. In Singapore, where no addition of ferrous sulfate to cement occurs, the chromate problems of construction workers have decreased (202). Changes in the blast furnace process have resulted in a lower chromate content, and the amount of chromate was found to be inversely related to the amount of slag in the cement. From 1983 to 1995 contact dermatitis from chromate in cement continued to fall in Singapore (203). However, from 1990 to 1995 chromate dermatitis increased, but not from cement; rather, the sources were leather, electroplating, welding, and metallic dyes.

The prognosis of occupational chromate dermatitis has been found to be poor (204). Even though 40% of workers with such a condition changed jobs to avoid chromate, 69% had persistent dermatitis (204). It has been recommended that on-site mixing of cement be done with ferrous sulfate to decrease dermatitis. This would increase cement costs 1% to 1.5% but protect those at greatest risk, in contrast to adding ferrous sulfate to premixed cement delivered to the work site (204).

Although chromium sensitivity has a reputation for intractability, the outcome of strict avoidance of further exposure to chromates was favorable in 72% of cases followed in Switzerland (205). Financial support of displaced workers was considered to be a factor in the more favorable outcome.

In addition to construction, chromate sensitization is an issue in the production of color television tubes (206). Ammonium chromate is used in production as a fixer and can cause occupational contact dermatitis.

SHOEMAKERS

A survey of 246 shoemakers found occupational contact dermatitis in 36 individuals (207). Irritant contact dermatitis was diagnosed in 20 (8.1%) and allergic contact dermatitis in 16 (6.5%). The most common allergens were p-tert-butylphenol-formaldehyde resin and mercaptobenzothiazole. Hyperkeratosis of the fingertips was the primary morphologic presentation.

OFFSHORE OIL WORKERS

Offshore oil workers are exposed to drilling mud. The composition of mud analyzed by Ormerod et al. (208) showed that inorganics and hydrocarbons make up the mud. The inorganics include aluminium, silicon, sulfur, potassium, calcium, barium, and iron. The hydrocarbons in the volatile phase of the mud are white spirit or low boiling point petroleum ether combined with paraffinic or naphthenic mineral oil. Fatty acid amines have been components of drilling mud, but in the last few years C16/C18 alpha olefins have become common additives, and cases of irritant contact dermatitis were seen from this component by Ormerod et al. (208).

AUTO MECHANICS

A survey of automobile mechanics found that 15% reported hand eczema (209). Patch tests performed on those mechanics with hand dermatitis found that 55% actually had irritant contact dermatitis. Only 19% had allergic contact dermatitis. The most frequent relevant reaction was to nickel, which was attributed to nickel-plated tools. One allergen not found on the standard screening series of allergens that proved helpful was *d*-limonene, which can be found in hand cleaners.

VIDEO DISPLAY TERMINALS

A variety of skin complaints have been blamed on video display terminals (VDTs). A systemic evaluation found a tendency for an increase in seborrheic dermatitis among such workers, which seems to relate to low levels of relative humidity rather than VDTs (210). A nonspecific erythema also seen among such workers correlated with perceived high work pace and inability to take rest breaks. No association was found with electrical or magnetic fields.

PERFORMING ARTISTS

In an investigation of opera house artists, 50% had a history of intolerance of cosmetics, but when patch tested, contact allergy was uncommon (211). The rate of fragrance allergy was similar in this profession to that commonly found among patch test clinic patients in general. However, fragrance sensitivity was overrepresented among the cosmetic intolerant group.

MUSICIANS

Recorders can be of boxwood, cedar, or rosewood construction. A 65-year-old man who played this instrument was found to be allergic to only his recorder made of boxwood (212). He had a hyperkeratotic eczema of his fingertips. Boxwood is from the *Buxus sempervirens* of the family Buxaceae.

Allergens found among musicians include rosin (colophony) to wax string instruments, nickel in chin rests, metallic parts of bows used on string instruments, cane reeds on woodwinds, and propolis in violin varnishes (213). Nonallergic skin changes found in musicians include soft tissue and bony changes, lip problems (hyperkeratosis and at times cheilitis), callus formation from repetitive trauma, and cutaneous hemorrhage from repetitive trauma (214). The repetitive trauma of musical instruments has caused conditions known as fiddler's neck, fiddler's fingers, drummer's digits, piano paronychia, pizzicato paronychia, guitar nipple, cellist's chest, and broken lips known as Satchmo's syndrome (named for Louis Armstrong) (215). Skin conditions can influence musicians' performances: Hyperhidrosis has caused musicians to change the instrument they play, xerostomia and hypersalivation can disable a wind player, and infections such as herpes labialis can impair brass and woodwind musicians (216).

REFERENCES

1. Fisher AA. Occupational, Industrial, and Plant Dermatology Symposium. San Francisco, March 26–28, 1979. Part 1: general considerations. *Cutis* 1979;24:143.
2. Fisher AA. Occupational, Industrial, and Plant Dermatology Symposium. Part 2: role of skin appendages, physical factors, pigment and malingering. *Cutis* 1979;24:249.
3. Owen CM, Gawkrodger DJ. Occupational dermatitis in Sheffield: a preliminary study. *Contact Dermatitis* 1999;40:223.
4. Holness DL, Nethercott JR. Comparison of occupational and non-occupational contact dermatitis. *Am J Contact Dermat* 1994;5:207.
5. Meding B, Swanbeck G. Occupational hand eczema in an industrial city. *Contact Dermatitis* 1990;22:13.
6. Holness DL, Nethercott JR. Is a worker's understanding of their diagnosis an important determinant of outcome in occupational contact dermatitis? *Contact Dermatitis* 1991;25:296.
7. Wall LM, Gebauer KA. A follow-up study of occupational skin disease in Western Australia. *Contact Dermatitis* 1991;24:241.
8. Kraus SM, Muselinovic NZ. Pre-employment screening for contact dermatitis among the pupils of a metal industry school. *Contact Dermatitis* 1991;24:342.
9. Fisher AA. *Contact dermatitis,* 3rd ed. Philadelphia: Lea & Febiger, 1986.
10. Kawai K, et al. Hyposensitization to urushiol among Japanese lacquer craftsmen: results of patch tests on students learning the art of lacquerware [Comments]. *Contact Dermatitis* 1991;25:290.
11. Reginella RF, Fairfield JC, Marks JG Jr. Hyposensitization to poison ivy after working in a cashew nut shell oil processing factory [Comments]. *Contact Dermatitis* 1989;20:274.
12. Rietschel RL, Klemm J, Thompson M. The influence of accommodation (hardening) on the response to irritants, allergens, and mediators of inflammation in humans. *Clin Res* 1982;30:605A.
13. Fisher AA. Occupational palmar psoriasis due to safety prescription container caps. *Contact Dermatitis* 1979;5:56.
14. White IR, Rycroft RIG. Low humidity occupational dermatosis—an epidemic. *Contact Dermatitis* 1982;8:287.
15. Meneghini CL, Angelini G. Occupational dermatitis artefacta. *Dermatosen* 1979;27:163.
16. Angelini G, Meneghini CL, Vena GA. Secretan's syndrome: an artefact edema of the hand. *Contact Dermatitis* 1982;8:345.
17. Robblee R. The dark side of worker's compensation: burdens and benefits in occupational disease coverage. *Ind Rel Law Rev* 1978;2:596.
18. Whitmore CW. Cutaneous impairment, disability and rehabilitation. *Cutis* 1970;6:989.
19. Goldsmith J. The new ethic: the doctor's responsibility for health on the job. *Environ Res* 1976;11:170.
20. Whitmore CW. Workmen's compensation. *Cutis* 1974;13:673.

21. Robinson Jr HM. Measurement of impairment and disability in dermatology. *Arch Dermatol* 1973;108:207.

22. Able EA. Mycosis fungoides and occupational exposure: is there an association? *Dermatol Clin* 1990;8:169.

23. Buckley WR. Lichenoid eruptions following contact dermatitis. *Arch Dermatol* 1958;78:454.

24. Canizares O. Lichen planus–like eruption caused by color developer. *Arch Dermatol* 1959;80:81.

25. Fry L. Skin disease from color developers. *Br J Dermatol* 1965; 77:456.

26. deGraciansky P, Boulle P, Quercy P, Cardol, J-L. Eruptions lichenoids et lichens plans vrais chez les ouvriers du developpement des films en couleurs. *Bull Soc Fr Dermatol Syphiligr* 1958;65: 498.

27. Knudsen E. Lichen planus-like eruption caused by color developer. *Arch Dermatol* 1964;89:357.

28. Roed-Petersen J, Menné T. Allergic contact dermatitis and lichen planus from black and white photographic developing. *Cutis* 1976; 18:699.

29. Marconi PMB, Campagna G, Fabri G, Schiavino D. Allergic contact dermatitis from colour developers used in automated photographic processing. *Contact Dermatitis* 1999;40:109.

30. Engasser PG. Leukoderma from hydroquinone? *J Am Acad Dermatol* 1982;7:134.

31. Frenk E, Loi-Zedda P. Occupation depigmentation due to a hydroquinone-containing photographic developer. *Contact Dermatitis* 1980;6:238.

32. Kersey P, Stevenson CJ. Vitiligo and occupational exposure to hydroquinone from servicing self-photographing machines. *Contact Dermatitis* 1981;7:285.

33. Goh CL. Allergic contact dermatitis and onycholysis from hydroxylamine sulphate in colour developer. *Contact Dermatitis* 1990;22: 109.

34. Soni BP, Sherertz EF. Contact dermatitis in the textile industry: a review of 72 patients. *Am J Contact Dermat* 1996;7:226.

35. Kiec-Swierczynski M. Occupational contact dermatitis in the workers employed in production of Texas textiles. *Dermatosen* 1982; 30:41.

36. Romaguera C, Grimalt F, Lecha M. Occupational purpuric textile dermatitis from formaldehyde resin. *Contact Dermatitis* 1981;7:152.

37. Dooms-Goossens A, et al. Dimethylthiourea, an unexpected hazard for textile workers. *Contact Dermatitis* 1979;5:367.

38. Wahlberg JE, Hogberg M, Skare L. Chloracetamide allergy in house painters. *Contact Dermatitis* 1978;4:116.

39. Hogberg M, Wahlberg JE. Health screening for occupational dermatoses in house-painters. *Contact Dermatitis* 1980;6:100.

40. Pedersen NB, Fregert S. Occupational allergic contact dermatitis from chloracetamide in glue. *Contact Dermatitis* 1976;2:122.

41. Liden C. Facial dermatitis caused by chlorothalonil in a paint [Comments]. *Contact Dermatitis* 1990;22:206.

42. Calnan CD. Acrylates in industry. *Contact Dermatitis* 1980;6:53.

43. Ezzelarab M, Hansson C, Wallengren J. Occupational allergy caused by 1,2-benzisothiazolin-3-one in water-based paints and glues. *Am J Contact Dermat* 1994;5:165.

44. Gruvberger B, Bjorkner B, Bruze M. Contact allergy to dichlofluanide in humans and guinea pigs. *Am J Contact Dermat* 1995;6:221.

45. Tobler M, Freiburghaus AU. A glove with exceptional protective features minimizes the risks of working with hazardous chemicals. *Contact Dermatitis* 1992;26:299.

46. Pigatto PD, et al. Are barrier creams of any use in contact dermatitis? *Contact Dermatitis* 1992;26:197.

47. Reynolds NJ, Peachey RD. Allergic contact dermatitis from a sulfosuccinate derivative in a hand cleanser. *Contact Dermatitis* 1990;22: 59.

48. Malten KE, et al. Nyloprint-sensitive patients react to NN′methylene bis acrylamide. *Contact Dermatitis* 1978;4:214.

49. Downham II TF, Birmingham DJ. Contact dermatitis to photographic print coating liquid. *Cutis* 1980;25:421.

50. Bastelain P-Y, et al. Sensitization to abietoformophenolic resin in printing ink. *Contact Dermatitis* 1980;4:145.

51. Windstrom L. Contact allergy to acrylate monomer in a printing plate. *Contact Dermatitis* 1982;8:68.

52. Malten KE. Cobalt and chromium in offset printing. *Contact Dermatitis* 1975;1:120.

53. Nethercott JR. Skin problems associated with multifunctional acrylic monomers in ultraviolet curing inks. *Br J Dermatol* 1978;98:541.

54. Castelain P-Y, Piriou A. New case of sensitization to Nyloprint. *Contact Dermatitis* 1978;4:310.

55. Pedersen NB, Chevallier M-A, Senning A. Secondary acrylamides in Nyloprint printing plate as a source of contact dermatitis. *Contact Dermatitis* 1982;8:256.

56. Pedersen NB. Allergy from NAPP. *Contact Dermatitis* 1980;6:35.

57. Bjorkner B, Dahlquist I, Fregert S. Allergic contact dermatitis from acrylates in ultraviolet curing inks. *Contact Dermatitis* 1980;6:405.

58. Milby TH, Epstein WL. Allergic contact sensitivity to malathion. *Arch Environ Health* 1967;15:89.

59. Hearn CED. A review of agricultural pesticide incidents in man in England and Wales. *Br J Industr Med* 1973;30:253.

60. Hjorth N, Wilkinson DS. Contact dermatitis. II. Sensitization to pesticides. *Br J Dermatol* 1968;80:272.

61. Kaloyanova E, Zielhuis RL. Documentation of international meetings: occupational health criteria for the evaluation of pesticides. *Int Arch Arbeitsmedizin* 1974;33:335.

62. Kleinman GD, West I, Augustine MS. Occupational disease in California attributed to pesticides and agricultural chemicals. *Arch Environ Health* 1960;1:118.

63. Rosival L, Jager KW. Documents of international meetings and activities: evaluation of various existing classifications of toxicity and hazard, as far as relevant for occupational exposure to pesticides. Report of an international workshop. *Int Arch Occup Environ Health* 1978;41:287.

64. Matsushita T, Nomura S, Wakatsuki T. Epidemiology of contact dermatitis from pesticides in Japan. *Contact Dermatitis* 1980;6:255.

65. Burry JN. Contact dermatitis from agricultural fungicide in South Australia. *Contact Dermatitis* 1976;2:289.

66. Fisher AA. Occupational, Industrial and Plant Symposium. Part 3: dermatitis in specific occupations. *Cutis* 1979;24:364.

67. Van Ketel WG. Allergic dermatitis to a new pesticide. *Contact Dermatitis* 1975;1:297.

68. Van Ketel WG. Sensitivity to pesticide benomyl. *Contact Dermatitis* 1976;2:290.

69. Schubert H. Contact dermatitis to sodium *n*-methyldithiocarbamate. *Contact Dermatitis* 1978;4:370.

70. Kleibl K, Rackova M. Cutaneous allergic reactions to dithiocarbamates. *Contact Dermatitis* 1980;6:348.

71. Matsushita T, Arimatsu Y, Nomura S. Experimental study on contact dermatitis caused by dithiocarbamates maneb, zineb and their related compounds. *Int Arch Occup Environ Health* 1976;37:169.

72. Cole DC, Carpio F, Math JJM, Leon N. Dermatitis in Ecuadorean farm workers. *Contact Dermatitis* 1997;37:1.

73. Fregert S. Allergic contact dermatitis from pesticides captan and phaltan. *Contact Dermatitis Newsletter* 1967;2:11.

74. Cottel WI. Difolatan. *Contact Dermatitis Newsletter* 1972;11:252.

75. Camarasa G. Difolatan dermatitis. *Contact Dermatitis* 1976;2:127.

76. Morris GE. Dermatoses from phenylmercuric salts. *Arch Environ Health* 1960;1:53.

77. Calnan CD. Dithianone sensitivity. *Contact Dermatitis Newsletter* 1969;3:119.

78. Bousema MT, Wiemer GR, Van Joost T. A classic case of sensitization to DD-95. *Contact Dermatitis* 1991;24:132.

79. Grace CT, Ng SK, Cheong LL. Recurrent irritant contact dermatitis due to tributyl tin oxide on work clothes. *Contact Dermatitis* 1991; 25:250.

80. Rycroft RJG. Contact dermatitis from organophosphorus pesticides. *Br J Dermatol* 1977;97:693.

81. Edmundson WF, Davies JE. Occupational dermatitis from naled. *Arch Environ Health* 1967;15:89.

82. Fregert S. Allergic contact dermatitis from the pestiade Rodannitrobenzene. *Contact Dermatitis Newsletter* 1967;1:4.

83. Peachey RDG. Skin hazards in farming. *Br J Dermatol* 1981;105:45.

84. Sharvill DE. Reaction to paraquat. *Contact Dermatitis Newsletter* 1971;9:210.

85. Samman PD, Johnston ENM. Nail damage associated with handling paraquat and diquat. *Br Med J* 1969;1:818.

86. Spencer MC. Herbicide dermatitis. *JAMA* 1966;198:1307.

87. Watanabe S. Contact dermatitis due to the herbicides PCP and MCPB. *Jpn J Clin Dermatol* 1070;24:945.

88. Cronce PC, Alden HS. Flea collar dermatitis. *JAMA* 1968;206:1563.

89. Lamberg S, Mulrennan JA. Deet bullous eruption resembling a blistering insect eruption. *Arch Dermatol* 1969;100:582.

90. Fisher AA. Contact urticaria due to medicaments, chemicals and foods. *Cutis* 1982;30:168.

91. Laubstein H. Kontaktekzem durch ein Rodentizid. *Berfusdermatosen* 1962;10:154.

92. Nishioka K, Kozuka T, Tashiro M. Agricultural miticide (BPPS) dermatitis. *Skin Res* 1970;12:15.

93. Wahlberg JE. Yellow staining of hair and nails and contact sensitivity to dinobuton. *Contact Dermatitis Newsletter* 1974;16:481.

94. Brasch J, Hessler H-J, Cristopher E. Occupational (photo) allergic contact dermatitis from azaperone in a piglet dealer. *Contact Dermatitis* 1991;25:258.

95. Kumar A, Freeman S. Photoallergic contact dermatitis in a pig farmer caused by olaquindox. *Contact Dermatitis* 1996;35:249.

96. Schuader S, Schroeder W, Geier J. Olaquindox-induced airborne photoallergic contact dermatitis followed by transient or persistent light reactions in 15 pig breeders. *Contact Dermatitis* 1996;35:344.

97. Susitaival P, et al. Hand eczema in Finnish farmers: a questionnaire-based clinical study. *Contact Dermatitis* 1995;32:150.

98. Kanerva L, Toikkanen J, Jolanki R, Estlander T. Statistical data on occupational contact urticaria. *Contact Dermatitis* 1996;35:229.

99. Nurse DS. Dermatitis danger to dairy farmers. *Med J Aust* 1978;1:223.

100. Black H. Analysis of routine battery results in Aukland skin clinic. *Contact Dermatitis Newsletter* 1972;12:323.

101. Lintum JC, Nater JP. Contact dermatitis caused by rubber chemicals in dairy workers. *Berufdermatosen* 1973;21:16.

102. Quirce S, et al. Occupational dermatitis in a ewe milker. *Contact Dermatitis* 1992;27:56.

103. Huriez CL, Martin P, Lefebvre M. Sensitivity to dichromate in a milk analysis laboratory. *Contact Dermatitis* 1975;1:247.

104. Mitchell JC, et al. Allergic contact dermatitis from Frullania and Compositae. *J Invest Dermatol* 1970;54:233.

105. Mitchell JC, Dupuis G. Allergic contact dermatitis from sesquiterpenoids of the Compositae family of plants. *Br J Dermatol* 1971;84:139.

106. Storrs EJ, Mitchell JC, Rasmussen JE. Contact hypersensitivity to liverwort and the Compositae family of plants. *Cutis* 1976;18:681.

107. Mitchell J, Rook AI. *Botanical dermatology—plants injurious to the skin.* Vancouver: Greenglass, 1979.

108. Thune P. Allergy to lichens with photosensitivity. *Contact Dermatitis* 1977;3:213.

109. Paulsen E. Occupational dermatitis in Danish gardeners and greenhouse workers. Part 2: etiological factors. *Contact Dermatitis* 1998;38:14.

110. Bruze M, Bjorkner B, Hellstrom AC. Occupational dermatoses in nursery workers. *Am J Contact Dermatitis* 1996;7:100–3.

111. Paulsen E, Skov PS, Andersen KE. Immediate skin and mucosal symptoms from pot plants and vegetables in gardeners and greenhouse workers. *Contact Dermatitis* 1998;39:166.

112. Pigatto PD, et al. Occupational atopic contact dermatitis from Rhizoglyphus. *Contact Dermatitis* 1991;25:193.

113. Ashworth J, Curry FM, White IR, et al. Occupational allergic contact dermatitis in east coast of England fishermen: newly described hypersensitivities to marine organisms. *Contact Dermatitis* 1990;22:185.

114. Piraccini BM, et al. Occupational contact dermatitis to coffee. *Contact Dermatitis* 1990;23:114.

115. Fregert S. Registration of chemicals in industries slimicides in the paper-pulp industry. *Contact Dermatitis* 1976;2:358.

116. Fisher AA. Formaldehyde: some recent experiences. *Cutis* 1976;17:665.

117. Fregert S. Allergic contact dermatitis from formaldehyde in paper. *Contact Dermatitis Newsletter* 1974;15:459.

118. Black H. Contact dermatitis from formaldehyde in newsprint. *Contact Dermatitis Newsletter* 1971;10:242.

119. Estlander T, Jolanki R, Kanerva L. Occupational allergic contact dermatitis from 2,3-epoxypropyl trimethyl ammonium chloride (EPT-MAC) and Kathon LX in a starch modification factory. *Contact Dermatitis* 1997;36:191.

120. Liden C, Karlberg A-T. Colophony in paper as a cause of hand eczema. *Contact Dermatitis* 1992;26:272.

121. Calnan CD. Carbon and carbonless copy paper. *Acta Derm Venereol* (Stockh) 1979;59:27.

122. Hjorth N. Contact dermatitis from cellulose acetate film. *Berufsdermatosen* 1964;12:86.

123. Calnan CD, Connor BL. Carbon paper dermatitis due to nigrosine. *Berufsdermatosen* 1975;20:248.

124. Carver JW. Typewriter ribbon and carbon inks. *Am Ink Maker* 1942;20:22.

125. Calnan CD. Unsolved problems in occupational dermatology. *Br J Dermatol* 1981;105:3.

126. Menné T, Asnae G, Hjorth N. Skin and mucous membrane problems from "no carbon required" paper. *Contact Dermatitis* 1981;7:72.

127. Rycroft RJG, Calnan CD. Occupational dermatology. *Dermatol Digest* 1979;18:21.

128. Murray R. Health aspects of carbonless copy paper. *Contact Dermatitis* 1991;24:321.

129. Marks Jr JG. Allergic contact dermatitis from carbonless copy paper. *JAMA* 1981;245:2331.

130. Harman RRM, Sarkany I. Studies in contact dermatitis XI. Copy paper dermatitis. *Trans St John Hosp Dermatol Soc* 1960;44:37.

131. Jensen M, Roed-Petersen J. Itching erythema amongst post office workers caused by a photocopying machine with wet toner. *Contact Dermatitis* 1979;5:389.

132. Mijnssen GAW, Verspyck X. Dermatitis from Ozalid and Radex copy paper. *Contact Dermatitis Newsletter* 1967;2:152.

133. Gianotti F, Meneghini GD. Observations concernant certaines dermatites eczemateuses par contact chez les travailleurs affects à la fabrication des papiers sensible. *Dermatologica* 1966;132:106.

134. Foussereau J, Benezra CR. *Les eczémas allergiques professionnels.* Paris: Masson et Cie, 1970.

135. Sengel PD, Khelladi A, Foussereau J. Allergie professionnelle au papier diazo dans l'industrie textile. *Derm Veruf Umwelt* 1979;27:178.

136. Van der Leun JC, et al. Photosensitivity owing to thiourea. *Arch Dermatol* 1977;113:1611.

137. Fisher AA. Allergic eczematous contact dermatitis due to thermofax paper. *Arch Dermatol* 1958;77:741.

138. Degos R, Lepine J, Akhoundzadeh H. Sensibilisation cutanée due à la manipulation de papier "reprographic." *Bull Soc Française Dermatol Syphiligraph* 1968;75:595.

139. Sheard CP, Spoor HJ, Abel R. Contact dermatitis from "high speed duplicator" papers. *Arch Dermatol* 1958;77:435.

140. Hasegawa J, Lerit F, Bluefarb SM. Contact dermatitis due to Thermo-Fax paper. *JAMA* 1958;166:1173.

141. Kendrick FJ. Dermatitis caused by a copying paper. *Arch Dermatol* 1958;77:334.

142. Kanerva L, et al. Contact dermatitis from telefax paper. *Contact Dermatitis* 1992;27:12.

143. Wikstrom K. Allergic contact dermatitis caused by paper. *Acta Derm Venereol* (Stockh) 1969;49:547.

144. Jordan WP, Bourlas M. Contact dermatitis from typewriter correction paper. *Cutis* 1975;15:594.

145. Guin JD. Contact dermatitis to perfume in paper products. *J Am Acad Dermatol* 1981;4:733.

146. Keith I, Erich W, Bush IM. Toilet paper dermatitis. *JAMA* 1969;209:269.

147. Larsen WG. Sanitary napkin dermatitis due to the perfume. *Arch Dermatol* 1979;115:363.

148. Parks TD. Perfume dermatitis. *JAMA* 1969;210:559.

149. Tacke J, Schmidt A, Fartasch M, Diepgen TL. Occupational contact dermatitis in bakers, confectioners and cooks: a population-based study. *Contact Dermatitis* 1995;33:112.

150. Fisher AA. Hand dermatitis—a baker's dozen. *Cutis* 1982;29:214.

151. Baker EW, Wharton GW. *Acarology.* New York: Macmillan, 1952.

152. Wütrich B. The cause of bakers' eczema. *Hautarzt* 1970;21:214.

153. Young E. Dyshidrotic (endogenic eczema). *Dermatologica* 1964;129:306.

154. Hjorth N. Occupational dermatitis in the catering industry. *Br J Dermatol* 1981;105:37.

155. Herxheimer H. The skin sensitivity to flour of bakers' apprentices: a final report of a long-term investigation. *Acta Allergy* 1973;8:42.

156. Jarvinen KAJ, et al. Unsuitability of bakery work for a person with atopy: a study of 234 bakery workers. *Ann Allergy* 1979;42:192.

157. Fisher AA. Urticarial and systemic reaction to contact varying from hair bleach to seminal fluid. *Cutis* 1977;19:715.

158. Odom RB, Maibach H. Contact urticaria: a different contact dermatitis. *Cutis* 1970;18:672.
159. Cronin E. *Contact dermatitis.* London: Churchill Livingstone, 1980.
160. Morren M-A, et al. α-amylase, a flour additive: an important cause of protein contact dermatitis in bakers. *J Am Acad Dermatol* 1993;29:723.
161. Kanerva L, Vanhanen M, Tupasela O. Occupational allergic contact urticaria from fungal but not bacterial alpha-amylase. *Contact Dermatitis* 1997;36:306.
162. Kanerva L, Vanhanen M. Occupational protein contact dermatitis from glucoamylase. *Contact Dermatitis* 1999;41:171.
163. Fisher AA. Cutaneous reactions to sorbic acid and potassium sorbate. *Cutis* 1980;25:350.
164. Malten KE. Four bakers showing positive patch tests to a number of fragrance materials which can be used in flavors. *Acta Derm Venereol* (Stockh) 1979;59:117.
165. Kanerva L, Estlander T, Jolanki R. Occupational allergic contact dermatitis from spices. *Contact Dermatitis* 1996;35:157.
166. Figley KD. Karaya gum hypersensitivity. *JAMA* 1940;114:109.
167. Camarasa JMB, Alomar A. Contact dermatitis from a karava seal ring. *Contact Dermatitis* 1980;6:139.
168. Fisher AA, Dooms-Goossens A. Persulphate hair bleach reactions. *Arch Dermatol* 1976;112:1407.
169. Calnan CD, Shuster S. Reactions to ammonium persulphate. *Arch Dermatol* 1963;88:812.
170. Lindemavr H, Drobil M. Contact sensitization to benzoyl peroxide. *Contact Dermatitis* 1981;7:137.
171. Roed-Petersen J, Hjorth N. Contact dermatitis from antioxidants: hidden sensitizers in topical medications and foods. *Br J Dermatol* 1976;94:233.
172. Kahn G, Phanuphak P, Claman HN. Propyl gallate-contact sensitization and orally induced tolerance. *Arch Dermatol* 1974;109:506.
173. Brun R. Eczame de contact à un antioxidant de la margerine (gallate) et changement de métier. *Dermatologica* 1970;140:390.
174. Heime VA, Fox G. Baker's eczema through chromium compound in flour. *Derm Beruf Umwelt* 1980;28:113.
175. Crotlin E, Kullavanijaya P. Hand dermatitis in hairdressers. *Acta Derm Venereol* (Stockh) 1979;59:48.
176. Wahlberg JE. Nickel allergy in hairdressers. *Contact Dermatitis* 1981;7:358.
177. Black MM, Russel BJ. Shampoo dermatitis in apprentice hairdressers. *J Soc Occup Med* 1973;23:120.
178. Wahlberg JE. Nickel allergy and atopy in hairdressers. *Contact Dermatitis* 1975;1:161.
179. Wilkinson DS, Hambly EM. Prognosis of hand eczema in hairdressing apprentices. *Contact Dermatitis* 1978;4:63.
180. Marks R, Cronin E. Hand eczema in hairdressers. *Aust J Dermatol* 1977;18:123.
181. van der Walle HB, Brunsveld VM. Dermatitis in hairdressers. Part 1: The experience of the past 4 years. *Contact Dermatitis* 1994;30:217.
182. Majoie IML, von Blomberg BME, Bruynzeel DP. Development of hand eczema in junior hairdressers: an 8-year follow-up study. *Contact Dermatitis* 1996;34:243.
183. Dahlquist E, Fregert S, Gruvberger B. Release of nickel from plated utensils in permanent wave liquids. *Contact Dermatitis* 1979;5:52.
184. Warshawshki L, Mitchell JC, Storrs F. Allergic contact dermatitis from glyceryl monothioglycolate in hairdressers. *Contact Dermatitis* 1981;7:351.
185. Temesvari LE, Varkonyi V. Contact urticaria provoked by egg. *Contact Dermatitis* 1980;6:143.
186. Rudzki E, Grzywa Z. Contact urticaria from egg. *Contact Dermatitis* 1977;3:103.
187. Lynde CW, Mitchell JC. Patch test results in hairdressers, 1973–81. *Contact Dermatitis* 1982;8:302.
188. Majoie IML, Bruynzeel DP. Occupational immediate-type hypersensitivity to henna in a hairdresser. *Am J Contact Dermat* 1996;7:38.
189. Aguirre A, et al. Positive patch tests to hydrogen peroxide in 2 cases. *Contact Dermatitis* 1994;30:113.
190. Kanerva L, et al. Occupational allergic contact dermatitis from potassium persulfate. *Contact Dermatitis* 1999;40:116.
191. Cronin E. Formaldehyde is a significant allergen in women with hand eczema. *Contact Dermatitis* 1991;25:276.
192. Krogsrud NE, Larsen AI. Grapeseed oil as a safe and efficient hand cleansing agent. *Contact Dermatitis* 1992;26:208.
193. Koh D, Foulds IS, Aw TC. Dermatological hazards in the electronics industry. *Contact Dermatitis* 1990;22:1.
194. Seidenari S, et al. Contact sensitization among ceramics workers. *Contact Dermatitis* 1990;22:45.
195. Lear JT, et al. Transient re-emergence of oil of turpentine allergy in the pottery industry. *Contact Dermatitis* 1996;35:169.
196. Barbaud A, Mougeolle JM, Schmutz JL. Contact hypersensitivity to arsenic in a crystal factory worker. *Contact Dermatitis* 1995;33:272.
197. Kanerva L, et al. Occupational allergic contact dermatitis caused by nitroglycerin. *Contact Dermatitis* 1991;24:356.
198. Hausen BM. Occupational allergic contact dermatitis from ethyl chloro oximido acetate [published erratum appears in *Contact Dermatitis* 1993 May; 28(5):312]. *Contact Dermatitis* 1992;27:277.
199. Conde-Salazar L, et al. Occupational allergic contact dermatitis in construction workers. *Contact Dermatitis* 1995;33:226.
200. Geier J, Schnuch A. A comparison of contact allergies among construction and nonconstruction workers attending contact dermatitis clinics in Germany. *Am J Contact Dermat* 1995;6:86.
201. Roto P, Sainio H, Reunala T, Laippala P. Addition of ferrous sulfate to cement and risk of chromium dermatitis among construction workers. *Contact Dermatitis* 1996;34:43.
202. Goh CL, Gan SL. Change in cement manufacturing process, a cause for decline in chromate allergy? *Contact Dermatitis* 1996;34:51.
203. Wong SS, et al. Occupational chromate allergy in Singapore: a study of 87 patients and a review from 1983 to 1995. *Am J Contact Dermat* 1998;9:1.
204. Halbert AR, Gebauer KA, Wall LM. Prognosis of occupational chromate dermatitis. *Contact Dermatitis* 1992;27:214.
205. Lips R, Rast H, Elsner P. Outcome of job change in patients with occupational chromate dermatitis. *Contact Dermatitis* 1996;34:268.
206. Ali SA. Occupational dermatitis in the manufacture of color television tubes. *Am J Contact Dermat* 1997;8:222.
207. Mancuso G, Reggiani M, Berdondini RM. Occupational dermatitis in shoemakers. *Contact Dermatitis* 1996;34:17.
208. Ormerod AD, Dwyer CM, Goodfield MJ. Novel causes of contact dermatitis from offshore oil-based drilling muds. *Contact Dermatitis* 1998;39:262.
209. Meding B, Barregard L, Marcus K. Hand eczema in car mechanics. *Contact Dermatitis* 1994;30:129.
210. Bergqvist U, Wahlberg JE. Skin symptoms and disease during work with visual display terminals. *Contact Dermatitis* 1994;30:197.
211. Farm G, Karlberg AT, Liden C. Are opera-house artistes afflicted with contact allergy to colophony and cosmetics? *Contact Dermatitis* 1995;32:273.
212. van Neer FJMA, van Ginkel CJW. Allergic contact dermatitis from a boxwood recorder. *Contact Dermatitis* 1997;36:305.
213. Fisher AA. Dermatitis in a musician. Part 1: allergic contact dermatitis. *Cutis* 1998;62:167.
214. Fisher AA. Dermatitis in a musician. Part 2: injuries to skin, soft tissue, and bone from musical instruments. *Cutis* 1998;62:214.
215. Fisher AA. Dermatitis in a musician. Part 3: injuries caused by specific musical instruments. *Cutis* 1998;62:261.
216. Fisher AA. Dermatitis in a musician. Part 4: physiologic, emotional, and infectious problems in musicians. *Cutis* 1999;63:13.

USEFUL READINGS

Dermatology

Adams RM. *Occupational skin disease.* Philadelphia: WB Saunders, 1990.
Cronin E. *Contact dermatitis.* Edinburgh: Churchill Livingston, 1980.
Foussereau J, Ezra Benezra J, Maibach H. *Occupational contact dermatitis.* Philadelphia: WB Saunders, 1982.
Maibach HI, Gellin GA, eds. *Occupational and industrial dermatology.* Chicago: Year Book Medical Publishers, 1982.

Schwartz L, Tulipan L, Birmingham DJ. *Occupational diseases of the skin,* 3rd ed. Philadelphia: Lea & Febiger, 1957.

General Occupational

Browning E. *Toxicity of industrial metals.* London: Butterworth, 1961.

Clayton GD, Clayton FE. Patty's industrial hygiene and toxicology, vols 2 and 3. New York: John Wiley & Sons, 1991.

Encyclopedia of occupational health and safety, vols 1 and 2. Geneva: International Labor Office, 1983.

Proctor NH, Hughes JP, Fischman ML. *Chemical hazards of the workplace.* Philadelphia: JB Lippincott Co, 1988.

Ramazzini B. *Diseases of workers* (first published in 1700). New York: Hafner Publishing Co, 1974.

Rom WN. *Environmental and occupational medicine.* Boston: Little, Brown and Company, 1982.

Zenz C, ed. *Occupational medicine.* Chicago: Year Book Medical Publishers, 1975.

Technical

Hawley GG. *The condensed chemical dictionary,* 10th ed. New York: Van Nostrand Reinhold, 1983.

Kirk-Othmer encyclopedia of chemical technology, 3rd ed. New York: Wiley-Interscience, 1983.

CHAPTER 26

Contact Dermatitis in Health Personnel

Physicians, nurses, dentists, veterinarians, pharmacists, and laboratory workers in histology and biologic chemistry are included in this group. The most common type of contact dermatitis in this group is an irritant dermatitis from frequent hand washing with various harsh, alkaline soaps, detergents, and disinfectant solutions. Such frequent washing produces a dry, fissured, pruritic dermatitis that readily becomes secondarily infected and eczematized. Persons with an atopic background in this group often develop intractable hand dermatitis (see Chapter 18). Health care personnel with hand dermatitis should use a mild, unscented soap free of all antiseptics and deodorants.

Reports of occupational dermatitis in hospital workers vary from 12% to 21% of workers affected. In one such study in Italy, the primary problem was found to be irritant contact dermatitis 95% of the time (1). Younger women were most likely to have hand eczema, and the most common irritants were chlorhexidine gluconate, glutaraldehyde, and glove powder. As is common in occupational contact dermatitis, atopy was a significant risk factor for the development of hand eczema.

Benzalkonium chloride (alkylbenzyldimethylammonium chloride), a quaternary ammonium cationic detergent, is widely used as a preoperative skin disinfectant and sometimes for the disinfection of surgical instruments. It is used in the treatment of burns, ulcers, wounds, and infected dermatoses. Benzalkonium chloride is also present in many cosmetics, deodorants, mouthwashes, dentifrices, lozenges, and ophthalmic preparations. It has produced allergic contact dermatitis in surgical personnel who handle instruments soaked in the antiseptic and who apply it as a preoperative skin disinfectant (2). Table 26.1 lists commercially available solutions containing benzalkonium chloride that must be avoided by surgeons and others sensitized to this chemical.

Two physicians were reported to have become sensitized to benzalkonium chloride from handling instruments soaked in the disinfectant for cold sterilization. They developed allergic conjunctivitis subsequently from the presence of benzalkonium chloride in ophthalmic solutions. The detergent is the most commonly used preservative in ophthalmic medications, solutions for contact lenses, and "artificial tears" (3).

> **Surgeons with hand dermatitis should avoid use of "medicated" and vitamin E soaps.**

Huriez et al. (4) reported that allergic contact sensitivity to topically applied quaternary ammonium compounds is not uncommon in France. These investigators suggested that such allergic sensitivity may produce generalized reactions from the systemic administration of drugs chemically related to topically applied quaternary ammonium compounds. Such medications include the cholinergic agents, hypotensive drugs (e.g., tetraethylammonium chloride), neuromuscular blocking agents (e.g., decamethonium bromide), or heparin antagonists (hexadimethrine bromide).

Patch testing with benzalkonium chloride should be performed with a 1:1,000 aqueous solution because higher concentrations may produce nonspecific irritant reactions (5).

SURGEONS

Surgical "scrubs" of the hands often precipitate atopic dermatitis with superimposed contact dermatitis of the hands in surgical personnel who have been free of atopic dermatitis since childhood.

Hexachlorophene is still a popular preoperating scrubbing agent. Many surgeons complain of dryness of the skin from this agent, which is a primary irritant reaction. Allergic reactions to hexachlorophene are rare. Cross-contact sensitivity and photocontact sensitivity to hexachlorophene have been observed in guinea pigs with primary photosensitivity to tetrachlorosalicylanilide and tribromosalicylanilide. It is not yet generally accepted that hexachlorophene is a primary photosensitizer, although such photosensitivity has been reported (6).

> **Hexachlorophene is present in Burdeo (Hill Pharmaceuticals) and Phisohex (Winthrop).**

TABLE 26.1. *Benzalkonium Chloride in Over-the-Counter Preparations*

Bactine Antiseptic/Anesthetic First-Aid Spray (Miles Laboratories)
Clens (Alcon/BP)
Mediconet (Medicone)
Medi-Quik (Lehn & Fink)
Mercurochrome II (Becton-Dickinson)
NTZ (Consumer Products Division, Winthrop)
Prefrin Liquifilm (allergen)
Prescription preparations
　Amino-Cerv (Milex)
　Cetylcide Solution (Cetylite)
　Florida Foam Improved (Hill Dermaceuticals)
　Ivy-Chex (nonaerosol) (Bowman)
　Zephiran Chloride 1:750 (Winthrop)
　Zephiran Chloride Spray (Winthrop)
　Zephiran Chloride Tinted Tincture (Winthrop)

Vitamin E

Several physicians and surgeons have developed allergic contact dermatitis from the use of so-called vitamin E soaps and hand lotions. There is a mistaken notion that topical vitamin E can somehow "improve" the skin. Although the systemic administration of vitamin E almost never produces any allergic reaction, various topical preparations can cause allergic dermatitis.

Betadine

Betadine Skin Cleanser and Surgical Scrub (Purdue Frederick) are rarely the cause of allergic contact dermatitis in health care personnel and may be substituted for hexachlorophene or deodorant soaps by physicians (7).

Patients have experienced chemical burns from povidone-iodine, usually after prolonged skin contact (8). Immediate hypersensitivity manifests as generalized urticaria, and angioedema can occur after application to wounds (9). Contact dermatitis has also been reported from povidone-iodine, although it is very uncommon (10).

Rubber Gloves

Any hand dermatitis that stops abruptly above the wrists should be considered as stemming from sensitization to ingredients in rubber gloves until proved otherwise (11).

Allergic hypersensitivity to such rubber chemicals as mercaptobenzothiazole, tetramethylthiuram, and isopropyl paraphenylenediamine present in the standard series are among the most common causes of allergic contact dermatitis in surgeons (12). Latex itself has become a problem as well and is discussed in Chapter 31 on rubber allergy and is briefly reviewed here.

Natural Rubber Latex

The prevalence of natural rubber latex (NRL) occupational allergy ranges from 8% to 17% and latex-induced asthma from 2.5% to 6% (13). Contact urticaria from natural rubber latex has been reported in 2.8% to 10.7% of European health care workers. In Finland, incidence rates are available rather than prevalence rates. Among laboratory assistants, the incidence of NRL allergy is 1.0 per 10,000 employed workers. Among cleaners who commonly wear rubber gloves, the incidence is only 0.5 per 10,000 workers. NRL allergy is found in 0.12% of unselected Finns prior to surgery. The incidence of NRL allergy in Finland among medical and nursing personnel is 1.8 per 10,000. It was 3.9 per 10,000 physicians, 2.2 per 10,000 for nurses, and 6.0 and 11.8 per 10,000 dentists and dental assistants, respectively (14).

The recent epidemic of latex sensitivity has led to surveys of health workers as to glove-related problems (glove related problems are discussed in detail in Chapter 31). In one such study, 37% of health workers reported skin symptoms with glove use (15). Of this group, 2% described contact urticaria–like symptoms, 10% eczematous dermatitis, and 24% an unclassifiable skin intolerance from gloves. These same investigators carefully evaluated patients with glove complaints by prick tests with multiple latex extracts as well as RAST testing (16). Less than 10% of medical workers reporting intolerance of latex gloves proved to be latex sensitive. Some patients identified as RAST positive were accepted as being latex sensitive even though they exhibited no symptoms on direct exposure to latex.

Part of the difficulty of understanding NRL allergy is the complexity of latex sap. More than 240 separate proteins have been identified by electrophoresis (17). Fewer than 25% of latex proteins are immunogenic, and the proteins that cause reactions are different in different populations (18). Among medical professionals, prohevein (20 kd) and hevein (4.7 kd) are the prevalent antigenic proteins, whereas children with multiple operations more frequently react to a 27 kd protein and rubber elongation factor (14 kd).

The reactions to NRL include urticaria, conjunctivitis, rhinitis, asthma, abdominal cramping, diarrhea, hypotension, and anaphylaxis (17). The most severe reactions have occurred with mucosal exposure. Glove powder can act as a carrier for NRL, giving rise to airborne elicitation of symptoms (19).

Presently, 19 new cases of contact urticaria/100,000 health care workers per year is occurring (20).

In her comprehensive review, Warshaw (21) has proposed a diagnostic algorithm.

A lack of standardized skin prick test materials and RAST tools that do not detect all cases make establishing a rapid and certain diagnosis challenging. To establish the presence of immediate hypersensitivity, the physician can cut a finger off a latex glove and have the patient moisten the finger and wear the dampened latex for 15 to 30 minutes to check for reactions. If no reaction occurs, the exercise can be repeated with a whole glove. Some authors have expressed concern about the safety of such testing, but patient history as to the nature of symptoms normally experienced when wearing gloves can guide the level of risk that wear testing actually poses.

A strong history of latex glove intolerance manifested by rapid onset of pruritus within minutes of donning gloves suggests immediate hypersensitivity. This is not always the case. Armstrong et al. (22) reported such a patient who was a nurse who did not develop respiratory symptoms when exposed to latex gloves. Her prick test to high-protein latex and to her gloves specifically was negative. A wet latex glove was tolerated with only pruritus and no whealing, except that when the patient was allowed to rub her hands in response to the pruritus, then and only then did whealing occur. A diagnosis of dermographism was made. Vinyl gloves did not provoke dermographism. Physical urticaria can closely mimic latex allergy. Thomson and Wilkinson (23) reported three additional cases of dermographism mimicking latex glove allergy. These cases highlight the need for an accurate diagnosis when a health care worker's career is at stake.

The cost of health facilities changing to nonlatex glove use is considerable. However, the costs to the institution of 1% of health care workers becoming fully disabled or 2% partially disabled has been estimated to exceed the cost of changing to a nonlatex environment (13).

> **Any eruption that stops abruptly at the wrists should be considered due to rubber gloves until proven otherwise; this is particularly true among surgeons.**

Hand Dermatitis in Orthopedic Surgeons from Acrylic Bone Cement

Acrylic bone cement, a mixture of polymethyl methacrylate and methyl methacrylate (acrylic monomer), is used for fixation of prostheses to bone in surgical procedures on the hip joint. The brochure describing the bone cement contains the following statement: "The liquid component (methyl methacrylate monomer) is a powerful lipid solvent. It should not be allowed to come into direct contact with sensitive tissues or be absorbed by the body. Also, it should not be permitted to come in contact with rubber, including rubber gloves."

Ironically, a surgeon cannot prevent the cement from coming into contact with rubber gloves, because rubber gloves are the only type of gloves used regularly in the operating room (24). The manufacturer of the bone cement recommends, "The surgeon [should] wear two pairs of rub-

ber gloves when handling the cement directly and discard these for a fresh pair immediately after he [or she] has finished putting the cement in place." It is thought that this is sufficient protection for an operator unless he or she is sensitive to the methyl methacrylate monomer. If, however, sensitization to acrylic monomer has occurred, sufficient cement penetrates the gloves to produce allergic contact dermatitis (25).

Some surgeons who have become sensitized to the bone cement have an assistant perform the part of an operation requiring handling of bone cement; the sensitized surgeon then completes the operation.

> **The acrylic bone cement used by orthopedic surgeons penetrates rubber gloves, causing not only dermatitis but also prolonged paresthesia of the surgeons' fingers.**

Allergic contact dermatitis of the hands from acrylic bone cement is accompanied usually by marked dryness and fissuring of the skin (26).

Another unique feature of allergic contact dermatitis caused by acrylic monomer is a distressing paresthesia of the fingertips in the form of a burning sensation, tingling, and slight numbness. The paresthesia may persist for several weeks after the dermatitis has subsided. Fisher (27) also saw this type of paresthesia in two orthodontists who became sensitized to acrylic monomer in bonding cement. The prolonged paresthesia caused by the monomer may be due to the fact that acrylic monomer is a powerful solvent that readily penetrates damaged skin and thus produces inflammation of the nerve endings in the fingers (28). One report described paresthesia persisting for at least 3 months in a patient who was allergic to a hydroxyethyl methacrylate compound (29).

Because the gloves currently available do not protect the hands from acrylic monomer, only the development of a "no-touch" technique will enable the orthopedic surgeon to utilize bone cement with instruments. Sufficient protection will be provided by avoiding direct contact of the gloved hands with the cement. A new potential problem in orthopedic personnel and patients was reported from plaster casts reinforced with melamine-formaldehyde resin. These casts are waterproof, but technicians applying them may become sensitized, as may patients. A 10% melamine-formaldehyde resin in petrolatum patch test is used diagnostically (30).

NURSES

Aside from exposures while in pursuit of their medical duties, nurses may be exposed to detergents, other cleansers, and alcohol that can lead to dryness and eczematization of their hands. Such irritated skin may be more readily sensitized than nonirritated skin to the medications and chemicals that nurses handle in their work.

When a nurse has intractable hand dermatitis, patch tests should be performed with the chemicals and medications listed under housewife's eczema and under eczema in the professional group. In addition, it may be useful to perform patch tests with streptomycin, penicillin, and chlorpromazine.

Streptomycin

This drug is an especially important occupational hazard to nurses and a frequent cause of allergic contact sensitization (31). The allergic dermatitis may first be noted at the tips of the thumb and the index and middle fingers where there is contact with streptomycin from a leaking syringe or needle. Prolonged contact in the sensitized individual may produce deep fissures and hyperkeratoses with superimposed eczematization. Once dermatitis has developed, several weeks of treatment may be required before the hands return to normal, even if contact with streptomycin is avoided.

For patch test purposes, a 2.5% aqueous solution of streptomycin is used. In most instances, sensitized individuals show a strongly positive patch test reaction. Occasionally the reaction is negative, but a scratch test may produce an urticarial wheal within 15 minutes, which may remain for 1 hour or so and be replaced by a papule or vesicle after 24 to 48 hours. Although scratch testing with streptomycin is a relatively safe procedure, the intracutaneous test is hazardous and may cause a generalized urticaria and anaphylactoid shock. Desensitization to streptomycin is dangerous and usually fails.

> **Nurses with hand dermatitis may be tested with streptomycin, penicillin, chlorpromazine, and glutaraldehyde in addition to the routine screening series.**

Penicillin

Allergic sensitization to penicillin may be initiated by external contact with various forms of penicillin, and dermatitis may be produced in sensitized individuals by contact with penicillin used for injections or by handling syringes contaminated with it. Allergic contact sensitivity to penicillin is combined usually with the immediate anaphylactic variety. Inhalation of penicillin from powder or aerosols or molds may produce asthma and anaphylactoid shock in individuals with contact sensitivity.

Patch tests may be performed with penicillin powder, ointment (500 U/g) or topical medications. The usual positive reaction occurs in 24 to 48 hours. In sensitive individuals, however, within a half hour an immediate reaction may occur consisting of an erythematous wheal, sometimes with pseudopods (32). A positive patch test reaction of the delayed type may be significant, because the allergic eczematous contact sensitivity is accompanied frequently by the immediate anaphylactic reaction. If there is a compelling need for penicillin in a patient who has a positive patch test reaction to it, scratch and intracutaneous tests must be performed to determine the presence or absence of the immediate type of sensitivity before systemic administration is attempted. Furthermore, systemic administration to an individual with a positive patch test reaction can produce a severe eczematous contact-type dermatitis medicamentosa, which may be widespread and disabling.

> **Medical personnel who have allergic contact sensitivity to penicillin often develop the immediate anaphylactic variety as well.**

Nurses and others with known sensitivity to penicillin must avoid handling all preparations containing this drug. Desensitization is hazardous and should be attempted with caution.

Chlorpromazine (Thorazine)

This drug is a common cause of contact dermatitis in nurses who inject it (33). Pharmacists and others who handle chlorpromazine powder or tablets may also become sensitized (34,35). Three types of sensitivity are seen with the phenothiazine drugs (36):

1. The usual allergic contact eczematous variety in which the covered patch test reaction is positive.
2. A photoallergic reaction in which the covered patch reaction is negative when the drug is used alone but becomes positive when the patch test site is irradiated.
3. A photoallergic reaction in combination with an allergic eczematous contact-type sensitization in which the patch test reaction is positive with the phenothiazine derivative alone, but a stronger response is elicited if the site is irradiated with a suberythematous dose of ultraviolet rays or exposed to strong sunlight for 20 minutes.

> **Thorazine and other phenothiazines may produce both allergic eczematous dermatitis and persistent photoallergy.**

The increased sensitivity of the skin to light sometimes persists for months. The patient sensitized to chlorpromazine, therefore, should avoid exposure to sunlight for at least several weeks after recovering from the dermatitis. If exposure is unavoidable, a sunscreen should be used to protect the involved skin.

Sensitivity to chlorpromazine may cause cross-reactions with other phenothiazine drugs, such as prochloroperazine, chlorpromethazine, pramazine, and promethazine hydrochloride (Phenergan).

Maclofenoxate

This injectable analeptic central nervous system stimulant can produce allergic contact dermatitis in nurses who inject their patients with the medication known as Lucidril in France (37).

Famotidine

Contact dermatitis of the hands occurred in a nurse handling famotidine, an H_2-receptor antagonist. An aqueous 10 mg/mL patch test was positive, and there were no cross reactions to ranitidine or cimetidine (38).

Required Vaccinations among Medical Personnel

US Occupational Safety and Health Administration regulations require personnel who handle body fluids to be offered hepatitis B immunization. Pruritic nodules lasting 1 to 2 years have occurred after subcutaneous injections of hepatitis B vaccine (Hevac B). An allergic reaction to aluminum hydroxide present in Hevac B leads to these granulomatous reactions, which contain aluminum crystals. A 1% aluminum chloride acetate or acitotartrath patch test is superior to aluminum hydroxide (39).

Prolonged reactions to Heptavac containing thimerosal have also been reported in health personnel receiving subcutaneous injections (40). It has been noted that thimerosal-sensitive patients tolerated intramuscular immunization without incident in contradistinction to subcutaneous injections (41). It has been estimated that 16% of Japanese who receive vaccinations containing 0.01% thimerosal will become sensitized (42). These individuals will be at risk for piroxicam photosensitivity via thiosalicylate allergy induction (42).

DENTISTS

Dentists frequently have combined irritant and allergic hand dermatitis (43). The tips and volar aspects of the fingers and the palms may become dry, fissured, and hyperkeratotic from exposure to both irritants and sensitizers. The fingers may become leathery, with loss of fine tactile perception. When the dorsal aspect of the fingers and hands become involved, erythema, edema, and vesiculation may occur. Patch tests are valuable not only in distinguishing between an allergic and an irritant hand dermatitis, but also in quickly pinpointing responsible allergens (44).

A strongly positive patch test reaction alerts the dentist to the risk of contacting even minute amounts of a material. Dentists protest frequently that they hardly touch or rarely use a chemical that produces a positive reaction, but it must be emphasized that a single exposure in a sensitized individual may produce a dermatitis that persists for a week or more. Even exposure once weekly may produce a chronic dermatitis. The dentist must not only avoid contact with the sensitizer but also become aware of the guises under which it may appear and the chemicals that cross-react with it.

Topical (Surface) and Injectable Local Anesthetics

Dentists, in particular, are frequently sensitized to local anesthetics because they are exposed in two ways: (a) by rubbing on the gum surface with the finger before the era of glove wearing, a solution, spray, or ointment containing a "caine," before the injection of the local anesthetic or for treating various conditions in the mouth, such as relief of ulcers or traumatic injury; and in the form of gauze packs or ointment for postextraction sockets (more than half of the agents listed for surface application in current accepted dental remedies contain benzocaine and many contain tetracaine; benzocaine and tetracaine are both p-aminobenzoic acid derivatives, which are sensitizers) and (b) by injecting a "caine" compound into the buccal areas. Skin contact is due to the leakage of the solution spilling over on the fingers used in retraction or holding the syringe.

Irritant Dermatitis in Dentists

Probably the most common causes of dermatitis among dentists are soaps, detergents, and other cleaners. In addition, the acids used in direct bonding agents and preventive fluoride treatments expose the dentists to strong irritants.

> **Dentists are exposed to irritants in soaps, detergents, cleaners, disinfectants, fluxes, plaster of paris, acids, fluorides, and bonding agents.**

The grinding, polishing, and buffing of metal alloys may release chromium that can produce a characteristic lesion, which is the chrome node appearing over the joints of fingers, eyelids, and face. Usually small painless ulcers, 2 to 4 mm in diameter, deep and firm, with slow healing, are apparent.

Dental Allergens

Dental personnel are exposed to many contact allergens, as shown in Table 26.2.

Dental Technicians

Skin problems related to work were reported by 36% of dental technicians, and most suspected plastic based materials in a survey of 1,132 such workers (45). Patch tests were per-

TABLE 26.2. *Contact Allergen Exposure in Dental Personnel*

Acrylates	Essential oils
Amalgrams (mercury)	Eugenol
Anesthetics, local	Peppermint
Antibiotics	Wintergreen
Bonding agents	Impression compounds
Acrylic	Rosin
Epoxy	Soldering fluxes
Disinfectants	Hydrazine
Cresol	Rosin
Formaldehyde	Wax (carnauba)
Halogenated salicyanilides	
Hexachlorophene	
Mercury	
Thymol	

formed on 55 examined workers, and allergic contact dermatitis was diagnosed in 64%, with irritant contact dermatitis seen in 24%. The most common allergen was 2-hydroxyethyl methacrylate, followed by ethylene glycol dimethacrylate and methyl methacrylate. Fingertip dermatitis was present in almost all of the allergy cases, and dorsal hand eczema was the most common presentation in irritant reactions.

Acrylic Monomer

In the United States, 95% of dentures are made of acrylic resin by mixing the acrylic liquid monomer methyl methacrylate with polymethyl methacrylate powder (46). Polymerization and hardening of the resin may take place by heating or by self-curing at room temperatures. For self-curing acrylic resins, polymerization of the mixture of liquid monomer and polymethyl powder is induced with an organic peroxide and an accelerator or promoter. The self-cured resin normally contains much more residual monomer than does the heat-cured resin.

As a rule, dentures are cured by heat, but when the dentist has to repair or build up a portion of the denture, the self-curing acrylic resin is used. In addition, self-curing acrylic material is used extensively in creating small temporary bridges, crowns, and fillings.

> **Uncured acrylic monomer is a sensitizer; when completely polymerized, acrylic compounds no longer produce dermatitis.**

Acrylic monomer alone is a powerful sensitizer, but the polymer and the heat-cured resin are not. Enough residual acrylic monomer is present in the self-cured portion of a denture, however, to cause reactions on the skin and the oral mucosa in sensitized individuals.

Excessive exposure of the dentist to acrylic monomer may cause not only an allergic contact eczematous reaction but also dryness and fissuring of the fingertips by a defat-

ting action on the skin. It is, therefore, advisable for dentists with hand dermatitis to avoid direct contact with liquid acrylic monomer and self-cured dentures and acrylic teeth. Dentists with marked allergic sensitivity to the acrylic monomer, proved by strong patch-test reactions may, nevertheless, wear heat-cured acrylic dentures.

It must be remembered, however, that the acrylic monomer is a strong solvent that readily penetrates rubber gloves.

Acrylic resin sealers and adhesives may produce hand dermatitis in sensitized individuals.

Patch Tests with Acrylic Monomer

Patch tests may be performed with 10% acrylic monomer in olive oil. Because some monomers contain benzoyl peroxide (test 10% in petrolatum) and hydroquinone (test 2% in petrolatum), patch tests with these chemicals should also be done to determine whether a positive reaction is due to the monomer or these additives.

Methyl methacrylate monomer usually produces a delayed eczematous patch test reaction in sensitized dental personnel. Occasionally, however, an allergic contact urticaria is produced, in which case an urticarial wheal will be produced at the patch test site within an hour.

Formaldehyde

Exposure to this disinfectant occurs during sterilization of dental instruments and is used for the reduction of ammoniacal silver nitrate.

Members of the medical and allied professions may be exposed to formaldehyde when it is used for sterilizing purposes, as a disinfectant, or as a fixing solution for tissues. Formaldehyde is not only a powerful sensitizer but also a potent primary irritant. A strong solution of formaldehyde can coagulate the protein of the skin and produce necrosis and scarring. Prolonged contact, even with weak solutions, may cause extreme dryness of the skin with fissuring. Formaldehyde solution (formalin) may cause the nails to become discolored, soft, or brittle. Paronychia and even suppuration of the matrix may follow exposure to this chemical.

When an allergic sensitization to formaldehyde solution occurs, the dermatitis may become widespread. In sensitive individuals, the mere presence of formaldehyde gas in a room in which a bottle of it was previously opened is sufficient to cause dermatitis. A minute amount of formaldehyde on thermometers, instruments, slides, and biopsy containers is also sufficient to produce dermatitis in sensitized individuals. Few patients are this exquisitely sensitive to formaldehyde. Flyvholm et al. (47) found most lose their reactivity between 5,000 and 10,000 ppm formaldehyde. They did not find any formaldehyde-sensitive patients who reacted to less than 250 ppm.

Mercury

Aside from producing eczematous dermatitis, metallic mercury from a mercury amalgam can produce a granulomatous response.

Dental Bonding Agents

Dental "bonding" is now popular. The bonding employs the use of an epoxy resin and a methacrylate. At present, BIS-GMA (2,2 bis (4(2-hydroxy-3 methacryloyoxy-propyloxy) phenyl-)-propane is the chemical generally used for almost all bonding. The term "BIS-GMA" refers to the reactants bisphenol A and glycidyl methacrylate.

Dental bonding exposes the dentist to BIS-GMA, a combination of bisphenol A (epoxy resin) and glycidyl methacrylate.

Unless the dentist practices a "no touch" technique, he or she will readily become sensitized to the epoxy resin or the methacrylate.

The bonding plastic is generally combined with quartz, lithium aluminum silicate, glass, or silicon dioxide to modify the physical properties of the resin. The size of these particles is generally 0.04 to 40 μm.

Contacto (bonding material) is free of methyl methacrylate and epoxy resin. Contacto contains hydroxyl groups and acrylic resins; it may be obtained from General Orthodontic Labs. Inc., P.O. Box 298, W.O.B., West Orange, NJ 07052.

Dental Impression Materials

Allergic reactions to dental impression materials have been reported by van Ketel (48), Cronin (49), Nally and Storrs (50), and van Groeningen and Nater (51). Dentists handling these materials may develop allergic contact dermatitis, and patients may develop stomatitis after impressions taken with Impregum material. The sensitizers appear to be the Impregum catalyst, methyl dichlorobenzene sulfonate.

Van Ketel (48) reported that a dentist with a contact dermatitis of his hands was allergic to these catalysts as shown by the fact that tests with 1% Impregum catalyst in acetone was strongly positive, whereas five other catalysts showed no positive reactions. The dentist did not react to Permlastic (Kerr-Sybron Corp., Romulus, MI 48174), an impression compound.

The catalysts in dental impression compounds and crowns may produce contact dermatitis of the hands in dentists and stomatitis in patients.

Scutan—Used in Crowns and for Tooth Sealing

Scutan is an irreversible, stiff epimin plastic that polymerizes in the cold and hardens quickly; it is used for sealing teeth. The catalyst is methyl *p*-toluenesulfonate, and the solvent is dibenzyltoluene.

The catalyst may produce contact dermatitis in dentists' fingers (52). Testing may be done with 1% in acetone.

As an alternative for Scutan, Texton (SS White Ltd., 51 St. Arms Road, Harrow, Middlesex HA1 lLR, England) may be used. Texton, however, contains methyl methacrylate, which may be sensitizing.

Essential Oils

In dentistry, essential oils are used chiefly as pharmaceutical aids and as mild antiseptics and anodynes. Those oils to which the dentist is exposed and which are sensitizers include:

1. *Eugenol.* This pale-yellow liquid with a strong smell of carnation is employed in the widely used zinc oxide–eugenol dental cement. It may also be combined with rosin and zinc oxide. It is the essential chemical constituent of clove oil and is also present in cinnamon oil, perfumes, soaps, and bay rum. Individuals sensitized to eugenol should avoid exposure to such products. Eugenol is both a primary irritant and a sensitizer. For patch testing, a 5% solution in olive oil or petrolatum is used.

2. *Clove oil.* This oil is used mainly in dentistry as an anodyne. For patch tests, a 25% concentration in castor oil is used.

3. *Cinnamon oil* (cassia oil). This oil is an antiseptic and a flavoring agent. For testing, a 5% solution in olive oil is used. Vermouths that are flavored with it are also possible sources.

4. *Flavoring agents.* Oils of spearmint, peppermint, wintergreen (methyl salicylate), and menthol. These flavoring agents may be tested 2% in olive oil.

5. *Balsam of Peru.* This substance is used in dentistry as a component of cement liquids. It is tested as a 10% solution in petrolatum.

6. *Eucalyptus oil.* This oil is used mainly as a solvent for gutta percha in root canal fillings. It is tested as a 1% solution in alcohol.

Essential oils, particularly eugenol, cinnamon oil, and clove oil, may cross-react with balsam of Peru, benzoin, rosin, and vanilla and may be present in or cross-react with perfumes in soap and toilet water.

VETERINARIANS AND ANIMAL FEED HANDLERS

Veterinarians are exposed to many contact allergens that not infrequently produce contact dermatitis. Contact dermatitis, which is uncommon for veterinarians, may be due to exposure to bovine tuberculin and Tylosin, which is restricted to

TABLE 26.3. *A Patch Test "Series" for Veterinarians*[a]

Antibiotics
  Benzyl penicillin
  Bezathine penicillin
  Dihydrostreptomycin 0.1% pet
  Erthromycin 1% pet
  Oxytetracycline 10% pet
  Penethamate hydroiodide 1% pet
  Penicillin G 10,000 IU G pet
  Procaine penicillin
  Spiramycin (Rovamycin) 10% pet
  Streptomycin 1% pet
  Tylosin tartrate (Tylan) 10% pet
Benzocaine 5% pet
Bovine tuberculin 10% aq
Formaldehyde 1% aq
Mercaptobenzothiazole 1% pet
  (rubber gloves and antiseptic)
Merthiolate 0.1% pet
Piperazine 1% aq
Procaine 2% aq
Rubber gloves
Tuberculin 10% aq

[a]Aq, aqueous; Pet, in petrolatum.

veterinary use (53,54). In addition, veterinarians are exposed to the numerous contactants listed in Table 26.3 (55).

Spiramycin

This antibiotic is given intramuscularly to cows for mastitis, to pigs for enteritis, and to cats for respiratory infections. Dogs may be treated with capsules. Both spiramycin and Tylosin are added to the drinking water given to pigs with enteritis.

Penethamate Hydroiodide (Benzyl Penicillin-Diethylaminoethylester)

This antibiotic is used for local treatment of mastitis in cows as a 25% suspension in oil injected into the teat of the cow's udder. Penethamate cross-reacts with penicillin in about 50% of the cases (56).

Unique forms of veterinary contact dermatitis are caused by bovine tuberculin, for which cattle are tested at regular intervals, and by the antibiotic Tylosin, which is restricted to veterinary use.

Mercaptobenzothiazole

Adams (57) reported that mercaptobenzothiazole is found in the following veterinary medications:

Analan Ointment (Diamond Labs.) 2%
Caladerm Ointment (Diamond Labs.) 1.25%

Delcreo Penetram Skin Balm (Delson) 1%
Dr. Merrick's Sulfodene Preparation (Westchester) 1.25%
Happy Jack Skin Balm 1%
Legear Flea and Tick Powder (Le Gear) 1%
Mercaptocaine (Pitman-Moore) 2%

"Immediate" Contact Urticaria in Veterinarians

Hjorth (56) suggested that veterinarians should have scratch tests done with a cow's hairs, horse dander, and a pig's bristles. These allergens can produce dermatitis, hay fever, and asthma in sensitized veterinarians.

In addition, obstetric work with cattle is not unusual among veterinarians. Specific IgE and positive scratch tests to cow placenta extract have been demonstrated in veterinarians with hand eczema after a cow's delivery (58).

Rudzki et al. (59) summarized occupational dermatitis in veterinarians, stating that the most common causes of such dermatoses are antibiotics, procaine, bovine tuberculin, and irritation from obstetric work.

Malten (60) listed the numerous "pet" medications that can produce contact dermatitis in veterinarians and others who apply them to animals (Table 26.4).

Animal Feed Additives

Commercially prepared animal feed may contain several growth stimulants, hormones, vitamins, anti-infection agents, minerals, antioxidants, and metals that may lead to allergic contact dermatitis from the handling of these additives (61). The following feed additives have been reported to produce allergic contact dermatitis.

TABLE 26.4. *Animal "Pet" Medications*

Anesthetics
  Antibiotics
  Antihistamines
  Antimycotic agents
Antiparasiticides
  Alugan
  Benzyl benzoate
  Carbaryl
  Dichlorphos
  Fenchlorphos
  Fenithrothion
  Lindane
  Mesulphen
  Piperonyl butoxide
  Propoxur
  Pyrethrin I
  Rotenone
  Tetrachloruinphos
Antiseptics
Eye medications

Tylosin

Neldner (62) described a 13-year-old girl with an allergic contact dermatitis from Tylosin acquired by feeding this antibiotic to a pig. Tylosin is used as a growth promoter in feed for cattle and swine.

Additives to animal feed can cause allergic contact dermatitis. In this setting, vitamin B_{12} has been identified as a cause with a negative reaction to cobalt (63).

Dinitolmide (Zoalene)

Bleumink and Nater (64) reported a worker in a poultry food factory with an allergic dermatitis of the hands due to dinitolmide, which is added to chicken food to control outbreaks of coccidiosis. Dinitolmide is a dinitrobenzine derivative.

Nitrofurazone (Furacin)

Neldner (62) found that the cause of an allergic contact dermatitis in a hog rancher was due to nitrofurazone, which he used to treat a pig infected with salmonella. Nitrofurazone is also used as a growth promoter in feed, especially for cattle and swine. Nitrofurazone was once a popular remedy for the treatment of burns and stasis ulcers. So many instances of allergic sensitivity to this remedy occurred that its use has largely been abandoned.

Furazolidone and Furaltadone

Furazolidone is used both as an antibiotic in veterinary medicine and as an animal feed additive. When patch tested at 2% in petrolatum, false-negative reactions occur. The correct vehicle for testing is either PEG-400 or alcohol (65). No cross-reactions have been reported between furazolidone and nitrofurazone, nitrofurantoin, and furfural (65). A 1% petrolatum patch test to furaltadone tartrate was successful in detecting allergy to this feed additive (66).

Ethoxyquin (Santoquin)

Melhom and Beetz (67) recorded an allergic contact dermatitis due to sensitization to ethoxyquin used as an antioxidant in animal feeds. The patient was employed in the manufacture of compounded animal feed.

Burrows (68) pointed out that vitamins A and D_3, as supplied by the manufacturer, contain 5% ethoxyquin (6-ethyl-1,2-dihydro-2,2,4-trimethylquinoline) as an antioxidant preservative. These vitamins are usually diluted with cereal in a premix that dilutes the ethoxyquin to between 0.2% and 0.15%. Further dilution in the final meal would end with a finished product containing 0.0001% ethoxyquin from the vitamin sources. It should be remembered that ethoxyquin also appears in the meal from two other sources. Fish, bone-meal, and tallow have an antioxidant that is likely to be ethoxyquin.

Quindoxin

Burrows (68) reported that quindoxin (Grufas) is used in Great Britain and Ireland as an antioxidant preservative in vitamin additives and animal feed. Burrows showed that quindoxin is capable of inducing a photodermatitis at a low concentration.

Scott and Dawson (69) reported 17 farmers who acquired a photocontact dermatitis from exposure to quindoxin in animal feed as a growth-promoting factor. The patients all showed a dry, lichenified, fissured dermatitis of the exposed parts of the body "resembling a cement dermatitis." Photopatch tests were positive with quindoxin 0.1% in petrolatum. Quindoxin is also capable of producing allergic contact dermatitis in the absence of light.

Halquinol

This chemical is added to feeds for prevention and treatment of scours in pigs caused or complicated by *Escherichia coli* and Salmonella. Those people who add it are exposed to a high concentration. Halquinol is a chlorinated derivative of 8-hydroxyquinoline (oxine) consisting of the following three constituents, added in a 0.1% concentration to meal: 5,7-dichloro-8-hydroxyquinoline, 5-chloro-8-hydroxyquinoline, and 7-chloro-8-hydroxyquinoline.

Caplan (70) noted that animal feed additives can provoke not only irritant, allergic eczematous dermatitis and photodermatitis, but also dermatitis that is urticarial in nature. Direct contact with the animal feed is not necessary because a diffuse dermatitis through the airborne route can occur in farmers and mill workers.

Fisher (61) reported a patient who was allergic to ethylenediamine hydroiodide who also showed a cross-reaction to ethylenediamine hydrochloride, to which he had become sensitized by using original formula Mycolog cream.

Burrows (68) listed the numerous chemicals that may be added to animal feed (Table 26.5).

Dawson and Scott (71) reviewed the contact dermatitis in agricultural workers due to animal feed additives.

PHARMACISTS

Pharmacists have acquired an unusual type of "contact" psoriasis owing to the trauma of the friction of closing and opening "childproof" prescription container caps. In several instances that Fisher observed (27), such friction has localized psoriasis in the area of friction in pharmacists who have psoriasis elsewhere on their body: this is termed Koebner phenomenon (72).

TABLE 26.5. *Commonly Used Animal Feed Additives[a]*

Drug	Uses
Amprolium 10% aq sol	Growth promoter in feed (poultry); coccidostat
Arsanilic acid, 3-nitro-4-hydroxyphenyl-arsonic acid 10% mineral oil	Organic arsenicals; growth promoters in feed (cattle, swine, and poultry)
Bacitracin zinc test as is	Growth promoter in feed (swine)
Chlortetracycline hydrochloride, oxytetracycline 3% pet	Growth promoter in feed (swine and sheep); prevention of bacterial enteritis
Diethylstilbestrol 0.1% ethyl alc	Feed additive used in fattening cattle or treatment of anestrus
Ethoxyquin 1% pet	Antioxidant preservative in vitamins A and D_3 and many foods
Ethylenediamine, ethylenediamine dihydroiodide 1% pet	Feed additive; especially for cattle with "foot rot" or "lumpy jaw"
Medroxyprogesterone acetate 1% pet	Feed additive (cattle, dogs, and sheep); threatened abortion and synchronizing estrus and ovulation
Neomycin sulfate 20% pet	Feed additive (swine), especially in sow farrowing to prevent dysentery
Nitrofurazone, furazolidone (Furacin) 1% pet	Growth promoter in feed (cattle and swine); also for *Salmonella*
Penicillin (powder or ointment) test as is	Seldom used in feed; mainly for variety of diseases, especially mastitis in lactating cows[b]
Phenothiazine,[c] piperazine citrate, and thiabendazole 1% aq sol	Feed additive (cattle and swine) for worm control
Sulfacetamide, sulfamethazine test as is	Growth promoter in feed, especially pig starter; to prevent bacterial enteritis
Tylosin (Tylan) 1% aq sol	Growth promoter in feed (cattle and swine): for gram-negative infection, *Leptospira,* and coccidiosis

[a]Aq, aqueous; Pet, in petrolatum; sol, solution; alc, alcohol.
[b]Used intramuscularly.
[c]Photosensitizer.

> **The friction of removing and applying "child-proof" prescription caps can induce psoriasis of the palms in pharmacists.**

LABORATORY WORKERS

Table 26.6 lists the allergens in workers in chemistry and histology laboratories (73,74).

An unusual source of epoxy resin is immersion oil. Leica® immersion oil uses modified cyclohexyl epoxy resin, which can cause airborne contact dermatitis affecting the face and neck (75). An epidemic of immersion oil dermatitis with the new Leica formula was confirmed to be due to epoxy resin, and the presence of diglycidyl ether of bisphenol A was confirmed by HPLC (76).

An electron microscopy technician was found to be allergic to three epoxy components: diglycidyl ester of hexahydrophthalic acid, epichlorohydrin, and an allergen not pre-

TABLE 26.6. *Allergens in Laboratory Workers in Biologic Chemistry and Histology[a]*

Allergens	Test	Use
Acrylamide	5% pet	Polyacrylamide gel electrophoresis
Aniline (amino benzol)[b]	1% pet	Ziehl staining
Benzidine (para-diamino-diphenyl)[b]	1% pet	Demonstration of blood in feces
Congo red	2% pet	Amyloid
N,N'-dimethylparaphenylenediamine	1% pet	Neisseria gonorrhea staining
Epoxy resin	1% pet	Electronic microscope
Epoxy resin hardener	1% pet	Electronic microscope
Formaldehyde	2% aq	Fixator (bouin liquid)
Glutaraldehyde	0.5% aq	Fixator (bouin liquid)
Mercury ammoniated	2% pet	Chloremia titration
Methyl orange	2% pet	Determination of pH
Paraphenylenediamine	2% pet	Glucidograms coloring
Phenylhydrazine	2% pet	Research of osazones in urine
Picric acid (trinitrophenol)	2% pet	Creatine titration
Potassium dichromate	0.5% pet	Cleaning of glassware
Sudan III	2% pet	Lipid staining
Sudan IV	2% pet	Lipid staining

[a]Aq, aqueous; Pet, in petrolatum.
[b]May cross-react with paraphenylenediamine.

viously reported—epoxy propane. Epoxy propane is a transition solvent and chemically similar to epichlorhydrin (77). A 1% concentration in acetone was positive in a patient but negative in 20 controls.

A water laboratory worker developed hand, arm, and face dermatitis from exposure to hydroxylammonium chloride (78). This chemical is used in the manufacture of pharmaceuticals, in the production of surface coatings, in photography, and in rubber, textile, and plastics industries. It has been reported to be a sensitizer in diazo copy paper, and from chemical and photographic facilities.

Acrylamide

Individuals working with polyacrylamide gel electrophoresis may become sensitized even if latex or polyvinyl chloride gloves are worn, as the acrylamine goes through these glove types (79).

ALCOHOL

Although it is widely recognized that alcohol can dry and irritate the skin, the possibility of alcohol being a cutaneous sensitizer is usually overlooked. Externally applied alcohol is usually ethyl alcohol, which for this purpose is denatured or is unfit for drinking because of the addition of chemicals. For industrial use, 5% methyl alcohol or acetone is often added to denatured ethyl alcohol; for ordinary or medicinal use, about 40 chemicals are available for denaturing it. Most of these substances have a bitter taste or cause emesis. Rubbing alcohol is 70% ethyl alcohol with a denaturing agent. In alcohol used in cosmetics, the added chemicals are odorless and nontoxic. Denatured alcohols used for perfumes and other cosmetics often contain diethyl phthalate.

The most popular denaturing agents in rubbing alcohol include tartar emetic, salicylic acid, quinine sulfate, colchicum extract, brucine (an alkaloid resembling strychnine), quassia (the bitter principle of a Jamaica wood), and sucrose octa-acetate (an anhydrous adhesive used in lacquers). Isopropyl alcohol, which has a slight odor resembling that of acetone, may also be used as a denaturing agent. Pure ethyl alcohol is used in some hospitals, but coloring matter, such as methylene blue or amaranth pink (an azo dye used to color elixir phenobarbital), is added to discourage drinking it. Some individuals who have allergic contact sensitivity to alcohol may react to the ingestion of alcohol with a generalized erythema. Reports indicate that allergic reactions to the alcohols are not as rare as formerly believed (80–84).

> **The "denaturing" agents added to alcohol are rare sensitizers.**

Richardson et al. (84) reported an allergic eczematous contact dermatitis to a commercially available prepackaged alcohol sponge (Preptic Swab). The dermatitis appeared on the hands of nurses and at the sites of electrocardiogram electrode placement (where the sponges were used as conductors) on cardiac patients. Patch tests indicated that the allergen is probably a volatile substance added to sterilize the swab. The actual sensitizer was not discovered.

Contact Dermatitis Caused by Alcohol

Allergic contact dermatitis is caused occasionally by pure ethyl alcohol, and the allergic sensitivity extends usually to amyl, butyl, methyl, and isopropyl alcohols. The dermatitis may take the form of an eczematous eruption or, rarely, an erythematous flush or contact urticaria at the exposed sites (85,86). Alcohols, however, are usually irritant.

Systemic Contact Dermatitis

The ingestion of alcohol or even beer or wine by individuals sensitized by external contact to alcohol may be accompanied by extensive stomatitis, aphthous stomatitis, urticaria, angioedema, morbilliform eruptions, or a flare of eczematous dermatitis at sites affected previously by the external exposure to alcohol.

Van Ketel and Tan-Lim (87) reported an allergic eczematous contact dermatitis from alcohol. This patient also had positive reactions to beer, red wine, sherry, and acetone. Van Ketel and Tan-Lim stated that an external reaction to alcohol does not necessarily mean that systemic contact dermatitis will develop after drinking alcoholic beverages.

> **Although allergic contact sensitivity to alcohol may be accompanied by systemic reactions on ingestion of alcohol, such a sequence does not always occur.**

Testing for Allergic Alcohol Hypersensitivity

Alcohol may be tested undiluted. Two types of reactions may occur: (a) an immediate urticarial contact reaction, which occurs usually within 15 minutes after the topical application of alcohol in the form of a bright red erythema with or without urticarial elements, which may persist for 2 hours or more (it is advisable to test for contact sensitivity to alcohol first by the open patch test method and to keep the patient under observation for an hour or so); and (b) a delayed reaction, which may take place after 24 or 48 hours with the formation of an erythematous, eczematous patch at the patch test site. Occasionally, there is a combination of the immediate and delayed reaction (87).

> **Alcohol may produce immediate contact urticaria or a delayed eczematous dermatitis; the many denaturing agents added to alcohol are rare sensitizers.**

Additional discussions on reactions to alcohol are detailed in Chapter 30.

ALLERGIC GLUTARALDEHYDE DERMATITIS IN THE MEDICAL AND ALLIED PROFESSIONS

There are several reports of nurses who acquired allergic glutaraldehyde dermatitis from handling instruments sterilized with this compound (88–91). Also reported were a technician handling a renal dialysis unit and an inhalation therapy assistant who acquired allergic contact dermatitis from contact with glutaraldehyde used as a cold sterilizing agent (92,93). Table 26.7 lists the exposure to glutaraldehyde in medical, nursing, dental, and allied personnel.

Cases have been reported of X-ray technicians and radiologists with allergic glutaraldehyde dermatitis due to the presence of glutaraldehyde in X-ray film solution (94,95).

> **Cidex, a buffered glutaraldehyde solution used as a cold chemical sterilizer for surgical and dental instruments in a dialysis unit and pulmonary apparatus, has caused allergic contact dermatitis.**

Belani and Priedklans (96) described an "epidemic" of serious laryngeal injury associated with endotracheal intubation. Glutaraldehyde used for sterilization was suspected. Since the introduction of single-use disposable endotracheal tubes, there have been no further cases of "pseudomembranous laryngotracheitis." Cidex may be obtained from any large hospital that uses it for sterilization, particularly for inhalation therapy. The following companies produce Cidex: Union Carbide, Ethicon, Arbrook, Matheson, Coleman, and Bell. Patch testing may be performed with 1% Cidex or 1% unbuffered glutaraldehyde in aqueous solution.

TABLE 26.7. *Exposure to Glutaraldehyde in Medical and Allied Professions*

Cold sterilizing solution
  Buffered (Cidex)
    Renal dialysis
    Pulmonary apparatus
Embalming
Tissue fixative
X-ray film solution

The Nature of Glutaraldehyde

Glutaraldehyde (1,5-pentanedial), an aliphatic dialdehyde that forms colorless crystals, is soluble in water, alcohol, ether, and similar organic solvents. It is available most frequently as 50% aqueous solution. It is used in a 2% water solution as a cold sterilizer, especially in hospital-medical work for sterilizing instruments, bronchoscopes, cystoscopes, and anesthetic equipment; in renal dialysis units for sterilizing forceps; and by patients at home for sterilizing their artificial kidneys.

Relation of Cidex to Glutaraldehyde

Cidex is a 2% acidic glutaraldehyde that is stable for long periods if stored in a cool place. When the buffering agent sodium bicarbonate is added, the resultant alkaline solution undergoes polymerization and loses its antimicrobial activity within 2 to 3 weeks. This alkaline Cidex is more active and quicker to take effect than the acidic glutaraldehyde.

Unbuffered solutions of glutaraldehyde are stable for long periods of time, have a mildly acid pH and a negligible odor, and are not potently antimicrobial; however, when Cidex becomes buffered to an alkaline pH of 7.5 to 8.0 upon the addition of sodium bicarbonate, the glutaraldehyde is "activated" and its antimicrobial (sporocidal, bactericidal, viricidal, and fungicidal) activity greatly enhanced for periods of up to 14 days.

Activated glutaraldehyde (Cidex) retains the skin-sensitizing properties of pure glutaraldehyde. Furthermore, the relatively strong irritant effect of pure glutaraldehyde on the eyes, nasal passages, upper respiratory tract, and even the pulmonary area make Cidex an important occupational hazard.

Glutaraldehyde is a moderately irritant dialdehyde that readily polymerizes; it is available at 99%, 50%, and 25% solutions. It is used as a sterilizing solution, tissue fixative, embalming fluid, and for tanning clothing and shoe leather because it enhances the resistance of the hide to sweat. Glutaraldehyde increases the water resistance of wallpaper and hardens photographic gelatin; it is used as an intermediate in the manufacture of resins and dyes and is prescribed for plantar hyperhidrosis, onychomycosis, and warts.

Therapeutic Uses of Glutaraldehyde

The therapeutic uses of glutaraldehyde are shown in Table 26.8.

TABLE 26.8. *Therapeutic Uses of Glutaraldehyde*

Antifungal agent
Bullous diseases
Hyperhidrosis
Warts

The Use of Glutaraldehyde for Hyperhidrosis

Jordan et al. (97) reported on a man who developed an allergic contact hypersensitivity from the use of glutaraldehyde for hyperhidrosis of the soles. Maibach (98) stated that glutaraldehyde is an effective topical therapeutic agent for patients with hyperhidrosis of the soles. A usage test was performed on the soles and antecubital fossae of six previously documented glutaraldehyde-sensitive patients. All had negative usage test reactions to 25% glutaraldehyde on the soles. When tested on the antecubital fossae with 2.5% glutaraldehyde, however, they developed a severe dermatitis within 48 hours. Clearly there is a striking variation in the way in which glutaraldehyde-sensitive patients tolerate or react to its use in two diverse anatomic sites.

The Use of Glutaraldehyde as an Antifungal Agent

Glutaraldehyde has been shown to have antifungal properties (99). Jordan et al. (97) reported a man who developed an acute contact dermatitis from the use of glutaraldehyde for onychomycosis.

Glutaraldehyde as a Therapeutic Agent for Warts

The use of glutaraldehyde for warts occasionally has been marked by irritation, but apparently no allergic reactions have been encountered from such use.

Glutaraldehyde as a Therapeutic Agent for Bullous Disease

Comaish (100) reported that topical glutaraldehyde decreased skin friction and enhanced resistance to friction injury produced at a given load in short-term experiments. A single application produces a detectable effect for up to 3 days. These observations partly explain glutaraldehyde's known antiperspirant action; however, similar observations have been made with dead skin *in vitro*. It is suggested that glutaraldehyde and similar substances may be useful when a reduction in friction trauma is necessary, such as in case of epidermolysis bullosa and porphyria cutanea tarda.

Des Grosseilliers and Brisson (101) stated that in two patients with localized epidermolysis bullosa (recurrent bullous eruption of the hands and feet or Weber-Cockayne syndrome), experimentally induced blisters were studied histopathologically. The blisters showed cleft formation in the suprabasal layers of the epidermis. Therapy with topically applied 10% glutaraldehyde was found to be beneficial, but the irritant and skin-sensitizing side effects of this chemical proved to be a limiting factor for its use.

These authors concluded that the therapeutic use of topical glutaraldehyde presents three general shortcomings: (a) The solution causes brown discoloration of the soles; (b) because of its chemical composition and instability, the preparation must be kept refrigerated to remain therapeutically effective for a 1-month period, and a new supply of the solution must be prepared every month; and (c) glutaraldehyde is an irritant and a potential skin sensitizer, and the development of an allergic contact dermatitis in a patient precludes further extensive use of this therapy.

Gordon (102), in commenting on Des Grosseilliers and Brisson's article, stated that because allergic reactions to glutaraldehyde are rare, and because no specific treatment exists for localized bullous epidermolysis, the treatment with glutaraldehyde should not be discarded. Furthermore, the brown discoloration can be minimized by use of a 2% solution of glutaraldehyde, and three baths will remove the stain.

Gordon also advocated the use of glutaraldehyde for herpes zoster and simplex and pseudomonas infections.

Industrial Exposure to Glutaraldehyde

Table 26.9 lists such exposure.

Glutaraldehyde Tanned Leather Shoes

There are no reports of shoe dermatitis developing from glutaraldehyde-tanned leather shoes. Jordan et al. (97) studied three patients with allergic hypersensitivity to glutaraldehyde. Although all of them had positive patch test reactions to glutaraldehyde-tanned leather, none of them had shoe dermatitis. Even the patient with hyperhidrosis was not sensitized by the use of glutaraldehyde.

Fisher (27) observed, however, one glutaraldehyde-sensitive nurse whose white shoes tanned with glutaraldehyde produced a contact dermatitis of the feet.

> **Industrial exposure to glutaraldehyde, including leather tanned objects, rarely produces allergic contact dermatitis; glutaraldehyde and formaldehyde do not cross-react.**

Weaver and Maibach (103) reported that a liquid fabric softener, containing 500 ppm. of glutaraldehyde, used to launder T-shirts provoked no reaction in 14 glutaraldehyde-sensitive subjects who wore them for 2 weeks. In another usage test, six glutaraldehyde-sensitive subjects applied 25% aqueous glutaraldehyde to their soles twice daily for a week without ill effect, whereas a 2.5% concentration ap-

TABLE 26.9. *Industrial Exposure to Glutaraldehyde*

Clothing
Hardening of photographic gelatin
Increase in water resistance in wallpaper
Intermediate in resin and dyes
Liquid fabric softener
Tanning of leather

plied to the antecubital fossae caused a severe dermatitis within 2 days.

Does Glutaraldehyde Cross-react with Formaldehyde?

Cronin (49) stated that cross-reactions between glutaraldehyde and formaldehyde did not occur in her patients. Test results with formaldehyde were negative in all the glutaraldehyde-sensitive patients but one, a renal dialysis assistant reported by Neering and van Ketel (92), who was in contact with both formaldehyde and glutaraldehyde and had positive reactions on patch testing. Maibach (98) found that 20 patients with positive patch test reactions to 1% aqueous glutaraldehyde all had negative reactions to 2% aqueous formaldehyde.

Garcia (104) reported a man who had positive reactions to both glutaraldehyde and formaldehyde. This was not unusual because he was extensively exposed to formaldehyde in his work as a prosecutor's assistant; apparently, however, he had never been exposed to glutaraldehyde.

In Fisher's series of six formaldehyde-sensitive persons (27), none showed cross-reactions to glutaraldehyde.

REFERENCES

1. Stingeni L, Lapomarda V, Lisi P. Occupational hand dermatitis in hospital environments. *Contact Dermatitis* 1995;33:172.
2. Afzelius H, Thulin H. Allergic reactions to benzalkonium chloride. *Contact Dermatitis* 1979;5:60.
3. Fisher AA, Stillman MA. Allergic contact sensitivity to benzalkonium chloride. *Arch Dermatol* 1972;106:169.
4. Huriez C, et al. Frequence des sensibilisations aux ammoniums quaternaire. *Semin Hop Paris* 1965;72:106.
5. Wahlberg JE. Two cases of hypersensitivity to quaternary ammonium compounds. *Acta Derm Venereol* (Stockh) 1962;42:230.
6. Morikawa F, et al. Some problems on the appraisal of the skin safety of hexachlorophene. *J Soc Cosmet Chem* 1974;25:113.
7. Marks Jr JG. Allergic contact dermatitis to povidone-iodine. *J Am Acad Dermatol* 1982;6:473.
8. Corazza M, Bulciolu G, Spisani L, Virgili A. Chemical burns following irritant contact with povidone-iodine. *Contact Dermatitis* 1997; 36:115.
9. Lopez Saez MP, et al. Acute IgE-mediated generalized urticaria-angioedema after topical application of povidone-iodine. *Allergol Immunopathol* (Madr) 1998;26:23.
10. Erdmann S, Hertl M, Merk HF. Allergic contact dermatitis from povidone-iodine. *Contact Dermatitis* 1999;40:331.
11. Fisher AA. Contact dermatitis in surgeons. *J Derm Surg* 1975;1:3.
12. Rudzki E. Occupational dermatitis among health service workers. *Dermatosen* 1979;27:112.
13. Phillips VL, Goodrich MA, Sullivan TJ. Health care worker disability due to latex allergy and asthma: a cost analysis. *Am J Public Health* 1999;89:1024.
14. Jolanki R, et al. Incidence rates of occupational contact urticaria caused by natural rubber latex. *Contact Dermatitis* 1999;40:329.
15. Wrangsjo K, Osterman K, Van Hage-Hamsten M. Glove-related skin symptoms among operating theatre and dental care unit personnel (I). Interview investigation. *Contact Dermatitis* 1994;30:102.
16. Wrangsjo K, Osterman K, van Hage-Hamsten M. Glove-related skin symptoms among operating theatre and dental care unit personnel (II). Clinical examination, tests and laboratory findings indicating latex allergy. *Contact Dermatitis* 1994;30:139.
17. Ownby DR. Manifestations of latex allergy. *Immunol Allergy Clin North Am* 1995;15:31.
18. Kurup VP, Murali PS, Kelly KJ. Latex antigens. *Immunol Allergy Clin North Am* 1995;15:45.
19. Truscott N. The industry perspective on latex. *Immunol Allergy Clin North Am* 1995;15:89.
20. Kujala V. A review of current literature on epidemiology of immediate glove irritation and latex allergy. *Occup Med* (Lond) 1999;49:3.
21. Warshaw EM. Latex allergy. *J Am Acad Dermatol* 1998;1.
22. Armstrong DKB, Smith HR, Rycoroft RJG. Glove-related hand urticaria in the absence of Type I latex allergy. *Contact Dermatitis* 1999;41:42.
23. Thomson KF, Wilkinson SM. Localized dermographism: a differential diagnosis of latex glove allergy. *Contact Dermatitis* 1999;41: 103.
24. Fisher AA. Hypoallergenic surgical gloves and gloves for special situations. *Cutis* 1975;15:797.
25. Pegum J, Medhurst FA. Contact dermatitis from penetration of rubber gloves by acrylic monomer. *Br Med J* 1971;2:141.
26. Fries JB, Fisher AA, Salvati EA. Contact dermatitis in surgeons from methylmethacrylate bone cement. *J Bone Joint Surg* 1975;57a:547.
27. Fisher AA. *Contact dermatitis,* 3rd ed. Philadelphia: Lea & Febiger, 1986.
28. Bohling HG, Borchard U, Drouin H. Monomeric methylmethacrylate acts on desheathed myelinated nerve and on node of Ranvier. *Arch Toxicol* 1977;38:307.
29. Fisher AA. Paresthesia of the fingers accompanying dermatitis due to methylmethacrylate bone cement. *Contact Dermatitis* 1979;5:56.
30. Ross JS, Rycroft RJG, Cronin E. Melamine-formaldehyde contact dermatitis in orthopaedic practice. *Contact Dermatitis* 1992;26:203.
31. Sidi E, Longueville R, Hincky M. *Occupational eczema in therapists.* Springfield, IL: Charles C Thomas Publisher, 1958.
32. Blanton WB, Blanton FM. Unusual penicillin hypersensitivities. *J Allergy* 1953;24:405.
33. Calnan CD, Frain-Bell W, Cuthbert JW. Occupational dermatitis from chlorpromazine. *Trans St John Hosp Derm Soc* 1962;48:49.
34. Lewis GM, Sawicky HH. Contact dermatitis from chlorpromazine. *JAMA* 1955;157:909.
35. Goodman D, Cahn MM. Contact dermatitis to phenothiazine drugs. *J Invest Dermatol* 1959;33:27.
36. Epstein S. Allergic photo contact dermatitis from promethazine (Phenergan). *Arch Dermatol Syph* 1960;81:175.
37. Fousseraeu J, Lantz JP. Allergy to maclofenoxate in nurses. *Contact Dermatitis Newsletter* 1972;6:231.
38. Monteserín J, Conde J. Contact eczema from famotidine. *Contact Dermatitis* 1990;22:290.
39. Cosnes A, Flechet M-L, Revuz J. Inflammatory nodular reactions after hepatitis B vaccination due to aluminum sensitization. *Contact Dermatitis* 1990;23:65.
40. Rietschel RL, Adams RM. Reactions to thimerosal in hepatitis B vaccines. *Dermatol Clinics* 1990;8:161.
41. Aberer W. Vaccination despite thimerosal sensitivity. *Contact Dermatitis* 1991;24:6.
42. Osawa J, et al. A probable role for vaccines containing thimerosal in thimerosal hypersensitivity. *Contact Dermatitis* 1991;24:178.
43. Samitz MH, Schmunes E. Occupational dermatoses in dentists and allied personnel. *Cutis* 1969;5:180.
44. Calnan CD, Stevenson CJ. Studies in contact dermatitis (XV). Dental materials. *Trans St John Hosp Derm Soc* 1963;18:24.
45. Rustemeyer T, Frosch PJ. Occupational skin diseases in dental laboratory technicians (I). Clinical picture and causative factors. *Contact Dermatitis* 1996;34:125.
46. Fisher AA. Allergic sensitization of the skin and oral mucosa to acrylic denture materials. *JAMA* 1954;156:238.
47. Flyvholm MA, et al. Threshold for occluded formaldehyde patch test in formaldehyde-sensitive patients: relationship to repeated open application test with a product containing formaldehyde releaser. *Contact Dermatitis* 1997;36:26.
48. van Ketel WG. Reactions to dental impression materials. *Contact Dermatitis* 1977;3:55.
49. Cronin E. Impregum (dental impression material). *Contact Dermatitis Newsletter* 1973;13:362.
50. Nally FS, Storrs J. Hypersensitivity to dental impression material. *Br Dental J* 1973;134:244.
51. van Groeningen G, Nater J. Reaction to dental impression materials. *Contact Dermatitis* 1975;1:373.

52. Malten KE. Recently reported causes of contact dermatitis due to synthetic resins and hardeners. *Contact Dermatitis* 1979;5:11.
53. Hjorth N, Schonning L. Occupational dermatitis from tuberculin among veterinary surgeons. *Contact Dermatitis Newsletter* 1968;4:64.
54. Hjorth N, Weismann K. Occupational dermatitis among veterinary surgeons caused by spiramycin and Tylosin. *Contact Dermatitis Newsletter* 1972;12:320.
55. Hjorth N. Battery for testing veterinary surgeons. *Contact Dermatitis* 1975;1:122.
56. Hjorth N. Occupational dermatitis among veterinary surgeons caused by penethamate. *Berufsdermatosen* 1967;15:163.
57. Adams RM. Mercaptobenzothiazole in veterinary medications. *Contact Dermatitis Newsletter* 1974;16:514.
58. Prahl P, Roed-Petersen J. Type I allergy from cows in veterinary surgeons. *Contact Dermatitis* 1979;5:33.
59. Rudzki E, et al. Occupational dermatitis in veterinarians. *Contact Dermatitis* 1982;8:72.
60. Malten KE. Therapeutics for pets as neglected causes of contact dermatitis in housewives. *Contact Dermatitis* 1978;4:296.
61. Fisher AA. Allergic contact dermatitis in animal feed handlers. *Cutis* 1975;16:201.
62. Neldner KH. Contact dermatitis from animal feed additives. *Arch Dermatol* 1972;106:722.
63. Rodriguez A, Echechipia S, Alvarez M, Muro MD. Occupational contact dermatitis from vitamin B_{12}. *Contact Dermatitis* 1994;31:271.
64. Bleumink E, Nater JP. Allergic contact dermatitis to dinitolmide. *Arch Dermatol* 1973;108:423.
65. deGroot AC, Conemans JMH. Contact allergy to furazolidone. *Contact Dermatitis* 1990;22:202.
66. Vilaplana J, Grimalt F, Romaguera C. Contact dermatitis from furaltadone in animal feed. *Contact Dermatitis* 1991;22:232.
67. Melhom HC, Beetz D. Das Antioxydans Aethoxyquin als berufliches Ebenzatogen bil einer futtermitteldosierer. *Berufsdermatosen* 1971;19:84.
68. Burrows D. Contact dermatitis in animal feed mill workers. *Br J Dermatol* 1975;92:167.
69. Scott KW, Dawson TAJ. Photo contact dermatitis arising from the presence of quindoxin in animal feeding stuff. *Br J Dermatol* 1974;90:543.
70. Caplan RM. Contact dermatitis from animal feed additives. *Arch Dermatol* 1973;107:18.
71. Dawson TAJ, Scott KW. Contact eczema in agricultural workers. *Br Med J* 1972;1:469.
72. Lorenzetti OJ. Occupational dermatitis-prescription container caps. *Contact Dermatitis* 1975;1:53.
73. Cronin E. Picric acid dermatitis. *Contact Dermatitis* 1975;1:64.
74. Grimalt F, Romaguera C. Cutaneous sensitivity to benzidine. *Dermatosen* 1981;29:95.
75. Downs AMR, Sansom JE. Airborne occupational contact dermatitis from epoxy resin in an immersion oil used for microscopy. *Contact Dermatitis* 1998;39:267.
76. Le Coz C-J, et al. An epidemic of occupational contact dermatitis from an immersion oil for microscopy in laboratory personnel. *Contact Dermatitis* 1999;40:77.
77. Morris AD, Ratcliff J, Dalziel KL, English JS. Allergic contact dermatitis from epoxy propane. *Contact Dermatitis* 1998;38:57.
78. Estlander T, Jolanki R, Kanerva L. Hydroxylammonium chloride as sensitizer in a water laboratory. *Contact Dermatitis* 1997;36:161.
79. Dooms-Goossens A, Garmyn M, Degreef H. Contact allergy to acrylamide. *Contact Dermatitis* 1991;24:71.
80. Wasilewski C. Allergic contact dermatitis from isopropyl alcohols. *Arch Derm Venereol* (Stockh) 1968;98:502.
81. Fregert S, et al. Alcohol dermatitis. *Arch Dermatol* 1969;49:493.
82. Fregert S, et al. Hypersensitivity to secondary alcohols. *Acta Derm Venereol* (Stockh) 1971;51:271.
83. Hicks R. Ethanol, a possible allergen. *Ann Allergy* 1968;26:64.
84. Richardson D, et al. Allergic contact dermatitis to "alcohol" swabs. *Cutis* 1969;5:1115.
85. Fregert SK, et al. Dermatitis from alcohols. *J Allergy* 1963;34:404.
86. Martin-Scott I. Contact dermatitis from alcohol. *Br J Dermatol* 1960;72:372.
87. van Ketel WG, Tan-Lim KN. Contact dermatitis from ethanol. *Contact Dermatitis* 1975;1:7.
88. Sanderson KV, Cronin E. Glutaraldehyde and contact dermatitis. *Br Med J* 1968;3:820.
89. Skog E. Sensitivity to glutaraldehyde. *Contact Dermatitis Newsletter* 1968;4:79.
90. Harman RRM, O'Grady KJ. Contact dermatitis due to sensitivity to Cidex (activated glutaraldehyde). *Contact Dermatitis Newsletter* 1972;11:279.
91. Lyon TC. Allergic contact dermatitis due to Cidex. *Oral Surg* 1971;32:895.
92. Neering H, van Ketel WG. Glutaraldehyde and formaldehyde allergy. *Contact Dermatitis Newsletter* 1974;16:518.
93. Gordon HH. Glutaraldehyde contact dermatitis. *Contact Dermatitis Newsletter* 1974;15:442.
94. Zach RG. How prevalent is glutaraldehyde sensitivity? *Consultant* 1980;6:116.
95. Fisher AA. Reactions to glutaraldehyde with particular reference to radiologists and x-ray technicians. *Cutis* 1981;28:113.
96. Belani KC, Priedklans J. An epidemic of pseudo membranous laryngotracheitis. *Anesthesia* 1978;47:530.
97. Jordan WP, Dahl MV, Albert HL. Contact dermatitis from glutaraldehyde. *Arch Dermatol* 1972;105:94.
98. Maibach HI. Glutaraldehyde: cross-reaction to formaldehyde. *Contact Dermatitis* 1975;1:326.
99. Dabrowa N, Landau JW, Newcomer VD. Antifungal activity of glutaraldehyde in vitro. *Arch Dermatol* 1972;105:55.
100. Comaish S. Glutaraldehyde lowers skin friction and enhances skin resistance to acute friction injury. *Acta Derm Venereol* (Stockh) 1973;53:455.
101. Des Grosseilliers JP, Brisson P. Localized epidermolysis bullosa: report of two cases and evaluation of therapy with glutaraldehyde. *Arch Dermatol* 1974;109:70.
102. Gordon HH. Glutaraldehyde therapy for epidermolysis bullosa. *Arch Dermatol* 1974;110:297.
103. Weaver LE, Maibach HL. Dose response relationships in allergic contact dermatitis: glutaraldehyde-containing liquid fabric softener. *Contact Dermatitis* 1977;3:65.
104. Garcia RL. Delayed hypersensitivity reaction to glutaraldehyde and formaldehyde. *Bull Assoc Milit* 1972;21:11.

CHAPTER 27

Dermatitis Due to Cutting Oils, Solvents, Petrolatum, and Coal-Tar Products

METALWORKING FLUIDS

The various industrial oils and fluids are shown in Table 27.1. These metalworking fluids are used throughout industry to cool and lubricate metalworking operations, for example, machining and grinding.

When hard materials such as metal are cut, so much heat is generated that a metal-cutting tool can become welded to the metal being cut (workpiece). Metalworking fluids are therefore directed at the interface between cutting tool and workpiece. By reducing friction and conducting away heat, the fluid cools the cutting process (1). Table 27.2 lists the three main types of metalworking fluids (2).

Insoluble Fluids

Skin exposure to neat (insoluble) oils can cause oil acne or folliculitis and, when prolonged, hyperpigmentation, keratoses, and cancer of the scrotum and other exposed skin. Eczematous dermatitis, rather than folliculitis, occurs occasionally and is usually irritant in etiology. Allergens added to neat oils may cause allergic contact dermatitis.

Soluble Fluids

Oil-in-water emulsions used for metalworking are commonly called "soluble oils." They contain not only emulsifiers, such as petroleum sulfonates and carboxylic acid soaps, but also corrosion inhibitors, phase stabilizers, extreme pressure additives, antifoams, dyes, and microbiocides. Oil acne does not occur, and keratoses and epithelioma are rare.

Eczematous eruptions are common with exposure to soluble oils. Clinically, the early stages of soluble-oil dermatitis may be characterized by the appearance of a fine follicular erythema. This appears to be a follicular eczema rather than a pustular folliculitis as seen with neat oils. Later stages of soluble-oil dermatitis are characteristically patchy, papular, and eczematous, and sometimes resemble discoid eczema over the backs of the hands or forearms. Vesicular palmar and finger eczemas are found rarely in soluble-oil dermatitis and, if present, can be associated either with allergic sensitization or with an underlying endogenous eczema.

Aqueous (Synthetic) Fluids

These fluids also commonly produce eczematous eruptions. Thirty percent of machinists heavily exposed to these fluids may acquire a dermatitis (1).

Allergic versus Irritant Reactions to Cutting Fluids

Arndt (3) stated that allergic contact dermatitis due to such oils is rare and, when it is reported, has been related to corrosion inhibitors, bacteriostatic agents, breakdown products, and nickel salts or chromates from machined metals. Rudzki et al. (4) reported that 6 industrial oils, 2 basic oils, and 18 oil additives used frequently in Poland were tested on 125 patients with suspected oil dermatitis. Allergic skin reactions were not noted with any of these oils or additives. Gellin (5) stated that primary irritant dermatitis and not allergic contact dermatitis is presently the major skin disorder among machinists and other workers handling cutting fluids and that prolonged immersion in watery or oil solutions produces the irritant dermatitis. Samitz and Katz (6) and Samitz (7) also found that instances of allergic contact sensitivity in association with cutting oil preparations are uncommon and when reported are related to bactericides, rust inhibitors, nickel salts, and chromates.

Shah et al. (8) sent a questionnaire to 64 patients who had contact dermatitis from metalworking fluids. Fifty-one responded to the survey. There was no difference in the outcome between those who gave up their occupation and those who continued to work with the fluids, indicating a poor prognosis. Biocides were the most common allergen found in the group.

Hodgson (9) reported that 50% of cutting oil eczemas were allergic in nature. He found that the dilution of sensitizing chemicals in the final cutting oil lubricant often obscured identification of the specific allergen.

TABLE 27.1. *Industrial Oils and Fluids*

Cooling emulsions
Cutting compounds
Drilling fluids
Grinding fluids
Lubricating fluids
Metalworking fluids

In his material, the following contact allergens produced allergic contact dermatitis of the hands in those working with cutting oils: antimicrobials, chlorocresol, dichlorophene, formaldehyde, trisnitrol, triazine, antioxidants, azo dyes used as coloring agents, hydrazine, and deodorizers such as pine oil and balsam of Peru.

> **The insoluble fluids, the so-called neat oils, produce oil acne, keratoses, and carcinomas; the "soluble" and "synthetic" fluids produce eczematous eruptions, mostly of the primary irritant variety and occasionally of the allergic variety.**

A cutting oil used in automobile seat manufacturing produced contact dermatitis in 12 workers who were machine operators (10). The chlorinated paraffin fraction of the oil was responsible. Half of the workers were also sensitive to epoxy resin. Because pure chlorinated paraffin was negative, an additive related to epoxy was suspected to be the actual allergen. Epoxy-related additives that have been found in cutting oils include glycidyl ester of hexahydrophthalic acid and Epoxide 7.

TABLE 27.2. *Make-up of the Various Types of Metalworking Fluids*

Insoluble fluids (neat oils)
    Additives
    Mineral, animal, or vegetable oils
    Sulfur, chloride, and phosphorus
Soluble oils (oil in water)
    Amine coupler
    Emulsifiers (sulfate, rosin)
    Germicides
    Oils
    Surfactants (carboxylic soaps)
    Water
Synthetic fluids (aqueous solutions)
    Amines
    Anti-foaming agents (silicone)
    Bacteriocides
    Deodorizers
    Dyes
    Fatty acids
    Soaps
    Water softeners

Patch Testing with Cutting Fluids

The three types of cutting fluids may be tested, as is, undiluted, although they may show irritant reactions to such testing. Dilution, to avoid irritancy, may give false-negative reactions to allergens in the fluid. Patch tests with the "routine" patch test series may occasionally detect the sensitizer in a cutting fluid (2).

Ethylenediamine Hydrochloride versus Amines in Cutting Oils

Angelini and Meneghini (11) reported that two engineers with dermatitis due to synthetic coolants had positive reactions to ethylenediamine and thought that this implied a cross-sensitization reaction with amines in the fluids.

Camarasa and Alomar (12) reported three cases of hand dermatitis eczema in metallurgical workers. All three workers, who improved greatly when away from work, had positive patch test results with the cutting fluids used in their work, as well as with ethylenediamine from the "standard" series.

Allergic reactions to ethylenediamine may signify cross-reactions with the other polyamines found in cutting oils—ethylenediamine (EDA), diethylenetriamine (DETA), triethylenetetramine (TETA), dipropylenetriamine (DPTA), tetraethylenepentamine (TEPA), diethylaminopropylamine (DEAPA), and trimethylhexamethylenediamine (TMDA). In a personal communication, Fregert (13) stated that he had seen cross-reactions between ethylenediamine, diethylenetriamine, and triethylenetetramine but was not certain if these are true cross-sensitizations, because the compounds may contain traces of the other two.

Triethanolamine

Certain synthetic cutting oils contain varying amounts of mineral oil with the fatty amine triethanolamine used as an emulsifying agent. Triethanolamine is also used widely in cosmetics. Suurmond (14) showed cross-reactions between triethanolamine and other tertiary amines, such as promethazine.

> **Patch tests may be performed with undiluted cutting fluids; the synthetic aqueous solutions are most likely to give a soaplike irritant reaction.**

Monoethanolamine

Soluble cutting oils (water soluble) can cause irritant contact dermatitis, and biocides added to such products can cause allergic contact dermatitis. Monoethanolamine (2-aminoethanol) is present in some soluble oils and is a rare cause of allergic contact dermatitis. A 2% in petrolatum concentration is adequate for patch testing, as it was negative in 50 controls and positive in a patient reported by Bhushan et al. (15).

Alkanolamineborates

Alkanolamineborates are used as metalworking fluids and can cause both irritant and allergic contact dermatitis (16). They are water-based fluids, and, because of their alkalinity, it is necessary to dilute them with an acidic buffer. The use concentration of these chemicals is in the range of 10% to 30%, and their primary function is corrosion inhibition.

Oleyl Alcohol

Contact allergy to cutting fluids can come from sources such as monoethanolamine and less commonly from oleyl alcohol (17). Oleyl alcohol is added to cutting fluids to improve the solubility of other components of the final formula. This rare allergen can also be seen as a contaminant in cetyl and stearyl alcohol.

Formaldehyde

Angelini and Meneghini (11) reported two cases of dermatitis in patients who were allergic to formaldehyde due to coolants. Formaldehyde had been added to used synthetic fluid after recovery as an antibacterial agent.

Grotan BK

Grotan BK is a "triazine" industrial bacteriocide, added worldwide to water miscible, metalworking fluids of the oil-in-water emulsion ("soluble oil") and synthetic types. Water miscible fluids provide cooling and lubrication for metalworking processes such as cutting and grinding. Bacterial growth in these fluids, which occurs particularly at oil-water interfaces, can cause problems of foul odor, metal corrosion, and emulsion breakdown. The active ingredient of Grotan BK is a hexahydro-1,3,5-tris(2-hydroxyethyl)-s-triazine. The recommended concentration of Grotan BK in a metalworking fluid is 0.15%. The triazine molecule liberates formaldehyde under certain conditions but, according to the manufacturers, this does not explain the antibacterial effect of Grotan BK. There is some controversy as to whether Grotan BK is a strong or weak sensitizer (18–21).

Patch tests may be performed with a 1% aqueous solution. Sensitivity to triazine bacteriocide may become more widespread because it is now being used in shampoos and cosmetics.

Phenolic Compounds

These antimicrobial agents, which include cresols, phenols, hexachlorophenes and dichlorophenes, bisphenols, and chlorinated phenols, are added to cutting oils to prevent bacterial growths that may break the emulsions in producing an offensive odor. It should be noted that the bisphenols are photosensitizers, and chlorinated phenols may produce leukoderma.

Mercaptobenzothiazole is present in cutting fluids as an anticorrosion, antibacterial, and antifungal agent.

Mercaptobenzothiazole (MBT)

Fregert and Skog (22) reported that allergic contact dermatitis in seven patients had an obvious connection with exposure to cutting oil containing MBT. The patients showed positive test reactions to MBT, which is used to prevent corrosion, especially of copper and tin, by lowering the pH of cutting oil. Mercaptobenzothiazole is present in the biocide Vancide TH as an antibacterial and antifungal agent.

Patch testing with routine screening patch test series is valuable in detecting allergens in the cutting fluids such as MBT, ethylenediamine, formaldehyde, and lanolin.

Six of Fregert's seven patients sensitive to MBT showed negative reactions to the cutting oil itself. Without testing the ingredients separately, their dermatitis would have been considered due to the primary irritant effect.

Sodium Pyrithione (Sodium Omadine)

Sodium pyrithione may be used in semisynthetic and synthetic oils, and contact dermatitis from exposure to this product has been reported (23). This material may also be encountered in water-based printers' ink and common antidandruff shampoos. A 0.3% aqueous solution has been recommended for patch testing.

Hydrazine

In the metal industry, there is wide exposure to hydrazine as a cleaning agent to prevent oxidation and corrosion of metallic surfaces. Hovding (24) reported that hydrazine shows cross-sensitization with Apresoline, isonicotinic acid hydrazide, phenylhydrazine, and Nardel. Two patients in the series reported by Rudzki et al. (4) were allergic to hydrazine.

Lanolin

The lanolin present in wool grease is used as an antirust compound in some cutting oil fluids and may cause allergic dermatitis in lanolin-sensitive persons.

Deodorant Agent

Pine oil, perfumes, and balsam of Peru may be added to industrial oils to reduce offensive odors. Hodgson (9) studied 50 patients with hand dermatitis from exposure to metalworking fluids. The most common positive reactions to pine oil, perfumes, and balsam of Peru were caused by pine oil, which produced four instances of allergic hand dermatitis.

Metals

Samitz and Katz (6) and Samitz (7) found that under ordinary working conditions in which grinding fluids were used, spot testing did not reveal the presence of nickel or chromates. Laboratory studies, however, showed that nickel can be leached from the machined metals. Dimethylglyoxime (DMG) was used to test for the presence of nickel, and diphenyl carbazide (DPC) for chromates. Machinery, wipe rags, work benches, and lathe scrap yielded repeated negative results when tested directly. Ashed sam-

TABLE 27.3. *Nonallergic Dermatoses from Cutting Oils*

Folliculitis
Hyperpigmentation
Irritant contact dermatitis
Keratosis
Leukoderma
Mechanical injury from metal fragments
Oil acne
Phototoxic dermatitis
Postinflammatory pigmentary changes
Scrotal cancer

TABLE 27.4. *Potential Oil and Cooling Fluid Additives[a]*

Ingredient	Patch test concentration (%)
Abietic acid	10
4-chloro-3-cresol (PCMC)	1
4-chloro-3-xylenol (PCMX)	0.5
Dichlorophene	0.5
2-phenylphenol (Dowicide 1)	1
Propylene glycol	5
Triethanolamine	2
4-*tert*-butylbenzoic acid	1
1,2-benzisothiazolin-3-one	0.05
Hexahydro-1,3,5-tris(2-hydroxyethyl)triazine (Grotan BK)	1
Bioban P 1487—consists of 70% 4-(2-nitrobutyl)moropholine and 20% 4,4-2-ethyl-2-nitro-trimethylene)dimorpholine in the commercial product	1
Chloroacetamide (Hibitane)	0.2
N-methylol chloroacetamide (Grotan HD)	0.1
1H-benzotriazol	1
Ethylenediamine dihydrochloride	1
Mercaptobenzothiazole	1
Zinc ethylenebis (dithiocarbamate)	1
Triclosan (Irgasan DP 300)	2
1-aza-3,7-dioxa-5-ethylbicyclo(3,3,0)octane (Bioban CS-1246)	1
4,4-dimethyloxazolidine 3,4,4-trimethyloxazoline (Bioban CS-1135)	1
2-hydroxymethyl-2-nitro-1,3-propandiol (Tris nitro)	1
Thiomersal	0.1
Hydrazine sulfate	1
Trichlorocarbanilide	1
Formaldehyde	1
Amerchol L 101	100
Dipentene	1
Sodium omadine	0.1
2-bromo-2-nitropropane (Bronopol)	0.25
Coconut diethanolamide	0.5
5-chloro-2-methyl-4-isothiazolon-3-one (Kathon CG)	0.02
1,2-dibromo-2,4-dysianobutane (Tektamer 38)	0.1

[a]From Nethercott JR, Holness DL. Contact dermatitis associated with exposure to oils and coolants. In: Menné T, Maibach HI, eds. *Exogenous dermatosis: environmental dermatitis.* Boca Raton, FL: CRC Press, 1991, p. 367. Used with permission.

ples of new and used cutting oil and of oil-wipe rags were similarly tested. The presence of neither nickel nor chromium was demonstrated.

Because the problem of nickel and chromate contamination and associated skin contact is potentially serious, Samitz and Katz (6) studied its application to workers using cutting oils. Surveys conducted in two plants revealed no instances of nickel or chromate dermatitis due to cutting oils. The nickel concentrations, however, discovered in their laboratory studies exceeded the sensitizing safety limit concentration of these metals. Correlation of these studies with actual exposure conditions to determine if contact dermatitis can result has not been done as yet.

Because Samitz and Katz (6) could not detect any nickel with the dimethylglyoxime spot test, it is unlikely that enough nickel is "leached" out by the grinding process to be clinically significant. Einarrson et al. (25) found increased cobalt content in used cutting fluids, but he was not certain of this discovery's clinical significance. Table 27.3 lists the nonallergenic dermatoses from cutting oils.

Interpretation of Patch Test Results

Testing with original versus "used" industrial oils diluted 1 to 25 in aqueous solution, a positive patch test reaction to the used "dirty" oil and not to the original oil would imply that additives such as corrosion inhibitors, bacteriostatic agents, or break-down products including nickel salts or chromates are the sensitizers. Because a positive patch test reaction to either the original or the used oils may be primarily irritant in nature, the tests should be repeated on three normal controls. Table 27.4 lists potential oil and cooling fluid additives (26).

Role of Bacteria in Cutting Fluids

Bactericides are added to protect against rancidity and preserve the cutting fluid emulsions. According to Rycroft, bacteria that grow plentifully in soluble oils are not usually directly pathogenic to humans (1). They may have a role in making a soluble oil more irritant, although this has not been proved.

Geretzki (27) reported that a list has been compiled showing pathogenic agents that can be isolated from oils (24). Under certain conditions, cutting oil may prove to be a pool of pathogenic agents.

It should be noted that the antimicrobial agents and biocides listed in Table 27.5 are used to prevent rancidity of the cutting fluids rather than to protect the worker.

OCCUPATIONAL ACNE

Occupational acne consists of two main varieties: one caused by petroleum and its derivatives and coal-tar products and the other, chloracne, due to halogenated aromatic hydrocarbons (Tables 27.6 and 27.7). Table 27.8 lists certain environmental factors that may influence the severity

TABLE 27.5. *Antibacterial Agents (Biocides) Registered for Use in Metalworking Fluids[a]*

Bioban P-1487 (IMC Chemical Group Inc.)	0.1% pet
Busan 85 (Buckman Laboratories Inc.)	1% pet
Captax, dermacid, mertax, and thiotax	1% pet
Chloroxylenol (Ottasept)	1% pet
Dowicid 1	1% pet
Dowicid A (Dow Chemical Co.)	1% pet
Dowicid 1 (Dow Chemical Co.)	1% pet
Dowicil 75 (Dow Chemical Co.)	2% pet
Formalin	2% aq
G-4	2% pet
G-11	0.5% pet
Givgard DXN (Givaudan Corp.)	1% pet
Grotan BK (Lehn & Fink Industrial)	1% pet
Grotan HD2 (Lehn & Fink Industrial)	1% pet
Kathon 886-MW (Rohm and Haas Co.)	0.025% pet
Merthiolate	0.1% pet
Onyxide 200 (Olin Corp.)	1% pet
Ottafact	0.01% pet
p-tertiary butyl phenol	2% pet
Preventol D-2 and D-3	2% pet
Proxel CRL (ICI United States Inc.)	0.1% pet
Resorcinol phthalen	1% alcohol
Rosin	20% pet
Sodium-Omadine (Olin Corp.)	0.1% pet
Triadine-10 (Olin Corp.)	1% pet
Tris-Nitro (IMC Chemical Group Inc.)	1% pet
Vancide 51 (RT Vanderbilt Co. Inc.)	1% pet
Vancide TH (RT Vanderbilt Co. Inc.)	1% pet
XD-8254 DBNPA (Dow Chemical Co.)	1% pet
Zinc Omadine (Olin Corp.)	0.1% pet

[a]Aq, aqueous; Pet, in petrolatum.

of occupational acne (28,29). Table 27.9 lists the differential diagnosis of chloracne.

Oil Acne

Oil acne or oil folliculitis consists of numerous comedones, follicular papules, and pustules in areas of heavy oil exposure, such as the extensor surfaces of the arms and thighs and under oil-soaked clothing. Pustules and furuncles may also appear.

> **Relatively mild occupational acne may be caused by crude and cutting oils, coal-tar oils, pitch, and creosote; halogenated aromatic chemicals can produce chloracne, which is a severe acneiform eruption sometimes accompanied by serious toxic effects.**

TABLE 27.6. *Oil and Tar Acne*

Coal-tar products	Petroleum and its derivatives
Coal-tar oils	Crude oil and fractions
Creosote	Cutting oils
Pitch	

TABLE 27.7. *Halogenated Aromatic Compounds (Chloracnegens)*

Contaminants of polychlorophenol compounds, especially herbicides (2,4,5-T and pentachlorophenol) and herbicide intermediates (trichlorophenol)
    2,3,7,8-tetrachlorodibenzo-*p*-dioxin (TCDD)
    Hexachlorodibenzo-*p*-dioxin
    Tetrachlorodibenzofuran
Contaminants of 3,4-dichloroaniline and related herbicides (Propanil and Methazole)
    3,4,3′,4′-tetrachloroazoxybenzene (TCAOB)
    3,4,3′,4′-tetrachloroazobenzene (TCAB)
Polyhalogenated biphenyls[a]
    Polybromobiphenyls (PBBs)
    Polychlorobiphenyls (PCBs)
Polyhalogenated dibenzofurans[a]
    Polybromodibenzofurans, especially tetrabromodibenzofuran
    Polychlorodibenzofurans, especially tri-, tetra-(TCDF), penta-, and hexachlorodibenzofuran
Polyhalogenated naphthalenes[a]
    Polybromonaphthalenes[b,c]
    Polychloronaphthalenes
Other
    1,2,3,4-tetrachlorobenzene (experimental)
    Dichlobenil (Casoron)—herbicide (clinical only)
    DDT (Crude trichlorobenzene)[c]

[a]The polychlorodibenzofurans and hexachloronaphthalenes may occur as contaminants in some PCBs.
[b]The polybromonaphthalenes may occur as contaminants in some PBBs.
[c]Not confirmed as chloracnegens.

With improved engineering and less heavy contact with oils, oil acne is not as prevalent as in the past. The people who are most often affected are machinists using insoluble cutting oils; workers in coal-tar plants who handle heavy coal-tar distillates and coal-tar pitch; auto, truck, and aircraft mechanics; roofers, oil-well drillers; coke-oven workers; petroleum refiners; rubber workers; textile mill workers; and road-maintenance workers. Melanosis and photosensitivity also may occur in these individuals.

Certain halogenated chemicals are potent acnegens that can produce chloracne (30–32). Most cases result from chloronaphthalenes and diphenyl contamination (PCBs), herbicides, herbicide intermediates, flame retardants,

TABLE 27.8. *Miscellaneous and Contributing Causes to Occupational Acne*

Bromides and iodides
Friction
Gram-negative folliculitis in swimming pools
Greasy cosmetics
Harsh detergents
Heat

and isomers of chlorodibenzodioxins and chlorodibenzofurans, which are the fly ashes and flue gases of industrial incinerators.

The polychloronaphthalenes, which were used primarily in insulating waxes, dielectrics, and wood preservatives, have now been replaced. The PCBs are now restricted to closed-system applications to avoid environmental contamination.

The contaminant 2,3,7,8-tetrachlorodibenzo-*p*-dioxin (TCDD) is a potent acnegen formed during the synthesis of trichlorophenol, an intermediate in the synthesis of the herbicide 2,4,5-T and also hexachlorophene.

Poisoning with TCDD may be acute, with nausea, vomiting, headache, and mucosal and skin irritation. The initial cutaneous reaction is comparable to a chemical burn, usually from a combination of trichlorophenol, TCDD, and sodium hydroxide, and is not chloracne. Chloracne is often the first and most constant finding of the *chronic* stage of TCDD poisoning. Systemic disorders may appear and include porphyria cutanea tarda, hyperpigmentation, and hypertrichosis without porphyria.

Bleiberg et al. (30) reported that 29 patients, who worked in a chemical factory engaged in the manufacture of 2,4-dichlorophenol (2,4-D) and 2,4,5-trichlorophenol (2,3,5-T), and who exhibited features of chloracne, were studied for the presence of porphyria cutanea tarda. In 11 cases, urinary uroporphyrins were elevated (30).

Chloracne may be accompanied by porphyria cutanea tarda.

TABLE 27.9. *Differential Diagnosis of Chloracne*

	Age	Sites	Clinical appearance
Acne vulgaris	Greatest involvement between ages 13 and 26	Face, neck, chest, and back to waist	Comedones, papules, pustules, cysts, and scars
Folliculitis	Any age	Any area, especially arms, dorsa of hands, thighs, and under oil-soaked clothing	Black comedones, papules, pustules, and melanosis
Chloracne	Any age	Face, especially neck, ear lobes, shoulders, abdomen, genitalia, and legs	Straw-colored cysts, numerous comedones and milia, papules, and often pruritus

At least two chlorobenzene compounds have been identified as chloracnegens (31). They are formed either as trace contaminants during the synthesis or further conversion to herbicides of 3,4-dichloroaniline, the starting material for the synthesis of several commercially important herbicides.

Taylor (32,33) reported several outbreaks of chloracne (mostly unreported in the medical literature) that occurred among workers exposed to azo and azoxybenzenes. In one small chemical plant, chloracne developed in more than 90% of the workers.

Features of Chloracne

1. Straw-colored cysts are characteristic. Comedones are often present involving every follicular orifice in affected areas. Pruritic inflammatory pustules and abscesses also occur, as in acne vulgaris. Although exposed body areas typically are involved, there may be lesions in covered areas. Edema of the eyelids and conjunctivitis may occur. A brownish discoloration of the nails may be present.

2. Chloracne lesions may continue to appear after all exposure to the inciting chemical has ceased.

3. Hyperpigmentation may follow exposure to TCDD or PCBs. Acute burns with marked facial edema and erythema with subsequent development of hyperkeratosis and chloracne may develop after explosions occurring during trichlorophenol production. "Cable rash" resembling photosensitivity preceded chloracne from exposures to cables insulated with various mixtures of chlorinated naphthalenes and biphenyls.

4. Although chloracne occurs typically from external cutaneous contact, ingestion or inhalation may be important.

5. Hirsutism, hyperpigmentation, and increased skin fragility are also common, suggesting systemic involvement with porphyria cutanea tarda, especially when the exposure is to TCDD.

6. Direct skin contact is probably the most common way chloracne develops, but inhalation and ingestion also may be responsible.

7. The wives and children of workers may also develop chloracne from contact with contaminated clothing and tools.

8. Dibenzodioxins are potent teratogens that depress cell-moderated immunity and that have several long-range, dose-related toxicologic effects in laboratory animals, including tumor induction. PCBs, PBBs, and TCDD can also modify tumor initiation in laboratory-animal oral and skin assays.

9. The low acnegenic threshold of these chemicals is illustrated by several reports of the families of plant workers in whom chloracne developed, even though they had never been in or near the factory; exposure occurred when work clothes or tools were brought home.

10. In mild, isolated cases, differentiation from acne vulgaris may be difficult or impossible.

TABLE 27.10. *Possible Systemic Complications of Chloracne*

Hepatotoxicity
Peripheral neuritis
Porphyria cutanea tarda
Possible carcinogenicity
Possible immune suppression

11. Prevention and control of chloracne require a totally enclosed manufacturing process with no opportunities for direct skin contact, ingestion, or inhalation of the chemical. The only other alternative is alteration of the chemical synthetic process to eliminate exposure to the contaminant chloracnegens.

12. Possible systemic complications of chloracne are listed in Table 27.10.

Therapy of Chloracne

Oil folliculitis is best treated by avoiding contact with oils and grease, by wearing oil-impervious aprons, or by environmental control. The wearing of gloves is usually hazardous in machinists and should be avoided. Work clothing should be changed frequently. Local acne medications (benzoyl peroxide gels or retinoic acid, tretinoin creams or gels) and oral antibiotics (tetracycline or erythromycin) are frequently helpful, along with other acne therapy.

In severe cases, chloracne is refractory to therapy with the usual methods used to treat acne vulgaris. Oral tetracylines, acne surgery (manual expression of comedones and cysts with a comedone extractor), and topical retinoic acid preparations are beneficial. Dermabrasion may be helpful later for severe scarring. Excellent results in various keratinizing disorders and in acne vulgaris (severe conglobate acne) have been achieved with the oral, synthetic retinoid, 13-*cis*-retinoic acid (isotretinoin or Accutane). A trial of this drug is warranted in severe cases of chloracne.

SOLVENT DERMATITIS

Solvents are responsible for an estimated 6% to 20% of cases of occupational dermatitis (34).

The organic solvents are indispensable in modern manufacturing processes. They are used to dissolve and thin lacquers, varnishes, and paints and to act as solvents for rubber and natural and synthetic resins. They are also used in the dry-cleaning industry and in the manufacture of organic dyes, artificial silk, glues, and cements. They act as extractives for fats, waxes, oils, and perfumes.

The physical properties of solvents influence the injurious effects they have on the skin. In general, the more poorly absorbed solvents cause more skin damage and the fewest systemic symptoms. The saturated hydrocarbon solvents and the paraffin series of solvents are stronger skin irritants than those derived from the aromatic series. The irritant effect decreases as the boiling point increases. The concentration, duration of exposure, and degree of occlusion of the area are also relevant. More irritation may be caused by washing with soaps and detergents and immersion in water.

All solvents can cause dermatitis by dissolving the natural protective barrier of oil on the skin. Some solvents are noticeably irritating on contact, but others cause no particular pain even while they are penetrating or defatting the skin.

A chronic fissured eczema results when the skin comes in frequent contact with solvents, as in washing grease from the hands or when cloths moistened with solvents are used for cleansing or degreasing. Solvents dissolve and remove the surface lipids, the lipid material in the stratum corneum, and the fatty fraction of cell membranes. The percutaneous absorption of water and other substances is increased through this defatting action. Solvents may also damage the stratum corneum cells themselves.

The most frequent cause of occupational dermatitis by solvents is the practice of washing with a solvent. Workers whose occupation requires them to wash with a solvent include painters, who use paint thinners and turpentine; plastic workers, who use acetone; printers, who use typewash; auto mechanics, who use gasoline and kerosene; and dry cleaners, who use trichloroethylene, perchloroethylene, and Stoddard solvent.

Employees usually clean their hands with available solvents. The workers use a variety of solvents, for example, petroleum, coal-tar derivatives, chlorinated hydrocarbons, alcohols, ketones, and turpentine, to remove materials such as ink, tar, glue, gum, cement and other mucilaginous and viscous substances, grease, oil, stain, lacquer, and varnish.

The active ingredients in paint strippers are solvents. Almost all paint strippers contain methylene chloride. Other solvents found in strippers include toluol (toluene), methanol, ethanol, acetone, and mineral spirits. Solvents may also damage the peripheral nervous system. The symptoms caused by this nerve damage are numbness, tingling sensations, weakness, and paralysis in the arms and legs. Solvents may also produce a lymphangitis when they enter into a fissure or laceration and pass through the dermis and into the lymphatics.

> **Solvents produce not only dry fissured dermatitis but also chemical lymphangitis and peripheral neuropathy.**

The prevention of solvent dermatitis involves educating workers in the importance of wearing protective clothing while using solvents as cleaning agents, or, preferably, not using solvents at all. Skin contact should be avoided while moving metal parts into and out of degreasing solutions. Clothing on which solvent has been spilled should be removed as soon as possible. Solvent-proof rubber gloves under solvent-proof sleeves closed at the wrist should be worn. If protective clothing cannot be worn, solvent-resistant barrier creams may be applied.

Gloves should be worn when using paint removers. Ordinary dishwashing gloves or surgical gloves will dissolve in paint remover. Neoprene-natural latex blend gloves such as those sold by Playtex International Corp. will withstand paint remover for a reasonable time. When steel wool is used with the paint remover, cotton gloves should be placed over the neoprene-latex gloves to protect the gloves from abrasion so that they will last longer.

Gloves made of Viton (Du Pont) rubber polymers protect against most solvents. Such gloves may be obtained through Godfrey Safety Equip. Co. Inc., 140 Greenwood Avenue, Midland Park, NJ 07432.

Alcohol Solvents

The following alcohol solvents may be tested "as is" undiluted:

1. Ethanol (denatured, ethyl or grain alcohol, spirit of wine, cologne spirit, ethyl hydroxide, and ethyl hydrate)
2. Methanol (wood or methyl alcohol, carbinol, and wood spirit)
3. N-propyl alcohol
4. Isopropyl alcohol (rubbing alcohol, 2 methyl-1-propanol, isopropylcarbinol, and 1-hydroxymethyl-propane)
5. Isobutyl alcohol
6. Isoamyl alcohol (fusel oil)

Kurwa (35) pointed out that contact sensitization to primary alcohols such as ethanol and methanol usually occurs from occupational exposure, as in nurses, doctors, and laboratory technicians, and occasionally from cosmetic use. Some cases have been recorded in which ingestion of alcohol has produced a reaction in the mouth; in others, asthma, angioedema, and urticaria were aggravated by drinking alcoholic beverages.

Isopropyl alcohol is used extensively in general and hospital practice in the form of prepacked swabs for cleansing the skin before injections are given.

Fregert et al. (36) demonstrated that patients with hypersensitivity to primary alcohols (in which the carbon atom attached to the hydroxyl group is also attached to two hydrogen atoms) are also hypersensitive to secondary alcohols (the hydroxyl group that is attached to a carbon atom linked to two other carbon atoms).

Allergic contact dermatitis to alcohols can be of the delayed, eczematous variety and the urticarial type (37–41). (See also the section on alcohol dermatitis in Chapter 26.)

> **Alcohol may produce both a delayed, eczematous contact dermatitis and an immediate contact urticaria.**

Berlin et al. (42) reported a woman who experienced eye and respiratory irritation with erythema of the face and swollen eyelids when in buildings that had been recently painted with water-based paints. She was patch test positive to Euxyl K 400 0.1% in petrolatum and to the solvent 2-(2-butoxyethoxy)ethanol (BEE). The BEE, also known as diethyleneglycol mono-*n*-butyl ether, was blamed for the symptoms. The authors noted one other case of allergy to the similar compound butoxyethoxyethyl acetate.

In patch testing with volatile organic solvents, Vail (43) showed that the highly volatile antigen-containing compounds, applied as is in an open patch test, evaporate so rapidly that they do not penetrate the stratum corneum in sufficient concentration to evoke a reaction. It is, therefore, advisable to use a modified open patch test, that is, covering the test area several minutes after application of the solvent in order to allow the solvent to penetrate the stratum corneum. Such evaporation, however, does not take place when the organic solvents are tested in olive oil; the usual patch test procedure may be used.

Aliphatic Hydrocarbons

Aliphatic hydrocarbons may be tested 50% in olive oil. These compounds refer to any organic compound that has an open chain of carbon atoms, whether normal or forked, saturated or unsaturated. Besides their use as solvents, these chemicals are also used as follows:

Pentane—Use: in thermometers, as an anesthetic
N-hexane—Use: determining refractive index of materials: filling for thermometers instead of mercury, usually with a blue or red dye
Benzine (petroleum naphtha, ligroin, petroleum ether, and petroleum benzine)
Petroleum naphtha (see Benzine)
Gasoline (petrol, motor spirits, and benzine)—Use: fuel, in paint mixing and rubber cements
Diesel—May contain enough water to support the growth of microorganisms; therefore, biocides may be added to diesel. Kathon FP is one such biocide, which has caused contact dermatitis. Positive patch tests were found to methylchloroisothiazolinone and 2-methyl-4-isothiazolin-3-one (44). This is the same combination found in Kathon CG.

　Dyes added to diesel have been thought by the public to possibly be responsible for rashes, but patch tests have not confirmed this. Rather, the more environmentally friendly diesel fuels that contain low concentrations of aromatic compounds and a lower sulfur content than traditional high viscosity, high aromatic and sulfur content oils are more irritating than the older product (45).
VMP naphtha—Use: varnishes and paint thinner
Mineral spirits (petroleum spirits and ligroin)
Stoddard solvent (white spirits)

Kerosene (kerosine, coal oil, and range oil) (paraffin—British term)—Use: kerosene lamps, flares, and stoves; as a degreaser and cleaner; and in insecticides

In the southern part of the United States, kerosene is used extensively for curing tobacco, heating, cooking, and in more remote rural areas for lighting. Fregert (46) reported a case of mercury dermatitis due to kerosene contaminated with mercury. Barnes and Wilkinson (47) described an eruption similar to that of toxic epidermal necrolysis without systemic symptoms in a boy whose clothing became contaminated with kerosene.

Aromatic Hydrocarbons

The chemicals included under the heading of aromatic hydrocarbons are a small segment in the broad category of organic solvents. They are classified as aromatics because of the presence of the benzene ring in their chemical structure.

Benzene (benzol, cyclohextriene, phenyl hydride, coal naphtha, phene, and benzole)—Test 5% olive oil. Use: manufacture of medicinal chemicals, dyes and many other organic compounds, artificial leather, linoleum, oil cloth, airplane dopes, varnishes, and lacquers; as solvent for waxes, resins, and oils

　Skin contact with liquid benzene may cause erythema and blistering, with prolonged or repeated contacts responsible for the development of a dry, scaly dermatitis. Any evaluation of exposure must also consider the absorption through the skin following contact with liquid benzene (48).
Coal-tar naphtha (naphthalene)—Test "as is." Use: dyes and moth repellent
Nitrobenzene 1 (nitrobenzol, oil of mirbane, and oil of bitter almonds)—Test 25% olive oil

　Tetrahydronaphthalene (tetralin) should be tested at 2.5% in olive oil, as higher concentrations were reported to cause irritant reactions (49).

　Aniline is obtained from the reduction of nitrobenzene, and the two chemicals are often used in the same industrial process. This compound is used in shoe dyes and as an artificial flavor in foods, soaps, and perfumes because its odor is like that of oil of bitter almonds. It is a volatile, yellowish fluid also used for refining lubricating oils and the manufacture of pyroxylin compounds.
Toluene (toluol, methylbenzene, phenylmethane, and methylbenzol)—Test 50% olive oil. Use: manufacture benzoic acid, benzaldehyde, perfumes, explosives, dyes, and many other organic compounds; also as a solvent in the extraction of various principles from plants
Styrene (cinnamene, cinnemenol, cinnamal, phenethylene, phenylethylene, styrol, styrene monomer, styrolene, and vinyl benzene)—Test 1% olive oil. Use: manufacture of synthetic rubber, modifier of alkyd acrylic and polyester resins, extractive of storax balsam, preparation of compound tincture of benzoin, and fixative for soap in the cosmetic industry

Styrene liquid is sometimes used in acrylic resin powder to form a denture. Polystyrenes may be used for denture material. Styrene not only is a synthetic industrial compound but can also occur in nature, for example, in raspberries.

Sjoberg et al. (50) described contact allergy to styrene with cross-reaction to vinyltoluene.

Xylene (xylol and dimethylbenzene)—Test 50% olive oil. Use: raw material for production of benzoic acid, phthalic anhydride, isophthalic and terephthalic acids, as well as their dimethyl esters used in the manufacture of polyester fibers; manufacturing dyes and other organics: sterilizing catgut; with Canada balsam as oil immersion in microscopy; cleaning agent in microscope technique

Altman (51) described allergic contact urticaria due to xylene. Testing with 1% and 100% xylene revealed an immediate, acute, urticarial patch (25 mm) to the 100% xylene and, in 15 minutes, a similar but smaller, urticarial patch (15 mm) to the 1% xylene. All other patches were negative. Three controls were negative to the 1% and 100% xylene.

Chlorinated Hydrocarbons

Carbon tetrachloride (tetrachloromethane and perchloromethane)—Test 10% olive oil. Use: as fire extinguisher; for cleaning clothing; for rendering benzin nonflammable; as azeotropic drying agent for wet spark plugs in automobiles; as solvent for oils, fats, lacquers, varnishes, rubber waxes, and resins; for extracting oils from flowers and seeds; for exterminating destructive insects; as solvent; for starting material in manufacture of many organic compounds

Chloroform Test 40% olive oil. Use: as solvent for fats, oils, rubber, alkaloids, waxes, gutta-percha, resins; as cleansing agent; in fire extinguishers to lower the freezing temperature of carbon tetrachloride; in the rubber industry

Ethylene dichloride (1,2-dichloroethane, symdichloroethane, ethylene chloride, glycol dichloride, and β-dichloroethane)—Test 50% olive oil. Use: solvent for fats, oils, waxes, gums, resins, and particularly for rubber: irritation of respiratory tract and conjunctiva, corneal clouding, equilibrium disturbances, narcosis, and abdominal cramps

Methylene chloride (dichloromethane, methylene dichloride, and methylene bichloride)—Test 1% acetone. Use: solvent for cellulose acetate: degreasing and cleaning fluids, and as a paint stripper

Methyl chloroform (1,1,1-trichloroethane)—Test 1% olive oil. Use: in cold-type cleaning; also in cleaning plastic molds. Caution: irritating to eyes, mucous membranes, and, in high concentrations, narcotic

Occupational allergic contact dermatitis to methyl chloroform was detected with concentrations down to

0.01% in olive oil (52). In the United States, 3 million workers per year are exposed to this solvent (52).

Trichloroethylene (trichloroethene, trilene, trethylene, and tri-clene)—Test 50% olive oil. Use: widely used as a dry-cleaning agent in compounds such as Du Pont Dry Cleaner, Glamorene Rug Cleaner, Tri-Clene Dry Cleaner, Tread Metal Cleaner, and Triad Metal Polish

Trichloroethylene is also used to degrease metal, as a solvent for oils, resins, sulfur, and phosphorus, and medicinally as a wound cleanser and for relief of angina pectoris. It may sensitize the patient to alcohol. A combination of alcohol ingestion and trichloroethylene exposure may produce an "aldehyde syndrome," with flushing of the skin, nausea, and vomiting. Alcohol-induced flushing has also been reported by skin absorption of dimethylformamide (53). This organic solvent caused such flushing in 19 of 102 workers up to 4 days after exposure and also caused contact dermatitis (53).

An irritant reaction may occur from contaminated clothing, also an exfoliative dermatitis or scarlatiniform eruption may result from contact with trichloroethylene (54,55).

Epstein (56) reported that epichlorhydrin used as a stabilizer in trichloroethylene can cause an allergic contact dermatitis in metalplate workers. Patients were tested 0.01% in alcohol (56).

Chlorinated hydrocarbons may produce irritant, allergic, and acneiform eruptions.

Perchloroethylene (tetrachloroethylene, carbon dichloride, and ethylene tetrachloride)—Test 25% olive oil. Use: dry cleaning and degreasing metals

Exposure to perchloroethylene causes flushing of the skin with ingestion of alcohol. This reaction is similar to an Antabuse reaction.

Sparrow (57) reported a 19-year-old male who had a connective-tissue type of disease similar clinically to vinyl chloride disease. It is suggested that this may have been caused by abnormal sensitivity to perchloroethylene to which he was exposed in his occupation.

Tetrachloroethane (1,1,2,2-tetrachloroethane, sym-tetrachloroethane, acetylene tetrachloride, and ethanetetrachloride)—Test 1% olive oil. Use: nonflammable solvents for fats, oils, waxes, resins, cellulose acetate, rubber, copal, phosphorus, sulfur, as solvent in certain types of Friedel-Crafts reactions or phthalic anhydride condensations; in the manufacture of paint, varnish, and rust removers; in soil sterilization, weed killer, and insecticide formulations; in the determination of theobromine in cacao; as immersion fluid in crystallography; in the biologic laboratory to produce pathologic changes in the gastrointestinal tract, liver, and kidneys; intermediate in the manufacture of trichloroethylene and other chlorinated hydrocarbons that have two carbon atoms

Esters

Esters are formed by a reaction of an alcohol and an acid. These esters are rare sensitizers.

Methyl acetate Test 10% olive oil. Use: solvent for nitrocellulose, acetylcellulose, and many resins and oils; manufacture of artificial leather

Ethyl acetate (acetic ether and vinegar naphtha)—Test 5% methyl ethyl ketone. Use: artificial fruit essences; solvent for nitrocellulose, varnishes, lacquers, and airplane dopes; manufacture of smokeless powder, artificial leather, photographic films and plates, artificial silk, perfumes; cleaning textiles

Isopropyl acetate—Test 10% olive oil. Use: solvent for cellulose derivatives, plastics, oils, and fats; in perfumery

Amyl acetate (isoamyl acetate, pear oil, banana oil, amyl acetate ester, and pentyl acetate)—Test 10% olive oil. Use: in alcohol solution as a pear flavor in mineral waters and syrups; as solvent for old oil colors, for tannins, nitrocellulose, lacquers, celluloid, and camphor; swelling bath sponges; covering unpleasant odors, perfuming shoe polish; manufacture of artificial silk, leather or pearls, photographic films, celluloid cements, waterproof varnishes, bronzing liquids, and metallic paints; dyeing and finishing textiles. A special grade of the amyl acetate has been used for burning in the Hefner lamp serving as a photometric standard.

Glycols

The glycols may be tested 5% in alcohol.

Ethylene glycol (1,2-ethanediol, glycol alcohol, glycol, and EG)—Use: antifreeze in cooling and heating systems; in hydraulic brake fluids; industrial humectant; ingredient of electrolytic condensers (where it serves as solvent for boric acid and borates); solvent in the paint and plastics industries; in the formulation of printers' inks, stamp pad inks, and inks for ballpoint pens; softening agent for cellophane; stabilizer for soybean form used to extinguish oil and gasoline fires; in the synthesis of safety explosives, glyoxal, unsaturated ester–type alkyd resins, plasticizers, elastomers, synthetic fibers (terylene and dacron), and synthetic waxes, and lens-cutting industry.

There are two reports of ethylene-glycol sensitivity (58,59). In both instances, the dermatitis occurred from exposure to ethylene glycol used to bathe glass lenses while they were being cut. In one instance, there was primary sensitization to ethylene glycol with cross-sensitivity to propylene glycol (59).

Most glycol ethers were found to be either nonirritating or only mildly irritating when studied by Draize testing and nonsensitizers by guinea pig maximization (60). Two glycol ethers were irritants: 2-butoxyethanol and isopropoxyethenol.

Cellulosolve (2-ethoxy ethanol, ethyl cellosolve, ethylene glycol, and monoethyl ether)—Use: solvent for nitrocellulose, lacquers, and dopes; in varnish removers, cleansing solutions, dye baths; finishing leather with water pigments and dye solutions; increasing stability of emulsions

Methyl cellosolve (ethylene glycol monomethyl ether and 2-methoxy ethanol)—Use: solvent for low-viscosity cellulose acetate, natural resins, some synthetic resins, and some alcohol-soluble dyes; in dyeing leather, sealing moisture-proof cellophane; in nail polishes, quick-drying varnishes and enamels, and wood stains. Readily absorbed through the skin

Butyl cellosolve (ethylene glycol monobutyl ether and 2-butoxyethanol)—Use: solvent for nitrocellulose, resins, grease, oil, and albumin; dry cleaning

Ketones

Ketones are substances with the characterizing atom group —CO—, linking two carbon atoms. The ketones apparently are not sensitizers.

Acetone (2-propanone, dimethyl ketone, beta-ketopropane, and pyroacetic ether)—Test 10% olive oil. Use: solvent for fats, oils, waxes, resins, rubber, plastics, lacquers, varnishes, rubber cements, manufacture of methyl isobutyl ketone, mesityl oxide, acetic acid (ketene process), diacetone alcohol, chloroform, iodoform, bromoform, explosives, aeroplane dopes, rayon, photographic films, isoprene; extraction of various principles from animal and plant substances; in paint and varnish removers; purifying paraffin; hardening and dehydrating tissues

Methyl ethyl ketone (buranone, 2-buranone, MEK, ethyl methyl ketone)

Methyl butyl ketone (2-hexanone, *N*-buryl methyl ketone, propyl acetate, MBK)

Methyl isobutyl ketone (hexone, isopropylacetone, 4-methyl-2-pentanone, MIBK)—Test as is. Use: solvent for gums, resins, nitrocellulose; in the surface coating industry; manufacture of smokeless powder; colorless synthetic resins

Miscellaneous Solvents

N-methyl-2-pyrrolidone. This solvent was reported to cause acute irritant contact dermatitis in 10 of 12 workers after 2 days of exposure (61).

d-limonene. The oil of several citrus, caraway, dill, and celery is now being used as an environmentally friendly alternative to halogenated hydrocarbons in up to 95% concentration. Uses include degreasing metals before painting, as a hand cleaner, as a substitute for xylene, and as a solvent for asphalt, heavy oil, and rosin (62). Allergic potential increases with air oxidation (62).

In guinea pigs *d*-limonene of high purity is not a sensitizer, but when exposed to air, oxidized *d*-limonene contains limonene oxide, carvone, and hydroperoxides, which can lead to sensitization (63).

Phenyl-alpha-naphthylamine (PAN). This substance has been incorporated into fire-resistant grease used on conveyor belts at a 1% concentration (64). PAN produced contact dermatitis confirmed by testing at 1% in petrolatum. PAN did not cross-react with phenyl-beta-naphthylamine or di-beta-naphthyl-*p*-phenylenediamine (63).

Carbon disulfide (carbon bisulfide and dithiocarbonic anhydride)—Test 10% olive oil—Use: in the manufacture of rayon, carbon tetrachloride, xanthogenates, soil disinfectants, electronic vacuum tubes; solvent for phosphorus, sulfur, selenium, bromine, iodine, fats, resins, and rubbers

Tetrahydrofuran (diethylene oxide and tetramethylene oxide)—Test 10% olive oil. Use: solvent for high polymers, especially polyvinyl chloride; as reaction medium for Grignard and metal hydride reactions; in the synthesis of butyrolactone, succinic acid, 1,4-butanediol diacetate; solvent in histologic techniques; may be used under US Federal Food, Drug and Cosmetic Act for fabrication of articles for packaging, transporting, or storing of foods if residual amount does not exceed 1.5% of the film

Dioxane (1,4-diethylene dioxide, diethylene ether, 1,4-dioxane, and para-dioxane)—Test 0.5% aqueous. Use: solvent for cellulose acetate, ethyl cellulose, benzyl cellulose, resins, oils, waxes, oil and spirit-soldyes, and many other organic as well as some inorganic compounds

Fregert (65) reported an allergic contact dermatitis from dioxane in a solvent for cleaning metal parts.

Turpentine (gum turpentine, oil of turpentine, spirit of turpentine, gum spirit, pine resin gum, wood turpentine, and sulfate wood pulp waste)—Oil of turpentine, a variable mixture of numerous terpenoid compounds, is derived from various sources, such as balsam of pine trees, and is a by-product in the manufacture of sulfate cellulose. The main components are alpha-pinene, beta-pinene, delta-3-carene, and dipentene (limonene). These are monoterpenes with a common chemical formula of $CH_{10}H_{16}$.

According to Pirila et al. (66), practically all oils of turpentine contain large amounts of 2-pinene. However, the 3-carene content varies in different types, being high (30% to 40%) in most sulfate oils and low or negligible in many balsam oils, for example, French oil of turpentine. The eczematogenic effect of 3-carene depends on its hydroperoxide content.

Hjorth and Wilkinson (67) confirmed that with turpentine the patch test reactions provoked by the same dilution are related to the source, the method of manufacture

(sulfate process or gum distillation), the amount of delta-3-carene present, and the concentration of peroxides formed during storage. These factors vary, as do the relative quantities of alpha-pinene and beta-pinene present. Because some patients may be sensitized by alpha-pinene and others by delta-3-carene, turpentine for testing should contain both of these ingredients and a suitable concentration of their peroxides.

The principal sensitizer in turpentine is the oxidation product of the terpene delta-3-carene, which can be tested 0.3% in petrolatum; old, oxidized turpentine is more irritating and sensitizing than the fresh variety.

Pirila et al. (66) used a mixture of 3-carene, 2-pinene, and limonenes containing 1% peroxides in olive oil for testing turpentine sensitivity.

Turpentine is both a primary irritant and a sensitizer. As an irritant, it usually acts by defatting the skin and causing dryness and fissuring. It is universally used as a cleanser for removing paints and waxes and is one of the most common causes of hand eczema.

Turpentine is an oleoresin obtained from various species of pine. The oleoresin contains a volatile oil (oil of turpentine), which is responsible for its properties and is the form generally used. The irritating and sensitizing property of turpentine varies greatly with the country of origin.

Opportunity for contact with turpentine is widespread, both in industry and elsewhere. It may be applied externally in the form of liniments, ointments, and "rubbing" compounds, and in some countries it is prescribed internally as an anthelmintic and laxative. Other compounds containing turpentine include varnishes, lacquers, floor waxes, cleansers, shoe and floor polishes, paint thinners, printers' ink, dry-cleaning preparations, and various adhesives, including adhesive tape. The skin of citrus fruits contains oleoresins related to turpentine. Topical agents containing turpentine include Mentholatum, Penetro Analgesic Rub, Cloverine Salve, Minard Liniment, Sloan's Liniment, Johnson's Anodyne, and Vicks Vaporub.

Old, oxidized turpentine is more irritating and sensitizing than is the freshly made product. When turpentine is allowed to stand, especially with exposure to light, oxidation results in the formation of formic acid and aldehydes, which may be irritating to the skin. Pinenes and limonene, which are also formed in the oxidation process, may cause allergic sensitization and cross-react with the oils in orange peels and other essential oils.

The terpenes in turpentine have also been incriminated as active sensitization agents. Similar terpenes are present in citrus fruits and celery, and the possibility of cross-reaction must be kept in mind. Cross-sensitivity reactions may also occur between turpentine and ragweed oleoresin, chrysanthemum, pyrethrum, and various balsams, such as those of pine, spruce, and Peru. Wood tars in general have been found to co-react with fragrance mix 43% of the time and balsam of Peru 31% of the time (68). This suggests a shared fragrance material may be present. Coreactions between wood tar and coal tar occurred only 18.5% of the time (68).

The residue remaining after distillation of crude oil of turpentine is rosin, or colophony, which consists mainly of abietic acid and 1-pinearic acid. Rosin obtained from turpentine is present in many adhesives and may cause dermatitis in sensitized individuals (see Chapter 22).

> **Turpentine may cross-react with ragweed oleoresin, chrysanthemum, pyrethrum, and the balsams of pine, spruce, and Peru.**

Cronin (69) reported that oil of turpentine has become an infrequent allergen in Europe because of its replacement by other solvents. In the United States, however, oil of turpentine is still widely used, particularly as a paint remover, and still causes both irritant and allergic reactions. *Olive oil*—This oil is generally safe for patch test purposes and is widely used as a diluent for other solvents in this chapter. However, when used on stasis dermatitis, allergic contact dermatitis may occur; 13 cases were reported within a 4-year period (70). While tests of multiple brands of olive oil were positive, individual tests to the nine components of olive oil listed in the Merck Index were negative (70).

REFERENCES

1. Rycroft RJG. Cutting fluids, oils and lubricants. In: Maibach HI, Gellin GA, eds. *Occupational and industrial dermatology.* Chicago: Year Book Medical Publishers, 1982, p. 233.
2. Fisher AA. Allergic contact dermatitis of the hands due to industrial oils and fluids. *Cutis* 1979;23:131;134,138, passim.
3. Arndt KA. Cutting fluids and the skin. *Cutis* 1969;5:143.
4. Rudzki E, Grzywa Z, Gajewski A. Attempt of preparing an industrial oils test series. *Berufsdermatosen* 1977;25:10.
5. Gellin GA. Cutting fluids and skin disorders. *Industr Med Surg* 1970; 39:65.
6. Samitz MH, Katz SA. Skin hazards from nickel and chromium salts in association with cutting oil operations. *Contact Dermatitis* 1975;1: 158.
7. Samitz MH. Effects of metalworking fluids on the skin. *Prog Dermatol* 1974;8:11.
8. Shah M, Lewis FM, Gawkrodger DJ. Prognosis of occupational hand dermatitis in metalworkers. *Contact Dermatitis* 1996;34:27.
9. Hodgson G. Eczemas associated with lubricants and metalworking fluids. *Dermatol Digest* 1976;10:11.
10. Scerri L, Dalziel KL. Occupational contact sensitization to the stabilized chlorinated paraffin fraction in neat cutting oil. *Am J Contact Dermatitis* 1996;7:35.
11. Angelini G, Meneghini CL. Dermatitis in engineers due to synthetic coolants. *Contact Dermatitis* 1977;3:219.
12. Camarasa JM, Alomar A. Ethylenediamine sensitivity in metallurgic industries. *Contact Dermatitis* 1978;4:178.
13. Fisher AA. *Contact dermatitis,* 3rd ed. Philadelphia: Lea & Febiger, 1986.
14. Suurmond D. Patch test reactions to phenergan cream, promethazine and triethanolamine. *Dermatologica* 1966;133:503.
15. Bhushan M, Craven NM, Beck MH. Contact allergy to 2-aminoethanol (monoethanolamine) in a soluble oil. *Contact Dermatitis* 1998;39:321.
16. Bruze M, et al. Occupational allergic contact dermatitis from alkanolamineborates in metalworking fluids. *Contact Dermatitis* 1995;32: 24.
17. Koch P. Occupational allergic contact dermatitis from oleyl alcohol and monoethanolamine in a metalworking fluid. *Contact Dermatitis* 1995;33:273.
18. Rycroft R. Is Grotan BK a contact sensitizer? *Br J Dermatol* 1978; 99:346.
19. Keczke K, Brown PM. Hexahydro, 1,3,5, tris (2-hydroxyethyl) triazine, a new bacteriocidal agent as a cause of allergic contact dermatitis. *Contact Dermatitis* 1976;2:92.
20. Harke HP. The sensitizing effect of preservatives for coolants [Letter]. *Contact Dermatitis* 1977;3:51.
21. Poitou P, Marignac B. Sensitizing effect of Grotan BK in the guinea pig. *Contact Dermatitis* 1978;4:166.
22. Fregert S, Skog E. Allergic contact dermatitis from mercaptobenzothiazole in cutting oil. *Acta Dermatovener* (Stockh) 1962;42:235.
23. Tosti A, Piraccini B, Brasile GP. Occupational contact dermatitis due to sodium pyrithione. *Contact Dermatitis* 1990;22:118.
24. Hovding G. Occupational dermatitis from hydrazine hydrate used in boiler protection: cross sensitization to a presoline, isoniazid and phenelzine. *Acta Derm Venereol* (Stockh) 1967;47:293.
25. Einarsson O, et al. Chromium, cobalt and nickel in used cutting fluids. *Contact Dermatitis* 1:182, 1975.
26. Nethercott JR, Holness DL. Contact dermatitis associated with exposure to oils and coolants in exogenous dermatosis: environmental dermatitis. In: Menné T, Maibach HI, eds. *Exogenous dermatoses: environmental dermatitis.* Boca Raton, FL: CRC Press, 1991:365.
27. Geretzki P. Pyodermia in metalworking industry [German]. *Dermatosen* 1982;30:116.
28. Taylor JS. The pilosebaceous unit. In: Maibach HI, Gellin GA, eds. *Occupational and industrial dermatology.* Chicago: Year Book Medical Publishers, 1982, p. 131.
29. Adams RM. Plastics other than epoxies. In: Maibach HI, Gellin GA, eds. *Occupational and industrial dermatology.* Chicago: Year Book Medical Publishers, 1982, p. 289.
30. Bleiberg J, et al. Industrially acquired porphyria. *Arch Dermatol* 1964;89:793.
31. Crow KD. Chloracne—an up to date assessment. *Ann Occup Hyg* 1978;21:297.
32. Taylor JS. Environmental chloracne: update and overview. *Ann NY Acad Sci* 1979;320:295.
33. Taylor JS. Occupational dermatoses: method of James S. Taylor, M.D. In: Conn HF, ed. *Current therapy.* Philadelphia: WB Saunders, 1979, p. 635.
34. Orris L, Tesser M. Dermatoses due to water soaps, detergents and solvents. In: Maibach HI, Gellin GA, eds. *Occupational and industrial dermatology.* Chicago: Year Book Medical Publishers, 1982, p. 25.
35. Kurwa AR. Contact dermatitis from isopropyl alcohol. *Contact Dermatitis Newsletter* 1970;8:168.
36. Fregert S, et al. Hypersensitivity to secondary alcohols. *Acta Derm Venereol* (Stockh) 1971;51:271.
37. Ludwig E, Hausen BM. Sensitivity to isopropyl alcohol. *Contact Dermatitis* 1977;3:240.
38. Stotts J, Ely WJ. Induction of human skin sensitization to ethanol. *J Invest Dermatol* 1977;69:219.
39. Jensen O. Contact allergy to propylene oxide and isopropyl alcohol in a skin disinfectant swab. *Contact Dermatitis* 1981;7:148.
40. Rilliet A, Hunziker N, Brun R. Alcohol contact urticana syndrome (immediate-type hypersensitivity): case report. *Dermatologica* 1980; 161:361.
41. Karvonen J, Hannuksela M. Urticaria from alcoholic beverages. *Acta Allerg* 1976;31:167.
42. Berlin K, Johanson G, Lindberg M. Hypersensitivity to 2-(2-butoxyethoxy)ethanol. *Contact Dermatitis* 1995;32:54.

43. Vail JT Jr. False-negative reaction to patch testing with volatile compounds. *Arch Dermatol* 1974;110:130.
44. Bruynzeel DP, Verburgh CA. Occupational dermatitis from isothiazolinones in diesel oil. *Contact Dermatitis* 1996;34:64.
45. Fischer T, Bjarnason B. Sensitizing and irritant properties of 3 environmental classes of diesel oil and their indicator dyes. *Contact Dermatitis* 1996;34:309.
46. Fregert S. Sensitization to mercury in kerosene and exacerbation from red tattoo. *Contact Dermatitis* 1975;1:255.
47. Barnes RL, Wilkinson DS. Epidermal necrolysis from clothing impregnated with paraffin. *Br Med J* 1973;4:466.
48. Gasper AL. Aromatic hydrocarbons. *Occupational Medicine, Current Concepts* (NYS Dept Health) 1980;3:1.
49. Heine A. Is tetrahydronaphthalene an allergen? *Contact Dermatitis* 1991;24:303.
50. Sjoborg S, et al. Contact allergy to styrene with cross reaction to vinyltoluene. *Contact Dermatitis* 1982;8:207.
51. Altman AT. Facial dermatitis. *Arch Dermatol* 1977;113:1460.
52. Ingber A. Occupational allergic contact dermatitis from methyl chloroform (1,1,1-trichloroethane). *Contact Dermatitis* 1991;25:193.
53. Cox NH, Mustchin CP. Prolonged spontaneous and alcohol-induced flushing due to the solvent dimethylformamide. *Contact Dermatitis* 1991;245:69.
54. Bauer M, Rabens SF. Trichloroethylene toxicity. *Int J Dermatol* 1977;16:113.
55. Bauer M, Rabens SF. Cutaneous manifestations of trichloroethylene toxicity. *Arch Dermatol* 1974;110:886.
56. Epstein E. Allergy to epichlorohydrin masquerading as trichloroethylene allergy. *Contact Dermatitis Newsletter* 1974;16:475.
57. Sparrow GP. A connective tissue disorder similar to vinyl chloride disease in a patient exposed to perchloroethylene. *Clin Exp Dermatol* 1977;2:17.
58. Dawson TA. Ethylene glycol sensitivity. *Contact Dermatitis* 1976;2:233.
59. Hindson C, Ratcliffe G. Ethylene glycol in glass lens cutting. *Contact Dermatitis* 1975;1:386.
60. Zissu D. Experimental study of cutaneous tolerance to glycol ethers. *Contact Dermatitis* 1995;32:74.
61. Leira HL, et al. Irritant cutaneous reactions to *N*-methyl-2-pyrrolidone (NMP). *Contact Dermatitis* 1992;27:148.
62. Karlberg AT, Magnusson K, Nilsson U. Air oxidation of *d*-limonene (the citrus solvent) creates potent allergens. *Contact Dermatitis* 1992;26:332.
63. Chang Y-C, Karlberg A-T, Maibach HI. Allergic contact dermatitis from oxidized *d*-limonene. *Contact Dermatitis* 1997;37:308.
64. Carmichael AJ, Foulds IS. Isolated naphthylamine allergy to phenyl-alpha-naphthylamine. *Contact Dermatitis* 1990;22:298.
65. Fregert S. Allergic contact dermatitis from dioxane in a solvent for cleaning metal parts. *Contact Dermatitis Newsletter* 1974;15:438.
66. Pirila V, et al. On the chemical nature of the eczematogens in oil of turpentine (V). Pattern of sensitivity to different terpenes. *Dermatologica* 1969;139:183.
67. Hjorth N, Wilkinson DS. Turpentine sensitivity. *Br J Dermatol* 1968;80:22.
68. Roesyanto ID, van den Akker TW, van Joost TW. Wood tars allergy, cross-sensitization and coal tar. *Contact Dermatitis* 1990;22:95.
69. Cronin E. Oil of turpentine—a disappearing allergen. *Contact Dermatitis* 1979;5:308.
70. Malmkvist Padoan S, Pettersson A, Svensson A. Olive oil as a cause of contact allergy in patients with venous eczema, and occupationally. *Contact Dermatitis* 1990;23:73.

CHAPTER 28

Dermatitis Due to Gases and Propellants

Tear gas, ethylene oxide, and propellants may produce irritant and allergic contact dermatitis.

DERMATITIS DUE TO TEAR GASES (LACRIMATORS)

The term "tear gas" includes not only gases but also liquids and solids that at ordinary temperatures give off vapors that produce so much irritation of the conjunctivae with lacrimation and photophobia that the affected individual is temporarily blinded and can more readily be subdued (1).

Most of the tear gases used by military and law enforcement officers are synthetic organic compounds. Citizens in the United States, and elsewhere, may carry tear gas, or "pepper spray," containing oleoresin of capsicum (2).

The Chemical Nature of Tear Gases

Chloracetophenone

This lacrimator, known in the United States as CN, was first used in World War I and has become a tear gas weapon used worldwide by the military and the police. Chloracetophenone ($C_6H_5COCH_2Cl$) is made by chlorinating acetic acid to form monochloracetic acid, which is further chlorinated with sulfur monochloride and chlorine gas to form chloroacetyl chloride. This compound is treated with benzene in the presence of aluminum chloride. It consists of colorless crystals that melt at 59°C and smells like apple blossoms (3,4).

Mace

Chloracetophenone is available in a compound called Mace, which is an acronym derived from the chemicals methylchloroform and chloracetophenone. Methylchloroform, a solvent, is 1,1,1-trichlorethane (5). Mace also contains kerosene. The chemical mixture is dissolved in an ether-alcohol combination and emitted under pressure from a grenade cartridge by one of the freons.

A billy club that sprays Mace out of its end is also available.

CS

This term refers to the lacrimator *ortho*-chlorobenzylidene malonitrile (6), a white powder that is often combined with ethyl bromacetate, a dispersing agent. The letters are rumored to represent Carson and Stoughton, the chemists who invented the chemical. It has been used in thermal grenades by the United States military in Vietnam, by American police in domestic disturbances, and by British forces in the north of Ireland.

Recently, CS has become available in the United States in aerosol form.

Miscellaneous Synthetic Tear Gases

Much less widely used lacrimators include the following:

Brombenzyl cyanide ($C_6H_5CHBrCN$) is known as CA in the United States and as Chamite in France
Ethyliodoacetate ($CH_3ICOOC_2H_5$) is the British SK
Bromacetone (CH_3COCH_2Br) is the American BA, the French Martinite, and the German B-Stoff
Xylyl bromide ($C_6H_4CH_3CH_2Br$) is the German T-Stoff
Benzyl iodide ($C_6H_5CH_2I$) is the French Fraissite
Ethyl bromoethanoate ($CH_2BrCOOC_2H_5$)
Phenyl carbylamine chloride ($C_6H_5CNCl_2$)
Benzyl bromide ($C_6H_5CH_2Br$) is the French Cyclite
Acrolein (CH_2CHCHO) is the French Papite
Bromo-methyl ethyl ketone ($BrCH_2COC_2H_5$)
Chloracetone (CH_3COCH_2Cl) is the French Tonite
Iodoacetone (CH_3COCH_2I) is the French Bretonite

Oleoresin of Capsicum

For some time, the US government has issued aerosol sprays containing this oleoresin to postal carriers for repelling animals, particularly dogs. Similarly, individuals may arm themselves with capsicum aerosols in containers varying in size from that of a lipstick to a fountain pen.

The oleoresin is a dark red, extremely acrid and pungent liquid that is extracted from cayenne pepper pods with alcohol or ethyl ether. It irritates the conjunctivae and the nasal and oral mucosa and can be classified as a tear gas or lacrimator. Although organic synthetic lacrimators do not affect dogs and other animals as much as they do humans, the oleoresin of capsicum is an efficient repellent for both man and beast.

Cayenne pepper *(Capsicum frutescens),* from which the oleoresin of capsicum is extracted, is distributed worldwide and has the following names in different countries: *pimenton* (Spain); *poivre rouge* (France); *cayennepferrer* (Germany); *kajennepeppar* (Sweden); *cayennepeper* (Holland); *pepe di caienna* (Italy); *pimentao-de-caiena* (Portugal); *kayenski pyerets* (Russia); *la-chiao* (China); and *filfil ahmar* (Arabic). In Japan, cayenne pepper is not known, but the closely related chili pepper *(togarashi)* is available. Cayenne pepper may colloquialy be called Guinea pepper, Spanish pepper, African pepper, and chilies or bird pepper (7).

> **Tear gases (lacrimators), whether synthetic or natural, such as oleoresin of capsicum, can produce both irritant and allergic dermatitis.**

Primary Irritant Reactions to Tear Gases

All lacrimators in high concentrations are powerful skin irritants and can produce first- and second-degree chemical burns. Third-degree burns with ulceration may result, particularly with CS, in the presence of moisture and occlusion. Stinging and erythema are produced when CS is wetted.

Mace dermatitis in particular can cause disfiguring depigmentation of black skin, which may persist for many months.

Technicians and others handling lacrimators, particularly CS, may acquire an irritant dermatitis, especially where there is constriction from wearing apparel, such as at the neck and waist, or in intertriginous areas, such as the axillae and vulva (8).

Irritant and possible allergic contact dermatitis may be severe in those on the wrong end of riot control sprays containing CS. One report from France found an average of 6 days was needed in the hospital following exposure (9).

> **The irritation from CN and other chlorinated lacrimators may be due to the release of hydrochloric acid from such compounds.**

Industrial Contact Dermatitis Due to Tear Gas

Shmunes and Taylor (10) reported that 25 of 28 workers in a chemical plant manufacturing *ortho*-chlorobenzylidene malonitrile (CS) gave a history of dermatitis involving the arms and neck. Two of 25 workers showed positive patch test reactions when tested with a 1:1,000 dilution of CS in olive oil. The study reveals that in the industrial setting, a significant sensitizing potential exists, but irritancy was the major factor in the production and perpetuation of the dermatitis.

Kanerva et al. (11) reported two cases of sensitization to CN and CS in workers following only one accidental exposure.

An awareness of the possible cutaneous responses to this chemical is advisable in view of its use by the military and by civilian authorities in the United States, as well as its adoption as the active ingredient in personal protective devices.

Localized Occupational Dermatitis in Police Officers from Tear Gas

Tear gas is supplied to police in canisters and holsters. Occasionally, such canisters may leak or become self-activated, and discharge the tear gas. Such localized dermatitis occurs usually on the hip near the belt line of the police officer who is wearing a can of Mace.

> **Police officers may acquire an irritant or allergic dermatitis on their hip near the belt line from leaking or self-discharging tear gas canisters or holsters.**

The manufacturers of chemical Mace aerosol tear gas projectors state that the projectors should be carried with the firing actuator downward in the pocket to make them less conspicuous and to reduce the chances of accidental discharge. It is important to have the firing actuator in the lock or safe position when carrying the projector to reduce the chance of an accidental discharge.

Allergic Contact Dermatitis from Tear Gases

Allergic contact dermatitis from chloracetophenone has been reported occasionally since as early as 1942 (12–15). It has been emphasized that the CN in Mace is a potent sensitizer, which cross-reacts with dichloracetophenone but not with *para*-chloracetophenone or bromoacetophenone. Although CS is also a sensitizer, it is not as potent as CN.

Allergic contact dermatitis from synthetic tear gas is typical eczematous dermatitis, often accompanied by marked edema. Contact sensitization to the oleoresin of capsicum is not common, but it suggests the possibility that ingestion of foods containing capsicum (spicy and ethnic foods, such as Mexican and Chinese) may produce an eczematous contact–type dermatitis. Diffuse erythema has been reported from the ingestion of capsicum.

Patch Testing with Tear Gases

Great care must be taken in performing patch tests with tear gases, because the minimum irritating concentration is as low as 1 part in 100,000.

Patch tests with tear gases should be started with a 1:100,000 dilution.

In Mace, CN is present in a 0.9% concentration. Patch tests may be performed with chemical Mace diluted 1 part with 100 parts acetone, which gives a 0.009% concentration of chloracetophenone. This concentration is not an irritant under a closed patch test and is sufficient to produce a positive allergic eczematous patch test reaction in sensitized individuals.

Patch tests with CS should be commenced with a 1:100,000 dilution in acetone. (It should be noted that CS dissolves with difficulty.) The other tear gases should be tested in a 1:100,000 dilution in ethanol to determine a concentration that is not irritating under a closed patch.

Capsicum may be tested in a 1% solution in ethanol.

Management of Tear Gas Dermatitis

In sensitized individuals, Mace must be removed from the skin with soap and water within a few minutes or dermatitis is inevitable. The lacrimator CS should also be removed with water as soon as possible. Although dry skin is unharmed initially by it, prolonged exposure may produce first- and second-degree burns and even ulceration. As soon as the individual begins to wash the powder off, a burning sensation and erythema occur but usually subside in an hour or so.

Barrier creams and petrolatum do not offer much protection from tear gas. Plastic clothing, including plastic helmets and visors, are the best protective devices available.

The treatment of primary irritation, burns, or allergic dermatitis from the tear gases is similar to the treatment of these conditions from other causes.

The US Surgeon General's report concerning chemical Mace states: "It is generally agreed that flushing of the agent with water from the contact point is the most effective treatment and that the application of salves, creams, or ointments should be discouraged since these substances aid in localizing the active material at the site of injury."

Tear gas should be flushed off with water; creams and ointments should be avoided because they localize the active material at the site of injury.

ETHYLENE OXIDE DERMATITIS

The most common types of cutaneous reactions to ethylene oxide gas are irritant reactions or burns, which may at times be severe. There are also a few reports of allergic reactions to this gas.

The Nature of Ethylene Oxide Sterilization

Ethylene oxide is a colorless, gaseous, simple epoxy compound whose sterilizing ability depends on its inherent toxic effect on all living cells. This is most likely because of ethylene oxide's ability to replace a hydrogen atom in protein molecules with hydroethyl (alkyl group), a process known as alkylation. Because this process is irreversible, the cell is killed. It is important, therefore, to remove all traces of ethylene oxide from the item sterilized before it comes into contact with human tissues. In addition, it is genotoxic (16).

Contact with inadequately aerated products sterilized with ethylene oxide can produce severe irritant dermatitis and burns; on rare occasions, an allergic reaction to ethylene oxide may occur.

Gaseous ethylene oxide has become one of the major sterilizing agents of medical equipment and materials. Sterilization can be accomplished at low temperatures and humidity, thus avoiding damage to heat- or moisture-sensitive materials, as might occur with autoclave sterilization. Its highly diffusive nature and its permeability make it possible to sterilize through hermetically sealed plastic wrapping films, shipping cartons, and containers.

The ethylene oxide gas sterilization process consists of two essential parts: (a) sterilization by ensuring penetration of a sufficient concentration of the gas into all parts of load and (b) aeration until one is certain that all gas residues are eliminated from the sterilized items.

The Ethylene Oxide Subcommittee of the American National Standards Institute recommends the following precautions be taken to avoid the hazards of ethylene oxide sterilization:

1. Polyvinyl chloride or rubber materials sterilized with ethylene oxide should not be used within 7 days following sterilization, if stored at room temperatures.
2. Polyethylene (3 to 5 mL) and paper wrap are the best packaging materials. Nylon and polyvinylidine chloride are less permeable to ethylene oxide.
3. Polyvinyl chloride objects that have been gamma-irradiated should not be resterilized with ethylene oxide because large amounts of ethylene chlorohydrin will be formed.

4. "Disposable" items should be discarded after use because the by-products of later ethylene oxide sterilization may include ethylene chlorohydrin, which is a severe skin irritant.
5. Water droplets should be removed from material to be sterilized, to prevent the formation of ethylene glycol, a powerful irritant.

Ethylene oxide gas sterilization is indicated for equipment (e.g., ventilators) that is too bulky for steam sterilization and for certain plastics, whereas syringes, instruments, drapes, gowns, rubber, and some heat-resistant plastics can all be steam sterilized.

It should be emphasized that the key to safety with ethylene oxide is proper aeration following sterilization.

Irritant Dermatitis and Burns from Ethylene Oxide

La Dage (17) reported a severe facial irritation from excess ethylene oxide in anesthesia masks. Hanifin (18) described six cases of contact dermatitis that were traced to residual ethylene oxide in prepacked nitrofurazone dressings. Ippen and Mathies (19) observed three workers who suffered from third-degree burns of the hands, forehead, axillae, periumbilical region, and the genitalia after cleaning a storage container that had traces of ethylene oxide. These authors suggest that, if an industrial case is seen, immediate treatment should be to rinse the affected area with water under pressure, such as may be obtained from using a hose. Contaminated garments should also be cleaned thoroughly.

Biro et al. (20) and Fisher (21) reported that 19 hospitalized women suffered postoperatively from severe burns of the buttocks and back from contact with reusable surgical gowns and drapes that had been sterilized with ethylene oxide and had not been properly aerated. Initially, an "epidemic" of bullous impetigo was suspected. Severe irritant reactions to detergents and antiseptics were also considered. The burned skin resembled a localized form of toxic epidermal necrolysis.

Testing samples of reusable gowns that had been worn by the patients showed that the amount of ethylene oxide residue varied from 3,600 ppm ethylene oxide to 10,800 ppm ethylene oxide. The safe level for ethylene oxide gas recommended by both the Health Industries Association (HIA) and the Z-79 Committee of New York Mount Sinai Hospitals is 200 ppm (maximum). The levels of residual ethylene oxide in the implicated gowns were thus determined to be 16 to 50 times the safe level for skin contact. Percutaneous absorption of ethylene oxide can be significant, especially under occlusion (16).

Occupational Exposure to Ethylene Oxide

Sporadic reports of irritant contact dermatitis (ICD) to ethylene oxide (ETO) have been published. A group of pharmaceutical workers in Israel, totalling 9 of 34 exposed persons, developed ETO ICD from overalls that were improperly aerated after ETO sterilization (22). A level of 500 ppm ETO was found in the garment bags. All patients developed severe pruritus, vesicles, and erythema around the wrists, which resolved after about 3 weeks. Hospital workers are not uncommonly affected, as discussed in a report by Romaguera and Vilaplana (23). The four workers were exposed to ETO from a leaking sterilizing unit. Patch tests were not performed in either case.

Taylor (24) reviewed the effects of industrial exposure to ethylene oxide. He stated that cutaneous exposure to ETO usually occurs during production of the liquid chemical or as a result of its use as a gas sterilizing agent. Because of its importance as an industrial compound, ETO is among the top chemicals produced in the United States. It is used widely as a raw material in the synthesis of many organic chemicals, as a solvent and plasticizer in the production of high-energy fuels, and in large quantities for the manufacture of ethylene glycol, the main ingredient of permanent antifreeze.

Taylor (24) pointed out that ETO (C_2H_4O) is a clear, colorless liquid below its boiling point of 10.7°C; above this temperature it is a clear, colorless gas with a sweetish odor. Its freezing point is -111.3°C. Ethylene oxide is miscible with water in all proportions. The explosive decomposition of ETO vapors is a major industrial hazard. As little as 3% ETO vapor in the air will support combustion and will be violently explosive if confined. When ETO is used as a sterilizing agent, this hazard is prevented by dilution of the vapor with various inert gases.

If liquid ETO is spilled directly on the skin, it should be allowed to vaporize before being washed with water. All clothing contaminated with liquid ETO should be removed at once, especially shoes and gloves, and washed immediately with large quantities of water. First aid for acute inhalation exposure and protective measures to prevent exposure are available from local poison control centers and usually from hospital safety offices.

Liquid ethylene oxide on the skin should be allowed to vaporize before washing it off; the pure anhydrous liquid is not injurious to the skin.

The hazards associated with production of ETO—well known to industrial toxicologists—include cutaneous burns, allergic contact dermatitis, mucosal irritation, acute inhalation toxicity, explosions, and fire. Pure anhydrous liquid ETO does not produce primary injury to the dry skin of workers, but solutions of ETO have a vesicant action and may cause conjunctivitis if splashed in the eye. Burns are more likely to occur when the solution is held in contact with the skin by clothing, gloves, and shoes. In common with other cutaneous irritants, repeated exposure may result in delayed allergic contact hypersensitivity.

TABLE 28.1. *Hazards from Industrial Exposure to Ethylene Oxide*

Allergic contact dermatitis
Acute inhalation toxicity
Cutaneous burns (irritant contact dermatitis)
Explosions
Fire
Mucosal irritation

TABLE 28.3. *Hazards from Ethylene Oxide Sterilization of Medical Equipment*

Hazard	Equipment
Anaphylaxis	Plastic and rubber tubing (hemodialysis)
Cutaneous burn	Rubber gloves and masks
Hemolysis	Plastic tubing
Tracheal inflammation	Endotracheal tubes

Acute inhalation toxicity to high concentrations may manifest as mucosal irritation and pulmonary edema. Lower concentrations of vapor result in delayed nausea and vomiting. A threshold limit value of 50 ppm ETO by volume in air is said to offer an adequate margin of safety from ostensible systemic effects.

Table 28.1 lists the hazards to industrial exposure, according to Taylor (24). Table 28.2 lists medical supplies sterilizable by ethylene oxide, and Table 28.3 lists hazards from ethylene oxide sterilization of medical equipment.

Allergic Reactions to Ethylene Oxide

Sexton and Henson (25) first experimentally produced allergic contact dermatitis to ETO. Dolovich and Bell reported a product of ethylene oxide gas with demonstration of IgE and IgG antibodies and hapten specificity. Their patient, on chronic hemodialysis, developed severe allergic reactions after exposure to articles such as plastic tubing and hemodialysis supplies that had undergone cold sterilization with ETO gas. It was shown that human serum albumin, exposed to ethylene oxide in the usual sterilization procedure, selectively elicited positive skin tests and *in vitro* histamine release.

Poothullil et al. (27) studied a patient who developed an anaphylactic reaction to ETO, and Bronk and van Ketel (28) described a patient with a postoperative delayed allergic contact reaction from a reusable operating room lift mat

TABLE 28.2. *Medical Supplies Sterilizable by Ethylene Oxide*

Hospital central supply sterilizers
  1. Telescopic instruments: bronchoscopes and endoscopes
  2. Plastic goods: catheters, syringes, gloves, petri dishes, parts for heart-lung machines, and renal dialysis units
  3. Rubber goods: tubing, surgical gloves, catheters, sheeting, and anesthesia face masks
  4. Instruments: knives, needles, and speculae
Commercial sterilizers
  1. Supplies listed above
  2. Drugs and medication: anesthetic, otic, and ophthalmic solutions; surgical jellies; and nitrofurazone dressings
  3. Implantable devices: sutures, prostheses, valves, and pacemakers

that had been sterilized with excessive ETO. Positive patch tests to ethylene oxide–sterilized patches and polyethylene glycol 300 were obtained. It is suggested that the allergic dermatitis could also be due to polyethylene glycol, a polymer of ethylene oxide and water.

The Spanish investigators Romaguera and Grimalt (29) and Alomar et al. (30) also reported allergic reactions from face masks sterilized with ETO.

The breakdown products of ETO are ethylene glycol and ethylene chlorohydrin. The allergic reactions to ETO may possibly be due to these breakdown products.

> **Under conditions of effective sterilization, ethylene oxide forms ethylene glycol and ethylene chlorohydrin; the skin reactions, however, are probably due to ethylene oxide itself, rather than to these by-products.**

Compounds Related to Ethylene Oxide

Ethylene Glycol

This glycol is used in antifreeze solutions as a solvent and in lacquer, adhesives, resins, inks, and stains. Allergic reactions have been reported in its use in eyeglass lens manufacture. Patch testing is best performed with 3% in alcohol (31).

Ethylene Chlorohydrin (Chloroethanol)

Ethylene chlorohydrin is a toxic solvent in polymers, lacquers, and insecticides. Wahlberg and Boman (32) stated that it can be absorbed through the skin.

Cellosolves (Methyl, Ethyl, Butyl, and Diethyl)

These cellosolves are monoalkyl ether of ethylene glycol, which are readily absorbed through the skin and can therefore produce poisoning by absorption as well as by inhalation. They are also strong solvents for paints, varnishes, plastics, and dyes and can cause defatting and drying of the skin.

Patch Testing for Allergic Reactions to Ethylene Oxide

Romaguera and Grimalt (29) showed that their patient was allergic to ethylene oxide by exposing gauze to ethylene oxide. The gauze was ventilated for 8 hours and produced a strong reaction (+++) in the patient. The gauze that ventilated for 24 hours had the same reaction, but the gauze that was properly ventilated for 48 hours produced no reaction.

Similarly, Alomar et al. (30) showed that in their patient, gauze and all materials sterilized with ethylene oxide at 24, 48, and 72 hours of ventilation showed positive reactions of ++ and +++ at 92 hours. Twelve controls tested simultaneously gave negative results.

They then tested a piece of gauze that had been sterilized with ethylene oxide in another machine from another sterilization department and obtained the same +++ positive reaction despite 48 hours of ventilation.

One gauze sterilized 48 hours beforehand was introduced into a sterile glass tube with 15 mL of double distilled water, and 48 hours later a patch test with the water showed a ++ positive reaction at 96 hours.

Shupack et al. (33) reported patch materials that rapidly lose ethylene oxide, such as fabric or rubber, produced few reactions even at ethylene oxide levels as high as 5,000 ppm. A patch material that loses ethylene oxide more slowly in polyvinyl chloride (PVC) film produced reactions at ethylene oxide levels above 1,700 ppm. The patch materials that retained ethylene oxide the longest were thick PVC blocks, and petrolatum applied to Webril pads produced the most reactions. When the ethylene oxide level in those materials approximated 1,000 ppm or higher, skin reactions usually appeared after 4 to 8 hours' contact. The level of reactivity among the volunteers was quite consistent. One subject, however, who developed sensitivity to ethylene oxide, showed a mild delayed reaction to approximately 1,000 ppm of ethylene oxide in PVC. Because little or no reaction developed to the patches containing ethylene oxide by-products, ethylene oxide itself can be assumed to be the toxic agent. The experiments support the conclusion that the lowest level of ethylene oxide that produces skin irritation in nonsensitized subjects approximates 1,000 ppm, when retained in slow-airing material against the skin for 4 hours or more.

> Materials such as fabrics and rubber, which rapidly lose ethylene oxide, produce few reactions even with high levels of ethylene oxide.

PROPELLANT DERMATITIS

Halogenated hydrocarbons (freons), which were widely used in the past, have now been largely replaced either voluntarily or because of government restriction, because they have been shown to cause damaging effects on the earth's ozone layer. The following propellants are commonly used: propane, butane, isobutane liquified petroleum gases (LPGs), compressed gases (e.g., nitrogen or carbon dioxide), and gelled propellants.

Deodorant Spray Allergy Due to Freons

Occasional case reports of allergy to freons have been published.

Three patients with an acute eczema in the axillae after the use of a deodorant spray were investigated by van Ketel (34). All three patients reacted positively to (open) patch tests with the propellant Freon 11 (trichloromonofluoromethane). One patient also reacted to Freon 12 (dichlorodifluoromethane). Of the other two patients, one developed an eczematous eruption after ethyl chloride had been sprayed onto the skin before biopsy was taken. Patch tests with ethyl chloride were performed on the other two patients and were found to be positive.

A single case report from Switzerland discussed a 30-year-old woman with patch test proven allergic contact dermatitis to both ethyl chloride and Freon 12 (CFC 12), which was caused by use of these agents in a medical aerosol (35).

> Freon propellants 11 and 12 may show cross-reactions with ethyl chloride.

Methylene Chloride (Dichlormethane, Carene)

This chemical may be added to freon sprays or may be used as an aerosol propellant by itself. It is a solvent and a degreasing agent and is a mild skin irritant because it can release hydrochloric acid in small amounts.

Trichloroethane (Methyl Chloroform)

This chemical may also be added to some freon sprays. It is a chlorinated hydrocarbon solvent and is used in the synthesis of many organic compounds.

Fowler (36) reported a case of contact urticaria in an eyeglass factory worker caused by trichloroethane. Immediate patch tests were positive, with negative delayed hypersensitivity tests. Ingber (37) reported a case of a metalworker exposed to trichloroethane used for cleaning metal plates. Positive patch tests were seen at 1%, 0.1%, and 0.01% in olive oil with five negative controls.

Feminine "Hygiene" (Deodorant) Sprays

Feminine hygiene sprays, a euphemism for female genital deodorants, are more delicately called abroad "intimate" or "intime" sprays. These sprays are packaged mainly in an aerosol form consisting essentially of a fragrance, an emollient, and a propellant. Some sprays, in addition, contain an antibacterial agent. These sprays have enjoyed an enormous sale in recent years, although their superiority over soap and water has been questioned (38).

Vulvitis and dermatitis produced by the sprays have been reported, principally by gynecologists, without distinguishing between irritant and allergic reactions (39–41). Gowdy (41) stated that 26 instances of dermatitis were reported to the US Food and Drug Administration (FDA), principally the irritant variety, but surmised that some of the reactions may have been due to "allergic" reactions to hexachlorophene or perfumes. There is no mention of patch testing procedure in these 26 cases. Gowdy also cited three instances of the reaction in the genital area of the "consorts" of women who had used the sprays.

> **Irritant dermatitis of the penis and scrotum may occur in the male sexual partner if the feminine hygiene spray is applied just before intercourse.**

Fisher (42) reported that 30 women were patch tested to the individual ingredients in 12 different feminine hygiene sprays that had produced a vulvar and inguinal or thigh dermatitis. In addition, two men were tested who had acquired penile and scrotal dermatitis after having sexual intercourse with women who used the sprays just prior to sexual intercourse.

Four positive patch test reactions were obtained. The specific ingredients that produced the positive patch test reactions and caused an allergic contact dermatitis and vulvitis from their presence in the sprays were benzethonium chloride, chlorhexidine, isopropyl myristate, and perfume.

Ingredients in Feminine Hygiene Sprays (Table 28.4)

Bacteriostats

Hexachlorophene. Prior to the FDA ban, hexachlorophene was the preferred bacteriostat in most US products. At one time, as many as 40 different sprays contained hexachlorophene. It is ironic that the "banned" hexachlorophene

TABLE 28.4. *Ingredients of Feminine Hygiene Sprays*

Bacteriostats (rarely used at present)
  Chlorohexidine
  Chloroxylenol
  Hexachlorophene (banned in United States)
  Methylbenzethonium chloride
  Triclosan
Emollients
  Glycerides
  Myristates
  Polyoxethylene derivatives
Perfumes
Propellants
  Fluorinated hydrocarbons

was the "safest" antibacterial agent from the standpoint of allergenicity. In a previous study, Fisher (43) had shown that hexachlorophene was a rare sensitizer.

Most manufacturers have not replaced the hexachlorophene with another antibacterial agent, with the hindsight explanation that antibacterial agents did not really contribute to the effectiveness of the feminine hygiene sprays.

Benzethonium chloride. This quaternary ammonium compound, which may show cross-reactions with benzalkonium chloride, is also a rare sensitizer (44). Its presence in a roll-on deodorant produced an allergic axillary dermatitis (45). In our series this agent produced an allergic reaction in one woman and one man.

Triclosan. At one time, a few feminine hygiene sprays contained triclosan (Irgasan DP 300), a diphenyl ether that is marketed in more than 200 different products throughout the world. In the United States, at least 20 formulations contain this bacteriostat; these include toilet soap bars, surgical scrub soaps, and underarm deodorants. It should be noted that the cloflucarban (Irgasan CF 3) in Safeguard soap is chemically unrelated to triclosan.

Chlorhexidine. This bacteriostat is present in several European feminine hygiene sprays. One of our patients who purchased a feminine hygiene spray abroad gave a positive patch test reaction to this chemical.

Perfumes

The fragrance of perfume components are selected with care because some perfume ingredients are irritants when applied to mucous tissues. Some brands of deodorant sprays use both a conventional perfume compound and an encapsulated perfume that releases the fragrance slowly over a longer period of time.

It is of interest to note that the patient in this series who was allergic to the perfume in the feminine hygiene spray also showed a strongly positive patch test reaction to balsam of Peru (46).

Propellants

The propellants previously used were the fluorinated hydrocarbons. These include trichloromonofluoromethane (Freon 11), dichlorodifluoromethane (Freon 12), and tetrafluoromethane (Freon 14). The propellants were rare sensitizers but were probably the most common cause of an irritant dermatitis when the spray is applied too closely to the vulvar area.

> **Feminine hygiene sprays held too close to the body may readily cause dermatitis due to irritation by the propellant.**

Emollients

A wide variety of emollients act as the carrier for the bacteriostat and the perfume. Among the preferred emollients are fatty esters such as isopropyl myristate and palmitate, fatty alcohols (including lauryl and myristyle), glycerides, and polyoxethylene derivatives of both fatty esters and fatty alcohol. These are rare sensitizers as noted in Chapter 17.

REFERENCES

1. Fisher AA. Dermatitis due to tear gases (lacrimators). *Int J Dermatol* 1970;9:91.
2. Hu H, Fine J, Epstein P, et al. Tear gas: harassing agent or toxic chemical weapon. *JAMA* 1989;262:660–663.
3. Stein AA, Kerwin WE. Chloracetophenone (tear gas) poisoning: a clinicopathological report. *J Forensic Sci* 1964;9:379.
4. Schwartz I, Tulipan L, Birmingham DJ. *Occupational diseases of the skin,* 2nd ed. Philadelphia: Lea & Febiger, 1957:466.
5. Fisher AA. Mace, a modern acronym and an ancient nomenclature. *JAMA* 1970;212:320.
6. Gleason MN, et al. *Clinical toxicology of commercial products,* 3rd ed. Baltimore: Williams & Wilkins, 1969:301.
7. Rosengarten F. *The book of spices.* Wynnewood, PA: Livingston Publishing, 1969:129.
8. Penneys NS, Israel RM, Indgin SM. Contact dermatitis due to 1-chloracetophenone and chemical mace. *N Engl J Med* 1969;281:413.
9. Parneix-Spake A, et al. Severe cutaneous reactions to self-defense sprays. *Arch Dermatol* 1993;129:913.
10. Shmunes E, Taylor JS. Industrial contact dermatitis. *Arch Dermatol* 1973;107:212.
11. Kanerva L, Tarvainen K, Pinola A, et al. A single accidental exposure may result in a chemical burn, primary sensitization, and allergic contact dermatitis. *Contact Dermatitis* 1994;31:229–235.
12. Frazier CA. Contact allergy to mace. *JAMA* 1976;236:2526.
13. Natrop KHE, Pinzer B, Hornk K. Skin lesions due to tear gas. *Hautschaden Tranengas Dermatol Monatsschr* 1975;161:678.
14. Holland P, White RG. The cutaneous reactions produced by o-chlorobenzyl-idenmalononitrile and w-chloroacetophenone when applied directly to the skin of human subjects. *Br J Dermatol* 1972; 86:150.
15. Ingram JT. Dermatitis from exposure to tear gas. *Br J Dermatol* 1942;54:319.
16. Wester R, Hartway T, Serranzana, et al. Human skin in-vitro percutaneous absorption of gaseous ethylene oxide from fabric. *Food-Chem-Toxicol* 1997;35:513–515.
17. La Dage LH. Facial "irritation" from ethylene oxide sterilization of anesthesia face mask. *Plast Reconstr Surg* 1970;45:179.
18. Hanifin JM. Ethylene oxide dermatitis. *JAMA* 1971;271:213.
19. Ippen H, Mathies V. Protracted chemical burns (ethylene oxide). *Berufsdermatosen* 1970;18:6.
20. Biro L, Fisher AA, Price E. Ethylene oxide burns: a hospital outbreak involving 19 women. *Arch Dermatol* 1974;110:924.
21. Fisher AA. Post-operative ethylene oxide dermatitis. *Cutis* 1973;12: 177.
22. Lerman Y, Ribak J, Skulsky M, et al. An outbreak of irritant contact dermatitis from ethylene oxide among pharmaceutical workers. *Contact Dermatitis* 1995;38:280–281.
23. Romaguera C, Vilaplana J. Airborne occupational contact dermatitis from ethylene oxide. *Contact Dermatitis* 1998;39:85.
24. Taylor JS. Dermatologic hazards from ethylene oxide. *Cutis* 1977;19: 189.
25. Sexton RJ, Henson EV. Experimental ethylene oxide human skin injuries. *Arch Ind Hygiene Occup Med* 1950;2:549.
26. Dolovich J, Bell B. Allergy to product(s) of ethylene oxide gas: demonstration of IgE and IgG antibodies and hapten specificity. *J Allergy* 1978;62:30.
27. Poothullil J, Shimizu A, Day RP, Dolovich J. Anaphylaxis from the products of ethylene oxide gas. *Ann Intern Med* 1975;82:58.
28. Bronk WJ, van Ketel WG. A possible case of delayed hypersensitivity to ethylene oxide. *Clin Exp Dermatol* (Oxford) 1981;6:4.
29. Romaguera C, Grimalt F. Irritant dermatitis from ethylene oxide. *Contact Dermatitis* 1980;6:351.
30. Alomar A, Camarasa JMB, Noguera J, Aspinolea F. Ethylene oxide dermatitis. *Contact Dermatitis* 1981;7:205.
31. Dawson TAJ. Ethylene glycol sensitivity. *Contact Dermatitis* 1976; 2:233.
32. Wahlberg JE, Boman A. 2-chloroethanol—percutaneous toxicity of a solvent. *Dermatology* 1978;156:299.
33. Shupack JL, Andersen SR, Romano SJ. Human skin reactions to ethylene oxide. *J Lab Clin Med* 1981;98:723.
34. van Ketel WG. Allergic contact dermatitis from propellants in deodorant sprays in combination with allergy to ethyl chloride. *Contact Dermatitis* 1976;2:115.
35. Bircher A, Hampl K, Hirsbrunner P, et al. Allergic contact dermatitis from ethyl chloride and sensitization to dichlorodifluoromethane (CFC 12). *Contact Dermatitis* 1994;31:41–44.
36. Fowler JF. Contact urticaria to 1,1,1-trichloroethane. *Am J Contact Dermatitis* 1991;2:239.
37. Ingber A. Occupational allergic contact dermatitis from methyl chloroform (1,1,1-trichloroethane). *Contact Dermatitis* 1991;25:193.
38. Feminine hygiene sprays remain controversial despite FDA action. (Medical News) *JAMA* 1972;219:449.
39. Kaye BM. Hazards of feminine hygiene sprays for women. *JAMA* 1970;212:2121.
40. Davis BA. Irritancy from feminine hygiene sprays. *Obstet Gynecol* 1970;36:812.
41. Gowdy JM. Feminine deodorant sprays. *N Engl J Med* 1972;287:203.
42. Fisher AA. Allergic reaction to feminine hygiene sprays. *Arch Dermatol* 1973;108:801.
43. Fisher AA, et al. Allergic contact dermatitis due to ingredients of vehicles. *Arch Dermatol* 1971;104:286.
44. Fisher AA, Stillman MA. Allergic contact sensitivity to benzalkonium chloride. *Arch Dermatol* 1972;106:169.
45. Shmunes E, Levy EJ. Quaternary ammonium compound contact dermatitis from a deodorant. *Arch Dermatol* 1972;105:91.
46. Hjorth N. *Eczematous allergy to balsams.* Copenhagen: Munksgaard, 1961:194.

CHAPTER 29

Plastic (Synthetic Resin) Dermatitis

Malten (1) reviewed dermatologic problems in the production and processing of plastics. With relatively few exceptions, they appear to be safe in production and processing if used with strict precautions. Uncured plastics are used increasingly in different industries and are responsible for a growing number of dermatoses. Fully cured or synthetic plastics polymerized by the addition of curing agents, stabilizers, catalysts, and plasticizers are rarely implicated.

GENERAL CONSIDERATIONS

Plastics consist of large numbers of long chainlike molecules made from small molecules (called monomers) linked together. These chainlike molecules are called polymers, and the process of linking the monomers together is called polymerization. In thermoplastics, the polymers lie side by side and can move when heated to fill different shapes. In thermosetting plastics, the long polymeric molecules are joined together or "cross-linked" by smaller molecules or by heat. The process of turning thermoplastics into thermosetting plastics by cross-linking is called curing. Heating thermosetting plastics does not change their shape.

Plastics are polymerized by the addition of curing agents, stabilizers, plasticizers, and catalysts. Accelerators and antioxidants are often added. Any of these chemicals may be irritants or sensitizers.

Plastics Commonly Causing Dermatitis

Epoxy resins and phenol-formaldehyde plastics cause allergic and irritant dermatitis. Carbamidformaldehyde and acrylic plastics cause allergic reactions. Polyester plastics produce irritant and rarely allergic dermatitis.

Plastics Rarely Causing Dermatitis

Polypropylene, polyurethane, Teflon, furene, polycarbonates, silicones, carbonyls, coumarone, cellulose derivatives, polystyrene, polyvinyl chloride (PVC), polypropylene chloride (PPC), polyvinyl acetate (PVA), polybutadiene nitrile alkyds, and polyethylene are rare causes of dermatitis.

Additives That Are Common Sensitizers

Phthalates (such as dibutyldioctyl), maleates, cobalt naphthenate, benzoyl peroxide, dimethylaniline, and toluenesulfonic acid commonly cause dermatitis. Sensitizers used in both plastics and rubber include naphthylamines, paraphenylenediamine derivatives, mercaptobenzothiazole, phenols, and epoxy resin hardeners.

Synthetic resins in the solid cured or fully polymerized state rarely cause dermatitis. The finished product is remarkably free of irritating or sensitizing properties. In the manufacture of these synthetic resins, however, there are many opportunities for contact with uncured resins, catalyzers, and modifiers, all of which may be skin irritants and sensitizers that readily produce dermatitis unless precautions are taken to protect the worker. In particular, epoxy resin systems have produced many instances of dermatitis.

> **Solid, completely polymerized resins rarely cause dermatitis. Incompletely cured resins may be irritants and sensitizers. The sawing and grinding of solid resins, however, may release sensitizers and irritants.**

It is possible that the sawing and grinding of completely polymerized resins may cause depolymerization with the release of chemicals that can cause irritation or sensitization. Such synthetic resin dust or grindings should be handled with the same precautions as those used with the unpolymerized chemicals.

Outside of industry, dermatitis due to synthetic resins is likely to occur only when the general population is exposed to the resins in the liquid or incompletely cured state, such as epoxy resin glues and adhesives, acrylic monomers used

TABLE 29.1. *Abbreviations for Names of Plastics*

Thermoplastics

ABS	Acrylonitrile/butadiene/styrene	acrylonitrile/butadiene/styrene plastic, ABS plastic
A/S/A	Acrylonitrile/styrene/acrylate	acrylonitrile/butadiene; acrylate plastic
CA	Cellulose acetate	
CAB	Cellulose acetate butyrate	
CAP	Cellulose acetate propionate	
CN	Cellulose nitrate	celluloid
E/P	Ethylene/propylene	
E/TFE	Ethylene/tetrafluoroethylene	
E/VAC	Ethylene/vinyl acetate	
FEP	perfluoro (ethylene/propylene), tetrafluoroethylene/hexafluoropropylene	
PA	Polyamide	polyamide
PB	Polybutylene	
PBTP	Polybutylene terephthalate	
PC	Polycarbonate	polycarbonate
PCTFE	Poly(chlorotrifluoroethylene)	
PE	Polyethylene, polyethene	ethylene plastic polyethylene
PELD	PE with low density	
PEMD	PE with medium density	
PEHD	PE with high density	
PETP	Poly(ethylene terephthalate)	
PEUHD	Polyethene, high density, high molecular	
PIB	Polylsobutylene	
PMMA	Poly(methyl methacrylate)	poly(methyl methacrylate)
POM	Polyoxymethylene	polyoxymethylene
PP	Polypropylene	propylene plastic polypropylene
PPO	Polyphenyleneoxide	
PPS	Polyphenylenesulfide	
PS	Polystyrene	styrene plastic, polystyrene
PTFE	Polytetrafluoroethylene	
PVAC	Poly(vinyl acetate)	vinyl acetate plastic, poly(vinylacetate)
PVAL	Poly(vinyl alcohol)	
PVB	Poly(vinyl butyral)	
PVC	Poly(vinyl chloride) nonrigid, flexible-plasticized rigid—normally not plasticized	vinyl chloride plastic, poly(vinyl chloride)
PVDC	Poly(vinylidene chloride)	vinylidene chloride plastic, poly(vinylidene chloride)
PVDF	Poly(vinylidene fluoride)	
PVFM	Poly(vinyl formal)	
SAN	Styrene acrylonitrile	styrene/acrylonitrile plastic
S/B	Styrene/butadiene	
SI	Silicone	silicone plastic

Thermosetting plastics and thermosets

EP	Epoxy resin	epoxy plastic
MF	Melamine-formaldehyde resin	
PF	Phenol-formaldehyde resin	
PUR	Polyurethane	urethane plastic
UF	Urea-formaldehyde resin	
UP	Unsaturated polyester	

to make artificial fingernails, and nail lacquer containing formaldehyde resins.

Synthetic resins producing dermatitis in the general population include:

1. **Acrylic nails and uncured acrylic dentures**
2. **Epoxy and formaldehyde resin glues and cements**
3. **Nail lacquer-toluene sulfonamide resin**

Patch Testing with Synthetic Resins

Tests with the chemicals involved in the manufacture of these resin systems must be performed with caution to avoid severe reactions. The correct concentrations and the proper vehicles for patch tests are still being evaluated. In the following discussion, suggestions are given for concentrations and for suitable vehicles. The solvents or vehicles should be chosen with care. Many resins can be incorporated in petrolatum (pet) for test purposes. Solvents generally useful include acetone, olive oil, and ethyl methyl ketone.

TABLE 29.2. *Resin Plasticizers*

Benzyl benzoate	5% pet[a]
Dibutyl phthalate	5% pet
Paratoluene sulfonamide	2% pet
Triacet	3% pet
Tricresyl phosphate	5% pet
Triphenyl phosphate	5% pet

[a]Pet = in petrolatum.

Acetone is a readily available unreactive solvent for the epoxy, polyester, and polyurethane monomers and prepolymers. When used as a solvent for urethane prepolymers, the acetone must be reasonably free of moisture. Because it is volatile, fresh solutions must be made for each patch test series.

Fregert (2) has suggested abbreviations for the names of plastics, as shown in Table 29.1. Table 29.2 lists common resin plasticizers with their patch test concentrations.

VINYL PLASTICS

The vinyl polymers (polyvinyl chloride, polyvinyl acetate, and polyvinyl alcohol) are not sensitizers, but certain additives may cause dermatitis. These polymers are thermoplastics. Table 29.3 lists the various additives that may sensitize and also the concentration for patch testing (3).

Saran and Other Vinyl Plastics

Saran, the generic name for certain polyvinylidene resins, may be used in belts, suspenders, and raincoats. Saran Wrap is used for occlusive dressings and may produce miliaria and maceration, particularly in patients who have atopic dermatitis. Dermatitis due to Saran Wrap has been reported (4). Plastics closely related to saran include the following polyvinyl resins: Elastiglass, Flamenol, Koroseal, Kogene, Korogel, and Vinylite Q.

TABLE 29.3. *Patch Testing with Vinyl Resins and Additives*

Vinyl resins	10% aq[a]
Additives	
Plasticizers	
Dibutyl phthalate	5% pet[a]
Diethyl phthalate	5% pet
Dioctyl phthalate	5% pet
Stabilizers	
Dibutyl tin dilaurate	0.5% pet
Dibutyl tin maleate	0.5% pet
Epoxy resin	2% pet
Ultraviolet light absorbers	
Benzophenones	1% pet
Resorcinol monobenzoate	1% pet
Aldehydes	
Glyoxal (dialdehyde)	1% aq

[a]Aq = aqueous; Pet = in petrolatum.

There have been reports of contact dermatitis caused by watchbands, garters, and suspenders made of Elastiglass, which is a vinyl acetate and a chloride polymerization product. The dermatitis in these cases was ascribed to traces of the plasticizer or stabilizer (dibutyl tin maleate or dibutyl sebacate) that was not removed properly during the production of Elastiglass (5).

Plastic mittens and tablecloths made of vinyl plastic may produce allergic contact dermatitis (6). Allergic skin reactions to epoxy resins used as plasticizers and stabilizers in polyvinyl chloride films have also been reported (7). PVC is used in leather cloth for clothes, shoes, upholstery packaging tags, and electrical insulation.

Hindson and Lawlor (8) reported an allergic reaction to glyoxal, a dialdehyde used in vinyl acetate to form an aqueous emulsion of an adhesive. This resin emulsion system is used in the manufacture of paints, adhesives, carpet backing, paper backing, wallpaper finishing, and as a plastic additive. A 10% aqueous solution of the resin emulsion gave a positive reaction, as did a 10% aqueous solution of the glyoxal.

Phthalates

Schulsinger and Mollgaard (9) reported seven cases of contact dermatitis in children due to identification bracelets made of polyvinyl chloride plastic. Patch tests with the bracelets were negative in the five cases tested. It is concluded that the reactions were irritant due to some unknown chemical in the bracelets. The authors stated that the most widely used plasticizer in PVC, phthalates, must have low sensitizing properties, as only one positive patch test was found in 1,532 patch tests with phthalate mK, performed as a joint study by the International Contact Dermatitis Research Group.

Two cases of contact dermatitis to the mouse attached to computers were found to be due to phthalates present in the plastic (10). One patient was sensitive to diethyl phthalate and the other to dimethyl phthalate, both tested at 5% in petrolatum. The manufacturers confirmed the presence of phthalates in the mice, and a cloth over the mice was preventive. Diethyl phthalate is used in most cellulose ester plastic commonly used to manufacture eyeglasses and hearing aids. Contact dermatitis to diethyl phthalate has been reported from these sources (11). Alternative materials that lack diethyl phthalate are Optyl (epoxy resin) and Perspec (methyl methacrylate) (11). The allergens in eyeglasses were reviewed by Nakada and Maibach (12). The allergens break down into metals, plastics, plasticizers, solvents, UV stabilizers, antioxidants, dyes, and waxes. The plastics include butyl acrylate, cellulose acetate, epoxy resin, and phenol-formaldehyde. The plasticizers include abietic acid, diethyl phthalate, tricresyl phosphate, triphenyl phosphate, and tritolyl phosphate. UV stabilizers include resorcinol monobenzoate and phenyl salicylate. Another source of allergy to plastic eyeglass frames is colophony, which is used to polish the plastic (13).

Fisher (14) reported plastic identification bracelets as a cause of PVC dermatitis in infants.

Toxic Vinyl Chloride Disease

Walker (15) reported that angiosarcoma of the liver and acroosteolysis (Raynaud's phenomena, lytic lesions of bone, and sclerodermatous skin changes) are recognized as occupational hazards in men engaged in the process of polymerization of vinyl chloride to PVC.

Over a 1-year period, 30 men from a local PVC plant were treated for symptomatic complaints of coldness and paresthesia of the hands or feet. Additional symptoms included undue fatigue, muscle and joint pains, dyspnea, and impotence. A severe but variable acrocyanosis of the hands and feet was observed in at least 10 patients. Radiologic bone changes were demonstrated in only two men, and these alterations were minimal. Skin histology revealed fragmentation of the elastic tissue in the dermis and abnormal staining of the collagen. Sclerodermatous skin changes were not present.

Arteriograms in the more severely affected patients demonstrated narrowing of the digital vessels. Finger blood flow and skin temperature fell dramatically when the patients were subjected to cool environments. Immunologic investigations in 20 patients revealed cryoglobulins or cryofibrinogen in 14 patients. Respiratory investigations suggested a perfusion impairment that is unexplained as yet.

Ward et al. (16) stated that a metabolite of vinyl chloride binds to plasma or tissue protein to form an antigen that is the possible toxin in toxic vinyl disease.

> **Toxic vinyl chloride disease, an occupational hazard in the manufacture of polyvinyl chloride, consists of Raynaud's phenomena, lytic disease of bone, and scleroderma.**

EPOXY RESINS

The epoxy resins probably cause more instances of occupational dermatitis, both in the United States and in other countries, than do any other chemicals introduced in recent years.

> **There are many types of epoxy resins, with most being based on the use of bisphenol A and epichlorohydrin to produce 4,4'-isopropylidenediphenol-epichlorohydrin resins, ranging in molecular weight from 340 to above 12,000, and from a liquid to high melting solid with increasing molecular weight.**

The versatile epoxy (epoxide or ethoxylene) resins are used widely in manufacturing electrical equipment for enclosing transformers, condensers, and other components, in automobile plants for tool and die casting, in paints for surface coating, and in aircraft and other industries for adhesive purposes.

Ingredients of Epoxy Resin Systems

In the manufacture and use of epoxy resins, individuals may acquire dermatitis from one or more of the following chemicals, which may be incorporated in the epoxy resin system:

Blends of other resins
Catalytic agents consisting of amines and anhydrides, which are called converters, hardeners, or curing agents
Fillers
Pigments
Plasticizers
Reactive diluents
Solvents
Uncured epoxy resin (liquid or solid)

The most frequently encountered sources of occupational dermatoses from epoxy resins have been diglycidyl ether of bisphenol A, which is the standard screening substance, 4,4'-diaminodiphenylmethane phenyl glycidyl ether and o-cresyl glycidyl ether (17). A series of compounds and patch test concentrations have been recommended (Table 29.4) (17).

Uncured Epoxy Resins

A typical uncured epoxy resin is obtained by the condensation of epichlorohydrin and p,p'-isopropylidenediphenol (bisphenol A). Other epoxy resins are condensates consisting of a mixture of polyglycidyl ethers. Epoxy resins are of little use in the form in which they are supplied to the market. They must be further polymerized or cured by the addition of curing agents, such as amines, amides, anhydrides, or inorganic fluoride compounds. Cured epoxy resins are hard, relatively insoluble materials that are nonirritating and nonsensitizing.

For patch testing purposes, bisphenol A may be used in a 1% concentration in pet. Bisphenol A is, at present, a standard patch testing substance. It must be emphasized that a negative reaction to bisphenol A does not rule out epoxy dermatitis, because the epoxy dermatitis may be due to curing agents.

About 75% of epoxy resins used worldwide are based on diglycidyl ether of bisphenol A. Allergic contact dermatitis has also been reported with other resins including heterocyclic dimethylhydantoin epoxy resin, phenol novolate epoxy resin, and brominated epoxy resin (18). These latter substances are found in electrical insulation, coil winding and cleaning of work sites, respectively.

TABLE 29.4. *Test Substances (see footnotes for suppliers) Used in Patch Testing of Patients Exposed to Epoxy Resin Compounds*

Test substance	Concentration % (w/w) in pet
Epoxy resins (ER)	
Standard epoxy resin (DGEBA-ER)[a]	1
CA epoxy resin (CA-ER)	
Araldit CY 184[b]	1
Lekuthern X100[b]	1
Amine hardeners (AHs)	
Ethylenediamine (EDA)[c]	1
Diethylenetriamine (DETA)[d]	1
Triethylenetetramine (TETA)[c]	0.5[e]
4,4′-diaminodiphenylmethane (MDA)[c]	0.5
Isophoronediamine (IPDA)[f]	0.5
Reactive diluents (RDs)	
n-butyl glycidyl ether (BGE)[f]	0.25
phenyl glycidyl ether (PGE)[f]	0.25
o-cresyl glycidyl ether (o-CGE)[f]	0.25
Allyl glycidyl ether (AGE)[g]	0.25
Butanediol diglycidyl ether (BDDGE)[g]	0.25
Hexanediol diglycidyl ether (Grilonit RV 1812)[g]	0.25
Neopentyl glycol diglycidyl ether (Grilonit RV 1815)[g]	0.25
Glycidyl ester of synthetic fatty acids (Cardura E 10)[g]	0.25
Glycidyl ether of aliphatic alcohols (Epoxide 8)[g]	0.25
Others	
Bisphenol A[c]	1
Epichlorohydrin[h]	0.1–0.3[h]
BIS-GMA[d]	2
BIS-MA[d]	2

Adapted with permission from Jolanki R, Kanerva L, Estlander T, et al. Occupational dermatoses from epoxy resin compounds. *Contact Dermatitis* 1990;23:172.

[a]Epikon Oy, Helsinki, Finland (from 1984 to Sept. 1985) Chemotechnique. Diagnostics AB, Malmo, Sweden (since Sept. 1985).

[b]See Ref. 4 (included in patch tests since Sept. 1985).

[c]Chemotechnique Diagnostics AB, Malmo, Sweden; during 1984 Epikon Oy in 7 patients and both suppliers in 17 patients.

[d]Chemotechnique Diagnostics AB.

[e]TETA of Chemotechnique Diagnostics AB diluted in water.

[f]Trolab, Hermal-Chemie Kurt Herrmann, Hamburg, Germany (included in patch tests since Sept. 1985).

[g]See Ref. 7 (included in patch tests since Sept. 1985).

[h]Epikon Oy (0.3% pet in 25 patients) from 1984 to Sept. 1985; Trolab since Sept. 1985 (0.1% pet).

> **Epoxy resin dermatitis can be due either to bisphenol A, which is present in the standard patch test tray, or to one of numerous "curing" agents that are not in the standard tray.**

Catalysts and Curing Agents

These chemicals speed the polymerization of epoxy resin. Liquid epoxy compounds can be cured to form hard, insoluble products by polymerization in the presence of catalysts or by polyaddition with cross-linking agents containing active hydrogen atoms. These curing agents or hardeners may act at either room or elevated temperatures and have been divided into the following four categories:

1. Amine hardeners (e.g., aliphatic polyamines and aminopolyamides)
2. Acid hardeners (e.g., polycarboxylic acids and dicarboxylic acid anhydrides)
3. Aldehyde condensation products (e.g., phenol, melamine, and urea-formaldehyde resins)
4. Inorganic or organic metallic compounds (e.g., boron trifluoride, titanium acid ester, and aluminum alcoholate)

Of this host of chemicals, amine hardeners appear to be the most potent sensitizers.

Epoxy Amine Hardeners

The amines are used particularly when the epoxy resin is cured, catalyzed, or self-hardened at room temperature.

These agents are usually aliphatic amines, such as diethylenetriamine, triethylenetetramine, and metaphenylenediamine, an aromatic amine hardener. In the uncombined state, they are caustic and can produce severe burns on contact with the skin. In addition, they can cause a severe allergic contact dermatitis characterized by severe redness, edema, and itching of the exposed parts. The aliphatic hardeners, diethylenetriamine and triethylenetetramine, are powerful water-soluble skin irritants. Airborne allergic contact dermatitis has been reported from the widely used hardener isophoronediamine (3-aminomethyl-3,5,5-trimethylcyclohexylamine). A 0.5% pet patch test concentration was used (19).

For patch testing purposes, a 0.1% aqueous solution may be used if no published reports are available. Even at this low concentration, controls should be used to make certain that positive results are not due to a primary irritant effect. Patch testing with "amine" hardeners may also be done with a 1% concentration in pet.

> **The amine epoxy "hardeners" or curing agents are powerful irritants and potent sensitizers. In addition, epoxy resin diluents, solvents, modifiers, and plasticizers can cause dermatitis.**

Other Hardeners

Another class of epoxy hardeners is the phthalic anhydrides. Kanerva et al. (20) reported a patient who was allergic to methylhexahydrophthalic anhydride. This compound and methyltetrahydrophthalic anhydride have been associated with contact urticaria and immunologically mediated respiratory disease. Their patient had coexistent immediate and delayed hypersensitivity.

Occupational Contact Urticaria

Hardeners for epoxy resins include dicarboxylic anhydrides. Inhalation of such compounds has led to urticaria, and skin contact with methylhexahydrophthalic anhydride and methyltetrahydrophthalic anhydride caused contact urticaria in patients with only airborne exposure (21).

Polyfunctional aziridine hardener (PFA), which is used in paints, primers, lacquers, and other protective coatings, has caused both contact urticaria and contact dermatitis (22). PFA hardener is synthesized from ethyleneimine or propyleneimine and a multifunctional acrylate such as pentaerythritol triacrylate or trimethylolpropane triacrylate (TMPTA). PFA hardener has been found as a contaminant in some TMPTA. In cases of dermatitis, no reactions were found to the materials from which PFA hardener is synthesized. A 1% aqueous concentration of PFA hardener is recommended for patch testing. Aziridine hardeners are associated with polyurethane plastics. One product demon-

strated to contain such chemicals is Neocryl CX 100, which contains TMPTA derivatives (23).

The epoxy hardener 2,4,6-tris(dimethylaminomethyl) phenol is a sensitizer but is not commonly found on commercially available resin series. Brooke and Beck (24) found a 0.5% concentration free of irritant reactions in 50 controls and suitable for identification of allergy.

Amine hardeners were a source of contact dermatitis in a Finnish painter (25). Over the years he was followed, he reacted to multiple hardeners, one of which had not previously been reported to cause contact dermatitis: tetraethylenepentamine.

Dermatitis rather than urticaria occurred after airborne exposure to the epoxy resin hardener 3-amino-methyl-3,5,5-trimethylcyclohexylamine (26). A patch test concentration of 1% in petrolatum is recommended.

Blends of Other Resins

Epoxy resins may be blended with urea-formaldehyde, phenol-formaldehyde, and melamine-formaldehyde resins, all of which are potential sensitizers and irritants.

Nonindustrial Exposure to Epoxy Resins

Epoxy glues are becoming increasingly popular for household use. They are made available in two parts, the hardener and the resin. The labels on the containers state that ingredients contacting the skin should immediately be removed with soap and water. It is claimed that the versatile epoxy glues can cement anything to anything. Artists and sculptors find many uses for these glues, and some have acquired epoxy resin dermatitis.

> **Epoxy resins may be present in household adhesives and glues and be blended with formaldehyde and with polyvinyl resins.**

Table 29.5 lists a standard epoxy resin series. It should be emphasized, however, that patch testing with the various epoxy resins in a "routine" series may fail to detect epoxy

TABLE 29.5. *Standard Epoxy Resin Patch Test Series[a]*

Araldite 670 (CIBA) (low molecular weight epoxy resin)	1% pet
Araldite 6060 (CIBA) (high molecular weight)	1% pet
Bisphenol A	1% acetone or pet
Epon 828 (Shell) (low molecular weight epoxy resin)	1% pet
Epon 1001 (Shell) (high molecular weight)	1% pet

Pet = in petrolatum
[a]Range: from molecular weight 340 to above 1,200.

resin sensitivity unless one tests with the patient's own sample of epoxy resin and with one of many epoxy hardeners or diluents.

Allergic contact stomatitis occurred from acrylic dental filling materials, Concise and Concise Composite (27). The patient was also allergic to epoxy resin from the standard tray. In Concise materials, the main acrylic compounds are triethylene glycol dimethacrylate and 2,2-bis-[4-(2-methacryloxypropoxy)phenyl]propane (bis-GMA). Because both epoxy resin and bis-GMA are derivatives of bisphenol A, it is likely that the positive patch test to epoxy resin was due to cross-sensitivity to the bisphenol A derivatives in the Concise.

Taylor (28) identified the source of epoxy resin positive patch tests in three children who had been wearing certain sizes of Sears, Roebuck and Co. Toughskin or Roughouser jeans with knee patches. Each child had eczema about the knees and also had positive patch tests to pieces of knee patches. Epon 828 (4,4-isopropyledene diphenylepichlorhydrin) was added to the knee patch adhesive as an adhesion promoter. One child had a positive patch test to Epon 828 at a dilution of 1:20,000. Sears substituted a nonepoxy adhesive for the knee patch of its jeans (28).

Approximately 5% to 10% of the underwear produced in Japan is said to be treated with an epoxy-lanolin softener (29).

Low and High Molecular Epoxy Resins

The low molecular resins Epon 828 and Araldite 670 are more potent sensitizers than the high molecular variety such as Epon 1001 or Araldite 6060. The low molecular epoxy resins have a lower viscosity and have a much greater ability to wet and penetrate the skin than do the higher variety.

It is mainly the epoxy resin oligomer of molecular weight 340 that is responsible for epoxy resin allergy (30). Occasionally, however, an epoxy resin of high molecular weight may produce sensitization, and some products regarded as safe because of high average molecular weight may contain significant quantities of the molecular weight 340 oligomer (31). When this oligomer and the oligomer of molecular weight 624 are absent, the product can usually be regarded as safe for practical purposes. This opens up opportunities for the primary prevention of epoxy resin sensitization.

The lower the molecular weight of an epoxy resin, the greater the allergenic potential.

Dahlquist and Fregert (32) proposed that when the face and eyelids are involved in an epoxy dermatitis, it is probable that there has also been sensitization to the curing agent or hardeners. The volatility of epoxy resin is so low that it is unlikely that sufficient fumes are in the air to involve the face. This indicates the importance of patch testing patients with suspected epoxy resin dermatitis with the hardeners. A greater emphasis on patch testing with the hardeners that the patient has actually used should enable further preventive recommendations to be made.

Epoxy resin curing agents, because they are more volatile than epoxy resin itself, are more likely to produce facial dermatitis than is the resin.

Table 29.6 lists some epoxy resin trade names and their producers. A spot test for the presence of epoxy resins may be valuable, because not all producers will divulge the contents of their products.

Spot Test for Bisphenol A Type Epoxy Resin with Sulfuric Acid Procedure

Dissolve the sample (about 0.1 g) in 2 mL of concentrated sulfuric acid by heating to 40° to 50°C on a water bath (33). Dilute, if necessary, with concentrated sulfuric acid until the color intensity is similar to that of 0.1 mole $\times$ 1^{-1} potassium dichromate solution (orange). With the aid of a glass rod, streak a drop of the epoxy resin solution across a piece of filter paper. If bisphenol A type of epoxy resins are present, the streaks will turn purple within 1 minute; the color eventually turns blue. A control test on an epoxy resin of the bisphenol A type should be carried out at the same time.

In this test both cured and uncured epoxy resins of bisphenol A type react positively. The sensitivity of this test is reduced in the presence of substances that darken in concentrated sulfuric acid. Such materials are other binders, for example, fish oil, tung oil, oiticica oil, linseed oil treated with cyclopentadiene, rosin, rosin esters, and some phenolic resins. They turn pink to red, which may cause confusion. Dilution to an approximate color makes the test specific for epoxy resins of bisphenol A type.

There are several reports of allergic contact dermatitis due to epoxy resin curing agents (Table 29.7) and diluents (Table 29.8) (34–39).

Reactive diluents used in epoxy resin systems include the glycidyl ethers. de Groot (39) identified three chemical plant employees who were sensitized to alpha-naphthyl glycidyl ether and p-fluorphenyl glycidyl ether. A patch test concentration of 1% in petrolatum was positive in all sensitized workers. A guinea pig maximization assay of alpha-naphthyl glycidyl ether sensitized all 20 animals. Other reactive diluents that have been reported to cause contact dermatitis are listed in Table 29.8.

Marble workers who were exposed to both epoxy resin and reactive diluents developed contact dermatitis more commonly to the diluent than the resin (40). The most frequent diluent was ortho-cresyl glycidyl ether in 10 of 22

TABLE 29.6. *Some Epoxy Resin Trade Names and Procedures*

Balkamp E-Pox-Cement
  Balkamp, Inc.; Mfr., Woodhill Chemical
Balkamp E-Pox-E Glue
  Balkamp, Inc.; Mfr., Woodhill Chemical
Balkamp E-Pox-E Steel
  Balkamp, Inc.; Mfr., Woodhill Chemical
Browning Silaflex Point-Fast Adhesive
  Browning
Carter's Epoxy Cement
  Carter's Ink
Colma Bonding Compound
  Sika Chem.
Colma-Dur, Regular and Gel
  Sika Chem.
Colma Kote M
  Sika Chem.
Colma Penetrating Grout
  Sika Chem.
Colma Sol
  All colors except green
  Sika Chem.
Colma Surface-Kote
  Sika Chem.
DAP One-Part Flexiseal
  DAP
DAP One-Part Flexiseal
  DAP
Duratite Epoxy Glue
  DAP
Enterprise Epox-Eze
  Laundry tub and appliance finish
  Enterprise Paint Mfg.
Epoxite
  Waterproofer
  Boyle-Midway
Epoxybond Paste
  Atlas Minerals & Chemicals Div.
Epoxybond Putty
  Atlas Minerals & Chemicals Div.
Jewel "Tile Like" Epoxy Enamel
  Jewel Paint & Varnish Co.
Kabo 612 Coating
  Knight, M.A.
Kentile Adhesive No. 9
  Epoxy type
  Kentile

LePage's Epoxy Glue
  LePage's
Magicolor New Look Epoxy Finish
  Enterprise Paint Mfg.
Mira-Plate Chemical Resistant Epoxy-Harbor Green
  O'Brien Corp.
Mira-Plate Clear
  Epoxy coating
  O'Brien Corp.
Plasti-Kote Epoxy Super Durable Spray Paint
  Plasti-Kote
Pratt's Spreader-Sticker
  Pratt, G.G.
PRC 940 Patching and Surfacing Compound
  Products Research
Safe Step
  Corrosion resistant and antislip finish
  Lester Labs.
Sears Craftsman Epoxy Cement 9-8059
  Sears, Roebuck
Super Everwear Gym Finish
  Uncle Same
Ten-Set
  Epoxy adhesive and putty; general use
  Fibre Glass-Evercoat
Troxymite
  Texas Refinery
Tuffy "C"
  Corrosion resistant finish
  Lester Labs.
USG Epoxy Block Filler Activator
  U.S. Gypsum
Velsicol Chlorendic Anhydride
  Fire retardant paints, epoxy curing agent, and specialty esters
  Velsicol
Weldwood Epoxy Cement
  Adhesive
  U.S. Plywood-Champion Papers Inc.
Wilhold Clear Epoxy Adhesive
  Wilhold Glues, Inc.
Wilhold Epoxy Cement for Concrete
  Wilhold Glues, Inc.
X-Pando Trav Mar
  Waterproofing basement wall; general adhesive

TABLE 29.7. *Epoxy Curing Agents or "Hardeners"*

Amino resin	1% pet
Diethylenetriamine (aliphatic polyamine hardener)	1% pet
Esterification with fatty or rosin acids	1% pet
Ethylenediamine hydrochloride	1% pet
Ketamines	1% pet
Lewis-type acids	1% pet
Metaphenylenediamine (aromatic amine hardener)	2% pet
Phenolic resin	1% pet
Phthalic anhydride (epoxy resin hardener)	1% pet
Triethylenetetramine (aliphatic polyamine hardener)	1% pet

Pet = in petrolatum.

TABLE 29.8. *Reactive Epoxy Diluents*

Allyl glycidyl ether
1,4-butanediol diglycidyl ether
n-butyl glycidyl ether
Cardura E10 (glycidyl ether or synthetic fatty acids)
o-cresyl glycidyl ether
Epoxide 7 (glycidyl ethers of aliphatic alcohols with predominantly C8 and C10 alkyl groups)
Epoxide 8 (glycidyl ethers of aliphatic alcohols with predominantly C12 and C14 alkyl groups)
1,6-hexanediol diglycidyl ether
Neopentyl glycol diglycidyl ether
Phenyl glycidyl ether

workers. In this same group, only four patients reacted to epoxy resin.

At times a product will produce contact dermatitis, but upon product analysis it has been found that the ingredients are not the stated ingredients and the contaminant present in the material is the actual allergen. This is somewhat common in the plastic/acrylate type of resin systems. A case of this type was reported by Dooms-Goossens et al. (41). A 43-year-old man who worked in the plastics industry was allergic to epoxy silane, but the actual allergen was a contaminant allyl glycidyl ether, which is a reactive epoxy diluent.

An aircraft factory worker developed urticaria and angioedema when working around epoxy resins (42). Delayed-type patch tests were negative, but patch tests applied for 30 minutes, removed, and read showed immediate whealing from epoxy resin 1% in petrolatum, phenyl glycidyl ether 0.25% in petrolatum, and cresyl glycidyl ether 0.25% in petrolatum. In discussing his case, Sasseville (42) pointed out that aliphatic polyamine hardeners, phthalic anhydrides, and epoxy resins have caused immediate reactions. The reactive diluents, which are highly volatile, was an unexpected additional finding.

The fact that patients sensitized to ethylenediamine hydrochloride from exposure to original formula Mycolog Cream may show cross-reactions with certain "amine" hardening agents is important (35,43,44).

Lachapelle and Lachapelle-Ketelaer (45) reported cross-sensitivity between an isophorone amine and isophorone disocyanate.

Table 29.9 shows the numerous exposures from the use of epoxy resins. Epoxy resin dermatitis has been described from a pacemaker and from a hemodialysis set (46,47). There are several reports of epoxy resin adhesives and glues that have produced unusual forms of contact dermatitis (48–50).

Fregert et al. (51) traced a hand dermatitis in a patient who had a contact dermatitis of the hands due to an unhardened epoxy resin that he had applied to certain sign boards. These authors emphasized that epoxy resin hardened at room temperature is seldom if ever completely cured.

Prevention of Epoxy Resin Dermatitis

Sigfrid Fregert, who made outstanding contributions to the study of various types of contact dermatitis, suggested that the following criteria should be met to help prevent epoxy resin dermatitis (International Symposium in Lund, Sweden, 1977):

1. Epoxy oligomer of molecular weight 340 should not be included, or at least only in a low concentration.
2. Epoxy oligomer of molecular weight 624 should probably be present only in a low concentration.
3. Reactive diluents should be of the high molecular weight type, probably over 1,000.
4. Hardeners should be of the adduct type and should not contain remains of aliphatic amines. It is probable that even polyaminoamides are free from risk when they do not contain remains of aliphatic amines.

Estlander et al. (52) found that the epoxy chemical bisphenol A can be found in some PVC gloves. Although bisphenol A is a nonsensitizer in the guinea pig maximization test, it is a weak sensitizer in humans and caused glove dermatitis in the patients of Estlander et al. Gas chromatography confirmed the presence of bisphenol A in the glove.

FORMALDEHYDE RESINS

Formaldehyde may be combined with the chemicals listed in Table 29.10 to produce various types of resins. Individuals allergic or sensitive to a formaldehyde-based resin may react either to formaldehyde alone or, more commonly, to the monomers themselves. Many such persons do not have positive patch test reactions to formaldehyde; thus, formaldehyde cannot be used reliably for screening.

> **Many individuals with allergic hypersensitivity to a formaldehyde resin are not allergic to formaldehyde itself.**

TABLE 29.9. *Uses of Epoxy Resins*

Adhesives
  All-purpose, aircraft, electrical, constructional, domestic, ceramic, metallic, waterproof, furniture, furnace gaskets, fiberglass, and metal cements
Product finishing
  Aircraft, road and bridge coating, appliance finishes, appliance primers, automotive primers, can and drum linings, chemical resistant finishes, pipe and tank linings, flame retardants, industrial floorings, equipment (marine, masonry finished), and wall panel coatings
Laminates
  Structural, electrical, and fibrous reinforcements, and filament windings
Electrical
  Encapsulations for transformers, coils, and motors
Polyvinyl chloride films in which epoxy resins have been used as stabilizers and plasticizers
  For example, in plastic gloves, adhesive tapes, plastic panties, handbags, chamber pots, and beads in necklaces
Miscellaneous industrial
  Applications: toolings and die casting, model making, jigs and fixtures, molding and patterns, marine varnishes, artistic and sculptural use

TABLE 29.10. *Types of Formaldehyde Resins*

Cashew nut shell oil
Melamine
Phenols (including *p*-tert-butylphenol)
Resorcin
Urea (dimethylene urea)

The various formaldehyde resins may be tested 5% to 10% in pet.

Phenol-Formaldehyde Resins

The phenols listed in Table 29.11 are used in phenol-formaldehyde resins. Besides formaldehyde, furfural may be used to produce "phenoplasts."

Products such as paper laminates and Bakelite are examples of phenol-formaldehyde resins. Fregert (53) reported that Bakelite may produce both allergic and irritant dermatitis. Two patients gave a positive patch test to Bakelite powder 10% in pet.

> **Bakelite, a phenol-formaldehyde resin, may produce allergic reactions. The Bakelite powder can produce an irritant reaction.**

p-tert-Butylphenol-Formaldehyde Resins

These resins are used in many adhesive and glue formulations, particularly in shoes, and are common sensitizers (53–60). As a rule, the sensitizing agent in these phenol-formaldehyde resins is the p-tert-butylphenol and not the phenol or formaldehyde.

Occupational groups at greatest risk are adhesive workers, plywood and box makers, foundry workers, dental personnel, brake-lining workers, textile manufacturers and handlers, insulation makers, leather finishers, automobile industry workers, and shoemakers.

Table 29.12 lists the wide variety of exposure to p-tert-butylphenol. An unusual case of occupational aphonia and dyspnea with type 1 and type 1 hypersensitivity to p-tert-butylphenol-formaldehyde in glass-wool was described by Kalimo et al. (61).

p-tert-butylphenol has proved to be a depigmenting agent in several patients (59,62,63). p-tert-butylphenol, by itself, may be tested 1% in pet. The resin may be tested 10% in pet.

> **There is wide exposure to p-tert-butylphenol, which is not only a potent sensitizer but also a depigmenting agent both in industry and among consumers.**

TABLE 29.11. *Phenols Used in Phenol-Formaldehyde Resins*

Alkyl phenols	Phenol
Bisphenol A	Resorcinol
Cresol	Xylenol
p-tert-phenylphenol	

TABLE 29.12. *p-tert-Butylphenol: Uses and Where Found*

Antioxidant and heat stabilizer in neoprene cements
Color film developers
Demulsifier for oil field drilling use
Deodorants and commercial disinfectants
Duplicating paper
Germicide detergents
Insecticides
Intermediate for rubber antioxidants
Intermediate in manufacture of varnish and lacquer resins
Leather articles laminated with neoprene contact cement
Motor and synthetic oils
Plasticizer for cellulose acetate
Printing inks
Resins to give latex glues initial adhesive force
Rubber cements, especially in shoes
Stabilizer in some cellulose ester plastics

p-tert-butylcatechol (PTBC) has been incorporated into both acrylic and polyester prosthetic devices. It was also found in Thermo-Fax paper in the 1950s and in PVC manufacturing, where occupational leukoderma can occur (64). Styrene frequently contains PTBC at a final concentration of 0.005% in cured resin, which has been reported to cause dermatitis (64).

Edwards and Edwards (65) reported that a Styrofoam flotation device known as "spoodles" due to a physical resemblance to noodles caused eight cases of axillary dermatitis, three of which were patch tested to the device with positive results. They incriminated polystyrene as the allergen, but no chemical analysis for contaminate or uncured resins was done. One of their patients exhibited contact urticaria to the patch test as well as delayed vesicular reaction.

Use of a standard group of allergens to screen for plastic and glue sensitization was evaluated in 839 patients over a period of 7 years (66). Only 52 had any reaction to this collection of 31 allergens, and the most prevalent was p-tertiary-butylphenol-formaldehyde resin (9 cases). There were 7 cases of diaminodiphenyl methane sensitivity and 5 colophony sensitive cases. The yield with this series of allergens supplied by Chemotechnique was quite low.

The standard patch test material p-tert-butylphenol formaldehyde resin can be a clue to sensitization to p-tert-butyl catechol. Zimerson and Bruze (67) were able to identify p-tert-butyl catechol as present in some brands of p-tert-butylphenol formaldehyde resin. Phenyl formaldehyde resin–sensitive patients were found to be commonly allergic to 2-methylol phenol and at times to other closely related methylol phenols (68).

The resin systems in marking pens can cause contact dermatitis (69). Ingredients identified include ninhydrin, arochean (phenolic formaldehyde maleic anhydride resin), 2-hydroxy-5-tert-butyl benzylalcohol, and 2,6-bis(hydroxymethyl)-4-tert-butylphenol. The latter compound is thought to cross-react with the common screening allergen 4-tert-butylphenol formaldehyde resin.

Urea-Formaldehyde Resins

These thermosetting resins are used in the products listed in Table 29.13. The urea-formaldehyde resins are commonly used as textile finishes. Allergic reactions to these finishes are rare except when extreme conditions such as heat, water, chloride, and alkali produce dimethyl- or urea-containing compounds that are contact sensitizers.

In addition, formaldehyde may be released from certain inferior urea-formaldehyde press plates and isolating foams (70). Hjorth and Fregert (71) reported that of 67 patients sensitized by urea-formaldehyde, 51 (76%) also reacted to formaldehyde.

A case of contact urticaria due to formaldehyde in a urea-formaldehyde resin adhesive has been reported (72).

> Urea-formaldehyde resins may cause textile dermatitis by breaking down and releasing formaldehyde. Sensitivity to the resin and formaldehyde is often associated.

Melamine-Formaldehyde Resin

Melamine-formaldehyde is a rare sensitizer. It is used extensively in tableware because the polymerized resin has good heat and water resistance and does not stain readily.

There is one report of an orthopedic cast reinforced with melamine-formaldehyde resin that produced a formaldehyde dermatitis in several patients (73). Fregert (74) described formaldehyde dermatitis from gypsum molds containing melamine-formaldehyde. Romaguera et al. (75) reported purpura from formaldehyde-urea-melamine resin.

Cashew Nut Oil–Formaldehyde Resin

Cashew nut oil has been combined with formaldehyde to form brake linings and clutch facings.

Patch Testing with Formaldehyde Resins

The following concentrations and vehicles are suggested for patch test procedures:

1. Phenol-formaldehyde resins 10% in pet
2. *p*-tert-butylphenol-formaldehyde resin 10% in pet
3. *p*-tert-butylphenol 10% in pet
4. Formaldehyde 2% in water
5. Hexamethylenetetramine 1% in pet
6. Furfuraldehyde 5% in water

ACRYLIC PLASTICS

The widely used acrylic resins, like the epoxy resins, may produce many instances of allergic and irritant dermatitis.

General Uses of Acrylic Resins

Possible exposures to acrylic compounds are listed by Malten (70) in Table 29.14. Acrylates and methacrylate compounds are used in leather finishing, as a textile size, in adhesives, paints, oil additives, utensils, artificial joints, lenses, and windows, and to produce artificial rubber and synthetic fibers. Moreover, diacrylates can be used as cross-links between polycondensates of unsaturated polyesters, for example, electron beam copolymerization in spray paints to multiple large surfaces such as doors, or in the production of photopolymer printing plates. Bullous irritant reactions in workers in the platemaking industry may be due to the irritant effect of tetraethylene glycol diacrylates. These diacrylates can also produce allergic reactions in sensitized persons who were unable to continue their work even when protected by gloves. The 4-H glove (Safety 4A/S 95 Lundtofte Gardsuen, P.O. Box 238, DK 2800, Lyngby, Denmark) has been recommended for protection against acrylates (76). This same glove has been found to be effective in epoxy resin exposure for up to 8 hours (77).

Ethyl acrylate has been used for decades as a basic material in compounding perfumes, but the Research Institute for Fragrance Materials discourages its use for this purpose.

TABLE 29.13. *Uses of Urea-Formaldehyde Resins*

Bottle caps	Surface coatings
Electric fittings	Textile resins
Isolating foams	Wood glues
Press plates	

TABLE 29.14. *Possible Exposures to Acrylic Compounds*

Construction adhesive, sealer, and stopper	Paint, adhesive, and additive to concrete
Cosmetics	Hair spray, fragrance, dentifrice, nail polish, and insecticide
Medical	Eye, dental, vascular prostheses, heart valve, artificial joint, contact lens, eyeglasses, adhesive plaster, wound spray, infusion system, and splint
Printing	Ultraviolet curable ink, photopolymer and flexographic printing plate
Textile	Fiber, finish (and on leather)
Utensils	Plexiglas, veneer, and synthetic rubber
Miscellaneous	Plastic foam, molecular sieve, gel electrophoresis, additive to lubricant, mineral sedimentation, soil improver, and water purification

Glycidyl methacrylate may give reactions to methacrylate-sensitive patients as well as to those sensitized to epoxy resins. The same holds true for a diacrylate ester of an epoxy resin (e.g., diglycidyl ether of bisphenol A), a member of a new class of products that may be called epoxy acrylate resins and that may be used for applications involving ultraviolet light or electron beam–initiated cross-linking.

> **"Epoxy acrylate" compounds, in which cross-linking is accomplished by ultraviolet light or electron beam, expose workers to both epoxy and acrylate sensitization.**

Malten (70) lists the known acrylic compound sensitizers shown in Table 29.15.

Use of a screening series of 30 acrylates in 275 patients over a 10-year period of time in Finland revealed that the most commonly encountered allergenic substances were 2-hydroxyethyl acrylate (12%), 2-hydroxypropyl methacrylate (12%), and 2-hydroxyethyl methacrylate (11%) (78). This should not be taken to imply that these substances are the most allergenic, as frequency of use and likelihood of contact with skin or mucous membranes have a controlling influence in the type of patient seen in patch test clinics.

The ingredients declared on material product safety data sheets can be unreliable in terms of a full disclosure of the true components of acrylic resins. Henriks-Eckerman and Kanerva (79) used gas chromatography and mass spectrometric methods to analyze 10 acrylic products.

Windshields are repaired with acrylates, and contact dermatitis to common acrylate allergens has been seen in workers exposed to this material. Hydroxyethyl methacrylate is one of the allergens likely to be found in this setting (80).

Chemists are exposed to novel compounds and concentrations of compounds that may not occur widely in the environment. A 31-year-old chemist developed contact dermatitis to glycidyl methacrylate and ethoxyethyl acrylate used to make textiles and paper water resistant (81). A concentration of 0.05% in acetone was positive to both compounds, and nitrile gloves were protective if used for no more than 1 day.

Acrylic Nails

The original concerns about acrylic nails focused on methyl methacrylate. Freeman et al. (82) reported four cases of acrylic nail–related changes consisting of nail fold, fingertip, and hand dermatitis, as well as face and neck reactions and dystrophic nails and fingertip paresthesias. Three of their cases were due to ethylene glycol dimethacrylate, and these cases did not react to methyl methacrylate.

A study of 11 patients with acrylate allergy associated with artificial nails found the most frequent sensitizers to be ethyl acrylate, 2-hydroxyethyl acrylate, ethylene glycol dimethacrylate, ethyl alpha cyanoacrylate, and triethylene glycol diacrylate (83).

Nail polish is usually associated with toluenesulfonamide-formaldehyde resin, now known as tosyl amine formaldehyde resin. Substitutes for this sensitizer have been introduced. One such material is methyl acrylate, which when present in nail polish has been identified as a cause of contact dermatitis by Kanerva et al. (84). This acrylate does not cure completely, and free monomer is still present in the hardened state.

Circuit Boards

The manufacture of circuit boards involves the use of silk-screen application of inks. Allergens identified in this process include diaminodiphenylmethane, 2-hydroxyethyl methacrylate, and triglycidyl isocyanurate (85). The latter is a trifunctional epoxy compound made from epichlorohydrin and isocyanuric acid. It is a hardener in thermosetting one-component polyester powder coatings, and it has been patch tested at a concentration of 0.1% to 10% w/w in petrolatum.

Open versus Closed Systems

Acrylic polymerized products manufactured in closed systems are usually not irritants or sensitizers. Polymerization

---

TABLE 29.15. *Acrylic Compound Sensitizers*[a]

Acrylamide
Acrylated epoxy resin
Acrylated polyester
Acrylonitrile
Butanediol diacrylate
Butyl acrylate
n-butyl acrylate
tert-butyl acrylate
Butyl methacrylate
Diethylene glycol dimethacrylate
Dipentaerythritol monohydroxypenta-acrylate
Ethyl acrylate
2-ethylbutyl acrylate
2-ethylhexyl acrylate
Ethyl methacrylate
Glycidyl acrylate
1,6-hexanediol diacrylate
Hexahydro- 1,3,5-triacrylol-*s*-triazine
2-hydroxyethyl methacrylate
1-hydroxypropyl methacrylate
Methyl methacrylate
N-methylol acrylamide
N,N'-methylenebis (acrylamide)
N-tert-butyl maleamic acid
Pentaerythritol triacrylate
Tetraethylene glycol dimethacrylate
Trimethylolpropane triacrylate

[a]Patch test 1% in acetone, petrolatum, or olive oil.

reactions of acrylates and diacrylates, however, are exceptions to the general safety rule because they can be produced in "open" systems. Thus, chain reactions can be interrupted and restarted again with acrylates, as, for example, in the manufacture of dental prostheses. Close contact with methyl methacrylate and benzoyl peroxide may thus cause contact dermatitis in dental technicians.

Initiators

Acrylates often include initiators to propagate the production of free radicals needed for chain production. One such compound is 2,2′-azobis(2-amidinopropane) dihydrochloride [AAPH], which caused an outbreak of dermatitis in workers manufacturing this substance. Eight cases of dermatitis were reported by Takiwaki et al. (86). Both 1% and 5% aqueous solutions of AAPH were positive in all eight cases and negative in six controls. AAPH is also being used in biomedical research concerning lipid peroxidation and antioxidants.

Another free radical donor is methyl ethyl ketone peroxide. This cross-reacts with benzoyl peroxide, and both irritant and allergic contact dermatitis can result from exposure. Keratitis is another potential exposure hazard of methyl ethyl ketone peroxide. This chemical is used in plastic resin systems such as fiberglass-reinforced plastics (87).

Table 29.16 lists the various components of most acrylic resin systems.

Ultraviolet-Cured Acrylates in the Printing Industry

The usefulness of the acrylates to the printing industry comes about because certain acrylic compounds can be made to polymerize almost instantaneously by exposure to ultraviolet light. They can therefore be used both in quick-drying inks and in the rapid production of printing plates from photographic negatives. Polymerization by ultraviolet light in one instance dries the ink and, in the other, hardens the plate where the photographic negative allows light through. Reports of allergic contact dermatitis have come from both applications. In almost all cases the acrylate involved did not cross-react with methyl methacrylate and irritated the skin, necessitating patch test concentrations sometimes as low as 0.1% to avoid false-positive reactions. Individuals with negative patch tests to acrylates have been

reported as having a phototoxic dermatitis from mixed isomers of amyl dimethylaminobenzoate, which are used as absorbers of ultraviolet light to initiate the reaction. Manufacturers have had to alter their formulations to exclude certain low molecular weight acrylates in order to decrease the dermatitis hazard from these new materials.

Ultraviolet (UV)-cured inks are based on three components (Table 29.17). The first component is a reactive base prepolymer with terminal acrylate groups that may make up 80% of the formulation. They are usually acrylated polyesters, acrylated polyethers, acrylated urethanes, or acrylated epoxy resins. The second component is a photoinitiator, often benzophenone, benzoin, or a chlorinated aromatic compound. The third component is the multifunctional acrylic monomers (MFAs) that are used as diluents with cross-linking properties to bind together the acrylated resins (88).

The popularity of the UV-cured inks has grown because they are efficient and simple to use. Exposure to ultraviolet light rapidly cured the liquid solution into a plastic coating, eliminating the need for heating or the use of a solvent evaporator. Ultraviolet light stimulates a photoinitiator that leads to the formation of free radicals and the creation of an acrylated polymer.

The first step in the curing process is the absorption of ultraviolet radiation by one or more photoinitiators such as benzophenone. The absorption of UV radiation results in the generation of free radicals, which, in turn, causes polymerization of the resin in which the pigments are incorporated and thus cures the ink film.

The polyfunctional acrylic monomers should be regarded as relatively potent allergic sensitizers, and care should be taken accordingly to minimize their contact with the skin in their industrial use. Measures that appeared effective in preventing the occurrence of further dermatitis include employee education, the use of impervious protective gloves, the expeditious removal of contaminating material from the skin using mild soap and water, daily showering, frequent washing of potentially contaminated skin areas, prompt removal of contaminated clothing, separation of clean and contaminated clothing, frequent changes of uniform, protective shielding against splashing from mills and rollers, and an effective vapor exhaust and ventilation system.

TABLE 29.16. *Components of an Acrylic Resin System*

Acrylic monomers
Colors (cadmium sulfide used in dentures)
Catalysts
  Benzoyl peroxide
  Methyl ethyl ketone peroxide
Inhibitor
  Hydroquinone
Plasticizer
  Dimethyl phthalate

TABLE 29.17. *Acrylate Inks: Light-Sensitive or UV Cured Acrylates: Components of UV Cured Inks*

Multifunctional acrylic monomers (MFAs) (these bind
  together acrylate resins)
Photoinitiator
  Benzophenone, benzoin, or chlorinated aromatic
    compound
Reactive base prepolymer with terminal acrylate group:
  acrylated polyesters, polyethers, urethanes, or epoxy
  resins

There are several reports of allergic reactions to the various acrylic compounds used in ultraviolet-cured inks (88–93).

Phototoxic Reactions Associated with Ultraviolet-Cured Acrylic Inks

Emmett et al. (94) described four workers employed in the manufacture of ultraviolet-cured inks who complained of photosensitivity characterized by an intense burning sensation during sun exposure. Dermatitis developed on exposed areas in three of these workers following sun exposure. Six compounds used as photoinitiators in the ink formulations were found to absorb solar ultraviolet radiations. Two preparations of mixed isomers (ortho and para) of amyl dimethylaminobenzoate were found to be phototoxic.

These responses could be prevented in two subjects by the application of a 10% sulisobenzone sunscreen prior to sun exposure. Two other photoinitiators, Michler's ketone and thioxanthone, were phototoxic *in vitro* but not after topical application *in vivo*.

The phototoxic reactions, observed with the two industrial preparations of undiluted mixed isomers of amyl dimethylaminobenzoate, were considered surprising as purified amyl *p*-dimethylaminobenzoate is demonstrably effective as a sunscreen at a 5% concentration. No phototoxicity was observed in these employees when a 5% concentration of amyl *p*-dimethylaminobenzoic acid was applied.

The silk-screen process has evolved to the point that silk is no longer a part of the process. Dacron and polyester stencils have largely replaced silk. Also in the process, photomechanical UV-cured acrylates are used. Goossens et al. (95) reported on a man exposed to Saatigraf in the printing of athletic shirts. He washed off UV-irradiated screens and was found allergic to ethylene glycol dimethacrylate and bis-GMA (an epoxy acrylate). He also reacted to tripopylene glycol diacrylate.

Undiluted amyl dimethylaminobenzoate, used as a photoinitiator in ultraviolet cured inks, can be phototoxic, whereas a 5% concentration is an effective sunscreen.

Acrylate in Printing Plates

Various acrylates are used to make printing plates. Positive patch tests were obtained to 2-hydroxyethyl methacrylate (0.1% in alcohol), diethylene glycol dimethacrylate (1% in methyl ethyl ketone), and tetraethylene glycol dimethacrylate (1% in methyl ethyl ketone) (96).

Tetraethylene glycol dimethacrylate, acting as an irritant and a sensitizer, caused an outbreak of dermatitis in a newspaper plant (97). Beurey et al. (98) recommended 0.5% to 0.1% of the resin for patch testing with these compounds.

Airborne contact dermatitis occurred from urethane diacrylate used as part of an ultraviolet-cured ink process in printing of lottery tickets (99).

Anaerobic Adhesives

Anaerobic sealants are liquid, thermosetting industrial adhesives that polymerize rapidly in the absence of air (100). Chemically, they are based primarily on esters of acrylates and methacrylates. Anaerobic adhesives are packaged in small volumes in low molecular weight polyethylene containers. The free passage of oxygen through the container walls inhibits cure during shipping and storage. These single component adhesives also contain initiators, accelerators, and other additives.

Loctite Corp. controls approximately 90% of the American market and 70% to 80% of the foreign markets in anaerobic sealants. Some Loctite products are marketed in a numbered series (Nos. 200 to 700). The 200, 300, 500, and 600 series are anaerobic; the 300 series includes polyurethane anaerobics. Most Loctite anaerobic adhesives are sold for industrial use, but some might reach consumers through the Loctite Permatex line, sold in automotive stores and by K-Mart (M Hauser, personal communication, Dec. 1983).

Anaerobic adhesives are used for locking screws firmly in position, as gaskets, as paper sealants, and for retaining and mounting cylindrical parts, particularly in the automotive industry.

Most cases of contact allergy from anaerobic sealants have emanated from Europe. Allardice (102), Magnusson and Mobacken (103), and Jansen (104) each reported hand dermatitis among European automotive assembly workers handling acrylic or methacrylic acid ester adhesives. The acrylic formation in Magnusson and Mobacken's cases was made by Loctite Corp. Cronin (105) reported three men and one woman who were allergic to dimethacrylate screw sealants. Cronin described the dermatitis as affecting principally the pulps of the fingers, causing a dry, scaly eczema, which was chronic and uncomfortable rather than incapacitating. The eczema was overlooked as being allergic, and many months elapsed before the patients were referred for patch testing. Positive patch tests in Cronin's patients included dimethacrylate ester (5%) and tri- (5%), tetra- (1%), and polyethylene glycol dimethacrylate (5%).

In 1982, Dempsey (106) in the United States described two cases of allergic hand eczema from Loctite compounds and one case from Sta-Loc 1250 Green anaerobic sealant and Sta-Loc 600 Redi-Form Gasket. The allergen in Loctite 306 was polyurethane dimethacrylate and in the Sta-Loc product was glyceryl methacrylate: Each allergen was positive at 1%. One patient was tested with ethyl and methacrylate, each at 1%, and was positive to both.

Mathias and Maibach (107) saw three electronic assembly workers with eczema of the fingers who were allergic to polyethylene glycol dimethacrylate found in an anaerobic sealant. Onycholysis developed in one worker, and no cross-reactions to methyl methacrylate developed. This again emphasizes the necessity for patch testing with the specific resin to which an individual has been exposed. In some instances, disposable plastic gloves and careful handling techniques (e.g., application of sealant to the screw socket rather than the screw) may permit affected individuals to continue work duties with the sealant. Automatic dispensing devices are used in some operations.

> **Anaerobic adhesives, acrylates that polymerize in the absence of air, are irritants and sensitizers.**

New materials continue to be used as acrylic sealants. An anerobic sealant contact dermatitis is most commonly traced to dimethacrylates, but 1-acetyl-2-phenylhydrazine has also been reported (108). This latter substance should be tested at 1% in pet.

IV Infusion Sets

Needles are secured to plastic supports for IV infusion sets, and contact dermatitis has occurred from the glues used to secure the two parts. Allergens include epoxy resin and phenoxypoly(ethyleneoxy)acrylate. The latter is a component of Loctite 302. This UV-cured glue has several other components that have also caused contact dermatitis in IV infusion sets, including isobornyl acrylate, betacarboxyethyl acrylate, and 1-benzoylcyclohexanol. Brand names of infusion sets that contain these allergens include Cliniset, Clini Soft, and Disetronic. An alternative that does not use glue is Pureline Basic, also known as Disetronic Infusion Set Plus (109).

Pressure-Sensitive Adhesives

The term "pressure-sensitive adhesive" (PSA) refers to a type of adhesive that, when in a dry state, adheres to a variety of surfaces merely by application of light bond pressure (1,93,110–131). PSAs were first developed in the mid-1800s for use on surgical tapes. The products that utilize PSAs are listed in Table 29.18 (29); today, the major markets are the tape and label industries. All of these products are combinations of two components: backing and the adhesive. Several backing materials are used, and tapes may be subdivided according to their construction into the following categories: fabric, paper, nonwoven fabric, plastic films (e.g., PVC, cellophane, matte acetate, polyester, and polyoleifin), aluminum foil, reinforced, two-faced, and transfer tapes. PSAs are usually classified by the chemical nature of the elastomer (111) (Table 29.19). Natural rubber was the first elastomer used in PSAs and is the most commonly used today, followed closely by acrylates. Major applications for natural rubber adhesives include packaging, masking, electrical, and double-sided tapes; examples of double-sided tapes are carpet tapes and tapes for holding insoles to the last in women's shoes.

There are several methods of applying PSAs (111): (a) organic solvent solutions, (b) water-based emulsions, (c) hot melts, and (d) radiation (UV or electron beam). Solvent-based PSAs predominate. Solvent-based adhesives consist typically of various elastomers in conjunction with tackifiers, plasticizers, ultraviolet inhibitors, fillers, antiozonants, and antioxidants (113). Examples of recipes for both rubber and acrylic solvent-based PSA are shown in Tables 29.20 and 29.21. See Table 29.22 for an example of a water-based PSA emulsion. Heskel et al. (115) list other PSA formulations. In acrylic PSAs, the most commonly used monomers are 2-ethylhexyl acrylate, butyl acrylate, ethyl acrylate, and acrylic acid. Some nonacrylic monomers, such as vinyl acetate, are also used frequently to modify the

TABLE 29.18. *Major Uses for Pressure-Sensitive Adhesives*

Labels
Tape
  Appliances
  Building electrical
  Corrosion protection
  Hospital and first aid
  Office and graphic arts
  Packaging and surface protection
  Shoe industry
  Splicing
Miscellaneous products
  Ceiling and floor tiles
  Disposable diaper tabs
  Graphic artwork
  Imitation wood grain
  Medical and sanitary products
  Protective maskings
  Wall and shelf covering

From Nakayama H, et al. As referenced by Malten KE, Nater JP, van Ketel WG. *Patch testing guidelines.* Nijmegen, Netherlands: Dekker and Van de Vegt, 1976:91.

TABLE 29.19. *Pressure-Sensitive Adhesives in the United States*

Types of elastomer	% of use
Natural rubber	46
Acrylates	34
Styrene-butadiene-rubber (SBR)	10
Block copolymers (SBS and SIS)	6
Others (polychloroprene, polyurethane, and vinyls)	4

From Hagan JW, Stueben KC. Pressure sensitive adhesives. In: Schneberger GL, ed. *Adhesives in manufacturing.* New York: Van Nostrand Reinhold, 1982:189.

SBS = styrene-butadiene-styrene; SIS = styrene-isoprene.

TABLE 29.20. *Rubber-Based Pressure-Sensitive Adhesive for High-Temperature Masking Tape*

Formulation	Parts per million
Crude rubber	50
GRS	50
Octyl phenol formaldehyde heat-curing resin	20
ZnO	60
Diethylene glycol ester of dihydroabietic acid	110
Antioxidants	2

From Hagan JW, Stueben KC. Pressure sensitive adhesives. In: Schneberger GL, ed. *Adhesives in manufacturing.* New York: Van Nostrand Reinhold, 1982:189.
GRS = government rubber styrene; ZnO = zinc oxide.

TABLE 29.22. *Recipe for Pressure-Sensitive Adhesive Emulsion*

Ingredient	Parts by weight
Nonylphenol ethylene oxide condensate (97% by weight oxyethylene units)	22.4
Sodium acetate	1.0
Water	465.0
Sodium metabisulfite (in 10 parts water)	0.9
Ammonium persulfate (in 10 parts water)	0.45
Vinyl acetate	83.6
2-ethylhexyl acrylate	352.0
Acrylic acid	4.4

From Hagan JW, Stueben KC. Pressure sensitive adhesives. In: Schneberger GL, ed. *Adhesives in manufacturing.* New York: Van Nostrand Reinhold, 1982:189.

polymer properties. Many other compounds have been used in the synthesis of acrylic PSAs; some are used in substantial quantities, others in small amounts for special purposes. Almost any conceivable monomer that is able to undergo vinyl polymerization has been mentioned in the voluminous patent literature (Table 29.23) (110).

Following a positive patch test from a PSA (e.g., a piece of a tape or label tested closed for 48 hours), testing with the standard screening tray may point to an allergen such as rubber, colophony, or epoxy resin. It may be necessary, however, to treat with the specific PSA components, including the specific rosin (colophony) derivative used in the PSA formulation. It is possible some industrial PSAs, not normally intended for skin contact, might irritate the skin following a 48-hour patch test occlusion.

> **Pressure-sensitive adhesives, adhering by application of light pressure, are used on adhesive tapes and labels that contain natural rubber or acrylates. Irritant and allergic reactions, contact urticaria, and red dermographism may be produced by such adhesives.**

TABLE 29.21. *Solvent-Based Acrylic Pressure-Sensitive Adhesive Formulation*

Formulation	Parts per million
Copolymer based on:	
2-ethylhexyl acrylate	590
Acetone	300
n-butyl acrylate	290
Benzene	130
Methyl acrylate	100
Glycidyl methacrylate	20
p-toluene sulfonic acid dried, cured 3 min at 100°C	5

From Hagan JW, Stueben KC. Pressure sensitive adhesives. In: Schneberger GL, ed. *Adhesives in manufacturing.* New York: Van Nostrand Reinhold, 1982:189.

Acrylic Medical Pressure-Sensitive Adhesives

Single component adhesives were developed to avoid the allergic reactions and irritability associated with rubber-based adhesives. These adhesives are usually formed by combinations of an acrylic ester monomer with a polar monomer. The acrylic ester monomer is replaced occasionally with an acrylic monomer combined with another type of monomer, such as vinyl acetate. These acrylic-based adhesive tape glues are less allergenic than the rubber-based glues, because the amounts of uncured monomers are negligible in the acrylic tapes (116). The reason for this may be that technical improvements have been made in manufacturing pressure-sensitive adhesive tapes. Several years ago, the adhesives were made by the polymer solution method that allowed accumulation of solvent impurities, low molecular fragments, and small quantities of monomers in the end product. Solution polymerization has been replaced currently by emulsion polymerization, which results in more complete polymerization, resulting in a lower concentration of reactive low molecular weight substances in the final adhesive. Only water and a detergent are needed in the production of aqueous acrylic dispersions rather than toxic, highly flammable solvents (117).

Recent reports have identified Curad adhesives as containing 2-ethylhexyl acrylate (2-EHA) (115–118) and alkyl maleamic acid, a polar monomer. The alkyl group in the maleamic acid is derived from tertiary amines whose alkyl groups range from C_8 to C_{16} with an average of C_{12} (dodecyl maleamic acid). No tackifiers or plasticizers are used, resulting in a polar, high molecular weight polymer. During this reaction, approximately 98% of the monomers are converted to a polymer. The polymer is washed, dissolved in solvent, coated on a vinyl film, and heated to remove potentially sensitizing solvents and residual monomers (115).

Heskel et al. (115) reported two patients with eczematous reactions to Curad brand medical adhesive plastic bandages who were found to be allergic to the *N*-dodecyl maleamic acid monomer (5% in pet). Vehicle-specific patch test reactions also occurred from *N*-octodecyl maleamic acid (1%

TABLE 29.23. *Monomers Used for Pressure-Sensitive Acrylic Adhesives*

Comonomer	Comonomer
Acrylates	*Diacrylates*
methyl	dimethylaminoethyl
ethyl	1,6-hexanediol
n-propyl	diethylene glycol
butyl	triethylene glycol
pentyl	tetraethylene glycol
isopentyl	glycol
2-methylbutyl	*Triacrylates*
n-hexyl	diethylene glycol
2-ethylbutyl	trimethylolpropane
methylpentyl	*Methacrylates*
heptyl	methyl
2,4-(methyl)pentyl	butyl
octyl	pentyl
2-ethylhexyl	hexyl
n-decyl	octyl
n-undecyl	2-ethylhexyl
n-dodecyl	*n*-nonyl
tridecyl	*n*-decyl
lauryl	*n*-dodecyl
stearyl	lauryl
10-cyclohexyl undecyl	isobornyl
fusel oil	hydroxyethyl
6-methoxy	hydroxypropyl
methoxyethyl	2-hydroxypropyl
ethoxyethyl	3-hydroxypropyl
methoxybutyl	cyanoethyl
hydroxyethyl	dimethylaminoethyl
hydroxypropyl	*t*-butylaminoethyl
4-hydroxybutyl	glycidyl
butanediol	benzophenone glycidyl
tetrahydrofurfuryl	3-(3,4-dichlorophenoxy)-2-hydroxypropyl
abitol	3-(2,4,6-trichlorophenoxy)-2-hydroxypropyl
cyanoethyl	3-(2,3,4,5-tetrachlorophenoxy)-2-hydroxypropyl
dimethylaminoethyl	3-(pentachlorophenoxy)-2-hydroxypropyl
diethylaminoethyl	10-chlorodecyl
glycidyl	sodium-2-sulfoethyl
benzophenone glycidyl	trimethoxysilylpropyl
3-chloro-2-hydroxypropyl	2-sulfoethyl
3-(3,4-dichlorophenoxy)-2-hydroxypropyl	*Dimethacrylates*
3-(2,4,6-trichlorophenoxy)-2-hydroxy-propyl	ethylene glycol
3-(2,3,4,5-tetrachlorophenoxy)-2-hydroxypropyl	1,3-butylene glycol
3-(pentachlorophenoxy)-2-hydroxypropyl	
triethylene glycol	maleic acid
polyethylene glycol	maleic anhydride[a]
dimethylaminoethyl	methyl maleate
Trimethacrylates	dibutyl maleate
trimethylolpropane	di-(2-ethylhexyl)maleate
Tetramethacrylates	bis-(2-hydroxyethyl)maleate
pentaerythritol	maleic acid amide
Acrylamides	maleic acid diamide
acrylamide	maleic nitrile
N-methylol	maleic dinitrile
N,N'-dimethyl	*Fumaric acid derivatives*
N-t-butyl	fumaric acid
N,N'-diacetonyl	diisopropyl fumarate
noctyl	di-*n*-butyl fumarate
t-octyl	di-sec-butyl fumarate
N-t-C$_9$	diamyl fumarate
N-t-C$_{12}$	*n*-hexyl fumerate
N-[(2-ethylhexoxy)methyl]	di-2-ethylbutyl fumarate
diacetone	diisoamyl ethylene difumarate
diacetophenone	di-*n*-octyl fumarate

continued

TABLE 29.23. *Continued*

Comonomer	Comonomer
2-isocyanate	di-2-ethylhexyl fumarate
2-acrylamido-2-methylpropanesulfonic acid	didodecyl fumarate
Methacrylamides	di-"Cellosolve" fumarate
methacrylamide	bis-(2-hydroxyethyl) fumarate
N-methylol	polypropylene glycol fumarate
N,N'-diacetonyl	fumaric acid amide
N-(*n*-butoxymethyl)	fumaric acid diamide
N-*t*-C$_{12}$	furmaric acid nitrile
2-isocyanate	furmaric acid dinitrile
Acrylimides	*Crotonic acid derivatives*
trimethylamine	crotonic acid
Methacrylamides	glycidyl crotonate
trimethylamine	*Itaconic acid derivatives*
triethylamine	itaconic acid
tributylamine	itaconic anhydride
1,1-dimethyl-1-(2-hydroxypentyl)amine	half esters of itaconic acid
1,1-dimethyl-1-(2-hydroxydecyl)amine	*Citraconic acid derivatives*
1,1-dimethyl-1-(2,3-dihydroxypropyl)amine	citraconic acid
1,1-dimethyl-1-(2-hydroxy-3-phenoxypropyl)amine	citraconic anhydride
1,1-dimethyl-2-(2-hydroxy-3-isopropoxypropyl)amine	half esters of citraconic acid
Methacrylic acid	*Maleamic acid derivatives*
Acrolein	butyl maleamic acid
Acrylonitrile	*t*-octyl maleamic acid
Methacrylonitrile	dibutyl maleamic acid
Maleic acid derivatives	di-(2-ethylhexyl) maleamic acid
vinylidiene chloride	primene maleamic acid
vinyl acetate	*Vinyl compounds*
vinyl propionate	vinyl chloride
vinyl butyrate	allyl glycidyl ether
vinyl 10-phenylundecanoate	triallyl cyanurate
vinyl toluene	triallyl isocyanurate
vinyl benzoate	*Styrene derivatives*
sodium vinyl sulfonate	styrene
methyl vinyl ketone	α-methylstyrene
vinyl naphthalene	*t*-butylstyrene
N-vinyl succinimide	*Lactones*
2-vinyl pyridine	β-propiolactone
N-vinylimidazole	γ-butyrolactone
4-vinyl pyridine	δ-valerolactone
N-vinyl pyrrolidone	ϵ-caprolactone
N-vinyl piperidone	diketene
N-vinyl caprolactam	*Betaines*
Vinyl ethers	3-[(12-acryloxyethyl)dimethylammonium] proprionate betaine
vinyl methyl ether	3-[(12-acryloxyethyl)dimethylammonium] propane sulfonate betaine
vinyl ethyl ether	3-[(12-methacryloxyethyl)dimethyl-ammonium]propionate betaine
vinyl butyl ether	*Isocyanates*
vinyl octyl ether	methylenebisphenyl-4–4'-diisocyanate
divinyl ether	acrylic acid-2-isocyanate ester
2-chloroethyl vinyl ether	polyisocyanate prepolymers
Allyl compounds	*Miscellaneous*
tetraallyloxyethane	1,2-bis(dimethylamino)-2-hydroxypropane
diallyl succinate	3-methacryloxypropyltrimethoxysilane
tetraallyl silicate	

From Satas D. Acrylic adhesives. In: Satas D, ed. *Handbook of pressure-sensitive adhesive technology.* New York: Van Nostrand Reinhold, 1982, Chapter 13, p. 660, with permission.
[a]Combined with methyl vinyl ether in some denture adhesives.

aqueous and alcohol but not 1% in pet), undecyl polyethylene oxymaleic acid ester (1% aqueous and alcohol but not 1% in pet), and octylmaleic acid ester (1% in pet but not 1% aqueous and alcohol). Two patients of Heskel et al. (115) were patch test negative to 3-EHA.

In 1975, Jordan (118) reported seven volunteers who developed contact sensitivity to Curad adhesives that were used to hold testing materials in place during the course of predictive patch testing. All seven volunteers were allergic to 2-EHA (5% in olive oil); three also reacted to *N*-tert-butyl maleamic acid (1% in pet), whereas none reacted to the remaining two acrylate components (acrylonitrile 5% in olive oil and ethyl acrylate 5% in olive oil). Several slightly different acrylic and methacrylic compounds produced no reactions in these patients. *N*-tert-butyl maleamic acid is not used in Curad adhesives, and Jordan's subjects may have demonstrated a cross-reaction to a chemical in the same generic class as dodecyl maleamic acid. Jordan's patients tolerated another adhesive tape (Dermicel Hypoallergenic Cloth Tape; Johnson & Johnson, New Brunswick, NJ).

Allergens in PSAs include rosin (colophony), lanolin, rubber accelerators and antioxidants, acrylates, *N*-dodecyl maleamic compounds, thiourea compounds, turpentine, and hydroquinones.

Scanpore tape also contains 2-EHA (117). In one guinea pig study, sensitized animals failed to show reactions to Scanpore tape because the concentration of free penetrable 2-EHA was so low (117).

With guinea pig test methods, monoacrylates are more potent sensitizers than corresponding monomethacrylates, and this is reflected in human experience (117). The allergic tendency of acrylic ester monomers decreases as the size of the acrylic ester group increases. The di- and tri-acrylate esters are potent allergens whose frequency of sensitization increases as the number of unsaturated groups in the monomer increases (1,93,115,119–121).

Other acrylic glues used in adhesive tape include cyanoacrylates and tetraethylene glycol dimethacrylate. When methyl 2-cyanoacrylate polymer, used as a medical adhesive, degrades, one of the products is formaldehyde (1).

Backing (Facing) of Medical Pressure-Sensitive Adhesives

Fregert et al. (116) reported 28 patients, reacting to an adhesive tape (Leukoflex-Beiersdorf AG, Hamburg) used in routine patch testing, who had positive patch test reactions to diphenylthiourea (DPTU) and phenylisothiocyanate (PITC) present in the PVC backing (not the adhesive) of the tape. These 28 positive reactors represented 1.1% of 2,491 patients who were routinely tested with DPTU 1% (w/w) in pet. Fifteen of the 28 had positive patch tests to higher dilu-

tions, one at 0.000001% (w/v) of DPTU. PITC was positive at 0.1% (v/v) in acetone and in four patients at 0.0001% (v/v). Some of the subjects also had positive reactions to diethyl- or dibutylthiourea, thiram mix, colophony, or abitol. DPTU is a heat stabilizer in the PVC and is partly decomposed to PITC. The two substances were also found in a PVC blister package for salt and pepper shakers. DPTU is permitted in PVC for food packing in the United States, Germany, Austria, and Italy. As a result of Fregert's report, DPTU was removed from the tape backing. It has not been established, however, if other sensitizers are present in the PVC used as backing (116). DPTU was also reported to be present in another unnamed European plastic tape (122).

Foussereau et al. (132) described a patient who reacted to polythene in the patch unit and was sensitive to colophony and abietic acids. Similar reactions have occurred with the Al-test.

Patch Testing with Acrylic Compounds

Cavelier et al. (133) reported that the irritancy of the whole group of acrylates makes them difficult compounds with which to patch test. Concentrations that are too high irritate and even actively sensitize (134). In order to avoid too low a dilution, the patch test concentrations recommended may be on the borderline of irritancy, and reactions are difficult to interpret.

Thus, methyl methacrylate monomer may be tested 1% in olive oil or pet, whereas pentaerythritol triacrylate should be tested 0.2% in pet. The hazards of patch testing with too high a concentration include an increased likelihood of sensitization. Kanerva et al. (135) reported that 14% (3 of 21) patients screened for acrylate allergy were actively sensitized by the patch test procedure. A 0.5% concentration of ethyl acrylate, 2-hydroxyethyl acrylate, and 2-hydroxypropyl acrylate was incriminated, and the concentration was lowered to 0.1%. When a patient became sensitized by the 0.1% concentration, these three acrylates were dropped from the screening series of (meth)acrylates (135).

In general, begin patch test with the acrylates in 0.5% concentration. Even a 1% concentration may occasionally irritate or sensitize.

Acrylic Bone Cement Used in Orthopedic Prostheses

Malten (70) lists the components of acrylic bone cement, which is used in artificial hip and knee operations (Table 29.24).

Many orthopedic surgeons and surgical personnel have developed allergic contact dermatitis of the hands from exposure to the methyl methacrylate monomer, which passes through rubber gloves (136–138).

TABLE 29.24. *Components of Orthopedic Acrylic Bone Cement*

Monomer liquid
Inhibitor: hydroquinone and ascorbic acid
   Mixture of various acrylates and methacrylates
   Multifunctional acrylates and methacrylates cross-linkers
   Plasticizer: dibutyl phthalate and triphenyl phosphate
   Radical donor: benzoyl peroxide
   Solvent: trichloroethylene, methylene chloride, ethylene chloride, and chloroform
   Ultraviolet radiation absorber
     (In some cases, promoter is used instead of radical donor, which is then present in the polymer powder.)
Polymer powder
   Antibiotics
     (In some cases radical donor is used instead of promoter, which is then present in the monomer liquid.)
   Colorants
   Promoter: dimethyl-*p*-toluidine, cobalt naphthenate
   Mixture of various polymers

Malten (70), as preventive measures, advises mixing the orthopedic cement mechanically, using a spatula for application, and wearing two cotton gloves and another rubber glove over the operation gloves. These three pairs of gloves should be removed as soon as possible and discarded. Contaminated instruments should be cleaned immediately, first with dry cotton balls, then with cotton balls wet with an appropriate solvent (methyl ethyl ketone or alcohol). Skin contamination should be cleaned locally in the same way, and the hands should be washed with ample soap and water.

> **The acrylic monomer in bone cement passes readily through rubber gloves.**

Fisher (137) reported that paresthesias in the involved fingers of the medical personnel sometimes lasted months after discontinuation of contact with the cement. Monomethyl methacrylate, after it penetrates the skin, may have an untoward effect on naked myelinized nerve fibers and on the Ranvier nodes (139). Acrylamide neurologic effects have also been described (140). Such effect on the peripheral nervous system in individuals with acrylic monomer dermatitis of the hands may explain the prolonged burning and tingling sensations that accompany the dermatitis.

Raw material for acrylic-type synthetic fibers has caused irritant and allergic contact dermatitis with paresthesia in some but not all of those affected (141). The substance responsible was acrylonitrile, which should be tested at 0.1% in pet (141).

> **Acrylic monomer penetration of the skin can produce persistent paresthesia of the fingers in surgical and dental personnel due to damage to peripheral nerve fiber.**

Lack of Reaction to Acrylic Bone Cement in Artificial Joint Rejection

Although many surgical personnel become sensitized to acrylic bone cement and develop allergic dermatitis, Fisher (142) did not encounter patients in whom sensitization occurred after the operation or patients in whom the rejection of an artificial joint could actually be traced to such sensitization.

There is some question as to whether rejection of an artificial joint might be due in some cases to insufficient fixation or to a delayed-type allergic reaction. Delayed-type allergy to methyl methacrylate monomer has been found rarely in patients undergoing hip surgery (143), perhaps because the sensitizers in these cements come in contact initially with the bloodstream (144). This situation may promote the production of suppressor cells (145).

> **Acrylic monomer sensitization in patients rarely, if ever, occurs from the acrylic bone cement. Rejection of an artificial joint does not seem to occur from acrylic monomer sensitization.**

Hydroxyethyl (Meth)Acrylate

Both hydroxyethyl acrylate (HEA) and hydroxyethyl methacrylate (HEMA) have been the source of acrylate problems among medical and dental-related fields. 2-hydroxyethyl acrylate was found to be the primary sensitizer in Lowicryl embedding medium (146). Protection was afforded by 4-H gloves but not vinyl or latex gloves (146). The hydropad of a transcutaneous electrical nerve stimulation (TENS) unit caused contact dermatitis due to its HEMA content (147). Likewise, 2-HEMA in Scotchprep Dentin Adhesive and Scotchbond 2 Light Cure Dental Adhesive led to allergic contact dermatitis in three dental nurses and three dentists (148).

Acrylic Resin System Components

The resin accelerator *N,N'*-dimethyl-paratoluidine has been widely used and is reported as a cause of burning, sore mouth in patients with acrylic dental plates (149,150). A 1% to 5% pet patch test concentration has been used. Benzoyl peroxide is a common curing agent and has also been a source of prosthesis dermatitis (151).

Plastics frequently contain ultraviolet light-absorbing materials to protect them from photodegradation. One such material, Tinuvin (P-(2-(2-hydroxy-5-methylphenyl) benzotriazole)) has been added to spandex, ostomy bags, and plastic watch straps and is also in cosmetics. In spandex, its concentration drops >80% with washing. No cross-reactions have been noted to other benzotriazoles, and patch tests at 0.01%, 0.1%, 1.0%, and 5.0% in pet have all been positive (152). Solol is another photoprotectant

TABLE 29.25. *Cyanoacrylate Glue Composition*

Ethyl cyanoacrylate	90.6%
Hydroquinone	0.4%
Organic sulfonic acid	Trace
Polymethyl methacrylate	9.0%

used in plastics. It is also known as phenyl salicylate, which is a sunscreen at 230 to 330 nm, and is used as an antiseptic and intestinal disinfectant as well as an occasional ingredient in some skin creams (153). Plastic safety glasses have been found to cause contact dermatitis due to the presence of this allergen (153).

Cyanoacrylate Glues (Crazy Glue, Super Glue)

The composition of one such glue is shown in Table 29.25. These glues contain no solvents. Their viscosity is fairly high, at 2,000 to 3,000 cps. These glues are known to be irritating to the eyes and respiratory tract when vaporized, but allergic reactions are considered unlikely because of the immediate bonding of the acrylate to surface keratin.

The liquid glues are hygroscopic but do not mix with water; the rapid polymerization reaction with water is exothermic. Nylon, vinyl, or rubber gloves should not be used, but polyethylene or polypropylene gloves are satisfactory.

Cyanoacrylates polymerize readily in air at room temperature and are used as adhesives for metal, rubber, glass, and plastics, and also in surgery to bind tissues and to seal wounds. Cyanoacrylates bond strongly to keratin, and isobutyl cyanoacrylate, which polymerizes when moist, has been used to fix vertebral discs and to prevent leakage from ileostomy appliances.

Workers using cyanoacrylates may complain of irritation and discomfort of their faces.

> **Irritation from cyanoacrylate adhesive may occur due to low humidity. Accidental bonding of the skin and gluing together of the eyelids have occurred from Crazy Glue.**

Calnan (154) reported patients with a slight irritant facial contact dermatitis and eye irritation, which was attributed to a vapor generated from a cyanoacrylate glue when spoiled parts of the glue were heated during soldering. The complaints were dropped after the humidity of the environmental air was raised. What would have been present in the vapor as alkyl cyanoacrylate monomer became polymerized by the water content of the air to an inert material.

Ethyl cyanoacrylate is used as a contact adhesive for metal, glass, rubber, plastics, and textiles. It is used to seal human tissues and is commonly referred to as super glue. When contact dermatitis is suspected, the monomer may

polymerize on Finn chambers and give false-negative reactions. Suspension in petrolatum retards the polymerization and allows the use of Finn chambers to detect the allergy. A concentration of 0.032% to 10% has been found adequate (155).

Only a few cases of contact dermatitis due to cyanoacrylates have been reported. Belsito (156) found three patients who were allergic to ethyl cyanoacrylate in artificial nail "wraps," and Tombs et al. (157) reported finger and eyelid dermatitis from occupational use of ethyl cyanoacrylate used to glue on artificial hairs. Tombs et al. pointed out that most of the cases previously reported have commonly been on areas of thin stratum corneum, such as behind the ears (158) or, as in their experience, the eyelids. A 10% concentration in pet is used for patch testing. Artificial nails made of cyanoacrylate glue have caused dermatitis in clients of nail salons as well as in nail technicians. Cases are relatively infrequent. One worker achieved adequate protection by wearing polypropylene gloves (159). Contact dermatitis to ethyl cyanoacrylate has also been reported to mimic small plaque parapsoriasis (160).

First-Aid Treatment for Skin Bonded with Cyanoacrylate Adhesive

Human skin can become accidentally bonded to itself by a cyanoacrylate adhesive. One manufacturer states, "In the event of such an accident, surgery should never be necessary to separate the bonded skin—simple first aid procedures are the best treatment." Do not try to pull the bonded surfaces apart with a direct opposing action. Immerse the surfaces in warm, soapy water. Peel or roll the surfaces apart by using a blunt edge such as a spoon handle. Wash adhesive off the skin with soap and water. Another manufacturer advises the use of acetone to dissolve the adhesive bond.

Margo and Trobe (161) noted that cyanoacrylate adhesives have been used for a wide range of industrial and domestic purposes since they were first commercially introduced almost three decades ago. Recently, their widespread availability in plastic containers resembling ophthalmic medicinal dispensers in size and shape has created a new consumer safety problem. Three patients mistakenly instilled cyanoacrylate adhesives into the eyes, resulting in firm upper-to-lower lid adhesion and transient keratoconjunctivitis. In one patient, the "tarsorrhaphy" had to be undone with scissors. Adequate prevention of these accidents can be achieved only by changing the packaging of glues so that it will not resemble the containers used for ophthalmic medications.

CELLULOSE ESTER PLASTICS

These plastics are used in eyeglass frames, hearing aids, steering wheels, toothbrush and hairbrush handles, tool handles, pens, and toys. In addition, the following are cellulose products: cellophane, rayon, cellulose nitrate (celluloid), collodion, pyroxylin, gun cotton, and cellulose film.

These products, particularly eyeglass frames, may produce both irritant and allergic reactions (162).

Industrial sensitization readily develops in workers exposed to the additives used in the manufacture of the cellulose ester plastics. More rarely, the finished products can produce allergic contact dermatitis.

Jordan and Dahl (162) found the principal sensitizers in these plastics to include the following:

1. *Resorcinol monobenzoate.* An ultraviolet absorber, which may cross-react with balsam of Peru but not with resorcinol. This chemical is not widely used at present.
2. *Azobenzene dyes*
3. p-*tert-butylphenol.* A sensitizer and depigmenting agent used for heat stabilizing.
4. *Ethylene glycol monoethyl ether acetate.* A solvent used to weld nosepads to eyeglass frames and laminate plastic sheets.
5. *Plasticizers.* The phthalates are the most common plasticizers in cellulose ester plastics and are rare sensitizers. The plasticizer triphenyl phosphate, which is used for cellulose acetate and nitrocellulose, has been found to cause allergic contact dermatitis in a plastic glue. A 5% in pet concentration is recommended for testing (163).

Table 29.26 lists the materials that should be used for patch testing individuals suspected of having allergic dermatitis from cellulose ester plastic.

Contact dermatitis from cellulose plastics is rare. When such dermatitis occurs, it is usually due to the additives.

Hamada and Horiguchi (164) reported a baker who was allergic to sodium carboxymethyl cellulose (CMC), used in making cakes. A patch test with 2% CMC in pet was positive. Carboxymethyl cellulose is an anionic cellulose polymer, synthesized from purified cellulose and sodium chloracetate; CMC is used to enhance viscosity of foods and cosmetics and as a bulk laxative and gastric antacid.

POLYESTER RESINS

There are many uses for polyester resins, ranging from casting and laminating to the manufacture of bathtubs to automobile bodies. Most of the workers at risk for contact dermatitis are employed in the manufacturing industries. The incidence of allergic sensitization is small compared with the extensive skin contact that occurs among these workers. Dermatitis results usually from irritation by solvents and fiberglass. The irritating components or inclusions of the polyester plastics are polybasic acids (phthalic anhydride), polybasic alcohols (propylene glycol), styrene (vinyl benzene), fiberglass, and acetone. The chief sensitizers are peroxide catalysts and cobalt (165–167).

Table 29.27 lists the ingredients of a polyester resin system and the concentration for patch testing. The unsaturated polyester is a condensation product of an unsaturated dibasic acid and glycol that may be tested 10% in acetate.

> **The finished, completely polymerized polyresins are not, as a rule, dermatologic hazards.**

TABLE 29.26. *Patch Tests for Cellulose Ester Plastic Sensitivity*

Substance	Percentage in vehicle
Cellulose acetate flakes	As is
Cellulose acetate flakes	10% in methyl ethyl ketone (MEK)
Cellulose acetate plastic	As is
Cellulose acetate propionate plastic	As is
Cellulose acetate butyrate plastic	As is
Carbon black	1% pet
Black dye mixture	1% pet
Solvent yellow 3 (Color Index No. 11160)	1% pet
Solvent red 26 (Color Index No. 26102)	1% pet
Other colorants of black dye mixture	1% pet
Ethylene glycol monoethyl ether acetate	5% in MEK
Potassium acid oxalate	0.5% aq
p-tert-butylphenol	2% pet
Dimethyl phthalate	As is
Diethyl phthalate	As is
Tricresyl phosphate	5% pet
Triphenyl phosphate	5% pet
Phenyl salicylate	2% pet
Resorcinol monobenzoate	1% pet
2,2'-dihydroxy-4,4'-dimethoxybenzophenone	1% in MEK

aq = aqueous; pet = in petrolatum.

TABLE 29.27. *Patch Testing Polyester Resin Systems*

Unsaturated polyester resin 10% in acetone
Cross-linking agents
  α-methylstyrene 1% pet
  Methyl methacrylate 5% pet
  Styrene (vinyl benzene) 1% in olive oil
  Vinyl toluene 1% in olive oil
Inhibitors
  Hydroquinone 5% pet
  Quinone 5% pet
  p-tert-butylcatechol 1% in acetone
Organic peroxide catalysts
  Benzoyl peroxide 5% pet
  Cumene hydroperoxide 0.5% pet
  Cyclohexanone peroxide 0.5% pet
  Methyl ethyl ketone peroxide 0.5% pet
Activators (accelerators)
  Cobalt naphthenate 5% pet
  Cobalt octate 5% pet
  Diethylaniline 10% in alcohol
Ultraviolet energy absorbers
  Benzophenone 5% pet
  Benzotriazoles 1% pet
Reinforcers
  Fiberglass—do not patch

Pet = in petrolatum.

Products such as Dacron (polyester fiber) and Mylar (polyester film) have not caused dermatitis. Exposure to chemicals in the manufacture of polyresin systems, however, can produce dermatitis, particularly the irritant variety.

Burrows and Campbell (168) reported on spin finishes, liquid dressings applied to synthetic fibers in the course of manufacture to facilitate their processing. Fourteen cases of dermatitis possibly due to spin finishes were found in a factory that manufactured polyester yarns. Patch testing with all of the constituents of the spin finishes being used during the period excluded any allergic cause. A direct irritant effect from the oils and surfactants was probably responsible.

Triglycidyl isocyanurate is used primarily in polyester coatings as a hardener, but it is also found in electrical insulation, inks, adhesives, and circuit boards. To identify this allergen in a paint factory worker, 5% in methyl ethyl ketone was used (169).

Polystyrenes

Polystyrene is available as sheets that can be cut and shaped, as molding pellets that can be fused, as foam sheets (Styrofoam) that can be cut with hot wire cutters, and as expandable polystyrene beads for foam molding. Cutting or sewing of factory-fresh or large slabs of Styrofoam releases the colorless, odorless gas methyl chloride and can release any trapped styrene monomer. In small amounts, methyl chloride can cause symptoms of drunkenness; in large amounts, it can cause dizziness, staggering, and even death. Open flames should be avoided when using expandable polystyrene beads because they contain flammable pentane gas. Some styrene cements used in cement Styrofoam contain styrene monomer.

> **Cutting large slabs of polystyrene foam may release toxic methyl chloride and irritating styrene monomer.**

Styrene (Vinyl Benzene, Styrol)

This chemical, sometimes used to modify polyester monomer, is an unsaturated hydrocarbon obtained from storax (styrax) balsam. Styrene may have an irritating, drying, and defatting effect on the skin, but it rarely produces allergic dermatitis. Because storax is used in the preparation of compound tincture of benzoin, in perfume, and as a fixative for soaps, allergic sensitization to styrene carries with it the possibility of cross-reaction with benzoin compounds and some soaps. Styrene can be removed from the skin with acetone. For patch testing purposes, either 1% styrene in olive oil or 2% styrene in pet can be used. One percent styrene in butyrolactone may also be used.

Styrene is used in the manufacture of synthetic rubber, as a modifier of alkyd acrylic and polyester resins, as an extractive of storax balsam in the preparation of compound tincture of benzoin, and as a fixative for soap in the cosmetic industry.

Styrene liquid is also sometimes used in acrylic resin powder to form dentures. The polystyrenes may also be used for denture material. Styrene not only is a synthetic industrial compound, used in polyester and other resins, but can also occur in nature, for example, in raspberries, in which it is formed by enzymatic decarboxylation of cis-cinnamic acid. It is also present in storax. Styrene may cross-react with benzoin compounds, certain soaps, and vinyl toluene (170), and may produce occupational dermatitis (171).

> **Styrene, used to modify polyester and acrylic resins, is present in raspberries and in storax, used to prepare tincture of benzoin and as a soap fixative.**

POLYURETHANES (ISOCYANATE RESINS)

Table 29.28 lists the occupational exposures to isocyanates that are chemicals with the general formula R-(N=C-O)n. They react with hydroxyl groups of polyols and form polyurethane. The isocyanates used in industry include several compounds. The most common is toluene diisocyanate (TDI) (172). TDI is a strong irritant but is not a common sensitizer.

TDI and 4,4′-diphenylmethane diisocyanate (MDI) can both be patch tested at 1.5% in pet. In a series of six patients sensitive to polyurethane, binding agents TDI and MDI were the most commonly identified as causative (173). Also of note is 1,6-hexamethylene diisocyanate (HDI). Sensitivity to diaminodiphenyl methane may also be found (173).

When airborne patterns of contact dermatitis are commonly seen with epoxy resins, isocyanates are a rare cause

TABLE 29.28. *Occupational Exposure to Isocyanates*

Adhesive workers
Casts for splints
Foundry core binders
Insulation workers
Lacquers
Organic chemical synthesizers
Paints
Polyurethane flexible and rigid foams
Polyurethane sprayers
Ship welders
Spray painters
Surface coatings
Synthetic rubber
Toluene diisocyanate (TDI)
Wire coating workers

of this pattern of dermatitis. One such case was due to a polyurethane resin in a glue used to make sandpaper for belt sanders (174). The patient was sensitive to MDI and TDI.

Emmet (175) reported that at least eight persons, employed as molders in the manufacture of polyurethane plastics in a small factory, developed dermatitis within 6 months. Three employees who were examined had eczematous eruptions on exposed areas. Patch testing on two employees revealed positive reactions to methylene bis(4-cyclohexylisocyanate), 1% in pet, and to methylenedianiline, 1% in olive oil. These concentrations were not irritating when tested on four normal volunteers. The distribution of the eruption suggested that airborne materials may have elicited the allergic contact dermatitis. After the institution of rigid hygienic measures to avoid further skin contact, no further instances of dermatitis occurred over the ensuing year.

Dicyclohexylmethane-4,4'-diisocyanate, also known as Desmodur W, PICM, reduced MDI (RMDI), saturated MDI, or methylene bis(4-cyclohexylisocyanate), is used in wool processing. In this use, contact dermatitis occurred when wool saturated with this chemical was handled by a 47-year-old textile worker. Fully cured resin was nonallergenic (176).

Both methylenedianiline and methylene bis appear to be strong allergic sensitizers under appropriate conditions of exposure. Whereas the diisocyanates are strong pulmonary sensitizers and relatively weak cutaneous sensitizers, the reverse may be true of the aliphatic diisocyanates (45,177).

Isocyanates are associated with occupational asthma, and in less than half of the cases with positive bronchial challenge test will a positive IgE-mediated reaction be found. Contact urticaria is not commonly reported with these agents, but Kanerva et al. (178) reported contact urticaria from diphenylmethane-4,4'-disocyanate (MDI) in a carpenter exposed to MDI in a polyurethane glue. They speculated that contact urticaria is more common than reported and their case was IgE-mediated.

The isocyanates in polyurethane resins are weak cutaneous sensitizers but are strong pulmonary allergens. The "amine" catalysts used in polyurethane resins are strong skin sensitizers.

Verdich and Skoven (179) reported that polyurethane plastics are made by reacting polyols (polyether alcohols) with a diisocyanate. The chemical reaction is catalyzed with tertiary amines (triethylamine, triethylenediamine, and similar compounds).

This patient showed a positive reaction to Desmophen, a polyether alcohol, used in the manufacture of polyurethane plastic from mixing a polyether alcohol in an open barrel. A patch test with Desmophen, as is, was strongly positive. Typical polyurethane resin components include Rigithane 112, Rigithane Catalyst C-112-R2, and Solithane 113.

Rigithane 112 (Thiokol Chemical Corp.)

For patch testing purposes, a 1% concentration of Rigithane prepolymer in alcohol or acetone should be used. Toluene, xylene, chloroform, and methylene chloride are also suitable solvents.

Rigithane Catalyst C-112-R2

This urethane resin catalyst may be tested in a 10% aqueous solution.

Solithane 113 (Thiokol Chemical Corp.)

The Solithane prepolymer may be patch tested in a 1% concentration in alcohol or acetone.

The Solithane catalysts include the following:

Solithane Catalyst C-113-300 (tertiary amine catalyst), which may be tested in a 1% alcohol solution
Diethylethanolamine (tertiary amine catalyst), which may be tested in a 0.5% aqueous solution
Solithane Catalyst C-113-328 (tertiary amine catalyst), which may be tested in a 10% aqueous solution
Methyl morpholine (tertiary amine catalyst), which may be tested in a 0.1% aqueous solution
Triethylenediamine (tertiary amine catalyst), which may be tested in a 0.1% aqueous solution

In addition to the above catalysts, cobalt, naphthenate, and tin are sometimes used as catalysts. In general, the concentrations for patch testing polyurethane compounds are as follows:

1. TDI 1% in pet
2. Methylene bis(4-cyclohexylisocyanate), 1% in pet
3. The catalyst methylenedianiline, 0.1% in olive oil
4. The catalyst triisopropanolamine, 0.5% in pet

Skin contaminated with isocyanates and other polyurethane components should be cleansed immediately and thoroughly with isopropyl alcohol.

Prevention of Irritation from Liquid Isocyanates

The liquid monomer can produce a marked inflammatory reaction characterized by edema and redness if it is not removed immediately from the skin. Contaminated skin, therefore, should be washed copiously and thoroughly with water, and the affected area should be treated with 30% isopropyl alcohol and should then be washed with soap and water.

All contaminated clothing should be removed, preferably in a safety shower.

FIBERGLASS

Nature of Fiberglass and Fiberglass Dermatitis

Glass fibers are prepared usually in one of two forms: wool fibers or textile fibers. Wool fibers are of varying lengths, whereas textile fibers are continuous filaments of yarns. The elements of fiberglass are shown in Table 29.29. Nearly all glass fibers are coated with binders, lubricants, or coupling agents that serve to bind individual fibers together, to protect the fiber surface, or to serve as a bonding agent if the fibers are to be eventually incorporated into a matrix of resins. Among the chemicals used for this purpose are phenyl-formaldehyde resins, urea-formaldehyde resins, melamine-formaldehyde resins, polyvinyl acetate, silicones, dyes, starch, epoxy resins, ammonium hydroxide, and mineral oils. Despite the addition of these materials, allergic sensitization is rare because these resin systems are in the fully cured state prior to human exposure (180).

Workers in composite plastic production develop predominantly irritant contact dermatitis based on data collected over 20 years by Tarvainen et al. (181). They found that 49% of their cases were irritant contact dermatitis predominantly to synthetic mineral fibers (e.g., fiberglass). Allergic contact dermatitis was seen in 42% of workers and was mainly epoxy resin dermatitis. Contact urticaria was present in 9%, mostly due to natural rubber latex.

The handling of glass fibers may cause an intense pruritic reaction, because fine particles and glass dust may readily penetrate the skin and cause a characteristic miliarial eruption consisting of small, erythematous follicular papules. Other skin lesions, including purpura, telangiectasis, folliculitis, urticaria, and linear erosions in the skin creases, may also be produced, particularly in fair-complexioned individuals with dry skin. In addition, paronychia may result from the penetration of glass spicules beneath the nail fold (182).

> **Fiberglass dermatitis is usually irritant in nature, consisting of folliculitis, petechiae, telangiectasia, urticaria, and linear erosions.**

> **In general, individuals with fair skin and blue eyes, who itched severely in a "rubbing" test with glass fibers, reacted severely to fiberglass exposure.**

Workers involved in the manufacture of glass fibers may also develop a pustular, follicular acneiform eruption from hydrogenated vegetable oils and coating emulsions. In addition, glass fibers and resins may coat and interfere with the porosity of leather footwear, often producing maceration and dermatitis of the feet.

Glass fiber particles may penetrate clothing and underwear and may produce a dermatitis on covered portions of the body. Glass particles may be brought home and transferred from the worker's clothing and skin to other members of the family. This type of "contagious" glass fiber dermatitis may be mistaken for scabies.

The washing of clothing contaminated with fiberglass in a washing machine with the family underwear may produce a family "epidemic" of itching (183). A cautionary label warning the consumer not to wash fiberglass products with other clothing is needed (184).

Elby and Jetton (185) reported a case of school desk dermatitis due to a primary irritant contact reaction to fiberglass present in reinforced plastic chairs and school desks.

> **The inclusion of fiberglass curtains or clothing contaminated with fiberglass in a washing machine with family wash may produce an "epidemic" of dermatitis closely resembling scabies.**

Fiberglass made from a mixture of polyvinyl alcohol, polyethylene glycol, acetic acid, and organosilane solution (Dow Corning Z-6032 silane) was produced in a facility where eight workers developed dermatitis on part areas exposed to the material (186). Four of the eight were found patch test positive to the organosilane, which was positive in all four at 0.3% aqueous. A contaminant in the organosilane was suspected to be the actual allergen, but this was not definitively ascertained.

Variations in Fiberglass Dermatitis

Some workers handling fiberglass suffer from dermatitis as long as they are exposed to it. Others become "hardened" with continual exposure to fiberglass and eventually no longer develop dermatitis from contact with it. Similarly, when fiberglass spicules from fiberglass curtains contaminate clothing in a washing machine, certain members of the family are more affected than others.

Bjornberg et al. (187) studied 98 workers who were patch tested with glass fibers and six chemical irritants in a glass-

TABLE 29.29. *Makeup of Fiberglass*

Substance	% in fiberglass (approximate)
Cullet (glass)	30
Sand	25
Borax	15
Sodium aluminum silicate	15
Soda ash	10
Dolomite (magnesium carbonate)	5
Limestone	5
Sodium nitrate (saltpeter)	1

wool factory. A rubbing test was done with the fibers and with Trafuril.

Trafuril is an ester of nicotinic acid that is a histamine-releasing agent when rubbed into the skin. The subjects with strong patch test reactions to one quality of fiber also reacted strongly to the other types of fibers, but they did not show any increased sensitivity to other tests. The subjects with intense skin reactions to rubbing with the fibers showed an increased skin reactivity to the patch tests with fibers. These subjects had fair skin and blue eyes. In another study, these authors reported that 33 workers at a glass-wool factory were tested (patch test with glass fibers and chemical irritants, epicutaneous tests with Trafuril, and intracutaneous tests with histamine) before starting work at the factory. They were then retested after at least 4 weeks of exposure to glass fibers (188). No statistically significant differences in the intensity of the skin reactions before and after exposure were found. Thus, no general increased irritancy of the normal skin was induced by the continuous exposure to glass fibers.

The hypothesis could thus not be confirmed that continuous exposure to glass fibers might induce an irritable state of the normal skin and might increase reactivity to irritants.

Bjornberg et al. (189) also studied workers in a glass-wool factory who were divided into three comparable groups: those with persistent troublesome itching from the fibers, those without itching, and those who had become "hardened" to the itching. The three groups were compared with respect to the results of patch testing with glass fibers and six chemical irritants, a rubbing test with fibers and six chemical irritants, and the Trafuril test. Anamnestic data with respect to atopy, itching from wool and synthetic fibers, sweating, and reactions to the sun were evaluated, as was also the general skin pigmentation. No statistically significant differences between the three groups were found in respect to any of these tests or factors except for a subjectively increased sensitivity in the rubbing test with fibers for the itching group. It is possible that similar itch-provocation tests might be useful for preemployment assessment to predict severe occupational itching from glass fibers.

Eczematous Nature of Certain Fiberglass Dermatoses

In some individuals, fiberglass dermatitis has a distinctly nummular eczema-like appearance, and at times even a more widespread eczematous reaction may occur that closely resembles a diffuse allergic contact dermatitis. Cuypers et al. (190) studied a control group of 36 normal persons who were patch tested with glass fibers. The tested filaments had a length of about 3 to 5 mm and a diameter of 9 to 13 μm. The glass fibers were obtained from the normal production process and had been coated with cured epoxy resin. A control group of 29 normal persons was tested with the same type of fibers from which the epoxy finish had been burned off. Another group of 36 persons was patch tested with coated and uncoated ultra-small glass globules

with a diameter of 10 to 50 μm. On every person, five patch tests with the same material were done. They were removed after 1, 5, 24, 48, and 72 hours. On the coated fibers, 12 of 36 tested people reacted with either a 1+ or 2+ reaction. On the uncoated fibers, a reaction could be noted in 10 of 29 persons.

The patch tests with coated as well as uncoated glass globules all gave negative results. A total of 60 biopsies were performed in those cases in which a 1+ or 2+ reaction was noted. The histologic examination of the biopsies showed no difference between the reactions on coated and uncoated fibers. The skin reactions to glass fiber showed, besides microtraumatic changes, several histologic characteristics of an eczematous reaction like spongiosis and perivascular lymphocytic infiltration. It was concluded that the microtraumatic influence of fiberglass spicules may produce histologic reactions of an eczematous nature closely mimicking an allergic contact dermatitis.

> In cases of fiberglass dermatitis, scrapings from the lesions, treated with 20% potassium hydroxide and examined microscopically, may show the presence of glass fibers.

Dermatitis Due to Fiberglass Resin Finishes

As a rule, the formaldehyde and epoxy resins applied to certain glass fibers are completely cured and do not produce allergic contact dermatitis. Occasionally, however, dermatitis caused by these resin finishes have been reported (191).

Kalimo et al. (61) described a patient who had both immediate type 1 and delayed type 4 hypersensitivity reactions to p-tert-butylphenol-formaldehyde resin in glass fiber finishes, and who developed aphonia without skin symptoms in connection with exposure to glass wool.

The patient, a 46-year-old truck driver, had been employed by a glass-wool delivery firm since 1972. The driver's work was to load and deliver glass-wool rolls (masses of glass fibers resembling wool), used for thermal insulation and air filters.

A significant patch test reaction was obtained with p-tert-butylphenol-formaldehyde resin. An urticarial reaction was seen in 60 minutes at the site of application, and in 3 days a delayed type 4 reaction also developed. The patient's own glass-wool material was tested repeatedly with identical immediate and delayed type skin reactions. Tests with the same wool in 10 control persons were not due to irritation of the wool. Formaldehyde caused no reaction.

Lucas (192) stated that fiberglass dermatitis is the most important cause of mechanical irritant contact dermatitis and the "spread" of the dermatitis within family groups through the cross-contamination of clothing with glass spicules from curtains or other fibrous glass items during washing. This cause of pruritus should always be suspected when several family members begin almost simultaneous complaints of intense itching. Contaminated work clothes can also serve as a source. In several instances, Lucas (192) traced the apparent source to commercially operated self-service coin laundries. Apparently, fibrous glass articles are often washed in such public facilities, and sufficient carry-over is present to contaminate the clothing of the next customer using the machine. Such items should be washed separately from other clothing items and in a basin or tub that can be rinsed thoroughly after use. Rubber gloves should be worn in the procedure.

> **Fiberglass irritant dermatitis may be complicated by an urticarial and an eczematous reaction that may mimic an allergic reaction clinically and histologically.**

ROCKWOOL

Nature of Rockwool and Rockwool Dermatitis

Rockwool is a type of mineral wool made by blowing a jet of steam through molten rock (such as limestone or siliceous rock) or through slag and is used for heat and sound insulation in the building industry. Such "wool" is usually transparent and glass in appearance and has thin, sharp fibers of different diameters. Mineral oil, a silicone compound, and phenyl-formaldehyde resin may be added. The resin is then cured by heat. Mineral cotton, silicate cotton, and slag wool are other names for rockwool.

The two varieties of dermatitis that develop from rockwool are mostly irritant in nature. Rockwool, which is produced from slag, often contains free lime and can produce a severe diffuse irritant reaction particularly on wet or perspiring skin. The other is a more or less punctate or follicular eruption that can become eczematous due to penetration of the sharp spicules.

Rockwool may cause severe itching and skin reactions on direct contact with the skin. Many workers seem to become hardened to this material, and the itching abates despite constant contact with it. These skin reactions are mostly looked on as a primary irritant contact dermatitis induced mechanically by the fibers.

> **Rockwool is also known as mineral cotton, silicate cotton, and slag wool. Rockwool dermatitis, irritant in nature, may be diffuse on wet skin, but punctate or follicular on dry skin.**

Bjornberg and Lowhagen (193) patch tested 225 eczematous patients with rockwool. A total of 25 (11%) had posi-

tive 2+ or 3+ reactions. Rockwool powder without spicules did not produce any patch test reactions. The authors concluded that the typical sharp properties of the fibers produce these skin reactions mechanically. The reactions often have the macroscopic appearance of a true allergic response. Even microscopically, some showed subcorneal bullae with spongiosis and dermal mononuclear infiltrate. In some reactions, spongiosis dominated the picture, and in others a dermal infiltrate was present without epidermal changes.

In a later study, Bjomberg and Lowhagen (194) reported that 25% of 315 subjects exhibited skin reactions when patch tested with mineral wool. Coating of the mineral fibers with phenyl-formaldehyde did not influence the skin reactions. The reactions seem to be induced mechanically, as the mineral without the fibers did not give any reactions. No allergic reactions to the chemical additives were demonstrated. Macroscopically, the reactions may stimulate an allergic response; microscopically, they seem to be toxic, sometimes with a prominent spongiosis.

ACKNOWLEDGMENTS

Parts of this chapter were originally contributed by James S. Taylor, MD, in the third edition of this book as Chapter 37, Adhesives, Gums, and Resins.

REFERENCES

1. Malten KE. Recently reported causes of contact dermatitis due to synthetic resins and hardeners. *Contact Dermatitis* 1979;5:11.
2. Fregert S. Abbreviations for names of plastics. *Contact Dermatitis* 1982;8:214.
3. Harris DK. Some hazards in the manufacture and use of plastics. *Br J Ind Med* 1959;16:233.
4. Osbourn RA. Contact dermatitis caused by Saran Wrap. *JAMA* 1964; 188:1159.
5. Morris GE. Vinyl plastics; their dermatological and chemical aspects. *AMA Arch Ind Hyg* 1953;8:535.
6. Templeton HJ. Contact dermatitis from plastic mittens. *Arch Dermatol Syphilol* 1950;61:854.
7. Fregert S, Rorsman H. Hypersensitivity to epoxy resins used as plasticizers and stabilizers in polyvinyl chloride (PVC) resins. *Acta Dermato-Venereol* 1963;43:10.
8. Hindson C, Lawlor F. Allergy to glyoxal in a polyvinyl resin emulsion. *Contact Dermatitis* 1982;8:213.
9. Schulsinger C, Mollgaard K. Polyvinyl chloride dermatitis not caused by phthalates. *Contact Dermatitis* 1980;6:477.
10. Capon F, et al. Occupational contact dermatitis caused by computer mice. *Contact Dermatitis* 1996;35:57.
11. Oliwiecki S, Beck MH, Chalmers RJG. Contact dermatitis from spectacle frames and hearing aid containing diethyl phthalate. *Contact Dermatitis* 1991;25:264.
12. Nakada T, Maibach HI. Eyeglass allergic contact dermatitis. *Contact Dermatitis* 1998;39:1.
13. Thorneby-Andersson K, Hansson C. Allergic contact dermatitis from colophony in waxes for polishing spectacle frames. *Contact Dermatitis* 1994;31:126.
14. Fisher AA. *Contact dermatitis,* 2nd ed. Philadelphia: Lea & Febiger, 1973:139.
15. Walker AE. Preliminary report of vascular abnormality occurring in men engaged in manufacture of polyvinyl chloride. *Br J Dermatol* 1975;93:22.

16. Ward AM, Udnoon S, Watkins J, et al. Immunological mechanisms in the pathogenesis of vinyl chloride disease. *Br Med J* 1976;1:936.
17. Jolanki R, Kanerva L, Estlander T, et al. Occupational dermatoses from epoxy resin compounds. *Contact Dermatitis* 1990;23:172.
18. Kanerva L, Jolanki R, Estlander T. Allergic contact dermatitis from non-diglycidyl-ether-of-bisphenol-A epoxy resins. *Contact Dermatitis* 1991;24:293.
19. Guerra L, Vincenzi C, Bardazzi F, et al. Contact sensitization due to isophoronediamine. *Contact Dermatitis* 1992;27:52.
20. Kanerva L, et al. Delayed and immediate allergy caused by methyl-hexahydrophthalic anhydride. *Contact Dermatitis* 1997;36:34.
21. Tarvainen K, et al. Immunologic contact urticaria due to airborne methylhexahydrophthalic and methyltetrahydrophthalic anhydrides. *Contact Dermatitis* 1995;32:204.
22. Kanerva L, et al. Occupational allergic contact dermatitis and contact urticaria caused by polyfunctional aziridine hardener. *Contact Dermatitis* 1995;33:304.
23. Hansson C, Ezzelarab M, Sterner O. Isolation and structural determination of two new haptens in an aziridine hardener. *Am J Contact Dermatitis* 1994;5:216.
24. Brooke R, Beck MH. Contact allergy to 2,4,6-tris(dimethyl-aminomethyl)phenol. *Contact Dermatitis* 1998;38:284.
25. Kanerva L, Jolanki R, Estlander T. Occupational epoxy dermatitis with patch test reactions to multiple hardeners including tetraethylenepentamine. *Contact Dermatitis* 1998;38:299.
26. Patussi V, Kokelj F, Buttazzi P. Occupational airborne contact dermatitis due to 3-amino-methyl-3,5,5-trimethylcyclohexylamine. *Contact Dermatitis* 1995;32:239.
27. Nijnemaki A, et al. Allergic stomatitis from acrylic compounds. *Contact Dermatitis* 1983;9:148.
28. Taylor JS, et al. Contact dermatitis to knee patch adhesive in boys' jeans: a nonoccupational cause of epoxy resin sensitivity. *Cleve Clin Q* 1983;50:123.
29. Nakayama H, et al. As referenced by Malten KE, Nater JP, van Ketel WG. *Patch testing guidelines.* Nijmegen, Netherlands: Dekker and Van de Vegt, 1976:91.
30. Fregert S, Thorgeirsson A. Patch testing with low molecular oligomers of epoxy resins in humans. *Contact Dermatitis* 1977;3:301.
31. Bokelund F, Fregert S, Trulsson L. Sensitization from epoxy resin powder of high molecular weight. *Contact Dermatitis* 1980;6:144.
32. Dahlquist I, Fregert S. Allergic contact dermatitis from volatile epoxy hardeners and reactive diluents. *Contact Dermatitis* 1979;5:406.
33. Fregert S, Trulsson L. Simple methods for demonstration of epoxy resins of bisphenol A type. *Contact Dermatitis* 1978;4:69.
34. Dahlquist I, Fregert S. Contact allergy to Cardura E and epoxy reactive diluent of the ester type. *Contact Dermatitis* 1979;5:121.
35. Rudzki E. Dermatitis from epoxy resin, triethylenetetramine and ethylenediamine. *Contact Dermatitis* 1978;4:53.
36. Goransson K. Allergic contact dermatitis to an epoxy hardener: dodecenyl-succinic-anhydride. *Contact Dermatitis* 1977;8:277.
37. LaChapelle JM, Tennstedt D, Dumont-Fruytier M. Occupational allergic contact dermatitis to isophorone diamine (IPD) used as an epoxy resin hardener. *Contact Dermatitis* 1978;4:109.
38. Dahlquist I, Fregert S. Contact allergy to the epoxy hardener Isophoronediamine (IPD). *Contact Dermatitis* 1979;5:120.
39. de Groot AC. Occupational contact allergy to alpha-naphthyl glycidyl ether. *Contact Dermatitis* 1994;30:253.
40. Angelini G, et al. Occupational sensitization to epoxy resin and reactive diluents in marble workers. *Contact Dermatitis* 1996;35:11.
41. Dooms-Goossens A, et al. Contact allergy to allyl glycidyl ether present as an impurity in 3-glycidyloxypropyltrimethoxysilane, a fixing additive in silicone and polyurethane resins. *Contact Dermatitis* 1995;33:17.
42. Sasseville D. Contact urticaria from epoxy resin and reactive diluents. *Contact Dermatitis* 1998;38:57–8.
43. Fisher AA. Cross-reactions between epoxy resin "amine" hardeners and ethylenediamine. *Cutis* 1976;17:839.
44. Van Hecke E. Ethylenediamine sensitivity from exposure to epoxy resin hardeners and Mycolog cream. *Contact Dermatitis* 1975;1:344.
45. Lachapelle JM, Lachapelle-Ketelaer MJ. Cross-sensitivity between isophorone diamine (IPD) and isophorone diiocyanate (IPDI). *Contact Dermatitis* 1979;5:55.
46. Anderson KE. Cutaneous reaction to an epoxy coated pacemaker. *Arch Dermatol* 1979;115:97.
47. Mork NJ. Contact sensitivity from epoxy resin in a hemodialysis set. *Contact Dermatitis* 1979;5:331.
48. Malten KE. Tracing back a positive reaction to epoxy resin. *Contact Dermatitis* 1977;3:217.
49. Hambly EM, Wilkinson DS. Unusual presentation of epoxy resin sensitivity. *Contact Dermatitis* 1978;4:114.
50. Bjorkner B. Allergic contact dermatitis from (foxy) epoxy. *Contact Dermatitis* 1980;6:499.
51. Fregert S, Persson K, Trulsson L. Allergic contact dermatitis from unhardened epoxy resin in a finished product. *Contact Dermatitis* 1979;5:277.
52. Estlander T, Jolanki R, Henriks-Eckerman M-L, Kanerva L. Occupational contact dermatitis to bisphenol A. *Contact Dermatitis* 1999;40:52.
53. Fregert S. Irritant dermatitis from phenolformaldehyde resin powder. *Contact Dermatitis* 1980;6:493.
54. Adams RM. "Spontaneous flare" to *p*-tert-butyl-phenol formaldehyde resin. *Contact Dermatitis* 1975;1:321.
55. Foussereau J, Cavelier C, Selig D. Occupational eczema from para-tertiary-butylphenol formaldehyde resins: a review of the sensitizing resins. *Contact Dermatitis* 1976;2:254.
56. Mobacken H, Hersle K. Allergic contact dermatitis caused by para-tertiary-butyl-phenol-formaldehyde resin in watch straps. *Contact Dermatitis* 1976;2:59.
57. Burrows D, Rycroft RJ. Contact dermatitis from PTBP resin and tricresyl ethyl phthalate in a plastic nail adhesive. *Contact Dermatitis* 1981;7:336.
58. Romaguera C, Grimalt F. Occupational leukoderma and contact dermatitis from paratertiary-butylphenol. *Contact Dermatitis* 1981;7:159.
59. Correcher BL, Perez AG. Dermatitis from shoes and an amputation prosthesis due to mercaptobenzthiazole and paratertiary butyl formaldehyde resin. *Contact Dermatitis* 1981;7:275.
60. Fregert S. Contact allergy to phenoplastics. *Contact Dermatitis* 1981;7:170.
61. Kalimo K, Saarni H, Kytta J. Immediate and delayed type reactions to formaldehyde resin in glass wool. *Contact Dermatitis* 1980;6:496.
62. Malten KE. Paratertiary butylphenol depigmentation in a "consumer." *Contact Dermatitis* 1975;1:181.
63. Saruta T, Nakamizo Y. Leukoderma due to paratertiary butylphenol (Japanese). *Rinsho Derma* (Tokyo) 1975;16:161.
64. Macfarlane AW, Yu RC, King CM. Contact sensitivity to para-tertiarybutyl-catechol in an artificial limb. *Contact Dermatitis* 1990;22:56.
65. Edwards EK Jr, Edwards EK Sr. Unusual cutaneous reaction to polystyrene in an otherwise healthy population. *Contact Dermatitis* 1998;38:50.
66. Tarvainen K. Analysis of patients with allergic patch test reactions to a plastics and glue series. *Contact Dermatitis* 1995;32:346.
67. Zimerson E, Bruze M. Demonstration of the contact sensitizer *p*-tert-butylcatechol in *p*-tert-butylphenol formaldehyde resin. *Am J Contact Dermatitis* 1999;10:2.
68. Bruze M, Zimerson E. Cross-reaction patterns in patients with contact allergy to simple methylol phenols. *Contact Dermatitis* 1997;37:82.
69. Hagdrup H, Egsgaard H, Carlsen L, Andersen KE. Contact allergy to 2-hydroxy-5-tert-butyl benzylalcohol and 2,6-bis(hydroxymethyl)-4-tert-butylphenol, components of a phenolic resin used in marking pens. *Contact Dermatitis* 1994;31:154.
70. Malten KE. Old and new, mainly occupational dermatologic problems in the production and processing of plastics. In: Maibach HI, Gellin GA, eds. *Occupational and industrial dermatology.* Chicago: Year Book Medical Publishers, 1982:255.
71. Hjorth N, Fregert S. Sensitivity to formaldehyde and formaldehyde resins. *Contact Dermatitis Newsletter* 1967;2:18.
72. Jakovljevicova E. Professional urticaria caused by urea-formaldehyde resin [Czech]. *Cesk Dermatol* 1976;51:323.
73. Logan WP, Perry H. Cast dermatitis due to formaldehyde sensitivity. *Arch Dermatol* 1972;106:717.
74. Fregert S. Formaldehyde dermatitis from a gypsum-melamine resin mixture. *Contact Dermatitis* 1981;7:56.

75. Romaguera C, Grimalt F, Lecha M. Occupational purpuric textile dermatitis from formaldehyde resins. *Contact Dermatitis* 1981;7:152.

76. Fisher AA. A glove for protection against acrylates. *Am J Contact Dermatitis* 1990;1:149.

77. McClain DC, Storrs FJ. Protective effect of both a barrier cream and a polyethylene laminate glove against epoxy resin, glyceryl monothioglycolate, frullania, and tansy. *Am J Contact Dermatitis* 1992;3:201.

78. Kanerva L, Jolanki R, Estlander T. 10 years of patch testing with the (meth)acrylate series. *Contact Dermatitis* 1997;37:255.

79. Henriks-Eckerman M-J, Kanerva L. Product analysis of acrylic resins compared to information given in material safety data sheets. *Contact Dermatitis* 1997;36:164.

80. Bang Pedersen N. Allergic contact dermatitis from acrylic resin repair of windscreens. *Contact Dermatitis* 1998;39:99.

81. Matura M, et al. Glycidyl methacrylate and ethoxyethyl acrylate: new allergens in emulsions used to impregnate paper and textile materials. *Contact Dermatitis* 1995;33:123.

82. Freeman S, Lee M-S, Gudmundsen K. Adverse contact reactions to sculptured acrylic nails: 4 case reports and a literature review. *Contact Dermatitis* 1995;33:381.

83. Koppula SV, Fellman JH, Storrs FJ. Screening allergens for acrylate dermatitis associated with artificial nails. *Am J Contact Dermatitis* 1995;6:78.

84. Kanerva L, Lauerma A, Jolanki R, Estlander T. Methyl acrylate: a new sensitizer in nail lacquer. *Contact Dermatitis* 1995;33:203.

85. Jolanki R, Kanerva L, Estlander T, Tarvainen K. Concomitant sensitization to triglycidyl isocyanurate, diaminodiphenylmethane and 2-hydroxyethyl methacrylate from silk-screen printing coatings in the manufacture of circuit boards. *Contact Dermatitis* 1994;330:12.

86. Takiwaki H, Arase S, Nakayama H. Contact dermatitis due to 2,2′-azobis(2-amidinopropane) dihydrochloride: an outbreak in production workers. *Contact Dermatitis* 1998;39:4.

87. Bhushan M, Craven NM, Beck MH. Contact allergy to methyl ethyl ketone peroxide and cobalt in the manufacture of fiberglass-reinforced plastics. *Contact Dermatitis* 1998;39:203.

88. Bjorkner B. Sensitization capacity of acrylated prepolymers in ultraviolet curing inks tested in the guinea pig. *Acta Dermato-Venereol* 1981;61:7.

89. Nethercott JR. Skin problems associated with multifunctional acrylic monomers in ultraviolet curing inks. *Br J Dermatol* 1979;98:541.

90. Bjorkner B, Dahlquist I, Fregert S. Allergic contact dermatitis from acrylates in ultraviolet curing inks. *Contact Dermatitis* 1980;6:405.

91. Bjorkner B. Allergenicity of trimethylol propane triacrylate in ultraviolet curing inks in the guinea pig. *Acta Dermato-Venereol* 1980;60:528.

92. Emmett EA, Kominsky JR. Allergic contact dermatitis from ultraviolet cured inks: allergic contact sensitization to acrylates. *J Occup Med* 1977;19:113.

93. Emmett EA. Contact dermatitis from poly-functional acrylic monomers. *Contact Dermatitis* 1977;3:245.

94. Emmett EA, Taphorn BR, Kominsky JR. Phototoxicity occurring during the manufacture of ultraviolet-cured ink. *Arch Dermatol* 1977;113:770.

95. Goossens A, Coninx D, Rommens K, Verhamme B. Occupational dermatitis in a silk-screen maker. *Contact Dermatitis* 1998;39:40.

96. Malten KE, van der Meer-Roosen CH, Seutter E. Nyloprint-sensitive patients react to N,N′-methylene bis acrylamide. *Contact Dermatitis* 1978;4:214.

97. Malten KE, Bende WJM. 2-hydroxy-ethyl-methacrylate and di- and tetraethylene glycol dimethacrylate: contact sensitizers in a photoprepolymer printing plate procedure. *Contact Dermatitis* 1979;5:214.

98. Beurey J, Mougeolle JM, Weber M. Accidents cutanes des résines acryliques dans l'imprimerie (Cutaneous manifestations due to acrylic resins used in printing [French]). *Ann Dermatol Venereol* 1976;103:423.

99. Guimaraens D, Gonzalez MA, Del Rio E, Conde-Salazar L. Occupational airborne allergic contact dermatitis in the national mint and fiscal-stamp factory. *Contact Dermatitis* 1994;30:172.

100. Malten KE. Dermatological problems with synthetic resins and plastics in glues. *Berufs-Dermatosen* 1984;32:81.

101. [no note 101]

102. Allardice JT. Dermatitis due to an acrylic sealer. *Trans St John's Hosp Dermatol Soc* 1967;53:86.

103. Magnusson B, Mobacken H. Contact allergy to a self-hardening acrylic sealer for assembling metal parts. *Berufs-Dermatosen* 1972;20:199.

104. Jansen K. Zur Haufigkeit unt Prophylaxe Allergischer Kontaktekzeme durch Acrylat-Klebstoffe. *Berufs-Dermatosen* 1975;23:183.

105. Cronin E. *Contact dermatitis*. Edinburgh: Churchill Livingstone, 1980:3.

106. Dempsey KJ. Hypersensitivity to Sta-Lok and Loctite anaerobic sealants. *J Am Acad Dermatol* 1982;7:779.

107. Mathias CGT, Maibach HI. Allergic contact dermatitis from anaerobic acrylic sealants. *Arch Dermatol* 1984;120:1202.

108. Foulds IS, Koh D. Contact allergy to 1-acetyl-2-phenyl-hydrazine in a dimethacrylate adhesive. *Contact Dermatitis* 1991;25:251.

109. Busschots AM, Meuleman V, Poesen N, Dooms-Goossens A. Contact allergy to components of glue in insulin pump infusion sets. *Contact Dermatitis* 1995;33:205.

110. Satas D (ed). *Handbook of pressure-sensitive adhesive technology*. New York: Van Nostrand Reinhold, 1982.

111. Hagan JW, Stueben KC. Pressure sensitive adhesives. In: Schneberger GL, ed. *Adhesives in manufacturing*. New York: Marcel Dekker, 1982:353.

112. Butler GL. Natural rubber adhesives. In: Satas D, ed. *Handbook of pressure-sensitive adhesive technology*. New York: Van Nostrand Reinhold, 1982:189.

113. Korcz WH. Block copolymers. In: Satas D, ed. *Handbook of pressure-sensitive adhesive technology*. New York: Van Nostrand Reinhold, 1982:220.

114. Schlademan JS. Tackifier resins. In: Satas D, ed. *Handbook of pressure-sensitive adhesive technology*. New York: Van Nostrand Reinhold, 1982:353.

115. Heskel NS, Samour CM, Storr FT. Allergic contact dermatitis from dodecyl maleamic acid in Curad adhesive plastic bandages. *J Am Acad Dermatol* 1982;7:747.

116. Fregert S, Trulson L, Zimerson E. Contact allergic reactions to diphenylthiourea and phenylisothiocyanate in PVC adhesive tape. *Contact Dermatitis* 1982;8:38.

117. Waegemaekers TLH, Van Der Walle HB. The sensitizing potential of 2-ethylhexyl acrylate in the guinea pig. *Contact Dermatitis* 1983;9:372.

118. Jordan WP. Cross-sensitization patterns in acrylic allergens. *Contact Dermatitis* 1975;1:13.

119. Rycroft RJG. Contact dermatitis from acrylic compounds. *Br J Dermatol* 1977;96:685.

120. Eisen HN, Tahchnik M. Elicitation of allergic contact dermatitis in the guinea pig. *J Exp Med* 1958;108:773.

121. Marks JG, Bishop ME, Willis WF. Allergic contact dermatitis to sculptured nails. *Arch Dermatol* 1979;115:100.

122. Frenk E. Irreversible depigmentierung der haut als folge eines akuten kontaktekzems auf heftpflaster. *Hautarzt* 1980;31:639.

123. Calnan CD. Diethyldithiocarbamate in adhesive tape. *Contact Dermatitis* 1978;4:61.

124. Cronin E. Sensitivity to zinc diethyldithiocarbamate in adhesive plaster. *Contact Dermatitis Newsletter* 1972;11:286.

125. Murphy JC, Reit AE, January HL. Cutaneous hypersensitivity to adhesive and Scotch tapes. *J Invest Dermatol* 1958;31:45.

126. Karlberg AT, Boman A, Wahlberg JE. Allergenic potential of abeitic acid, colophony and pine resin-HA. *Contact Dermatitis* 1980;6:481.

127. Cronin E, Calnan CD. Allergy to hydroabeitic alcohol in adhesive tape. *Contact Dermatitis* 1978;4:57.

128. Ducombs G. Allergy to colophony. *Contact Dermatitis* 1978;4:118.

129. James WD. Allergic contact dermatitis to a colophony derivative. *Contact Dermatitis* 1984;10:6.

130. Rasmussen JE, Fisher AA. Allergic contact dermatitis to a salicylic acid plaster. *Contact Dermatitis* 1976;2:237.

131. Calnan CD. Colophony dermatitis from insulated tools. *Contact Dermatitis Newsletter* 1972;11:281.

132. Foussereau J, et al. L'allergie à la colophane des rondelles en polyethylene des patch tests. *Bull Soc Fr Dermatol Syphiligr* 1971;78:604.

133. Cavelier C, Jelen G, Herve-Bazin B, Foussereau J. Irritation et allergie aux acrylates et methacrylate. Premiere partie: monoacrylates et monomethyacrylates simples (Irritation and allergy to acrylates

and methacrylates. Part 1: polyfunctional acrylic monomers [French]). *Ann Dermatol Venereol* 1981;108:549.

134. Cavelier C, Jelen G, Herve-Bazin B, Foussereau J. Irritation et allergie aux acrylates. Deuxieme partie: monomeres acryliques polyfonctionels (Irritation and allergy to acrylates and methacrylates. Part 2: polyfunctional acrylic monomers [French]). *Ann Dermatol Venereol* 1981;108:559.

135. Kanerva L, Estlander T, Jolanki R. Double active sensitization caused by acrylics. *Am J Contact Dermatitis* 1992;3:23.

136. Pegum JS, Medhurst FA. Contact dermatitis from penetration of rubber gloves by acrylic monomer. *Br Med J* 1971;2:141.

137. Fisher AA. Acrylic bone cement sensitization and dermatitis. *Cutis* 1973;12:333.

138. Fries JB, Fisher AA, Salvati EA. Contact dermatitis in surgeons from methyl methacrylate bone cement. *J Bone Joint Surg* 1975;57A:547.

139. Bohling HG, Borchard U, Drouin H. Monomeric methylmethacrylate (MMA) acts on desheathed myelinated nerve and on the node of Ranvier. *Arch Toxicol* 1977;38:307.

140. Edwards PM. Filling in the acrylamide picture. *Br J Ind Med* 1975; 32:31.

141. Bakker JG, Jongen SMJ, vanNeer FCJ, et al. Occupational contact dermatitis due to acrylonitrile. *Contact Dermatitis* 1991;24:50.

142. Fisher AA. *Contact dermatitis,* 3rd ed. Philadelphia: Lea & Febiger, 1986.

143. Monteney E, Oleffe J, Donkerwolke M. Methylmethacrylate hypersensitivity in a patient with cemented endoprosthesis: a case report. *Acta Orthop Scand* 1978;49:554.

144. Pahuja K, Lowe H, Chand K. Blood methyl methacrylate levels in patients having prosthetic joint replacement. *Acta Orthop Scand* 1974;45:737.

145. Polak L. Recent trends in the immunology of contact sensitivity: II. *Contact Dermatitis* 1978;4:256.

146. Tobler M, Wüthrich B, Freiburghaus AU. Contact dermatitis from acrylate and methacrylate compounds in Lowicryl® embedding media for electron microscopy. *Contact Dermatitis* 1990;23:96.

147. Marren P, DeBerker D, Powell S. Methacrylate sensitivity and transcutaneous electrical nerve stimulation (TENS). *Contact Dermatitis* 1991;25:190.

148. Kanerva L, Turjanmaa K, Estlander T, et al. Occupational allergic contact dermatitis caused by 2-hydroxyethyl methacrylate (2-HEMA) in a new dentin adhesive. *Am J Contact Dermatitis* 1991;2:24.

149. Tosti A, Bardazzi F, Piancostelli E, et al. Contact stomatitis due to *N,N*-dimethyl-para-toluidene. *Contact Dermatitis* 1990;22:113.

150. Nerschueren GLA, Bruynzeel DP. Allergy to *N,N*-dimethyl-*p*-toluidine in dental materials. *Contact Dermatitis* 1991;24:149.

151. Vincenzi D, Camelli N, Vassilopoulou A, et al. Allergic contact dermatitis due to benzoyl peroxide in an arm prosthesis. *Contact Dermatitis* 1991;24:66.

152. Arisu K, Hayakawa R, Ogino Y, et al. Tinuvin® P in a spandex tape as a cause of clothing dermatitis. *Contact Dermatitis* 1992;26:311.

153. Fimiani M, Casini L, Bocci S. Contact dermatitis from phenyl salicylate in galenic cream. *Contact Dermatitis* 1990;22:239.

154. Calnan CD. Cyanoacrylate dermatitis. *Contact Dermatitis* 1979;5: 165.

155. Bruze M, Bjorkner B, Lepoittevin J-P. Occupational allergic contact dermatitis from ethyl cyanoacrylate. *Contact Dermatitis* 1995;32: 156.

156. Belsito DV. Contact dermatitis to ethylcyanoacrylate-containing glue. *Contact Dermatitis* 1987;17:234.

157. Tombs RR, Lepoittevin J-P, Duprepaire F, et al. Ectopic contact dermatitis from ethyl cyanoacrylate instant adhesives. *Contact Dermatitis* 1993;28:206.

158. Pigatto PD, Giacchetti A, Altomare GF. Unusual sensitization to cyanoacrylate ester. *Contact Dermatitis* 1986;14:193.

159. Fitzgerald DA, Bhaggoe R, English JSC. Contact sensitivity to cyanoacrylate nail-adhesive with dermatitis at remote sites. *Contact Dermatitis* 1995;32:175.

160. Shelley ED, Shelley WB. Chronic dermatitis simulating small plaque parapsoriasis due to cyanoacrylate adhesive used in fingernails. *JAMA* 1984;252:2455.

161. Margo CE, Trobe JD. Tarsorrhaphy from accidental instillation of cyanoacrylate adhesive in the eye. *JAMA* 1982;247:660.

162. Jordan WP, Dahl MV. Contact dermatitis from cellulose ester plastics. *Arch Dermatol* 1972;105:880.

163. Camarasa JG, Serra-Baldrich E. Allergic contact dermatitis from triphenyl phosphate. *Contact Dermatitis* 1992;26:264.

164. Hamada T, Horiguchi S. Allergic contact dermatitis due to sodium carboxymethyl cellulose. *Contact Dermatitis* 1978;4:244.

165. Adams RM. Polyester resins. In: Maibach HI, Gellin GA, eds. *Occupational and industrial dermatology.* Chicago: Year Book Medical Publishers, 1982:291.

166. Key MM, Discher DP. Polyester resins: their dermatologic aspects in industry. *Cutis* 1966;2:1.

167. Bourne LB, Milner FJ. Polyester resin hazards. *Br J Ind Med* 1963; 20:100.

168. Burrows D, Campbell HS. Contact dermatitis to polyester spin finishes. *Contact Dermatitis* 1980;6:362.

169. Wigger-Alberti W, Hofmann M, Elsner P. Contact dermatitis caused by triglycidyl isocyanurate. *Am J Contact Dermatitis* 1997;8:106.

170. Sjoborg S, Dahlquist I, Fregert S, Trulson L. Contact allergy to styrene with cross reaction to vinyltoluene. *Contact Dermatitis* 1982;8:207.

171. Fregert S. Outbreak of irritant dermatitis from dial-lyl-phthalate (and styrene) in polyester resin. *Contact Dermatitis Newsletter* 1971;10: 234.

172. Mowe G. Health risks from isocyanates. *Contact Dermatitis* 1980; 6:44.

173. Estlander T, Keskinen H, Jolanki R, et al. Occupational dermatitis from exposure to polyurethane chemicals. *Contact Dermatitis* 1992; 27:161.

174. Schroder C, Uter W, Schwanitz HJ. Occupational allergic contact dermatitis, partly airborne, due to isocyanates and epoxy resin. *Contact Dermatitis* 1999;41:117.

175. Emmett EA. Allergic contact dermatitis in polyurethane plastic moulders. *J Occup Med* 1976;18:802.

176. Thompson T, Belsito DV. Allergic contact dermatitis from a diisocyanate in wool processing. *Contact Dermatitis* 1997;37:239.

177. Malten KE. 4,4′-diisocyanato dicyclohexyl methane (Hylene W): a strong contact sensitizer. *Contact Dermatitis* 1977;3:344.

178. Kanerva L, Grenquist-Norden B, Piirila P. Occupational IgE-mediated contact urticaria from diphanylmethane-4,4′-diisocyanate (MDI). *Contact Dermatitis* 1999;41:50.

179. Verdich I, Skoven I. Allergic contact dermatitis from Desmophen, a polyether alcohol. *Contact Dermatitis* 1979;5:120.

180. Fisher AA. Fiberglass vs mineral wool (rock-wool) dermatitis. *Cutis* 1982;29:412, 415–416, 422 *passim.*

181. Tarvainen K, et al. Occupational dermatoses from the manufacture of plastic composite products. *Am J Contact Dermatitis* 1995;6:95.

182. Heisel EB, Hunt FE. Further studies in cutaneous reactions to glass fibers. *Arch Environ Health* 1968;17:705.

183. Possick PA, Gellin GA, Key MM. Fibrous glass dermatitis. *Am Ind Hyg Assoc J* 1970;31:12.

184. Fisher BK, Warkentin JD. Fiber glass dermatitis. *Arch Dermatol* 1969;99:717.

185. Eby CS, Jetton RL. School desk dermatitis. Primary irritant contact dermatitis to fiberglass. *Arch Dermatol* 1972;105:890.

186. Heino T, Haapa K, Manelius F. Contact sensitization to organosilane in glass filament production. *Contact Dermatitis* 1996;34:294.

187. Bjornberg A, Lowhagen GB, Tengberg JE. Relationship between intensities of skin test reactions to glass-fibres and chemical irritants. *Contact Dermatitis* 1979;5:171.

188. Bjornberg A, Lowhagen GB, Tengberg JE. Does occupational exposure to glass-fibres increase the general skin reactivity to irritants? *Contact Dermatitis* 1979;5:175.

189. Bjornberg A, Lowhagen GB, Tengberg JE. Skin reactivity in workers with and without itching from occupational exposure to glass fibres. *Acta Dermato-Venereol* 1979;59:49.

190. Cuypers JMC, Hoedemaeker PJ, Nater PJ, de Jong MC. The histopathology of fiberglass dermatitis in relation to von Hebra's concept of eczema. *Contact Dermatitis* 1975;1:88.

191. Dahlquist S, Fregert S, Trulsson L. Allergic contact dermatitis from epoxy resin finished glass fiber. *Contact Dermatitis* 1979;5:190.

192. Lucas JB. Common industrial dermatoses. *Cutis* 1974;13:33.

193. Bjornberg A, Lowhagen GB. Patch test reactions to rockwool. *Contact Dermatitis* 1975;1:242.

194. Bjornberg A, Lowhagen GB. Patch testing with mineral wool (rock-wool). *Acta Dermato-Venereol* 1977;57:257.

CHAPTER 30

Contact Dermatitis from Food Additives and Dyes

CONTACT DERMATITIS FROM FOOD ADDITIVES

About 400 additives are included in the US Food and Drug Administration's list of additives "generally recognized as safe," except for large groups of natural flavors and oils. To be on this list, an additive must have been in use before 1958 and must have met certain safety specifications. Additives brought into use since 1958 must be approved individually. Substances are removed occasionally from the list by the FDA in light of new evidence.

Many additives to foods, cosmetics, and topical medications can produce contact dermatitis, including preservatives, antioxidants, dyes, flavoring agents, "spoilage retarders," "dough conditioners," "flavor protectors," and "cloudiness preventatives" (1) (Table 30.1).

The dermatitis that these chemical additives produce can be of several varieties, including irritant dermatitis, allergic eczematous contact dermatitis, and contact urticaria, both allergic and nonspecific in nature. The most common food additive dermatitis is a hand dermatitis in certain sensitized individuals, particularly homemakers, food handlers, bakers, and cooks. Often the same agents have also proved to be sensitizers in topical medications and cosmetics (2–4).

> **The labels on packaged foods reveal a bewildering host of chemical additives, some of which are sensitizers used in cosmetics and topical medications.**

Preservatives and Flavors Added to Foods

Table 30.2 lists the preservative antibacterial and antimold agents that are added to many foods. Of these preservatives, the parabens and sorbic acid are the most common causes of contact dermatitis.

The Parabens

These agents are used not only in many topical medications and cosmetics but also in many foods. Thus, methylparaben and propylparaben may be added in the amount of 1,000 parts per million to tomato pulp, puree, catsup, pickles, relishes, fruit juices, syrups, jams, marmalades, fruit jellies, mincemeat, milk preparations, soft drinks, and candy, and packaged fish, meat, and poultry. The ingestion of paraben-containing foods does not seem to produce flares in paraben-sensitive individuals.

Sorbic Acid

This preservative food additive is unique in that it can rarely produce both allergic eczematous contact dermatitis in sensitized individuals and a nonspecific contact urticaria in 5% of the population (5).

Sorbic acid may be added to flour, particularly in the making of rye bread. Fisher (6) reported one baker who had an eczematous contact dermatitis of the hand from hypersensitivity to sorbic acid and positive patch test reactions to sorbic acid and potassium sorbate and to flour.

Another baker developed an immediate reaction consisting of redness and slight itching of hands when he came in contact with flour containing sorbic acid. His 48-hour patch test gave negative results. However, he developed an immediate wheal from the application of 5% sorbic acid in petrolatum. This is a "nonspecific" contact urticaria from sorbic acid.

Clemmensen and Hjorth (7) also observed contact urticaria in 18 of 20 kindergarten children following the intake and accidental perioral application of mayonnaise salad dressing. In healthy adult controls, stinging tests and closed 20-minute patch tests with the salad dressing were positive in 9 out of 12 and 4 out of 10 cases, respectively. Twenty-minute "open" tests with the different components of the salad dressing were positive only to sorbic acid and benzoic acid. Urticaria was provoked by inunction of the salad dressing periorally in two healthy boys. Serial 20-minute closed patch testing with varying concentrations of sorbic acid in 91 patients and benzoic acid in 41 patients gave almost identical results. The response was only partially blocked by antihistamine applied locally before test-

TABLE 30.1. *Food Additives*

Additive	Comment
Benzoyl peroxide	Flour "improver"
Butylated hydroxyanisole	Oxidizer—prevents rancidity
Butylated hydroxytoluene	Oxidizer—prevents rancidity
Calcium disodium EDTA	Stabilizer, chelating agent
Calcium propionate	Antimold for bread
Chlorophyll	Color for pastry
Citric acid	Preservative
Dodecyl gallate	Antioxidant
Dyes, certified	Cause urticaria
Flavoring agents and spices	Cause contact dermatitis
Gum arabic (acacia)	Cream and cheese additive
Gum benzoin	Antioxidant
Karaya	Pastry filler
Lauryl and propyl gallate	Antioxidant
Lanolin	Chewing gum
Monoglycerol citrate	Preservative
Nordihydroguaiaretic	Antioxidant
Paraben	Preservative
Polysorbate	Preservative
Potassium persulfate	Sprayed on some fruits
Propylene glycol alginate	Filler
Sodium benzoate	Preservative
Sodium bisulfite	Antioxidant
Sodium silicon aluminate	Lump preventer in cake mix
Sorbic acid	Preservative
Tetramethylthiuram	Sprayed on bananas
Tocopherols	Antioxidant
Tragacanth	Vegetable gum filler

ing. The authors pointed out that nonimmunologic mechanisms are probably responsible for the transient reaction, and no restriction in the extensive use of sorbic acid or benzoic acid as preservatives in food should be considered. Lahti et al. (8) showed these types of reactions to be inhibited by prostaglandin-inhibiting agents, such as aspirin and indomethacin.

Fisher (5) observed the same type of nonspecific erythema and urticarial response in many individuals using a hydrocortisone cream containing sorbic acid as a preservative. In such individuals, it is preferable to use hydrocortisone ointment to avoid this uncomfortable stinging effect from the sorbic acid in the hydrocortisone cream, or to use a hydrocortisone cream free of sorbic acid.

Eating salad dressings containing sorbic acid may produce a transient nonallergic urticaria of the lips and perioral area in many individuals.

TABLE 30.2. *Preservatives Added to Foods*

Benzoic acid	Monoglycerol citrate
Calcium propionate	Parabens
Citric acid	Sodium benzoate
Guaiac gum	Sorbic acid

TABLE 30.3. *Antioxidant Food Additives*

Ammonium persulfate (flour color improver used in some European countries)
Benzoyl peroxide (flour color improver)
Butylated hydroxyanisole (BHA)
Butylated hydroxytoluene (BHT)
Dodecyl gallate
Gum benzoin
Lauryl and propyl gallate
Nordihydroguaiaretic acid (NDGA)
Sodium bisulfite
Vitamin E (tocopherols)

Antioxidants in Foods

Table 30.3 lists the antioxidants that may be used in various foods to prevent a common type of food spoilage—an undesirable change in color or flavor caused by oxygen in the air. For example, sliced fresh apples and peaches turn brown when exposed to air, and fatty foods, such as mayonnaise and lard, become rancid if kept unprotected too long. Both of these conditions are caused by oxidation and can be retarded by using antioxidants.

The darkening of some fruits and vegetables is known as "enzymatic browning." If foods containing certain enzymes are cut, bruised, or overripe and are exposed to air, the tissues turn brown. Apples, apricots, bananas, cherries, peaches, pears, and potatoes contain such enzymes. Antioxidants prevent or delay this enzymatic browning.

Oxidation also causes the rancid taste and odor that sometimes develop in fats, oil, mayonnaise, and lard. Processed foods that contain these materials are thus protected with antioxidants from possible oxidation in order to maintain their best flavor during storage.

At present, antioxidants, such as butylated hydroxyanisole and butylated hydroxytoluene, are replacing gum benzoin. These antioxidants, which may also be present in cosmetics, can be tested 2% in petrolatum for patch test purposes.

Antioxidants that are added to foods to prevent undesirable changes in color and flavor and to prevent spoilage may also be present in cosmetics.

With a few exceptions, the lipid-soluble antioxidants are phenols. Those favored by industry are butylated hydroxytoluene (BHT), butylated hydroxyanisole (BHA), nordihydroguaiaretic acid (NDGA), esters of gallic acid (propyl-, octyl-, and dodecyl-gallate), and tocopherols. NDGA is not used extensively in the United States.

Butylated Hydroxyanisole (BHA)

Other names for this antioxidant include Tenox GHA (Eastman), 2-*t*-butyl-4-methoxyphenol, 4-methoxy-2-*t*-

butylphenol, Embanox (May & Baker), and Nipantiox 1-F (Nipa).

BHA is used as an antioxidant for oils and fats either alone or with a gallate and a synergist, such as citric or phosphoric acid. It may be dissolved in many oils at room temperature or warmed slightly. BHA dissolves readily in molten fats.

Up to 200 ppm of BHA or BHT, or a mixture of these, may be used for the preservation of fixed oils, fats, or vitamin oil concentrates in pharmaceutical practice and food. Up to 100 ppm of BHA or BHT may be added to essential oils used in food; its use is not allowed in essential oils of the British Pharmacopeia.

BHA is used in a wide variety of products, including beverages, ice cream, candy, baked foods, gelatin, soup bases, potatoes, glazed fruits, potato flakes, dry breakfast cereals, dry yeast, dry mixes for desserts and beverages, shortening, smoked dry sausage, and emulsions as stabilizers for shortenings.

Roed-Petersen and Hjorth (9), in a search for contact sensitivity to antioxidants, patch tested consecutive patients referred with eczematous dermatitis. Six cases of allergic contact sensitivity to NDGA were observed. Three had been sensitized by one brand of cream containing 0.1% NDGA; in three other patients, the source of sensitization could not be traced.

Four patients had positive patch tests to BHA or BHT. In two cases, the positive patch tests were relevant because both patients remained asymptomatic when antioxidants were avoided in foods. They both had acute flares of vesicular eczema on the fingers after oral administration of small amounts.

The incidence of allergic hypersensitivity to the antioxidants BHA and BHT is low. Patients, once sensitized, may exhibit systemic skin and vascular reactions when they eat foods containing these agents.

Butylated Hydroxytoluene (BHT)

This antioxidant, which is substituted for toluene, has several names: Catalin CAO-3 (Ashland), DBPC, 2,6-di-*t*-butyl-*p*-cresol, Ionol (Shell), Ionol CP (Shell), Tenox BHT (Eastman), 4-methyl-2,6-di-*t*-butyl-phenol, Annulex BHT, Embanox BHT (May & Baker), Topanol OC, and O (ICI).

BHT, like BHA, is used as an antioxidant for oil and fats. In foods, BHT may be used to a 0.02% concentration, whereas in cosmetics it is used in a 0.01% to 0.1% concentration.

Reactions from Ingestion of the Antioxidants BHA and BHT

Fisherman and Cohen (10) reported that a group of patients developed a "positive sequential vascular response" to

TABLE 30.4. *Products Containing BHT Divided into Product Categories, Based on 440 products Registered March 1990 (typical concentrations are stated only for categories with clear trends and 10 or more registered products)*

Product category	No. of products*	Typical concentration
Paints and lacquers (1- and 2-component)	141	< 25 ppm
Hardeners for 2-component paints, glues, fillers, etc.	100	< 10 ppm
Binders for paints, glues, fillers, etc.	34	0–2000 ppm
Adhesives/glues	33	200–1000 ppm
Toiletries	31	200–1000 ppm
Industrial oil and grease (including cutting fluids)	23	300–10,000 ppm
Fillings and mouldings	23	< 25 ppm
Cleaning agents	11	< 200 ppm
Printing/offset products (inks, stabilizers, etc.)	9	—
Thinners and solvents	8	—
Flooring materials	5	—

*Some products are registered in two or more product categories. Categories with fewer than four products were omitted. Used with permission from Flyvolm, M-A., and Menné, T. Sensitizing risk of butylated hydroxytoluene based on exposure and effect data. *Contact Dermatitis* 23:341, 1990.

BHA and BHT. These patients, upon ingestion of BHA and BHT, had an intensification of rhinitis and asthma. Other symptoms noted on challenge were marked diaphoresis, somnolence, headaches, occasionally high retrosternal pain radiating to the back, flushing, and suffusion of the conjunctivae. In addition, all of the BHA-BHT patients, when tested with aspirin in doses of 100 mg, not only did not exacerbate clinically, but they often improved.

One investigation of BHT found none of 1,336 patients patch tested to be positive to 2% BHT in petrolatum (11). Other uses for BHT are given in Table 30.4. The table lists the product category only.

Sodium Bisulfite in Salads

Epstein (12) described hand eczema in a salad maker caused by Veg-White, an antioxidant used to prevent discoloration of fruits and vegetables in salads. The specific sensitizer in this preparation was sodium bisulfite. Patch tests can be performed with a 1% aqueous solution of sodium bisulfite.

Patch tests with sodium bisulfite must be interpreted with care because many test results are irritant in nature. Several controls should always be tested. Toxic effects from the ingestion of sodium bisulfite in foods have been reported recently (13–15).

Gallates (Gallic Acid Esters)

The esters most commonly used as antioxidants are the propyl, octyl, and dodecyl esters. The latter two are easily soluble in fats. Propyl ester is more soluble in water than in fats. These antioxidants are often used in the cosmetic and food industry, particularly in bakery goods and frying oils. In guinea pigs all three gallates are moderate to strong sensitizers, with dodecyl being the strongest (16). A 0.3% concentration in petrolatum is recommended for patch testing. Octyl gallate, when mixed with heated chicken fat, has caused an airborne contact dermatitis (17).

Lauryl Gallate

Brun (18) reported contact dermatitis in a baker due to lauryl gallate present as an antioxidant in margarine.

Postendorf (19) speculated that the topical application of cosmetics and pharmaceuticals containing gallates may produce dermatitis in certain individuals, "perhaps because they are sensitized by gallates in foodstuffs."

Oral Symptoms and Additives

Lip swelling and oral ulceration are symptoms that at times can be caused by food additives. Menthol, peppermint oil, dodecyl and octyl gallate, and butylated hydroxyanisole were identified as causative factors in five patients reported by Lewis et al. (20). For menthol and peppermint oil, restrictions were placed on toothpaste, mouthwashes, inhalers, and confections. For the gallates, margarine, oils, cosmetics, and lip balms were restricted. Butylated hydroxyanisole sensitivity was treated with avoidance of margarine, fats, soups, sauces, cakes, and pastries.

Peppermint Oil

The ingredients in peppermint oil include menthol, menthone, menthyl esters (acetate and isovalerate), l-limonene, pinene, phellandrene, and cineole. Wilkinson and Beck (21) emphasized the role of menthol as an allergen in peppermint oil and noted that menthol joins l-limonene, alpha-pinene, and phellandrene as causes of contact dermatitis.

Detection of menthol and peppermint oil allergy may be missed if patch test readings are not taken beyond day 4. Fleming and Forsyth (22) found day 5 to be the correct time to read for these allergens.

Morton et al. (23) reported 12 cases of allergy to peppermint oil and/or menthol sensitivity in patients with burning mouth syndrome, recurrent oral ulceration, or lichenoid oral reactions. Avoidance of the identified substance was clearly beneficial in at least half of these individuals.

Cinnamon Dermatitis

Malten (24) reported several bakers with contact dermatitis and identified cinnamon as the causative agent. It should be noted that cinnamon and balsam of Peru often cross-react. Fisher (25) observed a baker with allergic hypersensitivity in whom hand dermatitis flared whenever he drank vermouth containing cinnamon. This patient also developed a cheilitis from the use of a cinnamon-containing toothpaste.

Spices used in cooking may produce systemic contact dermatitis (26).

> **Sensitization to cinnamon, which cross-reacts with balsam of Peru, may cause a "systemic" contact dermatitis when vermouth is ingested and may produce cheilitis from the use of toothpaste containing cinnamic aldehyde.**

Tocopherols or Vitamin E

These natural substances are themselves rather prone to oxidation and are therefore not quite as suitable as the synthetic antioxidants already mentioned. Yet they are widely used as a result of the urge to produce pure natural foodstuffs. The smell of oxidized tocopherols is slightly reminiscent of fish, which can be a disadvantage in some foods. Most vegetable oils in their natural state contain considerable amounts of tocopherols, for example, 0.1% to 0.01%. Animal fats also contain tocopherols, but to a far lesser degree.

It is worthwhile to note that there are no reports of allergic reactions from the ingestion of vitamin E. Topical application of vitamin E, however, can readily produce allergic contact dermatitis. Thus, so many cases of dermatitis were produced by Mennen's "E" deodorant that it was withdrawn from the market. In addition, patients who pierce vitamin E capsules and rub the contents into their skin or apply various vitamin E creams or topical agents not infrequently acquire allergic contact dermatitis (see Chapter 10).

> **Ingested tocopherols (vitamin E) do not cause allergic reactions. Topical applications, however, have sensitized many individuals.**

Topical vitamin E may also cause contact urticaria (see Chapter 16).

Nordihydroguaiaretic Acid (NDGA)

This antioxidant, no longer used in food in the United States, is used in pharmaceutical and cosmetic preparations.

It may be made synthetically or extracted from guaiac and desert plants. Roed-Petersen and Hjorth (9) reported allergic reactions to this antioxidant.

Anise

Cakes baked with anise caused contact dermatitis in two women reported from Seville who were proven to be sensitive to the allergen in anise: anethole (27). The chemical name for anethole is 1-methoxy-4-(1-propenyl)benzene, and it is closely related to eugenol, but cross reactivity does not occur.

Garlic

Contact dermatitis to garlic has been associated with fingertip dermatitis but caused a pompholyx pattern of dermatitis when ingested orally as a commercially available garlic extract to treat hyperlipidemia (28). A 5% aqueous patch test to garlic extract was positive. Cooked garlic did not cause a reaction, as this denatures the allergens diallyldisulfide, allylpropyldisulfide, and allicin.

Miscellaneous Additives

Sesame

Sesame oil in food and cosmetics caused urticaria from ingestion and skin contact in two French patients (29). Prick tests were positive to crushed sesame seeds, sesame oil, or their own products.

Cashew

Allergen may be added to foodstuff and provoke systemic reactions that clinically display flexural, groin, and/or buttock erythema. Hamilton and Zug (30) reported this type of reaction in a Toxicodendron-sensitive patient who ingested a pesto sauce that contained raw cashew nuts. When cashew nuts are roasted, the allergen is inactivated, but the pesto had the raw nuts.

Emulsifying Agents in Foods

Propylene Glycol

Propylene glycol is the only emulsifying agent (Table 30.5) that has been shown to be a sensitizer. Individuals sensitized to propylene glycol from topical agents may exhibit a "systemic" contact dermatitis when they eat foods containing this emulsifier (31). Many prepared food salads contain propylene glycol. Table 30.6 lists some of the foods that contain significant amounts of propylene glycol.

TABLE 30.5. *Emulsifying Agents in Foods*

Cholic acid
Desoxycholic acid
Discetyl tartaric acid esters of mono- and diglycerides
Glycocholic acid
Mono- and diglycerides
Monosodium phosphate derivatives of above
Ox bile extract
Propylene glycol
Taurocholic acid

Propylene Glycol Dermatitis Due to Ingestion of Certain Foods

Fisher (31) reported three women, with exquisite allergic hypersensitivity to propylene glycol, who were certain that otherwise unexplained flares of their dermatitis were caused by the ingestion of foods containing propylene glycol. These women implicated the propylene glycol–containing foods shown in Table 30.6 as the cause of their flare-ups.

Flares of dermatitis were produced in two patients who deliberately ate propylene glycol–containing foods. Patch tests with the implicated foods gave negative results, however.

Hannuksela and Forstrom (32) performed double-blind tests with ingestion of capsules containing propylene glycol. Eight of 10 patients sensitive to a 2% propylene glycol patch test and seven of 28 sensitive to 10% to 100% patch tests exhibited an examthum 3 to 16 hours after ingestion of 2 to 15 mL of propylene glycol.

> **Propylene glycol, an emulsifying agent in many foods, particularly salad dressings, will produce a "systemic" contact dermatitis when ingested by propylene glycol–sensitive individuals. This is in contrast with paraben-sensitive patients, who do not "flare" when they ingest paraben-containing foods.**

TABLE 30.6. *Foods Containing Propylene Glycol*

Bakers Coconut
Dream-Whip Whipped Topping Mix
Duncan Hines cake mixes
Durkee Coconut
Durkee Real French Fried Onions and Potato Sticks
Hellman's Big H (sandwich mix)
Jello Cheesecake Mix
Kraft Thousand Island, Creamy Cucumber, Russian
  Dressing
Mountain Dew Beverage
Pepperidge Farms—pineapple n'cream, strawberry
  n'cream, and most of its frosted cakes
Pfeiffer Russian, cole slaw, French dressing
Pillsbury Plus cake mixes
Sara Lee chocolate n'cream layer, strawberry n'cream layer
  cake, French cheesecake, chocolate Bavarian, and
  strawberry cheesecake
Wise Butter Flavored Popcorn

TABLE 30.7. *Stabilizers in Foods*

Acacia (gum arabic)	Ghatti gum
Agar-agar	Guar gum
Ammonium alginate	Potassium alginate
Calcium alginate	Sodium alginate
Carbo bean gum	Sterculia (or karaya) gum
Chondrus extract	Tragacanth

Stabilizers in Foods

Table 30.7 is a list of food stabilizers. Some of the stabilizers also include waxes and gums, guaiac, guar, karaya, acacia (gum arabic), tragacanth, benzoin, spermaceti, carnauba, and beeswax; the last four are used to glaze confectionery. Acacia (gum arabic) is used in chocolate drinks, creams, French dressing, malt liquors, milk, mustard, pickles, cheese, ice cream, and sherbet. Guaiac gum is used as a preservative for fats and oils, guar gum for a preservative in milk products. Guar gum is also used as a stabilizer and as a thickening and film-forming agent for cheese, salad dressings, ice cream, and soups, and as a binding and disintegrating agent in tablet formulations in suspensions, emulsions, lotions, creams, and toothpastes.

Because some of these waxes and gums cross-react with balsam of Peru, routine patch testing with balsam of Peru may be valuable in discovering the cause of hand dermatitis in food handlers.

Karaya Gum Dermatitis

A baker complained that whenever he prepared meringue pies he developed a dermatitis on his hands. It was learned that karaya gum is used as a pastry filler and stabilizer of the meringue. Potassium sorbate is sometimes also used as a preservative in meringue. Patch testing revealed a positive reaction to karaya gum, which is a rare sensitizer. Karaya, a vegetable gum derivative, is also used widely in hair-waving lotions, denture adhesive powders, and furniture polishes, and as a cement for ileostomy appliances. It may occasionally produce allergic reactions from such exposure (33). (See also Chapter 11.)

Bleaching Agents to "Improve" Flour

The "persulfates" in Europe and occasionally benzoyl peroxide, in the United States, added to flour have produced contact dermatitis in bakers (34,35).

Ammonium Persulfate Reactions

Ammonium persulfate was previously used in certain European countries as a flour "improver" to render the flour white. This flour "improver" was especially used in Greece. In the United States, this chemical has never been used in flour but is used widely in hair bleaches to enhance the bleaching action of hydrogen peroxide. Interestingly, a woman who formerly baked bread in Greece and who had acquired a severe hand dermatitis from the presence of ammonium persulfate in flour developed a severe reaction and a flare-up of her hand dermatitis when she had her hair bleached in the United States (34).

Ammonium persulfate may not only produce an eczematous contact dermatitis, but in certain persons severe urticaria and anaphylactic shock may occur.

Cronin (36) stated that in the 1920s ammonium and potassium persulfates and benzoyl peroxide were added to flour to inhibit proteolytic enzymes from attacking the gluten films that surround the carbon dioxide bubbles that form during fermentation and make bread light. Both chemicals are sensitizers, and their introduction increased the incidence of baker's eczema. Persulfates, thought to be the greater hazard, were banned first in Switzerland, Belgium, and Denmark, and in 1957, in Germany, where persulfate sensitivity had become a considerable problem. After their use was prohibited in Germany, the incidence of baker's eczema fell.

Ammonium persulfate and benzoyl peroxide are still used to make flour in the Netherlands and Britain, but, although benzoyl peroxide is still widely used, many millers have replaced the persulfates with potassium bromate, which is equally efficient and easier to handle.

> **Ammonium persulfate, a "booster" hair-bleaching agent, was formerly used in Europe to bleach flour to improve its color.**

Benzoyl Peroxide Dermatitis

A young baker had acquired a contact dermatitis of the hands from the presence of benzoyl peroxide used as a flour bleach. When he applied a benzoyl peroxide acne preparation to his face, a severe facial dermatitis developed in addition to a flare-up of his hand dermatitis (4).

Irritant and Allergic Hand Dermatitis in Bakers Due to Food Additives

Table 30.8 lists the food additives to flour, bread, or pastry that can produce a nonspecific irritant dermatitis. Thus,

TABLE 30.8. *Food Additive Irritants That Bakers May Encounter*

Acetic acid
Ascorbinic acid (flour improver)
Bleaching agents
Calcium acetate and sulfate
Emulsifying agents
Lactic acid
Potassium bicarbonate
Potassium iodide and bromate
Yeast

TABLE 30.9. *Food Additive Allergens in the Baking Industry*

Allergen	Patch test concentration
Benzoyl peroxide	1% pet
Potassium bromate	5% in water
Cinnamon oil	0.5% pet
Limonene, oil of	1% alcohol
p-amino-azo-benzene	0.25% pet (indicator for azo dyes)
Eugenol	5% pet
Vanilla (alcoholic extract)	10% in acetone
Sorbic acid	5% pet
Karaya gum (sterculia gum)	As is
Ammonium persulfate (Europe)	1% in water

Pet = in petrolatum.

most instances of hand dermatitis in bakers that Fisher (37) observed were due to nonspecific dermatitis from various irritants, such as wet, sticky dough, sweetening agents, and various flavors. Soaps and detergents used for cleansing the hands are also often the cause of irritant bakers' dermatitis. In such instances, patch tests give negative results.

Bakers may also react to enzymes added to flour to facilitate the rising of dough. These additives also make bread lighter and extend shelf life. The enzymes used include alpha- and beta-amylase, cellulase, proteases, and lipoxygenases. Alpha-amylase has been identified as a cause of hand eczema and respiratory allergy (rhinitis and asthma) in bakers (38). Of 32 bakers tested, 7 were found to have immediate hypersensitivity and 2 had delayed hypersensitivity.

Table 30.9 lists the allergen food additives encountered by bakers and the concentration for patch test purposes.

Insecticide Sprays on Fruits

Table 30.10 lists insecticides that may adhere to foods. Such insecticides may produce contact dermatitis in those handling such fruits.

Miscellaneous Food Additives

Quillaja is used as a foaming agent for soft drinks, and sodium alginate is listed for a wide variety of foods. Aluminum sulfate, admittedly a rare skin sensitizer, is permitted in canned fish, pickles, relishes, and starch.

Colors Added to Foods

Several "natural" and 10 synthetic organic dyes are permitted in the United States. Citrus Red No. 2 and Sunset Yel-

TABLE 30.10. *Insecticides Sprayed on Fruits*

Potassium persulfate (many fruits)
Tetramethylthiuram disulfide (bananas)
Thiabendazol (citrus fruits)

low have formulas that indicate possible cross-reactions with paraphenylenediamine and sulfanilamide. The synthetic colors are permitted for the dyeing of oranges, apples, jam, butter, cheese, and fish.

Chlorophyll may be added to certain pastries.

Citrus Red No. 2, used to color Florida oranges, may cross-react with clothing dyes (39).

Curcumin

A pasta worker whose job it was to add food color to pasta and collect the fresh pasta from the machine was found allergic to curcumin food color (40). Curcumin is used to color butter, margarine, cheese, spaghetti, macaroni, and liqueurs. *Curcuma longa* is the source for turmeric, which is derived from the rootstock of the plant. The *Curcuma* rootstock is also the source for curcumin, the yellow food dye that produced positive patch test responses down to 0.001%. This is also a component of curry powder, and the patient reacted to curry powder at 1% concentration. She also reacted to ginger which is from *Zingiber officinale*, a member of the same family as *Curcuma longa*.

> **Florida oranges may be dyed with Citrus Red No. 2, which may cross-react with clothing dyes, paraphenylenediamine, and sulfanilamide. California oranges are not dyed.**

Potato Chip Dermatitis

Inman (41) traced three cases of contact dermatitis of the hands occurring in a potato chip factory that were due, respectively, to cheese powder, wheat filler, and onion powder.

Metals in Foods

Most foods contain traces of metals, including nickel and chromium (Table 30.11). Ethylenediamine tetra-acetate (EDTA) is added to many foods to chelate such metals. It must be emphasized that EDTA is not a sensitizer and does not cross-react with ethylenediamine hydrochloride, which is a notorious sensitizer.

Nickel may be added to act as a catalyst in hydrogenating fats. In addition, it has been reported that the ingestion of

TABLE 30.11. *Metals in Foods**

Aluminum sulfate
Chromium (from water)
Cobalt
Nickel (may also be added to hydrogenated fats)

*Ethylenediamine tetra-acetate (EDTA) is often added to foods to chelate these metals.

nickel in foods could produce pompholyx and flares of nickel dermatitis in sensitized individuals (42).

Sulfates in Foods

Sodium lauryl sulfate is used in egg white, sodium sulfate is added to biscuits and tuna fish, and sodium thiosulfate is added to table salt. The hands of food handlers with atopic or eczematous skin may be irritated by these sulfates. Aluminum sulfate is a permitted additive in canned fish, pickles, relishes, and starch.

Halogens in Foods

It should be noted that vegetable oil for citrus-flavored beverages is "brominated," and calcium iodate is used for some bakery products. Such iodine or bromine additives may produce "fixed" drug eruptions or eruptions of a pustular nature.

Several patients developed a pustular eruption from eating kelp in a salad or in vitamin preparations.

Kelp as a dietary supplement or present in vitamins contains sufficient iodine to produce iodide eruptions and flares of acne.

Norwegian Kelp Tablets are described as a dietary supplement. Each tablet is said to contain "0.225 mg of iodine, which supplies 22.5% of the Adult Minimum Daily Requirement in a base of organically grown alfalfa, for which no nutritional claims are made."

Kelp, a giant brown seaweed, is one of the largest algae and may grow as long as 300 feet. The ashes of this seaweed are used as a source of iodine and sometimes potash (43).

Silicates as Anticaking Agents

The silicates listed in Table 30.12 have not been implicated as contact allergens.

Synthetic Flavoring Agents

Table 30.13 lists these agents, many of which are sensitizers.

TABLE 30.12. *Anticaking Agents*

Aluminum calcium silicate
Calcium silicate
Magnesium silicate
Sodium aluminosilicate
Sodium calcium aluminosilicate
Tricalcium silicate

TABLE 30.13. *Synthetic Flavoring Substances*

Acetaldehyde
Acetoin
Aconitic acid
Anethole
Benzaldehyde
N-butyric acid
d- or *l*-carvone
Cinnamaldehyde
Citral
Decanal
Diacetyl
Ethyl acetate
Ethyl butyrate
Ethyl vanillin
Eugenol
Geraniol
Geranyl acetate
Glycerol tributyrate
Limonene
Linalool
Linalyl acetate
1-malic acid
Methyl anthranilate
3-methyl-3-phenyl glycidic acid ethyl ester
Piperanol
Vanillin

FOOD DYES AND COLORS

Dyes added to foods, drugs, cosmetics, and textiles may produce contact dermatitis.

Dyes and various colors are added to foods for the following reasons: (a) to ensure uniform color; (b) to replace colors changed by preservatives, various processes, heat, light, and cold; and (c) to augment color of pale foods.

Table 30.14 lists the various natural colors that may be added to foods; Table 30.15 lists synthetic dyes that may be added to food. Allergic contact dermatitis from such food dyes and colors is rare; however, three of the food dyes listed in Table 30.16—amaranth, Sunset Yellow, and tartrazine—have been implicated as causing contact urticaria and purpura. Another dye, neococcine (a carrine red dye), has been similarly implicated (44–49).

FD&C food dyes, particularly FD&C No. 5 (tartrazine), may produce urticaria, particularly in aspirin-sensitive individuals.

TABLE 30.14. *"Natural" Food Colors*

Anthocyanins	Flavonoids
Carotenoids	Metals
Chlorophyll	Turmeric spice

TABLE 30.15. *Food Synthetic Dyes*

Anthraquinone	Quinolene
Azo	Triarylmethane
Artificial caramel	Xanthene
Indigoid	

The food dyes that produce urticaria often occur in aspirin-sensitive individuals (47,50).

Nature of FD&C Azo Food Dyes

Food, Drug and Cosmetic (FD&C) azo dyes, derived from coal tar, are "certified." "Certification" refers to lack of toxicity and not to allergenicity. These dyes rarely cross-react with paraphenylenediamine and are widely used to color many foods, including gelatin desserts, oleomargarine, other edible fats and oils, maraschino cherries, sausage casings, frozen desserts, carbonated beverages (FD&C Blue No. 2 is used for special grape shades), candy and confectionery products, bakery products, spaghetti, and puddings.

The incidence of hypersensitivity to FD&C dyes in the general population is not known. An association, however, between hypersensitivity to aspirin and tartrazine has been described (48–58). Juhlin et al. (47) reported that seven of eight aspirin-sensitive patients were also allergic to tartrazine. Smith (51) found two of five aspirin-sensitive patients to be allergic to tartrazine. On the other hand, Samter and Beers (52), in 1967, reported 3 of 40 aspirin-sensitive patients to also be allergic to tartrazine. The following year, these authors (53) reported 14 of 182 aspirin-sensitive patients to also be allergic to tartrazine. The reported incidence of aspirin hypersensitivity varies among different authors but seems to be in the range of 1% to 5% of the population, the higher percentage found in patients with asthma (55,56). It would appear that tartrazine hypersensitivity is relatively uncommon, although it probably occurs with greater frequency in individuals with a documented history of allergy.

Food Dyes

Mitchell (39) tested with a food-dye series shown in Table 30.16 (39). (See also Chapter 17.) He found that a chef with

TABLE 30.16. *Food Dye Patch-Test Series*

Test 2% petrolatum	
Amaranth	Fast green
Benzyl violet	Indigotine
Brilliant blue	Ponceau SX
Citrus Red No. 2	Sunset Yellow
Erythrosine	Tartrazine

a foot dermatitis, who was mistakenly tested with a food patch test series, was found to react to Citrus Red No. 2 that apparently cross-reacted with the dye in his socks, which remained unidentified. Citrus Red dermatitis is rare. Bandmann and Nasemann (57) observed sensitization to a Ponceau (Red 6R) in a pastry cook. Citrus Red is now used to color Florida oranges, but not the California variety.

> **Citrus Red No. 2, a food dye that is added to Florida oranges but not to California oranges, like other food dyes is a rare sensitizer.**

DERMATITIS DUE TO DYES USED IN DRUGS

Pharmaceutical manufacturers add dyes to the liquid or solid formulation, the tablet coating, or the hard gelatin capsule of most of their products for purposes of drug identification and dosage form differentiation. These are valid reasons for the addition of coloring agents in drugs, and their continued inclusion is a necessity. Some manufacturers have employed vegetable dyes to color their products, but these agents have fallen into relative disuse because of a lack of stability resulting in a loss of uniformity of color.

For this reason, most companies now use one or more of the FD&C azo dyes (-N=N-group) that are derived from coal tar. These include FD&C Red No. 2, Red No. 3, Red No. 4, Blue No. 1, Blue No. 2, Violet No. 1, Green No. 3, Yellow No. 3, Yellow No. 5, Yellow No. 6, Yellow No. 10, and Yellow No. 11.

In addition to the pure FD&C dyes, various combinations of two or more may be employed to produce another color (e.g., Velo Dark Green dye contains FD&C Yellow No. 5). FD&C Lake dyes are also used, prepared by extending, on a substratum of alumina, a salt prepared from one of the water-soluble, pure FD&C dyes by combining the color with aluminum or calcium. Drug and Cosmetic dyes, such as D&C Red No. 40, are added occasionally to pharmaceutical products as coloring agents. This group, unlike the pure FD&C dyes, is not used to color food products. FD&C Red No. 2, Red No. 4, Blue No. 1, Yellow No. 5, and Yellow No. 6 are the dyes that have been used most frequently in drugs.

Several dyes used in pharmaceutical products have demonstrated the potential for inducing allergic reactions in hypersensitive patients. It should be noted that the population at large is exposed to potentially allergenic FD&C dyes in foods to a greater extent than in drugs. This reflects the obviously greater ingestion of food compared with drugs, as well as the greater amounts of dye included in food products compared with drugs. In addition, foods contain potentially allergenic vegetable dyes rarely present in pharmaceutical preparations. Nevertheless, a problem resulting from coloring agents in drugs has been identified and cannot be disregarded.

> **FD&C azo dyes in pharmaceuticals may produce urticaria, purpura, asthma, and fixed drug eruptions.**

Chafee and Settipane (54) in 1974 reported a case of recurrent asthma due to tartrazine. Tartrazine was finally implicated when the patient noted an exacerbation of symptoms upon taking 1.25-mg tablets of Premarin (conjugated estrogen), which also contain this dye. After elimination of tartrazine-containing products, the patient did well.

Criep (45) in 1971 reported a case of nonthrombocytopenic vascular purpura resulting from hypersensitivity to tartrazine in an adult. The patient gave a history of repeated episodes of bleeding into the skin and from various mucous membranes following ingestion of the dye.

Testing for Reactions to Dyes in Drugs

Lockey (48) described sublingual testing with diluted samples of pure FD&C dyes to challenge the patient and reported the technique in detail. The patient was observed for 20 minutes following sublingual administration for signs of hypersensitivity. Feingold (44) employed a method of clinical screening to diagnose and treat suspected allergy to FD&C dyes. Patients were divided into four groups based on their pattern of allergy and skin testing, and various elimination diets were prescribed for each group, in an attempt to identify and isolate offending allergens.

Juhlin et al. (47) administered tartrazine in an oral solution and observed patients for signs of hypersensitivity. Allergic patients responded significantly to quantities as little as 0.75 mg. (The amount of tartrazine present in various pharmaceutical preparations is variable, but may range from 0.002 mg to greater than 2.5 mg per dosage unit in those preparations that contain the dye.)

Michaâlsson et al. (49) were able to provoke purpuric reactions in their hypersensitive patients by administering allergenic dyes orally in colorless gelatin capsules. A topical vasodilator was applied to a skin test site, causing a localized nonpurpuric erythema before dye administration. In some trials, purpura developed only in this test area upon ingestion of the allergenic dye. In others, purpura was more widespread. Dyes to which the patient was not hypersensitive produced no purpura.

Fiedelman and Martens (50) suggested full disclosure in labeling of all additives present in drugs. This would help prevent exposure in those patients with known hypersensitivity to coloring agents, but would do little to prevent the occurrence of new cases. Another solution is the removal of coloring agents from certain drugs, particularly those used frequently in the treatment of atopic patients (e.g., antihist-

amines, antiasthmatics, and corticosteroids). As an alternative, pharmaceutical companies could selectively produce dye-free preparations for those patients with known or suspected hypersensitivity to coloring agents. Indeed, for this reason, tartrazine has been removed from one antiasthmatic preparation that is available both with and without dye (Marax syrup and Marax DF syrup).

> **Dye-sensitive individuals, atopics, and aspirin-sensitive patients should take pharmaceuticals free of dyes.**

In addition to their inclusion in medication meant for oral administration, coloring agents may be present in topical preparations. Often, hospital pharmacies will add coloring agents to solutions that were originally dye-free for purposes of identification. These preparations may cause contact dermatitis in hypersensitive individuals, a reaction not uncommonly seen after application of cosmetics that contain allergenic dyes.

D&C Yellow No. 11

D&C Yellow No. 11 (CAS No. 8003-22-3) is the FDA designation for a color additive certified for use in drugs and cosmetics. The dye component is principally 2-(2 quinolyl)-1,3-in-dandione, synthesized by the condensation of quinoline with phthalic anhydride at 200°C in the presence of zinc. The dye substance is also known as CI Solvent No. Yellow 33, CI No. 47,000, Quinoline Yellow SS, Quinoline Yellow Base, Quinoline Yellow Spirit Soluble, Waxoline Yellow T, and Arlosol Yellow SS.

Rapaport stated that quinazaline yellow SS (D&C Yellow No. 11), a quinoline chemical, elicited interest because of a potential for sensitization (58–61). This is an FDA-approved dye that is used widely in cosmetics. However, D&C Yellow No. 10, a closely related quinoline chemical, is more widely used in cosmetics and topical preparations, and there has been some concern about possible cross-sensitization between these two drugs.

Noster and Hausen (63) reported one case of occupational allergic contact dermatitis due to D&C Yellow No. 11 that was present in colored smoke used in a detonator. The authors attempted sensitization experiments on guinea pigs but were unsuccessful. Börkner and Magnusson (64), studying D&C Yellow 11 in 1981, commented on its use in spirit, lacquers, polystyrenes, polycarbonates, polyamides, acrylic resins, cosmetics, colored smokes, and hydrocarbon solvents. They patch tested 88 subjects with a 1% preparation in polyethylene glycol and found four positive patch test responses at 72 hours. One subject had a cross-reaction to D&C Yellow No. 10 when patch tests to that dye were carried out.

These dyes are used extensively to impart a green-yellow shade to cosmetics and topical preparations. More than 300 cosmetic preparations incorporate D&C Yellow into their formulas; usage of D&C Yellow No. 10 is even more widespread. In 1977, in the United States alone, 8.16 tons of D&C Yellow No. 10 and 2.23 tons of D&C Yellow No. 11 were used. Although in Europe D&C Yellow No. 10 is used as a food-coloring agent, especially in soft drinks, in the United States its use is not allowed in foods but is, however, allowed in drugs.

> **D&C Yellow No. 11, a quinolene dye, used widely in cosmetics, pharmaceuticals, and industry, may show cross-reactions with quinolene compounds used in topical and oral drugs, such as vioform, chloroquin, and ethoxyquin.**

Many other quinolines are used in medical products. Oral drugs, for example, iodochlorohydroxyquin, chloroquin, oxolinic acid (an antimicrobial used for urinary tract infections), and oxamniquine (an antischistosomal drug), are typical. In addition, coccidiostat, an animal feed, and ethoxyquin, an antioxidant in animal feed, have widespread usage and similar formulas. The contents of all of these preparations allow for the possibility of cross-reaction between the yellow dyes and chemically related topical and oral drugs.

Jordan (62) reported that a patient with D&C Yellow No. 11 sensitivity developed an allergic dermatitis from a yellow Irish Spring Soap containing this dye. She did not react, however, to green Irish Spring Soap.

> **D&C Yellow No. 11 is present in yellow Irish Spring, Pink Dove, and Caress bath soaps. D&C Yellow No. 11 does not cross-react with D&C Yellow No. 10.**

Pink Dove and Caress also contain Yellow D&C No. 11. Rapaport (58) stated that Yellow D&C No. 11 does *not* cross-react with Yellow D&C No. 10. This investigator was able to sensitize 15 subjects of a panel of 56 (27%) to Yellow D&C No. 11. Some of these patients, however, did not show any reactions on retesting. They could also use cosmetics containing the dye without difficulty. There were no cross-reactions with D&C No. 10. Rapaport commented that much stress is given to prophetic patch testing in terms of predicting difficulties with topically applied chemicals. Some of the chemicals in cosmetics are weak sensitizers, and detailed prophetic patch testing is necessary to seek out sensitization. Some subjects who showed positive sensitization patch test patterns 2 years earlier did not show positive reactions again to repeated insult patch tests after this

rest period. Only 50% of the subjects showed positive reactions on repeated insult patch testing 2 years later. Long-term usage of the dyes in great amounts on large areas of the body does not induce dermatitis, even though a positive patch test reaction was noted in several of the subjects. Positive prophetic patch test reactions to new or existing chemicals usually imply allergenicity for positive patch test subjects on environmental contact. Possibly contact was not maintained for a long enough period in this study.

Jordan (62) stated that the eliciting of a dye allergy from showering with a soap and his predictive tests show that D&C Yellow No. 11 is a significant allergen.

Palazzolo and DiPasquale (65) found a high sensitization frequency in guinea pigs with predictive testing with D&C Yellow No. 11.

> **Predictive tests in humans and guinea pigs indicate that D&C Yellow No. 11 is a potent allergen. Predictive testing with this dye, however, does not always correlate with clinical experience, because some patients sensitized by predictive testing use cosmetics containing the dye without reacting to them.**

PHOTOTOXIC DYES

Table 30.17 lists phototoxic dyes. (See also Chapter 23.) The phototoxic reaction may be dependent on oxygen or visible light (66).

Neutral Red

This dye is no longer used for the treatment of herpes simplex because not only it has proved ineffective, but it is also a contact sensitizer.

Mitchell and Stewart (67) reported that a woman developed allergic contact dermatitis from neutral red chloride that had been applied to the skin for herpes simplex of the nose in three episodes over 3 months. She also had contact dermatitis of the skin of the foot from contamination with the dye. The patient's patch test to the dye, which she had used in a 3% aqueous solution, was strongly positive. A patch test given to five control subjects was negative.

Dahlquist and Fregert (68) reported neutral red added as a pH indicator to a quaternary ammonium salt solution produced an allergic contact dermatitis.

TABLE 30.17. *Phototoxic Dyes*

Acridine orange	Methylene blue
Acriflavine	Neutral red
Dibromofluorescein	Rose Bengal
Disperse blue 35	Toluidine blue
Eosin	

Conant and Maibach (69) also reported allergic contact dermatitis from neutral red, as did Goldenberg and Nelson (70), from its use in the treatment of herpes genitalis.

> **Neutral red, a phototoxic and contact allergen dye, has not proven to be effective in the treatment of herpes simplex.**

"NATURAL" DYES

People first turned to plants for dyes. Among the best known and most widely used were woad (*Isatis tinctoria*) and indigo (*Indigofera tinctoria*), which gave a blue color. Yellows were provided by safflower (*Carthamus tinctorius*) and curcuma (*Curcuma ssp.*); madder (*Rubia tinctorium*), henna (*Larosonia*), and annatto (*Bixa orellana*) gave reddish hues.

Dyestuffs of animal origin were apparently developed later. It is interesting that all of these dyes were in the red color range, such as the Tyrian purple of the purpura shellfish (*Murex* spp., *Purpura* spp.) and carmine or crimson from the insects kermes (*Kermococcus vermilius*) and cochineal (*Dactylopius coccus*) (71).

The increasing mechanization of the textile industry in Europe from about the middle of the eighteenth century resulted in enormous growth in production and demanded large amounts of chemical aids, such as bleaches, detergents, and dyestuffs. This demand created the basis of the chemical industry. Originally, the chemical industry was very much textile-oriented but was only able to supply bleaches and detergents. Consequently, the cultivation of plants or insects yielding natural dyestuffs grew into a big business. Madder was produced in great quantities in southern Europe, but indigo, logwood, cattu, annatto, and cochineal had to be imported in large amounts (72).

The birth of synthetic organic chemistry replaced nearly all the traditional dyes of botanic and animal origin, but cochineal has managed to survive up to the present, even if only on a moderate scale. It is no longer used in the textile industry, even though no synthetic dye has yet surpassed it in brilliance or fastness, but it costs more. The use of cochineal today is restricted to food, drinks, cosmetics, and pharmaceutical products.

> **Synthetic dyes have largely replaced dyes derived from plants and animals. Only henna (plant hair dye) and carmine (a red insect dye) are used to any extent.**

Carmine

Carminic acid, the red dye made by the cochineal insect, is the essential constituent of carmine. If we squash the body of a live cochineal insect, a dark red liquid (containing the blood and the internal organs) squirts out; the dye in the liquid is the cochineal carmine. The dried insects of the commercial cochineal have to be immersed in hot water, or other solvent, to extract the dye (73). Nowadays only Peru and the Canary Islands are producing cochineal in an organized industrial manner.

Following the invention and manufacture of synthetic red dyes, mainly aniline derivatives, the cochineal dyes were gradually ousted from the textile industry, not because the synthetic colors were superior in color or fastness, but because they were cheaper and could be delivered in any quantity. The only places remaining for these magnificent natural products were the food, drink, cosmetic, and pharmaceutical industries. Even there, the synthetic red dye called Red No. 2, also known as amaranth (a coaltar dye), proved to be a serious competitor to the more costly natural products (74). In the United States alone, about 1 million pounds of this synthetic dye, valued at up to $55 million, is used annually in about $10 billion worth of food, drugs, and cosmetics.

Most of us would be surprised to learn how wide the use of red coloring matter is in the food, drink, cosmetic, and drug industry. Cochineal carmine is used widely in the most diverse products, but the bulk goes into pork sausage, dried fish, shrimps, ice cream, jams, jellies, yogurt, fruit in syrup, alcoholic and soft drinks, chocolate fillings, sweets, cider, and vinegar. In addition, it is found in millions of pink and red medicinal pills, syrups, and cosmetic products (74). In all of these products, cochineal serves no directly beneficial purpose except to make the products more attractive; this it does very effectively (75).

> **Carmine is used widely in cosmetics, drugs, and many foods. In cosmetics it is said to be noncomedogenic, in contrast to the synthetic red dyes.**

Carmine appears to be a rare contact sensitizer. Sarkany et al. (76) reported that its use in lipstick produced allergic contact cheilitis in three patients.

REFERENCES

1. Fisher AA. Contact dermatitis from food additives. *Immunol Allergy Pract* 1983;10:316.
2. Fisher AA. Contact dermatitis due to food additives. *Cutis* 1975;16:961.
3. Mitchell JC. The skin and chemical additives to foods. *Arch Dermatol* 1971;104:329.
4. Fisher AA. Dermatitis of the hands from food additives. *Cutis* 1982;30:304.
5. Fisher AA. Cutaneous reactions to sorbic acid and potassium sorbate. *Cutis* 1980;25:350.
6. Fisher AA. Hand dermatitis—a "baker's dozen." *Cutis* 1982;29:214.
7. Clemmensen O, Hjorth N. Perioral contact urticaria from sorbic acid and benzoic acid in a salad dressing. *Contact Dermatitis* 1982;8:1.
8. Lahti A, et al. Acetylsalicyclic acid inhibits non-immunologic contact urticaria. *Contact Dermatitis* 1987;16:133.
9. Roed-Petersen J, Hjorth N. Contact dermatitis from antioxidants. *Br J Dermatol* 1976;94:233.

10. Fisherman EW, Cohen G. Chemical intolerance to butylated-hydroxyanisole (BHA) and butylated-hydroxytoluene (BHT) and vascular response as an indicator and monitor of drug intolerance. *Ann Allergy* 1973;31:126.

11. Flyvholm M-A, Menné T. Sensitizing risk of butylated hydroxytoluene based on exposure and effect data. *Contact Dermatitis* 1990; 23:341.

12. Epstein E. Sodium bisulfite. *Contact Dermatitis Newsletter* 1970;7: 115.

13. Riggs BS, Harchelroad FP Jr, Poole C. Allergic reaction to sulfiting agents. *Ann Emerg Med* 1986;15:77.

14. Prenner BM, Steven JJ. Anaphylaxis after ingestion of sodium bisulfite. *Ann Allergy* 1976;37:180.

15. Wolf SI, Nicklas RA. Sulfite sensitivity in a seven-year-old child. *Ann Allergy* 1985;54:420.

16. Hausen BM, Beyer W. The sensitizing capacity of the antioxidants propyl, octyl, and dodecyl gallate and some related gallic acid esters. *Contact Dermatitis* 1992;26:253.

17. deGroot AC, Gerkens F. Occupational airborne contact dermatitis from octyl gallate. *Contact Dermatitis* 1990;23:184.

18. Brun R. Eczema de contact à un antioxydant de la margarine (gallate) et changement de métier. *Dermatologica* 1970;140:390.

19. Postendorf J. Oxidative deterioration in cosmetics and pharmaceuticals. *J Soc Cosmet Chem* 1965;16:203.

20. Lewis FM, Shah M, Gawkrodger DJ. Contact sensitivity to food additives can cause oral and perioral symptoms. *Contact Dermatitis* 1995; 33:429.

21. Wilkinson SM, Beck MH. Allergic contact dermatitis from menthol in peppermint. *Contact Dermatitis* 1994;30:42.

22. Fleming CJ, Forsyth A. D5 patch test reactions to menthol and peppermint. *Contact Dermatitis* 1998;38:337.

23. Morton CA, et al. Contact sensitivity to menthol and peppermint in patients with intra-oral symptoms. *Contact Dermatitis* 1995;32:281.

24. Malten KE. Four bakers showing positive patch-tests to a number of fragrance materials, which can also be used as flavors. *Acta Derm Venereol* (Stockh) 1979;59:117.

25. Fisher AA. Contact dermatitis due to cinnamon and cinnamic aldehyde. *Cutis* 1975;16:383.

26. Neering H, van Ketel WG. Allergy from spices used in Indonesian cooking. International Symposium on Contact Dermatitis. Gentofte, Denmark, 1974.

27. Garcia-Bravo B, Perex Bernal A, Garcia-Hernandez MJ, Camacho F. Occupational contact dermatitis from anethole in food handlers. *Contact Dermatitis* 1997;37:38.

28. Burden AD, Wilkinson SM, Beck MH, Chalmers RJ. Garlic-induced systemic contact dermatitis. *Contact Dermatitis* 1994;30:299.

29. Pecquet C, Leynadier F, Saiag P. Immediate hypersensitivity to sesame in foods and cosmetics. *Contact Dermatitis* 1998;39:313.

30. Hamilton TK, Zug KA. Systemic contact dermatitis to raw cashew nuts in a pesto sauce. *Am J Contact Dermatitis* 1998;9:51.

31. Fisher AA. The management of propylene glycol-sensitive patients. *Cutis* 1980;25:24.

32. Hannuksela M, Forstrom L. Reactions to peroral propylene glycol. *Contact Dermatitis* 1978;4:41.

33. Camarasa JM, Alomar A. Contact dermatitis from a karaya seal ring. *Contact Dermatitis* 1980;6:139.

34. Fisher AA, Dooms-Gossens A. Persulphate hair bleach reactions: cutaneous and respiratory manifestations. *Arch Dermatol* 1976;112:1407.

35. Calnan CD, Shuster S. Reactions to ammonium persulphate. *Arch Derm* 1963;88:812.

36. Cronin E. *Contact dermatitis.* London: Churchill Livingstone, 1980:181.

37. Fisher AA. *Contact dermatitis,* 3rd ed. Philadelphia: Lea & Febiger, 1988:591.

38. Morren M-A, et al. α-amylase, a flour additive: an important cause of protein contact dermatitis in bakers. *J Am Acad Dermatol* 1993; 29:723.

39. Mitchell JC. Allergic contact dermatitis from a certified food dye presenting as "sock dermatitis." *Contact Dermatitis Newsletter* 1972;11: 247.

40. Kiec-Swierczyunska M, Krecisz B. Occupational allergic contact dermatitis due to curcumin food colour in a pasta factory worker. *Contact Dermatitis* 1998;39:30.

41. Inman PM. Dermatitis in a crisp factory. *Acta Dermatovener* (Stockh) 1965;45:295.

42. Fisher AA. Possible role of diet in pompholyx and nickel dermatitis: a critical survey. *Cutis* 1978;22:412.

43. Fisher AA. Water-related dermatoses: I. *Cutis* 1980;25:132.

44. Feingold BF. Recognition of food additives as a cause of symptoms of allergy. *Ann Allergy* 1968;26:309.

45. Criep LH. Allergic vascular purpura. *J Allergy* 1971;48:7.

46. Lockey S. Reactions to hidden agents in foods, beverages and drugs. *Ann Allergy* 1971;29:461.

47. Juhlin L, Michaâlsson G, Zetterstrom O. Urticaria and asthma induced by food-and-drug additives in patients with aspirin hypersensitivity. *J Allergy Clin Immunol* 1972;50:92.

48. Lockey S. Drug reactions and sublingual testing with certified food colors. *Ann Allergy* 1973;31:423.

49. Michaâlsson G, Pettersson L, Juhlin L. Purpura caused by food and drug additives. *Arch Dermatol* 1974;109:49.

50. Fiedelman W, Martens J. Hypersensitivity to tartrazine (FD&C Yellow No. 5) and other dyes present in pharmaceutical products. *Cutis* 1975;15:576.

51. Smith AP. Response of aspirin-allergic patients to challenge by some analgesics in common use. *Br Med J* 1971;2:494.

52. Samter M, Beers RF Jr. Concerning the nature of intolerance to aspirin. *J Allergy* 1967;40:281.

53. Samter M, Beers RF Jr. Intolerance to aspirin: clinical studies and consideration of its pathogenesis. *Ann Intern Med* 1968;68:975.

54. Chafee FH, Settipane GA. Aspirin intolerance. I: frequency in an allergic population. *J Allergy Clin Immunol* 1974;53:193.

55. Settipane GA, Chafee FH, Klein DE. Aspirin intolerance. II: a prospective study in an atopic and normal population. *J Allergy Clin Immunol* 1974;53:200.

56. Yuninger JW, O'Connell EJ, Logan GB. Aspirin-induced asthma in children. *J Pediatr* 1974;82:218.

57. Bandmann HJ, Nasemann T. Dermatitis to Ponceau Red 6R dye. *Berufsdermatosen* 1961;9:79.

58. Rapaport MJ. Allergy to yellow dyes. *Arch Dermatol* 1984;120:535.

59. Calnan C. FD and C Yellow 11 in lipstick. *Contact Dermatitis* 1975; 1:121.

60. Larson W. Cosmetic dermatitis due to a dye (D and C Yellow 11). *Contact Dermatitis* 1974;1:61.

61. Rapaport MJ. Allergy to D and C yellow dye 11. *Contact Dermatitis* 1980;6:364.

62. Jordan W. Contact dermatitis from D & C yellow 11 Dye in a toilet bar soap [letter]. *J Am Acad Dermatol* 1981;4:613.

63. Noster U, Hausen BM. Berufsdebingtes Kontaktekzem durch gelben Chinophthalonfarbstoff (solven Yellow 33: CI 47000) (Occupational dermatitis due to a yellow quinophthalone dye (solvent yellow 33: C.I. 47000)). *Hautarzt* 1977;29:153.

64. Börkner B, Magnusson B. Patch test sensitization to D & C Yellow No. 11 and simultaneous reaction to quinoline yellow. *Contact Dermatitis* 1981;7:1.

65. Palazzolo MJ, DiPasquale LC. The sensitization potential of D & C Yellow No. 11 in guinea pigs. *Contact Dermatitis* 1983;9:367.

66. Morikawa F, Fukuda M, Naganuma M, Nakayana Y. Phototoxic reaction to xanthine dyes induced by visible light. *J Dermatol* 1976;3:59.

67. Mitchell JC, Stewart WD. Allergic contact dermatitis from neutral red applied for herpes simplex. *Arch Dermatol* 1973;108:689.

68. Dahlquist I, Fregert S. Allergic contact dermatitis from neutral red in quaternary ammonium salt solution. *Contact Dermatitis Newsletter* 1967;2:16.

69. Conant M, Maibach HI. Allergic contact dermatitis due to neutral red [letter]. *Arch Dermatol* 1968;109:735.

70. Goldenberg RL, Nelson K. Dermatitis from neutral red therapy of herpes genitalis. *Obstet Gynecol* 1975;46:359.

71. Baker JT. Dyes of animal origin. *Endeavour* 1974;33:11.

72. Brunello F. *The art of dyeing in the history of mankind.* Vincenza: Neri Pozza, 1973.

73. Baranovits FLC. *Cochineal carmine: ancient dye with a modern role.* Reading, PA: Department of Zoology, University of Reading.

74. Fisher AA. Contact Dermatitis, 3rd edition. Lea & Febiger, Philadelphia, 1986, p. 600.

75. Pelham Wright N. A thousand years of cochineal. *Am Dyestuff Reporter,* 19 Aug 1963, p. 635.

76. Sarkany I, Meara RH, Everall J. Cheilitis due to carmine in lip salve. *Trans St John's Hosp Dermatol Soc* 1961;46:39.

CHAPTER 31

Allergy to Rubber

Rubber is an organic substance, obtained from natural sources or synthesized artificially, that has the properties of extensibility, stretchability, and toughness. Rubber acquired its name from its ability to erase pencil marks (1). Before the last decade of the last millennium, when one talked of rubber allergy, the usual causes were the chemical additives such as vulcanizers and antioxidants. Although these are still major causes of rubber allergy, the focus among health care workers and public alike has been type 1 allergy to natural rubber latex.

TYPES OF RUBBER

Natural Rubber

Natural rubber occurs in over 200 species of plants, including dandelions and goldenrod. Only two species are commercially significant: the *Hevea braziliensis* tree and the guayule bush, *Parthenium argentatum*. Today, the Hevea tree accounts for more than 90% of the world's natural rubber supply. *H. braziliensis* is cultivated primarily in Southeast Asia and West Africa. Each acre of about 150 trees will produce in 1 week enough latex for 1,500 pairs of surgical gloves. Trees need 6 to 8 years of growth before they are mature enough for harvesting. Harvesting the liquid natural rubber latex is accomplished by cutting a groove in the tree and collecting the "sap" in a cup. Coagulation rapidly occurs; to prevent this ammonia, thiurams or other preservatives are added to the collection vessels (2,3). The major hydrocarbon in rubber is cis-1,4-polyisoprene, which makes up 30% to 40% of natural latex.

Natural latex may be processed in the liquid form or allowed to dry into sheets. The term "natural rubber latex" (NRL) is used to describe products such as gloves and condoms formed from concentrated liquid natural latex. Dry rubber latex refers to natural latex that is processed into a solid "dry" form of sheets that are able to be stored or shipped for processing into other products.

Natural rubber latex is used in a variety of applications. Liquid NRL preparations are needed for producing dipped articles such as gloves, condoms, and balloons. The NRL sap is usually centrifuged to reduce water content. This process also reduces extractable latex protein (3).

> **Natural rubber latex, obtained principally from the *Hevea braziliensis* tree, is used in gloves, adhesives, condoms, and medical devices.**

Ammonia is the primary latex preservative added to prevent coagulation. Low ammonia latices are available and are preferred by some processors because of their lower odor and the elimination of the deammoniation step that may utilize formaldehyde. Low ammonia latex utilizes three secondary preservative systems: (a) sodium pentachlorophenate, (b) tetramethylthiuram disulfide (TMTD) and zinc oxide, and (c) sodium dimethyldithiocarbamate and zinc oxide (2).

Balata and Gutta-Percha

The rubber from the Hevea tree occurs only in the cis form, whereas both balata and gutta-percha occur in the trans forms. Balata is harvested from wild bushes and trees in Surinam and Guiana. Raw balata is high in dirt and resin and must be purified by a solvent extraction process. Gutta-percha is obtained from trees of the family Sapotaceae native to Malaysia, Borneo, and Sumatra.

Guayule

Guayule (*Parthenium argentatum*) is a member of the sunflower family, which grows in northern Mexico and the Big Bend area of Texas. In 1976, the Mexican government built an industrial plant in northern Mexico to extract rubber from wild guayule. There are no significant structural differences between guayule and Hevea rubber, but guayule contains a contaminate resin that must be removed. The resin chemically contains volatile essential oils: alpha-pinene, dipentene, and cadinene and nonvolatiles: carotenoids, parthen oils, dihydroxy diterpenes, palmitic acid, stearic acid, linoleic acid, linolenic acid, transcinnamic acid, hard wax, parthenyl cinnamate, and a shellac-like drying resin (3,4). Rodriguez et al. (5), using the guinea pig maximization test, identified a potent contact allergen in an acetone extract of the dried leaves of the plant; the sensitizer was a sesquiterpene cinnamic acid ester (guayulin A). A breeding program to find strains of guayule low in allergen content was suggested.

SYNTHETIC RUBBERS

The first synthetic rubbers were developed in the late 1920s. During World War II, the need for synthetic rubber spurred further research, leading to the synthesis of government rubber-styrene (GR-S), a butadiene-styrene polymer. Polyisoprene rubber (IR) is a synthetic that is very similar in structure to NRL. Other synthetic rubbers include butyl rubber, nitrile rubber, neoprene, polybutadiene, ethylene-propylene, silicone, urethane, thiokol, and Hypalon rubbers. In addition, compounds often thought of as plastics, such as polyethylene and polyvinyl chloride, have certain properties of rubber and may contain chemical additives used in rubber. These different rubbers all have varying qualities, such as chemical resistance, temperature tolerance, elasticity, and tear resistance, that make each more or less suitable for certain applications (Table 31.1).

TABLE 31.1. *Types of Natural and Synthetic Rubber*

Chemical form/name	Other names	Selected uses	Comments
Natural			
Cis-1,4-polyisoprene	Monomer of natural rubber NR, TSR, and MSR	Tire treads, especially for racing cars, buses, trucks, and airplanes; adhesives; autoengine mounts and suspension units; building foundations; bridge bearings	Good elasticity resilience and tack; low heat buildup; the larger the tire, the greater the proportion of natural rubber
Trans-1,4-polyisoprene latex	Gutta-percha and balata	Golf ball covers; sheeting; tubing; submarine cables	See text
Latex	Natural rubber latex	Dipped goods	See text
Synthetic			
Styrene butadiene	Synthetic, Buna S, SBR, and GR-S	Tires; industrial rubber products	The most widely used synthetic rubber; good abrasion and crack resistance; poor strength
Polyisobutylene-polyisoprene	Butyl, IIR and GR-I	Tubeless tires; inner tubes; auto components; wire and cable insulation; adhesives	Good thermal stability; low gas permeability; good ozone, weather, chemical, and moisture resistance; electrical insulator; incompatibility with natural rubber and the main synthetics
Polybutadiene (solution polymersterospecific)	Butadiene and BR	Tire treads; adds stength and flexibility to plastics; foams and footwear; outdoor rubber products	High abrasion and crack resistance; good thermal stability; low skid resistance when wet; mixed with SBR
Polychloroprene	Neoprene, CR and GR-M	Wires; cables; hose; protective clothing; gaskets; adhesives; surgical gloves; latex foam	High tensile strength and resistance to oxygen, ozone, oil, and tearing
Acrylonitrile-butadiene	Nitrile, Buna N, NBR, and GR-N (previously GR-A)	Gasoline fuel hoses; oil well parts; fuel cell liners; conveyor belts; shoe soles; blends with PVC for artificial leather and paper coating; water-proofer for fabrics; work gloves	Outstanding oil resistance that increases with acrylonitrile content but at expense of low temperature flexibility
Polyisoprene	IR	See natural rubber	Molecular shape similar to natural rubber; may replace natural rubber for most purposes, except when nonrubber constituents are advantageous
Polysulfide	Thiokol GR-P	Gasoline hose; printing rollers; fuel tank linings; protective coating; caulking and putty	Excellent resistance to organic solvents, greases and oils; low gas permeability
Ethylene-propylene	EPR	Tire side walls, hoses, conveyor belts, and molded goods	Excellent resistance to oxygen, ozone, acids, and alkalis; lightweight
Ethylene-propylene terpolymer	EPDM	Same as EPR	Same as EPR

World Rubber Production

Guin et al. have written an excellent review of the history, production, and uses of rubber (3). In 1990, about 15 million tons of rubber were produced worldwide, with NRL accounting for about one-third of that. About 72% of NRL goes into tires, 10% to latex-dipped goods, and the rest to industrial products, footwear, and adhesives.

Rubber products may be a mixture of natural and synthetic rubber containing many compounds used in synthetic plastics; although completely cured synthetic plastics rarely cause dermatitis, fully cured rubber often produces allergic dermatitis.

COMPOUNDING AND VULCANIZATION

Raw rubber in the dry state has few commercial applications. For most uses, the rubber must be modified, usually by the addition of vulcanizing (curing) agents and other materials, followed by vulcanization. The exceptions include such uses as crepe rubber shoe soles, rubber adhesives, and masking tape (6).

The main applications of rubber elastomers require that the polymer chains be cross-linked after being formed into the shape of the final product. After cross-linking of the polymer chains, which is called curing or vulcanization, the article is elastic.

In 1839, Charles Goodyear described the process of vulcanization using lead and sulfur. The process helped to overcome the weaknesses of untreated natural rubber that occur with aging. Vulcanization is an irreversible process and was employed originally to denote heating rubber with sulfur, but it has been extended to include any process, with any combination of materials, that produces this effect. About 4 to 5 pounds of additives go into each 100 pounds of finished rubber. The accelerators and antidegradants account for about 90% of these additives.

Accelerators speed up the slow process of vulcanization by acting as catalysts and undergoing chemical changes. Table 31.2 lists selected commercial accelerators, several of which are potent sensitizers that can produce dermatitis in sensitized individuals who use the finished rubber product (7). The major accelerators include thiurams and carbamates, which act quickly, guanidine and mercaptobenzothiazole, which act at moderate speed, and thioureas, which work more slowly. Table 31.3 lists several peroxide curing agents.

The benzothiazolesulfenamides prevent premature curing and are called delayed-action accelerators. They also donate sulfur for curing. Ethylenethiourea (2-imidazolidinethione) is used widely for special-purpose elastomers such as polychloroprene (neoprene) and polyepichlorhydrin (8).

Antioxidants and antiozonants prevent rubber from drying or cracking by preventing oxidation by atmospheric oxygen or by decreasing the effect of ozone (9). These substances are used widely in polymers (rubber, adhesives, and plastics), gasoline, lubricants, and food; cured rubber accounts for the major consumption. Selected chemicals are listed in Table 31.4. The paraphenylenediamine-type antioxidants are usually the most effective in rubber and are used in the largest volume. Most are discoloring and staining and are used in applications in which this property can be ignored. Phenolic antioxidants are less discoloring than amines and include many of the newer antioxidants. Butylated hydroxytoluene (BHT) is the most used.

Retarders prevent premature vulcanization of rubber compounds during mixing, calandering, and other processing steps (7) (Table 31.5). N-(cyclohexylthio)-phthalimide is the predominant agent used.

Other Additives

There are a number of other rubber additives, some of which are listed in Tables 31.6, 31.7, and 31.8. The antidegradants prevent oxygen, ozone, heat, and light from damaging rubber. Additives include aniline, creosols, hydroquinone, phenol, quinolones, naphthylamines, alkylamines, and phosphites. Paraphenylenediamine (PPDA) and its derivatives are the primary antioxidants.

Raw rubber is not elastic but is used in crepe rubber shoe soles, rubber adhesives, and masking tape; vulcanization makes the raw rubber stretchable.

Other categories of rubber compounding materials are listed below.

Flame retarders (e.g., antimony oxide, hydrated alumina, and zinc borate)
Fungicides and germicides (e.g., pentachlorophenates and chlorophenols)
UV absorbers and stabilizers (Table 31.8) (10)
Optical brighteners (e.g., xylenols)
Chemical and heat stabilizers (e.g., BHT and silicates)
Homogenizing agents (e.g., aliphatic-naphthenic aromatic resins)
Dusting, dipping, washing materials (e.g., barium stearate, calcium stearate, silicates, and zinc stearate)
Finishes (e.g., beeswax, paraffin wax, and polyurethanes)
Odorants (e.g., essential oils and fragrances)
Antistaining agents (e.g., activated carbon)

Polymerization materials (catalysts, dispersing agents, emulsifiers, modifiers, chain extenders, cross-linkers, reducing agents, accelerators, activators, inhibitors, shortstops, and terminators) include tall oil rosin, sodium lauryl sulfate, n-dodecyl mercaptan, peroxides, amines, potassium dimethyldithiocarbamate, and alkylaryl polyether alcohols. Reclaiming materials include terpene pine tar, charcoal,

TABLE 31.2. *Selected Commercial Accelerators and Curing Agents for Rubber*

Compound	Other names	Uses
Aldehyde-amine reaction products		
1. Hexamethylenetetramine	Methenamine, Hiprex, Mendelamine, HEXA, HMT, HMT-A	Slow accelerator for NR and SBR; for activating thiazoles and thiurams Urinary tract antibacterial
Benzothiazoles		
2. 2-mercaptobenzothiazole (MBT)	Captax, benzothiazolethione, Mertax, Thiotax, Sulfadene	Primary accelerator for NR and synthetic rubbers
3. Bis(2,2'-benzothiazolyl) disulfide (MBTS)		Primary and scorch-modifying secondary accelerator for NR and SBR
4. Zinc salt of 2-mercaptobenzothiazole (2[3H]-benzothiazolethione, zinc salt)		Primary accelerator for NR and synthetic rubbers; secondary accelerator for latex foam
Benzothiazolesulfenamides		
5. *N*-tert-butyl-2-benzothiazole-sulfenamide	NTBBTS, Santocure NS	Delayed-action accelerator for NR and synthetic rubbers
6. *N*-cyclohexyl-2-benzothiazolesulfenamide	Sufenax CB, Accelerator CZ Durax	Delayed-action accelerator for NR and synthetic rubbers
7. 2-(4-morpholinyldithio) benzothiazole	MOR	Accelerator and sulfur donor from NR and synthetic rubbers
Dithiocarbamates		
8. Bismuth dimethyldithiocarbamate		Accelerator for NR, IR, BR, and SBR at high temperature and speed for improved dynamic properties in NR and IR
9. Cadmium diethyldithiocarbamate	Ethyl Cadmate	Primary accelerator for NR, EPDM, and SBI
10. Copper dimethyldithiocarbamate	Methyl Cumate	Ultra-accelerator for SBR and IR
11. Selenium dimethyldithiocarbamate	Methyl Selenac	Accelerator and vulcanizing agent for NR, SBR, and IR
12. Sodium dibutyldithiocarbamate	Butyl Namate	For fast precure of latex
13. Tellurium diethyldithiocarbamate	Ethyl Tellurac	Provides high modulus vulcanizates of NR, SBR, NBR, and EPDM
14. Zinc di-*n*-butyldithiocarbamate		For EPDM and natural and synthetic latexes
15. Zinc dibenzyldithiocarbamate	Accelerator ZBED Robac ZBED Arazate	For the manufacture of butyl rubber cable insulation
16. Zinc diethyldithiocarbamate	Ethyl Ziram Ethyl Zimate	Primary accelerator for NR and synthetic rubbers
17. Zinc dimethyldithiocarbamate	Methasan Metazin Methyl Zimate Vancide MZ-96 ZM ZDMC	Accelerator for NR and synthetic rubbers
Dithiophosphates		
18. Copper *O,O'*-di-isopropylphoshphoro-dithioate		Nonblooming, slightly staining accelerator for EPDM; used in combination with other accelerators
19. Zinc *O,O'*-di-*n*-butyl phosphoRodithioate		Nonblooming, nonstaining accelerator for EPDM; used in combination with other accelerators
20. Zinc *O,O'*-di-isoproyl phosphorodithioate, biscyclohexylamine complex		Nonstaining accelerator for EPDM; provides good heat resistance and compression set
Guanidines		
21. 1,3-diphenylguanidine	DPG Melaniline Nocceler D Sanceler D Soxinol D Vulkacit D/C	Secondary accelerator for thiazoles, sulfenamides, and thiurams
22. Di-*o*-tolylguanidine	DOTG	Slow-curing accelerator for NR, SBR, and NBR; activates thiazole accelerators

continued

TABLE 31.2. *Continued*

Compound	Other names	Uses
Thioureas		
23. *N,N′*-dibutylthiourea		Accelerator for neoprene, EPDM, and chlorobutyl
24. *N,N′*-diethylthiourea (1,3-diethyl-2-thiourea) (*N,N′*-diethylthio-carbamide)	Pennzone E	For CR, EPDM, and chlorobutyl
25. Ethylenethiourea (2-imidazo-lidinethione)	Mercozen Mercaptoimidazoline Imidazoline-2-thiol Imidazolidimethione ETU	Nonstaining accelerator for CR and epichlorohydrin
26. Diphenylthiourea	Thiocarbanilide DPTU	Nonstaining secondary accelerator for CR and EPDM
27. Trimethylthiourea	Thiate-E, TMTU	Fast-curing accelerator for neoprene; gives low compression set
Thiurams		
28. Dipentamethylenethiuram disulfide	Robac PTD, PTD, dicy-clopentamethylene-thiuram disulfide	For the manufacture of latex-dipped gloves
29. Dipentamethylenethiuram hexasulfide	Sulfads Piperidine	Ultra-accelerator and sulfur donor for NR and synthetic rubbers; primary accelerator for Hypalon synthetic rubber and butyl
30. Dipentamethylenethiuram tetrasulfide		For Hypalon cable insulation; also used in nitrile and butyl rubbers
31. Dipentamethylenethiuram monosulfide		For chemically blown cellular rubber products from NR and SBR for the production of sulfurless-cured articles, which must be free from bloom
32. Tetrabutylthiuram disulfide	Tetrabutylthioperoxydicar-bonothioic diamide	
33. Tetraethylthiuram disulfide	Antabuse Tetraethylthioperoxydicar-bonothioic Diamide Disulfiram TETD	Excellent for fast-press cures; less scorching than TMTD; alcohol-abuse deterrent; immunomodulator
34. Tetramethylthiuram disulfide (TMTD)	Thiuram Vancide TM Thiurad TMTD	Excellent for fast-press cures; especially good for IIR and CR
35. Tetramethylthiuram monosulfide		Booster for thiazoles, especially in nitrile rubbers
Thiocarbamyl sulfenamide		
36. *N*-oxydiethylenethiocarbamyl-*N*-oxydiethylenesulfenamide		Primary accelerator for NR and synthetic rubbers; provides fast cure and scorch safety
Curing (vulcanizing) agents		
37. Alkylphenol-formaldehyde resin		Effective as resin curing agent for IIR; provides good heat resistance
38. Alkylphenol disulfides		Vulcanizing agent
39. *N,N′*-caprolactam disulfide		Nonblooming and nonstaining sulfur donor in the vulcanization of NR and synthetic rubbers
40. *p*-quinone bis(benzoylxime)		Less scorching than *p*-quinone-dioxime; an effective coagent of peroxide cure
41. 4,4′dithiobismorpholine	Morpholine *N-N* disulfide Sulfasan R	Vulcanizing agent for NR and synthetic rubbers; provides excellent heat aging
42. *p*-quinone dioxime	*p*-benzoquinone dioxime, Cyclohexadienedione dioxime, PQD	Used for vulcanizing IIR
43. Sulfur	Brimstone	For vulcanizing NR and synthetic rubbers

BR, butadiene rubber; CR, chloroprene rubber; EPDM, ethylene-propylene-diene terpolymer; IIR, polyisoprene rubber; IR, isoprene rubber; NR, natural rubber; SBR, styrene-butadiene rubber

Adapted from Taylor J. In Fisher's *Contact Dermatitis,* 4th ed. Williams & Wilkins, Baltimore, 1995, and Internet site: www.chemfinder.com. This list contains names of chemicals that may no longer be available.

TABLE 31.3. *Peroxide Curing Agents for Rubber**

Compound	Uses
1. Benzoyl peroxide	Cross-linking silicone and fluorosilicone elastomers
2. 1,1-bis(*t*-butylperoxy)-3,3,5-trimethylcyclohexane	Cross-linking SBR, NBR, EPR, EPDM, and silicones at low operating temperatures
3. Dicumyl peroxide	Nonsulfur curing agent for NR, IR, SBR, BR, NBR, EPDM, and CR
4. 2,5-dimethyl-2,5-bis(*t*-butylperoxy)-hexane	Vulcanization or cross-linking elastomers and polyolefins (e.g., EPDM, EPM, PE, and NBR)

*This list contains names of chemicals that may no longer be available.

Internet site: www.chemfinder.com.

aryl disulfide, tall oil acid–refined caustic soda, zinc chloride, and 4,6-ditertbutyl-*m*-cresol (1,3).

Solvents include commercial benzene, butyl alcohols, 1,1,1-trichloro-ethane, toluene, xylene, and ethylene glycol monobutyl ether.

Blowing agents are foam-producing agents used for cellular rubber, such as sponges and latex. Blowing can be compared to baking a cake with yeast; the blowing agent decomposes and causes the compound to expand, followed by curing. Inorganic substances, such as sodium or ammonium bicarbonate and ammonium nitrite, are used; they generally release carbon dioxide gas (Table 31.6) (8).

Peptizers, also called chemical plasticizers or softeners, soften rubber and lower the viscosity of uncured rub-

TABLE 31.4. *Selected Commercial Antioxidants and Antiozonants for Rubbers**

Chemical name	Other names
Amines	
1. Diphenyl-*p*-phenylenediamine	Age Rite DPPD[d]
	Benzenediamine, dianilinobenzene DPPD[b]
2. Di-beta-naphthyl-*p*-phenylenediamine	Age Rite White, DBNPD[a]
3. Phenyl-α-naphthylamine	Akrochem Antioxidant PANA
	Additin 30
	Naugard PAN
	N-phenyl-a-naphthyl-amine
4. 1,2-dihydro-2,2,4-trimethylquinoline	Age Rite Resin D[d] acetonanil
5. Zinc salt of 2-mercapto-4(5)-methyl benzimidazole	
6. 6-ethoxy-1,2-dihydro-2,2,4-trimethylquinoline	Ethoxyquin
7. *N*-isopropyl-*N*′-phenyl-*p*-phenylenediamine	NINP-PPDA
8. *N*-(1,3-dimethyl butyl)-*N*′-phenyl-*p*-phenylenediamine	
9. *N,N*′-bis(1,4-dimethylpentyl)-*p*-phenylenediamine	
10. *N*-phenyl-*N*′-cyclohexyl-*p*-phenylenediamine	CPPD
11. *p,p*-diaminodiphenyl methane	4,4-methylenebisbenzeneamine, DADPM, DAPM, diphenylmethane diamine
Phenols	
12. Butylated hydroxy toluene (2,6-di-tert-butyl *p*-cresol)	BHT[d]
13. 2,5-di-*t*-butyl-hydroquinone	
14. Tetrakis methylene (3,5-di-tert-butyl-4-hydrohydroxy-cinnamate)	Irganox 1010[c]
15. Bisphenolic	
16. 2,2′-methylene-bis-(4-methyl-6-(1-methyl-cyclohexyl)phenol)	Bis[2-hydroxy-5-methyl-3-(1-methylcyclohexyl)phenyl]methane
17. 2,5-di(tert-amyl)hydroquinone	Santovar A, 2,5-bis(1,1-dimethylpropyl)hydroquinone
18. 4,4′-thiobis(6-*t*-butyl-*m*-cresol)	Santonox
19. 4,4′-butylidenebis (6-*t*-butyl-*m*-cresol)	SWP
20. Butylated hydroxy anisole	BHA
21. 2-tert-butyl hydroquinone	TBHQ
22. 1,1,3-tris-(2-methyl-4-hydroxy-5-tert-butyl phenyl)butane	
23. 2,6-di-tert butyl-4-sec-butylphenol	
24. 2,2′ methylene bis(6-tert-butyl-*p*-cresol)	
Metal salts of dithioacids	
25. Nickel dibutyldithiocarbamate	
26. Nickel di-isobutyldithiocarbamate (contains 11.5–13.5% nickel)	Isobutyl Niclate[b]
27. Nickel dimethyldithiocarbamate	Methyl Niclate
Sulfides	
28. Dilauryl thiodipropionate	DLTD
	Didodecyl 3,3-thiodipropionate
29. Distearyl thiodipropionate	Dioctadecyl 3,3-thiodipropionate
30. Octodecyl B (3,5-*t*-butyl 4-hydroxyphenyl) propionate	Irganox 1076
31. Thiodipropionic acid	
Phosphites	
32. Tris(nonyl henol) phosphite	

Adapted from Internet site: www.chemfinder.com. This list contains names of chemicals that may no longer be available.

[a]Antiozonant.

[b]Antioxidant and antiozonant.

[c]Also antioxidant for plastics, especially polyolefins.

[d]Also antioxidant for plastics.

TABLE 31.5. *Retarders for Rubber**

Compound	Other name	Uses
1. Benzoic acid		Retarder for NR and synthetic rubbers
2. *N*-(cyclohexylthio) phthalimide (CTP)		Retarder for NR and synthetic rubbers; it works best with sulfenamide type accelerators
3. *N*-nitrosodiphenylamine (NDPA)		Staining retarder for NR and synthetic rubbers
4. Phthalic anhydride	PA	Nonstaining retarder for NR, SBR, and NBR
5. Salicylic acid		Retarder for NR and SBR; accelerator for W types of neoprene

*This list contains names of chemicals that may no longer be available. Adapted from Internet site: www.chemfinder.com.

ber (Table 31.7). Peptizers have been reported to produce allergic dermatitis from contact with the finished product (7,11).

Processing agents do not affect physical or performance properties of rubber. Some are low molecular weight polyethylenes. *N*,*N*′-ethylenebis(stearamide) functions as a mold-releasing agent and detackifier (6).

> **Of the numerous chemical additives to rubber, the accelerators that speed up vulcanization and the antioxidants that prevent rubber deterioration are the main sensitizers.**

Reinforcing agents and fillers for rubber include carbon black, zinc oxide, calcium carbonate, calcium silicate, silicon dioxide, clay, and magnesium carbonate (12).

Bonding agents are used for adhering rubber to reinforcing agents, such as glass, textile, or steel, as used in tires, hoses, and belts. Resorcinol, resorcinol-formaldehyde, 2-naphthol, and tetrachlorobenzoquinone are examples (6).

Reclaimed Rubber

Vulcanized rubber scrap (old tires and inner tubes), either natural or synthetic in origin, when reworked to render it suitable as a raw material, is termed "reclaimed rubber." There are three major methods of reclaiming rubber that involve mechanical, chemical and heat processing, and devulcanization of the old rubber. Goodyear has employed microwaves for this process. Some reclaiming chemicals are listed above under "Other Additives."

Tires, hoses, belts, molded and extruded goods, and asphalt products (roadway chip sealers, waterproofing membranes, crack-and-joint sealers, hot-mix binders, and roofing materials) consume about 80% of the rubber reclaim manufactured. Reclaimed rubber may be used in the tire carcass and sidewall compounds. Reclaimed natural rubber is used in cements, dispersions, and pressure-sensitive tape; butyl reclaim is used in tubes and inner liners for tires.

TABLE 31.6. *Blowing Agents for Rubber and Plastics**

Chemical name

1. Diazoaminobenzene
2. Benzenesulfonyl hydrazide
3. *p*-toluenesulfonyl hydrazide
   p,*p*′-oxybis(benzenesulfonyl hydrazide)
4. Azodicarbonamide
5. Dinitrosopentamethylenetetramine tetramine
6. *p*-toluenesulfonyl semicarbazide
7. Azodicarbonamide/DNPT blend

*This list contains names of chemicals that may no longer be available. Adapted from Internet site: www.chemfinder.com.

TABLE 31.7. *Rubber Peptizers (Chemical Plasticizers or Softeners)**

1. Thio-beta-naphthol
2. Pentachlorothiophenol
3. Zinc salt of pentachlorothiophenol
4. 2,2′-dibenzamidodiphenyl disulfide
5. Activated dithiobisbenzanilide
6. Zinc thiobenzoate
7. Phenylhydrazine
8. Oils/petroleum fractions[a]
9. Pine tars[a]
10. Resins (e.g., terpenes, rosin)[a]
11. Pitch[a]
12. Tetramethylthiuram disulfide[b]
13. Tetraethylthiuram disulfide[b]

*Compiled from Taylor J. in Fisher's *Contact Dermatitis*, 4th ed. Williams & Wilkins, Baltimore, 1995. This list contains names of chemicals that may no longer be available.
[a]Especially used for natural and SBR rubbers.
[b]Used for Neoprene GN rubber.

TABLE 31.8. *Selected Ultraviolet Inhibitors (Absorbers, Stabilizers) for Rubber**

Chemical composition	Trade name
1. 2-(5 chloro-2H-benzotriazol-2-yl)-6-(1,1,dimethylethyl)-4 methyl phenol	Tinuvin 326
2. 2(2′-hydroxy-5′-methylphenyl)-2H benzotriazole	Tinuvin P
3. bis(2,2,6,6-tetramethyl-4-piperidinyl) sebacate	Tinuvin 770
4. bis(1,2,2,6,6-pentamethyl-4-piperidinyl) (3,5-bis-(1,1,dimethyl ethyl)-4-hydroxy phenyl methyl) butyl propanedioic acid	Tinuvin 144
5. Resorcinol monobenzoate	Eastman Inhibitor RMB
6. Octadecyl 3,5-di-tert butyl-4-hydroxy hydrocinnamate	Irganox 1076
7. Tetrakis methylene (3,5-di tert-butyl-4-hydroxy hydrocinnamate)	Irganox 1010
8. Dimethyl succinate polymer with tetramethyl hydroxy-1-hydroxyl piperidine	Tinuvin 622LD

*This list contains names of chemicals that may no longer be available. Adapted from Internet site:www.chemfinder.com.

IMMEDIATE HYPERSENSITIVITY TO LATEX

Nutter (13), in 1979, and Förström (14), a year later, were the first to definitively report type 1 latex allergy. Since then, frequent reports of latex allergy have dramatically increased the awareness of this problem among health care workers as well as the general public. The US Food and Drug Administration issued a medical bulletin in 1991 identifying the risk of life-threatening anaphylaxis associated with latex contact (15). The American Academy of Dermatology has issued a position paper on latex allergy and has published a review of the topic by Warshaw (16,17).

Identification of the Allergen

At this time, identification and isolation of the allergen responsible for latex immediate hypersensitivity (IH) has not been fully accomplished. One of the difficulties is that different sources of raw material and different extraction and testing methods have been used. For example, various forms of latex, finished goods, and even rubber tree parts have been tested. Hamman (2), in an excellent reference paper on latex IH, suggests that factors such as latex harvesting and preservation methods, seasonal variation, and other factors may affect antigenicity. Further substantiating the concept that natural latex processing plays an active role in antigen development is the observation that workers handling raw natural latex are not known to suffer from latex IH (C Hamman, personal communication, 1993).

A number of different latex protein antigens have been identified, and several appear to be important in human allergy. It is possible that different patients will react to different antigens. Hevein, a 4.7kd protein, may be a major allergen in health care workers (18). Prohevein, a 20kd protein, contains similar antigens (19). Alenius et al. (20) stated that "rubber elongation factor" (14.6kd) is allergenic in 18% of their NRL immediate hypersensitivity patients.

Factors Influencing Latex IH

Many individuals that must frequently wear latex exam gloves report that the powder irritates the skin. To date, actual allergy to the powders, principally cornstarch, has been documented very rarely (21). However, it has been shown that cornstarch glove powder absorbs latex protein. This may increase the aerosolization of the latex allergen and enhance the development of respiratory symptoms (22).

Atopic individuals, especially those with hand eczema, appear to be at higher risk for developing latex IH. Also spina-bifida patients with meningomyelocele, possibly because of frequent operative and genitourinary latex exposure, are at high risk.

Why large numbers of cases have only been reported since the mid- to late 1980s has been debated. There are most likely multiple factors, but the main reason may be the entry into the marketplace of quickly and poorly made latex products coincident with the increased need for protection from HIV and other infectious diseases. Inexperienced manufacturers produced great quantities of latex products that may not have been well compounded or leached of allergens. Once individuals are sensitized by high allergen concentrations, even low levels of latex protein can cause a reaction.

> **Factors predisposing to latex immediate (type 1) hypersensitivity include atopy, frequent glove use, hand eczema, and having had multiple surgeries, especially as a child.**

Clinical Findings

The initial presentation of latex IH may be confused with irritant or allergic contact dermatitis by both the patient and physicians. Indeed, eczematous changes are almost always seen in the case of repeated latex exposure as occurs when wearing latex gloves. A critical point is to question the patient concerning whether itching, burning, swelling, or other symptoms occur within 1 hour or less of donning gloves or whether changes are noted only after chronic use. Also, other history of reactions to balloons, condoms, and so on, should be obtained. Even in the absence of positive history, patients with hand eczema who wear latex gloves frequently should be considered candidates for further investigation.

Respiratory and mucosal symptoms are the next most common complaint in latex IH. Symptoms may be mild to severe and even fatal. Repeated exposure may lead to worsening of the allergy.

The most severe findings occur when the route of exposure is mucosal or parenteral. Deaths have been reported due to latex anaphylaxis from exposure to barium enema tube cuffs. Exposure of a latex-sensitive patient to gloves during surgery, dental work, or vaginal or rectal examination may cause anaphylaxis.

Diagnosis

The diagnosis must first be suspected on clinical grounds. No test is both specific and sensitive, so several procedures may be required. Anti-latex IgE RAST tests are very specific and relatively sensitive, so these tests are the first step in making a diagnosis. Use of a blood test avoids the possibility of an adverse reaction to a skin test and may be obtained by practitioners unable to do skin testing. Patch, prick, or use tests may still be necessary, however, if the RAST is negative and clinical suspicion is high. Inasmuch as standard allergens are not now available, a test solution can be easily made, as noted in Table 31.9. Also, testing to pieces of latex gloves can be done. An algorithm for this is given in Table 31.10. Because testing may rarely provoke a severe reaction, resuscitation equipment should be near at hand.

It is important to note that latex allergy, despite its current popularity, still accounts for only a portion of reactions to rubber products. Additives such as accelerators and antioxidants are the causes of many, if not most, cases of rubber allergy. Therefore, even patients who are suspected of having latex IH should have "regular" patch testing to determine delayed hypersensitivity to these allergens. In addition, to further complicate the matter, Belsito (23) reported type 1 immediate reactions to carbamates.

TABLE 31.9. *Preparation of "Latex Allergen" for Skin Testing*

1. Place about 20 1-cm² pieces of latex glove in 5 ml of sterile saline.
2. Shake occasionally over a 2-hour period.
3. Transfer to a sterile, clean container without a rubber top.
4. Make a fresh supply weekly.

TABLE 31.10. *Algorithm for Skin Testing for Latex Allergy**

1. Closed patch test with either 1-cm² piece of latex glove or "latex solution" from Table 31.13, or both, for 20 minutes on forearm.
   If - ↓   If + ↳ Stop
2. Cut out one finger of the latex glove and place on patient's finger for 20 minutes (or less if symptoms develop).
   If - ↓   If + ↳ Stop
3. Place whole glove on patient's hand for 20 minutes or less if symptoms develop.
   If - ↓   If + ↳ Stop
4. Prick tests with "latex solution" on forearm using stylette or sterile needle to prick through a drop of the solution. Use histamine and saline positive, negative controls.
   If - ↓   If + ↳ Stop

Probably not latex allergic.

*Note: Pruritus and development of an urticarial wheal constitute a positive test. Resuscitative capability should be available.

Prevalence of Latex IH

Health care workers have the greatest likelihood of developing latex IH, other than the meningomyelocele patients noted above. Those with atopy and prior hand eczema are at highest risk. Several studies summarized by Hamman (2) have shown the prevalence overall in hospital-based physicians and nurses to be in the range of 5% to 10%. DeGroot et al. (24) studied laboratory workers in the Netherlands and found that 5.0% were NRL RAST positive and 8.3% were prick test positive.

Hamman et al. (25) tested 2,166 dental workers at national meetings with prick testing to glove extracts. Positive tests were found in 6.2%.

Ylitilo et al. (26) screened 3,269 children for latex allergy as part of a routine prick test panel. Positives were found in 55 (1.7%). Thirty (1.0%) were further positive with both RAST and glove use tests. A number of these children had not undergone surgery, and one-third were asymptomatic. In Spain, 29 of 100 children with myelomeningocele were latex allergic (27).

Special Considerations for Latex-Allergic Patients

As is always the case, avoidance of an allergen is the most reliable form of treatment. For those who must wear exam or surgical gloves, vinyl gloves can be used safely. For those who require more sensitivity of touch, the Tactyl 1 glove (Smart Practice Inc., 3400 East McDowell, Phoenix, AZ 85008; tel: 800-822-8956) or the Dermaprene glove

(Ansell Inc., P.O. Box 1252, Dothan, AL 36302; tel: 800-633-0909) may be useful.

Cross-reactivity in latex-allergic patients has been demonstrated to banana, kiwi, avocado, passion fruit, and chestnut, and occasionally to other fruits and nuts, but is apparently an uncommon occurrence (28).

Latex-allergic patients should inform their dentists and physicians of their problem, especially if undergoing obstetrical or surgical procedures, endoscopy, or barium enema exams. Contact with any latex-containing medical device, even an insulin syringe, can cause a reaction (29). Wearing a "medical alert" bracelet or necklace may be advisable in case the person is incapacitated.

Delayed Hypersensitivity to Latex

Wakelin et al. (30) tested 608 patients with various preparations of NRL. Only 24 reactions were seen, all ranked at ± or 1+. Of the nine 1+ reactions, six were felt to be due to concomitant thiuram allergy, and the other three faded at the second reading. The author's conclusions were that patch testing with NRL gave a very low yield and was not recommended for routine use.

In contrast, Wilkinson and Burd (31) reported that 7 of 117 patients (6.0%) with hand dermatitis and glove use were positive on patch testing with NRL. The tests were done with NRL containing no additives using 0.7% ammonia as an anticoagulant. Three of these seven had a negative prick test for latex IH. None reacted to rubber additives.

The reasons for this discrepancy are uncertain but may be due to patient selection and allergen factors. At this time, the value of testing for DH with NRL is uncertain.

EPIDEMIOLOGY OF RUBBER ADDITIVE SENSITIVITY

Although immediate reactions to NRL are now common, delayed hypersensitivity, also called cell-mediated sensitivity, has been recognized for many years. Rubber is a common cause of ACD, and in 1976 Malten et al. (32) stated the incidence of sensitization to rubber was increasing. The best data on the frequency of rubber sensitivity come from various patch test clinics throughout the world. The North American Contact Dermatitis Group (NACDG) reported on rates of patch test reactions over several time periods (Table 31.11) (33,34). The data suggest that allergy to the mercapto agents is declining, whereas reactions to the other substances are increasing. Both the thiurams and carbamates lead the list in each year analyzed. Most persons who react to carbamates also react to thiurams, most likely representing a true cross-reaction, because these two agents are chemically similar.

The most comprehensive recent review of rubber allergy was undertaken by Conde-Salazar et al. in Spain (35). Seven thousand patients were evaluated and 4,680 were tested over a 10-year period to five rubber mixes: thiuram mix, carba mix, black rubber mix, mercapto mix, and naphthyl mix. Of the 4,680 tested, 686 (14.7%) had one or more positives to rubber chemicals, 119 of these were allergic only to rubber additives. Almost half of the positives (336) were construction workers. A breakdown of the individual allergens is given in Table 31.12.

A German study showed a lower rate of rubber allergy than either Spain or North America (36). Only 3.8% of 3,851 reacted to one or more rubber allergens (thiourea and naphthyl mix were not used as screens on all patients). Although the total number of reactors was lower, relative proportions were similar, with thiuram positive in 72% and carba positive in 25%.

Age and Gender in Rubber Allergy

Allergy to rubber chemicals is usually more frequent in men than women. Presumably, much of this is due to the correlation between rubber allergy and work exposure. Conde-Salazar et al. (35) found that 18% of men and only 7% of women reacted to rubber allergen mixes. The NACDG has found statistically significant differences in rubber allergy between men and women as well (Table 31.13) (37). In this group, dermatitis of the hands and feet were more common in men than women, although face and neck dermatitis was more frequent in women.

TABLE 31.11. *Prevalence of Positive Patch Test Reactions to Rubber Chemicals (Based on Data from the North American Contact Dermatitis Group)**

Chemical	Year				
	1972	1982	1985	1996	1998
Black rubber mix 0.6%	NT	1.4%	1.4%	2.3%	1.5%**
Carba mix 3%	NT	3.8%	3.3%	5.7%	7.3%
MBT 1%	4.8%	4.8%	2.7%	2.1%	1.8%
Mercapto mix 1%	NT	2.5%	2.9%	2.2%	1.8%
Mixed thioureas 1%	NT	NT	NT	0.7%	1.3%
Thiuram mix 1%	4.2%	4.3%	3.9%	6.8%	6.9%

*Concentrations are in petrolatum.
** N-I-NP-PPDA tested instead of black rubber mix (34,37,80,81).
NT = not tested.

TABLE 31.12. *Distribution Positive Patch Test to Rubber Mixes in 686 Patients with Rubber Allergy**

Allergy	Number +	Association
Thiuram mix	569 (82.9%)	20% carba +
Carba mix	153 (22.3%)	76% thiuram +
Black rubber mix	122 (17.8%)	14% thiuram +
Mercapto mix	111 (16.0%)	14% thiuram +
Naphthyl mix	17 (2.5%)	18% black rubber +

*Adapted from Conde-Salazar, et al., ref. 35.

Rubber sensitivity is also well documented in children (38–40). Leyden and Kligman (38) found rubber chemicals were the most common contact allergens in children. Of 653 children tested with a standard battery, 98 had positive reactions, of which 41 were from thiuram or mercaptobenziothiazole (MBT). Veien et al. (39) reported five boys and four girls (11.7% of 77 children with one or more positive patch tests to all standard series chemicals) who reacted to rubber chemicals. Six of the nine reactions were considered currently relevant, although the sources were not listed.

> **Rubber sensitivity is common in children, particularly in shoes and particularly to mercaptobenzothiazole.**

MECHANISM OF CONTACT ALLERGY FROM RUBBER ADDITIVES

With the exception of a report of isoprene in a rubber factory and rare reports of delayed hypersensitivity to latex, ACD to rubber is not caused by the natural rubber latex itself (30–32,41). Rather, it is the chemical added in the manufacturing process that sensitizes (7,32,42–50). Allergens may be present in some chemical form in the final product, and both consumer and manufacturer are at risk of being sensitized. Thus, fully cured rubber products often cause allergic contact dermatitis (7). There are several possible explanations. According to Fregert (12), many of the rubber additives are decomposed partially or totally during vulcan-

TABLE 31.13. *Reactions to Rubber Allergens in Men and Women (Based on Data from the North American Contact Dermatitis Group)*

Allergen	Percent positive	
	Men (N = 2000)	Women (N = 2900)
Thiuram mix	4.2	5.9
Carba mix	3.8	2.8
Mercapto mix	2.8	1.5
MBT	3.2	1.3
Black rubber mix	2.1	1.6

MBT, mercaptobenziothiazole

ization, but others, such as antioxidants, are intended to be present in the cured product. Small quantities of accelerators and antioxidants may not be consumed in curing and may "bloom" or migrate to the surface (44). Contact allergy may be enhanced by local heat and sweating. Other reasons may include incomplete curing at lower temperatures, presence as an exposed chemical side group rather than in the linear structure of the rubber polymer, and the degradation of rubber by heat, friction, ozone, and other factors (51). Stankevich et al. (52) demonstrated the migration of thiuram and a mercapto compound (*n*-cyclohexyl-2-benzothiazolsulfenamide) from rubber in food containers (52).

OCCUPATIONAL RUBBER DERMATITIS

Contact dermatitis is common among rubber workers but is less frequent than among users of rubber (3,12,53). Prevalence rates from industrial studies are 3.1, 3.7, and 5.6 cases per 1,000 workers in Great Britain, Australia, and Finland, respectively. California's rate of 7 per 1,000 workers included plastics workers (51,54,55).

In a Finnish study, 56% of the cases represented irritant dermatitis, especially from solvents and bulk rubber. More than half of the allergic contact dermatitis cases were caused by PPDA compounds. Many workers acquired dermatitis through work that did not permit use of protective gloves. It was possible to transfer workers with PPDA who were handling black rubber to a job with colored rubber. Workers could often handle cured rubber if the dermatitis was caused by uncured rubber (54).

According to Schwartz et al. (44), Prosser White found hexamethylenetetramine (HMT) to be the most active cause of dermatitis in the rubber industry in the 1930s. HMT decomposes to formaldehyde and is both an irritant and a sensitizer. According to Adams (3), HMT is now rarely used in the manufacture of rubber except for textile adhesives but is primarily used as a catalyst for the production of phenolic resins.

Tires

It is often difficult to learn the identity of the additives in various rubber products. Tires represent such an example, with compounding formulas considered proprietary information by manufacturers. Although formulations vary among different manufacturers, the same additives are used in both natural and synthetic tire components. Cronin (42), in 1980, listed representative accelerators, antioxidants, retarders, peptizers, processing oils, and other additives used in the British tire industry.

Study of Tire Workers in the United States

The list of chemicals patch tested by Suskind, in his unpublished 1979 study of workers in a large US tire factory, gives a clue to some of the rubber additives used in the

United States tire industry (RR Suskind, Cincinnati, OH, personal communication, 1984). Suskind tested 502 employees with 36 rubber and 12 nonrubber materials. The rubber-related materials that elicited the most reactions and the number of employees reacting were 4,4'-dithiodimorpholine 1% in 45 employees, 4,4'-dithiodimorpholene 0.5% in 4 employees, oil-extended polybutadiene rubber in 11 employees, paraphenylenediamine 1% in 8 employees, diphenylguanidine 2% in 7 employees, nickel sulfate 2.5% in 7 employees, and n-cyclohexylthiophthalimide 1% in 8 employees (see also Tables 31.23 and 31.24).

Most of the reactions to nonrubber-related chemicals occurred from balsam of Peru 25% (in 17 people), potassium dichromate 0.5% (in 15 people), ethylenediamine 1% (in 10 people), and neomycin 20%.

The lists of rubber and nonrubber substances that Suskind tested provide epidemiologic information on chemical exposure in a tire production plant. With the exception of butyl rubber, nickel sulfate, neomycin, phenolformaldehyde resin, and n-cyclohexylthiophthalimide, at least half of all positive patch test reactions were associated with occupational or possibly nonoccupational dermatitis. The sources of occupational exposure to the nonrubber chemicals were not specified.

Other Cases of Contact Dermatitis from Tires

Most reports of contact allergy from tires are from paraphenylenediamine antioxidants. Bieber and Foussereau (56), in 1967, reported nine cases of n-isopropyl-n'-phenyl-paraphenylenediamine contact dermatitis, including four men who handled finished tires at work. Subsequently, Herve-Bazin et al. (57) studied 42 men who were sensitized to isopropylparaphenylenediamine (IPPD) by handling tires: 17 men in the tire manufacturing industry, 5 among tire dealers, and 20 men in the automobile transport and servicing sectors. All of the men were patch test positive to n-phenyl-n'-cyclohexyl-paraphenylenediamine (CPPD) and 37% to paraphenylenediamine. Fifteen men were tested with n-dimethyl-1, 3-butyl-n'-phenylparaphenylene-diamine (DMPPD), and all reacted to it.

> **Paraphenylenediamine-type rubber antioxidants have been reported as producing most cases of tire dermatitis; such rubber antioxidants are used more often in other countries than in the United States.**

Cronin (42) reported 20 men and 1 woman with rubber sensitivity acquired by handling finished tires between 1966 and 1976. The dermatitis affected the palms and flexor surfaces of the wrists and was easily mistaken for constitutional hand eczema. Patch test results were IPPD (19/19 positive), CPPD (14/18 positive), and PPDA (7/21 positive).

Fregert (58) reported a man with IPPD and CPPD sensitivity initially acquired from wearing black rubber gloves who subsequently developed dermatitis from contact with his car tires.

The incidence of sensitization from IPPD has been reduced in a British tire plant by automation in tire building and by limiting the amount of IPPD used to 2% or less of the total rubber mix (59).

Miscellaneous Occupational Rubber Allergies

Other cases are listed in Table 31.14. (See reference 4 for more detailed discussion of occupational rubber dermatitis.)

It is interesting to note that Conde Salazar et al. (35) found that almost half of 686 rubber allergic patients were construction workers. Presumably, this is due to use of rubber boots, gloves, and other protective gear. Rubber industry workers were not included in the study, because construction work was the only occupational rubber association.

In a recent NACDG report, MBT, mercapto mix, and thiuram mix reactors were more often to be occupationally exposed than otherwise (60). Individual occupations were not recorded in this study. Although carba mix and black rubber mix were also more often work-related, the difference was not statistically significant.

Cronin (42) correctly stated that most of the rubber additives, which are firmly entrenched in the rubber industry, have been used satisfactorily for years and are unlikely to be replaced soon. Subsequent studies of the rubber industry and commercial products have shown the current rubber patch test chemicals to be the major sensitizers. Because manufacturing requirements change, however, more efficient chemicals are found and prices vary. The numerous chemicals used in the rubber industry warrant surveillance for potential sensitivity. The thioureas are more recent examples (61–70). Another is 4,4-dithiodimorpholine (71), which was one of several chemicals that caused dermatitis in a Danish rubber factory. Subsequently, it was tested at 1% concentration in an investigation of 110 patients with contact dermatitis, and 6 had positive results.

TABLE 31.14. *Miscellaneous Causes of Occupational Rubber Dermatitis*

Object
Rubber bands
Rubber molds used in concrete forming
Cosmetic sponges
Bank note counters
Finger stalls
Earphones
Packing/sealing for tubes/pipes
Face masks (gas O_2)
Dairy equipment (tubes and hoses)
Aircraft seals, lining tubes, and tires
Motor vehicle parts
Automotive hoses

TABLE 31.15. *Selected Chemicals for Patch Testing with Rubber and Related Substances*

	Source H = Hermal, C = Chemotechnique, TT = True Test
Mercapto mix (contains 0.33% each)	H, C*, TT**
N-cyclohexyl-2-benzothiazolesulfenamide[a]	
2,2′-benzothiazyl disulfide[a]	
Morpholinylmercaptobenzothiazole	
Thiuram mix (contains 0.25% each)	H, C, TT
Dipentamethylenethiuram disulfide[b]	
Tetramethylthiuram disulfide[b]	
Tetramethylthiuram monosulfide[b]	
Tetraethylthiuram disulfide[b]	
PPD (black rubber) mix (contains 0.1% IPPD, 0.25% CPPD, and 0.25% DPPD)	C, TT
N-phenyl-N′-cyclohexyl-p-phenylenediamine	
N-isopropyl-N′-phenyl-p-phenylenediamine[b]	
N,N′-diphenyl-p-phenylenediamine	
Carba mix (contains 1% each)	C, TT
1,3-diphenylguanidine[a]	
Zinc diethyldithiocarbamate[a]	
Zinc dibutyldithiocarbamate[a]	
Mercaptobenzothiazole 2%	H, C, TT
Dodecylmercaptan 0.1%	C
2,2,4-trimethyl-1,2-dihydroquinoline 1%	C
Hydroquinone monobenzylether 1%	C
N-phenyl-2-naphthylamine 1%	H, C
Diaminodiaphenylmethane 0.5%	H, C
Hexamethylenetetramine (methenamine) 2%	H, C
Thioureas	
Diphenylthiourea 1%	H, C
Diethylthiourea 1%	C
Dibutylthiourea 1%	H, C
Thiourea 0.1%	H, C
Zinc dimethyldithiocarbamate 1%	C
Other	
Review of Tables 31.2 through 31.8 identifies other potentially sensitizing rubber additives.	
Patch testing is suggested with specific elastomer additives to which a patient is exposed.	

All concentrations are in petrolatum.
*2.0% pet. Contains morpholinylmercaptobenzothiazole.
**TT conc's are expressed in mg/cm²
[a]Tested separately at 1%.
[b]Tested separately at 19.

Table 31.15 lists some of the major current rubber chemicals and their patch testing concentrations. An example is dioctyl phthalate, a plasticizer identified as an allergen in a rubber worker (72).

A worker in a foam rubber plant developed a pustular reaction to hexafluorosilicate, a gelifier used to maintain the foam structure (73). Patch tests were negative. Testing on rabbits confirmed that the chemical is able to induce pustules, presumably a type of irritant response.

Sensitivity to components of synthetic elastomers should also be suspected. A student technologist was sensitized to Hylene W (4,4′-diisocyanate dicyclohexyl methane), an aliphatic monomer used in the manufacture of polyurethanes (74). Hypalon (chlorosulfonated polyethylene)

"20" and "30" rubbers, which contained epoxy resin as a stabilizer, sensitized a rubber worker who applied the polymer as a lacquer for rubber boots. Patch tests were positive to the two Hypalon rubbers and to epoxy resin (75).

Adams (76) suggested that mercaptobenzimidazole (MBI) be substituted for MBT because it is probably less allergic. This was substantiated by Foussereau et al. (77) Adams and Fregert observed that in subjects allergic to MBT, the MBI patch test was negative in 44 of 46 (about 95%) cases.

Rubber Allergy in Shoemakers

Mancu⬤ et al. (78) reported on rubber allergy in 240 workers at five factories in Italy. Only 16 (6.5%) had ACD. MBT and the adhesive paratertiary butylphenol formaldehyde resin were the main allergens. Workers assembling the shoes were at greatest risk for ACD.

PATCH TESTING WITH RUBBER MIXES

With the exception of mercaptobenzothiazole (MBT) and now N-I- paraphenylenediamine, the NACDG recommends that patch test screening for rubber allergy be performed with "mixes" of rubber chemicals rather than a single substance (79–83). This testing strategy is accepted worldwide (Table 31.15).

Early Mixes

There is considerable literature describing the use of mixtures in patch testing (84–88). Their usefulness lies in one patch covering several test substances. Bonnevie (84), in 1939, pioneered the use of patch test mixes employing four wood tars and also chrysarobin with anthrarobin. Hjorth (86), in 1963, employed mixes of wood tars, paraben esters, caines, and antibiotics. Nine rubber chemicals were incorporated into a mix by Gotz and Istvanovic (87) in 1963. Epstein (88), in 1967, reviewed the literature and reported his findings with mixes of caines, antihistamines, rubber chemicals, and antibacterial agents, respectively. He used a screening set of five mixtures containing a total of 23 chemicals in addition to 10 conventional single-substance patch tests. He found concordance between patch test–positive results in seven rubber-sensitive patients from a mix consisting of rubber chemicals (mercaptobenzothiazole [MBT]), tetramethylthiuram disulfide, and monobenzyl ether of hydroquinone each 1% in petrolatum) and from the individual chemicals. Less than half of his patch test–proven rubber-sensitive patients reacted to the mix, however, and he added thio-beta-naphthol and phenyl-beta-naphthylamine, each 1%, to broaden the scope of the rubber-additive screening. This new mix with five components gave frequent false-positive reactions and was discarded. These irritant reactions were caused by thio-beta-naphthol, which was found to be less irritant in the mix than when it was tested separately.

Current Mixes: Validation and Cross-Reactivity

Subsequent refinement of rubber patch test mixtures has occurred. To minimize irritant reactions, the concentration of the individual mix constituents was reduced to less than 1%; carba mix is an exception. Carba mix is the only rubber allergen mix that still gives a fairly high rate of irritant reactions. Almost always these dissipate by 48 hours after patch removal.

MBT Mix

Mitchell et al. (89), in 1976, reported the results of patch testing with MBT 1% in petrolatum and with MBT mix containing MBT and three derivatives, each at 0.25%. The results, showing 48 patients MBT positive and mix negative, suggested that the concentration of MBT in the mix was too low compared with MBT itself in the standard screen. Accordingly, MBT 1% petrolatum was retained separately in subsequent screening trays. In 1979, MBT was removed from the mix so that the concentration of the three remaining constituents could be raised from 0.25% to 0.333%. A subsequent 1982 evaluation of the new mix versus 1% MBT suggests that the mix will detect a small number of patients who are MBT negative but mix positive (90).

Fregert (91) studied the pattern of cross-reactions among the mercapto group of chemicals. He found that a combination of a benzene and a thiazole ring and a thiol group in the 2-position were necessary for cross-sensitivity. Cronin (42) tabulated the results of testing with separate constituents of mercapto mix. In both men and women the greatest number of reactions was to MBT, and in both sexes there was a decreasing incidence of reactions to morpholinyl MBT (MMBT), CBS, and dibenzothiazyl disulfide (MBTS). Hansson and Agrup (92) have shown, however, that what is put into a mix may not be what is still there when we do a patch test. They showed that, in reality, MBTS is the major chemical left in the MBT mix after only a few weeks storage time. This is due to the other mix ingredients reacting together to form the MBTS. Only about 25% to 30% of the other agents was present at the 3-week analysis.

Thiuram Mix

Van Ketel (93), in the Netherlands, found thiuram mix to be a good indicator of thiuram sensitivity (93); there was good correlation between testing with thiuram mix and its components. Tetramethylthiuram disulfide (TMTD) alone was not an adequate indicator of thiuram allergy. Van Ketel also found a much lower incidence of allergy to dipentamethylene thiuram disulfide (PTD) than that reported in England,

where PTD and tetraethylthiuram disulfide (TETD) are more frequent sensitizers than TMTD and tetramethylthiuram monosulfide (TMTM) (42). Other European investigators (94,95) have found that reactions to TMTM and TMTD were highest when components of the mix were tested. These variations between countries may reflect differences in usages by manufacturers for rubber goods.

Cronin (42) found the four thiuram mix chemicals do not always cross-react one with another. Malten et al. (32) list cross-reactions for thiuram mix components (a): 1) For TMTD—probably bisdimethyldithio-carbamate and bisdiethyldithiocarbamate (ZDC) (according to Malten et al., as soon as soap containing TMTD is used with water, TMTD decomposes to dimethyldithiocarbamate). TMTD also cross-reacts with TETD and TMTM, both components of thiuram mix; (b) for tetraethylthiuram disulfide-thiuram mix components TMTD and TMTM, and tetraethylthiuram monosulfide; and (c) for dipentamethylene-thiuram disulfide (PTD)—TMTD and TMTM.

Naphthyl Mix

Naphthyl mix was removed from the North American Contact Dermatitis Group's standard screening tray in 1979 because of a low rate of reactivity (JS Taylor, et al. Unpublished data on epidemiology of contact dermatitis in North America, 1976–1982, Task Force on Contact Dermatitis, American Academy of Dermatology, Evanston, IL). In 1980, Cronin (42) found phenyl-beta-naphthylamine (PBN) to be present in many types of tires, and some naphthyl compounds, such as PBN, were also present in rubber and plastic. She tested the separate constituents of the mix in about half of her mix-positive patients. Each of 9 reacted to dibetanaphthyl-p-diamine (DBNPD), and 7 of 11 were positive to PBN. Van Ketel (82), in 1983, also reported a low sensitization rate for naphthyl mix from the Netherlands. PBN is no longer manufactured in the United States or Germany because it is considered a carcinogen; however, India still may produce PBN (AJ Rizzer, Mobay Chemical Co., Pittsburgh, PA, personal communication).

Carbamates and Diphenylguanidine (Carba Mix)

In Cronin's experience (42), simultaneous reactions to thiuram mix and carba mix are not infrequent and occur probably because thiurams are derivatives of dithiocarbamates. At St. John's Hospital (London, England) she found that most of the patients reacting only to carba mix were males and that diphenylguanidine (DPG) was the most likely sensitizer; DPG, which is not a carbamate, is used more in industrial than in consumer rubber products. Doubtful reactions are more likely to occur with carba mix than with the other mixes. Subsequent testing with the separate components of the mix may clarify whether the weak response is an irritant or an allergic reaction. Malten et al. (32) list probable cross-reactions for carbamates as substances derived from thiocarbamate, which are used as pesticides.

PPDA Mix

The St. John's results of testing the separate constituents in most of the 53 patients positive to PPDA mix were isopropyl-paraphenylenediamine (IPPD) positive in 45 of 48, phenylcyclohexyparaphenylenediamine (CPPD) positive in 38 of 45, and diphenylparaphenylenediamine (DPPD) positive in 17 of 43 (42). Paraphenylenediamine itself was usually negative and so a poor detector of sensitization to this group of chemicals. Cross-reactions may also occasionally occur with the hair dye chemical paraminodiphenylamine (96). About 20% of those who react to PPDA mix may be allergic to certain textile dyes, especially the disperse dyes (see Chapter 19). (See the section Tires above for a discussion of other cross-reactions.) In response to uncertain availability and usage of some components of the mix, the NACDG in 1998 substituted the single agent *N*-isopropyl-*N*-phenylparaphenylenediamine (IPPPDA). It appears to be a less satisfactory allergen than the mix.

Mixed Thioureas

In response to the appearance of case reports of allergy to the thioureas in rubber materials, especially sporting goods and shoes, the NACDG began testing with a mix of di-alkyl thioureas in 1991. Other than case reports, there is not enough epidemiologic data to determine the significance of this allergen. The NACDG data are shown in Table 31.11.

Strategies for Patch Testing with Mixes

The rubber mixes allow patch testing of chemically closely related rubber chemicals (e.g., TMTD and TETD); phenylcyclohexyl PPD and diphenyl PPD) that frequently do not cross-react (Table 37.15). The 13 items in the four rubber mixes plus MBT in Table 37.15 allow the screening capacity of the standard tray to be increased greatly while conserving space. A weak positive reaction to one of the mixes may be due either to a mild irritant effect of the total mixture or to a weak allergy to one of the components. When in doubt about the significance of such a weak reaction, the components of the mix should be tested separately. Separate testing of the components should also be done if the patch test mix is negative (possibly because the components are not present in sufficient concentration to elicit a positive reaction) but rubber allergy is strongly suspected. In that case, it may be important to test with a thin shaving from the suspected rubber article or with other individual rubber chemicals suspected of causing the allergy. Bleached rubber syndrome should also be suspected when rubber dermatitis is suspected but patch tests to rubber chemicals are negative (97).

> Patch testing with rubber "mixes" allows the screening capacity of the standard patch test tray to be greatly increased while conserving space.

Patch Testing with Pieces of Rubber

Veien (98) reported results of patch testing with substances not in the standard series. These additional items were tested along with the standard tray chemicals. Specific rubber items eliciting relevant reactions among 24 patients included 17 gloves, 3 finger stalls, 2 rubber tubing, 1 rubber sponge, and 1 bra strap. The rubber allergies demonstrated by testing with items supplied by the patients themselves could, in many instances, have been identified by the standard series. Only 9 of the 17 patients reacting to gloves, however, had concomitant reactions to rubber chemicals.

THIOUREAS

Contact dermatitis from the thiourea rubber accelerators is being reported more frequently (Table 31.16). The most recent data from the NACDG found that 1.3% of 4,098 patients reacted to mixed dialkyl thioureas (1% pet).

Diethylthiourea (DTU) used in conjunction with hydrazine was reported to have caused dermatitis of the ears in two rubber workers. Patch testing to both chemicals was positive, but concentrations were not given (61).

DTU, present as an accelerator in neoprene foam weather strips used in a new car factory for hood and door seals, also caused an outbreak of dermatitis in 15 car assembly workers and mechanics. The rashes occurred primarily on the hands, forearms, and sometimes the face, corresponding to the sites of contact with the rubber. Workers who fitted the strips in another factory were not affected. This difference was explained by White and Vickers (62) according to the way the two groups of men came into contact with the seals. The fitters who applied them handled the strips only with their palms, whereas the assembly workers and mechanics touched the rubber with all parts of their hands and arms.

DTU was also the cause of hand dermatitis in a Danish factory cleaner who came in contact with an acidic detergent containing 0.4% DTU. Patch tests revealed DTU 1%

TABLE 31.16. *Thiourea and Derivatives: Nonrubber Exposures*

Diazo copy paper, especially blueprints, clothing patterns
Commercial detergents
Adhesive tapes
Paint and glue removers
Fruits and vegetables (metabolized from carbamate fungicides)

petrolatum positive; negative to dibutylthiourea (DBTU), thiuram mix, and carba mix (64).

Fregert (65) routinely patch tested 2,491 subjects with DTU 1% in petrolatum and found all were negative.

Diphenylthiourea (DPTU), which was found to be present in PVC adhesive tape backing, caused dermatitis in 28 people using the tape (65). Fregert (66) identified DPTU in other PVC objects and in certain brands of rubber gloves. According to Adams (3), DPTU is derived from aniline and carbon disulfide, and its use declined following the discovery of MBT in the 1920s.

Meding et al. (99) reported 11 cases of allergy to DPTU in rubber orthopedic knee or elbow sleeves. A range of symptoms, including dermatitis, purpura and urticaria, were seen. All seven that were tested reacted to DPTU 1% pet, six reacted to ETU 1% pet, and two reacted to carbamates. The DPTU was present in an adhesive used in the sleeves. ETU was apparently not present in the products, so it was probably a cross-reactor.

DBTU is used as an anticorrosive agent in metal pickling solutions and as a paint and glue remover. The latter was associated with allergic contact dermatitis of the hands in a machinist who handled plastics, paints, and solvents. DBTU was patch test positive at 0.2% and 0.1% pet (100).

Ethylenethiourea (ETU) sensitivity was reported in a factory worker sewing rubber products, such as fire-protection suits, equipment to make special doors water-tight, and equipment for handling and dumping oil at sea. Patch tests proved positive to rubber material from work, ETU in concentrations from 0.01% to 1% aqueous and Maneb (fungicide) 1% pet; negative to DBTU, DTU, DPTU, ethyleneurea, thiourea, carbamates, and ethylenediamine (68). Of 775 patients previously patch tested by Bruze and Fregert (68) to ETU 1% pet, one patient was positive. Maneb and other ethylenebisdithiocarbamate fungicides and slimicides may be metabolized to thioureas. Accordingly, carbamates and ETU may be found on or in fruits, berries, potatoes, and vegetables; whether sensitivity could be maintained by exposure to these low concentrations is uncertain (68).

The thiourea rubber accelerators may produce allergic contact dermatitis not only in rubber products but also in detergents, polyvinyl adhesive backings, metal anticorrosive agents, plastics, photocopy paper, and textiles.

Dimethylthiourea (DMTU) sensitivity was reported in a textile cutter with conjunctivitis and dermatitis of the eyelids, corners of the mouth, and nasal mucous membranes. There was a strong positive patch test to the textile cutting patterns she handled; these had been duplicated by diazo processing that contained DMTU. In another case, a construction designer had dermatitis of the hands, face, and neck from diazo copy paper. He reacted to DMTU, thiourea, and ammonium paper developers (101). Previous contact dermatitis reactions from diazo-sensitized paper have been attributed to nickel, chromates, p-methyl-aminophenol-sulfate (Metol), diazonium salts (present in unexposed paper), and color developers. Thiourea and derivatives are used in almost all kinds of photocopy paper as antioxidants to prevent discoloration. Diazo-sensitized paper without dimethylthiourea (Sepia) can be provided by GAF Corp. (69).

DBTU was the cause of airborne ACD in two patients with dermatitis on exposed surfaces. Both were exposed to BTU in a paint-removing solvent. The product is a strong irritant that may have predisposed to the development of the allergy (102).

Thiourea contact sensitivity was reported by Nurse (70) in a man exposed to paper used for printing architectural and printing plans. He was patch test positive to both undeveloped and developed paper, as well as Diazo 580 1% aqueous and thiourea 1% aqueous. The patient's hands were also sun sensitive, but photopatch testing was not performed. Sensitivity to thiourea was described by Van Der Leun et al. (103), in 1977, in two patients working with photocopy paper and presenting with photodermatitis. Patch testing with thiourea was positive, in one case with exposure of the test site to light and in the other without light exposure.

Ethylbutylthiourea (EBTU) contact allergy produced severe plantar foot dermatitis in 10 patients who wore Nike athletic shoes with insole material prepared by Spenco Medical Corp. The identification of EBTU as the allergen by Roberts and Hanifin in 1979 must be considered a classic example of the sleuthing sometimes required to identify a contact allergen (104). Spenco Corp. obtained the innersole material from Rubatex Corp., which assembled the nylon-foam rubber innersole with a neoprene-based adhesive obtained from General Adhesive and Chemical Co. EBTU was used as an accelerator in the adhesive and was supplied to General Adhesive by Pennwalt Corp. A new innersole without EBTU has been marketed since then in Spenco and Nike innersoles. None of these patients reacted to a large series of known rubber or adhesive allergens. Cross-sensitivity was later demonstrated between EBTU and other substituted thioureas: DTU, DBTU, DMTU, trimethylthiourea, and thiourea. No cross-reaction occurred with ethylene thiourea. This cross-sensitivity may be important because several of Robert's and Hanifin's original patients continued to have dermatitis after discontinuing the Nike shoes and alkylthioureas may be present in other shoes (100).

GLOVES—HOUSEHOLD, INDUSTRIAL, AND SURGICAL

The rubber product that most often causes dermatitis is gloves (12). Any patient with a diffuse or patchy eczema on the dorsum of hand and fingers and who wears rubber gloves may be sensitive to rubber. Although this typical pattern may have an abrupt cutoff above the wrist, the classical distribution of rubber glove dermatitis was seen in few of Cronin's patients (42). Many had a nonspecific pattern of hand eczema, and, in most patients, diagnosis could not have been made with certainty without routine patch testing. The eruption may mimic a photodermatitis.

Even when the patient is not allergic to rubber, the gloves may make an existing hand dermatitis worse from occlusion and maceration. To avoid this, thin, white cotton lining gloves worn inside unlined rubber or vinyl gloves are suggested. The cotton liners can be changed during long tasks. Wearing two pairs of gloves, however, is not always feasible in workers requiring fine touch or dexterity. It may be wise to always recommend vinyl or other special gloves to prevent rubber dermatitis in hand eczema patients without rubber allergy. The appendix gives a table of gloves recommended for those with rubber-additive allergy. Cronin (42) stated that gloves may give false-negative patch test reactions. According to Jordan (105), occlusion for 72 or 96 hours may be needed to elicit allergy to thin pieces of rubber, especially surgeons' gloves. Alternatively, be aware of a false-positive, irritant, "corner pressure effect" from testing thicker pieces of rubber or rubber shavings.

Knudsen et al. (106) studied several types of rubber household and surgical gloves for release of thiurams and carbamates. They found wide ranges of release of these chemicals, with household gloves generally releasing less than the surgical gloves. There was a definite correlation of being patch test positive to a glove and the amount of allergen released.

> **Label information giving levels of allergens released from rubber gloves would be very helpful for rubber allergic glove users.**

If patch testing with the glove is positive in the absence of a reaction from a standard tray rubber substance, another rubber chemical may be the culprit (108). Cronin (42) identified a patient allergic to the antioxidant methylcyclohexyl-dimethylphenol 1% that was present in a rubber glove. Most of Cronin's patients, however, were allergic to dipentamethylenethiuram disulfide (PTD) present in thiuram mix. Of 257 women and 91 men with rubber glove dermatitis, more than 80% of each group reacted to a thiuram. Ninety-six percent of the men reacted to thiuram mix, indicating it is essential to use several chemicals of a group, or a mixture of them, for testing.

According to Fisher (107,113), any hand dermatitis in a surgeon should be considered as stemming from sensitization to ingredients in rubber gloves until proved otherwise. Polano (109), in 1958, identified four surgeons and one nurse patch test positive to dioxydiphenyl 1% in ung. cetyl.

In 1973, Lintum and Nater (110,111) studied five surgeons with hand eczema; each reacted to rubber gloves and thiuram chemicals, and one was also sensitive to carbamates. In a study by Fisher (107) of 11 surgeons who acquired allergic contact dermatitis of the hands from surgical gloves, patch testing revealed that 7 had positive patch tests to mercaptobenzothiazole. The other four were allergic to various other rubber chemicals. In Great Britain, Cronin (42) identified the accelerator zinc diethyldithiocarbamate (ZDC) and the antioxidant polymerized 2,2,4-tri-methyl-1,2-dihydroquinolone as the chemicals in one widely used surgical glove.

A report from Oregon identified two antioxidants in latex exam gloves that caused isolated cases of ACD (112). Two patients reacted to 4,4′-thiobis (6-tert-butylmetacresol) (Lowinox 44536). One also reacted to BHA and BHT. Both were negative to rubber allergens but positive to gloves.

> **Rubber gloves are frequent causes of contact dermatitis.**

A good substitute for household use for those allergic to rubber is the Allerderm vinyl glove and similar products. Vinyl exam gloves are safe but lack elasticity and are therefore poorly suited to tasks requiring fine touch sensitivity. The Tactyl-1 glove, made of a plastic polymer, is safe for latex allergic as well as rubber accelerator positive patients and offers superior touch in contrast to vinyl.

Hand protection by gloves is also an important issue for industrial workers (107,114,115). The degree of protection afforded by various glove materials varies for different combinations of chemical agents and protective materials. The US National Institute for Occupational Safety and Health (114) studied the extent of penetration of solvents and carcinogens through gloves of various compositions. The manufacturers of industrial gloves can provide tables that list specific information on the choice of gloves for use in handling various chemicals.

Before prescribing gloves of any kind for industrial use, the industrial plant safety officer should be contacted to determine whether gloves can be worn safely. Gloves are contraindicated in certain occupations involving machine tool grinding or work with rapidly moving parts.

Other Glove Reactions

Endotoxins

Shmunes and Darby (116) reported dyshidrosis of the hands in a hospital phlebotomist. The source of the irritation, which occurred clinically and on usage tests 12 to 24 hours after wearing gloves (Micro Touch by Arbrook Inc.) for 10 to 20 minutes, was linked to bacterial endotoxin in latex gloves. Sterilization of the gloves by gamma irradiation increased endotoxin levels. When the bacterial count is elevated, the endotoxin is water soluble and is absorbed onto powder inside the gloves. Sweating under the gloves may enhance entry into the skin with subsequent dyshidrosis. No systemic symptoms were reported as may occur in cases of endotoxin reactions from contaminated biologicals intended for intravenous or intramuscular use.

Eyelid Dermatitis/Edema: "On Call" Dermatitis

Jordan (105) in an astute observation, described eyelid dermatitis in the absence of hand eczema in obstetric physicians and nurses who are allergic to rubber gloves. These personnel frequently use and then remove gloves after a few minutes. Brief contact with the eyelids allows the rubber accelerator (e.g., thiuram), which is leached into the donning powder, to remain on the eyelids; the rubber accelerator can be removed from the hands by washing.

Eyelid edema without hand eczema was reported by Calnan (71) to occur in a patient every time he was in contact with rubber. The reported attack occurred after laying a rubber-backed carpet. Penile edema was also present. Patch tests were positive to thiuram and carba mixes; scratch tests with the mixes were both negative.

DERMATITIS FROM CONSUMER RUBBER ARTICLES

Malten et al. (32) pointed out that contact with most rubber articles is casual, except for the wearing of rubber gloves. Rubber is therefore not suspected as a cause of dermatitis by the patient. Rubber sensitivity may be the entire cause of a dermatitis, or it may be superimposed upon a preexisting eczema. Rubber allergy often has no distinctive clinical pattern and cases will be missed unless patients are patch tested with standard tray rubber chemicals (42). A positive reaction to a rubber chemical is significant and is usually relevant (12). As Cronin (42) stated, the source of rubber contact can nearly always be identified and eliminated, either curing or alleviating the patient's eczema (see Tables 31.14, 31.16, 31.19, 31.24).

Condoms

Contact dermatitis from rubber condoms is usually easy to diagnose, because there is a clear relationship with intercourse and it is often accompanied by marked penile edema. In 1966, Hindson (117) reported 33 men and 2 women with dermatitis due to rubber condoms. The women presented with pruritus vulvae. In 1980, Cronin (42) identified English condoms as containing the accelerators zinc MBT, PTD, and ZDC and the antioxidant polytrimethylhydroquinolone. Condoms, like latex gloves, can cause immediate hypersensitivity in addition to ACD.

Fisher (7) identified two instances in which a preservative powder that had been dusted on the condom was the cause of dermatitis. Removal of the powder by washing allowed the patients to use the condom without acquiring dermatitis. In one instance, the powder contained 10% monobenzyl ether of hydroquinone. Fisher (7) reported that several of his rubber-sensitive patients found by trial and error that only certain brands of condoms produced dermatitis.

Severe penile dermatitis developed in a patient after 25 years of wearing a condom catheter (118). Allergy to thiuram and MBT was documented. Switching to a silicone device was curative.

Nonrubber condoms are Fourex Natural Lamb Skins (Schmidt) and Trojan Naturalamb (Young's Drug Products) made of processed sheep intestine (caecum). Both brands are made from raw materials obtained from abbatoirs in New Zealand. It should be noted that nonrubber condoms may not be completely protective against the spread of HIV (119).

The differential diagnosis of condom allergy includes pubic, scrotal, and groin dermatitis and vulvitis from other contraceptive agents, such as spermicidal jellies, creams, foams, diaphragms, and lubricants (120–122). Fisher (122) described connubial contact dermatitis from propylene glycol in K-Y Jelly and from feminine hygiene sprays. Vulvitis may also occur from irritants and sensitizers in douches, nail polish, nickel-plated zippers, sanitary napkin clasps, soaps, perfumes, clothing, and bubble baths (121).

Diaphragms and Pessaries

Fisher (7,120,121) mentioned the occurrence of vaginitis and vulvitis from rubber diaphragms and pessaries in rubber-sensitive individuals.

Tourniquet

Thiobetanaphthol, a peptizing agent added to rubber to facilitate its flow during molding, was identified as the sensitizer in a tourniquet applied to an arm before an intravenous injection (123).

Dialysis Unit

In an investigation of pruritic skin rashes in a hemodialysis unit, eight patients, four of whom had dermatitis, were patch test positive to various thiurams (124). It was postulated that thiurams were eluted from the hemodialysis apparatus and sensitized the patients, some of whom developed dermatitis.

Hot Water Bottle

Cronin (42) reported three patients who had contact dermatitis from hot water bottles. All three were patch test positive to MBT as well as the bottle. The dermatitis corresponded to the site of rubber contact. In an 81-year-old man with dorsal hand eczema, however, the cause of the dermatitis was initially covert. The positive MBT patch test was the clue to diagnosis, and it was eventually determined, with some difficulty, that he lay in bed with his hands under a hot water bottle.

Rubber Sheet

Cronin (42) also reported severe contact dermatitis in an incontinent man who always slept on a rubber sheet. He required hospitalization to clear the eczema, and on patch testing he reacted to the sheet and to dioxydiphenyl 1% in petrolatum.

Rubber-bulb Eyedropper

Eyelid dermatitis of 2 years' duration in a woman with a history of previous dermatitis from rubber gloves and elastic resolved after she stopped dispensing eyedrops from a bottle with a rubber bulb for the dropper. She was patch test positive to MBT 2% and negative to mercapto mix, the standard series and the ingredients of the eye solution. Calnan and Cronin (125) postulated that MBT was present in the rubber of one of the drop-bottle bulbs and that it may have contaminated the eyedrops, but the piece of rubber used for testing was probably too small to produce a reaction. They identified one similar previously reported case.

> **The rubber in many medical devices, such as in catheters, douche bulbs, drains, tourniquets, hot water bottles, and dialysis units, may produce dermatitis or urticaria.**

CPAP Straps

Individuals with sleep apnea may be treated with a continuous positive airway pressure device (CPAP). This involves wearing a breathing mask, held in place by rubber straps. Both Reynaerts et al. (126) and Scalf and Fowler (127) have reported thiourea allergy and dermatitis from the straps.

Swim Gear

Swim Goggles

Goette (128) reported a "raccoon-like" periorbital leukoderma from contact with swim goggles. The patient, a 12-year-old female, had worn the same goggles the preceding year without ill effects and then had reused them after the leukoderma had cleared without any ill effects. A toxic reaction is postulated to have occurred from chemicals that leaked from the goggles and were eventually exhausted. Three of the substances present in the goggles were identi-

fied: zinc bis(diethylcarbamodithioato-S,S'), phenol, 2,2'-methylene bis(6-(1-dimethylethyl)-4-methyl), and N,N'-diethylthiourea. Goette (128) stated that a representative of the Canadian manufacturer of the goggles was aware of 12 similar cases.

Two major brands of swim goggles, Speedo (Pro, Ultravision, Sprint, Anti-Fog, and Relay) and Hilco Swim N' Sun are made of black neoprene rubber with ethyl butyl thiourea as an accelerator (R Cash, Rubatex Corp., Bedford, VA, personal communication, 1984; T Bengston, North Vancouver, BC, personal communication, 1984; L Kindler and H Weis, Portland, OR, personal communication, 1984; L Sauve, International Forms Co., personal communication, 1994). The manufacturer of Speedo goggles (International Servisport Corp. Ltd., 200–445 Mountain Highway, North Vancouver, BC, Canada V7J 2L1) and the distributor of Hilco Swim N' Sun goggles (Hilsinger Corp., Plainville, MA 02762) will supply special air-blown neoprene goggles that do not contain EBTU but that do contain dibenzothiazyldisulfide (MBTS) to anyone allergic to the regular neoprene goggles. Both companies should be contacted directly. Other goggles made of silicone rubber are now available.

> **The rubber edges of swim goggles may produce a "raccoon-like" periorbital depigmentation.**

Swim Caps

Cronin (42) mentions that two of her patients with a history of swim cap dermatitis were sensitive to MBT. Speedo manufactures an all-silicone swim cap in addition to regular latex, siliconized latex, and Lycra swim caps.

Scuba Face Masks

Maibach (129) described a mini-epidemic of facial dermatitis among scuba divers using face masks containing IPPD. Patch testing was positive to thinly shaven 2-cm² patches of the rubber from the mask, as well as to IPPD 0.5% in petrolatum. Tuyp and Mitchell (130) reported a dermatologist who had a recurrent facial dermatitis after scuba diving and who had a positive patch test from IPPD.

Other Swim Gear

Speedo makes two types of nose clips that are dipped in latex rubber and an earplug made from Kraton, an SBS rubber block copolymer (131). Kick boards are usually made of styrofoam or other synthetic polymer (T Bengston, North Vancouver, BC, personal communication, 1984).

Adams (63) reported dermatitis in a diver from DTU incorporated into a rubber wet suit. There were positive patch tests to a piece of the wet suit and DTU 0.1% in petrolatum. The standard tray rubber allergens were negative. The diver wore a substitute suit without DTU for 8 years without recurrence, except on one occasion when he borrowed a friend's wet suit, resulting in a severe recurrence requiring hospitalization. Recreational divers with rubber allergy may be able to tolerate the Polar-Tec suit, which is made of Lycra with a fleece lining. Local dive shops can help locate this and other alternatives.

Clothing and Related Articles

Garters

Garter dermatitis has become a clinical rarity since the introduction of panty hose. In England, Cronin (42) identified the sensitizing chemicals as either a thiuram or MBT.

Surgical Support Stockings

For patients with allergy to rubber components of support hose, Jobst (Jobst Inc., Box 471048, Charlotte, NC 28247-1048) makes a special-order stocking with a spandex core. This may be an adequate alternative, depending on the pressure requirements of the disorder, for patients allergic to the latex core of regular Jobst stockings. Jobst recommends special-order white woven bobinette material for patients with dye allergy. These same alternatives may be used for arm supports.

Hair Net Elastic

Dermatitis due to elastic in hair nets may mimic seborrheic dermatitis. In such instances, wrap-around hair nets without elastic may be substituted; hair ribbons are another alternative (7).

Dress Shields

In 1960, Schulz and Hermann (132) reported 12 cases of dress shield eczema affecting the axillae. All 12 patients were patch test positive to 4,4'-dioxydiphenyl (DOD), and 6 of the 12 also reacted to other rubber chemicals. DOD has been implicated in contact allergy from condoms. Cronin (42) also reported a case in a man. Differential diagnosis of dress shield eczema includes contact allergy from clothing and antiperspirants (7).

Rubber Panties

In addition to irritation and maceration from occlusion in the diaper area, rubber panties have caused contact allergy (7). Most panties today are made of vinyl (132).

Brassieres

One case of allergy to the spandex rubber used in a brassiere was reported from Japan (133). The patient re-acted to 2-hydroxy-methyl-phenyl benzotriazole (Tinuvin-P) contained in the spandex; she did not react to other benzotriazoles.

Rubber Dental Plates

Rubber dentures are rarely, if ever, used today, but such dentures have caused stomatitis (7). Standard acrylic dentures are readily available substitutes (7). The reverse usually occurs, however, with rubber or vinyl dentures, serving as a possible substitute for acrylic allergy. Vulcanite rubber dentures contain only natural rubber, zinc oxide, and sulfur and undergo a slow cure; there are no other rubber additives (JM Rabb, Hygienic Corp., Akron, OH, personal communication, 1984).

Rubber Headrest

Women with rubber sensitivity have been reported to have developed an eruption resembling nuchal neurodermatitis from contact with the rubber kidney-shaped headrest attached to the shampoo tray in beauty parlors. Dermatitis was prevented by placing a plastic sheet or towel over the headrest (7). Many such headrests today are plastic.

Rubber Cosmetic Sponges

In 1950, Furman (134), Fisher (7), and Leider reported 26 women with cosmetic sponge contact dermatitis involving the face and especially the eyelids. Such cases are still routinely seen. Usually the patient suspects allergy to the cosmetics, but patch testing gives the correct answer. Alternatives for cosmetic application are tissues and brushes. An adhesive is used to hold the brush bristles in the holder, but this is an unlikely cause of dermatitis. Fisher (135), in 1993, reported three new cases of dermatitis from cosmetic sponges, all of which were caused by tetramethylthiuram.

Eyelash Curlers

In 1945, Curtis (136) reported eyelid dermatitis from phenyl beta naphthylamine after use of eyelash curlers with rubber edges. This type of eyelash curler is rarely used now (42). Plastic eyelash curlers without rubber edges are available as substitutes (7). A more recent report of eyelash curler allergy was due to PPDA mix components (137).

Dermatitis limited to the ears occurred in a Japanese woman who wore rubber earplugs in the bath (138). She was allergic to both MBT and thiurams.

Rubber Pillows and Cushions

Cronin (42) reported two cases of facial dermatitis traced to rubber pillows and one case of a man with a dermatitis, beginning on his buttocks and spreading to his groin, abdomen, and legs, that was caused by a sponge rubber cushion he used at work.

Balloons and Rubber Toys

Balloons may cause intermittent episodes of eczema involving the lips and lower half of the face and the cause may not be obvious to the patient or physician (42). Gaul (139) reported two cases that were traced to monobenzyl ether of hydroquinone. Cronin (42) described three patients each of whom was thiuram sensitive.

In the 1960s, dermatitis occurred on the face of 40% of the children playing with toys made of semisolid rubber called Flubber. Referred to as Flubberitis (7), the condition was thought to be an irritant dermatitis and folliculitis phenomenon caused by an oil used in the production of Flubber. These products, also sold as Roobly Rubber and Plubber, were easily molded into any shape, and their resiliency enabled them to be used as bouncing toys. Flubber was composed of partially polymerized butadiene and mineral oil (70:30 ratio) with minor amounts of polymerization catalysts, antioxidants, and stoppers. Patch testing was inconclusive (140,141).

Balloons contain natural rubber latex and therefore are common causes of NRL contact urticaria.

Squash Ball

Cronin (42) reported palmar dermatitis in a carpenter who played squash. He was patch test positive to PPD mix, and IPPD was confirmed by the manufacturers to be present in the ball.

Rubber Wishbone

Palmar eczema in two windsurfers was reported after contact with the rubber wishbone, which is held by the surfer to remain afloat. The wishbone is sometimes held continually over many hours. Both surfers were patch test positive to PPD mix. A substitution of aluminum for the black rubber was curative (142).

BLEACHED RUBBER SYNDROME

Jordan and Bourlas (97) reported six patients who reacted to the elastic of their bleached underwear but not to new unbleached elastic supplied by the manufacturer. The components of the elastic and standard tray rubber chemical were also patch test negative. Washing the elastic with full-strength commercial bleach (5% sodium hypochlorite in water), however, gave the patients allergic responses due to the effect of bleach on the rubber accelerator, zinc dibenzyldithiocarbamate (ZDC). Using superb detective work to identify the allergen, ZDC was made to react with bleach, and the resultant gum was extracted with diethyl ether.

Eight compounds were identified in the reaction mixture by gas chromatography/mass spectrometry. The individual components were tested on volunteers after sensitization to the reaction mixture was produced in 14 of 25 volunteers. One component, n,n'-dibenzylcarbamyl chloride, produced an allergic response in each sensitized volunteer.

In practice, a presumptive diagnosis of bleached rubber dermatitis can be made if the patient is patch test positive to rubber from his or her underwear and negative to the screening rubber allergens. Treatment is simple; the patients must buy new underwear, and no bleach should be added to the wash. All of Jordan's original patients remained free of this dermatitis without changing to other brands of underwear. Similar reactions may take place with other bleached rubber apparel such as sneakers (WP Jordan, personal communication).

> **Chemicals in underwear elastic or in rubber sneakers may be oxidized to become sensitizers by washing with bleaches containing sodium hypochlorite or Chlorox.**

RUBBER PURPURA AND LICHENOID DERMATITIS

Both Fisher (143,144) and Shmunes (145) reviewed purpuric contact dermatitis, including rubber purpura. Fisher (143) referred to the PPPP syndrome as an allergic dermatitis characterized by pruritus, petechiae, and purpura produced by IPPD. Cases have been reported associated with wearing elasticized underwear, rubber boots, a rubber diving suit, and a rubberized support bandage for the leg (143,144,146,147). The petechial, purpuric, eczematous dermatitis has been located typically at the exact sites of rubber contact with skin, but has also been generalized, similar to the eruption caused by sensitivity to carbromal and meprobamate (143,147,148). Positive patch tests have been recorded from IPPD and DPPD, and in one report concomitant reactions occurred from MBT, MBTS, and phenyl-beta-naphthylamine (PBN) (14). In some cases, the patch test sites have been purpuric (148,149). Fisher (150) saw a case of ACD that progressed to a pigmented purpura appearance from nylon stockings.

Shmunes (145) described a 59-year-old hat saleswoman with a severe purpuric eruption of the exposed areas of the face, neck, and arms. Patch testing to paraphenylenediamine produced a purpuric, eczematous response. During this investigation in 1977, Shmunes determined that IPPD was added to elastic material used in some elastic trim on undergarments in the United States.

Lichenoid pigmented contact dermatitis from IPPD has also been reported. Calnan (151) observed a case in a truck driver who contacted rubber tires, and Ancona et al. (148) described a case in a tire assembler.

Meding et al. (99) reported purpura in association with diphenylthiourea allergy.

> The rubber antioxidant *n*-isopropyl-*n*-phenyl-paraphenylenediamine may produce lichenoid and purpuric eruptions and may cross-react with oxidation-type hair dyes.

DEPIGMENTATION FROM RUBBER CHEMICALS

The first report of chemically induced leukoderma was by Oliver et al. (152) in 1939 from monobenzyl ether of hydroquinone (MBH), as an antioxidant used in rubber gloves. Half the workers wearing them were affected. After use of the gloves was discontinued, repigmentation began in some workers several months later, and within 3 years almost all the workers had regained their normal skin color. One of the commercial designations for MBH was Age Rite Alba, which is no longer manufactured by RT Vanderbilt Co. Inc. MBH is still available medically as a depigmenting agent and is sold as Benoquin by Elder Pharmaceutical Co., which is supplied by a small specialty chemical company. MBH is a potent depigmenting chemical contraindicated for bleaching discrete tan or brown spots (melasma and lentigines), and its only therapeutic application is the rare need to depigment normal skin in persons with extensive vitiligo. MBH may produce pigment loss at distant, untreated sites. It is also an allergen (90,139,153–155). Gaul (139) reported several severe cases of vesicular contact dermatitis from MBH. In 1984, van Ketel (154) observed sensitization from a depigmenting cream containing MBH, which was accompanied by sensitivity to hydroquinone. The hydroquinone applied earlier in an ointment may have induced the sensitivity.

Hydroquinone produces only local skin lightening and is used pharmacologically for melasma, postinflammatory hyperpigmentation, and similar disorders. Hydroquinone rarely produces complete depigmentation. It is a weaker allergen than MBH (156,157). Concomitant sensitivity to hydroquinone and *p*-methoxyphenol has been observed in the guinea pig (158).

Related chemicals producing depigmentation include monomethyl ether of hydroquinone (*p*-methoxyphenol or *p*-hydroxyanisole) and monoethyl ether of hydroquinone (*p*-ethoxyphenol) (63). Other depigmentors are listed by Gellin (159): *p*-tert-butylphenol, *p*-tert-butylcatechol, *p*-isopropylcatechol, *p*-octylphenol, *p*-nonylphenol, *p*-phenylphenol, *p*-tert-amylphenol, *p*-cresol, dimethylamine hydrochloride (MEDA), β-mercaptoethylamine hydrochloride (MEA)], physostigmine (Eserine), diisopropylfluorophosphate, and *n,n´,n″*-triethylenethiophosphoramide (Thio-TEPA). Paratertiary butylphenol caused 100 cases of local depigmentation from the use of bindi in India. Fifteen patients were patch tested, and all were negative (160).

> Hydroquinones used in the rubber industry may produce depigmentation of the skin.

NONRUBBER SOURCES OF RUBBER CHEMICALS

Many rubber chemicals may be present not only in rubber or adhesives, but also in other products, such as plastics, pesticides, oils, and organic dyes (12). Contact dermatitis has occurred from some of these sources.

MBT may be found in antifreeze (12), cutting oils (149), heavy duty greases (161), black tire paints (161), special detergents (161), pottery mold releasing fluid (162), photographic film emulsion (163), fungicides (12), and veterinary medications (164) (Tables 31.17 and 31.18). Salts of MBT, when used to prevent mildew in fabrics or as an algicide or slimicide, may not be as prone to cause ACD as MBT in rubber (165).

Thiurams are used extensively in fungicides (165) and have also been found in some oils and paints (161), animal repellents (161), seed disinfectants, soaps (12,166), and Antabuse (12,53) (Tables 31.19 and 31.20).

Other rubber chemicals with nonrubber uses include dithiocarbamates as lawn and garden fungicides (12,167), carbamates as heat stabilizers for polyethylene (161), paraphenylenediamine compounds as retarders for acrylates and as inhibitors or sweeteners in gasoline (161), diaminodiphenylmethane as a cross-linker in epoxy resins and polyurethanes (11), and antioxidants and other rubber additives in plastics (12). Boman et al. (168) reported a case of sensitivity from phenyl-alpha-naphthylamine present at 1% concentration in a grease used by an aircraft worker. Tables 31.21, 31.22, 31.23, and 31.24 contain partial lists of products that may contain carba mix and PPD mix chemicals. Morpholine may be present as an antioxidant in coolants, and trimethyldihydroquinoline may be used as an antioxi-

TABLE 31.17. *Mercaptobenzothiazole: Potential Exposures*

Adhesives
Black tires
Boots and shoes
Cleansers (auto cooling systems)
Clothes (rubberized fabrics, i.e., brassieres and girdles)
Cutting oils
Cements (contact, plastic, waterproofing, rubber, shoe, tile, and thermoplastic)
Detergents (granulated and tablets)
Fungicides
Greases (heavy duty)
Paints (black tire)
Photographic film emulsion
Rubber (accelerator)
Rubber products
Veterinarian medicaments

TABLE 31.18. *Partial List of Products That May Contain Mercaptobenzothiazole**

Analan Ointment
Aurimite
Betz Algacide (Tx-P)
Betz Slime-trol Rx-15, Rx-29, and Rx-35
Betz Slimicide D-2
Caladerm Ointment
Cal-pox Lotion
Delcreo Pentram Skin Balm
Dr. Merrick's Scratchhex for Dogs
Dr. Merrick's Sulfodene Preparation
Dr. Merrick's Scratchhex Medicated Powder for Dogs
Ear-rite
Gormel's Complete Rose Spray
Happy Jack Skin Balm
Legear Flea and Tick Powder
Mercaptocaine
Mobile Rubber Lubricant
NACAP (corrosion inhibitor)
Tree-top Spray
Vancide 26EC, 20S, 26, 51, and 61Z

*Some of these products may no longer be available.

dant in high pressure lubricants (FJ Storrs, Portland, OR, personal communication, 1983).

Thiuram and Carbamate Pesticides

Cronin (165) believed the thiuram and carbamate fungicides rarely sensitize. Schulz and Hermann (169) reported dermatitis in dock workers unloading produce treated with thiuram. Shelly (170) reported a golfer who developed dermatitis after contact with TMTD used as a fungicide on a golf course. The fungicide was applied to his skin for 15 minutes and produced a large eczematous reaction 30 hours later coupled with a generalized flare despite the continuance of systemic steroids. Cronin (165) mentioned a man who developed dermatitis after applying a thiuram insecticide in his garden. When patch tested, he reacted to TMTD and to three related thiurams. In 1981, Goitre et al. (171) from Italy stated that TMTD was used as an antifermenta-

TABLE 31.19. *Thiurams: Potential Exposures*

Adhesives (neoprene)
Antioxidant (polyolefin plastics)
Crepe soles (neoprene)
Disinfectants (seeds)
Fungicides
Germicides
Insecticides
Lubricating oils
Paints (neoprene)
Pesticides
Putty
Repellents (rabbits, rats, deer, and mice)
Rubber industry—accelerators for vulcanization of rubber; latex preservative
Soaps and shampoos

TABLE 31.20. *Fungicides and Animal Repellents That May Contain Thiuram**

ABCO T.F.—75 Turf Fungicide
Acti-Dione Thiram
Agway Thiram
Agway Thiram Parathion
Agway Thiram-Tinasad
Arasan 50 Red Thiram Seed Protectant
Arasan SF-M Thiram Seed Protectant
Arasan SF-X Seed Protectant
Arasan 42-S Thiram Fungicide and Repellent
Arasan 75 Thiram Seed Protectant
Balcite Special Herbicide
Bonide Rabbit and Deer Repellent
Bulb-Saver
Chaperone New Aerosol Rabbit and Squirrel Repellent
Chew-NOT Repellent—for rabbits, deer, and meadow mice
Earl Ferris Bulb Dust
Evershield T Seed Protectant
Gro Lawn Fungus Control
Henry Field's Gladiolus β Bulb Dust
Hopkins Special Granules
Kromad Turf Fungicide
Magic Circle Rabbit Repellent
Morgro Plus Fungicide
Niacide M4 Ethion 4 lead Arsenate 15 Dust Insecticide
Niagara Thiram Dust Fungicide
Niagara Thiram Wet Tablet Powder Fungicide
Nibble-Not Repellent for Rabbits, Deer, and Meadow Mice
Northrup King Hybrid Sweet Corn Seeds, Treated
Nott's Bulb-Saver
Patterson's Turf Fungicide
Pearson's Diel-Ram
Pearson's Melon β Pine Seed Protectant
Pearson's Moly-Stand
Pennwalt Thiram-PCNB
Pratt Animal Repellent
Protex-A-Plenty Stimusoy Seed Protectant
Proturf Fertilizer and Fungicide
Rootone with Fungicide for Better Rooting Control
Science Gladiolus and Bulb Dust
Science Seed Protectant
Scuttle-turf Fungicide
Superkill-Thiram Terraclor Cotton Fungicide
Terrsan-Thiram Organic Mercury Turf
Terrsan 75 Fungicide
Thiramad
Thiramad Plus Turf Fungicide
Thylate Thiram Fungicide
Turf Builder-Plus 1

*Some of these products may no longer be available.

tive agent in jams, fruits, and vegetables and also in cosmetics (soaps, deodorants, shampoos, creams, and face lotions).

Copeman (172), in 1966, recorded a case of toxic epidermal necrolysis (TEN) caused by cutaneous hypersensitivity to monosulfiram (tetraethylthiuram monosulfide), which was applied as a scabicide. The patient, who had been treated for rubber sensitivity 28 years previously, began developing the TEN within 3 hours of application of monosulfiram and later had a positive patch test to TMTD.

TABLE 31.21. *Partial List of Products That May Contain Carba Mix Chemicals**

1,3-diphenylguanidine
  Coast Pro Seal Accelerator
  Darex Activator Cover 700
  DPG Accelerator Regular
Diethyldithiocarbamate
  Camel Universal Cement 267
  Ethazate
Dibutyldithiocarbamate
  All Purpose Cement No. 514
  Bostik 2003 Part B
  Butazate 50D
  Butyl Zimate
  Kox All Purpose Cement
  Magicure Activator
  PSA—Paper—High Polymer
  Perma Lastic PL 5184
  Shoe Canvas, Lasting, Box Toe, Sock Heel Pad—Natural
    Rubber Latex
  2–17 Latex Adhesive

*Some of these products may no longer be available.

TABLE 31.22. *Partial List of Products That Contain Paraphenylene Diamine**

Cyzone I.P.
Eastozone 34
Fleezwx
Floxaone 3C
Nonox-2A
Sanoflex 36

*Some of these products may no longer be available.

TABLE 31.23. *Main Uses of Paraphenylenediamine and Related Chemicals in Industry*

Antioxidants in rubber industry (used to prevent
  deterioration; retards surface cracking and flaking)
Antiozonants
Retarder in manufacture of acrylates
May be in gasoline as inhibitor or sweetener

TABLE 31.24. *Items Reported to Cause Dermatitis from Ingredients of the Black Rubber Mix*

Rubber top of women's knee-high stockings
Shoe and boots
Rubber dental tip
Black rubber gloves
Tires
Scuba mask
Wind surfing boards
Rubber tip of walking stick
Police officer's black rubber truncheon
Squash ball
Rubber spectacle "chain"
Rubber fingerstalls
Rubber bank note counters
Underwear elastic

The carbamate fungicides Zineb and Maneb have also caused contact allergy (166,173,174). In the cases of Maneb allergy reported by Nater et al. (173), patch tests to standard tray carbamates and thiurams and Zineb were negative (173). Two of the three patients were positive to ammonium dithiocarbamate and one to sodium-ethylene-bis (dithiocarbamate). Adams and Manchester (167) reported a supermarket clerk allergic to Maneb and thiuram, but negative to Zineb.

Cronin (165) reported the results of testing of both Zineb and Maneb by the International Contact Dermatitis Research Group. There were three nonrelevant positives of 655 eczematous patients tested with Zineb 1% in petrolatum. Maneb was an irritant at 1% in petrolatum concentration with a reaction from 35 of 655 patients; one of these reactions in a florist with hand eczema was thought to be clinically relevant.

Methiocarb, also called 3,5-dimethyl-4-(methylthio)phenol carbamate, is an insecticide and molluscicide. It was found to be the cause of hand dermatitis in a flower farmer. Tests to the carbamate mix were negative. Methiocarb, trade name Mesurol, was tested at 0.5% pet (175).

Many rubber chemicals are also used in plastics, pesticides, oils, and organic dyes.

RUBBER, ANTABUSE, AND ALCOHOL

Thiuram-Alcohol Reactions

Erythema, urticaria, and pruritus may develop shortly after alcohol is consumed by persons who have ingested disulfiram (Antabuse, tetraethylthiuram disulfide). According to Webb (176) and van Ketel (177), this reaction, first observed in the rubber industry, was applied to the treatment of alcoholism. Administered by mouth or by subcutaneous implantation, disulfiram interaction with ethanol is based on the inhibition by disulfiram of the enzyme aldehyde dehydrogenase. This block in the metabolism of imbibed ethanol results in the accumulation of toxic levels of the substrate for this enzyme, acetaldehyde.

The alcohol-disulfiram reaction is nonallergic and occurs in all individuals so exposed. Topical exposure to thiuram can also produce an Antabuse reaction when drinking alcohol (169,178). Shelly (170) reviewed two cases, one of which was in a woman who experienced facial flushing every Sunday night after her bath. Bathing on weekdays had no such effect. Investigation revealed that she had cocktails only on Sunday and regularly used a thiuram-containing soap.

Erythematous skin reactions have also been reported in patients taking disulfiram and contacting alcohol-containing substances, specifically an aftershave lotion (179), an alcohol-containing tar gel used to treat psoriasis (180), and a beer-containing shampoo (181). Haddock and Wilkin (182) studied this phenomenon and found that erythema from topically applied alcohols was not statistically different before or after the patients were taking disulfiram. They postulated that topically applied alcohol leads to facial or generalized erythema as a result of a systemic rather than a local reaction, requiring a substantial amount of alcohol to enter the system.

> **Tetraethylthiuram disulfide, a rubber accelerator, is used as Antabuse to control alcoholism. The toxic Antabuse effect can be caused not only by ingestion of alcohol or Antabuse but also by topical exposure to these compounds.**

It is claimed that ingested ethanol can exacerbate lesions of allergic contact dermatitis from thiurams. The basis for this observation is Van Ketel's description (177) of three homemakers with tetramethylthiuram disulfide allergy who developed severe aggravation of eczema a few hours after consuming alcohol. Webb et al. (92) reported a patient who noted that the rash on the dorsa of his feet worsened with alcohol ingestion. The basis for these observations is obscure and deserves further study (3,183).

Antabuse Reactions in Thiuram-Sensitive Patients

Webb et al. (176) stressed that patients should be questioned carefully regarding possible rubber contact allergy prior to administration of Antabuse. They reported a severe, widespread dermatitis developing in a 32-year-old man 5 hours after beginning treatment with Antabuse. Similar systemic eczematous reactions have been reported by Wilson (184), Pirila (185), and Goitre et al. (171).

Lachapelle (183) reported allergic contact dermatitis in two persons with disulfiram implants that extended out onto the skin. Although one patient could tolerate disulfiram by mouth, oral administration to the other patient caused a widespread eczematous dermatitis. Van Hecke and Vermander (186) reported on a 35-year-old alcoholic man who developed an eczematous dermatitis of the extremities as well as at a 2-year-old disulfiram implantation site on his abdomen following treatment with 400 mg of disulfiram (Antabuse). Patch tests were positive to thiuram mix, TMTD, TMTM, TETD, and a crushed Antabuse tablet. Alcohol intolerance after an implant usually lasts no longer than 6 months.

Other reported Antabuse reactions are fixed drug eruptions and acne (44).

Antabuse "Reaction" in Nickel-Allergic Patients

Ingestion of disulfiram may provoke a flare-up of nickel dermatitis at sites previously contacted by nickel. Klein and

Fowler (187) reported an alcoholic who developed dermatitis on the wrist (watch) and abdomen (belt buckle) shortly after Antabuse was started. No nickel had recently contacted the areas, but prior dermatitis to nickel had occurred. Patch test was positive only to nickel (187).

Exposure to other chemicals can produce a flushing reaction when associated with alcohol ingestion. These chemicals include calcium cyanamide, trichloroethylene, and butyral doximine (188).

Treatment of Nickel Dermatitis with Disulfiram

Several reports from Europe and one from Fowler in the United States have indicated that disulfiram is effective in treating some nickel-allergic patients (see Chapter 35) (189).

REFERENCES

1. Rubber. In: *The new encyclopedia Britannica,* vol. 15, 15th ed. London: Macropaedia, 1982.
2. Hamann CP. Natural rubber latex protein sensitivity in review. *Am J Contact Dermatitis* 1993;4:4.
3. Adams RM, Goin J, Hamann C, Sullivan K. Natural and synthetic rubber. In: *Occupational skin disease,* 3rd ed. Philadelphia: WB Saunders, 1999, pp. 501–551.
4. St Cry DR. Rubber, natural. In: *Kirk-Othmer encyclopedia of chemical technology,* vol. 20, 3rd ed. New York: Wiley Interscience, 1982.
5. Rodriguez E, Reynolds GW, Thompson JA. Potent content allergen in the rubber plant guayule *(Parthenium argentatum). Science* 1981; 211:1444.
6. Barnhart, RR. Rubber compounding. In: *Kirk-Othmer encyclopedia of chemical technology,* vol. 20, 3rd ed. New York: John Wiley and Sons, 1982.
7. Fisher AA. Dermatitis from rubber, adhesives and gums. In: Fisher AA, ed. *Contact dermatitis,* 2nd ed. Philadelphia: Lea & Febiger, 1973.
8. Taylor R, Son PN. Rubber chemicals. In: *Kirk-Othmer encyclopedia of chemical technology,* vol. 20, 3rd ed. New York: Wiley Interscience, 1982.
9. Nicholas PP, Luxeder AM, Brooks LA, Hammes PA. Antioxidants and antiozonants. In: *Kirk-Othmer encyclopedia of chemical technology,* vol. 3, 3rd ed. New York: Wiley Interscience, 1978.
10. Korcz WH, St Clair DJ, Ewins Jr EE. Block copolymers. In: Satas E, ed. *Handbook of pressure sensitive adhesive technology.* New York: Van Nostrand Reinhold, 1982.
11. Sears JK, Touchette NW. Plasticizers. In: *Kirk-Othmer encyclopedia of chemical technology,* vol. 18, 3rd ed. New York: Wiley Interscience, 1982.
12. Fregert, S. *Manual of contact dermatitis,* 2nd ed. Chicago: Year Book Medical Publishers, 1981.
13. Nutter AF. Contact urticaria to rubber. *Br J Dermatol* 1979;101:597.
14. Förström L. Contact urticaria from latex surgical gloves. *Contact Dermatitis* 1980;6:33.
15. Food and Drug Administration. Allergic reactions to latex-containing medical devices. *FDA Med Bull* 1991.
16. Warshaw EM. Latex allergy. *JAAD* 1998;39:1–24.
17. Cohen D, Scheman A, Stewart L, et al. American Academy of Dermatology's position paper on latex allergy. *JAAD* 1998;39:98–106.
18. Gidrol X, Chrestin H, Tan HL, Kush A. Hevein, a lectin-like protein from *Hevea brasiliensis* (rubber tree) is involved in the coagulatiion of latex. *J Biol Chem* 1994;269:9278–9283.
19. Alenius H, Kalkkinen N, Lukka M, et al. Prohevein from the rubber tree *(Hevea brasiliensis)* is a major latex allergen. *Clin Exp Allergy* 1995;24:659–665.
20. Alenius H, Kalkkinen N, Yip E, et al. Significance of rubber elongation factor as a latex allergen. *Int Arch Allergy Immunol* 1996;109: 262–268.

21. Guin J, et al. Occupational protein contact dermatitis to cornstarch in a paper adhesive. *Am J Contact Dermatitis* 1999;10:83–88.
22. Seaton A. Latex as aeroallergen. *Lancet* 1990;336:808.
23. Belsito DV. Contact urticaria caused by rubber: analysis of seven cases. In: *Dermatology clinics,* Adams R, Nethercott J (eds.), vol. 8. Philadelphia: WB Saunders, 1990, pp. 61–66.
24. DeGroot H, DeJong NW, Duijster E, et al. Prevalence of natural rubber latex allergy (type I and type IV) in laboratory workers in the Netherlands. *Contact Dermatitis* 1998;38:159–163.
25. Hamann CP, Turjanmaa K, Rietschel R, et al. Natural rubber latex hypersensitivity: incidence and prevalence of type I allergy in the dental professional. *J Am Dent Assoc* 1998;129:43–54.
26. Ylitilo L, Turjanmaa K, Palosuo T, Reunala T. Natural rubber latex allergy in children who had not undergone surgery and children who had undergone multiple operations. *J Allergy Clin Immunol* 1997; 100:606–612.
27. Estornell-Moragues F, Nieto-Garcia A, Mazon-Ramos A, et al. Latex allergy in children with myelomeningocele: incidence and associated factors. *Actas Urol Esp* 1997;21:227–235.
28. DeCorres LF, et al. Contact urticaria: sensitization to chestnuts and bananas in patients with contact urticaria from latex. *Contact Dermatitis* 1990;23:277.
29. Towse A, O'Brien M, Twarog FJ, et al. Local reaction secondary to insulin injection: a potential role for latex antigens in insulin vials and syringes. *Diabetes Care* 1995;18:1195–1197.
30. Wakelin S, Jenkins R, Rycroft J, et al. Patch testing with natural rubber latex. *Contact Dermatitis* 1999;40:89–93.
31. Wilkinson S, Burd R. Latex: a cause of allergic contact eczema in users of natural rubber gloves. *JAAD* 1998;38:36–42.
32. Malten KE, Nater JP, van Ketel WG. *Patch testing guidelines.* Nijmegan, Netherlands: Dekker & van de Vegt, 1976.
33. Marks JG, Belsito DV, DeLeo VA, et al. North American Contact Dermatitis Group patch test results for the detection of delayed-type hypersensitivity to topical allergens. *JAAD* 1998;38:911–918.
34. Marks JG, Belsito DV, DeLeo VA, et al. North American Contact Dermatitis Group patch test results, 1996–1998. *Arch Dermatol* 2000;136:534–536.
35. Conde-Salazar L, et al. Type IV allergy to rubber additives: a 10-year study of 686 cases. *J Am Acad Dermatol* 1993;29:176.
36. Von Hintzenstern J, et al. Frequency, spectrum and occupational relevance of type IV allergies to rubber chemicals. *Contact Dermatitis* 1991;24:244.
37. Nethercott JR, et al. Patch testing with a routine screening tray in North America, 1985–1989: gender and response. *Am J Contact Dermatitis* 1991;2:130.
38. Leyden JJ, Kligman AM. Contact dermatitis to Neomycin sulfate. *JAMA* 1979;242:1276.
39. Veien NK, et al. Contact dermatitis in children. *Contact Dermatitis* 1982;8:373.
40. Levy A, et al. Contact dermatitis in children. *Contact Dermatitis* 1982;6:260.
41. Wyss M, et al. Allergic contact dermatitis from natural latex without contact urticaria. *Contact Dermatitis* 1993;28:154.
42. Cronin E. Rubber. In: Cronin E, ed. *Contact dermatitis.* New York: Churchill Livingstone, 1980.
43. Kortschak E. Rubber chemicals. *Aust J Dermatol* 1977;18:127.
44. Schwartz L, Tulipan L, Birmingham DJ. Dermatoses in the manufacture of rubber. In: *Occupational diseases of the skin.* Philadelphia: Lea & Febiger, 1957.
45. Foussereau J, Benezra C, Maibach HI. Rubber industry. In: *Occupational contact dermatitis.* Philadelphia: WB Saunders, 1982.
46. Schultheiss E. Gummi und Ekzem, Berufsdermatosen, Monographien, Band 3, Aulendorf, Cantor, 1959.
47. Bonnevie P, Marcussen PV. Rubber products as a widespread cause of eczema: report of 80 cases. *Acta Derm Vernerol* (Stockh) 1945;25:163.
48. Wilson HTH. Rubber dermatitis: an investigation of 106 cases of contact dermatitis caused by rubber. *Br J Dermatol* 1969;81:175.
49. Nurse DS. Rubber sensitivity. *Aust J Dermatol* 1979;20:31.
50. Song M, Degreef H, DeMoubeuge J, et al. Contact sensitivity to rubber additives in Belgium. *Dermatologica* 1979;158:163.
51. Feinman S. Rubber sensitivity. Unpublished review. Washington, DC: Consumer Product Safety Commission, 1984.
52. Stankevich VV, et al. Hygienic assessment of organosulfur accelerators for vulcanization of rubbers for the food industry. *Gig Sanit* 1980;10:88.
53. Fregert, S. Chemicals used in both rubber and plastic. *Contact Dermatitis Newsletter* 1971;9:204.
54. Kilpikari I. Occupational contact dermatitis among rubber workers. *Contact Dermatitis* 1982;8:359.
55. Varigos GA, Dunt DR. Occupational dermatitis: an epidemiological study in the rubber and cement industries. *Contact Dermatitis* 1981;7:105.
56. Bieber PL, Foussereau J. Role de deux amines aromatiques dans l'allergie au caoutchouc; PBN et 4010 NA, amines antioxidantes dans l'industrie due pneu. *Bull Soc Dermatol Syphil* 1968;75:63.
57. Herve-Bazin B, et al. Occupational eczema from *n*-isopropyl-*n'*-phenyl-paraphenylenediamine (IPPD) and *n*-dimethyl-1,3 butyl-*n'*-phenylpara-phenylenediamine (DMPPD) in tyres. *Contact Dermatitis* 1977;3:1.
58. Fregert S. Relapse of hand dermatitis after short contact with tires. *Contact Dermatitis Newsletter* 1973;7:351.
59. Munn A. In: Cronin E, ed. *Contact dermatitis.* New York: Churchill Livingstone, 1980.
60. Nethercott JR, et al. Patch testing with a routine screening tray in North America, 1987–1989: Occupation and response. *Am J Cont Derm* 1991;2:247.
61. Livesley B, Lambelle J. Perichondritis helicis: an industrial hazard—two case reports. *J Laryngol Otol* 1967;81:1063.
62. White WG, Vickers HR. Diethylthiourea as a cause of dermatitis in a car factory. *Br J Ind Med* 1970;27:167.
63. Adams RM. Contact allergic dermatitis in a wetsuit. *Contact Dermatitis* 1982;8:277.
64. Anderson KE. Diethylthiourea contact dermatitis from an acidic detergent. *Contact Dermatitis* 1983;9:146.
65. Fregert S, Trulson L, Zimerson E. Contact allergic reactions to diphenylthiourea and phenyl isothiocyanate in PVC adhesive tape. *Contact Dermatitis* 1982;8:38.
66. Fregert S, Dahlquist I, Trulson L. Sensitization capacity of diphenylthiourea and phenylisothiocyanate. *Contact Dermatitis* 1983;9:87.
67. Kanerva L, et al. Contact dermatitis from dibutylthiourea. *Contact Dermatitis* 1984;10:158.
68. Bruze M, Fregert S. Allergic contact dermatitis from ethylene thiourea. *Contact Dermatitis* 1983;9:208.
69. Dooms-Goossens A, et al. Dimethylthiourea, an unexpected hazard for textile workers. *Contact Dermatitis* 1979;5:367.
70. Nurse DS. Sensitivity to thiourea in plan printing paper. *Contact Dermatitis* 1980;6:153.
71. Calnan CD. Rubber sensitivity presenting as eyelid oedema. *Contact Dermatitis* 1975;1:124.
72. Shorvill DE. Reaction to dioctyl phthalate in a rubber worker. *Contact Dermatitis Newsletter* 1971;9:208.
73. Dooms-Goossens A, et al. Pustular reactions to hexafluorosilicate in foam rubber. *Contact Dermatitis* 1985;12:42.
74. King CM. Contact sensitivity to Hylene W. *Contact Dermatitis* 1980;6:353.
75. Kilpikari I, Home H. Contact allergy to Hypalon rubber. *Contact Dermatitis* 1983;9:529.
76. Adams RM. Possible substitution for mercaptobenzothiazole in rubber. *Contact Dermatitis* 1975;1:246.
77. Foussereau J. Allergy to MBT and its derivatives. *Contact Dermatitis* 1983;9:514.
78. Mancuso G, Reggiani M, Berdondini RM. Occupational dermatitis in shoemakers. *Contact Dermatitis* 1996;34:17–22.
79. Rudner EJ, et al. The frequency of contact sensitivity in North America, 1972–1974. *Contact Dermatitis* 1975;1:277.
80. Rudner EJ, et al. Epidemiology of contact dermatitis in North America. *Arch Dermatol* 1972;108:537.
81. Rudner E. North American group results. *Contact Dermatitis* 1977;3:208.
82. van Ketel WG. Low sensitization rate of naphthyl mix. *Contact Dermatitis* 1983;9:77.
83. Task Force on Contact Dermatitis (North American Contact Dermatitis Group). *Patch testing in allergic contact dermatitis.* Evanston, IL: American Academy of Dermatology, 1984.
84. Bonnevie P. *Aetiologie und Pathogenese der Ekzemkrankheiten.* Leipzig: Barth, 1981.
85. Mitchell JC. Patch testing in mixes. *Contact Dermatitis* 1981;7:98.

86. Hjorth, N. Routine patch tests. *Trans St Johns Hosp Dermatol Soc* 1963;49:99.

87. Gotz H, Istanovic N. Die Bedeutung von Gummi-allergenen insbesondere bei Bergleuten. *Hautarzt* 1963;14:345.

88. Epstein E. Simplified patch test screening with mixtures. *Arch Dermatol* 1967;95:269.

89. Mitchell JC, et al. Patch testing with mercaptobenzothiazole and mercapto-mix. *Contact Dermatitis* 1976;2:123.

90. Lynde CW, et al. Patch testing with mercaptobenzothiazole and mercapto mixes. *Contact Dermatitis* 1982;8:273.

91. Fregert S. Cross-sensitivity pattern of 2-mercaptobenzothiazole (MBT). *Acta Derm Venereol* (Stockh) 1969;49:45.

92. Hansson C, Agrup G. Stability of the mercaptobenzothiazole compounds. *Contact Dermatitis* 1993;28:29.

93. van Ketel WG. Thiuram mix. *Contact Dermatitis* 1976;2:232.

94. Conde-Salazar Gomez L., Gomez Urcuyo JF. Sensibilidad a los componentes de la goma en obreros de la construction. *Acta Dermosifiliograf* 1976;67:297.

95. Themido, R, Brandão, FM. Contact allergy to thiurams. *Contact Dermatitis* 1984;10:251.

96. Schonning L, Hjorth N. Cross sensitization between hair dyes and rubber chemicals. *Berufsdermatosen* 1969;17:100.

97. Jordan Jr WP, Bourlas MC. Allergic contact dermatitis to underwear elastic. *Arch Dermatol* 1975;111:593.

98. Veien NK. Patch testing with substances not included in the standard series. *Contact Dermatitis* 1983;9:304.

99. Meding B, et al. Allergic contact dermatitis from diphenylthiourea in Vulkan heat retainers. *Contact Dermatitis* 1990;22:8.

100. Roberts JL, Hanifin JM. Contact allergy and cross reactivity to substituted thiourea compounds. *Contact Dermatitis* 1980;6:138.

101. Torres V, et al. Occupational contact dermatitis to thiourea and dimethylthiourea from diazo copy paper. *Am J Contact Dermatitis* 1992;3:37.

102. Kanerva L, Estlander T, Alanko K, Jolanki R. Occupational airborne allergic contact dermatitis from dibutylthiourea. *Contact Dermatitis* 1998;38:347–348.

103. Van der Leun JC, et al. Photosensitivity owing to thiourea. *Arch Dermatol* 1977;113:1611.

104. Roberts JL, Hanifin JM. Athletic shoe dermatitis, contact allergy to ethyl butyl thiourea. *JAMA* 1979;241:275.

105. Jordan WP. 24-, 48-hour patch tests. *Contact Dermatitis* 1980;6:151.

106. Knudsen BB, et al. Release of thiurams and carbamates from rubber gloves. *Contact Dermatitis* 1993;28:63.

107. Fisher AA. Contact dermatitis in surgeons. *J Derm Surg Oncol* 1975;1:63.

108. Sidi E, Hincky M. Les eczémas aux gants de caoutchouc (étude de 102 cas). *Presse Med* 1954;62:1305.

109. Polano MK. Ekzem durch gummihand-schuhe. *Dermatologia* 1958;116:105.

110. Lintum JCA, Nater JP. Sensitization to rubber chemicals in different professions. *Contact Dermatitis Newsletter* 1973;14:396.

111. Nater JP. Uberempfindlichkreit gegen gummi. *Berufsdermatosen* 1975;23:161.

112. Rich P, et al. Allergic contact dermatitis to two antioxidants in latex gloves: 4,4′-thio bis(6-tert-butyl-meta-cresol) (Lowinox 44536) and butylhydroxyanisole. *J Am Acad Dermatol* 1991;24:37.

113. Fisher AA. "Hypoallergenic" surgical gloves and gloves for special situations. *Cutis* 1975;15:797.

114. NIOSH. *Proceedings and summary of the record of the NIOSH open meeting on chemical protective clothing.* Rockville, MD: National Institute for Occupational Safety and Health, 1981.

115. Liden C. Occupational dermatoses at a film laboratory. *Contact Dermatitis* 1984;10:77.

116. Shmunes E, Darby T. Contact dermatitis due to endotoxin in irradiated latex gloves. *Contact Dermatitis* 1984;10:240.

117. Hindson TC. Studies in contact dermatitis: (16): Contraceptives. *Trans St Johns Hosp Derm Soc* 1966;52:1.

118. Harmon CB, Connolly SM, Larson TR. Condom-related allergic contact dermatitis. *J Urol* 1995;153:1227–1228.

119. Fisher AA. Condom conundrums: part 1. *Cutis* 1991;48:359.

120. Fisher AA. Allergic reactions to contraceptives. *Cutis* 1974;13:337.

121. Fisher AA. Vulvitis due to contactants. *Cutis* 1974;13:725.

122. Fisher AA. Consort contact dermatitis. *Cutis* 1979;24:595.

123. Schamberg IL, Flesch P. Contact dermatitis from rubber caused by allergic sensitivity to thio-beta-naphthol. *J Invest Dermatol* 1953;21:59.

124. Pennys NS, Edwards LS, Katsikos JL. Allergic contact sensitivity to thiuram compounds in a hemodialysis unit. *Arch Dermatol* 1976;112:811.

125. Calnan CD, Cronin E. False positive reaction to mercaptobenzothiazole from rubber in eyedrop bottle. *Contact Dermatitis* 1981;7:283.

126. Reynaerts A, Bruze M, Erikstam U, Goossens A. Allergic contact dermatitis from a medical device, followed by depigmentation. *Contact Dermatitis* 1998;39:204–205.

127. Scalf LA, Fowler JF. Allergic contact dermatitis caused by dialkyl thioureas in a patient with sleep apnea. *Am J Contact Dermatitis* 1999;10:169–171.

128. Goette DK. Raccoon-like periorbital leukoderma from contact with swim goggles. *Contact Dermatitis* 1984;10:129.

129. Maibach HI. Scuba diver facial dermatitis: allergic contact dermatitis to n-isopropyl-n-phenylparaphenylenediamine. *Contact Dermatitis* 1975;1:330.

130. Tuyp E, Mitchell JC. Scuba diver facial dermatitis. *Contact Dermatitis* 1983;9:334.

131. Blue Book 1983. *Materials, compounding ingredients, and machinery for rubber.* New York: Bill Communications, 1983.

132. Schulz KH, Hermann WP. 4,4′-dioxydiphenyl als ursache von schweib blattekzemen. *Derm Woschenchr* 1960;141:124.

133. Arisu K, et al. Tinuvin® P in a spandex tape as a cause of clothing dermatitis. *Contact Dermatitis* 1992;26:311.

134. Furman D, Fisher AA, Leider M. Allergic eczematous contact–type dermatitis caused by rubber sponges used for the application of cosmetics. *J Invest Dermatol* 1950;15:223.

135. Fisher AA. Allergic contact dermatitis (caused by rubber cosmetic sponges) simulating cosmetic dermatitis. *Cutis* 1993;51:320.

136. Curtis GH. Contact dermatitis of eyelids caused by an antioxidant in rubber fillers of eyelash curlers. *Arch Dermatol* 1945;52:262.

137. McKenna KE, McMillan C. Facial contact dermatitis due to black rubber. *Contact Dermatitis* 1992;26:270.

138. Deguchi M, Tagami H. Contact dermatitis of the ear due to a rubber earplug. *Dermatology* 1996;193:251–252.

139. Gaul LE. Results of patch testing with rubber antioxidants and accelerators. *J Invest Dermatol* 1957;29:105.

140. Jacobziner H, Raybin HW. The rise and decline of flubberitis. *NY State J Med* 1963;1:2562.

141. Sauer GC. Flubber dermatitis. *Arch Dermatol* 1965;91:465.

142. Tennstedt D, Lachapelle JM. Windsurfer dermatitis from black rubber compounds. *Contact Dermatitis* 1981;7:160.

143. Fisher AA. Allergic petechial and purpuric rubber dermatitis: the PPPP syndrome. *Cutis* 1974;14:25.

144. Fisher AA. Purpuric contact dermatitis. *Cutis* 1984;33:346.

145. Shmunes E. Purpuric allergic contact dermatitis to paraphenylenediamine. *Contact Dermatitis* 1978;4:225.

146. Batschvarov B, and Minkov DM. Dermatitis and purpura from rubber in clothing. *Trans St Johns Hosp Dermatol Soc* 1968;54:178.

147. Calnan CD, Peachy RDG. Allergic contact purpura. *Clin Allergy* 1971;1:287.

148. Ancona A, Monroy F, Fernandez-Diez J. Occupational dermatitis from IPPD in tires. *Contact Dermatitis* 1982;8:91.

149. Fregert S, Skog E. Allergic contact dermatitis from mercaptobenzothiazole in cutting oil. *Acta Derm Venereol* (Stockh) 1962;42:235.

150. Fisher AA. Nonoccupational dermatitis to "black" rubber mix: part 2. *Cutis* 1992;49:229.

151. Calnan CD. Lichenoid dermatitis from isopropylaminodiphenylamine. *Contact Dermatitis Newsletter* 1971;10:237.

152. Oliver EA, Schwartz L, Warren LH. Occupational leukoderma: preliminary report. *JAMA* 1939;113:927.

153. Dorsey CS. Dermatitic and pigmentary reactions to monobenzylether of hydroquinone. *Arch Dermatol* 1960;81:245.

154. van Ketel WG. Sensitization to hydroquinone and the monobenzylether of hydroquinone. *Contact Dermatitis* 1984;10:253.

155. Lynde CW, Warshawski L, Mitchell JC. Patch test results with shoewear screening tray in 119 patients, 1977–1980. *Contact Dermatitis* 1982;8:423.

156. Adams RM. Depigmentation from occupational chemicals. In: *Occupational skin disease.* 3rd ed., Philadelphia: WB Saunders Co., 1999, pp. 15–20.

157. Jirasek L, Kalensky J. in Cronin (ed.) *Contact Dermatitis*, Churchill Livingstone: New York, 1980.
158. van der Walle HB, et al. Contact sensitization to hydroquinone and *p*-methoxyphenol in the guinea pig, inhibitors in acrylic monomers. *Contact Dermatitis* 1982;8:147.
159. Gellin GA. Pigment responses: occupational disorders of pigmentation. In: Maibach HI, Gellin GA, eds. *Occupational and industrial dermatology.* Chicago: Year book Medical Publishers, 1982.
160. Bajaj AK, Gupta SC, Chatterjee AK. Contact depigmentation from free paratertiary-butylphenol in bindi adhesive. *Contact Dermatitis* 1990;22:99.
161. Task Force on Contact Dermatitis (North American Contact Dermatitis Group). *Exposure lists—contact dermatitis antigens.* Evanston, IL: American Academy of Dermatology, 1982.
162. Wilkinson SM, Cartwright PH, English JSC. Allergic contact dermatitis from mercaptobenzothiazole in a releasing fluid. *Contact Dermatitis* 1990;23:70.
163. Rudzki, E, et al. Dermatitis from 2-mercaptobenzothiazole in photographic films. *Contact Dermatitis* 1981;7:43.
164. Adams RM. Mercaptobenzothiazole in veterinary medications. *Contact Dermatitis Newsletter* 1974;16:514.
165. Cronin E. Pesticides. In: *Contact dermatitis.* New York: Churchill Livingstone, 1980.
166. Dick DC, Adams RH. Allergic contact dermatitis from monosulfiram (Tetmosol) soap. *Contact Dermatitis* 1979;5:199.
167. Adams RM, Manchester RD. Allergic contact dermatitis to Maneb in a housewife. *Contact Dermatitis* 1982;8:271.
168. Boman A, et al. Phenyl-alpha-naphthyl-amine—case report and guinea pig studies. *Contact Dermatitis* 1980;6:299.
169. Schulz KH, Hermann WP. Tetramethylthiuramdisulfide, ein thioharnstoffderivat als Ekzemnoxe bei Hafenarbeitern. *Berufsdermatosen* 1958;6:130.
170. Shelly WB. Golf-course dermatitis due to thiram fungicide. *JAMA* 1964;188:415.
171. Goitre M, Bedello PG, Cane D. Allergic dermatitis and oral challenge to tetramethyl-thiuram disulphide. *Contact Dermatitis* 1981;7:272.
172. Copeman PWM. Toxic epidermal necrolysis caused by skin hypersensitivity to monosulfiram. *Br Med J* 1968;1:623.
173. Nater JP, Terpstra H, Bleumink E. Allergic contact sensitization to the fungicide Maneb. *Contact Dermatitis* 1979;5:24.
174. Kleibl K, Rácková M. Cutaneous allergic reactions to dithiocarbamates. *Contact Dermatitis* 1980;6:348.
175. Willems PW, Geursen-Reitsma AM, van-Joost T. Allergic contact dermatitis due to methiocarb (Mesurol). *Contact Dermatitis* 1997;36:270.
176. Webb PK, et al. Disulfiram hypersensitivity and rubber contact dermatitis. *JAMA* 1979;241:2061.
177. Van Ketel WG. Rubber, alcohol and eczema. *Dermatologica* 1968;136:442.
178. Gold S. A skinful of alcohol. *Lancet* 1966;2:1417.
179. Mercurio F. Antabuse-alcohol reaction. *JAMA* 1952;149:82.
180. Ellis CN, Mitchell AJ, Beardsley GR. Tar gel interaction with disulfiram. *Arch Dermatol* 1979;115:1367.
181. Stole D, King LE. Disulfiram-alcohol skin reaction to beer-containing shampoo. *JAMA* 1980;244:2045.
182. Haddock NF, Wilkin JF. Cutaneous reaction to lower aliphatic alcohols before and during disulfiram therapy. *Arch Dermatol* 1982;118:157.
183. Lachapelle JM. Allergic "contact" dermatitis from disulfiram implants. *Contact Dermatitis* 1975;1:218.
184. Wilson H. Side-effects of disulfiram. *Br Med J* 1962;2:1610.
185. Pirila V. Dermatitis due to rubber. Proceedings of the 11th National Congress of Dermatology. *Acta Derm Venereol* (Stockh) 1957;11:252.
186. van Hecke E, Vermander F. Allergic contact dermatitis by oral disulfiram. *Contact Dermatitis* 1984;10:254.
187. Klein LR, Fowler JF. Nickel dermatitis recall during disulfiram therapy for alcohol abuse. *JAAD* 1992;26:645–646.
188. Birmingham DJ. Occupational dermatoses. In: Clayton GD, Clayton FE, eds. *Patty's industrial hygiene and toxicology,* vol. 1, 3rd rev. ed. New York: John Wiley and Sons, 1978.
189. Fowler, JF: Disulfiram is effective for nickel allergic hand eczema. *Am J Contact Dermatitis.* 1992;3:175–182.

CHAPTER 32

Allergy to Gums, Rosin, and Natural Resins

Natural gums are produced principally in Africa or Asia and include seaweed extracts, plant exudates, gums from seed or root, and gums obtained by microbial fermentation. These resinous polysaccharides or their derivatives are completely water soluble or swell substantially in water (1). Gums are used in industry because their aqueous solutions or dispersions possess suspending and stabilizing properties. Gums may produce gels or act as emulsifiers, adhesives, flocculents, binders, film formers, lubricants, or friction reducers. The principal natural gums are listed in Table 32.1. Although karaya, acacia, and tragacanth are probably the most common sensitizers among them (2), such reports are infrequent. These gums may be used as is for patch testing.

KARAYA GUM

Karaya, or sterculia gum, is the dried extract of the *Sterculia urens* tree, which is now primarily cultivated in India. Gum karaya is the least soluble gum exudate; it is used in foods as a thickening and suspending agent and as a stabilizer in salad dressings, ice cream, sherbets, and frozen desserts, in which it prevents the formation of large ice crystals. Gum karaya is also used in cheese spread, sausages, meat products, and bakery goods.

A large proportion of karaya is used by the pharmaceutical industry as a bulk laxative. It is also used as a dental adhesive. Ulcerations, fibrous lesions, and accelerated bone resorption have been reported with inappropriate use of denture adhesives and ill-fitting dentures. In the paper industry, gum karaya is used as a binder for pulp in the preparation of long-fibered, lightweight papers. Gum solutions are used as thickening agents for printing dyes as well as textile sizes (3).

Karaya is an ingredient in some cosmetics, particularly hair-waving lotions. It may be used in toothpastes, powders, adhesives, and cement substances to make ostomy bags adhere to skin. Contact dermatitis from a karaya seal ring has been reported. Glycerin and parabenzoin (not listed in the *Merck Index*) were added. The patient was not tested to the individual components of the ring (4).

Respiratory allergy has been reported with cross-sensitivity to gum arabic and karaya gum (5).

GUM ARABIC

Gum arabic (acacia) is a dried exudate from a species of an acacia tree, produced only under the adverse conditions of lack of moisture, poor nutrition, and hot temperatures. Most commercial gum comes from a single species, *Acacia senegal,* in the Sudan and West Africa. It has wide and varied industrial uses but is normally a stabilizer and thickener in foods. It is used specifically as an adhesive in bakery icings and toppings, as a foam stabilizer in beer, and as a crystallization inhibitor in sugar syrups. Other uses are in the preparation of spray-dried flavors and in the preparation of pasta. Gum arabic has limited application in the cosmetic and pharmaceutical industries as a binder and emulsion stabilizer, but the main nonfood uses are in the formulation of inks and adhesives and in the textile industries, where it is used as a sizing agent (3). Acacia syrup is listed in the *US National Formulary* (6). Gum arabic has been reported to cause respiratory allergy, especially in the printing trades. Dermatitis has also been reported. A gum from cashew (*Anacardium*) may be used to adulterate gum arabic (5).

Three renal transplant recipients found to be hypersensitive to prednisone tablets had reacted to the tragacanth and acacia used in their manufacture. Their symptoms subsided when a formulation using methylcellulose was substituted (7).

Gum arabic adhesive may be preserved with formaldehyde, which was the cause of contact allergy in a lithoplater. Patch tests with gum arabic (as is) were positive (but negative at 1% and 10%), and formaldehyde (2%) was also positive (8). A similar case was reported due to 1,2-benzisothiazolin-3-1 used as a preservative in gum arabic (9).

GUM TRAGACANTH

Gum tragacanth is an exudate from several species of tree, of the genus *Astragalus,* found in the dry, mountainous regions of Iran, Syria, and Turkey. Tragacanth is used in cosmetics, particularly gum-based hair dressings, and in troches, toothpaste, depilatories, and other topical medications. It has been used as a bulk laxative, an excipient for pills and tablets, and as the basis of lubricants for catheters

TABLE 32.1. *Principal Natural Gums*

Gum	Source	Uses
Agara	*Rhodophyceae* seaweed extract	Food, dentistry, medicine, microbiology, laxatives
Carrageenan	*Rhodophyceae* seaweed extract	Food, cosmetics, pharmaceuticals, toothpastes
Guar gum	*Cyanaposis tetragonolibus* seed extract	Food, mining, papermaking, petroleum, production, laxatives
Gum arabic (acacia)	*Acacia senegal* plant exudate	Food, pharmaceutical, printing inks (see also text)
Gum karaya (sterculia)	*Sterculia urens* plant exudate	Food, pharmaceuticals, paperbinders, printing dyes, laxatives (see also text)
Gum tragacanth	*Astralagus* plant exudate	Food, cosmetics, pharmaceuticals, printing pastes, laxatives (see also text)
Locust bean gum	*Ceratonia siliqua* plant exudate	Food, cosmetics, papermaking, textile sizing
Xanthan gum	Microbial fermentation	Food, pharmaceuticals, petroleum production, cosmetic emulsifier
Algine	*Phaeophyceae* seaweed extract	Food, general industry, pharmaceuticals, laxatives
Gum ghatti	*Anogeissus latifolia* tree exudate	Food, emulsifier, adhesive, explosives, petroleum drilling, textiles
Tamarind gum	*Tamarindus indica* see extract	Food, textiles
Psyllium gum	*Plantago ovata* plant extract	Cosmetics, hair-setting, lotions, laxatives (see also text)
Quince seed gum	*Cydonia vulgaris* or *oblonga* seed extract	Cosmetics, hair-setting, lotions, laxatives, pharmaceutical emulsifier and stabilizer
Large gum	*Larix occidentalis* tree extract	Food, cosmetics, pharmaceuticals
Pectin	Extracts from cell walls of all plant tissues	Jam, jelly, and salad dressing additive

and surgical instruments, but such preparations must be sterilized (6). In the food industry, it is used as a thickening or stabilizing agent; in the textile industry as a sizing agent and print paste thickener; and as an emulsifier in furniture, floor, and auto polishes (3).

An immediate life-threatening allergic reaction in a 35-year-old woman was attributed to the tragacanth present in the beef burger that she was eating (6).

Contact dermatitis in a 4-year-old boy at the sites of electrocardiogram electrodes was due to tragacanth in the electrode jelly (6).

> **Gums are water-soluble, resinous polysaccharides that swell on addition of water. Karaya, acacia, and tragacanth are the principal sensitizers of these natural gums.**

Psyllium Gum

Anaphylaxis from psyllium in a laxative and airborne dermatitis and asthma in a psyllium factory worker have been reported (10,11). IgE antibodies to psyllium were found in both patients.

NATURAL RESINS

Natural resins are derived from many sources and have diverse properties. They are mainly oleoresins from tree saps and related fluids, and they occur secondarily from other sources such as insect exudations (shellac) and minerals

(Utah coal resin). Table 32.2 lists the major resins, their class (of industrial use), country of origin, source, and uses (12,13). Natural resins used in medicines, perfumes, and flavors are listed in Table 32.3. Another term applied to these resins is "copal" (a Mexican word meaning "incense"), which describes hard oleoresins, particularly of fossil origin; such resins are useful in varnish making. Copal resin is dug from the remains of trees long dead. Several plants yield copals, for example, *Agathis, Bursera, Canarium, Copaifera,* and *Hymenaea.* Contact sensitivity to copal occurs, and dermatitis has been seen in workers during its production (5). Copal became a designation for quality in an attempt to distinguish between botanic and commercial points of origin. It applies mainly to Congo, kauri, pontianak, and Manila resins. Amber and Utah coal resins may be the oldest of the copals (12).

Jost et al. (13) published a treatise on the nomenclature and chemistry of various resins that may be of interest to readers wishing to have a detailed understanding of these various substances. They also discussed 16 cases of allergic contact dermatitis from a Manila resin used in a surgical adhesive called Alpharopal. Interestingly, 13 of the 16 reacted to colophony (20% pet). Six reacted to abietic acid, and several cross-reactions with other resins were noted (13).

Allergic contact dermatitis or positive patch tests have been documented from most of these natural resins (designated in Tables 32.2 and 32.3 by an asterisk). Table 32.4 lists some pharmaceutical products containing some of these resins (benzoin, balsam of Peru, myrrh, and tolu balsam). Cashew nutshell oil, which is now used infrequently because of its high sensitizing capacity, contains approximately 90% anacardic acid and 10% cardol, but the compo-

TABLE 32.2. *Natural Resins*

Resin	Class	Country of origin	Source	Uses
Accroides (yacca)	—	Australia	*Xanthorrhoea* tree leaves	Paper and wallboard lacquer, wood mahogany stains, picric acid
Amber	—	Baltic shores	Fossils of *Pinus succinifera*	Ornamental beads and jewelry, rubefacient
Canada balsam*	—	United States and Canada	*Abies balsamera*	Microscope slide mounting, cement for optical glass, varnish
Cashew nutshell oil*	—	—	*Anacardium occidentale*	Varnish, cutting oils (use largely abandoned because of severe allergic contact dermatitis)
Chinese, Thai, and Japanese lacquer*	—	—	*Rhus verniciflua, Melanorrhea usitata*	Artwork, furniture lacquer
Congo	Amber, dark, white, and pale	Zaire	Fossil trees	Varnishes, flavors, perfumes, pharmaceuticals
Copals	—	South America	*Caesalpinacea*	Varnishes
Damar	Bativia, Singapore	Indonesia, India, Malaysia	*Dipterocarpaceae*	Resin modifier or nitrocellulose coatings
East India	Batu, black, pale macassar, and pale Singapore	Indonesia	Fossil trees	Coatings
Elemi, gum*	—	Philippines, India, Utah	*Burseraceae*	Solvent and plasticizer in lacquers, coatings
Gilsonite	—	Mineral	Mineral	Coatings
Kauri*	Brown, pale	New Zealand	Fossil trees	Coatings
Manila*	Boea, Loba, and Macassar, Philippines	Indonesia, Philippines	*Caraucariacean Agathis alba* tree	Coatings, polishes
Mastic, gum*	—	Greece	*Pistacia lenticus* tree (Anacardiaceae family)	Clear coatings over artistic paintings, Chinese medicines
Rosin*	Gum, tall oil, and wood	United States	Poinus tree	See section on colophony
Sandarac	—	Morocco	*Tetraclinis articulata* tree	Artistic coatings
Shellac*	—	India	Insect (*Kerria laca*)	Coatings, cosmetics
Utah coal resin	—	Utah	Mineral	Paint, medicine

*Allergic contact sensitivity has been reported.
From Refs. 2 and 3.

TABLE 32.3. *Natural Resins in Perfumes and Flavors*

Resins	Point(s) of origin	Source
Balm of Gilead (Mecca balsam)	Saudi Arabia and Abyssinia	*Commiphora opobalasmum* tree
Balsam of Peru*	Central America	*Myroxylon pereirae* tree bark
Balsam of Tolu*	Equatorial America	*Myroxylon punctatum* tree
Benzoin*	Thailand, Sumatra, and Java	*Styrax* tree
Copaiba**	West Indies and Brazil	*Copaifera landsdorfi* tree
Frankincense* (olibanum)	Saudi Arabia and environs	*Boswellia* tree
Guaiac*	West Indies and South America (north coast)	*Guaiacum officinale* tree
Labdanum	—	*Cistus ladaniferus* and related shrubs
Myrrh*	Saudi Arabia and East Africa	Commiphora tree
Opopanax* (sweet myrrh)	—	Commiphora tree, Burseraceae family
Storax**	Asia Minor	*Liquidambar orientalis* tree

*Allergic contact dermatitis or positive patch tests (some cross-reactions).
**Cross-reaction with benzoin derived from Styrax (Styracaceae).

sition varies (5,14). There are resorcinol derivatives that share a common molecular skeleton with the 3-pentadecyl phenols of poison ivy. In South America, timber from the cashew nut tree (*Anacardium occidentale*) is used for house and boat building. The tree, a native of Brazil, is grown principally for its nuts, oil, and gum. Cashew nutshell oil has been used in medicine as a rubefacient and vesicant. It has been found in many sources in industry: a preservative for fishing lines, an insect repellent, book bindings, gloss on vanilla beans, cloth markers, and varnishes and cutting oils. It has also been used in the manufacture of automobile brake pads, as a gum arabic substitute, and in combination with formaldehyde as a resin.

A Chinese orthopedic medicine meant to be used either topically or orally, has been reported to cause ACD. The product contains both myrrh and mastic gum, each at a 12.5% concentration. One patient reacted to mastic, one to myrrh, and one to both on patch testing. None reacted to balsam of Peru or colophony (15).

The history, chemistry, and allergic contact dermatitis from urushiol-containing Japanese lacquer has been reviewed by Mitchell and Rook (5). Dermatitis has been reported from a Chinese jar buried for 1,000 years. The Thai lacquer tree (*Melanorrhoea usitata*) contains thitsiol ($C_{23}H_{36}O_2$). Three cases were reported, two nonoccupational, from Bangkok. All reacted to 10% lacquer in pet. The Japanese lacquer contains urushiol ($C_{21}H_{32}O_2$) and the Vietnamese tree laccol ($C_{18}H_{26}O_2$) (16). Kawai et al. (17) reported that heating Japanese lacquer reduces its allergenicity.

TABLE 32.4. *Some Pharmaceutical Products That May Contain Selected Gums and Resins*

Karaya (sterculia) gum
  Inolaxine Granules (Dales; Farillon, both of Britain)
  Normacol Standard (Norgine, Britain) for constipation and colostomy control
  Tex (Simpla, Britain) for peristomal use in conjunction with gel and aluminum oxide basis
  Carbozine (Nu-Hope)
  Formula A Stretchable Karaya Washers and Sheets (United States)
  Karaya Gum (various)
  Trans-Plantar (Tsumura Medical)
  Other proprietary names
    a. Decorpa (also contains guar gum) (Britain, Belgium, France, Germany)
    b. Karagum (Australia)
    c. Normalax (Sweden)
Tragacanth gum
  Compound Tragacanth Paste (BPC 1954)
  Compound Tragacanth Powder (BP)—suspending agent for insoluble powders
  Tragacanth Mucilage (BPC 1973)
  Delsym 12-Hour Cough Relief (Fisons)
  Agora Raspberry and Marshmallow Stool Softener
  Gordobalm (Gordon) Liniment

continued

TABLE 32.4. *Continued*

Compound tincture of benzoin
  Toothache, cold sore, canker sore products
  a. Kakn-a Viscous Liquid (Blistex)
  b. Cold Sore Lotion (DeWitt) 1.2%
  Various ostomy skin protective products
  Sprays
  a. Benzoin Compound Spray (Norton; Vestric, both of Britain)
  b. Rikospray (Riker, Britain)
  c. Stuart Tinct Benzoin Co. Spray (Stuart, Britain)
  d. Aerozoin Spray (Graham Field)
  Compound Benzoin Tincture (USP and BP)
  Benzoin Tincture (BPC 1973)
  TinBen (ferndale)—skin protectant
  POD-Ben-25 (Palisades)
Balsam of Peru
  Diaper rash and prickly heat products
  a. Balmex products (Macsil)—baby powder, emollient lotion, and ointment
Hemorrhoidal products (astringent function)
  a. Wyanoid Suppositories (Wyeth) 30 mg
  b. Wyanoid Ointment (Wyeth) 1%
  c. Rectal Medicone Ointment (Medicone) 12.5 mg
  d. Rectal Medicone Suppositories (Medicone) 3.75 mg/g
  e. Hemorrin (Jeffrey Martin) Ointment (1.8%) and suppositories
  f. Blue-Gray Suppositories (Columbia Medical) 12 mg
  g. Hemorrhoidal HC Suppositories
Myrrh
  Odara Mouthwash (Lorvic)
  Astring-O-Sol Mouthwash (Winthrop)
  Teething Lotion (DeWitt)
  Gum Zor (DeWitt)
  Myrrh Tincture (BPC 1973)
Tolu Balsam
  Linctuses—pediatric compound Tolu Linctus (BP)
  Lozenges—Tolu basis for Lozenges (BPC 1959)
  Solutions—Tolu Solution (BP)
  Syrups—Tolu Balsam Syrup (USNF); Tolu Syrup (BP)
  Tincture—Tolu Balsam Tincture (USNF) and Tolu Tincture (BP 1959)
  Vicks Throat Lozenges
  Dr. Demi-Heal (Quality) diaper rash
  Proderm Topical (Don B. Hickman) Dressing for decubitus ulcers
  TinCoBen (Ferndale)
Acacia
  Dulcolax Tablets
  Agoral Raspberry and Marshmallow Stool Softener
  Dramamine Tablets

Canada balsam from the balsam fir tree caused dermatitis when used in perfumery (Table 32.2). A sensitized laboratory worker also showed positive patch test reactions to lavender oil, eucalyptus oil, clove oil, balsam of Peru, styrax, eugenol, isoeugenol, nerolidol, and farnesol (5).

ROSIN

Rosin (colophony) is a product of pine tree oleoresin (Table 32.2). Depending on the method of extraction, three kinds of colophony may be identified: (a) gum rosin, obtained by topping living trees and distilling the resin to yield turpentine oil and the gum resin residue; (b) wood rosin, a distillate from dead pine tree stumps; and (c) tall oil rosin (liquid rosin), a by-product of pulping pine wood (*tall* is the Swedish word for pine) (5,18,19). According to Mitchell and Rook (5), rosin produced in the United States is obtained from the longleaf pine *(Pinus palustris)* and the loblolly pine *(P. taeda)* of the south Atlantic and eastern Gulf states. European solder fluxes contain rosin from Portugal (20), and European standard patch test tray rosin is from China (21).

In the most recent data from the North American Contact Dermatitis Group, rosin (20% pet) gave positive patch tests in 2.0% of 3,443 patients (J Marks, personal communication, Hershey, PA, 1999). In Zurich in 1994, 3.6% of 1,062 patients were positive (22).

In 1988, the estimated total production of rosin was over 1.2 million metric tons. Gum rosin accounted for about 60% of this total, tall oil rosin 35%, and wood rosin the remainder. In the United States, tall oil accounts for three-fourths of the total rosin produced. Rosin used in paper products, rubber, adhesives, and inks accounts for the majority of the total rosin produced. China, Latin America, and Portugal produce much gum rosin, and Scandinavia, Russia, and the United States produce mostly tall oil rosin.

Rosin consists of about 90% resin acids and 10% neutral matter; of the resin acids, about 90% are isomeric with abietic acid. Gas chromatographic analysis of resin acids in colophony from different sources included varying amounts and distributions of dehydroabietic, neoabietic, pimaric, isopimaric, sandaracopimaric, palustric, tetrahydroabietic, and dehydroabietic acids (5,21). Rosin is used in a crude form, which is a soft, sticky, amber-colored material, or in chemically modified forms: hydrogenated, disproportionated, esterified, polymerized, as a salt, or reacted with maleic anhydride or formaldehyde (13).

Esterification of rosin reduces its allergenicity, as does hydrogenation (23). Cronin (24) reported patch test results of patients with colophony allergy at St. John's Hospital (London, England). Twenty-nine patients who were negative to a maleic ester of colophony reacted to colophony (each 20% in pet); 4 patients reacted to both, and 2 gave equivocal reactions to the ester and were negative to colophony.

Karlberg (25,26) has extensively studied rosin and has succeeded in identifying at least two allergenic chemicals present in both tall oil and gum rosin. She states that purified abietic acid is nonallergenic. However, abietic acid is easily oxidized by air unless special handling precautions are taken. A major oxidation product of abietic acid, 15-hydroperoxyabietic acid, is a strong allergen (27). Oxidation products of dehydroabietic acid are also allergenic (28). It is possible that previous reports of allergy to abietic acid were actually identifying allergy to the oxidation products present in patch test material. Walber (29), for example, found 9 of 15 patients who reacted to colophony also reacted to abietic acid (5% pet). Karlberg's data suggest that the allergens in tall oil and gum rosin are very similar, so that it is unlikely to matter which type is used for patch testing and which type a patient is exposed to.

Commercially modified rosins are more allergenic than natural rosins. Maleopimaric acid in modified rosin has been shown to be a strong sensitizer (30). It may be necessary to patch test with various modified rosin products because cross-reactivity with natural rosin may not always occur (31).

Hausen et al. (32), in guinea pig testing, further documented the allergenicity of several rosin oxidation products.

Hausen reviewed more than 60 articles reporting contact dermatitis to colophony; epidemiologic studies demonstrate an increasing number of cases since 1980 (32). A person has many opportunities to become exposed to colophony and modified products and thus sensitized to them. One of the largest single uses is in the sizing of paper and paperboard. Rosin is added to paper to increase its water resistance. It serves as a protective coating for glossy paper, price labels, plastics, and stickers and prevents feathering and spreading of ink. Small quantities of resin acids can be transferred from paper to articles packed in it, for example, food substances. Examples of other uses include the manufacture of soaps, varnishes, sealing wax, printing inks, driers (for paints), adhesives, binders, soldering fluxes, gloss oils for paints, pitch for lager beer casks, and rosining bows of violins and other string instruments. Rosin is used on the shoes of dancers and on floors of studios and stages to prevent slipping. A detailed list of potential sources of rosin exposure is provided in Table 32.5.

TABLE 32.5. *Source of Exposure to Rosin**

Adhesives, adhesive plasters, surgical incision drapes
Asphaltic products, emulsions, and foundry supplies
Brewery pitch (see Surface coatings)
Cardboard
Caulking compounds
Cements (linoleum, rubber, shoe, thermoplastic tile, and lens coating); cement air-entraining agents
Chewing gum
Clay: modeling clay
Cleaners and lubricants for leather and office machines, grease remover for clothes
Clothing (rosin-containing prewash)
Cosmetics (brilliantine, wax depilatories, eyeshadow, mascara, rouge, hair pomade, nail varnish, hair spray (rarely))
Dentistry: dressing† (dental and periodontal); dental cements (zinc-eugenol cement), liquids and cavity varnishes; impression pastes; sealing pulp canals as antiseptics‡
Fillers (putty and wood dough)
Fireworks
Flexible colloidion BP (not USP)

continued

TABLE 32.5. *(Continued)*

Glues, mastics, and sealants
Grease and lubricant thickener; axle grease
Insulations: electrical and thermal insulating tapes
Inks (ceramic, marking, mimeographic, printing) may contain rosin; water-fast colors in artist's pens
Jointing tapes
Linoleum, floor coverings; floor tiles; adhesive bedding and cement
Match tips
Medicants (human and veterinary); proprietary medicants, disinfectants, and insecticides; component
    of plasters, cerates, and ointments for its stiffening and adhesive qualities; preservative;
      depilating hair-pull wax (humans, packing house animals); dog repellent, diuretic (veterinary);
      wart removers
Flexible collodion BP (not USP)
Newspaper (see Paper)
Oils: tall oil, cutting oil, core oil
Opsite: surgical incision drape
Ostomy appliances
Paper: size for paper and paperboard, coating, finishing film, prevents feathering and spreading of
    ink; used on paper, glossy paper, price labels, plastics, stickers, and fax photographic paper
    (see Inks)
Patch test unit (see Polythene)
Pens: felt tip, artist's (see Inks)
Plastics: surface coating
Polishes (floor, furniture, metal, shoe, and car)
Polythene (polyethylene)
Printing (see Paper)
Rosins and derivatives: gum (may contain turpentine traces); wood and tall oil rosin; rosin oil, tall oil,
    rosinol, retinol, Abitol, and ester gums
Resins: adulterant or modifier of alkyd, synthetic, ester, metals, and phenolic resins
Rubber: tire-compounding aid, reclaiming agent, and emulsifier for synthetic rubber
Sawdust and resin of pine and spruce
Sealants, wood swellers
Shoes (adhesive)
Soaps: brown, clear (transparent), and yellow (soft laundry bar soaps (solubilizing and sudsing agent);
    soap water used with cutting oil
Soldering fluxes, soldering agents
Solvents
Strains
Surface coatings (lager beer casks, rustproof coatings, coatings for price labels and cans; see Paper);
    polish for roasted coffee beans
Tackifier (to prevent slipping)
    Athletic grip aids: wrestlers, gymnasts, ball players, bowlers; rosin bag for baseball players; handles for
      sports equipment—golf and tennis racquets
    Sticky fly papers
    Stringed instrument bows (violinist's rosin)
    Dancers' shoes; floor of studios and stages
    See Rubber
    Machine belts in industry
    Other nonslip applications
    Postage stamp glue
Tapes: medical, industrial (electrical insulating) (see Adhesives)
Varnishes: maleic resin adducts (rosin + maleic anhydride): used extensively in oil and spirit varnishes
    and lacquers
Waterproofing agents: cardboard, walls; oil cloth
Waxes (sealing, shoemakers, tree, grafting, car, floor, and furniture); wax modifications; physiotherapy
    wax (contaminated); zein compositions

*Rosin and its derivatives may be but are not always present.
†Derived from list supplied by John Mitchell, M.D.
‡Has been combined with chloroform, zinc oxide, or eugenol.

CLINICAL PRESENTATIONS OF ROSIN ALLERGY

It may be difficult to find the product responsible in an individual patient with a positive routine patch test reaction to rosin. Accordingly, Table 32.5 should be reviewed in detail with the patient. Farm (33) has extensively reviewed clinical aspects of rosin allergy. She studied 180 workers in a tall oil rosin factory and 132 members of an opera company who had extensive exposure to rosin. Only 7 (3.9%) and 3 (2.3%), respectively, reacted to rosin on patch testing. In another portion of her report, 10 of 13 patch test positive patients had a positive ROAT to 20% rosin applied for several days.

Evaporated colophony from soldering tin threads may cause facial dermatitis (34). Rosin has been documented as a cause of perioral dermatitis from chewing gum and hand eczema from newspaper (35,36).

Kanerva et al. (37) reported a female secretary with hand dermatitis that repeatedly worsened at work and cleared when away from the office. Allergy to rosin was documented. The rosin content of the fax paper was 1%. The patient also reacted to balsam of Peru.

Although cross-reactions between rosin and balsam of Peru are said to occur, Mitchell believes the evidence is scanty (J Mitchell, personal communication, December 1983). Malten lists other cross-reactions for rosin as oil of turpentine, wood tar, pine resin, and spruce resin. Cross-reaction with tea-tree oil (*Melaleuca*) has been reported (38).

Eight of 149 workers (5.4%) in the electronics industry in Singapore reacted to rosin in solder (39). Three patients reacted to rosin in the adhesive of a hydrocolloid dressing (DuoDerm or DuoDerm-E, Bristol-Myers-Squibb Co., Princeton, NJ) (40).

Rosin has been reported to cause allergy in lipsticks (41,42), lottery tickets (43), sawdust (44,45), floor polish (46), cardboard dust (46), depilatory wax (47), paper money (48), and bindi (49).

One of the main sources of rosin exposure is paper. Karlberg et al. (50) found that "environmentally friendly" paper made from mechanical pulp contains more rosin and is more allergenic than paper made from other pulps. A decrease in the manufacturing of paper from chemically treated pulps may be better for the ecology but may be worse for contact dermatitis sufferers.

Asthma may be caused by occupational exposure to colophony (6).

Zinc oxide apparently exerted an inhibitor, or "quenching," effect on allergic contact dermatitis reactions to rosin from adhesive tape in one study (51). Farm (33), however, found no such inhibition of rosin allergy by zinc oxide in seven subjects tested specifically for this.

BALTIC AMBER

Karlberg et al. (52) studied allergenicity of Baltic amber and determined that abietic acid and dehydroabietic acid are present in amber. Five of seven rosin-allergic patients reacted to amber (10% pet) on patch testing, but wearing an amber necklace produced no reaction (52).

SHELLAC

Shellac (Table 32.2) is a resinous excretion of the insect *Laccifer (Tachardia) lacca* exuded as a protective cover onto certain host trees. Shellac has irritant and sensitizing properties and has been removed from some cosmetics. Its main use is as a coating lacquer; other uses are in cosmetics, dental impression material, waxes, and cementing book covers. Pharmaceutical Glaze (*US National Formulary*) is a denatured solution containing 20% to 51% anhydrous shellac, prepared with alcohol (95%) or dehydrated alcohol; it may contain waxes and titanium dioxide as an opaquing agent (6).

Shellac and colophony both caused allergic cheilitis from a lipstick sealant (53). Shellac was tested at 100%, and 50 controls were negative. Eyelid dermatitis from shellac in mascara (tested at 20% in ethanol) has been reported (54).

BENZOIN

Benzoin is present in tincture of benzoin (10% alcohol) (Table 32.3). Compound tincture of benzoin contains 10% benzoin, 2% aloe, 8% storax, and 4% balsam of Tolu in ethyl alcohol. Arning's tincture contains tincture of benzoin, ammonium tumenol, anthrarobin, and ether.

Sources of exposure to benzoin have been listed as adhesives (preservative), cosmetics (nail polish, perfumes, and cuticle removers), inks, benzoinated lard (BPC 1954), antioxidants in creams, expectorants, throat lozenges, raw beeswax, bee glue, and water-repellent barrier creams. Many of these uses were discovered by Hjorth in 1961 (56). Benzoin is still used in medicine as an adhesive (either alone, as a tincture, or as an adhesive for another medicament, such as podophyllum), as a photoinitiator for acrylates, rarely in cosmetics, and as a skin-toughening agent in grease-paint makeup (55).

Benzoin may cross-react with balsam of Peru and related resins, including balsam of Tolu, styrax (storax) (56), myrrh, locust, galbanum, gamboge and olibanum, and other group-specific substances listed by Malten and Fisher (J Mitchell, personal communication, December 1983).

Benzoin may be a more frequent sensitizer than previously thought, especially when used as a medical adhesive, and should be used with caution for this purpose. Fowler has seen positive patch tests in both patients and medical personnel. Fairly severe local reactions and a generalized eruption have been reported with benzoin allergy (57,58). Hollister medical adhesive or Mastisol may be substituted with less chance of allergic reactions.

Hjorth (56) found 2.3% positive reactions among 1,421 consecutive patients patch tested with compound benzoin tincture USP. He also found that benzoin would react almost without exception in patients sensitive to balsam of

Peru. It may be patch tested in a concentration of 10% in alcohol. It may be useful to do an open patch test first; if the test is negative, proceed to a closed patch test to minimize severe reactions. Benzoin in petrolatum may give false-negative results.

> **All persons allergic to Balsam of Peru should be taught to avoid tincture of benzoin because of frequent cross-reactivity.**

Compound tincture of benzoin is known by at least 27 other names (e.g., Balsamum Equitus Sancti Victorius, Guttate Nader, and Jerusalem Balsam) (6). See Table 32.4 for a list of some over-the-counter products containing benzoin.

Podophyllum and cantharidin are two other resins used frequently in dermatology. Both are strong vesicants used for the treatment of warts and may produce severe irritant reactions. Severe systemic toxicity may occur if they are applied over large surfaces or to open areas (6).

> **Many natural resins contain oleoresins that are sensitizers. The ubiquitous rosin (colophony) is a pine tree oleoresin whose main sensitizing components are abietic acid and hydroabietyl alcohols. Tincture of benzoin, which is widely used, is not an uncommon sensitizer.**

REFERENCES

1. Teot AS. Resins, water soluble. In: *Kirk-Othmer encyclopedia of chemical technology,* 3rd ed. New York: Wiley Interscience, 1982; 20:207.
2. Nilsson DC. Sources of allergenic gums. *Ann Allergy* 1960;18:518.
3. Cottrell IW, Baird JK. Gums. In: *Kirk-Othmer encyclopedia of chemical technology,* 3rd ed. New York: Wiley Interscience, 1980;12:45.
4. Camarasa JMG, Alomar A. Contact dermatitis from a karaya seal ring. *Contact Dermatitis* 1980;6:139.
5. Mitchell J, Rook A. *Botanical dermatology.* Vancouver: Greenglass, 1979:66, 84, 145, 381, 385, 435, 521.
6. Martindale J. *The extra pharmacopoeia.* London: The Pharmaceutical Press, 1982:314.
7. Rubinger D, Friedlander M, Superstine E. Hypersensitivity to tablet additives in transplant recipients on prednisone. *Lancet* 1978;2:689.
8. Cooke MA, Wilkinson JF. Formalin sensitivity in gum arabic. *Contact Dermatitis Newsletter* 1973;13:379.
9. Freeman S. Allergic contact dermatitis due to 1,2-benzisothiazolin-3-one in gum arabic. *Contact Dermatitis* 1984;11:146.
10. Gauss WF, Alarie JP, Karol MH. Workplace allergenicity of a psyllium-containing bulk laxative. *Allergy* 1985;40:73–76.
11. Zaloga GP, Hierlwimmer UR, Engler RJ. Anaphylaxis following psyllium ingestion. *J Allergy Clinical Immunol* 1984;74:79–80.
12. Weaver JC. Resins, natural. In: *Kirk-Othmer encyclopedia of chemical technology,* 3rd ed. New York: Wiley Interscience, 1982;20:197.
13. Jost T, Sell Y, Foussereau J. Contact allergy to Manila resin. *Contact Dermatitis* 1989;21:228.
14. Schwartz L, Trulipan L, Birmingham DJ. Occupational diseases of the skin. 1957:555.
15. Lee TY, Lam TH. Allergic contact dermatitis due to a Chinese orthopaedic solution tieh ta yao gin. *Contact Dermatitis* 1993;28:89–90.
16. Kullavanijaya P, Ophaswongse S. A study of dermatitis in the lacquerware industry. *Contact Dermatitis* 1997;36:244–246.
17. Kawai K, Nakagawa M, Kawai K, Miyakoshi T, et al. Heat treatment of Japanese lacquerware renders it hypoallergenic. *Contact Dermatitis* 1992;27:244–249.
18. Widstrom L. Contact allergy to colophony in soldering flux. *Contact Dermatitis* 1983;9:205.
19. Arlt HG Jr. Tall oil. In: *Kirk-Othmer encyclopedia of chemical technology,* 3rd ed. New York: Wiley Interscience, 1983;22:531.
20. Ducombs G. Allergy to colophony. *Contact Dermatitis* 1978;4:118.
21. Karlberg AT, Boman A, Wahlberg JE. Allergenic potential of abeitic acid colophony and pine resin-HA. *Contact Dermatitis* 1980;6:481.
22. Bangha E, Elsner P. Sensitization to allergens of the standard series at the Department of Dermatology in Zurich 1990–1994. *Dermatology* 1996;193:17–21.
23. Karlberg AT, Boman A, Nilsson JLG. Hydrogenation reduces the allergenicity of colophony (rosin). *Contact Dermatitis* 1988;9:22.
24. Cronin E. *Contact dermatitis.* Edinburgh: Churchill Livingstone, 1980:3.
25. Karlberg AT. Air oxidation increases the allergenic potential of tall-oil rosin: colophony contact allergens also identified in tall-oil rosin. *Am J Contact Dermatitis* 1991;2:43.
26. Karlberg AT. Contact allergy to colophony: chemical identifications of allergens, sensitization experiments and clinical experiences. *Acta Derm Venereol* (Stockh) 1988;139[Suppl 1].
27. Karlberg AT, et al. Identification of 15-hydroperoxyabietic acid as a contact allergen in Portuguese colophony. *J Pharm Pharmacol* 1988; 40:42.
28. Karlberg AT, et al. Contact allergy to dehydroabietic acid derivatives isolated from Portuguese colophony. *Contact Dermatitis* 1988;19:166.
29. Wahlberg J. Abeitic acid and colophony. *Contact Dermatitis* 1978;4:55.
30. Karlberg AT, et al. Maleopimaric acid—a potent sensitizer in modified rosin. *Contact Dermatitis* 1990;22:193.
31. Hausen BM, Mohnert J. Contact allergy due to colophony (V). Patch test results with different types of colophony and modified-colophony products. *Contact Dermatitis* 1989;20:295.
32. Hausen BM, Krohn K, Budianto E. Contact allergy due to colophony (VH). *Contact Dermatitis* 1990;23:352.
33. Farm G. Contact allergy to Colophony. *Acta Dermato-Venereologica* 1997[Suppl 201].
34. *Handbook of nonprescription drugs,* 7th ed. Washington, DC: American Pharmaceutical Corp., 1982:73.
35. Satyawan I, Oranje AP, Van Joost TH. Perioral dermatitis in a child due to rosin in chewing gum. *Contact Dermatitis* 1990;22:182.
36. Lidén C, Larberg AT. Colophony in paper as a cause of hand eczema. *Contact Dermatitis* 1992;26:272.
37. Kanerva L, et al. Contact dermatitis from telefax paper. *Contact Dermatitis* 1992;27:12.
38. Selvaag E, Eriksen B, Thune P. Contact allergy due to tea tree oil and cross-sensitization to colophony. *Contact Dermatitis* 1994;31:124–125.
39. Hiok-Hee T, Madellynn Tsu-Li C, Chee-Leok, G. Occupational skin disease in workers from the electronics industry in Singapore. *Amer J Contact Dermatitis* 1997;8:210–214.
40. Sasseville D, Tennstedt D, Lachapelle JM. Allergic contact dermatitis from hydrocolloid dressings. *Amer J Contact Dermatitis* 1997;8:236–238.
41. Inoue A, Shoji A, Aso S. Allergic lipstick cheilitis due to ester gum and ricinoleic acid. *Contact Dermatitis* 1998;39:39.
42. Batta K, Bourke JF, Foulds IS. Allergic contact dermatitis from colophony in lipsticks. *Contact Dermatitis* 1997;36:171–172.
43. Pereira F, Manuel R, Gafvert E, et al. Relapse of colophony dermatitis from lottery tickets. *Contact Dermatitis* 1997;37:43.
44. Watsky KL. Airborne allergic contact dermatitis form pine dust. *Amer J Contact Dermatitis* 1997;8:118–120.
45. Meding B, Ahman M, Karlberg AT. Skin symptoms and contact allergy in woodwork teachers. *Contact Dermatitis* 1996;34:185–190.
46. Karlberg AT, Gafvert E, Meding B, et al. Airborne contact dermatitis from unexpected exposure to rosin (colophony): rosin sources revealed with chemical analyses. *Contact Dermatitis* 1996;35:272–278.

47. de-Argila D, Ortiz-Frutos J, Iglesias L. Occupational allergic contact dermatitis from colophony in depilatory wax. *Contact Dermatitis* 1996;34:369.

48. Koch P. Occupational contact dermatitis from colophony and formaldehyde in banknote paper. *Contact Dermatitis* 1995;32:371–372.

49. Koh D, Lee BL, Ong HY, et al. Colophony in bindi adhesive. *Contact Dermatitis* 1995;32:186.

50. Karlberg AT, Gafvert E, Liden C. Environmentally friendly paper may increase risk of hand eczema in rosin sensitive persons. *J Am Acad Dermatol* 1995;33:427–432.

51. Sóderberg TA, et al. Inhibitory effect of zinc oxide on contact allergy due to colophony. *Contact Dermatitis* 1990;23:346.

52. Karlberg AT, Boman A, Liden C. Studies on the allergenicity of Baltic amber. *Contact Dermatitis* 1992;27:224–229.

53. Rademaker M, Kirby JD, White IR. Contact cheilitis to shellac, Lanpol 5 and colophony. *Contact Dermatitis* 1986;15:307–308.

54. Scheman AJ. Contact allergy to quaternium-22 and shellac in mascara. *Contact Dermatitis* 1998;38:342–343.

55. Hoffman TE, Adams RM. Contact dermatitis to benzoin in grease paint makeup. *Contact Dermatitis* 1978;4:379.

56. Hjorth N. Balsam of Tolu, styrax and benzoin. *Acta Derm Venereol* (Stockh) 1961;41[Suppl 46]:61.

57. Coskey RJ. Contact dermatitis owing to tincture of benzoin. *Arch Dermatol* 1978;114:128.

58. Spott DA, Shelley WB. Exanthem due to contact allergen (benzoin) absorbed through skin. *JAMA* 1970;214:1181.

CHAPTER 33

Contact Leukoderma (Vitiligo) Hyperpigmentation and Discolorations from Contactants

LEUKODERMA (VITILIGO) FROM CONTACTANTS

Contact leukoderma, also called contact vitiligo or contact depigmentation, may be defined as a complete depigmentation usually without preceding inflammation. This is in contrast to postinflammatory hypopigmentation, which must by definition be preceded by inflammation and in which total depigmentation does not occur. Because of the frequent association with workplace exposure, contact leukoderma is sometimes called occupational leukoderma or vitiligo.

Contact leukoderma may be indistinguishable from idiopathic vitiligo. Fisher (1) suggested that some cases of idiopathic vitiligo may be due to unsuspected inhalation or ingestion of chemicals that produce contact leukoderma. Table 33.1 lists the chemicals capable of producing contact vitiligo.

Paratertiary Butylphenol

Exposure to paratertiary butylphenol (PTBP) is widespread in industry, and consumers who use synthetic leather, plastics, glues, and germicidal phenolic detergents can also be exposed to it. Table 33.2 lists the numerous ways in which individuals can be exposed to this phenolic compound.

Malten et al. (2), in a comprehensive review of "occupational vitiligo," pointed out that depigmentation may occur without preceding irritation, dermatitis, or burns. Malten (3), distinguishing between occupational vitiligo and contact vitiligo in a "consumer," reported a case of mild contact dermatitis on a man's left wrist and later on the right wrist, after he started wearing his watch on that side. This contact dermatitis was from the glue (called Bison Kit in the Netherlands), which contains *p*-tertiary butylphenol formaldehyde resin from which "free" PTBP is released and which produced the depigmentation. This deduction was made from the fact that PTBP is a monomer that forms synthetic adhesives by polymerizing with formaldehyde.

Some monomeric PTBP remains "free," however, in the final phenol formaldehyde resin.

Malten et al. (2) predicted that cases of occupational vitiligo can be expected in workers handling PTBP and its homologous substances in a variety of factories and occupations if measures are not taken from the beginning to avoid direct skin contact, inhalation, and ingestion of these chemicals.

Saruta and Nakamizo (4) reported occupational leukoderma on the neck, arms, hands, breast, abdomen, and hip of pharmaceutical workers exposed to PTBP. Histologic investigation of these parts of the body revealed remarkably vacuolated cells in the basal layers. Occlusive dressings of PTBP applied to the backs of black guinea pigs resulted in experimental leukoderma. In the normal skin of two patients, occlusive dressings with PTBP produced leukoderma not only in areas in direct contact with PTBP but also beyond the occluded areas.

Itoh et al. (5) theorized that PTBP may produce a "capillaritis" of the superficial skin vessels that can produce a more generalized distribution of PTBP beyond actual contact with the chemical.

The *bindi,* the circular mark worn on the forehead of Indian women, has an adhesive on the back that may be coated with PTBP. Skin contact with PTBP in the adhesive led to depigmentation without dermatitis (6,7). Some Indian synthetic wallets, commonly carried against the breast by Indian women, have also caused leukoderma. Analysis showed that monobenzyl ether of hydroquinone was the cause (8).

Alkyphenols

Calnan (9) reported occupational leukoderma from the alkylphenols. In workers in industrial plants producing alkylphenols, patches of leukoderma developed not only on exposed skin but also on areas covered by clothing. Inges-

TABLE 33.1. *Chemicals Capable of Producing Contact Vitiligo*

Diisoptopyl fluorophosphate
Hydroquinone
Mercaptoamines, such as N-(2-mercaptoethyl)-dimethylamine hydrochloride (MEDA) and β-mercaptoethylamine hydrochloride (MEA)
Monobenzyl ether of hydroquinone
Monoethyl ether of hydroquinone (p-ethoxyphenol)
Monomethyl ether of hydroquinone (p-methoxyphenol or p-hydroxyanisole)
N, N′, N″-triethylenethiophosphoramide (Thio-TEPA)
p-cresol
p-isoprophylcatechol
p-methylcatechol
p-nonylphenol
p-octylphenol
p-phenylphenol
p-tert-amylphenol
p-tert-butylcatechol
p-tert-butylphenol
Physostigmine (eserine)

tion and inhalation of vaporized phenols appear to have been responsible for a systemic effect on melanocytes.

Table 33.3 lists skin color changes from occupational chemicals.

Pigmentation of the Palms and Scalp from Phenolic Hair Tonics

Forman (10) reported pigmentation of the palms and scalp that was probably from proprietary hair tonics containing various phenols and phenolic derivatives.

> **The various phenols, quinoline, and the diphenyls are all capable of being photoactivated or condensed to form polynuclear quinonoid compounds that are often colored.**

TABLE 33.2. *Exposure to Paratertiary Butylphenol*

De-emulsifiers for oil field use
Deodorants
Duplicating paper
Formaldehyde resin CKR-1634
Germicidal phenolic detergent compounds
Insecticides
Latex glues
Motor oil additives
Paratertiary butylphenol formaldehyde resins
Plasticizers for cellulose acetate
Printing inks
Rubber antioxidants
Soap antioxidants
Synthetic oils
Varnish and lacquer resins
Valve plants

TABLE 33.3. *Skin Color Changes Due to Occupational Chemicals*

Yellow	Dichromate
	Dinobuton
	Fluorescein dye
	Glutaraldehyde
	4,4′-methylenedianiline: catalyst for epoxy and urethane resins
	Nitric acid
	Picric acid and picrates
	Sodium nitrite
Blue	Cobalt
	Indigo
	Oxalic acid in automobile radiator cleaners
	Silver nitrate in photographers
	Sulfadiazine silver (silvadene) in pharmaceutical workers and nurses in burn units
Brown	Chrysarobin and anthralin in pharmacists and nursing personnel
	Paraphenylenediamine in dye manufacture and photography developers
	Permanganates in bleach and dye makers, water purifiers, and paper pulp bleaches
	Phenothiazines (agricultural workers, veterinarians, and nurses)
Red	Soda ash
	TNT
Black	Mercury
	Osmium trioxide in histology technicians, incandescent lamp makers, organic chemical synthesizers, and platinum hardeners
	Gold from jewelry
Orange	Chlorine gas
	Phenothiazine
	Tetryl (trinitrophenylmethylnitramine)
Green	Copper dust in electrical workers, machinists, and copper smelters

Modified by personal communication with Dr. Robert Adams, Palo Alto, CA, 1998.

Paradoxical Pigmentary Effects of Topical Mercury Compounds

Mercury-containing topical agents have long been used as bleaching agents because mercury can displace copper from tyrosinase, inactivating the enzyme that plays a role in the synthesis of melanin (11). Repeated applications of mercury-containing ointments or cosmetics, however, may give rise to gray-brown pigmentation limited to areas to which it is applied, with accentuation in the skin folds. Burge and Winkelmann (12), using the electron microscope, demonstrated that melanin pigmentation increased secondarily to the presence of the metal.

> **Topical mercury compounds may act initially as bleaching agents, but prolonged use may result in hyperpigmentation.**

> There are many opportunities for exposure to paratertiary butylphenol, butylcatechol, and phenolic detergents at home and in industry, all of which can produce contact leukoderma (vitiligo).

TABLE 33.4. *Germicidal Phenolic Detergents Containing Paratertiary Butylphenol*

Product	Manufacturer
Bactophene	Sanfax Corp.
Microphene	Sanfax Corp.
O-Syl	Lehn and Fink Division, Sterling Drug
Phenocide	Center Chemicals

Paratertiary Butylcatechol

Gellin et al. (13) were among the first to recognize that some persons with "idiopathic vitiligo" may actually have an environmentally or occupationally induced leukoderma. Four workers at an assembly plant in Michigan developed leukoderma from exposure to paratertiary butylcatechol (PTBC). These workers had dermatitis on the upper limbs before the onset of leukoderma. Their depigmentation began as early as a few months to as late as 4 years after they started work in the assembly plant. In one patient, a man, leukoderma was confined to the hands and forearms, but in the other three patients, distant areas were also affected. One of these three patients, a woman, had depigmentation over 75% of her body surface.

When patch tested with PTBC, three of the four patients had eczematous positive patch test reactions. In one man, an area of depigmentation remained for over 20 months, even though the reaction had subsided.

Experimentally, the catechol derivative was found to induce varying degrees of irritation in six volunteer subjects and to cause depigmentation in black, but not albino, guinea pigs. The related chemical, PTBP, had the same effect.

Gellin et al. (13) stated that both PTBP and PTBC are structurally related to monobenzyl ether of hydroquinone, which has long been known to induce occupational leukoderma. Thus, it appears that many phenols and catechols are capable of depigmenting mammalian skin, especially with group substitutions at the *para* position. The investigators theorized that the mechanism of pigment loss is due to competitive inhibition of tyrosine oxidation, with a resultant cytotoxic effect on melanocytes.

Occupational exposure to coal tar and tar products led to allergic contact dermatitis to PTBC and subsequent progressive leukoderma (14). There was no cross-reactivity to PTBP in this case.

Depigmentation Caused by Phenolic Detergent Germicides

Kahn (15) reported that certain phenolic detergent germicides, used widely in hospitals and many households, may cause depigmentation of the skin. Such depigmentation occurred on the hands and forearms of five persons on the housekeeping staff of a Denver hospital, 6 months after they used the phenolic detergent-disinfectant O-Syl, containing PTBP, for cleaning. At about the same time, seven employees of an adjacent Denver hospital had a similar experience. Six months after introduction of the phenolic-disinfectant Ves-Phene, containing paratertiary amylphenol (PTAP), the skin on the patients' hands and arms also showed depigmentation.

Both PTBP and PTAP are found in many germicidal disinfectants. PTAP is also used in the manufacture of oil-soluble resins, in organic synthesis, as a plasticizer, and as a fumigant. A 1% PTAP sensitized 5 of 13 patients in this report, and the 6% solution irritated the skin of every person to whom it was applied. This agent is apparently more toxic to epidermal and bacterial cells than is PTBP. A 1% ethanolic PTAP solution produces depigmentation similar to that produced by 6% PTBP solution.

Tables 33.4 and 33.5 show the germicidal phenolic detergents that contain PTBP and PTAP, respectively.

Kahn found that these agents depigmented the skin of both patients and volunteers within 2 weeks without producing dermatitis. In three patients, depigmentation disappeared at the test site within 6 months. In the other two, it was still present more than 1 year after testing. The average onset of depigmentation was about 2 weeks.

In a discussion of the mechanism of pigment loss, Kahn found that phenolics remain in the skin long after application, and the reduction of pigment may be masked for weeks by melanin already scattered throughout the epidermis.

TABLE 33.5. *Germicidal Phenolic Detergents Containing Paratertiary Amylphenol*

Product	Manufacturer
Bactophene	Sanfax Corp.
Beaucoup	Huntington Laboratories
Chlorocide	Center Chemicals
Galahad	Puritan Chemical
Listophene	Enterprise Paint Mfg.
Matar	Huntington Laboratories
Microphene	Sanfax Corp.
Phenocide	Center Chemicals
Phenomycin	Franklin Division of Purex
Staphene	Vestal Laboratories
1-Stroke Vesphene	Vestal Laboratories
Tergisyl	Lehn and Fink Division, Sterling Drug
Tri-Kem	Airwick Industries
Ves-Phene	Vestal Laboratories
Ves-Phene O	Vestal Laboratories

HYDROQUINONE USES AND ABNORMAL REACTIONS

Hydroquinone, known by the various synonyms shown in Table 33.6, is used widely in industry as a reducing agent, as a photographic developer, and as an antioxidant or stabilizer for certain materials that polymerize in the presence of oxidizing agents. Thus, in acrylic and polyester resin systems, its presence prevents unintended spontaneous polymerization (16). Other occupational exposures are shown in Table 33.7. It is also used as a reagent for phosphate determination.

Hydroquinone dust is a mild primary irritant. Skin sensitization to the dry solid is rare but occurs on occasion from contact with its alkaline solutions. The skin may be depigmented by repeated applications of ointments of hydroquinone, but this virtually never occurs from contact with dust or dilute water solutions. Following prolonged exposure to elevated dust levels, brownish conjunctival stains may appear. These stains may be followed by corneal opacities and structural changes in the cornea, which may lead to loss of visual acuity (17). The early pigmentary stains are reversible, whereas the corneal changes tend to be progressive.

Depigmentation from Hydroquinone in Photographic Development

There are several reports of occupational leukoderma from exposure to hydroquinone developer in photography (18–21). The concentration of hydroquinone in the various photographic processes was probably over 7%.

At a dermatology meeting, Fisher (22) saw a high school student who developed contact vitiligo of the hands from exposure to hydroquinone in a school course on photographic development.

Occupational vitiligo from hydroquinone in photographic developers can occur in industry and in amateurs.

Depigmentation from "Bleaching Creams" Containing Hydroquinone

Numerous so-called bleaching creams (Table 33.8) containing hydroquinone are used widely in attempts to lighten hyperpigmented areas of the skin, such as melasma, freck-

TABLE 33.7. *Occupational Exposures to Hydroquinone*

Antioxidant makers
Bacteriostatic agent makers
Cosmetologists (artificial nails)
Dental personnel
Drug makers
Fur processors
Motor fuel blenders
Organic chemical synthesizers
Paint makers
Photographic developer makers
Plastic stabilizer workers
Rubber antioxidant
Stone coating workers
Styrene monomer workers

les, senile lentigines, and other forms of melanin hyperpigmentation.

Adverse reactions that have been reported in the past include rare instances of allergic reactions, erythema, and stinging sensations. However, a possible toxic reaction to hydroquinone has been noted in several patients (23,24). This toxic reaction may cause complete depigmentation of the treated areas instead of lightening of hyperpigmentation, which may result in a rather unsightly condition known as guttate hypomelanosis, and more widespread contact leukoderma. The possibility of such hydroquinone preparations inflaming latent idiopathic vitiligo must be considered.

A review of the literature and personal communications from various authorities (25–27) indicate that hydroquinone bleaching creams containing low concentrations of hydroquinone are safe and do not produce the depigmentation once seen with the use of monobenzyl ether of hydroquinone.

TABLE 33.8. *Bleaching Creams Containing Hydroquinone*

Alphaquin
Ambi (Kiwi Brands)
Artra (Plough)
Black and White (Plough)
Dr. Fred Palmer Skin Whitener
Eldopaque and Eldoquin (ICN)
Esoterica (USV Pharm)
Lustra (Medicis)
Melpaque (Stratus)
Melquin (Stratus)
Nadinola (Chattem)
NeoStrata AHA Gel
Neutrogena Melanex (Neutrogena)
Nuquin (Stratus)
Porcelana
Posner Skinona Cream
Solaquin Cream (ICN)
Viquin (ICN)
Ultra Glow
Ultraquin

TABLE 33.6. *Hydroquinone Synonyms*

1,4-benzenediol	Hydrochinone
Dihydroxybenzene	Hydroquinol
p-dihydroxybenzene	p-hydroxyphenol
p-diphenol	Quinol

Fisher (24) encountered four patients who had never used monobenzyl ether of hydroquinone but nevertheless acquired disfiguring leukoderma following the use of three popular bleaching creams containing 2% hydroquinone.

> Contact leukoderma from bleaching creams containing low concentrations of hydroquinone rarely occurs, is toxic, is not allergic in nature, and is not revealed by closed standard patch test procedures.

Role of Patch Testing with Hydroquinone

The few patients who developed leukoderma from hydroquinone bleaching creams had neither preceding inflammation nor a positive patch test reaction to 1% hydroquinone in petrolatum after 72 hours.

In one patient, "open testing" (rubbing 1% hydroquinone in pet into one site) produced hypopigmentation on normal skin. Such findings indicate that depigmenting action is not allergic but toxic in nature.

Hydroquinone may cross-react with resorcin and pyrocatechol.

Relation of Monobenzyl Ether of Hydroquinone to Hydroquinone

Van Ketel (28) stated that sensitization to monobenzyl ether of hydroquinone occurs rather frequently, whereas hydroquinone is regarded as a rather weak sensitizer. He reported that one of his patients showed sensitization to both hydroquinone and monobenzyl ether of hydroquinone. It is possible that sensitization to monobenzyl ether may be partially explained by hydrolysis to hydroquinone.

Butylated Hydroxytoluene Depigmentation

Vollum (29) reported two black children, one with psoriasis and one with eczema, who developed hypopigmentation after treatment with polyethylene film (polythene) applied over a corticosteroid ointment. The area of depigmentation was limited to the skin covered by the polyethylene. Analysis of the film showed that it contained butylated hydroxytoluene (BHT) as an antioxidant to prevent decomposition, and this seemed to be the responsible factor. In one patient, the skin gradually returned to normal 8 weeks after treatment was ceased; in the other, there was no sign of repigmentation 4 weeks after cessation of treatment.

Although there have been several reports of allergic contact dermatitis from this antioxidant in cosmetics and foods, there have been no other reports confirming depigmentation from BHT (30).

Tosti et al. (31) reported possible contact leukoderma in a ceramics worker heavily exposed to lacquers containing phenolic compounds, including phlobaphenes, stilbenes, flavonoids, and lignins.

Nonoccupational Vitiligo from Contactants

With the increasing use of synthetic leather and shoe adhesives containing PTBP, vitiligo of the feet, particularly in women, is to be expected.

Frenk and Kocsis (32) reported depigmentation from adhesive tape. One of the adhesive tapes studied was of polyvinyl chloride, with a natural rubber base adhesive containing a derivative of dihydroxydiphenylmethane.

Leukoderma from Adhesives

Neoprene adhesives and PTBP resin adhesives may produce leukoderma (33,34).

Maibach (personal communication) reported a case of depigmentation on the breast induced, presumably, by hydroquinone of monobenzyl ether present in breast prostheses ("falsies") worn by the patient.

Para-phenylenediamine

Taylor et al. (35) reported four cases of contact leukoderma from hair coloring agents. Another report detailed contact leukoderma with no dermatitis on the lip after use of a mustache coloring product containing para-phenylenediamine (PPDA). Patch test was negative to PPDA (36). A report of hair dye depigmentation from India discussed a patient with allergy to PPDA with positive patch tests. The test sites depigmented 3 months later (37).

Other Causes of Contact Vitiligo

Alta, a red solution used by some Indian women to color the feet, has been reported to occasionally cause depigmentation (38). Alta contains two azo dyes, Crocein Scarlet MOO and rhodamine B. Depigmentation occurred at patch test sites and also at the site of a patch test to PPDA.

Kanerva and Estlander (39) reported persistent (2.8 years) depigmentation at sites of patch testing with acrylates. The test substances were dental resins tested at use concentrations instead of being diluted as recommended.

Rubber "consumer" products, such as condoms, rubberized stockings, bandages, orthopedic splints (40), and cosmetic face sponges, can produce contact vitiligo (Table 33.9).

In a personal communication, Dr. Paul Kelley of Martin Luther King Jr. General Hospital, Los Angeles, reported that leukoderma may develop after intralesional injections of corticosteroids or use of Cordran tape. Pigment loss is usually temporary but may be permanent, and its cause is as yet unknown.

TABLE 33.9. *"Consumer" Products Producing "Nonoccupational" Vitiligo*

Acrylates
Adhesive tapes
Bindi
Cinnamic aldehyde in a toothpaste
Dyes: Para-phenylenediamine and alta
Germicidal phenolic detergents
Latex glues
Rubber products
 "Falsies," condoms, stockings, girdles, bandages, cosmetic face sponges
Shoes
Wristwatch bands

Perioral Leukoderma from Cinnamic Aldehyde

Mathias et al. (41) described a perioral leukoderma simulating vitiligo in a 25-year-old woman. A patch test to cinnamic aldehyde was positive; depigmentation was observed at the patch test site 3 months after the initial application. No changes in pigmentation occurred from a concomitant allergic patch test reaction to neomycin sulfate. A toothpaste containing cinnamic aldehyde was implicated; perioral hypopigmentation resolved when a toothpaste without cinnamic aldehyde was substituted. A repeated patch test to cinnamic aldehyde again showed depigmentation at the patch test site 3 months after application.

> Cinnamic aldehyde in a toothpaste produced perioral leukoderma and a delayed hypopigmented patch test reaction after 3 weeks.

Differentiation of Idiopathic and Contact Vitiligo

Fitzpatrick (42) indicated that vitiligo from contactants can readily be confused with the "idiopathic" variety. Histologic examination is of no help because melanocytes degenerate similarly in both conditions. Idiopathic vitiligo is usually permanent, whereas vitiligo from contactants may sometimes clear if the causative contactant is removed.

A careful history may reveal exposure to a depigmentary chemical listed in the tables. It should be emphasized that direct skin contact with these chemicals may not be necessary, because it is possible that inhalation or ingestion of sufficient amounts may also produce vitiligo.

Fitzpatrick (42) noted that "idiopathic" vitiligo may accompany other diseases, such as thyrotoxicosis, hyperparathyroidism, and pernicious anemia.

Frenk and Kocsis (32), in their case report of depigmentation from either a plastic strip or adhesive, stated they could distinguish contact vitiligo from the idiopathic variety by the presence in the electron microscope of "unusual clear cells." This has not been confirmed from other reports.

Fisher (43) stated that subtle ocular changes, such as pigment loss in the iris, may be found in idiopathic vitiligo. Presumably this would not occur in contact leukoderma.

> Contact vitiligo (leukoderma) and idiopathic vitiligo look alike under the microscope.

Experimental Reproduction of Contact Vitiligo

Gellin et al. (13) found that the experimental depigmentary effect of local open application of PTBP to black guinea pigs appeared to be vehicle dependent and seemed on occasions to be related to concomitant irritancy. PTBP in concentrations of 0.005, 1.5, and 10 g/100 mL of acetone was ineffective, although the two higher concentrations were irritating. With dimethyl sulfoxide or propylene glycol, a depigmentary (and irritating) effect of PTBP was seen only in the 10 g/100 mL solutions but not in the 1 or 5 g solutions, which were not irritant.

Similarly, experimental incubation in human volunteers is dependent upon strength, vehicle, method of external application (frequency, open or closed), and site of application. Kahn (15) reported that depigmentation (after closed patch testing on alternating days with 6% PTBP in alcohol) occurred after an average of 2 weeks.

> Because the leukoderma produced by chemicals is not allergic in nature but is a gradual toxic process, closed-patch testing for 48 to 72 hours may be of no help. Closed-patch testing for at least 2 weeks may reproduce the depigmentation.

Diminished Contact Sensitivity in Vitiliginous Skin

Uehara et al. (44) studied 30 patients with vitiligo (10 of the segmental type and 20 of the generalized type) who were sensitized with dinitrochlorobenzene (DNCB) in a normal skin site on the upper medial aspect of the arm. Challenge tests with DNCB were performed in vitiliginous patches and in normal skin sites. In vitiliginous patches, diminished contact sensitivity reactions to DNCB were noted in both groups of patients, whereas in normal skin sites, a normal delayed hypersensitivity response to the same antigen developed in the same patients. Tuberculin reactivity was not suppressed in vitiliginous lesions. The investigators suggested that diminished contact reactivity in vitiliginous skin might be due to functional changes in Langerhans' cells or to an alteration of carrier (skin) proteins in the lesions.

Nordlund et al. (45) made a similar observation of diminished reactivity to monobenzone in areas of vitiligo, and a similar lack of contact dermatitis occurred with airborne exposure to parthenium in India (vitiliginous areas of the lips and fingers remained uninvolved) (46). Similarly, a lack of dermatitis has been reported within areas of nevoid depigmentation despite surrounding textile dermatitis (47).

> **Diminished contact sensitivity in vitiliginous skin may result from functional changes in Langerhans cells.**

Prognosis and Treatment of Contact Vitiligo

Spontaneous repigmentation of affected areas may occur occasionally. In most instances, however, the depigmentation lasts indefinitely. Ehrenfeld (48) treated a hospital orderly who acquired depigmentation from washing instruments with a solution of O-Syl detergent. Employing the technique described by Fulton et al. (49), Ehrenfeld treated the patient by painting a solution of methoxsalen on the dorsum of the right hand and irradiating the area with a bank of UV lights. The PUVA treatments were performed at weekly intervals for 2 months. Pigment about the hair follicles on the proximal phalanges of the right hand began to form after six treatments. No such repigmentation occurred on the left hand, which had not been treated. Kahn (15), however, did not succeed in obtaining repigmenting in his cases of contact vitiligo with topical psoralens and sunlight.

Postinflammatory Pigmentary Changes

Gellin et al. (13) stated that increased pigmentation may be a postinflammatory response following contact dermatitis from diverse causes. Photosensitive reactions may follow contact with tar, pitch, and psoralens, or phytodermatitis may result from contact with celery, figs, or limes. (See chapter TK.) Physical damage from chemical and thermal burns may also be responsible. Postinflammatory hyperpigmentation may occur after some inflammatory skin diseases such as lichen planus or fixed drug eruption.

Decreased pigmentation may also be postinflammatory following contact dermatitis from various causes. It can result from physical damage inflicted by chemical and thermal burns, or it may occur after any inflammatory dermatosis such as psoriasis or contact dermatitis. Clinically, postinflammatory hypopigmentation manifests as a decrease in color, not total abscence of melamine, as is seen in leukoderma. Recovery to normal skin color is nearly universal once the inflammation has subsided.

> **Following contact dermatitis or thermal burns, hyper- or hypopigmentary changes may occur.**

Hypopigmentation or Hyperpigmentation from Rubber

Rubber compounds containing antioxidants, particularly hydroquinone, have long been known to produce leukoderma. Hamada and Horiguchi (50), however, reported chronic melanodermatitis from rubber caused by contact with the rubber peephole of a ship radarscope.

Bleehen and Hall-Smith (51) reported marked depigmentation of the skin in areas in direct contact with an elasticized brassiere containing spandex yarn. They suggested that the persistent skin depigmentation that occurred in this case is an isomorphic phenomenon due to friction and pressure from the brassiere in a patient with vitiligo.

> **Rubber compounds usually produce hypopigmentation, but melanodermatitis may occasionally be produced.**

Hydroquinone Damage to the Dermis from Bleaching Creams

South African dermatologists (52,53) reported an outbreak of exogenous ochronosis and colloid milium in patients who had used strong hydroquinone bleaching creams. These phenomena developed after a few years and took place when the melanocytes had overcome the bleaching influence. Sun exposure and thorough inunction of the cream were required for the more advanced changes. Analogous changes have been seen when the skin is exposed to certain crude fuels in persons who work in the sun; phenolic components in the fuels are suspected. Sarcoid-like reactions to the ochronotic material and to the lichenoid eruptions at the affected sites are also encountered.

> **Exogenous ochronosis, colloid milia, sarcoid-like reactions, and lichenoid eruptions have occurred in persons of dark skin color from prolonged use of strong (over 5%) hydroquinone bleaching creams.**

Hydroquinone Bleaching Creams Wrongly Used for Lentigo Maligna

A report (54) warns of the danger of mistakenly using such creams in superficial malignant melanomas. In one patient, use of such a depigmenting cream delayed surgical excision of a lentigo maligna for 1 year and allowed it to grow to considerable size. Depigmentation occurred in the center of the lesion, demonstrating that hydroquinone can affect abnormal as well as normal melanocytes.

> **Bleaching creams may delay the proper treatment of lentigo maligna and malignant melanoma.**

Paradoxical Nail Pigmentation with Hydroquinone

An orange-brown to chestnut-brown color may develop on the nail plate with application of hydroquinone over the distal fingertips. Oxidation of hydroquinone has been one explanation, and this may be observed with the cream itself upon prolonged exposure to air (55). A role for sunlight in the production of this pigmentation has also been suggested (56). These changes can be confused with heavy metal poisoning or half-and-half nails.

Benzene Hyperpigmentation

Dupre et al. (57) reported that a manual worker exposed to benzene derivatives developed blue to black spots confined to the hands, which represented pigmented granules in elastic and collagen fibers. This appears to be a new entity, probably a variant of exogenous ochronosis produced by professional contact with certain chemicals. Tinctorial or histochemical affinity of the ochronotic-like substance is not observed. The granules are found only inside connective tissue structures.

Cutaneous ochronosis from hydroquinone has been reported in the United States, even from over-the-counter products (58,59). However, because the concentration of hydroquinone in over-the-counter products may exceed a presumed 2% concentration, as noted previously, the concentration responsible may be similar to those in the South African cases.

Exogenous ochronosis may be caused by a number of chemicals, such as phenol, hydroquinone, and resorcinol, after repeated contact with the skin. The pigmentation probably represents either a polymer of the causative chemical itself or a polymer of homogentisic acid owing to interference with tyrosine metabolism.

Leukomelanosis from Piper Betle Leaves

A report from Taiwan discusses 15 patients with areas of mottled depigmentation and hyperpigmentation in the face (60). All had applied steamed leaves of the plant *Piper betle* (betle pepper) as a "treatment" for melasma or freckling. The patients observed stinging and erythema after leaf application. The authors stated that the leaves contain the essential oils chavical and chavibetal, which are phenolic derivatives. Patch testing was not performed.

REFERENCES

1. Fisher AA. Vitiligo due to contactants. *Cutis* 1976;17:431.
2. Malten KE, et al. Occupational vitiligo due to paratertiary butylphenol and homologues. *Trans St Johns Hosp Derm Soc* 1971;57:115.
3. Malten KE. Paratertiary butylphenol depigmentation in a "consumer." *Contact Dermatitis* 1975;1:181.
4. Saruta T, Nakamizo Y. Leukoderma due to paratertiary butylphenol. *Rinsho Dermatol* 1974;16:161.
5. Itoh K, Nishitani N, Hara I. A study of cases of leucomelanodermatitis due to phenyl phenol compounds. *Bull Pharm Res Inst* 1968;76:5.
6. Mathur AK, Srivastava AK, Singh A, Gupta BN. Contact depigmentation by adhesive material of bindi. *Contact Dermatitis* 1991;24:310.
7. Bajaj AK, Gupta SC, Chatterjee AK. Contact depigmentation from free paratertiary-butylphenol in bindi adhesive. *Contact Dermatitis* 1990;22:99.
8. Bajaj AK, Gupta SC, Chatterjee AK. Contact depigmentation of the breast. *Contact Dermatitis* 1991;24:58.
9. Calnan CD. Occupational leukoderma from alkylphenols. *Proc R Soc Med* 1973;66:258.
10. Forman L. Pigmentation of the palms and scalp probably due to proprietary hair tonics, containing various phenols and phenolic derivatives. *Br J Dermatol* 1977;93:718.
11. Levantin A, Almeyda J. Drug-induced changes in pigmentation. *Br J Dermatol* 1973;89:105.
12. Burge KM, Winkelmann RF. Mercury pigmentation. *Arch Dermatol* 1970;102:51.
13. Gellin GA, Possick PA, Perone VB. Depigmentation from 4-tertiary butyl catechol—an experimental study. *J Invest Dermatol* 1970;55:190.
14. Gawkrodger DJ, Cork MJ, Bleehen SS. Occupational vitiligo and contact sensitivity to para-tertiary butyl catechol. *Contact Dermatitis* 1991;25:200.
15. Kahn G. Depigmentation caused by phenolic detergent germicides. *Arch Dermatol* 1970;102:177.
16. Bentley-Phillips B, Bayles MAH. Butylated hydroxytoluene as a skin lightener. *Arch Dermatol* 1974;109:216.
17. US Department of Health, Education and Welfare, NIOSH. *Occupational diseases—a guide to their recognition.* Washington, DC: US Government Printing Office, 1977;249.
18. Kersey P, Stevenson CJ. Vitiligo and occupational exposure to hydroquinone from servicing self-photographing machines. *Contact Dermatitis* 1981;7:285.
19. Frenk E, Loi-Zedda P. Occupational depigmentation due to a hydroquinone-containing photographic developer. *Contact Dermatitis* 1980;6:238.
20. Duffield JA. Depigmentation of the skin by quinol and its monobenzyl ether. *Lancet* 1952;1:1164.
21. Das M, Tandon A. Occupational vitiligo. *Contact Dermatitis* 1988;18:184–185.
22. Fisher AA. *Contact dermatitis,* 3rd ed. Philadelphia: Lea & Febiger, 1986.
23. Smith TL. Depigmentation from 2% hydroquinone cream. *Schoch Lett* 1981;31:48.
24. Fisher AA. Can bleaching creams containing 2% hydroquinone produce leukoderma? *J Am Acad Dermatol* 1982;7:134.
25. Jimbow K, Obata H, Pathak MA, Fitzpatrick TB. Mechanism of depigmentation by hydroquinone. *J Invest Dermatol* 1974;62:436.
26. Spencer MC. Topical use of hydroquinone for depigmentation. *J Am Acad Dermatol* 1965;194:962.
27. Engasser P, Maibach HI. Cosmetics and dermatology: bleaching creams. *J Am Acad Dermatol* 1981;5:143.
28. van Ketel WG. Sensitization to hydroquinone and the monobenzyl ether of hydroquinone. *Contact Dermatitis* 1984;10:253.
29. Vollum DI. Hypomelanosis from an antioxidant in polyethylene film. *Arch Dermatol* 1971;104:70.
30. Fisher AA. Contact dermatitis to antioxidants in cosmetics and foods. *Cutis* 1976;17:21.
31. Tosti A, Gaddoni G, Piraccini BM. Occupational leukoderma due to phenolic compounds in the ceramics industry? *Contact Dermatitis* 1991;25:67–68.
32. Frenk E, Kocsis M. Depigmentation due to adhesive tape: ultrastructural comparison with vitiligo and vitiliginous depigmentation associated with a melanoma. *Dermatologica* 1974;148:284.
33. Calnan CD, Cooke MA. Leukoderma in industry. *J Soc Occup Med* 1974;24:59.
34. Wozniak KD, Hamm G. Allergisches Kontaktekzem und vitiligoartige Depigmentierungen durch parateritiares Butylphenol. *Berufsdermatos* 1977;25:215.

35. Taylor JS, Maibach HI, Fisher AA, Bergfeld WF. Contact leukoderma associated with the use of hair colors. *Cutis* 1993;52:273–280.

36. Brancaccio R, Cohen DE. Contact leukoderma secondary to paraphenylenediamine. *Contact Dermatitis* 1995;32:313.

37. Bajaj A, Gupta S, Chatierjee A, et al. Hair dye depigmentation. *Contact Dermatitis* 1996;35:56–57.

38. Bajaj AK, Panley RK, Misra K, et al. Contact depigmentation caused by an azo dye in alta. *Contact Dermatitis* 1998;38:189–193.

39. Kanerva L, Estlander T. Contact leukoderma caused by patch testing with dental acrylics. *Am J Contact Dermatitis* 1998;9:196–198.

40. Nabai H, Mehregan A. Rubber induced depigmentation secondary to a wrist splint. *Cutis* 1994;53:295–296.

41. Mathias CGT, Maibach HI, Conant MA. Perioral leukoderma simulating vitiligo from use of a toothpaste containing cinnamic aldehyde. *Arch Dermatol* 1980;116:1172.

42. Fitzpatrick T. Vitiligo. *Int J Dermatol* 1973;12:202.

43. Fisher A. Ask the experts: the role of ocular disturbances in the differentiation of idiopathic vitiligo from contact leukoderma. *Am J Contact Dermatitis* 1997;8:53.

44. Uehara M, Miyauchi H, Tanaka S. Diminished contact sensitivity response in vitiliginous skin. *Arch Dermatol* 1984;120:195.

45. Nordlund JJ, Ferget Z, Kirkewood J, Lerner AB. Dermatitis produced by application of monobenzone in patients with active vitiligo. *Arch Dermatol* 1985;121:141.

46. Singh KK, Srinivas CR, Balachandran C, Menon S. Parthenium dermatitis sparing vitiliginous skin. *Contact Dermatitis* 1987;16:174.

47. Srinivas CR, Singh KK, Balachandran C. Textile dermatitis sparing nevoid depigmentation. *Contact Dermatitis* 1987;16:235.

48. Ehrenfeld ID. Depigmentation due to phenolic detergent germicide: treated with methoxsalen and black-lite. *Arch Dermatol* 1971;104:216.

49. Fulton JE, Leyden J, Papa C. Treatment of vitiligo with topical methoxsalen and black-lite. *Arch Dermatol* 1969;100:224.

50. Hamada T, Horiguchi S. Chronic melanodermatitis due to the rubber peephole of a ship radarscope. *Contact Dermatitis* 1978;4:245.

51. Bleehen SS, Hall-Smith P. Brassiere depigmentation: light and electron microscope studies. *Br J Dermatol* 1970;83:157.

52. Findlay GH, Morrison JGL, Simson IW. Exogenous ochronosis and pigmented colloid milium from hydroquinone bleaching creams. *Br J Dermatol* 1975;93:613.

53. Findlay GH, DeBeer HA. Chronic hydroquinone poisoning of the skin from skin-lightening cosmetics: a South African epidemic of ochronosis of the face in dark-skinned individuals. *S Afr Med J* 1980;57:187.

54. Savin JA, Hardie RA. Proprietary depigmenting cream used wrongly for lentigo maligna. *Br Med J* 1981;282:1666.

55. Garcia RL, White JW Jr, Willis WF. Hydroquinone nail pigmentation [letter]. *Arch Dermatol* 1978;114:1402.

56. Coulson IH. "Fade out" photochromonychia. *Clin Exp Dermatol* 1993;18:87.

57. Dupre A, Bonafe J-L, Virabes R, Arquie M-T. Idiopathic pigmentation of the hands: professional exogenous ochronosis? New entity? *Arch Dermatol Res* 1979;266:1.

58. O'Donoghue MN, Lynfield YL, Derbes V. Ochronosis due to hydroquinone. *J Am Acad Dermatol* 1983;1:123.

59. Hoshaw RA, Zimmerman KG, Menter A. Ochronosislike pigmentation from hydroquinone bleaching creams in American blacks. *Arch Dermatol* 1985;121:105.

60. Liao Y, Chiang Y, Tsai T, et al. Contact leukoderma melanosis induced by the leaves of *Piper betle (Piperacene)*: a clinical and histopathologic survey. *J Am Acad Dermatol* 1999;40:583–589.

CHAPTER 34

Contact Urticaria

Contact urticaria (CU) is reported frequently. The wheal-and-flare reaction that appears where certain agents contact the skin may be allergic (immunologic) (ICU) or due to agents that produce a nonallergic (nonimmunologic) contact urticaria (NICU). Some contactants affect normal, intact skin, whereas others require damaged (eczematized or fissured) skin to produce urticaria (1–3). In the nonallergic variety, the reaction is produced without any previous sensitization and can be provoked in almost all exposed individuals. The allergic variety appears only in previously sensitized individuals. A third variety of contact urticaria is due to an uncertain mechanism, in which both allergic and nonallergic mechanisms can be found. For example, the stings and bites of arthropods that pierce the skin may initially produce nonimmunologic urticaria. Some individuals, however, become sensitized. Subsequent exposure to these arthropods produces an allergic urticaria.

> As a rule, nonimmunologic contact urticaria testing is done on normal intact skin. The allergic variety may require testing on scratched or previously eczematized skin.

Some contactants are "ambidextrous," in the sense that they seem capable of being primarily urticariogenic in most individuals, but in certain sensitized patients they can also produce delayed eczematous reactions (contact dermatitis).

NONIMMUNOLOGIC CONTACT URTICARIA (NICU)

This nonimmunologic type of urticaria, occurring without previous sensitization in nearly all individuals exposed, is the most common and potentially least serious form of contact urticaria because severe systemic reactions are not evoked (Table 34.1). A direct influence on dermal vessel walls or a nonantibody-mediated release of vasoactive substances such as histamine, slow-reacting substance A, and bradykinin is the probable cause (2). The fact that nonsteroidal anti-inflammatory drugs (NSAIDs), including as-

pirin, have an inhibitory effect on NICU suggests that prostaglandins may also play some role in the reaction.

Certain agents commonly used as preservatives, fragrances, or flavoring agents in foods, soft drinks, ice cream, chewing gum, soaps, shampoos, perfumes, mouthwashes, or pharmaceutical products, such as creams or ointments, are primary urticants in many normal people. These agents include the widely used benzoic acid, sodium benzoate, sorbic acid, cinnamic acid, cinnamic aldehyde, balsam of Peru, acetic acid, butyric acid, and ethyl-, butyl-, isopropyl-, or cetyl alcohol.

The strongest urticariogenic agents are benzoic acid, sorbic acid, cinnamic acid, and cinnamic aldehyde. Most individuals will react with a localized urticarial response less than 45 minutes after application of relatively high concentrations to intact skin, such as 5% in petrolatum. Lower concentrations considerably lessen the urticarial reactions, although many will still react with some degree of erythema.

Kligman (4) showed clearly that a given agent may cause NICU at one concentration and may produce only erythema or itching at lower concentrations. Ten volunteers developed NICU to benzoic acid 2%, sorbic acid 2%, and cinnamic aldehyde 0.5% after a 10-minute exposure to normal skin of the face. After a one to 5 dilution, all 10 reacted with only erythema without a wheal. Finally, with another five-fold dilution to 0.08% or 0.02%, respectively, several, but not all, reacted with pruritus only without objective skin findings. This may explain the frequent occurrence of facial irritation from some cosmetics and topical products with negative patch tests.

> Sorbic acid, benzoic acid, cinnamic acid, and cinnamic aldehyde are strong primarily urticariogenic agents that produce contact urticaria in most individuals, both atopic and nonatopic.

Lahti (2) found that most of the skin reactions in an open test to benzoic acid 5.0%, sorbic 2.5%, and cinnamic acid 5.0% in petrolatum appeared within 45 minutes and disap-

TABLE 34.1. *Agents That Can Produce Nonallergic Contact Urticaria*

Acetic acid	Dimethyl sulfoxide
Alcohol*	Insect stings†
Balsam of Peru*	Methyl nicotinate
Benzoic acid*	Moths†
Caterpillar hair†	Sodium benzoate*
Cinnamic acid*	Sorbic acid*
Cinnamic aldehyde*	Trafuril (nicotinic acid ester)
Cobalt chloride*	

*Can also produce delayed eczematous contact dermatitis.
†Can also produce allergic contact urticaria.

peared within 2 hours. The optimum time for recording the results was 40 to 45 minutes after the application of the test substance. Atopic persons were no more liable to get NICU from these substances than nonatopic individuals, and scratching or stripping the skin did not seem to alter the urticarial response.

The feeding of capsules with benzoic acid, sorbic acid, cinnamic acid, and sodium benzoate to patients resulted in objective symptoms in 15% and subjective symptoms in 33% of the 106 patients tested. Most of the reactions might have been nonspecific and comparable to placebo reactions. No correlation was seen between the reactivity in the skin test and that in the peroral test.

Rosenhall and Zetterstron (5) challenged 100 asthma patients with benzoic acid and elicited asthma, rhinitis, or urticaria in 47 of them.

PUVA has been shown to suppress NICU to benzoic acid and methyl nicotinate (6).

Shriner and Maibach (7) reported on regional and age-based variations in reactivity to benzoic acid. Elderly subjects reacted less vigorously than younger ones. Eight sites on the neck, face, and forearm were tested with benzoic acid 2.5% pet with greater to lesser reactivity in that order.

Test Method

The most common test for nonimmunologic contact urticaria is the open test, in which a small amount of test substance is applied to the volar aspect of the intact skin of the forearm. The result is recorded after 30 to 45 minutes. The patient should be off all NSAIDs and antihistamines for at least 48 hours. Lahti et al. (8) have shown that the best vehicle for testing substances for NICU is an alcohol-water or alcohol- propylene glycol mixture.

Dimethylsulfoxide (DMSO)

Dimethylsulfoxide is also known as Sulfinylbis(methane); methyl sulfoxide; SQ 9453; DMS-70, DMS-90; Deltan; Demasorb; Demavet; Demeso; Dermasorb; Solicur; Domoso; Dromisol; Gamasol 90; Infiltrina; Hyadur;

Somipront; and Suntexan. DMSO is used therapeutically as a local analgesic, an anti-inflammatory agent, and a promoter for percutaneous penetration of certain chemicals. Although not approved in the United States for use in humans, it is often used on horses, especially for treatment of inflamed joints and tendons. DMSO causes erythema or whealing on contact.

Stoughton and Fritsch (9) reported that DMSO 20% caused transient erythema at the site of application in most subjects. Real contact urticarial lesions are frequently caused by DMSO at higher concentrations (10). Because the response may occur upon first contact, the mechanism is classified as nonimmunologic in nature.

Industrial and veterinary grades of DMSO may not be safe for humans. Furthermore, according to *Drug Therapy* (1980;11:60), the US Food and Drug Administration has warned that, because it is such a powerful solvent, DMSO may act as a "carrier" for many internally poisonous substances that do not ordinarily get through the skin. Camphor and menthol, for example, which are present in many arthritis "rubs," are quite safe when applied topically but may cause unpleasant and dangerous effects when transported through the skin and into the bloodstream by the supersolvent DMSO.

Kellum (11) reviewed the literature on DMSO and reported that no allergic contact sensitization to DMSO ever developed in a study of several hundred people. When patch tests were occluded with plastic tape, however, the primary irritant effects of DMSO were greatly enhanced. Epidermal vesiculation, histologic evidence of epidermal cell death, and a perivascular dermal infiltrate were observed. With repeated and continuous applications of DMSO to the skin (90% concentration, daily continuous application with occlusion), "hardening" (acquired tolerance to irritating compounds) was achieved by the skin of most individuals within approximately 1 month.

> **Dimethylsulfoxide (DMSO), a strong urticariogenic solvent and therapeutic agent, is a primary irritant under patch test occlusion.**

Trafuril

In Europe, the tetrahydrofurfuryl ester of nicotinic acid (Trafuril, Ciba-Geigy, Basel, Switzerland) has been used as a rubefacient in inflammatory joint diseases and in the management of mild disorders of the blood circulation of the hands and feet (12,13). Trafuril probably exerts symptomatic relief due to a direct microcirculatory effect from the erythema or a wheal and flare that follows topical application in most individuals. The erythema or wheal and flare lasts usually from 2 to 4 hours. The reaction from Trafuril varies greatly in different individuals.

> **Trafuril, an ester of nicotinic acid, is used therapeutically in Europe. It is urticariogenic in most individuals, except most atopics.**

Trafuril is not used as a therapeutic agent in the United States. However, it is permitted to be used in animal experimentation.

Vaillancourt (14) tested 72 apparently healthy subjects with Trafuril and found a local hyperemic reaction with or without edema on the application site within 5 to 10 minutes in 69 subjects. This reaction was considered to be a normal response. Patients suffering from atopic dermatitis, acute rheumatic fever, and rheumatoid arthritis had a blanching reaction instead of urticaria and erythema.

Sorbic Acid

Sorbic acid, like benzoic acid, is a widely used antimicrobial agent and is a natural preservative occurring, for example, in berries of the mountain ash *(Sorbus)* (15). It is active against molds and yeasts and to a lesser degree against bacteria. Below pH 6.5 (optimal pH 4.5) it is used as a preservative for many pharmaceutical products and foods at a concentration of up to 0.2%.

Fryklof (16) noticed that creams and ointments containing sorbic acid caused erythema and slight itching and sometimes slight edema on the face in about half of the 20 persons tested. Hjorth and Trolle-Lassen (17) confirmed the results of Fryklof and reported erythema reactions in 18 of 26 persons tested. Rietschel (18) saw a female patient who had contact urticaria from shampoo containing sorbic acid. Rietschel's patient had both skin and respiratory symptoms and was sensitive to both sorbic acid and synthetic oil of cassia. The contact urticaria could only be elicited on intact skin of the face by open testing. The source of the patient's contactants was her shampoo and toothpaste.

> **Benzoic acid and sorbic acid, at concentrations usually used for preservatives (up to 0.2%), are able to elicit immediate skin reactions that vary from erythema to a clear contact urticarial wheal-and-flare response in some persons. Such a reaction produces stinging when used in therapeutic cream and may worsen the dermatitis that is being treated.**

Benzoic Acid

Benzoic acid occurs in balsam of Peru and balsam of Tolu, in many essential oils from flowers and spices, and in berries (cranberries and other berries) (19–21). It has antibacterial and antifungal properties and is commonly used as a preservative in acidic food products. Whitfield's ointment, containing benzoic acid 6% as an antifungal agent and salicylic acid 3%, can be used in the treatment of fungal infections of the skin (22).

Repeated applications of benzoic acid in petrolatum to the same skin site diminished the whealing gradually and finally abolished it in most cases. After the disappearance of reactivity to benzoic acid, the skin was fully capable of reacting to histamine (in the scratch test). This indicates that the decreasing reactivity to benzoic acid in repeated applications was due to the emptying of the storage of mediator(s) in the skin rather than to fatigue of the dermal vessels and thus caused a failure to react. NICU from benzoic acid is probably mediated by vasoactive substances other than histamine, because the reaction was not inhibited by oral antihistamine (hydroxyzine) before the test or by emptying the histamine storage in the skin with compound 48/80 (23).

According to Lahti (23), scratching the skin did not strengthen the reactions to benzoic acid. The absorption of benzoic acid from intact skin of the back is apparently sufficient for maximal contact urticarial reactivity, and therefore the damage done to the barrier of the corneal layer did not have any enhancing influence. The mechanical trauma itself could be why the contact urticarial response was diminished in some patients.

Severe systemic immediate allergic reactions have been reported after occupational handling of materials containing benzoic acid, showing that some of the compounds, which are capable of evoking nonallergic urticaria, may exceptionally also be true sensitizers under proper conditions (19).

NICU in the perioral area from sodium benzoate has been reported (24).

> **Scratching or stripping the skin does not enhance the contract urticarial reaction from benzoic acid or other nonimmunologic urticarial agents.**

Cinnamic Acid

Cinnamic acid has been found among the constituents of the essential oils of basil, Chinese cinnamon, Styrax, oil of cinnamon, coca leaves, and balsam of Peru (25). It is used as a flavoring and fragrance ingredient in pharmaceutical preparations, food products, and perfumery (26). Cinnamic acid has antibacterial and antifungal properties similar to those of benzoic acid. Contact urticaria from cinnamic acid 5% in petrolatum occurs in most normal individuals.

Cinnamic acid may be present in sunscreens that contain cinnamates. The stinging, burning sensation that occurs from the application of such sunscreens may be due to the primary urticariogenic properties of the esters of the cinnamic acid, such as menthyl and benzyl cinnamates. In addition, the coniferyl alcohol esters of cinnamic acid may be present not only in balsam of Peru, but also in balsam of Tolu and benzoin (gum benzoin).

Cinnamic Aldehyde

Cinnamic aldehyde is a constituent of cinnamon and is one of the substances responsible for the typical odor and flavor of this spice. Its oxidation occurs readily on exposure to air, yielding cinnamic acid. Cinnamic aldehyde is used as a flavoring agent in soft drinks, chewing gum, ice cream, baked goods, dentifrices, mouthwashes, and soaps.

Contact urticaria from cinnamic aldehyde has been reported by some authors. Nater et al. (27) found erythema and edema in three patients and erythema alone in three other patients from cinnamic aldehyde 10% in alcohol. Rudzki and Grzywa (28) noted immediate reactions to both balsam of Peru and cinnamic aldehyde in two patients. Cinnamic aldehyde is also a potent sensitizer, and delayed-type allergic contact dermatitis (ACD) caused by this substance has been described by many authors (29–31).

Cinnamic aldehyde at concentrations as low as 0.01% may evoke an erythematous response associated with a burning, tingling feeling of the skin (32). Such weak, transient reactions from cinnamic aldehyde–containing products are hardly clinically significant and probably go unrecognized by the consumer in most instances; however, mild adverse effects may be an intended positive selling point adding a "lively sensation" produced in the mouth for some oral hygiene products or chewing gums.

On patch testing, cinnamic aldehyde often causes an immediate stinging reaction with or without a visible wheal and flare. Patients may mistakenly believe this is an allergic reaction. The symptoms usually dissipate within a few hours of application of the patch.

Balsam of Peru

This balsam, which contains many aromatic substances, can produce both a nonallergic contact urticaria and delayed allergic contact dermatitis (20,33,34).

Forsbeck and Skog (35) state that closed patch tests with balsam of Peru gave rise to nine immediate reactions among 121 patients with different dermatoses and to 10 reactions among 57 patients with chronic urticaria. Among compounds of balsam of Peru, cinnamic aldehyde, cinnamic acid, benzoic acid, and benzaldehyde also gave the same reactions. The reactions, which could not be transferred passively with serum from patients, were abolished by antihistamine given before testing and by pretreatment with compound 48/80. Balsam of Peru and cinnamic aldehyde did not provoke new symptoms when given orally to patients.

Quenching Effect of Eugenol

Eugenol, when applied before cinnamic aldehyde, sorbic acid, or benzoic acid to intact skin, was capable of diminishing or "quenching" the subject's NICU response to these agents (36). The mechanism is unknown, but apparently is unrelated to histamine release. The same phenomenon does not occur with delayed hypersensitivity. The clinical ramifications of this phenomenon deserve exploration.

"STINGERS" AND NICU

The cosmetic industry is concerned with the sensory irritation interpreted as "stinging" by some individuals. Those with sensitive skin "stingers" may be unable to tolerate most topicals and cosmetics, wrongly believing that they are allergic to the products (37).

The application of 10% lactic acid to the nasolabial fold is one way to separate stingers from non-stingers. Coverly et al. (38) reported that the frequency of NICU to various agents such as DMSO and benzoic acid was no different in stingers and nonstingers, nor in males and females.

ALLERGIC (IMMUNOLOGIC) CONTACT URTICARIA

The usual criteria for regarding a reaction as allergic are (a) a history of previous exposure without symptoms, (b) the degree of specific sensitization, which tends to increase with further exposure; and as a rule, a low proportion of exposed subjects that are affected. An increasing number of chemicals are being reported as being responsible for immunologic contact urticaria.

The most common immediate immunologic mechanism is probably the one mediated by IgE. Nonspecific elevation of IgE has been reported frequently in association with immunologic contact urticaria, and IgE specific for the offending antigen has been found in some cases. Although the prevalence of nonimmunologic contact urticaria is the same in atopic and nonatopic individuals, it is likely that immunologic contact urticaria is more common among atopic patients (1). Urticaria, however, may also be caused by allergic mechanisms not requiring IgE; specific IgG and perhaps also IgM might be responsible by activation of the complement flow through the classical pathway (2).

> The prevalence of nonallergic contact urticaria is the same in atopic and nonatopic individuals, whereas allergic contact urticaria is probably more common in atopic individuals mediated through IgE, but other mechanisms may be involved.

Passive Transfer

This procedure in some instances may prove that a contact urticarial reaction is immunologic. Passive transfer is accomplished by injecting 0.1 ml of freshly obtained serum from the patient into the forearm of a human volunteer or into a test animal, such as a monkey. After 24 hours, 0.1 ml of the eliciting agent is applied topically to the injection site and to a contralateral saline control site. A positive result, indicated by a wheal-and-flare response only at the donor serum injection site, is considered proof of a reaction being mediated by humoral immunologic mechanisms.

At present, the "proof" of allergic contact urticaria is done mostly by direct *in vivo* testing of the patient's skin with the suspected contactant. It is hoped that in the future *in vitro* testing will help identify specific agents in food and other contactants that are the actual causes of allergic contact urticaria.

Allergic Contact Urticaria to Rubber

Immediate IgE-mediated contact hypersensitivity to natural latex, derived from the *Hevea brasiliensis* tree, has over the last few years become one of the most important "new" dermatologic afflictions, particularly among health care workers and certain patients. Respiratory symptoms are not uncommon. Rarely, contact urticaria to additives in rubber has also been reported (see Chapter 31 for a full discussion).

ALLERGIC CONTACT URTICARIA DUE TO FOODS

A number of foods have been shown to cause ICU. These are listed in Table 34.2. Usually, cases present as an occupational hand eczema, so careful questioning may be necessary to uncover the possibility of food ICU.

It should be stressed that in these cases of "immediate" food urticarial contact dermatitis the classic delayed 48-hour patch tests are negative, and therefore scratch or immediate patch tests with the raw foods may be necessary to prove the cause of this "immediate" contact food dermatitis.

TABLE 34.2. *Foods That Have Been Reported as Producing Contact Urticaria*

Apple	Meat (chicken, lamb,
Artichoke	turkey, beef, liver,
Asparagus	venison, and pork)
Bean	Milk
Beer	Paprika
Caraway seed	Peach
Carrot	Potato
Egg	Rice
Endive	Sesame seed and oil
Fish	Shellfish
Flour	Spices
Kiwi fruit	Strawberry
Lettuce and other salad greens	

At least three control subjects should also be tested when performing scratch tests with "whole" foods. A positive reaction in the patient that is not duplicated in three controls makes it likely that the reaction is allergic in nature. It appears that these patients with allergic contact urticaria due to food handling can usually eat such foods without experiencing a "flare" of the dermatitis. It is most likely that either cooking of the foods or the action of digestive juices denatures the protein components and renders the food "hypoallergenic" for these patients. At present, however, it is not clear whether the food antigens that allergists use in testing for allergic rhinitis, asthma, and gastrointestinal allergy are also the antigens that are responsible for the immediate allergic contact urticaria of hands from handling certain foods.

> **Testing for contact urticaria to foods usually requires application of the raw food to eczematized skin or to a scratch.**

Milk

Edwards (39) described contact urticaria that developed in a child as a reaction to cow's milk. After heating the milk to 80°C for 30 seconds, the child did not have a similar reaction. This 8-month-old girl presented with urticaria on the neck, perioral, and chest areas that had developed immediately after her diet was changed from an infant formula without iron to commercial, pasteurized cow's milk. A few minutes after first drinking warm cow's milk, the baby developed a red eruption on the face that disappeared after 30 minutes. There were no systemic manifestations of allergy.

Lecks (40) reported that a child developed a severe urticarial reaction of the diaper area with an anaphylactoid reaction from the use of Diaparene Neonatal Ointment, which contains a milk protein (casein). This case report is presented to alert pediatricians, allergists, and other practicing physicians of the hazards of using Diaparene Neonatal Ointment in infants and young children exquisitely sensitive to cow's milk proteins.

Egg

Rudzki and Gryzwa (41) described a patient with contact urticaria from egg. Temesvari and Varkonyi (42) had two patients who acquired contact dermatitis from egg. One patient was a beautician who used eggs in shampoo: She was allergic to both the white and yolk of raw eggs. The ingestion of the yolk of the egg produced generalized urticaria. The second patient, who was also a hairdresser, was allergic to the white of a raw egg on epicutaneous testing.

Ushijima et al. (43) reported that a 1-year-old boy had previously experienced transient red swelling of the lips after ingestion of raw egg white. He became hoarse and vomited immediately after he took some powder from medicines containing Leftose for the treatment of a common cold. About 20 minutes later, an urticarial rash developed on the peroral and mandibular regions where the vomited materials had accumulated. The rash disappeared spontaneously within 20 minutes. Leftose is a commercial name of lysozyme chloride, which is used as a medicine in Japan for the common cold, because of its mucolytic activity. Leftose is extracted from egg white, which contains a large amount of lysozyme.

The serum IgE level was within normal limits. The RAST score to egg white was 3. An open patch test with Leftose was positive, but the test with commercially obtained antigen of egg white was negative. The Prausnitz-Küstner reaction was performed and the patient's mother, and two healthy volunteers were used. Challenges with Leftose by topical and oral application were negative. Challenge with raw egg white by oral administration, however, induced a wheal-and-flare reaction. Prausnitz-Küstner reaction using heated serum failed to produce a positive reaction.

A diaper ointment containing casein produced contact urticaria and an anaphylactoid reaction in a milk-sensitized child, and a Japanese "cold" medicine containing lysozyme derived from egg white produced similar symptoms in an egg white–sensitive infant.

Potatoes

Sensitivity to potatoes may be so severe that merely rubbing the intact skin with a raw potato may cause a wheal to form (44–46). More often a strongly positive scratch test reaction to raw potato is obtained consisting of a large wheal within 20 minutes in sensitized individuals. Scratch tests with cooked potatoes usually give negative results. Potato sensitivity can cause "housewife's hand eczema" and can be classified as an "occupational allergy" in cooks. These patients who have allergic contact sensitivity can eat cooked potatoes without any reaction.

Pearson (45), who reported potatoes to be a cause of contact urticaria and asthma, demonstrated positive passive transfer and decreased respiratory function after potatoes were scraped by the patient and the fine liquid from the ruptured potato cells was inhaled.

Patients with allergic contact urticaria from potatoes may be so sensitive that merely rubbing a raw potato on intact normal skin may elicit a large wheal and flare.

Fish

Hjorth and Roed-Petersen (47) reported that some homemakers with atopic dermatitis remarked on an aggravation of their eczematic lesions after contact with fish, particularly white haddock and herring, that caused an itching erythema within 30 minutes after contact with the allergen. An open epicutaneous test with fish on the site of a preceding eczema produced a blister (dyshidrotic blister formation) in the sensitized patient. On normal skin (on which there was no preceding eczema) an open epicutaneous test with fish (mostly haddock) resulted in an urticarial reaction in patients on the contact site. Those patients noted that their eczema got worse in contact with fish and showed a higher IgE serum level with fish.

Mitchell (48) reported that a woman with chronic hand eczema attributed the dermatitis to handling fresh shrimp. Scratch tests were carried out on the forearm flexure to the flesh (edible portion) of the shrimp (Pandalus). The raw and the boiled shrimp flesh was applied to the scratch site without covering; a drop of sea water (millipore filtered) was applied to a scratch test site as a control. Five physicians served as concomitant controls.

"Immediate" reaction to raw fish may be not only in the form of a wheal and flare but also in "vesicular reactions" forming a dyshidrotic eczema.

Evidently some agent in uncooked shrimp flesh was capable of evoking localized contact urticaria, but only when the epidermal barrier was broken by a dermatitic reaction or by an experimental scratch. The agent is heat-labile. The contact urticarial reactions were rather slower to develop than is usual with standard scratch tests, possibly from slow release of the active agent from a solid piece of flesh.

Maibach (49) reported a female atopic food-service worker who had facial irritation that she thought was related to handling seafood. Testing on the arm and hand gave no reaction, but a wheal and flare developed when shrimp was applied to the forehead. This demonstrates the need to use extraordinary testing methods at times.

Hjorth and Weissmann (50) observed a positive scratch test to prawn in a 44-year-old sandwich maker; they also found that prawns produced irritant patch test reactions.

Lombardi et al. (51) cited the case of a 12-year-old boy with atopic dermatitis who acquired contact urticaria from cod. The patch test with pieces of raw cod and an intradermal test with antigenic extract of cod both provoked an immediate specific wheal reaction. Immersion of the boy's hands and forearms in a basin of water in which a cod had been washed was followed by the appearance of urticaria, first on the contact areas and almost immediately thereafter on the face. Results of the RAST were negative, as were those of the oral challenge, which was done three times in a double-blind test with gelatin capsules filled with 15 g of cooked cod or placebo.

Beck and Nissen (52) emphasized that atopic individuals have a higher frequency of contact urticaria to fish than do nonatopic individuals.

Squid (*Loligo japonica*) may also cause contact urticaria (53).

Dominguez et al. (54), in Spain, evaluated 29 children who all had IgE-mediated fish sensitivity. Although the children were avoiding fish in the diet, incidental contact with fish produced urticaria in all and respiratory symptoms in one.

Meat

The following meats have been reported as causing allergic contact urticaria, particularly in individuals with chronic hand dermatitis: chicken, lamb, turkey, calves' liver, beef, venison, and sausage (55–61).

Fisher and Stengel (57) reported a 50-year-old butcher who had chronic dermatitis of the hands for 6 years. History revealed that the dermatitis became worse when he handled the raw calves' liver. When the calves' liver was placed at the site of a scratch on the forearm, a large wheal and flare was produced in 15 minutes. Six control subjects showed no such reaction. Chicken liver did not produce a reaction.

Fisher (58) reported a 60-year-old woman who stated that her chronic hand dermatitis was made worse by wearing rubber gloves. Routine patch testing revealed positive patch tests to nickel and mercaptobenzothiazole.

The patient stated emphatically that whenever she prepared beef hamburgers the hand dermatitis flared severely. In addition, when she ate a medium rare beef hamburger her lips swelled and she developed fissuring of the angles of the mouth resembling perlèche. She did not have any symptoms, however, when she ate a well-done hamburger. The patient was tested on normal skin, and she had no reaction to beef, pork, or chicken. The three meats were then applied to normal skin of the back on which a small scratch had been made. Each meat was gently rubbed in with a Q-Tip. Within 15 minutes an urticarial wheal without any flare appeared at the site at which the beef had been applied. No reaction was obtained with the pork or chicken. No reaction to the scratch test sites with the raw beef was obtained in six controls. It was found subsequently that the patient did not react to cooked beef at a scratch test site.

Moseng (59) reported that a male butcher's assistant, who was feeding a machine daily with pig's gut (Taiwanese import) as part of sausage production, developed urticarial, crusted, erosive lesions mainly on the extremities. Eating hot dogs produced urticaria in the patient.

Usually individuals with CU to meat react to only one animal product. One case, however, has been reported where allergy (CU) to beef, lamb, horse, and pork meat co-existed. All were positive on scratch testing, but cooked meats could be eaten with no ill effect (62).

> **Testing for contact urticaria from meat usually requires a scratch site to elicit the wheal-and-flare reaction. The patient is usually allergic to only one specific type of meat.**

Fruit

Lombardi et al. (51) reported that a 14-year-old boy had an immediate positive reaction to both the patch (with evolution to delayed eczematous reaction) and intradermal tests with peach skin; the same results with the pulp of the fruit provoked no reaction. The RAST results were negative, and the patient tolerated repeated ingestion of peeled peach and capsules containing pulp and peel (20 g), whereas handling the fruit provoked immediate urticaria on the hands and glottal edema, which immediately resolved with steroid treatment.

Andersen and Lowenstein (63) reported the possibility of contact urticaria from handling apples. They stated that most of the patients with reactions to raw potatoes and apples are atopics. Patients without any evidence of atopy, however, may also develop immediate-type reactivity to protein-like materials. The authors found that cross-reactivity between various vegetables and fruit occurs.

One case of CU to strawberry was seen in a fruit picker (64). RAST testing was negative. Kiwi fruit was implicated as causing CU in an Italian woman (65). Rather than hand eczema, her complaints were cheilitis and stomatitis. CU to litchi fruit has been reported (66).

Latex-allergic patients occasionally experience cross-reactions from handling or eating certain fruits including banana, peach, and kiwi (67).

Green Vegetables

Krook (68) reported four patients, with occupational contact dermatitis to lettuce (*Lactuca sativa*), who had cross-sensitivity to endive (*Cichorium endivia*). One of the patients also had contact urticaria to lettuce and endive, and another reacted positively to scratch tests with these vegetables as a sign of immediate allergy. In two cases such immediate allergy was considered the cause of a vesicular, intense itching eruption within a few minutes of contact with fresh leaves of *Lactuca* on previously eczematous skin. The severe chronic dermatitis of the hands of these patients is ascribed to combined delayed and immediate allergy. Another salad green, *Eruca sativa*, has also been reported to cause CU (69).

Artichoke (70) and asparagus have been reported to cause CU (71).

Carrots

Munoz et al. (22) reported a case of urticaria and upper respiratory symptoms caused by contact with carrots. Scratch tests were positive.

Beans

The winged bean *(Psophocarpus tetragonolobus)* produced facial edema in a food chemist who worked extracting the bean oil (73). In addition to a strong reaction to this bean, he reacted weakly to soybean, which is related. No other positive patch or scratch tests were found, and the patient cleared after avoiding both beans. CU, dermatitis, and rhinitis were caused in one patient by dust from castor beans (74).

Rice

A young woman developed widespread urticaria and dyspnea after a wedding ceremony at which she had thrown rice (75). She had no problem eating cooked rice. Prick tests were positive to rice, with weak reactions to corn, peanut, and beans. Apparently, these other foods did not provoke symptoms.

Potato

An atopic individual with coexistent allergy to potato and latex has been reported. IgE to both was present. Both skin and respiratory symptoms occurred (76).

Beer

Van Ketel (77) reported contact urticaria from beer, but not from other alcoholic beverages. A 30-year-old woman, after entering a bar, noted that her face became red, swollen, and itchy after staying for 1 or 2 minutes. She showed the same symptoms in a room where visitors were drinking beer. After her husband had drunk a glass of beer, kissing him on the mouth provoked redness and itching of the lips and surrounding skin within a few minutes. When her husband drank any other alcoholic drink she tolerated kissing without any trouble. The patient herself tolerated drinking other alcoholic beverages very well. She refused to drink any kind of beer because on one occasion she developed shock after drinking a mouthful of beer.

A scratch test with beer was performed on the forearm. The reaction was positive in a few minutes and was strong after 20 minutes. The edema around the test site spread to the upper arm, which became swollen within 30 minutes after the test. These symptoms disappeared after 2 hours.

Plants and Seeds

Heygi and Dolezalova (78) described a female patient who was so allergic to caraway seeds that patch tests with this spice and the use of toothpastes and a soap containing caraway seed oil produced urticaria and syncope. Sunflower seeds, poppy flowers, mulberry pollen, lupin (pea), and gerbera have been reported to cause CU (79–83).

In a study of Danish gardeners, 35 of 105 (33%) tested had an immediate reaction to one or more plants. Most were atopic. Symptoms tended to be rather minor and short-lived (84).

Other Food-Related Allergens

Cellulase enzyme used in the production of starch and amylase can cause occupational CU (85–87).

Occupational CU has been reported from paprika (88).

Sesame seed oil has been reported to cause CU in two nonatopic subjects. In both cases, both CU from cosmetic products and generalized urticaria from foods with sesame seed or oil occurred (89).

ALLERGIC CONTACT URTICARIA FROM TOPICAL MEDICATIONS

Allergic contact urticaria may occur from the active ingredient in topical medications or from preservatives, solvents, and emulsifying agents in the topical medication.

Antibiotics

Most of the antibiotics shown in Table 34.3 that have produced contact urticaria have also produced anaphylactic reactions when tested in various ways.

Penicillin

Penicillin is no longer used topically in the United States because it is such a common and potent sensitizer. Maucher (90) and Haustein (91) produced urticaria followed by systemic allergic reactions in three patients with severe hypersensitivity to systemic penicillin by patch testing with penicillin. Boonk (92) has shown that "hidden contacts" with penicillin may produce contact urticaria.

Neomycin

This antibiotic, which is a common cause of delayed eczematous contact dermatitis, can also cause allergic con-

TABLE 34.3. *Antibiotics Capable of Producing Allergic Contact Urticaria*

Bacitracin*	Neomycin†
Cephalosporins	Penicillin†
Chloramphenicol†	Rifamycin
Gentamycin	Streptomycin*

*Intradermal test has produced anaphylaxis.
†Closed patch test has produced anaphylaxis.

tact urticaria and even anaphylactic shock when used topically, and even by a patch test procedure (90,93). Pippen (94) reported a patient with delayed hypersensitivity to neomycin in whom anaphylaxis developed after this chemical was applied inadvertently to a stasis ulcer (94).

> **Penicillin and neomycin may produce contact urticaria at a patch test site, as well as generalized urticaria in certain sensitized individuals.**

Bacitracin

Roupe and Strannegard (95) cited a case of anaphylactic shock after topical administration of an ointment containing bacitracin and neomycin. Antibacitracin reagins were demonstrated in sera from this patient with atopic dermatitis, and there is strong evidence that the anaphylactic reaction was due to hypersensitivity to bacitracin.

Comaish and Cunliffe (96) reported that bacitracin applied to a varicose ulcer may also produce an anaphylactic reaction; circulating antibacitracin reagins could be demonstrated, and intracutaneous testing may produce anaphylaxis.

Bjorkner and Moller (97), however, studied three patients allergic to bacitracin, all of whom also had positive tests to neomycin. After intracutaneous injection of bacitracin, the three patients showed a delayed eczematous reaction. A strong immediate wheal-and-flare reaction was also induced. This was inhibited by a simultaneous local injection of the antihistamine mepyramine, which also abolished the vascular response to histamine and to the histamine liberator polymyxin B. Depletion of cutaneous histamine by pretreatment with polymyxin B diminished the wheal and flare induced by bacitracin. The authors concluded that the vascular effects of intracutaneous bacitracin in human skin are due to a release of histamine. The immediate wheal and flare was the same in healthy controls as in the three patients with delayed hypersensitivity to bacitracin. Thus, the intracutaneous test with bacitracin did not disclose any signs of circulating reagins, as have been demonstrated in cases of anaphylaxis cited by Roupe and Strannegard (95) and Comaish and Cunliffe (96).

> **Intracutaneous bacitracin has been reported as producing anaphylaxis in bacitracin-sensitive patients. One study, however, reveals that intracutaneous bacitracin produces a wheal and flare in normal individuals.**

Haustein's case (91) of anaphylactic shock elicited by topical administration of bacitracin would implicate circulating reagins against bacitracin.

Streptomycin

Levene and Withers (98) demonstrated anaphylaxis to topical streptomycin. The patient had an anaphylactic reaction from intradermal testing. Rudzki et al. (99) described a nurse who worked in a tuberculosis sanatorium who developed a contact urticaria from streptomycin. Two minutes after several drops of streptomycin prepared for injection were placed on her forearm, a large wheal appeared; a few minutes later, rhinitis and lacrimation developed, which required hydrocortisone administration.

Chloramphenicol

Kosakava (100) cited a patient sensitized to chloramphenicol who had an anaphylactoid reaction from a closed patch test.

Cephalosporins

Tuft (101) studied an instance of contact urticaria that resulted from an acquired sensitization to cephalosporin compounds in a chemist. Patch tests elicited an immediate urticarial response. Similar control tests with other antibiotics gave negative results. Although the patient's primary complaint was urticaria, prolonged or excessive contact with the cephalosporin also caused coryza and syncope. There was, however, no recurrence of symptoms after the patient transferred to another laboratory in which he worked with other chemicals.

A number of cases of occupational CU to cefotiam dihydrochloride have been observed in Japan (102).

> **Closed patch testing with patients sensitized to penicillin, neomycin, or chloramphenicol may produce anaphylaxis. Intradermal testing with bacitracin and streptomycin may result in anaphylaxis.**

Rifamycin

Rifamycin is an antibiotic derived from *Streptomyces mediterranei*. It has twice been reported to cause CU after use on a cutaneous ulcer. In one instance anaphylaxis and shock occurred (103). In this case, an open test produced urticaria and a Prausnitz-Küstner test was positive, indicating a serum factor, probably IgE, was causative.

Gentamycin

Maucher (90) reported that patch testing with this antibiotic can produce an urticarial reaction in sensitized individuals.

TABLE 34.4. *Allergic Contact Urticaria: Miscellaneous Topical Medications*

Aescin
Aminophenazone
Benzocaine
Benzophenone
Chloramine-T
Chlorhexidine
Chlorocresol
Chlorpromazine
Cisplatin
Diphenylcyclopropenone, DNCB, SADBE
Lindane
Menthol
Nitrogen mustard (mechlorethamine)
Promethazine
Vitamin E oil

DNCB, dinitro chlorobenzene; SADBE, squaric acid dibutyl ester.

Miscellaneous Topical Medications (Table 34.4)

Table 34.4 lists other typical medications that have produced allergic contact urticaria.

Aescin

Aescin, an extract of the horse chestnut *(Aesculus hippocastanum)*, caused CU in a patient who was using a product cointaining this substance as a topical balm for knee pain. A prick test was positive but was negative in 10 controls (104).

Aminopyrine (Pyramidon)

Camarasa et al. (105) described an unusual case of contact urticaria. A boy had had a Cibalgine suppository inserted, which is composed of aminophenazone and allobarbital. The mother developed a strong, itching sensation on one hand immediately after touching her son upon his return from the operating room after a tonsillectomy. Within a few minutes, a pronounced edema of the face and eyelids commenced and became generalized to an alarming degree. She was admitted to an intensive care unit.

Patch tests with a Cibalgine suppository resulted in a 3+ urticarial reaction (wheal) after 5 minutes, which evolved into an acute generalized urticaria after a further 5 minutes, requiring treatment with epinephrine. Patch testing with the aminopyrine gave an immediate strong urticarial reaction. Testing with allobarbital was negative. The lymphocyte transformation test was positive for aminopyrine. The mechanism of transfer from the son's skin to the patient's hand remains unknown in this case.

Benzocaine

This topical anesthetic, which is not an uncommon cause of delayed eczematous contact dermatitis, can also on rare occasions produce contact urticaria.

Ryan et al. (106) reported that a 39-year-old man developed edema and vesiculation of the oral mucosa after the application of benzocaine (Hurricane) gel. Open testing demonstrated an immediate urticarial reaction. Closed patch tests were positive after 48 hours. The contact dermatitis was consistent with delayed-type hypersensitivity. The authors concluded that a nonimmunologic mechanism caused the contact urticaria because passive transfer was negative. The fact that passive transfer was negative does not necessarily mean, however, that a nonallergic mechanism was not involved, because passive transfer is not always successful and benzocaine does not produce urticaria in controls.

Rudner (107) described a 77-year-old woman who developed swelling of lips 2 days after applying Anbesol (alcohol, benzocaine, phenol, and iodine) pomade. There was no prior dermatitis or prior "caine" exposure. Anbesol was applied to the patient's forearm after her original lip lesion had cleared up. Several hours later, there was localized redness and swelling at the site of application of the Anbesol. The possibility exists that the reaction was due to benzocaine. Although passive transfer was not attempted, Rudner (107) concluded that this case was a classic example of immunologic contact urticaria.

Benzophenone

Ramsay et al. (108) found a man with a broad-spectrum light sensitivity who demonstrated simultaneously an urticarial and contact sensitivity to a preparation containing 5-benzoyl-4-hydroxy-2-methoxybenzene sulfonic acid (sulisobenzone). Both the benzophenone and the sulfonic acid parts of the molecule were required for elicitation of the contact dermatitis reaction, although benzophenone alone elicited only the urticarial reaction.

Chloramine-T

CU and rhinitis have been reported from use of this agent, which is a topical disinfectant. A hospital bath attendant in Finland with hand dermatitis from using a cleaner containing this agent had greatly elevated IgE antibodies to the agent. Allergic asthma can be caused by this agent also (109).

Chlorpromazine and Promethazine

Horio (110) described a 54-year-old woman who had a recurrent pruritic eruption in light-exposed areas. She had a combination of three types of hypersensitivity to chlorpromazine: allergic contact dermatitis, photocontact dermatitis, and immediate allergic photosensitivity. Immediate wheal reactions were found after long-wave ultraviolet light irradiation of photopatch test and intradermal injection sites with chlorpromazine. These responses were differentiated from phototoxic reactions. A positive passive transfer reaction was also observed.

Haustein (91) stated that promethazine produced shock and urticaria after patch testing with promethazine.

Chlorhexidine

Several reports of CU to chlorhexidine have been published (111–113). One person had both ACD and CU. The other developed respiratory symptoms as well as urticaria. Contact anaphylaxis has been reported from exposure to chlorhexidine during a skin graft procedure and from a wound care cleanser. In both cases, prick tests were positive (114,115).

Most cases have been reported in Japanese patients, the significance of which is uncertain (116).

Chlorocresol

This disinfectant, in an aviary incubator cleaning solution, caused CU in a 28-year-old worker (117).

Cisplatin

A nurse developed CU thought to be due to this anti-cancer drug. Open tests were positive to two platinum salts (118).

Diphenylcyclopropenone (DPC), Dinitrochlorobenzene (DNCB), and Squaric Acid Dibutyl Ester (SADBE)

DPC is used as a topical immunotherapeutic agent in the treatment of viral warts and alopecia areata. Tosti et al. (119) reported generalized urticaria in four patients using DPC for alopecia. Concentrations as low as 0.05% were enough to produce symptoms. A total of 127 patients were treated with DPC during this period. DNCB caused CU and dyspnea in one unrelated case also used for alopecia (120). Fowler has observed occasional instances of CU in patients treated with squaric acid immunotherapy for warts.

Vitamin E Oil Used Topically

Many individuals pierce vitamin E capsules and rub the contents into their skin to "remove" wrinkles and to improve the "tone" of the skin. Such efforts are, of course, in vain, because there is no therapeutic effect from such inunctions. Several patients have developed delayed allergic contact dermatitis and also contact urticaria from the application of vitamin E oil (121).

Mitchell (122) described two boys who developed localized then partially generalized urticaria from application of a vitamin E preparation for thermal burns. The mother had pricked a capsule of vitamin E and applied the oil from the capsule twice daily for 3 days; no covering was applied. One week after the last application, confluent papular erythema appeared around the burn site. This erythema became urticarial and disseminated widely on the trunk in a diffuse pattern, extending to a patchy pattern, but was maximal around the burn site. In addition, erythematous urticar-

ial wheals appeared on the face. The eruption faded during 1 week with peeling of the skin. Patch tests to the vitamin E and the vehicle were not carried out.

Menthol

Papa and Shelley (123) described a case of menthol hypersensitivity that produced a chronic urticaria and a diagnostic basophil response.

Nitrogen Mustard

Grunnet (124) studied a 36-year-old woman and a 16-year-old boy, both suffering from mycosis fungoides, who developed urticaria and an anaphylactoid reaction after topical whole body application of nitrogen mustard. Prick tests with nitrogen mustard solution produced a wheal-and-flare response. Both patients had previously been treated intermittently with total body applications of nitrogen mustard for 2 years and 1 year, respectively, without complications.

Daughters et al. (125) reported on a 68-year-old woman with mycosis fungoides en plaque who had severe dyspnea, urticaria, pruritus, and swelling of her hands 5 minutes after topical total body application of nitrogen mustard. In the preceding 5 years, she had been treated at least 100 times with this chemical topically without having allergic manifestations. Six weeks after her reaction, open epicutaneous application of nitrogen mustard produced a wheal-and-flare response at the test site. This was followed by signs of anaphylaxis.

Contact Urticaria Due to Vehicle Ingredients of Topical Medication

Various solvents and preservatives in topical medications listed in Table 34.5 may produce allergic contact urticaria.

Benzyl Alcohol

Edwards (126) presented a patient with immediate urticarial and delayed hypersensitivity to benzyl alcohol present in a sunscreen.

Emulgade F

This emulsifier, containing cetyl stearyl alcohol, was suspected of causing CU and anaphylaxis (127). Later patch testing reproduced the anaphylactoid symptoms.

TABLE 34.5. *Contact Urticaria—Vehicle Ingredients of Topical Medicaments*

Benzyl alcohol (sunscreen)	Petrolatum
Emulgade F	Polyethylene glycol
Monoamylamine	Polysorbate 60
Organic mercurials	Sorbitan sesquioleate
Parabens	

Monoamylamine

Tharp (128) reported that monoamylamine, an ingredient of tolnaftate (Tinactin) cream, produced both an immediate urticarial reaction and a delayed eczematous response. The monoamylamine in the Tinactin is an organic neutralizing agent that is being used specifically to adjust the pH of the cream so that it will thicken.

Organic Mercurials

Mercurochrome (thimerosal) has been reported to cause CU and anaphylaxis after use on superficial abrasions (129,130).

Mathews (131) studied a physician who had asthma and urticaria, which was traced to hospital-laundered bed linens and uniforms. Scratch tests with phenylmercuric propionate, present as an antibacterial fabric softener used in the hospital laundry, produced a wheal-and-flare response. Provocative inhalation tests produced asthma within 5 minutes.

Parabens

Henry et al. (132) stated that this preservative, which is a fairly common cause of delayed eczematous hypersensitivity, can also produce allergic contact urticaria, such as developed in a patient after topical application of paraben-containing compounds. Positive open patch test results and a positive passive transfer (Prausnitz-Küstner reaction) test demonstrated an immunologic mechanism for the patient's skin reaction.

Petrolatum

CU with a positive open application test and positive delayed patch tests to all allergens in petrolatum has been reported (133).

Polyethylene Glycol (PEG)

Fisher (134) reported that two patients had an immediate contact reaction from polyethylene glycol 400 used as a solvent in Tinactin and Lotrimin antifungal lotions. A third patient had a similar reaction to PEG 300 in Americaine Otic Solution. In all three instances, a wheal and flare occurred by rubbing in the PEG into the intact skin of the forearm of the sensitized patients.

Polysorbate 60

Maibach and Conant (135) studied an adult male patient who noted redness on his forehead when applying 1% hydrocortisone cream. Testing revealed that application of the hydrocortisone cream produced urticaria only on the forehead but not on the back or forearm. The chemical responsi-

ble in the cream was determined to be polysorbate 60, an emulsifying agent that is a mixture of stearate esters of sorbitol and sorbitol anhydrides, consisting predominately of the mono ester. It is also known as Tween 60 (ICI America), Polyoxyethylene 20 sorbitan monostearate, Emsorb 6905 (Emery), and Armotan-20 (Armak).

It should be noted that polysorbate 60 is not related to sorbic acid, which is a primary urticariogenic agent.

Sorbitan Sesquioleate

This emulsifier in a corticosteroid ointment has caused CU (136).

ALLERGIC CONTACT URTICARIA FROM VARIOUS METALS

Aluminum

An atopic woman with simultaneous CU and ACD to nickel and aluminum has been reported. Symptoms were controlled by chronic antihistamine use (cetirizine 10 to 20 mg/day) (137).

Iridium

A worker in an electrochemical factory developed CU to iridium. A prick test with iridium chloride was weakly positive, but a scratch test produced anaphylaxis. Testing with platinum, a potential contaminant of the iridium solution, was negative, as was testing in controls (138).

Nickel

Osmundsen (139) reported two patients in whom urticaria was elicited by contact with nickel-containing objects. A chamber-prick test with nickel sulfate 2.5% in petrolatum evoked a strong urticarial reaction in both patients. A 48-hour delayed patch test reaction was positive in these patients. In addition, a 20-minute patch test with nickel sulfate 2.5% in petrolatum or normal appearing skin on the forearm was negative. A chamber-prick test (material applied to a prick on the skin and covered by a Finn chamber) with nickel sulfate 2.5% in petrolatum elicited in 20 minutes a strong urticarial reaction with pseudopods and a large flare, measuring 8 by 15 cm. The patient experienced an intense itching starting about 1 minute after the application of the test material.

Chamber-prick tests with nickel sulfate 2.5% in petrolatum, performed in five patients with ordinary nickel dermatitis (and with positive 48-hour patch tests) and in three patients with chronic urticaria, revealed no immediate reaction. The author was not aware of any previous report on clinically relevant immediate reactions to nickel. These responses to nickel were apparently clinically relevant, but it is uncertain whether they are due to immunologic or nonimmunologic mechanisms. If an immunologic mechanism is accepted, immediate hypersensitivity is coexistent with delayed hypersensitivity to nickel (139).

Rhodium

Nakayama and Imai (140) reported that 17 of 50 workers at a major precious metal factory had suffered from contact urticaria, contact dermatitis, and asthma for the preceding 9 years. Scratch patch test for 1 hour using a Finn chamber revealed that 9 of 12 patients were sensitized with platinum and 7 of 12 patients with rhodium as far as the immediate-type hypersensitivity was concerned. A closed patch test for 48 hours revealed that the patients were sensitized to rhodium, platinum, and mercury.

Platinum

Osmundsen (139), Key (141), and Levene (142) investigated allergic contact urticaria from industrial exposures to platinum salts.

> The metals nickel, rhodium, iridium, and platinum can produce allergic contact urticaria.

NONALLERGIC CONTACT URTICARIA FROM METALS

The only metal that has been implicated in such a reaction is cobalt chloride. Cobalt chloride is often used as a color indicator in experimental sweat tests. It produces allergic contact dermatitis, tuberculin-like reactions, and urticaria when injected intradermally. Smith et al. (143) reported contact urticaria from cobalt chloride and suggested that histamine or other vasoactive substances are at least partially responsible for the reaction.

Contact urticaria from cobalt chloride is evidently not a rare event. The precise mechanism causing urtication is unknown, but it is suggested that cobalt chloride in an alcoholic solution induces the release of vasoactive amines from mast cells through a nonimmunologic means (144).

ALLERGIC CONTACT URTICARIA FROM VARIOUS CHEMICALS

Several types of chemicals have been implicated as causing an immunologic type of contact urticaria (Table 34.6). Key (141) stated that occupational urticaria is usually caused by inhalation of an allergenic material. Occasionally, however, chemicals can cause generalized urticaria by cutaneous contact and percutaneous absorption. Exposures that have been productive of occupational urticaria are shown in Table 34.7.

TABLE 34.6. *Allergic Contact Urticaria: Miscellaneous Contactants*

Acrylic monomer
Alcohol
Butyl-hydroxytoluene
Diethyltoluamide
Formaldehyde (leather) (spray starch)
Metals:
    Aluminum
    Iridium
    Nickel
    Platinum
    Rhodium
Oleylamide
Phenylmercuric propionate
Protein hydrolysates in hair conditioners
Sodium silicate
Spray starch
Terpinyl acetate
Vinyl pyridine
Woods
Xylene

Acrylic Acid

Although acrylates are common causes of ACD, acrylic acid is not thought of as a sensitizer. Acrylic acid, also known as 2-propenoic acid, is a basic monomer used in manufacturing more complex molecules. Fowler (145) reported a chemical laboratory worker who developed CU on exposed surfaces while at work. Respiratory symptoms did not occur. Imme-

TABLE 34.7. *Materials Causing Contact Urticaria in Industry*

Materials	Industrial exposures
Acrylic acid	Plastics workers
Aliphatic polyamines	Epoxy resin workers
Aminothiazole	Pharmaceutical workers
Ammonia	Ammonia workers
Castor bean pomade	Castor oil extractors, fertilizer workers, and farmers
Chlorothalonil	Nursery or forestry workers
Complex platinum salts	Platinum refiners
Epoxy resins and related hardeners	Plastics, aircraft, and electronics workers
Formaldehyde	Phenolic and amino resin workers, fumigators, and laboratory workers
Glyceryl thioglycolate	Hairdressers
Lindane insecticide	Workers and cotton dusters
Penicillin	Pharmaceutical workers and nurses
Sodium sulfide	Photographers, workers with dyes, tanning, and hides
Spices	Spice workers, bakers, and sausage makers
Sulfur dioxide	Paper mill workers
Trichloroethane	Glass and metal cleaners
Vinyl pyrilidine	Chemistry research workers
Xylene	Chemistry research workers

diate testing revealed severe pruritus and a 3-cm wheal within 60 seconds after application of acrylic acid in 2% olive oil. Six controls were negative. A typical 2+ patch test reaction was present at the site after 48 hours, although the material had been wiped off the arm after 2 minutes.

Alcohol

Ophaswongse and Maibach (146) have reviewed cutaneous reactions to alcohols. Both NICU and immunologic CU have been reported, primarily from ethanol. Exposure may occur in medical and restaurant personnel and from recreational use.

Fowler has seen a case of anaphylaxis induced by drinking champagne, with a positive prick test to grape (personal communication, Dr. Hobert Pence, Louisville, KY, 1998).

Chlorothalonil

This agent is an agricultural fungicide and wood preservative. A tree nursery worker suffered CU and respiratory symptoms from handling seedlings that were treated with it (147). Anaphylaxis was reproduced by patch testing.

Diethyltoluamide (DEET)

Maibach and Johnson (148) showed that Deet, a popular insect repellent, can cause an allergic contact urticaria syndrome.

Denatonium Benzoate (Denaturing Agent for Alcohol)

Bjorkner (149) reported that a 30-year-old maid developed asthma and pruritus after using an insecticidal spray (Pyrex). The same symptoms appeared with an alcoholic skin disinfectant (M-sprit) and other preparations denatured with denatonium benzoate (Bitrex). An open epicutaneous test (20 minutes) showed a wheal and erythema to Pyrex, M-sprit, and Bitrex diluted to 2×10^{-6} mg 1^{-1}.

Denatonium benzoate was first used as a denaturant for alcohol in toilet preparations in 1960. M-sprit consists of 70% ethanol in water; denatonium benzoate is a commonly used skin disinfectant in many Swedish hospitals.

Formaldehyde

Formaldehyde and related compounds are extremely common causes of ACD. CU from formaldehyde has been reported in a dialysis patient. Prick and patch tests were positive. Specific IgE was present (150). Formaldehyde vapors may also cause allergic asthma.

Gases

Ammonia and simple gaseous compounds have been shown to produce contact urticaria (151–153).

Glyceryl Thioglycolate

Although a common cause of ACD in hairdressers, CU is unusual. A case with positive prick test and negative patch tests has been reported (154).

Naphthylacetic Acid

This agent, used as a plant growth regulator, produced one case of CU (155).

Paraphenylenediamine (PPDA) and Other Dyes

Temesvari (156) reported that PPDA caused CU in three patients; two reacted to hair dye and one to colored cotton thread. Contact anaphylaxis has also been reported (157).

Basic Blue Dye No. 99 caused CU in an elderly woman from a semipermanent hair coloring product. The dye (CI 56059; CAS 68123-13-7) is an aminoketone (158).

Plastics

In one case plastic folders and PVC provoked strong urticarial reactions on unbroken skin after 20 minutes (139). These reactions correlated with the clinical history. The plastic materials that provoked the contact urticaria contained BHT or oleylamide. A 20-minute patch test with several articles of plastic (polyethylene and PVC) and with butylhydroxytoluene (BHT) 1% in ethanol elicited urticarial reactions. BHT is used as an antioxidant in plastic. Furthermore, open patch test with oleylamide (amide of oleic acid) 0.1% in ethanol elicited a strong urticarial reaction in 20 minutes. This chemical is used as a slipping agent in plastic.

A patient working with electronic components was proven to have CU to polypropylene used in capacitors (159).

Epoxy resin and the diluents phenylglycidyl ether and cresylglycidyl ether caused CU and respiratory symptoms in an aircraft factory worker. (160)

Phthalic anhydrides, epoxy resin hardeners, can also produce CU and respiratory symptoms. (161)

Polyfunctional aziridine, used as a cross-linker in epoxy systems, caused ACD in two and CU in one patient. (162)

Diphenylmethane-4,4-diisocyanate (MDI) caused CU in an atopic carpenter. RAST tests were positive to MDI and to related isocyanates. (163)

Protein Hydrolysates

These substances, which are derived from natural proteins such as collagen, keratin, and silk, are used to "repair" broken hairs or split ends. Niinimaki et al. (164) studied 11 hairdressers with hand dermatitis by prick testing them to 22 protein hydrolysates. All were atopic, and all reacted to Crotein Q, hydroxypropyl trimonium hydrolyzed collagen.

A nonoccupational case with anaphylactoid symptoms has also been reported in a nonatopic woman (165).

Sodium Silicate

Tanaka et al. (166) described an unusual combination of a primary irritant effect from sodium silicate with an allergic contact urticarial reaction and the production of ulcerative contact dermatitis. The patient had had recurrent ulcerative lesions on his left hand for 2 years. The ulcers were associated with chronic eczematous changes resulting from primary irritant contact dermatitis. The patient also had CU from sodium silicate. An immediate wheal-and-flare reaction was found 15 minutes after application of sodium silicate to a scratch test site. This response was not seen in healthy control subjects. The coexistence of primary irritant contact dermatitis and contact urticaria, both induced by sodium silicate, has not previously been described.

Solvents

Xylene

Altman (167) described an acute urticarial reaction to xylene in a patient who was allergic to this solvent in her work. More recently, cases have been reported in medical laboratory technicians and in several factory workers (168–170).

CU and a serum sickness–like reaction have been reported from exposure to a cleaning solvent used in a clothing factory (N355) containing xylene, cumene, and trimethylbenzene (171).

Methyl Ethyl Ketone (MEK)

An Australian painter showed a positive open patch test to MEK and had severe irritation from occupational contact (172).

Trichloroethane (TCE)

Fowler (173) reported a woman employed at an eyeglass manufacturer who developed urticaria on exposed surfaces when working with TCE cleaning glass lenses. Routine patch testing was negative. A positive 1-cm wheal developed after a 20-minute closed patch test on the forearm. Six controls were negative. The patient eventually had to change jobs because she could not find an area of the factory where she was free of symptoms.

Wood

Hausen (174) stated that some species of wood or wood shavings may produce nonimmunologic types of reactions, although immediate reactions based on immunologic mechanisms are more characteristic. Species that have induced

such immunologic reactions include obeche, larch, limba, and occasionally teak. A state of allergic sensitivity is proved by rubbing the patient's skin, moistened slightly before by water, with a piece of the suspected wood species 20 to 30 times on the forearm. By this process, urticarial reactions are produced within several minutes, yielding a large wheal and flare, while the nonoffending species remain negative.

Mukali wood (Aningeria robusta), a member of the Sapotaceae family, produced occupational asthma and CU in a woodworker (175).

ALLERGIC CONTACT URTICARIA FROM ANIMALS, INSECTS, THEIR APPENDAGES, AND SECRETIONS

Allergic contact urticaria may occur from animal hair, dander, saliva, serum, placenta, and even human seminal fluid (Table 34.8).

Rat Tails

Rudzki et al. (99) showed that a psychologist who experimented with rats developed urticaria, rhinitis, and conjunctivitis. He developed contact urticaria 5 minutes after his forearm touched a rat's tail.

Guinea Pigs

Rudzki et al. (99) described a nurse who developed contact urticaria from handling guinea pigs.

Saliva (Dog and Rat)

Calnan (176) reported a patient who acquired allergic CU from dog saliva. Fowler has seen a case in a veterinarian who reacted to dog saliva but not to dog hair.

Burrows (177) stated that in companies in which large numbers of rats are used experimentally, asthma, hay fever, and urticaria are common among research workers. The problem seems to occur particularly with rats. Those people

TABLE 34.8. *Allergic Contact Urticaria from Animals and Animal Products*

Saliva (dog, rat)
Hair
Seminal fluid (human)
Dander
Serum
Placenta
Jellyfish, Portuguese man-of-war
Bovine blood and amniotic fluid (cow)
Cockroach, mites, midges
Rat's tail
Guinea pig

carrying out experiments rather than the animal-house attendants are affected. This finding would suggest that the allergen is contained in internal secretions such as saliva rather than in hair or skin. This problem is so great in some laboratories that a labor problem is created.

Hair and Dander

Allergic contact urticaria was reported by Rudzki and Gryzwa (178) from animal hair, and Uehara and Ofuji (179) obtained positive patch test reactions to human dander in 120 of 181 (66%) patients with atopic dermatitis, in 2 of 28 (7%) patients with allergic contact dermatitis, and in 1 of 31 (3%) normal controls. The frequency of positive reactions was significantly higher in patients with atopic dermatitis. The reactions consisted of erythema and papules, which showed histologically an eczematous change at the upper parts of hair follicles. It is suggested that certain patients with atopic dermatitis exhibit contact hypersensitivity to human dander. Whether or not the hypersensitivity has any relationship to the pathogenesis of the dermatitis was not determined by this study.

Human Seminal Fluid

The first report of a case of an allergic reaction in a woman to male semen was published by Halpern et al. (180) in 1967. They showed that the condition was mediated by a skin-sensitizing antibody now known as IgE. Additional patients with allergy to seminal fluid have been reported in the literature (181–184). Mikkelsen et al. (185) reported a woman who acquired an urticarial and anaphylactic reaction to male semen. Skin tests with her husband's semen produced a wheal and flare. An IgE reaginic antiseminal plasma antibody was found. No agglutinating antibody for suspensions of washed spermatozoa was found when the husband's dead spermatozoa or living or dead spermatozoa of a group O donor were used.

Mathias et al. (186) studied a woman with atopic dermatitis who experienced anaphylactic episodes after intercourse with her husband, with subsequent exacerbations of her atopic dermatitis. Skin testing and an *in vitro* leukocyte histamine release assay established the diagnosis of immediate hypersensitivity to her husband's seminal fluid; delayed hypersensitivity to seminal fluid could not be demonstrated. Antigen was found in the seminal fluid of nonrelated men. Radioallergosorbent testing detected the presence of circulating IgE antibodies specific for seminal plasma protein. Immunotherapy with seminal plasma may have limited the severity of a subsequent reaction. Serum from the husband and nonrelated men also contained antigen that provoked histamine release from the patient's leukocytes *in vitro*. The antigen in serum was associated with the globulin fraction and had a temporal relationship to ejaculation, appearing within 12 hours of ejaculation and disappearing within 4 days.

Bovine Blood and Amniotic Fluid

Degreef (187) reported a case of protein contact dermatitis with positive RAST tests to fresh bovine blood and amniotic fluid in a veterinary surgeon who suffered for 2 years from itching skin lesions on his arms and face, which were aggravated when he performed a cesarean section on a cow.

The following RAST tests clinched the diagnosis:

1. Bovine amniotic fluid: 1,889 counts +++ (control: 380 counts)
2. Bovine blood: 1,623 counts +++ (control: 662 counts)
3. Bovine blood and amniotic fluid: 1,153 counts +++ (control: 372 counts)

Placenta of Cow

Schmidt (188) observed a "verified" case of contact urticaria of the immunologic type in a veterinary surgeon. After 2 years in his job, the patient started to feel itching localized to his arms and only occurring when he loosened the placenta from cows. The placenta is normally removed between 12 and 24 hours after delivery. He did not observe any trouble when working with horses, pigs, or other domestic animals. His total IgE in serum was 91 mg/ml, and he showed a positive RAST test to a cow but a negative RAST to a cat and a horse. With a prick test, a +++ reaction to cow was produced. The patient showed a 3-mm reaction to amniotic fluid and a large 25-mm reaction to chorion-allantoic fluid and to the placenta from a cow. As his reaction became worse, he had to leave his job as a veterinary surgeon.

Fowler observed a similar case in a veterinarian who developed CU when delivering calves and the placenta. Prick test to bovine vaginal secretions was positive.

Jellyfish and Portuguese Man-of-War

The stings of these coelenterates will produce a nonimmunologic linear papular urticaria in almost all individuals. Hartmann et al. (189) stated that the results of a preliminary screening of serum from patients varying in their reaction to envenomations indicate the potential of these toxin proteins to induce an allergic state in humans and illustrate the use of the RAST as a screening device to detect persons sensitive to coelenterate stings.

The coelenterate venom produces nonspecific damage to human skin and also lyses human basophils *in vitro*. This experiment demonstrates the immunogenicity of the toxins and their potential for inducing an allergic state, a previously unrealized aspect of coelenterate envenomation. Further discussion of this topic is found in Chapter 37.

Jellyfish and Portuguese man-of-war produce a nonallergic urticaria in practically all individuals. In a few, an allergic reaction and anaphylaxis may occur, as proved by the RAST test.

Insects

Cockroach

Zschunke (190) state that cockroaches are used to investigate insect hormones and analogous compounds. The aim of such research is to develop a new class of insecticide. This investigator observed dermatitis, urticaria, rhinitis, bronchitis, and asthma in four research assistants whose job was breeding cockroaches. These patients had patch tests with a cockroach extract on the volar aspect of the forearms. Dilutions of 1:1,000 produced wheals (diameter 5 to 10 mm) within approximately 15 minutes, which disappeared in about 30 minutes. Zschunke (190) concluded that dermatitis due to cockroaches should be classified as allergic contact urticaria.

Chironomid

These are small midges used by aquarists as fish food. A case of CU with positive prick test and IgE was reported (191).

Mites

Tetranychus urticae, a large mite, may be a frequent cause of CU and contact dermatitis in farm workers (192).

Contact of the intact skin with certain caterpillar hairs, moths, and plant nettles may produce a nonimmunologic contact urticaria.

ALLERGIC CONTACT URTICARIA DUE TO TEXTILES

Silk, wool, rubber, and nylon may produce allergic contact urticaria.

Rudzki (193) reported that, in 1928, a 7-year-old girl developed wheals similar to those from contact with nettles after putting on a silk coat. It was observed soon afterward that any contact with silk elicited similar symptoms, so she endeavored to avoid any contact with this material. Over the years, each contact with silk produced increasingly severe urticaria. At the age of 56 she was still allergic to silk. When silk was applied to the flexor aspect of her right forearm, a typical contact urticaria appeared.

Three divergent views are held as to the nature of the silk allergen: the silk fiber itself, the gum or glue (sericin) contained in raw silk, and the silkworm. The silkworm pupa contains 10 times more allergen than does the cocoon. Because there is undoubted sensitization to silk cloth that contains no pupa and relatively little sericin, some of the allergen must persist in finished silk (194).

Silk allergy may manifest itself as inhalant symptoms, urticaria, or dermatitis (195).

Wool

Many atopic individuals do not "tolerate" wool (i.e., woolen clothing exacerbates their itching). Some atopic individuals will occasionally acquire "itchy bumps," which somewhat resemble small urticarial wheals where woolen clothing is worn (196).

Spray Starch for Clothing

McDaniel and Marks (197) discovered that contact urticaria in a commercial spray starch for clothing was due to a dual sensitivity to formaldehyde and terpinyl acetate. A 20-year-old nonatopic woman had a 1-year history of pruritis and hives that occurred within minutes of wearing spray-starched clothes. New "wash-and-wear" clothes produced similar symptoms, but washed, unstarched clothes were worn without difficulty. Open tests were applied at different times to her forearm and back with the commercial spray starch and its ingredients. Within 15 minutes, urticaria was observed resulting from the spray starch, formaldehyde, and perfume. Further testing with 34 undiluted coded ingredients of the perfume produced hives that were due to one substance, later identified as terpinyl acetate, which was present in the perfume in a 0.25% concentration. The perfume and terpinyl acetate were formaldehyde-free, according to the manufacturer. A dozen control subjects had negative open test results to formaldehyde and terpinyl acetate.

Formaldehyde in Leather

Helander (198) described a patient who developed a contact urticaria after she handled leather used to make leather dresses that was found qualitatively to contain minimal amounts of formaldehyde. The patient worked as a carver and model setter in a factory that made leather dresses. She had had urticaria almost daily, most severely on the hands, and occasionally, edema of the lip. During the weekends and vacations when the patient had no contact with leather, there was no evidence of skin eruption. The patient had cut foreign leather that was found to contain minimal amounts of formaldehyde. The patient was transferred to another department in which she handles only domestic leather that does not contain formaldehyde.

The patient initially developed urticaria around a formaldehyde test site in less than 1 hour after the tests were applied; the urticaria became generalized in a few hours.

Nylon

Nylon was the apparent cause of CU in a nursing student (199). She reacted to nylon underpants and stockings. Extensive testing found an urticarial reaction to nylon above. No reaction was seen to dyes, finishes, or other materials. She was not atopic.

Tinofix S

Urticaria and anaphylaxis occurred in a 55-year-old man due to a textile finish used on his pants (200). Tinofix S is described by deGroot and Gerkens (200) as a condensation product of dicyandramide, formaldehyde, ammonium chloride, and ethylenediamine. The patient did not react to the individual ingredients, only to the Tinofix S.

CONTACT URTICARIA DUE TO COLD, HEAT, SUN, WATER, AND AIR

The various physical urticarias due to cold, heat, sun, and water may be immunologic and nonimmunologic in nature.

Cold Urticaria

Essential acquired contact cold urticaria is regarded as immunologic in nature. Lesions appear usually within minutes after contact, for example, with an ice cube. The passive transfer test is positive in about 50% of reported cases. The transferable agent has been suggested to be IgE or IgM (201,202).

Swimming in cold water or exposure to a cold wind may produce a shocklike syndrome, presumably due to histamine release. Kaplan et al. (201) stated that there is evidence that histamine may be involved in urticaria due to cold. Highet and Titterington (203) stated that the present evidence favors a major role for histamine and that a combination of hydroxyzine (Atarax), an H1 antagonist, and cimetidine (Tagamet), an H2 antagonist, is a good combination for suppressing cold urticaria erythema.

Although essential cold urticaria is considered immunologic in nature, there is also evidence that histamine may be involved and that a combination of Tagamet (an H2 antagonist) and Atarax (an H1 antagonist) is useful in the treatment of cold urticaria.

Heat Urticaria

This type of urticaria is considered to be nonimmunologic in nature. Despite numerous investigations, the pathophysiology of this syndrome has not been delineated. DeMoragas et al. (204) implicated the kininogen-kinin system and possibly histamine, whereas Daman et al. (205) suggested the activation of the alternative complement pathway in the genesis of increased vascular permeability in this rare type of contact urticaria.

Solar Urticaria

Solar urticaria is a rare physical urticaria. Various clinical, biophysical, biochemical, and immunologic studies have shown that the disease can be classified into several different types. Allergic, unknown, and protoporphyrin mechanisms have been suggested (206). Solar urticaria may occur after exposure to both ultraviolet and visible light; a range of reactions including syncope is possible (207).

Parrish et al. (208) stated that solar urticaria is characterized by rapid development of an urticarial reaction in areas of skin exposed to nonionizing electromagnetic radiation. The wavelengths responsible for this reaction usually fall between 290 and 700 nm. Mast cell degranulation is associated with the development of solar urticaria and elevated levels of histamine, and eosinophil and neutrophil chemotactic factors have been found in the venous blood draining the site of the reaction. The relative importance of these mediators in the production of urticaria is unknown and it is also quite possible that other mediators are involved in the reaction. The mechanisms by which nonionizing radiation produces mast cell degranulation and release of mediators is also not certain. In some cases, an antigen-antibody reaction, perhaps involving a reaginic antibody, appears to be important and sensitivity to radiation can be transferred to normal individuals. In other cases, however, there is little evidence for an immunologic pathogenesis.

Aquagenic Urticaria

In aquagenic urticaria, perifollicular hives appear on skin exposed to tap water or distilled water, saline, and the patient's own sweat or sebum (209,210). It has been proposed that a toxic histamine-releasing substance is formed through the combination of water and sebum.

Greaves (211) stated that aquagenic urticarial eruptions appear to depend on acetylcholine release from sympathetic cholinergic nerve endings and involve histamine release, at least in part from skin mast cells.

The pharmacologic basis of aquagenic urticaria was studied in two patients; this condition provides small circular wheals surrounded by bright red flares when skin comes into contact with water.

A solution of scopolamine, a potent anticholinergic agent, was applied to areas of skin, and the test sites were challenged with water. In four of five experiments, there was a complete blockade of water-provoked whealing, indicating that acetylcholine is involved in the genesis of aquagenic urticarial lesions. The acetylcholine is derived presumably from sympathetic cholinergic nerve endings in the affected skin.

Based on the evidence that acetylcholine is released when water penetrates the stratum corneum in aquagenic urticaria patients and that histamine is also released from degranulated mast cells in some patients, it is speculated that water may activate sympathetic cholinergic fibers to produce a depolarization that releases acetylcholine. Acetylcholine is a histamine liberator, so it could degranulate mast cells, releasing histamine and producing wheals.

A "skin-protective" foam, called Pro-Q in the United States and ProDerm elsewhere, has been anecdotally reported to provide dramatic relief from aquagenic urticaria in a child (personal communication, Thomas Skold, Ponsus Pharma, Stockholm, Sweden, 1999).

Atmoknesis

Bernhard (212) commented on the phenomenon, reported by some patients, that they itch upon removal of clothing and "exposure" to air. He termed this "atmoknesis," after the Greek roots *atmos* (air) and *knesis* (itching).

> **Aquagenic urticaria appears to depend on acetylcholine release from sympathetic nerve endings, which can be blocked by scopolamine at sites tested with water. Antihistamines control the pruritus but not the wheal and flare.**

COMBINED ECZEMATOUS AND URTICARIAL REACTIONS

There are many compounds that can produce an acute allergic contact urticarial reaction, which may be followed by a typical delayed type of eczematous reaction (Table 34.9). Such compounds will produce initially an immediate wheal-and-flare reaction within 30 to 45 minutes, followed by a delayed eczematous response at 48- to 72-hour readings (1,108,145).

Testing for immediate reactions on previously eczematous skin can result in prompt itching followed within a few minutes by either urticarial responses alone or combined with eruptions of vesicles and all macroscopic features of delayed eczematous dermatitis (48,68,213).

Some primarily urticariogenic compounds, such as sorbic acid, cinnamic aldehyde, and balsam of Peru, can produce a nonimmunologic contact urticaria in many individuals and delayed eczematous reactions in some patients.

> **Many compounds can produce an acute allergic contact urticaria followed by an allergic eczematous contact dermatitis in some individuals. Some primarily urticariogenic agents, such as sorbic acid, cinnamic aldehyde, and balsam of Peru, can produce nonallergic contact urticaria in many individuals but delayed allergic eczematous contact dermatitis only in a few.**

Vinyl pyridine has produced delayed eczematous contact dermatitis in one patient and allergic contact urticaria in another individual; both patients were engaged in chemical research (99,214).

Krook (68) reported a unique combined vesicular and urticarial eruption. Thus, in sensitized individuals, vegetables

TABLE 34.9 *Contactants That May Cause Combined Delayed Eczematous and Urticarial Reactions*

Acrylic acid	Lettuce
Ammonium persulfate	Metals:
Benzocaine	Nickel
Castor bean	Rhodium
Cinnamic aldehyde	Platinum
Endive	Rubber
Epoxy resin	Sorbic acid
Latex	Teak
Lemon perfume	Vinyl pyridine

such as lettuces, endives, and tomatoes may produce an immediate vesicular, intensively pruritic eruption within a few minutes of contact on previously eczematized skin. There is sometimes a combined urticarial and vesicular eruption due to these vegetables. A prerequisite for the appearance of the immediate vesicular reaction observed in some cases seems to be that the allergen comes into contact with previously damaged skin.

Hjorth and Roed-Petersen (47) stated that contacting certain proteinaceous foods, particularly fish, in open patch tests, may produce erythema and edema on normal skin after 20 minutes. Previously eczematous, now normal skin often responds with a crop of vesicles preceded by erythema and with itching 30 minutes after the application of the open test.

These authors suggest that contact with food protein can (a) cause a primary allergic dermatitis, termed protein contact dermatitis; (b) aggravate allergic and irritant dermatitis; and (c) cause a preexisting atopic dermatitis to flare.

> **Contact with certain foods can cause allergic contact urticaria on normal skin and an immediate vesicular eruption in the same patient on previously eczematous but now normal-looking skin.**

CU to natural latex may present as hand eczema that may be indistinguishable from allergic or irritant contact dermatitis.

Contact Anaphylaxis

Skinner and Fowler (116) have reviewed the reported causes of anaphylaxis precipitated by skin contact with an allergen. Natural rubber latex has been identified as an extremely important allergen able to cause contact anaphylaxis (see Chapter 31). Other agents implicated in contact anaphylactic episodes include bacitracin, rifamycin, neomycin, chlorhexidine, mercurochrome, Emulgade F (an emulsifier), chlorothalonil, formaldehyde, lidocaine, milk (casein), paraphenylenediamine, and castor bean (116,215).

AMMONIUM PERSULFATE—A CAUSE OF CONTACT URTICARIA OF UNCERTAIN MECHANISM

This type of contact urticaria refers to reactions elicited by chemicals for which neither an allergic nor a direct influence on vessels or release of vasoactive substances can be proven currently. Ammonium persulfate, an oxidizing agent used in hair bleaches, is the classic example. The fact that some individuals react on the first exposure and the finding of negative passive transfer attempts favor a nonimmunologic mechanism, whereas negative tests in most controls dispute the concept of direct release of vasoactive substances (216). The variety of reaction patterns, including toxic dermatitis, localized or generalized urticaria, rhinitis, asthma, and even vascular collapse, is puzzling.

Ammonium persulfate is used widely to "boost" peroxide hair bleaches to obtain a platinum blond effect. The persulfates can produce a variety of cutaneous and respiratory responses, including allergic eczematous contact dermatitis, irritant dermatitis, localized edema, generalized urticaria, rhinitis, asthma, and syncope (217). Some of these reactions appear to be truly allergic, whereas others appear to be due to the release of histamine on a nonallergic basis.

Patch tests may be performed with 2% to 5% aqueous solution of ammonium persulfate. Scratch tests may result in asthma and syncope. In some patients, merely rubbing a saturated solution of ammonium persulfate into the skin will evoke a large urticarial wheal. Hairdressers should be made aware that these ammonium persulfate hair bleach preparations may provoke severe reactions and should seek medical attention if the client complains of severe itching, tingling, a burning sensation, hives, dizziness, or weakness.

> **Ammonium persulfate used with peroxide to create a "platinum blond" color may produce contact urticaria and even anaphylactoid reactions in some individuals by an unknown mechanism.**

Calnan and Shuster (216) first reported that hair bleaches containing ammonium persulfate could produce a local urticarial reaction and a "generalized histamine reaction." They stated that it had not been determined whether the release of histamine from the skin was a direct action on the mast cells or by an immune mechanism.

Testing with Ammonium Persulfate

The method of testing with ammonium persulfate is the one suggested by Brun et al. (218) and Reiffers et al. (219) as follows: Put 0.4 g of dry persulfate in 20 ml vials, then close the vials with gum stoppers (like antibiotic vials). Inject 20 ml of water in each vial and keep them no longer than 1 day. Always use fresh 2% solution of ammonium persulfate.

> **Testing for ammonium persulfate hypersensitivity should be done with a fresh 2% aqueous solution. Resuscitation equipment should be available in event of a severe reaction.**

Prevention of Ammonium Persulfate Reactions with Prednisone and an Antihistamine

Patients who have moderately severe reactions after the use of ammonium persulfate consisting of mild urticaria and moderate edema of the forehead and the eyelids could prevent the reaction by the administration of 40 mg of prednisone and 12 mg of chlortrimetone on the night before a hair bleaching procedure. In addition, the prednisone and the antihistamine should be administered 1 hour before the ammonium persulfate is applied (121).

PRINCIPLES OF SKIN TESTING FOR CONTACT URTICARIA

The following procedures may be followed when it is suspected that a contactant may be producing contact urticaria.

1. Test the substance on normal skin that has apparently never before been the site of dermatitis.
2. If negative, test on previously affected skin even though the skin at present appears to be normal. Previously affected skin may remain for a long time in a state of increased responsiveness as compared with skin that has never been the site of dermatitis.
3. Testing on eczematous skin may be worthwhile, providing the tested area shows only light erythema, so that an urticarial reaction may be readily perceived on the eczematous skin.
4. If all these test procedures are negative, the suspected contactant should be rubbed gently into a small scratch.
5. It should be noted that, as a rule, those substances that produce NICU will show reactions on normal skin that has never been the site of dermatitis.
6. The use of controls is much more significant in immunologic CU than in the nonimmunologic variety. Thus, such nonallergenic contact urticants as sorbic acid and benzoic acid may only react in about half of the population. Tests for immunologic CU should be negative in at least three to five controls.
7. The upper back, the antecubital space, and the volar aspect of the forearm are suitable sites for testing. Some agents causing NICU, however, such as benzoic acid, may react only on the face and not elsewhere.

8. Precautions: Because anaphylactoid reactions may occur in highly allergic patients from skin testing, epinephrine and resuscitation equipment should be available.

9. Local and systemic NSAIDs inhibit NICU, and antihistamines may inhibit some forms of allergic contact urticaria (167).

PRETREATMENT ADJUNCTS TO TESTING FOR CONTACT URTICARIA

Blocking Agents

Pretreatment of the test site with 0.1 ml of atropine in 1:1,000 solution or lidocaine in 1:100 dilution indicates that a cholinergic mechanism is involved if blockade of the test site is achieved. The use of antihistamine agents via oral administration or via local pretreatment can provide evidence of a histamine-mediated reaction if successful inhibition of the skin test is achieved. Local anesthesia induced by lidocaine decreased the reactivity to benzoic acid significantly with concentrations of both 1.0% and 0.25% (220).

Compound 48/80

When compound 48/80 (Sigma Chemical Co., St. Louis, MO) is injected intradermally, mast cells at the site will release histamine and a hive will form. If 0.1 ml of a 0.05-mg/ml solution is injected into the same site on a patient's ventral forearm at 8-hour intervals, usually no response can be elicited by the third injection, as mast cells have been depleted of their histamine. Twenty-four hours after the initial injection, 0.1 ml of the incriminated substance is applied to the pretreated site and to a control site. If a typical wheal occurs at the control site but not at the prepared site, the response may, in part, be mediated by histamine. The refractory period of reactions mediated by histamine produced by compound 48/80 has been reported to last 2 to 6 days.

CONTACT URTICARIA STATISTICS

Kanerva et al. (221) presented comprehensive occupational statistics regarding CU in Finland from 1990 to 1994. Other than this report, and except for latex allergy, comprehensive data on prevalence of CU are woefully inadequate. Kanerva et al. found that 2,759 cases of occupational contact dermatoses were reported to the Finnish Register of Occupational Disease, of which 815 (29.5%) were CU. Women accounted for 70% of the cases. The top allergens were cow dander (362 cases); latex (193 cases); flour, grains, and feed (92 cases); foodstuffs (25 cases); and industrial enzymes (14 cases). Farmers and animal attendants were the most common occupational group with CU, followed by bakers, nurses, chefs, and dental assistants.

Katsarou et al. (222) studied the incidence of immediate reactions to patch test allergens of the European standard series. No attempt was made to differentiate NICU from allergic CU, but presumably the majority of reactions were of the NICU variety. Of 664 patients, balsam of Peru reacted in 113, fragrance mix in 112, paraben mix in 30, and clioquinol in 13. A total of 328 reactions were seen to the 24 test substances. Presence of atopy was not increased in the reactive group.

REFERENCES

1. von Krogh G, Maibach HI. The contact urticaria syndrome. *Semin Dermatol* 1982;1:59.
2. Lahti A. Non-immunologic contact urticaria. *Acta Derm Venereol* 1980;60[Suppl 91].
3. Odom RB, Maibach HI. Contact urticaria: a different contact dermatitis in dermatotoxicology and pharmacology. In: Marzulli FN, Maibach HI, eds. *Advances in modern toxicology,* vol 4. Washington, DC: Hemisphere Publishing, 1977.
4. Kligman AM. The spectrum of contact urticaria-wheals, erythema, and pruritus. *Derm Clin* 1990;8:57.
5. Rosenhall L, Zetterstron O. Asthmatic patients with hypersensitivity to aspirin, benzoic acid and tartrazine. *Tubercle* 1975;56:168.
6. Larmi E. PUVA treatment inhibits nonimmunologic immediate contact reactions to benzoic acid and methyl nicotinate. *Int J Dermatol* 1989;28:9.
7. Shriner D, Maibach H. Regional variation of nonimmunologic contact urticaria: functional map of the human face. *Skin-Phamacol* 1996;9:312–321.
8. Lahti A, Poutiainen AM, Hannuksela M. Alcohol vehicles in tests for non-immunological immediate contact reactions. *Contact Dermatitis* 1993;29:22.
9. Stoughton RB, Fritsch W. Influence of dimethylsulfoxide (DMSO) on human percutaneous absorption. *Arch Dermatol* 1964;90:512.
10. Kligman AM. Topical pharmacology and toxicology of dimethyl sulfoxide—part 1. *JAMA* 1965;193:796.
11. Kellum RE, ed. Selected reviews of the literature. *Arch Dermatol* 1966;93:135.
12. Schneider R. Erfahrungen mit Trafuril-Liniment. *Wien Med Wochenschr* 1953;103:30.
13. McCabe RJ. Studies with the local use of the furfuryl ester of nicotinic acid. *Arch Dermatol* 1956;74:522.
14. Vaillancourt de G. The cutaneous application of a nicotinic acid cream as a diagnostic aid in various rheumatic diseases. *Can Med Assoc J* 1954;71:283.
15. Windholz M, ed. *The Merck index: an encyclopedia of chemicals and drugs,* 9th ed. Rahway, NJ: Merck & Co, 1976.
16. Fryklof L-E. A note on the irritant properties of sorbic acid in ointments and creams. *J Pharm Pharmacol* 1958;10:719.
17. Hjorth N, Trolle-Lassen C. Skin reactions to preservatives in creams. *Am Perfum* 1962;77:43.
18. Rietschel RL. Contact urticaria from synthetic cassia oil and sorbic acid limited to the face. *Contact Dermatitis* 1978;4:347.
19. Pevny I von, Rauscher E, Lechner W, Metz D. Excessive allergie gegen Benzoesaure mit anaphylaktischem Schock nach Expositionstest. *Dermatosen* 1981;29:123.
20. Hjorth N. Eczematous allergy to balsams, allied perfumes and flavouring agents. *Acta Derm Venereol* (Stockh) 1981;41[Suppl 46]:216.
21. Juhlin L, Michaelsson G. Forbjudet och tillatet vid overkanslighet for konserveringsmedel och fargamnen. *Lakartidningen* 1973;70:1414.
22. Martindale W. *The extra pharmacopoeia,* 27th ed. Wade A, ed. London: The Pharmaceutical Press, 1977.
23. Lahti A. Skin reactions to antimicrobial agents. *Contact Dermatitis* 1978;4:302.
24. Munoz F, Bellido J, Moyano J, et al. Perioral contact urticaria from sodium benzoate in a toothpaste. *Contact Dermatitis* 1996;35:51.
25. Opdyke DLJ. Cinnamic acid. In: Monographs on fragrance raw materials. *Food Cosmet Toxicol* 1978;16[Suppl 1]:687.

26. Collins FW, Mitchell JC. Aroma chemicals. Reference sources for perfume and flavour ingredients with special reference to cinnamic aldehyde. *Contact Dermatitis* 1975;1:43.

27. Nater JP, De Jong MCJM, Baar AJM, Bleumink E. *Contact Dermatitis* 1977;3:151.

28. Rudzki E, Grzywa Z. Two types of contact urticaria and immediate reactions to patch-test allergens. *Dermatologica* 1978;157:110.

29. Calnan CD. Cinnamon dermatitis from an ointment. *Contact Dermatitis* 1976;2:167.

30. Magnusson B, Wilkinson DS. Cinnamic aldehyde in toothpaste: (1) clinical aspects and patch tests. *Contact Dermatitis* 1975;1:70.

31. Schorr WF. Cinnamic aldehyde allergy. *Contact Dermatitis* 1975;1:108.

32. Mathias CGT, Chappler RR, Maibach HI. Contact urticaria from cinnamic aldehyde. *Arch Dermatol* 1980;116:74.

33. Temesvari E von, Soos G, Podanyi B, et al. Contact urticaria provoked by balsam of Peru. *Contact Dermatitis* 1978;4:65.

34. Rudzki E, Grzywa Z. Immediate reactions to balsam of Peru, cassia oil and ethyl vanillin. *Contact Dermatitis* 1976;2:360.

35. Forsbeck M, Skog E. Immediate reactions to patch tests with balsam of Peru. *Contact Dermatitis* 1977;3:201.

36. Safford RJ, et al. Immediate contact reactions to chemicals in the fragrance mix and a study of the quenching action of eugenol. *Br J Dermatol* 1990;123:595.

37. Maes D, Marenus K, Smith W. Invisible irritation: a new look at product safety. *Cosmet Toilet* 1990;105:43–50.

38. Coverly J, Peters L, Whittle E, Basketter D. Susceptibility to skin stinging, non-immunologic contact urticaria and acute skin irritation: is there a relationship? *Contact Dermatitis* 1998;38:90–95.

39. Edwards EK. Contact urticaria to cow's milk. *Cutis* 1981;28:450.

40. Lecks HE. Anaphylaxis from milk protein in diaper ointment. *JAMA* 1980;244:1560.

41. Rudzki E, Gryzwa Z. Contact urticaria from egg. *Contact Dermatitis* 1977;3:103.

42. Temesvari E, Varkonyi V. Contact urticaria provoked by egg. *Contact Dermatitis* 1980;6:43.

43. Ushijima N, Miyanaga K, Yoshimura S, et al. Allergic contact urticaria to lysozyme. Report 6th International Symposium on Contact Dermatitis and Joint Meeting between ICRD and JCDRG, Tokyo, 1982.

44. Nater JP, Swartz JA. Atopic allergic reaction due to raw potato. *J Allergy* 1967;40:202.

45. Pearson RSB. Potato sensitivity. An occupational allergen in housewives. *Acta Allergol* 1966;21:507.

46. Cronin E. Immediate type hypersensitivity to potato. *Contact Dermatitis Newsletter* 1973;13:58.

47. Hjorth N, Roed-Petersen J. Berufsekzeme durch proteine. *Z Hautkr* 1975;50:851.

48. Mitchell JC. Contact urticaria from a shrimp, *Pandalus*. *Contact Dermatitis Newsletter* 1974;16:486.

49. Maibach HI. Regional variation in elicitation of contact urticaria syndrome (immediate hypersensitivity syndrome): shrimp. *Contact Dermatitis* 1986;15:100.

50. Hjorth N, Weissmann K. Occupational dermatitis in chefs and sandwich makers. *Contact Dermatitis Newsletter* 1972;11:300.

51. Lombardi P, Campolmi P, Giorgini S, Spallanzani P. Food contact urticaria. Report 6th international symposium on contact dermatitis and joint meeting between ICRG and JCDRG, Tokyo, 1982.

52. Beck HI, Nissen K. Contact urticaria to commercial fish in atopic persons. *Acta Dermatol* 1982;63:257.

53. Coverly J, Peters L, Whittle E, Basketter D. Susceptibility to skin stinging, non-immunologic contact urticaria and acute skin irritation: is there a relationship? *Contact Dermatitis* 1998;38:90–95.

54. Dominguez C, Ojeda I, Crespo J, et al. Allergic reactions following skin contact with fish. *Allergy-Asthma-Proc* 1996;17:83–87.

55. Hjorth N, Roed-Petersen J. Occupational protein contact dermatitis in food handlers. *Contact Dermatitis* 1976;2:23.

56. Maibach HI. Immediate hypersensitivity in hand dermatitis. Role of food-contact dermatitis. *Arch Dermatol* 1976;112:1289.

57. Fisher AA, Stengel F. Allergic occupational hand dermatitis due to calves' liver. An urticarial "immediate" type hypersensitivity. *Cutis* 1977;19:561.

58. Fisher AA. Allergic contact urticaria to raw beef—histopathology of the specific wheal reaction at the scratch test site. *Contact Dermatitis* (in press).

59. Moseng D. Urticaria from pig's gut. *Contact Dermatitis* 1982;8:135.

60. Jovanovic M, Oliwiecki S, Beck MH. Occupational contact urticaria from beef associated with hand eczema. *Contact Dermatitis* 1992;27:188.

61. Geyer E, Kranke B, Derhaschnig J, et al. Contact urticaria from roe deer meat and hair. *Contact Dermatitis* 1998;39:34.

62. Iliev D, Wuthrich B. Occupational protein contact dermatitis with type I allergy to different kinds of meat and vegetables. *Int Arch Occup Environ Health* 1998;71:289–292.

63. Andersen KE, Lowenstein H. An investigation of the possible immunological relationship between allergen extracts from birch, pollen, hazelnut, potato, and apple. *Contact Dermatitis* 1978;4:73.

64. Grattan CEH, Harman RRM. Contact urticaria to strawberry. *Contact Dermatitis* 1985;13:191.

65. Veraldi S, Schianchi-Veraldi R. Contact urticaria from Kiwi fruit. *Contact Dermatitis* 1990;22:244.

66. Giannattasio M, Serafina M, Guarrara P, et al. Contact urticaria from Litchi fruit. *Contact Dermatitis* 1995;33:67.

67. DeCorres L, et al. Contact urticaria. Sensitization to chestnuts and bananas in patients with contact urticaria from latex. *Contact Dermatitis* 1990;23:277.

68. Krook G. Occupational dermatitis from *Lactuca sativa* (lettuce) and *Cichorium* (endive). *Contact Dermatitis* 1977;3:27.

69. Pigatto PD. Ig-E-mediated contact and generalized urticaria from *Eruca sativa*. *Contact Dermatitis* 1991;25:191.

70. Quirce S, Tabar A, Olaguibel J, Cuevas M. Occupational contact urticaria syndrome caused by globe artichoke. *J Allergy Clin Immunol* 1996;97:710–711.

71. Sanchez M, Hernandez M, Morena V, et al. Immunologic contact urticaria caused by asparagus. *Contact Dermatitis* 1997;37:181–182.

72. Munoz D, et al. Anaphylaxis from contact with carrot. *Contact Dermatitis* 1985;13:345.

73. Lovell CR, Rycroft RJG. Contact urticaria from winged bean (*Psophocarpus tetragonolobus*). *Contact Dermatitis* 1984;10:314.

74. Kanerva L, Estlander T, Jolanki R. Long-lasting contact urticaria from castor bean. *J Am Acad Dermatol* 1990;23:351.

75. DiLernia V, Albertini G, Bisighini G. Immunologic contact urticaria syndrome from raw rice. *Contact Dermatitis* 1992;27:196.

76. Jeannet-peter N, Piletta-Zanin P, Hauser C. Facial dermatitis, contact urticaria, rhinoconjunctivitis, and asthma induced by potato. *Am J Contact Dermatitis* 1999;10:40–42.

77. van Ketel WG. Immediate type allergy to malt in beer. *Contact Dermatitis* 1980;6:279.

78. Heygi E, Dolezalova A. Urticarial reaction after patch tests of toothpaste with a subshock condition: hypersensitivity to caraway seed. *Cesk Dermatol* 1976;51:19.

79. Duran S, Delgado J, Gamez R, et al. Contact Urticaria from sunflower seeds. *Contact Dermatitis* 1997;37:184.

80. Gamboa P, Jaurequi I, Urrutia, et al. Allergic contact urticaria from poppy flowers. *Contact Dermatitis* 1997;37:140–141.

81. Munoz F, Delgado J, Palma J, et al. Airborne contact urticaria due to Mulberry (*Morus alba*) pollen. *Contact Dermatitis* 1995;32:61.

82. Gutierrez d, Conde A, Duran S, et al. Contact urticaria from *Lupin*. *Contact Dermatitis* 1997;36:311.

83. Estlander T, Kanerva L, Tupasela O, Jolanki R. Occupational contact urticaria and type I sensitization caused by gerbera. *Contact Dermatitis* 1998;38:118–120.

84. Paulsen E, Stahl-Skov P, Andersen K. Immediate skin and mucosal symptoms from pot plants and vegetables in gardeners and greenhouse workers. *Contact Dermatitis* 1998;39:166–170.

85. Kannerva L, Vahanen M, Tupasela O. Occupational contact urticaria from cellulase enzyme. *Contact Dermatitis* 1998;38:176–177.

86. Kanerva L, Vanhanen M, Tupasela O. Occupational contact urticaria from fungal but not bacterial alpha-amylase. *Contact Dermatitis* 1997;36:306–307.

87. Kanerva L, Tarvainen K. Allergic contact dermatitis and contact urticaria from cellulolytic enzymes. *Am J Contact Dermatitis* 1990;1:244–245.

88. Foti C, Carino M, Cassano N, et al. Occupational contact urticaria from paprika. *Contact Dermatitis* 1997;37:135.

89. Pecquet C, Leynadier F, Saiag P. Immediate hypersensitivity to sesame in foods and cosmetics. *Contact Dermatitis* 1998;39:313.

90. Maucher OM. Anaphylaktische reaktionen beim epicutantest. *Hautarzt* 1972;23:139.

91. Haustein UF. Anaphylactic shock and contact urticaria after the patch test with professional allergens. *Allerg Immunol* 1976;22:349.

92. Boonk WJ. Dermatologic hazards from hidden contact with penicillin. *Dermatosen* 1981;29:131.

93. Eriksen HC. Anaphylactic shock caused by neomycin treated with external cardiac massage. *Ugeskr Laeg* 1963;125:1077.

94. Pippen R. Anaphylactoid reaction after chymacort ointment. *Br Med J* 1966;5496:1172.

95. Roupe G, Strannegard O. Anaphylactic shock elicited by topical administration of bacitracin. *Arch Dermatol* 1969;100:450.

96. Comaish JS, Cunliffe WJ. Absorption of drugs from varicose ulcers: a cause of anaphylaxis. *Br J Clin Pract* 1967;21:97.

97. Bjorkner B, Moller H. Bacitracin: a cutaneous allergen and histamine liberator. *Acta Derm Venereol* (Stockh) 1973;53:487.

98. Levene G, Withers A. Anaphylaxis to streptomycin and hyposensitization. *Trans St Johns Hosp Dermatol Soc* 1969;55:184.

99. Rudzki E, Rebandel P, Rogozinski T. Contact urticaria from rat tail, guinea pig, streptomycin and vinyl pyridine. *Contact Dermatitis* 1981;7:186.

100. Kosakava M. Sub-Schock bei der Epikutan-probe mit Chloramphenicol. *Berufsdermatosen* 1977;25:134.

101. Tuft L. Contact urticaria from cephalosporins. *Arch Dermatol* 1975; 111:1609.

102. Shimizu S, Chen K, Miyakawa S. Cefotiam-induced contact urticaria syndrome. *Dermatology* 1996;192:174–176.

103. Mancuso G, Masara N. Contact urticaria and severe anaphylaxis from rifamycin SV. *Contact Dermatitis* 1992;27:124.

104. Escribano M, Munoz-Bellido F, Velazquez E, et al. Contact urticaria due to aescin. *Contact Dermatitis* 1997;37:233.

105. Camarasa JMG, Alomar A, Perez M. Contact urticaria and anaphylaxis from aminophenazone. *Contact Dermatitis* 1978;4:243.

106. Ryan ME, Davis BM, Marks Jr JG. Contact urticaria and allergic contact dermatitis to benzocaine gel. *J Am Acad Dermatol* 1980; 2:221.

107. Rudner EJ. Contact urticaria. *Int J Dermatol* 1979;18:418.

108. Ramsay DL, Cohen HJ, Baer RL. Allergic reaction to benzophenone. *Arch Dermatol* 1972;105:906.

109. Kanerva L, Alanko K, Estlander T, et al. Occupational allergic contact urticaria from chloramine-T solution. *Contact Dermatitis* 1997; 37:180–181.

110. Horio T. Chloropromazine photoallergy: coexistence of immediate and delayed type. *Arch Dermatol* 1975;111:1469.

111. Bergqvist-Karlsson A. Delayed and immediate-type hypersensitivity to chlorhexidine. *Contact Dermatitis* 1988;18:84.

112. Okano M, Nomura M, Hata S, et al. Anaphylactic symptoms due to chlorhexidine gluconate. *Arch Dermatol* 1989;125:50–52.

113. Wong WK, Goh CL, Chan KW. Contact urticaria from chlorhexidine. *Contact Dermatitis* 1990;22:51.

114. Cheung J, O'Leary J. Allergic reaction to chlorhexidine in an anesthetized patient. *Anaesth Intern Care* 1985;13:429–439.

115. Ohtoshi T, Yamauchi N, Tadokoro K, et al. IgE antibody mediated shock reaction caused by topical application of chlorhexidine. *Clin Allergy* 1986;16:155–161.

116. Skinner S, Fowler JF. Contact anaphylaxis. *Am J Contact Dermatitis* 1995;6:133–142.

117. Freitas JP, Brandao FM. Contact urticaria to chlorocresol. *Contact Dermatitis* 1986;15:252.

118. Schena D, Barba A, Costa G. Occupational contact urticaria to cisplatin. *Contact Dermatitis* 1996;34:220–221.

119. Tosti A, Guerra L, Bardazzi F. Contact urticaria during topical immunotherapy. *Contact Dermatitis* 1989;21:196.

120. VanHecke E, Santosa S. Contact urticaria to DNCB. *Contact Dermatitis* 1985;12:282.

121. Fisher AA. Urticarial and systemic reactions to contactants varying from hair bleach to seminal fluid. *Cutis* 1977;19:715.

122. Mitchell JC. Contact urticaria from a vitamin E preparation (vitamin E-vegetable oil) in two siblings. *Int J Dermatol* 1975;14:246.

123. Papa CM, Shelley WB. Menthol hypersensitivity: diagnostic basophil response in a patient with chronic urticaria, flushing and headaches. *JAMA* 1964;189:549.

124. Grunnet E. Contact urticaria and anaphylactoid reaction induced by topical application of nitrogen mustard. *Br J Dermatol* 1976;94:101.

125. Daughters D, Zackheim H, Maibach H. Urticaria and anaphylactoid reactions after topical application of mechlorethamine. *Arch Dermatol* 1976;94:101.

126. Edwards Jr EK. Allergic reactions to benzyl alcohol in a sunscreen. *Cutis* 1981;28:332.

127. Ring J, Galosi A, Przybilla B. Contact anaphylaxis from Emulgade F. *Contact Dermatitis* 1986;15:48.

128. Tharp CK. Contact urticaria. *Arch Dermatol* 1973;108:135.

129. Torres J, DeCorres F. Anaphylactic hypersensitivity to mercurochrome (Merbromium). *Ann Allergy* 1985;54:230–232.

130. Sanz P, Munoz F, Serrano C, et al. Hypersensitivity to mercuric fluorscein compounds. *Allergol Immunopathol* 1989;17:219–222.

131. Mathews KP. Immediate-type hypersensitivity to phenylmercuric compounds. *Am J Med* 1968;44:310.

132. Henry JC, Tschen EH, Becker LE. Contact urticaria to parabens. *Arch Dermatol* 1979;115:1231.

133. Grin R, Maibach H. Long-lasting contact urticaria from petrolatum mimicking dermatitis. *Contact Dermatitis* 1999;40:110.

134. Fisher AA. Immediate and delayed allergic contact reactions to polyethylene glycol. *Contact Dermatitis* 1978;4:135.

135. Maibach HI, Conant M. Contact urticaria to a corticosteroid cream: polysorbate 60. *Contact Dermatitis* 1977;3:350.

136. Hardy H, Maibach H. Contact urticaria syndrome from sorbitan sesquioleate in a corticosteroid ointment. *Contact Dermatitis* 1995; 32:114.

137. Helgesen A, Austad J. Contact urticaria from aluminum and nickel in the same patient. *Contact Dermatitis* 1997;37:303–304.

138. Bergman A, Svedberg U, Nilsson E. Contact urticaria with anaphylactic reactions caused by occupational exposure to iridium salt. *Contact Dermatitis* 1995;32:14–17.

139. Osmundsen PE. Contact urticaria from nickel and plastic additives (butylhydroxytoluene, oleylamine). *Contact Dermatitis* 1980;6:452.

140. Nakayama H, Imai T. Occupational contact urticaria, contact dermatitis and asthma caused by rhodium hypersensitivity. 6th International Symposium on *Contact Dermatitis* and Joint Meeting between ICRG and JCDRG. Tokyo, 21 May 1982.

141. Key MM. Some unusual allergic reactions in industry. *Arch Dermatol* 1961;83:3.

142. Levene GM. Platinum sensitivity. *Br J Dermatol* 1971;85:590.

143. Smith JD, Odom RB, Maibach HI. Contact urticaria from cobalt chloride. *Arch Dermatol* 1975;111:1610.

144. Maibach HI, Johnson H. Contact urticaria syndrome. *Arch Dermatol* 1975;111:726.

145. Fowler JF. Immediate contact hypersensitivity to acrylic acid. *Derm Clin* 1990;8:193.

146. Ophaswongse S, Maibach H. Alcohol dermatitis: allergic contact dermatitis and contact urticaria syndrome. *Contact Dermatitis* 1994;30:1–6.

147. Adams RM. *Occupational skin disease,* 2nd ed. Philadelphia: WB Saunders, 1990.

148. Maibach HI, Johnson HL. Contact urticaria syndrome: contact urticaria to diethyltoluamide immediate-type hypersensitivity. *Arch Dermatol* 1975;111:726.

149. Bjorkner B. Contact urticaria and asthma from detonium benzoate (Bitrex). *Contact Dermatitis* 1980;6:466.

150. Maurice F, Rivory J, Larsson P, et al. Anaphylactic shock caused by long term hemodialysis. *J Allergy Clin Immunol* 1986;77:594–597.

151. Combes FC, Morris GE. Contact sensitivity to inappreciable exposures. *Industr Med* 1956;25:289.

152. Morris GE. Urticaria following exposure to ammonia fumes. *AMA Arch Health* 1956;13:480.

153. Zschunke E. Occupational urticaria due to sulfur dioxide. *Berufsdermatosen* 1967;15:23.

154. Shelley W, Shelley E, Talanin N. Urticaria due to occupational exposure to glyceryl monothioglycolate permanent wave solution. *Acta Derm Venereol* 1998;78:471–472.

155. Camarasa J. Contact urticaria to naphthylacetic acid. *Contact Dermatitis* 1986;14:113.

156. Temesvari E. Contact urticaria from paraphenylenediamine. *Contact Dermatitis* 1984;11:134.

157. Pasche-Koo F, French L, Piletta-Zanin P. Contact urticaria and shock to hair dye. *Allergy* 1998;53:904–905.

158. Jagtman B. Urticaria and contact urticaria due to Basic Blue 99 in a hair dye. *Contact Dermatitis* 1996;35:52.

159. Tosti A, et al. Contact urticaria from polypropylene. *Contact Dermatitis* 1986;15:51.

160. Sasseville D. Contact urticaria from epoxy resin and reactive diluents. *Contact Dermatitis* 1998;38:57–58.

161. Kanerva L, Hyry H, Jolanki R, et al. Delayed and immediate allergy caused by methylhexahydrophylactic anhydride. *Contact Dermatitis* 1997;36:34–38.
162. Kanerva L, Estlander T, Jolanki R, Tarvainen K. Occupational allergic contact dermatitis and contact urticaria caused by polyfunctional aziridine. *Contact Dermatitis* 1995;33:304–309.
163. Kanerva L, Grenquist-Norden B, Piirila P. Occupational IgE mediated contact urticaria from diphenylmethane-4,4-diisopcyanate (MDI). *Contact Dermatitis* 1999;41:50–51.
164. Niinimaki A, Niinimaki M, Makinen-Kiljanen S, Hannukesala M. Contact from protein hydrolysates in hair conditioners. *Allergy* 1998;53:1078–1082.
165. Pasche-Koo F, Claeys M, Hauser C. Contact urticaria with systemic symptoms caused by bovine collagen in a hair conditioner. *Am J Contact Dermatitis* 1996;7:56–57.
166. Tanaka T, Miyachi Y, Horio T. Ulcerative contact dermatitis caused by sodium silicate: co-existence of primary irritant contact dermatitis and contact urticaria. *Arch Dermatol* 1982;118:518.
167. Altman AT. Facial dermatitis (xylene). *Arch Dermatol* 1977;113:1443.
168. Palmer KT, Rycroft RJG. Occupational airborne contact urticaria due to xylene. *Contact Dermatitis* 1993;28:44.
169. Goodfield MJD, Saihan EM. Contact urticaria to naphtha present in a solvent. *Contact Dermatitis* 1988;18:187.
170. Weiss R, Mowad C. Contact urticaria from xylene. *Am J Contact Dermatitis* 1998;9:125–127.
171. Mader R, Fowler J. Contact allergy to an organic solvent: immediate sensitivity and a serum sickness-like reaction. *Am J Contact Dermatitis* 1995;6:32–33.
172. Varigos GA, Nurse DS. Contact urticaria from methyl ethyl ketone. *Contact Dermatitis* 1986;15:259.
173. Fowler JF. Contact urticaria to 1,1,1-tricholoroethane. *Am J Contact Dermatitis* 1991;2:239.
174. Hausen B. *Woods injurious to human health—a manual.* New York: Walter de Gruyter, 1981.
175. Garces-Sotillos M, Blanco-Carmona J, Juste-Picon S, et al. Occupational asthma and contact urticaria caused by mukali wood dust. *J Investig Allergol Clin Immunol* 1995;5:113–114.
176. Calnan CD. Allergy to dog saliva. *Contact Dermatitis Newsletter* 1968;3:41.
177. Burrows D. Urticaria from rats. *Contact Dermatitis* 1979;5:122.
178. Rudzki E, Grzywa A. Two types of contact urticaria and immediate reactions to patch test allergens. *Dermatologica* 1978;157:110.
179. Uehara M, Ofuji S. Patch test reactions to human dander in atopic dermatitis. *Arch Dermatol* 1976;112:951.
180. Halpern BN, Ky T, Robert B. Clinical and immunological study of an exceptional case of reaginic type sensitization to human seminal fluid. *Immunology* 1967;12:247.
181. Levine BB, Siraganian RP, Schenkeim I. Allergy to human seminal plasma. *N Engl J Med* 1973;288:894.
182. Schultz KH, Schirren C, Kuepper I. Allergy to seminal fluid. *N Engl J Med* 1974;260:916.
183. Levine BB. Allergy to seminal fluid. *N Engl J Med* 1974;260:916.
184. Frankland AW, Parish WE. Anaphylactic sensitivity to human seminal fluid. *Clin Allergy* 1974;4:249.
185. Mikkelsen EJ, Henderson LL, Leiferman KM, et al. Allergy to human seminal fluid. *Ann Allergy* 1975;34:239.
186. Mathias CGT, Frick OL, Caldwell TM, et al. Immediate hypersensitivity to seminal fluid and atopic dermatitis. *Arch Dermatol* 1980;116:209.
187. Degreef H. Protein contact dermatitis with positive RAST tests to fresh bovine blood and amniotic fluid in a veterinary surgeon. 6th International Symposium on Contact Dermatitis and Joint Meeting between ICRG and JCDRG. Tokyo, 21–22 May 1982.
188. Schmidt H. Contact urticaria. *Contact Dermatitis* 1978;4:230.
189. Hartmann KR, Calton GJ, Burnett JW. Use of the radioallergosorbent test for the study of coelenterate toxin-specific immunoglobulin E. *Int Arch Allergy Appl Immunol* 1980;61:389.
190. Zschunke E. Contact urticaria, dermatitis and asthma from cockroaches. *Contact Dermatitis* 1978;4:313.
191. Galindo P, Melero R, Garcia R, et al. Contact urticaria from chironomids. *Contact Dermatitis* 1996;34:297.
192. Astarita C, Di-Martino P, Scala G, et al. Contact allergy: another occupational risk to *Tetranychus urticae. J Allergy Clin Immunol* 1996;98:732–738.
193. Rudzki E. Contact urticaria from silk. *Contact Dermatitis* 1977;3:53.
194. Urbach E, Gottlieb PM. *Allergy.* New York: Grune & Stratton, 1946.
195. Sheldon JM, Lovell RG, Mathews KP. A manual of clinical allergy. Philadelphia: WB Saunders, 1953.
196. Hambly EM, Levia L, Wilkinson DS. Wool intolerance in atopic subjects. *Contact Dermatitis* 1978;4:240.
197. McDaniel WR, Marks JG. Contact urticaria due to sensitivity to spray starch. *Arch Dermatol* 1979;115:628.
198. Helander I. Contact urticaria from leather containing formaldehyde. *Arch Dermatol* 1977;113:1443.
199. Dooms-Goossens A, et al. Contact urticaria due to nylon. *Contact Dermatitis* 1986;14:63.
200. DeGroot AC, Gerkens F. Contact urticaria from a chemical textile finish. *Contact Dermatitis* 1989;20:63.
201. Kaplan AP, Gray L, Shaff RE, et al. In vivo studies of mediator release in cold urticaria and cholinergic urticaria. *J Allergy Clin Immunol* 1975;55:394.
202. Wanderer AA, Maselli R, Ellis EF, Ishizaka K. Immunologic characterization of serum factors responsible for cold urticaria. *J Allergy Clin Immunol* 1971;48:13.
203. Highet AA, Titterington DM. Treatment of cold urticaria. *Br J Dermatol* 1979;101:51.
204. DeMoragas JM, Gimenez-Camarasa JM, Noguera J. Localized heat urticaria. *Arch Dermatol* 1973;108:684.
205. Daman L, Lieberman P, Ganier M, Hashimoto K. Localized heat urticaria. *Allergy Clin Immunol* 1978;61:273.
206. Horio T. Photoallergic urticaria induced by visible light: additional cases and further studies. *Arch Dermatol* 1978;114:1761.
207. Ramsey CA. Solar urticaria. *Int J Dermatol* 1980;19:233.
208. Parrish JA, Jaenicke KF, Morison WL, et al. Solar urticaria: treatment with PUVA and mediator inhibitors. *Br J Dermatol* 1982;106:575.
209. Tkach JR. Aquagenic urticaria. *Cutis* 1981;28:454.
210. Chalamidas SL, Charles CR. Aquagenic urticaria. *Arch Dermatol* 1971;104:541.
211. Greaves MM. Pharmacologic basis of aquagenic urticaria. Report of Annual Meeting of the European Society for Dermatologic Research. *Amsterdam Skin Allergy News* 1980;11:3.
212. Bernhard J. Nonrashes: Atmoknesis: pruritus provoked by contact with air. *Cutis* 1989;44:143.
213. Rothenborg HW, Menne T, Sjølin KE. Temperature dependent primary irritant dermatitis from lemon perfume. *Contact Dermatitis* 1977;3:37.
214. Foussereau J. Allergic eczema from vinyl-4-pyridine. *Contact Dermatitis Newsletter* 1973;11:26.
215. Fukunaga T, Kawagoe R, Hozumi R. Contact anaphylaxis to paraphenylenediamine. *Contact Dermatitis* 1996;35:185–186.
216. Calnan CD, Shuster S. Reactions to ammonium persulfate. *Arch Dermatol* 1968;88:812.
217. Fisher AA, Dooms-Goossens A. Persulfate hair bleach reactions. *Arch Dermatol* 1976;112:1407.
218. Brun R, Jadassohn W, Paillard R. Epicutaneous test with immediate type reaction to ammonium persulfate. *Dermatologica* 1966;133:89.
219. Reiffers J, Hunziker N, Brun R, et al. Unusual contact dermatoses. *Dermatologica* 1974;148:285.
220. Johansson J, Lahti A. Topical non-steroidal anti-inflammatory drugs inhibit nonimmunologic immediate contact reaction. *Contact Dermatitis* 1988;19:161.
221. Kanerva L, Toikkanen J, Jolanki R, Estlander T. Statistical data on occupational contact urticaria. *Contact Dermatitis* 1996;35:229–233.
222. Katsarou A, Armenaka M, Ale I, et al. Frequency of immediate reactions to the European standard series. *Contact Dermatitis* 1999;41:276–279.

CHAPTER 35

Contact Dermatitis and Other Reactions to Metals

As a group, metals are the most common contact allergens. Nickel is the most common cause of metal allergy, and in most series ranks as the most common of all screening allergens (1). Reactions to gold, chrome, cobalt, and organic forms of mercury are also frequently seen. Most other metals can cause some form of skin reaction, such as allergic or irritant dermatitis (1). The latest data from the North American Contact Dermatitis Group show that nickel was positive in 14.2% of 3,429 patients tested over a 2-year period, ranking first overall. Thimerosal (10.9%), gold (9.5%), and cobalt (9.0%) ranked fifth, sixth, and ninth in overal prevalence (2).

Allergic sensitivity to a metal is usually highly specific, and a cross-sensitivity reaction with other metals is exceptional. Many reports of cross-reactions between metals are actually co-reactions, which occur because of simultaneous exposure to two or more metals. This is particularly the case with cobalt, nickel, and chromium. For example, cement, which is a common cause of chromate allergy, also contains cobalt, which may contribute to allergic contact dermatitis (ACD) from cement.

Sensitization to trace metallic elements in detergents, tattoo marks, dental fillings, metallic foreign bodies, metals of orthopedic appliances, and foods may produce allergic metal dermatitis. Table 35.1 summarizes the various reactions to metals.

ACD to metal generally occurs only if the metal salts are in solution, as occurs with perspiration or exposure with bodily fluids. It is, therefore, possible for individuals who show marked allergic contact sensitivity to a chromate solution to be able to handle chrome-plated objects without difficulty, for example. Similarly, contact with stainless steel containing nickel usually does not produce nickel dermatitis in a nickel-sensitive individual, because the alloy binds the nickel so firmly that sweat cannot liberate nickel salts. In most cases with chronic exposure, however, eventually enough of the allergen will penetrate the skin and ACD will occur.

PLATED METALS

So-called plated metals consist of electrodeposited metallic coatings embracing various metals and alloys with widely varying physical and chemical properties (3). The metals range in hardness from soft materials, such as lead and tin, to those as hard as nickel and chromium. Chemically, these substances range in reactivity from electronegative (anodic) metals, such as zinc and cadmium, to the relatively inert nodal metals, exemplified by gold and platinum. In color, electrodeposited coatings vary from the white of zinc, cadmium, and silver, through the yellows of brass, and the greens and reds of the gold alloys, to the black of platinum black and black nickel. Liden et al. (4) tested a number of nickel-containing alloys. Many alloys and nickel liners under gold, silver, or chrome plating gave positive reactions in test subjects. This confirms that plating will not prevent nickel allergy in most cases.

Small, inexpensive metallic items, such as garter clips, zippers, and other cheap fasteners, generally are simply nickel-plated. Metallic watch bands and most costume jewelry are usually flashed with bright chromium (or some other electrodeposit, e.g., gold, silver, or rhodium) after nickel-plating. In general, the thin deposits of chromium and other metals over the nickel are not continuous but contain many microscopic discontinuities, sometimes referred to as pinholes or pores. The nickel in a chrome-plated object, for example, may come through the pinholes of the plated object after being dissolved out by sweat and produce dermatitis in individuals with allergic hypersensitivity to nickel. The extent to which the underlying nickel may be attacked by sweat will, of course, depend on the degree of porosity of the overlying metal coating. Accordingly, one cannot assume that the underlying nickel will not come through a chrome-plated object, even though it appears not to have been worn off.

Except for industrial plating, in which the chrome coating is used because of its own unique mechanical and

TABLE 35.1. *Reactions to Metals*

Miscellaneous reactions
   Metal fume fever—cadmium and zinc
   Metallic dust and moisture folliculitis—antimony spots
   Smelters itch—arsenic trioxide
   Coin rubbing dermatitis (çao-gio)
   Zinc "pox"
   Baboon syndrome
Primary irritant dermatitis and chemical "burns"
Allergic contact sensitivity
Systemic contact dermatitis
Granulomas
Erythema multiforme
Platinosis (asthma)
Pompholyx
Tattoo granulomas
Urticaria
Photosensitization dermatitis
   Cadmium sulfide in tattoos
   Chromates
   Cobalt
Pigmentation and discoloration
   Accidental tattoos
   Argyria (silver)
   Black dermographism
   Chrysiasis
   Hair: copper (green), cobalt (white), and silver (black)
   Iron siderosis, endogenous or exogenous
   Nails: mercury, lead, silver, and chromate
   Rusting
Lichen planus

chemical properties, chrome-plated objects generally carry a much thicker deposit of nickel than of chromium, the ratio generally being at least 100:1. Nickel-plated objects are pinkish white, whereas chrome plating imparts a bluish white color.

STAINLESS STEEL

The dermatologist, the allergist, and often the orthopedic surgeon are concerned with stainless steel because it may contain sensitizing metals, such as chromium, nickel, cobalt, and other trace metals.

Stainless steel is an iron-based alloy usually containing at least 12% chromium. Basically, the chromium content imparts the stainless property. The addition of nickel is said to create a hard, smooth surface, which increases resistance to corrosion, wear, and abrasion. Some stainless steels contain as much as 26% chromium; others contain as much as 37% nickel.

Various other ingredients may be added, such as molybdenum, magnesium, silicon, carbon, phosphorus, cobalt, and sulfur. The molybdenum helps prevent pitting by body chlorides.

The term "solid solution" as applied to stainless steel means that an element is dispersed homogeneously and is not a separate phase, such as a precipitant. When stainless steel is manufactured, all the metals are contained in a solution at a temperature of 2,400°C. As it cools, a crystalline lattice is formed, which locks in the various metals.

> Stainless steel is basically an iron-chromium solid solution alloy with nickel and other ingredients added to increase resistance to corrosion and pitting.

Liden et al. (5) showed that 27% of 565 metal hand tools available in Sweden released significant nickel as measured by the dimethylglyoxine test.

Corroded steel may show pit marks, which may be produced by acids and sodium chloride. Even though sodium chloride produces grains of stainless steel, the lattice framework is preserved with the metals locked into it. Rust may be formed when there is high humidity in the presence of salt, and chromic oxide may be formed, but its role in chrome sensitivity has not been established.

Stainless Steel Sutures

Several nickel-sensitive individuals have had stainless-steel sutures inserted for surgical procedures without a reaction. Ethicon stainless-steel sutures contain approximately 10% nickel.

METALS IN SOAP AND DETERGENTS

Ingber et al. (6) have shown that detergents and bleaches may be significant sources of chromium exposure. Of 38 detergents and surface cleaners and 12 bleaches, 90% of patients had over 1 ppm of chromium and 56% had over 7 ppm of chromium. Irritant effects from the cleaners may potentiate ACD from the low level of chromium. Palmolive dish washing liquid (Colgate-Palmolive, United States) was the highest, at 546 ppm (6).

Several European studies have stressed that nickel and chromium present in detergents are factors in the production of dermatitis, particularly hand eczemas, in individuals sensitized to these metals. Nickel was found in amounts as great as 9 mg/kg in Dutch phosphate-containing detergents (7). In order to eliminate nickel-sensitization from detergents, ethylenediamine tetra-acetate (EDTA) was added during manufacture, because the nickel-EDTA complex has no sensitizing properties (8). The Dutch investigators concluded that nickel in detergents plays a minor role in nickel dermatitis. A Spanish report, however, concluded that the amount of nickel and chromium in detergents is sufficient to account for the persistence of contact dermatitis due to these metals after the more obvious contacts have been eliminated (9). In a later report, also from Spain, 30 domestic detergents and cleaners were analyzed for cobalt and nickel. Of these, 78.6% showed "considerable" amounts of cobalt, and most also contained nickel. Whether the levels were high enough to cause ACD is uncertain (10).

Fisher performed the dimethylglyoxime spot test for nickel on several concentrated solutions of American detergents with negative results.

The source of nickel in American detergent compounds is the raw materials used in the manufacturing process, and the most likely source of chromates in trace quantities (up to 5 ppm) is principally phosphates (Professional Services Division, Procter & Gamble Co, personal communication).

Chromic acid or chromates may be added to brushless shaving creams to prevent rusting of razor blades.

> **Reports differ greatly as to the significance of nickel and chromates in detergents. It is uncertain if American detergents are able to cause nickel or chromate sensitization or dermatitis.**

METAL SALTS IN COSMETICS

The following metallic salts are permitted color additives, according to the US Food, Drug, and Cosmetic Act regulations:

- Iron oxide—brownish yellow and ochre
- Chlorophyllin copper complex—green
- Chromium oxides—olive and bluish green
- Cobalt blue—blue
- Lapis lazuli—reddish blue
- Ultramarine blue—reddish blue
- Manganese violet—violet
- Potassium ferrocyanide—yellow solution

> **Many metal salts are relatively safe color additives for cosmetics.**

Nickel may also be present in cosmetics as a contaminant. Because the facial, and especially the eyelid, skin is very sensitive, it would seem possible that metals in cosmetics could cause ACD there in very sensitive individuals. Cobalt and chromate are common sensitizers. Chromium allergy is usually due to hexavalent chromate, but trivalent chromium may cause allergy occasionally. Skin that is already dermatitic is at greater risk for further sensitization. Zugerman (11) reported a case of eyelid dermatitis due to yellow iron oxide. Considering the vast usage of color cosmetics, reactions to the coloring agents seem to be rare.

METAL SALTS IN HAIR DYES

Hair dyeing with metallic dyes is incompatible with permanent waving and coloring with the oxidation type of dyes.

The great popularity of such hair treatment has noticeably curtailed the use of the metallic dyes by women. Large quantities of all types of metallic dyes, however, are still used by men. In the United States, the most popular metallic dyes are lead, silver, and copper. Nickel is rarely used alone but may be combined with silver, iron, and copper. Silver dyes in the form of a 5% silver nitrate solution are still widely used at home and in beauty shops for dyeing eyebrows and lashes. Allergic reaction or argyria rarely occurs from the use of metallic silver hair dyes. In other countries, cobalt and manganese may be used as hair dyes.

> **Metallic salts in hair dyes are not toxic on intact skin and rarely cause dermatitis.**

The US Food, Drug, and Cosmetic Act imposes no restriction on the use of metallic hair dyes, because such products are generally considered harmless to the intact skin. Metallic dyes may be absorbed through abrasions, however, and produce toxic effects. Men who use metallic color restorers on mustaches should be warned about the danger of accidental ingestion.

Allergic reactions to metallic hair dyes are rare. In this sense, they are safer than the oxidation-type dyes.

METAL SALTS IN TATTOOS

Allergic reactions to metal salts used for tattooing are not infrequent. Mercury, chromium, cobalt, and cadmium have been reported as producing various types of reactions in tattooed areas in sensitized individuals (12).

The salts of tattoo metals that may have an allergic effect and the corresponding colors are as follows: (a) red—mercury sulfide (cinnabar and vermillion), (b) green—chromium and chromic oxide, (c) blue—cobalt aluminate, and (d) yellow—cadmium.

Mercury

In the form of red cinnabar in a tattoo, mercury may produce itching, swelling, and eczematous and granulomatous reactions in sensitized individuals. Often the red tattooed areas are quiescent for many years, then suddenly an acute allergic reaction occurs. In one instance, the red portions of a tattoo began to itch and swell following intradermal injections of a vaccine containing thimerosal, a complex organic mercurial compound used as a preservative (13). In another instance, Fisher observed an itchy swelling of the red areas in an individual who ingested calomel (mercurous chloride) and who showed a positive patch test reaction to ammoniated mercury and Mercurochrome. A generalized eczematous eruption may result from laceration of a tattoo in a mercury-sensitive patient (14). Aside from mercury sulfide, nonmetallic red colors in tattoos include an organic pigment (scarlet lake), carmine (dried insect bodies), cochinilla, and cadmium red (selenide).

Chromium

Chromium oxide powder is one of the principal green dyes used in tattooing. This powder is known as chrome green or Casalic green, and it is very stable, resistant to acids, and insoluble in water, alcohol, and acetone. Guignet's green is a closely related green pigment that contains a mixture of hydrous chromium oxides. Lowenthal (15) cited a case of persistent eczema of the extremities that did not clear until five green areas were excised from a tattoo on the arm.

Apparently, these chrome particles may lie latent in tattoos for 20 years or more, then suddenly produce an allergic eczematous dermatitis.

Chromium sesquioxide (viridian), emerald green, may also be used in tattoos. In addition, chlorinated copper (phthalocyanine) may be employed in green tattoos.

Cobalt

In the form of cobalt blue (azure blue and cobaltous aluminate), cobalt has been reported as causing a sarcoidal allergic reaction in areas in which it was used as a light blue tattoo pigment (16). A patch test with cobalt evoked a positive reaction, and cobalt was also demonstrated in the pathologically altered parts of the tattoo. A tattoo test with cobalt blue elicited an inflammatory tissue reaction. In some blue tattoos copper phthalocyanine may be used. Indigo is occasionally added.

Cadmium

This substance, in the form of cadmium sulfide, is sometimes used as a yellow pigment in tattoos, and these areas may itch and swell on exposure to sunlight. Experimental areas tattooed with cadmium sulfide showed an edematous reaction only when exposed to light of 3,800, 4,000, and 4,500 Å wavelengths (17). The swelling reaction to cadmium sulfide in yellow tattoos seems to be phototoxic. Occasionally, commercial red tattoo pigment shows traces of cadmium sulfide, which may induce a photosensitive reaction after exposure to sun (18). Aside from cadmium sulfide in yellow tattoos, chrome zinc and lemon yellow (chrome salts) may be present. Yellow ochre (hydrate of ferric oxide) may be added.

In one patient a reaction to a red tattoo was not caused by mercury or cadmium but to an azo dye in the tattoo (19).

In tattoos, mercury red, chrome green, cobalt blue, or cadmium yellow may produce localized or generalized eczematous eruptions in sensitized individuals. Granulomatous and photosensitive reactions can also occur.

Scutt and Gotch (20) list other tattoo colors that may or may not contain metals.

Black:

1. Logwood (containing chrome)
2. Black waterproof ink (containing charcoal suspended in ammoniacal solution containing phenol)

Brown:

1. Venetian red (hydrate of ferric oxide)
2. Cadmium salts

White:

1. Titanium or zinc oxide
2. Lead carbonate (flake white)

Purple:

1. Manganese

Nguyen and Allen (21) attributed itching in a purple tattoo to manganese, but they did not patch test the patient. Scutt and Gotch (20) warn that tattoos occasionally become inflamed and pruritic, only to clear without any therapy.

Tattoos occasionally become erythematous and pruritic, only to subside spontaneously.

Rubianes and Sánchez (22) reported one case of a woman who developed a granulomatous response to iron oxide used for cosmetic permanent eyebrow tattooing. The reaction developed 4 weeks after the implantation. Systemic corticosteroids were required to clear the reaction.

ACTION OF SODIUM CHLORIDE AND SWEAT ON METALS

A ring dermatitis due to primary irritation from the action of salt on jewelry alloys may be produced. The sodium chloride acting on the metal may come from sweat or from table salt that has become trapped between the ring and the finger. The salt discolors and corrodes the metal, which may produce a primary irritant type of dermatitis.

It is likely that, in most cases, disolution of metal in sweat or other liquids is important before clinical allergic manifestations will develop. A discussion of metals, alloys, and relationship to sweating has been published (23).

In addition, a greenish black smudge due to sulfur in the sweat of some people may be produced with all types of metallic jewelry. These persons should remove rings frequently and powder their fingers with an absorbent powder that is free of zinc oxide to prevent both black dermographism and sulfide discoloration.

> **Sweat and table salt trapped under a ring may produce an irritant dermatitis and dissolve out nickel and gold to produce an allergic dermatitis in sensitized individuals. A high sulfur content of sweat may also corrode metal and produce a greenish sulfide smudge.**

Relationship of Sweat to "Rusting"

A "ruster" is an individual who produces a corrosive effect by fingering a freshly polished metallic surface. Abnormally high concentrations of chloride ion in sweat are responsible for these adverse effects (24). Although patients ⌐ fibrosis of the pancreas may sweat profusely, ⌐vidence that "rusters" have pancreatic

⌐ized to nickel or gold acquire ⌐ach metallic objects only when ⌐ showing the importance of the ⌐t.

⌐occurs in workers in the precision en- ⌐urton et al. (25) pointed out that expe- ⌐ the precision engineering industry rec- ogniz⌐ ⌐ people secrete sweat that readily corrodes metal. Polished metal surfaces touched by these persons will show rusty fingerprints within a few days, causing unsightly blemishes on the metal. The rust can cause the malfunction of complex small components, such as the tumblers of locks and equipment used in the electronic industry. "Rusters" are often unable to wear gloves to protect the metal because of the high degree of manual dexterity required for the job. Such employees, once they are detected, may lose their jobs.

The following measures may enable the "ruster" to continue his or her work: (a) keeping as cool as possible by wearing light clothing; (b) remaining on a low-salt diet; (c) washing the hands frequently to remove sodium chloride from the surface of the skin; (d) removing sweat from the metal immediately after it is handled, because rusting begins quickly; and (e) using Drysol, which is aluminum chloride in alcohol, to help reduce palmar and finger sweating (26).

> **The sodium chloride content in the sweat of perspiring fingers of certain individuals is high enough to corrode and rust freshly polished metallic surfaces.**

> **A low-sodium diet, cool environment, and application of Drysol may control "rusting."**

METALS IN COINS

Coins contain other metals beside the metal from which they take their names.

The US Coinage Act, passed 23 July 1965, changed the composition of the dime, quarter, and half dollar. These denominations formerly contained 90% silver and 10% copper. All silver was eliminated from the dime and quarter, and the percentage was reduced substantially in the half dollar.

The dime and quarter are manufactured from strips composed of three layers of metal bonded together and rolled to the required thickness. This is called cladding. The face is 75% copper and 25% nickel, and the core is pure copper, which is visible on the edges of the coins.

> **Since 1965, US "silver" coins, such as dimes and quarters, have contained only nickel and copper. The half dollar still contains a small amount of silver.**

For students of numismatics and handlers of old coins who may be nickel-sensitive, it is of interest that nickel is present in the following US coins: (a) Flying Indian Head cent series, 1856 to 1864; (b) three-cent pieces, 1865 to 1888; (c) five-cent nickels, 1866 to date, except for those issued from 1942 to 1945.

Metal Dermatitis from Coins

Nickel dermatitis of the hands from normal handling of nickel coins rarely occurs because of inadequate exposure and the protection of the thick, horny layer of the palm. Fisher has observed two patients, however, with nickel dermatitis of the fingers due to unusual circumstances. One patient habitually carried coins in the finger portion of her glove; the other rubbed her nose with coins, producing dermatitis not only of the fingers but also of the side of the nose that resembled seborrheic eczema. Both sites cleared promptly when contact with nickel coins was avoided.

> **Adequate exposure to coins containing nickel can cause dermatitis of the hands in sensitized individuals.**

The thick, horny layer of the palmar aspect of the hands and fingers undoubtedly prevents many cases of dermatitis due to nickel coins at these sites. Prolonged contact, however, with pressure, such as pushing a baby carriage with a nickel-plated handle bar, can produce nickel dermatitis in sensitized women. Experimentally, when nickel coins were kept on the palms under occlusion for 24 hours, allergic dermatitis did occur in two nickel-sensitive individuals that Fisher tested.

Bang Pedersen et al. (27) found that much more nickel was released from coins in water and synthetic sweat than from nickel-plated metal. This indicates that silver-colored coins may be a more relevant source of allergen in everyday life than plated objects, apart from those objects that are in more or less permanent contact with the skin, such as zippers and earrings. It is thus possible that the contamination of the hands, as found in this study, is sufficient to maintain an already established eczema from nickel. Husain (28) stated that a palmar dermatitis developed in a patient due to coins.

Use of Coins for Patch Test for Nickel Sensitivity

Morgan (29) found that eight British patients with positive reactions to nickel sulfate reacted severely to simultaneous patch testing with English "silver" coins that contained an alloy of cupronickel. Similarly, 10 patients who were sensitive to nickel showed a true allergic eczematous reaction to contact with American nickel coins, which are also essentially a cupronickel alloy.

Fisher found that patch testing with nickel coins is a reliable method of ascertaining sensitivity to nickel, provided that US World War II–era nickels are not used, and that nonspecific pressure effects and papular, pustular reactions are not confused with true allergic eczematous reactions. Testing with coins often results in an inflammatory spot reaction because of irregularity and spurs, especially along the borders of the coins. In addition, one must not confuse nonspecific follicular, miliaria-type reaction to a coin. A true allergic reaction is normally accompanied by itching, erythema, papules, and small vesicles.

Patch testing with nickel coins, however, is not a substitute for testing with a standard allergen preparation and should not be used for routine diagnosis. It may be of some educational value to the patient.

"Therapeutic" Coin-Rubbing Dermatitis (ÇAO GIO)

Yeatman and van Dang (30) report that coin rubbing (çao gio) is the Vietnamese practice of rubbing the skin with a coin to alleviate various common symptoms of illness. The back, neck, head, shoulders, and chest are common sites of application. Although mimicking the lesions of trauma, it is not a harmful procedure and no complications are known. A survey of 50 Vietnamese living in the United States since 1975, showed marked distrust of American physicians, owed largely to actual or perceived criticism of çao gio. Acceptance of çao gio as a valid cultural practice will facilitate compliance and adequate medical follow-up.

Description of Çao Gio Methods

The back and chest are massaged with a medicated substance, such as mentholated ointment or oil. Firm downward strokes with a coin, comb, or spoon over the spine and ribs produce petechiae and ecchymoses. For headache, the head is massaged in a temporofrontal direction, and the skin between the eyebrows is pinched until reddened. For cough, nausea, and vomiting, the neck and chest are preferred sites, and the sternomastoid muscle is compressed at the point of its insertion into the sternum.

At first appearance, the patient may appear to be a "battered" or abused child (31–35). Yeatman and van Dang (30) believe, however, that cutaneous lesions resembling those seen in inflicted trauma, but produced by emotionally nurturant folk practices, should not be considered as harmful. They also believe that when treating Vietnamese patients, the physician should discuss the practice of çao gio in neutral, if not favorable, terms. The patient or parent may initially deny the practice. Better understanding and acceptance by the physician, however, should improve rapport, compliance, and subsequent appointment keeping.

Tan (36) stated that coin rubbing is also popular in Indonesia as part of traditional medicine and is known under several names, including kerok and kerik. Coin rubbing has a definite connection with China and is practiced frequently by the Chinese and those of Chinese ancestry, especially among the older generations.

Coconut oil or cajuput oil is usually used as a skin lubricant and is applied most often to the back and the neck and less frequently to the chest. Coconut oil seems to give a fast subjective sense of well-being if applied to patients who have colds and other influenza-like diseases, especially those who have fever and malaise. The oil is used as a home remedy for children as well as adults. The darker the color of the oil and the more ecchymoses that develop as a result of this rubbing, supposedly the greater the extent of the patient's cold.

> The production of ecchymotic dermatoses by coin rubbing (çao gio, kerok) as a therapeutic measure by Vietnamese, Chinese, and Indonesian patients has not resulted in any complications and should not be considered as a form of child abuse or "battering."

Ecchymoses from Native American Medical Technique

Seigle (37) stated that one of the practices by Navajo medicine men is literally to "suck out" problems (e.g., gallstones and headaches) that the patient may have. When the mouth is used in this way, annular ecchymotic areas develop over the parts of the body where the patient is treated (e.g., abdomen, neck, and arms).

Physicians who treat Native Americans are oriented to be supportive of traditional healing methods if they are performed in addition to modern medical practice. In cases in which patients must stay in the hospital, they are encouraged to have the medicine men perform a ceremony in the hospital room.

Medical care provided by the US Indian Health Service is free, whereas that offered by the medicine man is for a fee, either money or goods. For this reason, some patients value the traditional cure more than the service that is offered at the hospital. (Note: The production of ecchymosis by "sucking" is similar to that produced by "cupping," which was popular in the United States before the advent of antibiotics.)

Relationship between Cobalt, Nickel Allergy, and Other Metal Allergies

Kranke and Aberer (38) analyzed positive patch test reactions to metal in 11,516 patients. Their results are shown in Table 35.2. The most striking findings were that 95% of those allergic to palladium also reacted to nickel and that 79% of cobalt-allergic patients reacted to nickel.

In England, studies of chromate-sensitive patients in two different time periods showed that 41% and 34% of patients in the two groups also reacted to cobalt (39). The authors postulated that cosensitization to these two metals often results from cement exposure.

Rystedt (39) concluded that nickel sensitivity, in combination with irritant eczema, induces a high risk of developing cobalt allergy. From her investigation, it is not possible to conclude which are the primary and secondary events, but most facts indicate that nickel sensitivity followed by irritant dermatitis of the hands appears first, and that cobalt sensitivity is a secondary phenomenon. It is possible that a preexistent nickel allergy increases the risk of developing cobalt allergy, because of the high frequency of hand eczema among nickel-sensitive individuals. The cobalt allergy then seems to aggravate the hand eczema. All the hard-metal workers in Rystedt's study with simultaneous nickel and cobalt sensitivity had severe dermatitis of the hands. This dermatitis was more severe than in individuals who had only an irritant contact dermatitis.

In general, concomitant nickel and cobalt allergies have a strong association with severe hand eczema.

TABLE 35.2. *Metal Co-Reactivity*

(Percentage of patients allergic to other metals of those positive to the metal listed in the top line)

	Nickel	Cobalt	Palladium	Chromate
Nickel	—	78.9%	94.6%	39.6%
Cobalt	23.4%	—	36.2%	31.3%
Palladium	33.0%	42.5%	—	NS
Chromate	5.5%	14.7%	NS	—

NS, Not stated
Adapted from Kranke and Aberer, Ref. 38.

Eight hundred fifty-three hard-metal workers were examined and patch tested with 20 substances from their environment, including nickel and cobalt. Nickel sensitivity was found in 2 men and 38 women. Eighty-eight percent of the nickel-sensitive individuals had developed a jewelry dermatitis before use in the hard-metal industry or before the appearance of hand eczema. Twenty-nine percent of the hard-metal workers gave a history of slight irritant dermatitis. In the nickel-sensitized group, 40% had had severe hand eczema that generally appeared 6 to 12 months after starting employment. In 25% of the cases, nickel-sensitive individuals developed cobalt allergy, compared with 5% in the total population investigated.

The relationship of cobalt and nickel allergy was studied by Lammintausta et al. (40). An increase in positive patch tests to either metal was found in guinea pigs sensitized to both metals as compared to those sensitized with only one. For example, 4 of 13 sensitized only to nickel later had positive patch tests to nickel, whereas 7 of 13 that were first sensitized to cobalt and then to nickel later reacted to nickel.

Coexistence of cobalt and nickel allergy is common. Although the mechanism is not understood, it may be more than a simple co-reactivity.

PATCH TESTS WITH METALS AND THEIR SALTS

Table 35.3 lists the concentrations of metal salts recommended for patch test purposes.

In performing patch tests with metal salts, one must be careful not to interpret the pustular or follicular patch test reactions as allergic responses. Such reactions are not uncommon and should be considered as a nonspecific, primary irritant type of response.

A number of metal salts are now available commercially for patch testing (Table 35.3). If testing with nonstandardized materials, it may be more convenient to test in water rather than petrolatum. False-positive reactions may be more likely than with standardized allergens.

Negative Patch Test Reaction in Suspected Metal Dermatitis

Whenever an individual is suspected of having a metal hypersensitivity and the patch test response is negative, a careful investigation usually reveals that the patient is free of metal allergy. For example, many women are suspected of having nickel dermatitis because of an eruption in the garter area presumably due to a nickel-plated garter buckle or clasp. In several instances, a negative nickel test result was obtained, and further investigation revealed that the dermatitis was actually due to sensitivity to the rubber of the garter.

TABLE 35.3. *Suggested Patch Test Concentrations for Metals*[a]

	Source	Comments
Aluminum		
Aluminum metal	Hermal	
Aluminum chloride 2% pet	Chemotechnique	Irritant (?)
Arsenic		
Sodium arsenate 10% aq		Irritant (?)
Beryllium		
Beryllium sulfate 1% aq		Active sensitization
Beryllium chloride 1% pet		
Cadmium		
Cadmium chloride 1% pet	Chemotechnique	Irritant (?)
Chrome		
Potassium dichromate 0.25% pet	US, screening	
Potassium dichromate 0.5% pet	Europe, screening	
Cobalt		
Cobalt chloride 1% pet	Hermal, Chemotechnique, screening	Follicular purpura
Copper		
Copper oxide 5% pet	Chemotechnique	Nickel contamination (?)
Copper sulfate 2% pet	Chemotechnique	
Gold		
Gold sodium thiosulfate 0.5% pet	Hermal, Chemotechnique	Persistent positive
Gold sodium thiomalate 1.0% pet	Myochrisine	Persistent positive
Indium		
Indium sulfate 10% aq	Chemotechnique	
Iridium		
Iridium chloride 1% aq	Chemotechnique	
Iron		
Ferric chloride 2% aq		
Ferrous sulfate 5% pet		
Red iron oxide 2% pet	Chemotechnique	
Lead		
Lead acetate 0.5% aq		
Lead chloride 0.2% aq		
Manganese		
Manganese dioxide 10% pet		
Mercury		
Mercuric chloride 0.01% aq	Chemotechnique	
Ammoniated mercury 1% pet	Hermal, Chemotechnique	
Mercury metal 0.5% pet	Hermal	
Thimerosal 0.1% pet	Hermal Chemotechnique	
Amalgam 5% pet	Chemotechnique	
Molybdenum		
Ammonium heptamolybdenate 1% pet		
Nickel		
Nickel sulfate 2.5% pet	Hermal, Chemotechnique, screening US	
Nickel sulfate 5.0% aq	Hermal, Chemotechnique, screening Europe	If 2.5% negative
Palladium		
Palladium chloride 1% pet	Hermal Chemotechnique (2% pet)	
Platinum		
Ammonium tetrachloroplatinate 0.25% aq	Chemotechnique	
Ammonium hexachloroplatinate 0.1% aq	Chemotechnique	
Rhodium		
Rhodium sulfate 0.05% aq		
Rubidium		
Rubidium iodide 10% pet		
Silver		
Silver nitrate 1% aq	Chemotechnique	Staining, irritant (?), oxides when old

continued

TABLE 35.3. *(Continued)*

	Source	Comments
Tin		
Tin chloride 1% pet		
Titanium		
Titanium oxide 1% pet		
Vanadium		
Vanadium pentoxide 10% pet		
Zinc		
Zinc sulfate 2% pet		
Zinc pyrithione 1% pet	Chemotechnique	

*a*Aq, aqueous; pet, petrolatum.

Whenever nickel sensitivity is suspected but not confirmed by a positive patch test reaction, one must make certain that some other substance is not the cause of the dermatitis. Cobalt and gold especially may cause jewelry dermatitis, even in the absence of nickel allergy.

Some discordance in patch test reactivity is well known and is referred to by Rietschel as the "twinkling back" syndrome. Simonetti et al. (41) found a fairly high discordance with nickel sulfate (5% pet) in 612 consecutive patients. They tested allergens from two different suppliers and found that only 78% of patients reacted to both allergens, with almost equal numbers reacting to only one or the other test material. This illustrates the variability among patch test materials.

Seidenari et al. (42) studied 58 women with a history of nickel allergy but negative screening tests. On repeat testing, 6 (10%) exhibited a positive reaction, but 19 (21%) developed a positive reaction when the test site was occluded for one day before testing with an empty Finn chamber. Also, pretreatment of the test site with the surfactant sodium lauryl sulfate increased the number of positive reactions (43).

In contrast, the addition of a commercial detergent to nickel patch test materials in petrolatum did not significantly increase the test sensitivity (44).

False-negative patch tests in individuals with a history of metal allergy may occur. Pretreatment of the test sites with simple occlusion or with a surfactant may yield more positive results.

False-Positive Metal Patch Test Results

On several occasions Fisher has observed that if metal salts are tested close to each other, a strong positive patch test reaction to nickel will be accompanied by false-positive patch test reactions to the adjacent metal salts, particularly cobalt and copper. These same cobalt and copper salts often show a negative reaction when tested at least 6 inches from the nickel patch test site. Apparently, a strong positive nickel reaction creates a nonspecific hypersensitivity of the surrounding skin and induces false-positive reactions to the other metals.

Intradermal Testing with Metal Salts

Meneghini and Angelini (45) studied a group of patients with clinically evident contact dermatitis and with a history suggestive of contact with metals (patch test reactions to metals were negative). The positive reactions obtained in several cases indicate that intradermal tests may reveal specific sensitivities, which patch tests using standard concentrations are not always capable of demonstrating. Meneghini and Angelini claimed that the results of this study confirm that, in certain special situations and with easily soluble chemicals not irritant to the tissues, intradermal tests may demonstrate specific sensitivities that cannot be revealed by patch tests employing technically suitable concentrations. This is true not only of chromium, nickel, and cobalt, but also of other substances, such as penicillin, neomycin, rivanol, gentian violet, and those allergens that, are in the standard concentration, for example, sulfonamides (46–48). Meneghini and Angelini concluded that a positive reaction on intradermal testing should be considered evidence of low-grade allergic sensitivity not demonstrable on less sensitive patch testing.

In conclusion, it must be emphasized that the authors believe that although patch testing remains the main diagnostic tool in contact allergy, whenever the allergen can be injected into the skin, the intradermal test represents a sensitive and valid diagnostic technique, which is particularly useful in cases of low-grade allergic sensitivity that is not always demonstrable on patch testing in routine concentrations.

Marcussen (49) compared the diagnostic value of the patch and intradermal tests with particular reference to nickel hypersensitivity and concluded that the intradermal test with nickel sulfate, 1:10,000, appeared to be more sensitive and more specific than a patch test using 5% nickel sulfate. Marcussen also found that intradermal testing improves the diagnostic results in nickel allergy by approximately 14%. Marcussen, however, admitted that there was a closer conformity than expected with nickel sulfate, 1:10,000, and with patch tests with 5% nickel sulfate. He further stated that five nickel-sensitive patients showed negative patch test reactions and positive intradermal reactions with nickel sulfate, but four of these patients showed positive patch test reactions when they were retested.

Möller (50) also believes intradermal testing may be of occasional value, especially in cases of uncertain patch test reactions. He reviewed 49 patients with 78 equivocal reactions to chromate, cobalt, and/or nickel. Positive tests at 72 hours were seen in 24 of the 78 injections. Among 10 other patients suspected of metal allergy by history but with negative patch tests, only 3 reacted to ID testing (50).

In the opinion of Fisher and Fowler, intradermal testing with metal salts should be considered an investigative procedure at present, because there is no general agreement about its significance, advantages, or disadvantages.

Fisher has not observed individuals with allergic hypersensitivity to a metal or its salts in whom he was not able to obtain a positive patch test reaction.

Rather than performing intradermal testing in cases of presumed metal allergy and negative patch tests, pretreatment of the test site with occlusion or surfactant or even repeating the test with no modifications will yield more positive results. Adequate testing with a battery of various metals will identify isolated reactions to metals beyond nickel.

> **Patch tests with metals are so reliable that intradermal testing may be considered an investigative procedure. Intradermal tests with metals have no advantage over patch tests except for testing for sarcoidal reactions with certain metal salts.**

Testing for sarcoidal reactions to zirconium salts may be performed by rubbing the zirconium preparation into a test site prepared by multiple scratches or denuded by a dermal curet. In addition, an intracutaneous test may be performed with a 1:10,000 solution of sodium zirconium lactate.

GRANULOMATOUS REACTIONS TO METALS

Many metals are capable of inducing a granulomatous reaction when introduced into the skin of sensitized individuals. Mercury, chromates, and cobalt in tattoos often produce sarcoidal granulomas. Mercury granulomas of the skin can be caused by a broken thermometer. Beryllium may produce not only a localized but also a systemic sarcoidal reaction. Zirconium compounds, used in poison ivy medica-

tions, readily induce a granulomatous response. Silicon in powders can form granulomas in injured skin. Aluminum, an adsorbent in injectables, may produce granulomas at injection sites.

An intralesional injection of corticosteroids in the concentration of 5 to 10 mg/mL often causes involution of such metal granulomas.

> **Mercury, chromium, zirconium, beryllium, cobalt, and silicon can produce sarcoidal granulomas, which may be treated with intralesional corticosteroids.**

ROLE OF METALS IN BLACK DERMOGRAPHISM

Although Urbach and Pillsbury (51) clearly defined black dermographism 30 years ago, discussions at dermatologic meetings would indicate that the mechanism of black dermographism is still generally rather poorly understood. Black dermographism, the most common cause of skin discoloration from metal jewelry, literally means "black writing on the skin." The discoloration is a thin deposit of metallic powder produced by the friction of a metallic object on skin contaminated by powders or abrasives (52).

Black dermographism is really a misnomer because the phenomenon is not confined to the skin and is not physiologic. It is purely a physical phenomenon, which can readily be produced on paper or fabrics (53).

Black dermographism is explained on the basis of the relative hardness of powders dusted on the skin and of metals rubbing on it. (Hardness is defined as the capacity of a substance to abrade another.) By plotting common powders used in cosmetics and medications with metals used in jewelry, it is noted that zinc oxide and pumice are harder than nickel, iron, platinum, silver, gold, copper, and tin. Carbon is the hardest of all and is abundant in urban and industrial dust. Carbon is dirtying in itself and adds to the discoloration of metals by abrading them. In general, any powder listed in Table 35.4 will abrade any metal on the scale below it, and the effect will be streaks of color in the pattern of the friction (54).

Only stainless steel and chromium are harder than cosmetic powders and other makeup, and black dermographism cannot be produced with jewelry made of these cheaper metals. Often the more expensive the jewelry and the more precious the metal, the more discoloration produced by makeup. Twenty-four-karat (pure) gold and platinum readily produce black dermographism.

Calamine lotion, face powders containing zinc oxide, titanium dioxide and ferric oxide, and certain dentifrices (both toothpastes and powders) readily remove a fine metallic powder from jewelry and other metallic objects, staining the skin black. The powder is always black, because the particles are so fine that they do not reflect light.

TABLE 35.4. *Comparison of the Hardness of Metals and Powders*

Powders	Scale of Hardness	Metals
Carbon	10	
	9.5	Chromium
	7	Steel
Zinc oxide and pumice	5.5	
	5	Nickel
	4.5	Iron
	4	Platinum
Boric acid	3	Antimony
Magnesium and bismuth	2.5	Silver, gold, and copper
Kaolin, aluminum, and sulfur	2	Tin
Calcium salts	1.5	Lead
Talcum and zinc stearate	1	

Putting zinc oxide powder or pancake makeup containing it or titanium dioxide on the skin and rubbing with a gold or silver ring immediately produces black lines on the skin. No such effect is obtained with zinc stearate, which is a soft powder.

When an individual applies makeup to the face or body or uses a dentifrice (containing pumice), some of the substances may lodge under rings or other jewelry worn on the neck or wrist. In order to avoid black dermographism, metallic ornaments should be removed and the skin that will be in contact with the jewelry should be cleansed with soap and water to make certain that no makeup or dentifrice remains at these sites.

Rapson (55) thoroughly reviewed black dermographism related to gold.

Black dermographism from cosmetics or dentifrices is the most common discoloration under a ring. Another source of discoloration may be skin secretions and perspiration that contain sulfides and chlorides. These chemicals combine with the molecules of silver and copper that are usually present in a gold alloy to form black salts, such as silver chloride and copper sulfate. This reaction sometimes occurs only when a woman is pregnant, apparently because of changes in body chemistry.

In some maritime, semitropical climates the chlorides from the sea may combine with normal skin secretions to form corrosive chemicals.

> **Smudging or discoloration of the skin may be due to black dermographism or to chlorides and sulfides in the atmosphere or in sweat.**

Workers in rubber factories may be exposed to sulfides, which may tarnish rings. Heavy industrial smog is often thick with sulfides from the burning of low-grade, sulfur-laden coal and fuel oil or with other corrosive chemicals, such as phosphates. These air pollutants can attack gold alloys directly, even when jewelry is not being worn. When the tarnishing ring is slipped back on the finger, or a bracelet onto the arm, the thin film or tarnish rubs off in a black smudge.

> **Black dermographism is a physical phenomenon produced by friction of substances in cosmetics that are harder than nickel, gold, or silver, which remove fine metallic particles from jewelry and other metallic objects.**

CONTACT ALLERGY TO ALUMINUM

Aluminum is a fairly inert metal with a multitude of uses based on its strength and light weight. Irritant folliculitis from aluminum salts in antiperspirants is not unusual. Steinegeer (56) attributed unusual, transient grayish brown and blue skin lesions to air pollution from an aluminum factory. Hemmer et al. (57) routinely tested 1,922 patients with aluminum chloride hexahydrate (2% aq). Only four reacted (0.21%), and none of these reactions were reproducible with a dilution series.

Allergic granulomas and nodules have been reported in children following vaccinations containing aluminum and in adults after hepatitis B vaccination. Essentially, these reactions occur at the site of vaccination, although ACD to aluminum may occur elsewhere as well. Slater et al. (58) found aluminum hydroxide in granulomas by X-ray microanalysis. In a report from Denmark, 21 children developed granulomas, and all were positive on patch tests (59).

ACD to aluminum salts may occur from prior sensitization by vaccinations or hyposensitization injections or may arise rarely from exposure to deodorants or topical aluminum containing medications. Aluminum acetate in eardrops has caused allergic contact dermatitis (60). Considering the wide use of aluminum salts in antiperspirants, aluminum allergy is rare.

Aluminum allergy is usually detected on patch testing when virtually all the sites exhibit a reaction, usually with a prominent annular component corresponding to the Finn chamber edge. Aluminum chloride (2% aq) or other salts such as aluminum oxide (10% pet) can be tested for confirmation. Aluminum hydroxide apparently gives less accurate results and probably should not be used.

Patch Test Problems with Aluminum Finn Chambers

Although generally inert, the aluminum in Finn chambers may interact with metal salts in patch test preparations. Mercury salts were first reported to show this interaction (61). Nickel and cobalt in water may interact as well (62). However, because these metals are routinely tested in petrolatum rather than water, there is probably no practical consequence to the clinician.

Possible Systemic Contact Dermatitus from Aluminum in Toothpaste

Veien et al. (63) described 3 children with generalized itching, all positive to aluminum chloride 2% aq. They were all using the same toothpaste that contained 30% to 40% aluminum oxide.

ANTIMONY IRRITATION AND ALLERGY

Antimony and its compounds are used in alloys, type metal, batteries, foil, ceramics, safety matches, ant paste, textiles, and medicinals (such as tartar emetic, Fuadin, and antimony sulfide).

Antimony is strongly irritating to tissues, including mucous membranes. Chronic antimony poisoning is similar to chronic arsenic poisoning, with symptoms of itchy skin, pustules, stomatitis, and conjunctivitis.

Antimony may produce "antimony spots," an irritant folliculitis in freely perspiring workers exposed to antimony trioxide dust that is due to penetration of the dust into the sweat follicles (64). Three employees making antimony brazing rods developed pustules and papules from antimony dust and fumes (65). In addition, lichenoid and eczematous eruptions resembling atopic dermatitis may occur (66). Antimony trioxide (as is) gave positive reactions in 2 of 190 ceramics workers (67).

Antimony trioxide may be present in fireproof packaging, and antimony pentasulfides are used in fireworks and matches.

ARSENICAL CONTACT DERMATITIS

Contact dermatitis due to arsenic is rare in the general population, but not in industry. The roasting of lead, copper, gold, and cobalt ores that contain arsenic exposes the worker to arsenic trioxide (white arsenic). Arsenic exposure may also take place in the manufacture of insecticides, fungicides, weed killers, poisons used for baits, glasses, enamels, and alloys.

Irritant and allergic contact dermatitis may be produced. Folliculitis with secondary pyoderma and furunculosis is not uncommon. So-called smelter's itch, due to arsenic trioxide, occurs in smelt workers who may develop eczematous eruptions, folliculitis, furunculosis, and ulcerative lesions on the extremities and nasal septum. Birmingham and Key (68) described similar lesions in children exposed to arsenic trioxide in a mining community. The presence of sweat, excoriations, or wounds facilitates the formation of arsenical ulcers.

A 10% aqueous solution of sodium arsenate may be used for patch testing. Arsenic not infrequently produces nonspecific, pustular patch test reactions.

True allergic reactions to contact with arsenical compounds are rare. Holinquist (69) reported dermatitis from exposure to arsenic in a refinery. He obtained positive patch tests with nonirritant concentrations of arsenic compounds. Patients with arsenical keratoses and cancers from the use of Fowler's solution did not give positive patch tests with arsenical preparations.

Allergy to sodium arsenate (1% aq) caused dermatitis on exposed surfaces of a glass factory worker in France (70).

BERYLLIUM DERMATITIS AND GRANULOMAS

Beryllium is a light metal that forms an oxide and several soluble and insoluble solutions. It is used in the manufacture of alloys for electrical equipment and ceramics, and it is present in some phosphorus used in cathode ray tubes and a few fluorescent lights. It may be used in orthodontic devices. Soluble beryllium salts are easily hydrolyzed, with the formation of the free acids, causing severe irritations of the skin with papulovesicular eczematoid, weeping, and itchy lesions. When particles penetrate the skin, ulcers and necrosis may occur.

Curtis (71), after an exhaustive evaluation, reported 13 cases of beryllium dermatitis among workers in two beryllium extraction plants near Cleveland, Ohio. The criteria for establishing the dermatitis as an allergic eczematous type were fulfilled. Pure beryllium metal is insoluble with respect to the skin and sweat and therefore cannot be used for patch testing. Beryllium fluoride sensitizes the skin to a high degree, which accounts for the high incidence of dermatitis among these workers in the fluoride process of beryllium extraction. Beryllium sulfate and beryllium chloride have less capacity to sensitize the skin, and beryllium nitrate has little or none, according to these experiments.

For patch tests, a 1% aqueous unbuffered solution of beryllium sulfate or beryllium chloride is recommended.

When beryllium phosphors were widely used in fluorescent tubes, many instances of beryllium granulomas occurred after people had received cuts from the broken tubes (72–74).

Surgical excision was the only cure for beryllium granuloma before adrenocorticotrophic hormone (ACTH) or corticosteroid was found to bring about improvement (75,76). Fisher (77) reported the complete resolution of a beryllium granuloma after injury with a fluorescent tube by the use of 5% cortisone in Aquaphor.

In Europe, as late as 1967, fluorescent tubes were still reported as producing beryllium granuloma (78). In this report, a young man had cut his right ring finger on a broken fluorescent tube. Patch tests with beryllium sulfate 2% and beryllium nitrate 0.38%, 0.19%, and 0.019% gave positive results. A total dosage of nearly 2,000 mg of prednisone induced regression of the granuloma, but no sooner was the drug discontinued than deterioration set in. The granuloma was therefore extirpated. Five years later, the patch test reaction became positive again. Nevertheless, the operation had favorable clinical and functional results.

> **Some beryllium granulomas may respond to corticosteroid therapy, but often surgical excision becomes necessary.**

Jones Williams (79) presented a case report of a 48-year-old man who, following a relatively trivial finger injury, developed systemic chronic beryllium disease. Initially, he cut his finger on a grinding wheel contaminated with beryllium oxide. This injury developed into a chronic skin ulcer that failed to respond to steroids and 15 months later necessitated amputation of the affected finger. Noncaseating granulomas were present in the ulcer, and spectroscopic analysis revealed the presence of beryllium. The diagnosis was further confirmed by a positive patch test. Six months later, two granulomas together with beryllium containing nodules were removed from the lymphatics of the same forearm. The wounds healed, chest symptoms were absent, and there was no radiologic evidence of disease. The patient remained apparently well but in June 1970, nearly 7 years after the original injury, he presented with multiple firm nodules along the course of the lymphatics in the injured arm. Biopsy showed fibrous nodules with surrounding epithelioid cell granulomas that, on analysis, contained beryllium. Of even graver import are the radiologic findings of bilateral pulmonary mottling, evidence of impaired pulmonary function, and the presence of granulomas in a lung biopsy. It is probable that the recurring lymphatic lesions resulted from the original injury, but the chest lesions indicate an additional inhalation exposure.

Beryllium in Dental and Medical Devices

Recently, beryllium allergy has resurfaced after a scarcity of reports for many years. Haberman et al. (80) reported two cases of allergy induced by beryllium in a dental prosthesis. Both had positive patch tests only to beryllium (BeCl$_2$ 1% pet). In addition, a third patient had dermatitis localized to one arm in which he had an orthopedic implant for fracture stabilization. Again, the only reaction was to BeCl$_2$ but definate proof of beryllium in the implant could not be obtained. Vilaplana et al. (81) reported three cases of beryllium allergy, all with strongly positive patch tests to BeCl$_2$ (1% pet). One woman had oral stomatitis from beryllium in a denture, and a dental technician had hand dermatitis from working with beryllium. The third patient had dermatitis in the area of an orthopedic implant, but it was uncertain if the implant contained beryllium.

As is the case with other allergens that are not often used for testing, the true incidence of beryllium allergy is unknown, but it may be higher than is currently appreciated.

Chronic Beryllium Disease

Inhalation exposure to beryllium may produce pulmonary granulomas. Chronic beryllium disease is a systemic granulomatosis process that primarily affects the lungs, skin, and lymphatics. Reportedly, up to 16% of workers exposed to beryllium metal or dust may develop this condition that mimics sardoidosis (82).

BRASS AND BRONZE

Brass, which contains copper, zinc, tin, lead, and molybdenum, rarely causes allergic contact dermatitis. Lip trouble, among brass players, is usually due to irritant or pressure dermatitis. Some brass may contain traces of nickel. Bronze is an alloy of copper and tin. Traces of lead, phosphorous, nickel, and zinc may be present. Gun metal consists of bronze with zinc. The "gold leaf" that is claimed to be added to some eyeshadows is probably a fired bronze powder coated with stearic acid.

CADMIUM COMPOUND REACTIONS

In modern industry, cadmium is an important metal. It is used as a corrosion inhibitor, as a neutron brake in atomic piles, as a stabilizer in plastics, in dry batteries, in dye production, in soldering and welding, and in photochemistry. The toxic effects of cadmium due to the inhalation of cadmium oxide (metal fume fever) are common. Such inhalation may produce respiratory tract inflammation, pulmonary edema, and decreased sense of smell. Renal toxicity may occur. Cadmium chloride does not appear to be a sensitizer in industry (83–86).

Cadmium Red (Cadmium Selenide) in Dentures and Cooking Utensils

A mixture of cadmium selenide and cadmium sulfide may be used as the pink pigment in acrylic resin. Pure Cadmium Selenide Red No. 1124 is used for the coloring of lucite dentures. Pure cadmium selenide reds are insoluble in perspiration, in natural water, and in dilute hydrochloride acids present in gastric juices. Cadmium red is soluble in muriatic acid. Cadmium reds are nonabsorptive through the skin. Although cadmium reds are classified as poisonous and cannot be used in food colors, they can be used as ingredients in the manufacture of dental rubber, enameled ware, and cooking utensils, or in the production of toys or tinware. In the manufacture of enameled ware, cadmium reds are not affected unless the enamel is destroyed by acids.

Kaaber et al. (87) stated that cadmium red is not a sensitizer.

> 1. **Cadmium oxide in industry may produce "metal fume fever," an inhalation pulmonary reaction.**
> 2. **Cadmium chloride is not a sensitizer in industry but may be phototoxic in tattoos.**
> 3. **Cadmium selenide (cadmium red) is not a sensitizer in dentures or kitchen utensils.**

A large German study found many questionable or positive patch tests to cadmium chloride (1% pet) in 719 patients (88). There were 198 reactions, but only 6 were graded 2+ or 3+. The remainder were felt to be nonspecific irritant reactions, and in the authors' opinion, the stronger reactions were not relevant. The same authors later performed a dilution study and recommend testing with cadmium chloride 0.5% pet, but only in those with a likely exposure to cadmium (89).

CARBON DERMATOSES

Carbon occurs in the pure state as the diamond and as graphite. It is used in electricity as the carbon arc through which the current is conducted and in carbon arc lighting and welding and in batteries.

Friedman (90) reported that the graphite in "lead" pencils produced an allergic dermatitis. Carbon black, consisting of finely divided amorphous forms of carbon, is used in pigments in rubber products and as filtering agents. Capusan and Mauksch (91) stated carbon black plant workers developed fissured hyperkeratoses of the palms and black tattoos of the hands and forearms.

CHROMATE

Chromium is ubiquitous; it is the fourth most common material in the earth's crust. Chromium is distributed widely in both the earth and the sea, and is more abundant than cobalt, copper, zinc, molybdenum, lead, nickel, and cadmium. Widespread exposure to chromium compounds is therefore not surprising. Chrome currently is the fifth most common metal allergen (see Table 35.9). In contrast to other metals, allergy to chrome has been stable or declining in most reports.

Clinical Features of Allergic Eruptions Caused by Chromates

Such eruptions tend to be insidious and persistent and are prone to relapse. Although the eruption may at times be acute and show oozing, it has a greater tendency to be dry, to fissure, and to lichenify. Chromate eruptions may mimic nummular eczema, atopic dermatitis, neurodermatitis, dry forms of dermatophytosis, and primary irritant reactions. Widespread chromate dermatitis may resemble ragweed dermatitis. Once chromate sensitivity has been established, the dermatitis tends to become more severe and more extensive and takes longer to clear with each exposure, even when there is prompt removal from contact with the chemical (92,93).

Chronicity of Chromium Dermatitis

Burry and Kirk (94) are quite pessimistic, labeling chromate-sensitized industrial workers "chrome cripples." In studies of contact dermatitis in southern Australia, they observed manual workers who had been sensitized by an obvious source of chromium or chromate salts and had been disabled by continuous or recurrent dermatitis, a few becoming virtually unemployable.

These investigators found that only minute quantities of chromium or chromate salts need be present in the environment to cause dermatitis in sensitized subjects. The contamination of factories and other workplaces by cement dust or chromate salts in solution (e.g., in diesel engine coolants) provides a constant source of allergen. The authors suggested that "[c]omplete responsibility for the dermatitis should always remain on the shoulders of the original employer's insurance company covering the [worker] at the time of sensitization. This would allow the disabled work[er] to experiment in a variety of tasks until he found one in which he was able to work free of dermatitis."

Burrows (95) found that only 8% of patients with chromate sensitivity from cement were free of dermatitis 10 to 13 years after the initial eruption. Breit and Turk (96) stated that a review of the available literature (97,98) showed that the prognosis for the dichromate-allergic patient was poor. They suggested that the only way to improve the situation was to prevent sensitization by strict avoidance of prolonged contact with dichromate-containing material.

Even with avoidance of chrome, however, many individuals develop chronic eczema. Since 1981, ferrous sulfate has been added to cement in Denmark (99). Despite this, 12 of 17 workers with allergic hand eczema in 1981 suffered from chronic hand eczema in 1987. This occurred despite early retirement or change in occupation (100).

Prevention of Cement Dermatitis

Fregert et al. (100) found that ferrous sulfate could be added to cement to reduce water-soluble hexavalent chromate to trivalent chromate, which is much less allergenic. Avnstorp (101) compared cement workers in 1981, before Denmark began adding ferrous sulfate to cement, to new workers in 1987. Significantly fewer workers (6/227) in 1987 had positive patch tests to chromate compared to 1981 workers (20/190). In contrast, in Australia, where iron sulfate is not added to cement, no change in the incidence of occupational chromate dermatitis was seen in 1989 compared to 1980 (102).

In a follow-up Danish study in 1996, of 4,511 consecutive patch test patients, 79 were allergic to chromate. Only 10 were related to cement contact, and 7 of these had been sensitized before 1981 (103). In contrast, in England, where ferrous sulfate is not used in cement, there was no difference in positive patch test rates between 1983 and 1993 (104).

Unfortunately, for this technique to be effective, the iron sulfate must be added to fresh cement. In stored cement, the iron sulfate oxidizes to an inactive form. Also, this adds about 1% to the cost of the cement. Nonetheless, the benefits in reducing not only medical costs and work absenteeism but also the discomfort of chronic eczema, would seem to suggest the benefit would outweigh the problems.

Chromate dermatitis tends to become chronic and lichenified, particularly from industrial exposure.

Chrome-Tanned Leather Articles

After cement and related construction materials, leather is the next most common source of chromate allergy, except in certain occupational settings.

Chrome tanning is used particularly for light, flexible leathers, such as shoe uppers, and leather for other wearing apparel. The chromates are the principal cause of allergic dermatitis from leather articles.

Fisher's review of 20 patients with dichromate sensitivity revealed that only 4 of them had shoe dermatitis. These four also suffered from hyperhidrosis. Apparently, sweat is necessary to leach the chromates from leather and produce dermatitis in chromate-sensitive patients.

Freeman (105) reported that in 55 patients with shoe allergy, 23.6% were caused by chromate. This was second only to rubber allergens as a whole (43.6%). There is a distinct international difference in causes of shoe allergy. In a report from India, 75% of cases were due to chromate, perhaps because of higher humidity and temperature there, resulting in more perspiration (106).

Leather gloves must be avoided in workers with chromate sensitivity.

Shoe dermatitis caused by chromate sensitivity is associated with hyperhidrosis.

Control of sweating may permit chromate-sensitive patients to wear chrome-tanned shoes without difficulty.

Less Common Sources of Exposure to Chromates

Chromium compounds have been long recognized for their primary irritant corrosive effects on the skin and for their potent skin-sensitizing properties and ability to produce allergic contact dermatitis. In occupational exposure, both effects are common, but in the general population, the allergic contact dermatitis is seen almost exclusively.

Chromates in Bleaching Agents

Javelle water (eau de javelle), a disinfecting and bleaching agent, is essentially a solution of sodium hypochlorite and sodium chloride. Sufficient potassium dichromate may be added (as a coloring and stabilizing agent) to cause dermatitis in dichromate-sensitive individuals (107).

In contrast, of 20 household bleaches in common use in the United States, only 2 were found to contain detectable chromate (108). In these two, the level was between 0.1 and 0.3 ppm, which is probably inadequate for allergy elicitation.

Chromates in Detergents

Phosphate-containing detergents have chromium salts, which may produce dermatitis in chrome-sensitive individuals (109). Ingber et al. (6) found significant levels of chromium in some detergents on the Israeli market.

Brushless Shaving Cream

This is essentially a vanishing cream to which a lubricant has been added, forming an oil-in-water emulsion. Chromic acid or chromates may be added to prevent rusting of razor blades.

Chromated Catgut

Tritsch et al. (110) reported an experiment with five chrome-sensitive individuals on whom implanted threads of chromic plain catgut produced a granulomatous inflammation with secondary involvement of the epidermis. Harp strings were shown to produce contact dermatitis in musicians (111).

The general population is exposed to chromates in leather, matches, glue, paint, detergents, chromic catgut, bleaches, and cement.

Chrome-Plated Materials

These metallic objects rarely cause allergic dermatitis, probably because of relative insolubility in sweat. This is in sharp contrast to nickel-plated objects, which are a common cause of allergic contact dermatitis.

Fregert (112) suggested that chromate-sensitive patients avoid the use of metal cigarette lighters, which may be chromium-plated. It has been Fisher's experience, however, that individuals with even a high degree of hypersensitivity to chromates can handle chrome-plated objects without difficulty.

Chromates in Matches

Both in the United States and elsewhere, some matchheads contain chromates (113). Perspiring fingers touching unlit matches may readily dissolve chromates from matchheads. In addition, the flame and fumes from a lit match may contain considerable amounts of the chemical. After the flame has been extinguished, the charred matchhead still contains traces of chromates and, when placed in pockets, may contaminate pocket linings with chromates. Book matches may similarly contaminate pockets (114). Otitis externa may be caused by cleansing or scratching the ear canal with matches in sensitized individuals.

Samitz (MH Samitz, personal communication) extracted matchheads with sulfuric acid and tested the filtrate for hexavalent chromium with alcoholic diphenyl carbazide. Positive results in paper book matches were found in four out of seven domestic brands. Wood stick matches in three samples from Italy, Japan, and Sweden gave positive results for the presence of dichromates.

Hide Glues Containing Chrome

Morris (115) cited several instances of allergic eczematous dermatitis in chrome-sensitive individuals caused by contact with hide glues. Such glues are made by detanning chrome-tanned leather scraps in acids or in lime.

Epoxy Resin Adhesive Containing Chrome

A tile layer developed ACD to chromate (116). The epoxy flooring adhesive was found to contain cement as a filler.

Chrome Alloys

Chromate dermatitis may occur in the manufacture of chrome alloys. Dermatitis that occurs from contact with the finished alloy, however, is usually due to metals other than chrome, particularly nickel.

"Blackjack Disease" Caused by Chromates

Fregert et al. (117) reported an unusual occupational hazard of professional gamblers, roulette buffs, and card players—"blackjack disease," a dermatitis caused by exposure to chromium salts used for dyeing green felt or baize, which covers the gambling tables. These investigators stated that although the exact amount of chromates adhering to a player's hands after playing cards on a green felt tabletop is unknown, there is probably sufficient chromate to produce dermatitis in chromate-sensitive individuals (118,119).

Chromium in Food and Dietary Supplements

Burrows (119) stated that minute quantities of chromium are also found in food: dairy products (mean 0.10 $\mu g/g$), meat and fish (mean 0.11 $\mu g/g$), vegetables (mean 0.03 $\mu g/g$), fruits (mean 0.02 $\mu g/g$), and grains (mean 0.04 $\mu g/g$). The highest concentrations in food occur in thyme (10.00 $\mu g/g$), black pepper (3.3 $\mu g/g$), and cloves (1.50 $\mu g/g$). Animal diets contain higher amounts (e.g., dog food pellets have 4.24 $\mu g/g$). Vegetation unlikely to be eaten, such as leaves of trees, contains higher quantities; for example, wild cherry leaves have 0.57 $\mu g/g$ and pasture grass, 1.30 $\mu g/g$. Cigarettes contain 0.39 $\mu g/g$, and drinking water, 0 to 0.112 ppm. Total human body content is about 6 mg of chromium; there is a higher concentration in infants, and animals generally have very much higher concentrations (120).

The following foods are high in chromates and should be avoided by chromate-sensitive individuals: potatoes, mushrooms, onions, apples, watercress, frozen peas, canned plums, prunes, corn, baked beans, whole-grain flour, whole egg, spices, tea, beer, wine, cocoa, and chocolate.

Burrows (119) stated that small quantities of potassium dichromate taken orally will produce an exacerbation of chromium dermatitis (121,122). This is surprising, in view of the findings of Donaldson and Barreras (120), who showed that most chromium is changed in the acid media of the stomach to trivalent chromium and not absorbed.

A severe exacerbation of dermatitis occurred in a bricklayer given a homeopathic drug that resulted in an intake of 60 μg of dichromate daily (123).

Fowler (124) reported a man with scattered, generalized dermatitis of recent onset and patch tests positive only to chromate. The man reported that several weeks before the onset of the dermatitis, he began taking the dietary supplement chromium picolinate. The dermatitis resolved soon after he quit taking the supplement. Chromium picolinate is purported to be helpful in weight loss and control of blood sugar in diabetics, but adequate clinical trials are currently lacking.

Role of Chromates in Industrial Dermatitis

Table 35.5 lists the great variety of industrial exposures to chromates (125). The following occupations are particularly well known for their risk to employees of chromium dermatitis: cement work, chromium plating, dyeing, printing, photography, work using antirust agents, and work with wood impregnated with chromium (119).

In addition, chromium dermatitis has been reported from the following (125–140): defatting solvent, food laboratories, oil from galvanized sheet metal, postage stamps, coolant oils, offset printing, blackjack green baize tabletops, milk testing, TV screens, shoes, quick lime, magnetic tapes, detergents, and bleaches and boiler linings.

Automobile Industry

Primer paints containing zinc chromate have caused many cases of allergic contact dermatitis among sensitized workers (141). Hexavalent chromate used as a chromate dip to prevent corrosion of nuts and bolts used in automobile assembly has been reported as another cause (142). Adequate rinsing of the nuts and bolts decreases the hazard. Chromium may be present in automobile antifreeze.

Ceramics Industry

Enamelers and decorators in the ceramics industry may occasionally react to chromates, although other metals, including nickel, cobalt, and red iron oxide, are more common allergens (67).

Foundry Industry

In addition to cement, foundry sand may be contaminated with chromates by the addition of chromium magnesite bricks, which are used as refractory material in the steel furnace.

Pulp Industry

Fregert et al. (143) reported sensitization to chromium and cobalt in the processing of sulfate pulp.

TABLE 35.5. *Occupational Exposures to Chromates*

Acetylene workers	Ink makers
Aniline workers	Linoleum workers
Artificial flower makers	Lithographers
Automobile industry workers	Marble colorers
Battery (dry) makers	Match-factory workers
Bleachers	Mixers (rubber)
Blueprint makers	Mordanters
Builders	Musicians (harpists)
Candle (colored) makers	Paint makers
Carbon printers (photography)	Painters
Cement makers	Paper hangers
Ceramic workers	Paper makers
Chrome workers	Paper money makers
Chromium platers	Pencil (colored) makers
Color makers	Photoengravers
Colorers (marble)	Photographic workers
Compounders (rubber)	Photogravure workers
Crayon (colored) makers	Pottery workers
Cutting oil makers	Printers
Dye makers	Pulp makers
Dyers	Railroad employees (diesel locomotives)
Electroengravers	Rubber workers
Electroplaters	Rustproofers
Enamel makers	Stainless steel and other chrome alloy makers
Enamelers	Tannery (chrome) workers
Etchers	Television makers
Explosives (ammonia and pyroxylin) workers	Textile printers
Firefighters	Vulcanizers
Floor tile installers	Wallpaper printers
Foundry workers	Waterproofers (paper and textiles)
Frosters (glass and pottery)	Wax ornament workers
Furniture polishers	Welders
Glass colorers	Woodworkers (handling wood impregnated
Glass polishers	with chromated zinc chloride)
Glaze workers (pottery)	

Railroad Industry

Sodium dichromate is added to diesel locomotive radiator fluids as an antioxidant to prevent rusting of radiators and pipelines. Inasmuch as many workers acquired chromate dermatitis from this source in the past, various substitute antioxidants, such as borates and nitrates, have been tried, unsuccessfully.

Building Repair Industry

Spackle compounds, which are plaster-like mixtures used to repair defects in walls, contain chromates (144).

Chromates in Corundum

Corundum used in glass polishing may contain chromates (145).

Chrome Plating

Lee and Goh (146) reported that 71% of chrome platers from 17 factories had chrome ulcers, dermatitis, or both or had scars from old ulcers. Mucosal irritation, mostly of the throat, was present in 57%. Workers in "hard" chrome plating, where the plating is thicker for industrial uses, were more likely to have mucosal irritation, whereas "bright" chrome (for decorative use) workers had a higher incidence of skin ulcers.

Welding Industry

Gases and fumes from welding, especially those from the welding of chromium steel alloys, may contain large amounts of not only chromium oxide but also hexavalent chromium (147). Exposure may produce allergic contact dermatitis in individuals who are sensitized to chromates. Shelley (148) reported a flare-up of a chrome dermatitis of the palms resulting from the inhalation of fumes from acetylene welding by a patient with a markedly positive patch test reaction to a 0.25% aqueous solution of potassium bichromate.

Zugerman (149) reported chromium dermatitis in arc welders. One of his patients was so sensitive to chromates that he was unable to work in any part of the plant without developing a cutaneous eruption.

Television Manufacturing Industry

Stevenson (135) studied patients with hand dermatitis who made color TV screens. Of 26 workers with hand dermatitis engaged in this process, 18 had chrome sensitivity.

Ammonium dichromate was used in making color television screens to produce cross-linking of light-sensitized polyvinyl alcohol. This enables fluorescent compounds (in turn red, green, and blue) incorporated in the polyvinyl alcohol to adhere to the screen. Although protective clothing and gloves were worn, examination of patients with a Wood's light showed persistence of the fluorescent compounds on the hands and nail folds even after repeated washing of the hands. Wood's lamp examination explained eczema of the wrists and feet; fluorescence of wristwatches and protective rubber overshoes revealed the presence of contamination with the fluorescent materials containing chromates.

Table 35.6 lists substances and industries that should be avoided by persons sensitive to chromates.

Patch Tests with Potassium Dichromate

Patch testing with potassium dichromate is generally carried out in the United States by using a concentration of 0.25% in petrolatum. In the past, 0.5% had been used, but this resulted in many irritant false-positive reactions. This also may have resulted in an erroneous diagnosis of chromate allergy if the investigator was unaware of the propensity for irritant reactions. European studies have shown that using a 0.375% concentration may be helpful but still results in false-positives (150). Nonetheless, European researchers prefer to use the 0.5% concentration, then attempt to determine relevance on clinical grounds.

A study of 54 individuals found a linear correlation between reactivity and concentration in patients known to be allergic to chromate (151). Using the T.R.U.E. test system,

TABLE 35.6. *Substances and Industries to Be Avoided by Chromate-Sensitive Individuals*

1. Chrome-plated metal—probably will not cause difficulty
2. Leather (most shoe, belt, and other chrome-tanned leather)
3. Construction industry (cement, mortar, plaster, drywall)
4. Bleaching agents (dichromate as coloring and stabilizing agent, javelle water)
5. Matchheads
6. Cosmetics (chromium oxide-green)
7. Tattoos (chromium oxide and Casal's or Guignet's green)
8. Glues (hide glues from detanning leather straps)
9. Automotive industry:
   a. Primer paints (zinc chromate)
   b. Dips to prevent corrosion of nuts and bolts
   c. Welding with chrome alloys
10. Foundries (chromates are added to sand for bricks)
11. Antioxidants for radiators and pipelines for diesels
12. Building repair (spackle)
13. Rustproofing (protection of iron against corrosion and rusting; also used in coolants and grinding emulsions)
14. Cutting oils
15. Catgut (chromated)
16. Paints and enamels (chromate pigments—especially green, orange, and yellow)
17. Detergents (phosphate-containing detergents usually have chromium)
18. Etching agent
19. Electroengraving of copper

which provided for a high degree of control of allergen concentration, various dilutions of both chrome VI and chrome III were tested.

Testing with potassium dichromate 0.5% may give irritant false-positive reactions, which the inexperienced patch tester may misinterpret. In the United States, most of the standard series therefore contains the 0.25% concentration.

Forty-one percent reacted only to the 0.25% concentration, 41% reacted to 0.05%, and one reacted to 0.001%. This suggests that for screening purposes the 0.25% concentration, although occasionally giving a false-positive irritant reaction, is suitable. Testing at a lower level will miss many reactions, whereas more irritancy will occur at a higher concentration.

Kosann et al. (152) studied a 6-hour versus 48-hour patch test to chromate and found the shorter testing was unreliable.

Cement as it is ordinarily used is a primary irritant under a patch test. When it is diluted enough to avoid being a primary irritant, the chromium concentration may be so reduced that a positive patch test reaction will not be obtained, even if the patient has been sensitized to chromates. It therefore seems advisable to test with dichromate directly when chromate sensitivity is suspected.

Chromium Valences and Contact Dermatitis

In lymphocyte stimulation tests, both trivalent and hexavalent chrome are capable of giving a strong positive response (153). The reason that trivalent chrome is clinically less important is probably due to its very poor skin penetration compared to hexavalent chrome.

Hexavalent chromate is the most powerfully sensitizing chromate because of its solubility and capacity to penetrate the skin.

---

1. **Metallic chromate with zero valence is not a sensitizer.**
2. **Trivalent chrome is a very rare sensitizer.**
3. **Hexavalent chromium is a strong sensitizer because of its solubility and capacity to penetrate the skin.**

In the work by Nethercott et al. (151), 54 patients allergic to hexavalent chromate were tested with higher levels of trivalent chromate with only a few reactions. The calculated minimum elicitation threshold (MET) for chrome VI was $0.076 \mu g/cm^2$ and for chrome III was over $33 \mu g/cm^2$.

Chrome Ulcers

Chromates may have a corrosive, necrotizing effect on living tissue, forming ulcers, or "chromeholes" (154). Chrome ulcers on the skin and the perforation of the nasal septum are still common in workers exposed to strong chromate solutions in tanning, electroplating, and chrome production. Chrome ulcers generally occur on exposed areas of the body, chiefly on the hands, forearms, and feet, and they develop readily at the site of insect bites and other injuries. In the presence of chrome dust or vapors, ulceration of the nasal septum often occurs.

The typical chrome ulcer is a crusted, painless lesion. Removal of the adherent crust reveals a punched-out ulcer, 2 to 5 mm in diameter, with a thickened, indurated, undermined border and a base that is covered with exudate. Ulcers of the nasal septum may be painless, but with continued exposure or trauma, the lesions may extend to the underlying tissues and become painful. These lesions usually heal with an atrophic scar in several weeks if further chrome exposure is carefully avoided. No known therapy accelerates the process (154).

Chrome ulcers are produced by hexavalent salts and are independent of an allergic reaction.

Samitz (155) recommended that 10% ascorbic acid in an ointment be applied to the nasal septum for the prevention of chrome ulcers in exposed individuals. In addition, he stated that prompt washing of the exposed skin with an "antichrome solution," such as sodium pyrosulfite, or simply with water helps to diminish the degree of ulceration.

Burrows (119) stated that in Great Britain an ointment of lanolin and soft paraffin is used on exposed skin to prevent chrome ulcerations.

Hexavalent chrome is ulcerogenic, but trivalent chrome is not (119). Apparently the oxidizing properties of hexavalent chromium compounds cause denaturation of the proteins of the skin. This process continues until all the hexavalent chromium is reduced to the trivalent state.

The corrosive, necrotizing action of the chromate ion on living tissue is independent of its sensitizing properties. Perforation of the nasal septum and chrome ulcers of the skin occur in individuals who are not necessarily allergic to the chromates (154).

CEMENT DERMATITIS AND BURNS

Nature of Portland Cement

The original portland cement is named for the Isle of Portland, Dorset, England.

Modern portland cement is a type of hydraulic cement whose essential constituents are tricalcium silicate and dicalcium silicate, with varying amounts of alumina, tricalcium aluminate, and iron oxide. The pH is usually above 12, which is in the range of a strong alkali.

Table 35.7 shows the average composition of regular portland cement, which contains large amounts of calcium oxide in combination with silicon dioxide (SiO_2) and aluminum oxide (Al_2O_3). Because excess calcium oxide, which is alkaline, can be formed during the processing of the raw materials in the manufacture of portland cement, these cements can have varying degrees of alkalinity. Calcium oxide, known as lime, combines with water to form calcium hydroxide and, secondarily, sodium and potassium monoxide, which in the presence of water convert to sodium and potassium hydroxide. Severe burns and ulcerations can occur when this wet cement comes into close contact under pressure with the skin.

Cement can also produce an irritant dermatitis from its alkaline, hygroscopic, and abrasive properties. Allergic dermatitis can occur from the ubiquitous presence of hexavalent chromates in cement in patients who have become sensitized to this metallic salt. The chrome salt is an accidental contaminant of cement and is not an "additive" in the usual sense. Indeed, the earth's entire crust contains chromates in some amounts.

Fresh concrete contains about 15% cement. Mortar used for bricklaying and plaster often contains cement.

Cement Dermatitis and the Chromates

Not only construction workers, but also artists and do-it-yourself home builders are exposed to cement and the hazards of cement dermatitis.

The main sensitizers in cement are the dichromates, but other metals, such as nickel and cobalt, may be present. Reports constantly appear from various countries indicating that cement continues to produce many cases of chromate dermatitis (156,157,158). Soluble chromates have been identified in most of 25 samples of British cement.

Many workers may develop cement dermatitis, including masons, tile setters, and cement workers. Not infrequently, such dermatitis is persistent and tends to become widespread.

TABLE 35.7. *Average Composition of Regular Portland Cement*

Calcium oxide (CaO) 64%
Silicon dioxide (SiO_2) 21%
Aluminum oxide (Al_2O_3) 5.8%
Iron oxide (FeO_3) 2.9%
Magnesium oxide (MgO) 2.5%
Alkali oxides 1.4%
Sulfur oxide (SO_3) 1.7%

The varieties of cement dermatitis:

1. **Allergic contact dichromate sensitivity**
2. **Allergic dermatitis to cobalt or nickel**
3. **Alkaline and hygroscopic irritant dermatitis**
4. **Silica particles irritant dermatitis**
5. **Cement burns**

It is likely that the irritant effect and the alkaline content of cement interfere with the skin's defenses, permitting penetration and sensitization to the dichromates in cement to take place more readily. Not infrequently, individuals develop cement dermatitis after having worked with cement for many years without difficulty.

The incidence of cement dermatitis is highest among workers handling wet cement on small building jobs. In cement factories and on large-scale building jobs, the filling of cement and the mixing and placing of concrete are usually done mechanically, reducing contact with cement by the workers.

Some cement has been reported to contain, in addition to chromium, cobalt and nickel. Hypersensitivity to cobalt and nickel may produce cement eczema under such circumstances. Patch tests, therefore, should be performed not only with dichromate but also with nickel and cobalt in suspected cement dermatitis.

Cement Burns Resulting in Necrotic Ulcers Due to Kneeling on Wet Cement

Fisher (159) reported two cases of severe burns, with resulting ulceration and necrosis of the skin of the knees and legs caused by kneeling on premixed cement. In both instances, portland premixed cement had been poured onto the ground to make patios. Neither patient was a professional in the handling of cement.

To smooth out the poured cement, which was uneven and lumpy, both patients had knelt down on their knees in order to facilitate the smoothing process with a board. The wet cement readily penetrated the patient's clothing and produced third-degree chemical burns of the knees and adjacent areas, necessitating hospitalization, debridement of the burn areas under anesthesia, and application of skin grafts.

In neither case had the patients been warned that wet cement should not be allowed to come in contact with the skin.

Rowe and Williams (160) described a 66-year-old white man who spent 2 hours kneeling in wet ready-mixed cement. When he got up, he noticed that the skin over both shins was of a "peculiar green color," which gradually darkened during the next two days to a "deep purple blue." The resultant painful burns and ulcerations required hospitalization and applications of split-thickness grafts.

Hannuksela et al. (161) presented six patients who had been making a floor by leveling wet cement in a kneeling position. They all developed nearly identical curved ulcers on both sides of both patellae. The subjects were not aware of the irritating properties of fresh wet concrete. The features common to these six cases were a 2- to 6-hour exposure to calcium lye, insufficient protection that allowed the clothes to get wet, and pressure on the exposed areas. Immediately after stopping work, the patients noticed that the exposed skin was red; deep ulcers developed within 12 hours.

Warnings should be given by those who deliver or sell premixed cement to nonprofessional users that care should be taken not to allow the wet cement to make contact with skin (162).

There appears to be fairly general agreement that direct skin contact, prolonged contact time, and pressure on exposed areas by kneeling or by persistent contact of cement against the skin by rubber boots, polythene sheeting, or rubber gloves are the conditions necessary for wet portland cement to cause an acute ulcerative contact dermatitis.

Ready-mixed concrete as delivered to the site can be both more difficult to spread and marginally more alkaline than freshly mixed concrete. Wide fluctuations in alkalinity from batch to batch, however, are unlikely. Ready-mixed concrete is generally made in highly automated batching plants, where batching mistakes are very unlikely because they are specifically guarded against (163). There are two main types of ready-mixed concrete: central mixed and transit mixed. With the first type, mixing is done at the plant and the drum on the truck merely agitates the mixture (2 to 6 rev/min). With the second type, batching only is done at the plant and mixing occurs on the truck (4 to 16 rev/min). Usually only 70 revolutions at mixing speed are required. Maximum haulage for central mixed concrete is usually 10 miles or half an hour (164), but distance and time can be increased by using transit mixing. None of the reports in the literature to date comment on which type of mixing was used in burn cases, but these details may be important to ascertain in future cases, if further light is to be shed on the etiology of cement burns.

Users of premixed cement should be warned that skin contact with wet cement can result in burns.

Burns from Hardened Concrete

Stoermer and Wolz (165) reported that cement burns from contact with wet premixed cement is not uncommon. However, the available literature does not show reports of dermatitis caused by hardened concrete. They reported two patients who acquired "cement burns" by unloading concrete building stones from a truck. It was raining at the time, and their clothes were wet. In this case, particles of concrete stones were eluted with distilled water, and the pH value was 11.2. No additional chemicals were used in the cement.

Burns from dry hardened concrete have been reported in patients carrying hardened concrete blocks in the rain.

Chrome Contamination of the Environment

Environmental chromium contamination has become a topic of interest in areas where chromite ore processing formerly occurred. Soil levels of up to 100 ppm chrome VI and 19,000 ppm chrome III have been reported in areas where slag has been used as landfill. The concern has been primarily because chrome VI may be an inhalation carcinogen. The risk of contact dermatitis and skin ulceration is also a potential problem, and cleanup standards based on the cutaneous risk have been proposed. Based on threshold studies of levels of chrome needed to produce a positive patch test, along with presumed bioavailability of chrome in soil, it is likely that only a very few of the most highly sensitive individuals could develop ACD from environmental exposure (151,166).

Specific Treatments for Chromate Dermatitis

In addition to the usual treatment of ACD, several options for prevention and treatment of chromate allergy have been proposed. Sodium dithionate (also known as sodium sulfoxylate or sodium hydrosulfite) has been used in the chrome industry to "neutralize" chrome splashes on the skin (167). This is said to considerably diminish the incidence of chrome ulcers.

Romaguera et al. (168) devised a "barrier cream" for use in chromate allergy. The composition included tartaric acid, silicone, glycine, and other ingredients. Theoretically, the ingredients act as chelators and also reduce chrome VI to chrome III, which is less allergenic. The authors reported good results in a majority of chrome-allergic construction workers. Further studies with this compound may be warranted.

Miyachi et al. (169) reported that Dapsone (100 mg/day) improved hand eczema in five cement workers. Theoretically, the Dapsone reduced tissue superoxide radicals that may have led to clinical improvement. A controlled trial of this agent has not been performed as yet.

Chemical Test for Chromates

The object is placed in hot water to extract any chromium present. The solution is acidified with diluted hydrochloric acid. Then a 1% alcoholic solution of diphenyl carbazide is added. The development of a persistent red color is specific for hexavalent chromium salts. The test is sensitive to 10 ppm.

COBALT DERMATITIS

Cobalt is a silver gray, magnetic, brittle metal, which is widely used in additives to produce blue color in porcelain, glass pottery, and enamels. Probably the most common source of exposure is nickel-plated objects, which almost always contain cobalt. Nickel and cobalt are so similar chemically that it is not possible to separate these metals completely at a reasonable cost.

Cobalt may be detected (in the presence of 1,000 times as much nickel) by using a 1% aqueous solution of 2-nitroso-1-naphthol-4-sulfonic acid at pH 7 to 8, which produces a red coloration.

Allergic cobalt dermatitis was thought to be more common in Europe than in the United States, possibly because of the presence of cobalt in European detergents and of sufficient amounts in European cement to sensitize construction workers and those who work with clay and pottery.

This concept probably developed because for many years the North American Contact Dermatitis Group (NACDG) did not routinely test with cobalt (NACDG Patch Test Studies 1987–1989, unpublished observation). However, current data show the rates of patch test reactions in North America to be similar to European studies (170–172) (Table 35.8).

Another fallacy is that cobalt allergy almost always occurs in concert with nickel allergy. In fact, this is not true, even though most metal objects that contain cobalt also contain nickel. NACDG data from 1992–1993 indicated that 20 (40%) patients positive to cobalt were negative to nickel (unpublished data). Edman (173) similarly found 23 of 73 (32%) cobalt-positive patients not allergic to nickel.

Marcussen (174) described a cobalt-sensitive patient with a dermatitis resembling that produced by nickel. Many of his cobalt-sensitive patients did not show a hypersensitivity to nickel. Marcussen believed that cobalt hypersensitivity may be responsible for a typical clinical picture hitherto described as nickel dermatitis. He concluded that diagnostic patch tests should always include both nickel and cobalt.

Vitamin B$_{12}$ and Cobalt Dermatitis

Price and MacDonald (175) stated that allergy to vitamin B$_{12}$ (cyanocobalamin), a cobalt-containing compound, was recognized in two patients shown to be sensitive to cobalt on patch testing by Rostenberg and Perkins (176) and Fisher (177). They reported a case of recurrent cheilitis in a patient who was found to be allergic to cobalt and who ingested vitamin B$_{12}$ tablets regularly. The patient developed an acute stomatitis of the hard palate when her dentist unwittingly fitted a denture containing a chrome cobalt alloy.

Fisher (177) reported one cobalt-allergic patient that was correlated with an allergic reaction to vitamin B$_{12}$ in injectable Berubigen (Upjohn). (One ml of Berubigen contains 43.4 μg of cobalt.) This cobalt-sensitive patient gave a positive patch reaction to 2% aqueous solution of cobalt chloride and to the vitamin B solutions in the strengths of 100 and 1,000 μg per milliliter. In addition, there were positive delayed scratch and intradermal reactions to the vitamin B$_{12}$ solutions. The patient noted that, following each injection of vitamin B$_{12}$, the injected area became red, tender, and pruritic, but not eczematous. Oral ingestion of vitamin B$_{12}$ produced similar flares in the sites of previous injections. The patient also had an intractable hand eczema. Although this patient initially showed no patch test reactions to nickel, the third patch test apparently sensitized her, and she became strongly positive to it.

> **Vitamin B$_{12}$, a cobalt-containing compound, may be a source of cobalt sensitization. Injection or ingestion of the vitamin may produce flares of dermatitis in sensitized individuals.**

In one reported case there was a delayed tuberculin reaction to intradermal injection, but not to subcutaneous and intramuscular injections, of vitamin B$_{12}$ (Cobione), a cobalt-containing compound (178).

Kelensky and Schwank (179) described hypersensitivity to cobalt in a cream (Perilacin) used for hyperhidrosis. Patch tests were positive to cobalt, and in one patient, vitamin B$_{12}$ produced positive epicutaneous and intradermal test reactions.

Cobalt in Hair Dyes

Cobalt may be used with a developer to produce light brown shades of hair. First featured by Roux of Paris, cobalt nitrate is used either alone or in mixtures with silver and ammonium compounds. The developer is pyrogallol with or without other phenolic compounds and iron salts.

Cobalt Diet

Table 35.9 lists some foods thought to be high in cobalt.

Occupational Cobalt Dermatitis

Some of the described industrial exposures to cobalt include the following.

Industries Using Hard Metals

As reported in Skog (180), cobalt is employed as a binding agent to make hard metal, which consists of metal carbides and a binding agent that are presented and sintered into plates.

TABLE 35.8. *Prevalence of Metal Allergy[a]*

| | | Test Substances | | | | | | | | | | | |
| Study | Concentration (%) | Nickel | | | | Chromate | | | | Cobalt | | | |
		Total tested	Total + (%)	M + (%)	F + (%)	Total tested	Total + (%)	M + (%)	F + (%)	Total tested	Total + (%)	M + (%)	F + (%)
NACDG, 1998	2.5	3,429	14.2	NR	NR	3,440	2.8	NR	NR	4,095	9.0	NR	NR
Hong Kong, 1987–1998	5	437	10.5	NR	NR	437	0.9	NR	NR	437	7.8	NR	NR
NACDG, 1996	2.5	3,108	14.3	NR	NR	3,106	2.0	NR	NR	3,087	8.0	NR	NR
NACDG, 1972	2.5	1,200	11%	NR	NR	1,200	7.6	NR	NR	NR	NR	NR	NR
Denmark, 1984 hand eczema	5	141	NR	6.5%	26.3%	141	NR	4.5%	7.7%	141	NR	8.7%	1.1%
Denmark, 1985–1986	5	2,166	15.6%	5.1%	20.7%	2,166	4.3%	5.0%	3.9%	2,166	4.6%	1.6%	6.1%
Eastern Europe, 1982	5	2,400	7.3%	2.1%	10.5%								
Netherlands 1984–1986	5	1,785	14.8%	3.2%	20.8%	1,785	4.6%	6.2%	3.8%	1,785	7.7%	4.7%	9.3%
Saskatoon 1983–1987	2.5	542	17.4%	8.5%	23.1%	542	6.1%	6.1%	6.1%	NR	4.7%		
West Germany, 1977–1983	5	11,962	9.2%	2.6%	13.7%	11,962	4.3%	5.1%	3.7%	11,962	4.7%	3.0%	5.9%
Toronto, 1983–1987	2.5	447	11.9%	7.7%	16.9%	NR	NR	NR	NR	NR	NR	NR	NR
	5	629	10.5%	5.1%	16.7%	NR	NR	NR	NR	NR	NR	NR	NR

[a]NACDG, North American Contact Dermatitis Group; NR, not reported; M, male; F, female.
Note: All allergens tested in petrolatum potassium dichromate 0.5 (Europe & Canada) and 0.25% (NACDG), cobalt chloride 1% at all centers. From Reference 1.

TABLE 35.9. *Foods High in Cobalt*

Apricots	Coffee
Beans	Liver
Beer	Nuts
Beets	Scallops
Cabbage	Tea
Cloves	Whole-grain flour
Cocoa and chocolate	

Wolfram carbide (a tungsten compound) and the carbides of titanium, nobilium, and tantalum are frequently used.

Hard metal is characterized by a high degree of wear resistance. Consequently, it is used for rock drills, cutting tools, drawing, pressing and stamping tools, and mechanical parts exposed to heavy strain.

Hard metal dusts may produce primary irritant dermatitis with folliculitis or a chronic lichenified eczema. In addition, allergic eczematous contact dermatitis may develop, which is often due to the cobalt.

Fischer and Rystedt (187) reported that hard metal contains about 10% cobalt. Eight hundred fifty-three hard-metal workers were examined and patch tested with substances from their environment. Initial patch tests with 1% cobalt chloride showed 62 positive reactions. Allergic reactions to cobalt were reproduced in 9 men and 30 women by means of secondary serial dilution tests. Hand etching and hand grinding, which are traumatic to the hands, involved the greatest risk of cobalt sensitization. Twenty-four women, who had probably been sensitized by hard-metal work, had cobalt allergy and a simultaneous nickel allergy. They had probably been sensitized to nickel before their employment, then became sensitized to cobalt by hard-metal work, although cosensitization to jewelry or metal-working could occur.

Carbide Industry

McDermott (182) reported that cobalt is a common binding component in all grades of carbide. Pneumoconiosis and allergic sensitization from such cobalt-carbide compounds can occur.

Polyester Resin Industry

Cobalt naphthenate is commonly used in the manufacture of polyester resin. Several instances of allergic contact dermatitis were encountered in Great Britain that were attributed to workers handling cobalt naphthenate in polyester synthesis (183).

Paint Industry

Cobalt siccatives or driers, which are present in certain paints, have been reported as producing allergic contact sensitivity in paint factory workers (184). These are organic cobalt naphthenate or cobalt-resinate based on linseed oil.

Cement Industry

Although the cobalt content of cements may be low (less than 0.01%), cement workers in Holland have become sensitized to cobalt (185).

Industrial exposure to cobalt includes hard metals, polyester resins, paints, cements, pottery, ceramics, pigments, glass alloys, lubricating oils, inks, and animal feeds.

Two building workers in Cuba also had isolated cobalt allergy due to cement contact (186).

Marcussen (174) found two patients with cobalt hypersensitivity with coincident hypersensitivity to dichromate (174). Both of these cement workers had typical cement dermatitis characterized by dry, lichenified eczema of the hand, arms, and feet. Because these patients had positive patch test reactions to both dichromate and cobalt, it would be difficult to determine what role the cobalt hypersensitivity played in the production of the cement dermatitis.

In a 5-year study of 449 construction workers, cobalt was the second most common allergen (20.5%) after chromate (42.1%) (158).

Bricklaying

Camarasa (187) found that a high percentage of bricklayers in Barcelona showed hypersensitivity to both chromium and cobalt, but he noted that hypersensitivity to cobalt does not appear in patients allergic to chromium and working in other occupations. DeFonseca (188) concluded that cobalt has a higher sensitizing power than nickel and that sensitization to chromium augments sensitivity to cobalt.

Mueller and Breucker (189) found that in most of their 79 cobalt-sensitive patients, the most frequent cause of dermatitis was cement (29%), and that when these patients showed reactions to chromium and nickel, the sensitization was due to simultaneous exposure to the three metals and not to cross-reactions.

Combined reactions to cobalt, nickel, and chromium are not uncommon and do not represent cross-reactions but simultaneous, distinct, and specific sensitizations.

Plastics Manufacturing

Cobalt-containing catalysts may be used in plastics manufacturing. Allergy to cobalt in workers has been reported (190,191). Allergy to epoxy compounds in these workers is much more common, however. Cobalt naphthenate has been reported to cause ACD, with a negative patch test to cobalt chloride (192).

Pottery Workers

Dermatitis from exposure to wet clay containing cobalt may occur (193). Cobalt dermatitis from dry clay or finished wares is rare. Cobalt may be added to clay to neutralize the yellow color produced by impurities.

Cobalt is present in pigments used for amateur painting of pictures, china, and enameling. The dried paint or enamel is not an allergen. Cobalt is also used as a drying agent in linseed oil and printing inks.

Manufacture of Alloys Containing Cobalt

Alloys containing cobalt include alnico, duralumin, nobilium, permalloy, stellite, ticonium, and vitallium. Allergic dermatitis in workers making alloys of cobalt has been shown by patch tests to be due in some instances to the dust of metallic cobalt (93). The dust also has been reported as causing asthma. It is believed that a dusty atmosphere containing metallic cobalt particles favors a sensitization to cobalt.

Miscellaneous Industries Using Cobalt

Currently, cobalt is used extensively in the carbide, glass, ceramic, enamel, electrical, and pigment industries. It may also be used in printing inks and in animal feeds. Cobalt in animal feeds has caused allergy in a Finnish pig farmer and an English animal feed worker (194,195). Cobalt-2-ethylhexoate caused hand dermatitis in an offset printer (196). Two of the ink driers he worked with contained this chemical. Inks, paints, and varnishes may contain cobalt and other heavy metal catalysts, which help speed the drying process.

Cobalt chloride is an ingredient of the adhesive mixture used for some flypapers and hair dyes (197).

Unusual Urticarial Reaction to Cobalt

Nurnberger and Arnold (198) reported Quincke's edema as a manifestation of a cobalt allergy due to sensitization by cobaltous shell splinters in the arm. Injection of a cobalt-iron preparation was followed by a refractory bilateral periorbital edema. Patch testing showed a "monovalent" allergy to cobalt.

> **Cobalt dermatitis may result from exposure to substances containing the metal, such as hair dyes, flypaper, shell splinters, antiperspirant creams, crayons, and fertilizers.**

Photosensitization Dermatitis Due to Cobalt

Camarasa and Alomar (199) reported a bricklayer with a chronic and severe eczema, combined with a chronic papular dermatosis in sun-exposed areas, associated with multiple sensitivities. Chromate, mercaptobenzothiazole, and parabens sensitized the patient in the usual way, but cobalt produced a reaction only after light exposure. This last fact justifies a new approach to those bricklayers suffering from dermatitis in areas exposed to sunlight and when their clinical course proves to be unsatisfactory or unexplained.

Romaguera et al. (200) found that four patients with chronic photocontact dermatitis were sensitive to cobalt salts. They presented as cases of contact dermatitis from cement or pig fodder with persistent lesions on exposed areas. Only two of them had standard patch test–positive reactions to chromate and cobalt, but all showed positive photo patch tests to cobalt. Photo-oxidation tests proved that cobalt salts are photosensitizing. The patients' chronic actinic dermatitis was due to exposure to cobalt salts.

> **Spanish investigators report photo-contact dermatitis from cobalt.**

Patch and Intradermal Testing with Cobalt

A "reaction" peculiar to cobalt patch tests has been described by Storrs (FJ Storrs, M.D., personal communication). This consists of a "cayenne pepper" speckled appearance of the patch site without edema or uniform erythema, apparently due to a poral reaction. This is not an allergic reaction.

Allenby and Basketter (201) found that of six cobalt-allergic patients who reacted to cobalt chloride 1% aq, only one reacted to 0.1% aq. As long as the poral reaction is kept in mind, testing at 1% would seem reasonable.

In the past, intradermal testing with cobalt and other metal salts has been performed. Marcussen (202) outlined some of the difficulties with interpreting these tests, including impurity of the testing material and nonspecific immediate urticarial reactions. Currently, intradermal testing with metal salts is felt to be unnecessary, except in research protocols.

> **Intradermal tests with cobalt may give nonspecific urticarial reactions. A positive patch test reaction may be more specific.**

COPPER DERMATITIS

Copper, a common component of alloys and plating materials, may rarely be the offending agent in patients with metal dermatitis, particularly when patch testing excludes more commonly involved metals, such as nickel, chromium, mercury, cobalt, and gold (203).

The rarity of allergic reactions to copper seems to be borne out, because in the 1970s and 1980s the Allergy Department of the New York Skin and Cancer Unit had been able to authenticate only three cases of allergic reactions to metallic copper or its salts. Researchers there studied a patient with a combined allergic reaction to gold and copper, agreeing with Epstein that multiple metal allergies in one individual are due to separate and simultaneously induced sensitivities by each offending metal. It must be remembered, however, that because routine testing with copper salts is not carried out, the true incidence of copper allergy may be underestimated, just as was done with gold in the past.

In the past, when copper salts were being used for iontophoresis for fungal infections on severely eczematized feet, no instances of dermatitis due to these salts were reported, proving how rarely sensitization to copper occurs.

Exposure to copper salts may take place from contact with insecticides, fungicides, food processing procedures, fertilizers, and mordants used in fur dyeing (204).

D'Alibour's solution contains copper sulfate, zinc sulfate, and camphor water. Concentrated solutions of copper sulfate are caustic and produce primary irritation. Copper and copper alloy in silver metallic jewelry corrode readily on the skin, and, in the presence of adequate concentration of salt, a primary irritation is produced.

A report from India implicated copper allergy as a cause of orodynia and lichen planus in three dental patients. Unfortunately, patch test and clinical details were not given (205).

Copper is ubiquitous in all US coinage except the zinc-coated steel pennies of 1943. In Saltzer's case (203) of copper sensitivity, a penny, a nickel, and a dime provoked erythema and vesiculation at the patch test site within 24 hours (203).

> **Allergic reactions to copper are rare. In the presence of salt, copper corrodes readily on the skin to form a primary irritant dermatitis. Patients with marked copper hypersensitivity may react positively to a penny, nickel, or dime, all of which contain copper.**

So-called copper itch, which is caused by a dust of copper precipitate, is probably due to the presence of arsenic in the mixture (204). Cohen (206) reported toxic effects from copper dust, which include upper respiratory irritation, "metal fever," ulceration, and perforation of the nasal septum.

Dermatitis Due to Copper Intrauterine Devices

One widely used contraceptive method is the copper intrauterine device (IUD). Copper metal in contact with biologic substrates is highly reactive. The copper ions thereby produced also have biologic effects. Thus, this device is a pharmacologic agent.

The biologic evidence, most clearly shown with laboratory animals, is that the copper IUD has its contraceptive effect by inhibiting implantations (207). The copper-containing intrauterine device was developed to overcome such undesirable side effects as metrorrhagia, pain, and expulsion, common to previous appliances. The CU-7 brand of intrauterine copper contraceptive (Searle) has a plastic component composed of polypropylene homopolymer with barium sulfate added to render it radiopaque. Its shape approximates the number 7. Coiled around the vertical limb is pure virginal electrolytic copper wire. This wire provides a surface area of 200 mm².

Barranco (208) reported the first case of eczematous dermatitis due to a copper IUD. Another case was described by Forck et al. (209). Both cases were verified by patch testing.

Barkoff (210) stated that a 24-year-old woman developed an acute urticarial reaction secondary to a copper intrauterine contraceptive device. Allergy to copper was proven by scratch tests. The condition cleared with removal of the intrauterine device.

> **Copper-containing intrauterine devices have been reported as causing eczematous and urticarial eruptions.**

Dry et al. (211) tested for allergy to copper by patch tests in 69 women who were using copper IUDs and 50 young women who did not use any IUD. These 119 women also tested to nickel. Patch tests were performed with a 5% solution of copper sulfate and with a 10% glycerol solution of nickel sulfate. The tests were read immediately after removal of the patches after 48 hours of application.

The one positive test to copper was observed in a woman with known previous allergy to copper. She developed generalized dermatitis 8 days after placing the IUD. Replacement by Lippes loop (no copper involved) resulted in a rapid and definitive improvement.

Romaguera and Grimalt (212) also reported contact dermatitis from a copper-containing intrauterine contraceptive loop.

Karlberg et al. (213) noted that copper is a very rare sensitizer. After reviewing over 100 cases published before 1983, they accepted only four cases as true copper allergy, and 20 as probably relevant. The largest series was that of Dhir et al. (214), who found 10 workers allergic to copper sulfate in a furniture polish. However, they did not test for nickel or other allergy.

Van Joost et al. (215) pointed out that nickel and copper allergy may coexist, and both may be significant.

Unusual Reactions to Copper

Pande and Gupta (216) reported a 17-year-old boy who developed thrombo-cytopenic purpura after ingesting 1% copper sulfate solution (2 mg/day) given for vitiligo. This probably represented an allergic rather than a toxic reaction. Reid (217) reported that within 2 hours of having a premolar tooth temporarily filled with black copper cement, a woman became almost completely covered with an itching urticarial rash. In this instance, the patient had already suggested that she might be allergic to certain dental cements. The rash subsided after a few hours, although mild skin irritation persisted for 2 or 3 days.

GOLD

Before the late 1980s, there were scattered case reports of gold allergy, but most references, including previous editions of this book, suggested that gold allergy was rare (218–221). There are probably two reasons for this misconception. First, testing for gold allergy was rarely done and if done may have been inadequate because of poor allergens. Second, gold is metalurgically inert and therefore was thought to be immunologically inert.

Obviously, gold allergy is anything but rare, as has been established in numerous patch test centers in the last decade. Prevalence of positive patch test reactions to gold has been as high as 9.5% in large series, and numerous papers have been published discussing various features of gold allergy. The NACDG from 1996 to 1998 tested over 4,000 patients and found 9.5% were positive to gold sodium thiosulfate (0.5% pet) (2). Gold was the sixth most frequent allergen. Similarly, Bruze et al. (222), from Sweden, reported prevalence of about 9% in consecutive patients. A number of other studies from Europe and Asia have reported rates anywhere from 1% to 23%.

In the early 1990s some investigators were concerned that many gold patch test reactions seemed to lack relevance. However, as more data accumulates, cases previously thought to be lacking in relevance have been shown to be caused by gold contact. For example, Fowler (223), in 1988, reported two women with eyelid dermatitis and gold allergy. Since then, statistical analysis has confirmed the association in Sweden and North America (222). The NACDG found that of 388 gold-allergic patients, 7.5% had eyelid dermatitis (unpublished observation). In addition to dermatitis, lichen planus, both oral and cutaneous, is sometimes associated with allergy to gold (or other metals) in dental work (see Chapter 36) (224).

The vast majority of gold-allergic patients are women, probably because of greater jewelry usage. Also, most have gold dental work (crowns or fillings), although most have no oral symptoms (222,225).

Patch Testing for Gold Allergy

Fowler (226) reviewed various published reports of gold allergy. Gold chloride, also called trichloride, is composed of gold in dilute hydrochloric acid. This acid compound may predispose to irritant reactions. The best agent for patch testing is gold sodium thiosulfate (0.5% pet), also known as sodium thiosulfatoaurate. Gold sodium thiomalate (injectable therapeutic gold) may also be used. Potassium dicyanoaurate is used in the electronics industry and may cause ACD and irritant contact dermatitis (ICD). It is not a reliable patch test allergen. Gold leaf is also not a reliable patch test allergen, because it is poorly soluble.

> Allergic gold dermatitis may become papular and persistent. Patch tests for gold allergy should include gold salts because gold leaf, metallic gold, and gold scrapings may yield false-negative reactions in gold-sensitive patients. A positive gold patch test may persist for months.

A German study confirmed that gold sodium thiosulfate at 0.5% pet versus 0.25% pet was twice as likely to yield positive results (227).

Experimental Gold Allergy

Gold chloride was found to be a strong sensitizer in a human maximization test (228). However, to date there have been no reports of successful sensitization to gold in animals, according to Bruze and Andersen (229). This study demonstrates the frequent inadequacy of animal predictive tests in identifying human allergens.

Noneczematous Persistent Papular Gold Eruptions

Allergic gold dermatitis may be a "dermal" type of contact dermatitis characterized by minimal eczematous epidermal changes and by marked dermal involvement (230).

Shelley and Epstein (231) emphasized that allergic gold dermatitis may be manifested as a chronic papular eruption. Bowyer (232) reported that an allergic eczematous patch test to gold may become papular and that such a papular patch test will show a "dermal" infiltrate when examined histologically.

The so-called allergic "dermal" contact dermatitis produced by gold, neomycin, nickel, and ragweed is an allergic contact dermatitis in which the eczematous element is minimal or absent. The eruption remains edematous and erythematous throughout its course. Histologically, there is a normal epidermis or an epidermis with little spongiosis. There is usually edema and a dense perivascular small, round cell infiltrate in the dermis. "Dermal" contact dermatitis is combined occasionally with the usual papulovesicular eczematous variety, in which case, one can usually demonstrate both a positive patch and an intracutaneous reaction with the specific allergen.

Petros and Macmillan (233) reported that a contact sensitivity to gold developed in a patient 6 months after she had her ears pierced and started wearing gold earrings. The patient developed pruritus, soreness and swelling of the earlobes, as well as irritation and pruritus under her gold wedding band. A biopsy from one of the ear lesions showed a dense infiltration of the dermis with lymphocytes and plasma cells. There were no significant changes in the epidermis.

Suzuki (234) may have found one reason for the persistence of clinical findings in some cases of gold ACD. In this study, small microfragments of gold were found in the skin by X-ray microanalysis long after earrings were removed. In another study, five of eight patients developed persistent papules at intradermal gold test sites, which lasted up to 20 months (235). X-ray microanalysis revealed gold in tissue macrophages.

Metallic gold in jewelry and dental appliances can readily produce allergic dermatitis and stomatitis. Sweat, saliva, pressure, and friction may be required to produce a reaction from metallic gold.

In a letter published in the *Journal of the American Medical Association* in 1974, Fisher (236) pointed out:

> Even the use of pure gold earrings is not quite safe following ear piercing. While allergic gold sensitization from ear piercing is much rarer than nickel sensitization, it is, nevertheless, a definite hazard. Incidentally, gold dermatitis tends to be persistent, sometimes lasting for several months, even though there is no further contact with gold.
>
> Sensitization to both nickel and gold can be avoided by piercing the ears with a stainless steel needle (18 to 20 gauge) and inserting stud earrings of stainless steel that give a negative reaction for a spot test for nickel. The only way to be certain that the stud earrings are free of nickel is to do the dimethylglyoxime test for the presence of free nickel. I have found that most of the inexpensive gold earrings contain sufficient nickel to give a dimethylglyoxime positive test. The stainless steel earrings are left in place for 3 weeks until the channel is completely epithelialized, after which time any earrings may be inserted.

Malten and Mali (237) theorized that, because metallic gold is corroded only by substances such as halogens or alkaline cyanides that are not present in the body, gold dermatitis is probably not based on an ordinary allergic mechanism, but on "an enzymatic interference in a biochemically deviant individual," as described by Rostenberg. The reac-

tions to gold that Fisher observed, however, appear to be a true allergic variety of the "dermal" type. There is speculation that the persistence of the dermatitis may be due to the persistent presence of gold in the dermis.

Gold Ring Dermatitis

In some instances, dermatitis from a ring is due to a primary irritation from trauma, accumulated detergents, or the corrosive action of salts on the ring. Allergic gold ring dermatitis does occur commonly.

Comaish's case (238) of allergic gold ring dermatitis showed that both the dermatitis and the positive gold patch test reaction persisted for several months after exposure to the gold had ceased. Repeated patch tests with scraping from the ring (18 karat) and pure gold leaf were negative at 48 to 72 hours. Patch testing with gold chloride (chloroauric acid, 2%) showed a strongly positive eczematous response at 48 hours. Redness and infiltrated papules persisted at the site for more than 2 months but were fading at 3 months.

Lack of reaction to ring scrapings and gold foil is typical and indicates that testing with gold salts in gold allergy is important.

Rytter and Schubert (239) showed a primary sensitization after wearing a gold ring for 18 months. A positive test was obtained with very low solutions of sodium gold thiosulfate, and a lymphocyte transformation gave a positive result.

Nature of White Gold

According to the US Treasury Department, white gold is a gold-base alloy with sufficient alloying constituents to give a white color. Palladium, to the extent of 10% in the alloy, gives an excellent white gold; a cheaper alloy contains 10% nickel and 5% zinc. As the gold content is lowered, other alloying constituents may be used; thus, in 14 and 18 karat alloys, nickel, copper, zinc, and silver are among the elements to be found

The dimethylglyoxime test readily detects the presence of nickel in metallic gold. Whenever allergic dermatitis from a gold ring is suspected a dimethylglyoxime test and patch tests with gold sodium thiosulfate, copper sulfate, nickel sulfate and palladium chloride should be performed to determine which metal is the culprit.

White gold ring dermatitis may be due to the presence of nickel, gold, copper, or palladium.

So-called jeweler's gold is in reality "jeweler's metal" that contains copper, zinc, and tin.

Systemic Gold Reactions

Systemic therapy with gold, for rheumatic and/or dermatologic diseases, is often complicated by cutaneous adverse effects. Lichenoid eruptions and dermatitis are both seen. British investigators, using lymphocyte transformation assays to gold and nickel, found that patients with lichenoid reactions often showed positive tests to gold but those with dermatitis often reacted to nickel. Nickel is a significant contaminant of the injectable gold tested (Myochrisin, Rhone-Poulenc) (240). Möller et al. (241) found positive gold patch tests in 7 of 20 candidates for gold therapy and therefore recommend testing all prospective patients before starting chrysotherapy. In another 10 gold-allergic patients given intramuscularly (IM) gold, flares of previous test sites and transient fevers were noted (242).

Chrysiasis

The deposition of gold in the skin, leading to blue-gray pigmentation, is termed chrysiasis. This occurs after the therapeutic administration of gold, usually for rheumatoid arthritis. It rarely occurs with cumulative doses under 50 mg/kg and is common with doses above 150 mg/kg (243). Miller et al. (244) studied a case of chrysiasis and identified gold microparticles in the superficial dermis.

Gold Schnapps Syndrome

Russell et al. (245) reported three patients with lichenoid eruptions and gold allergy provoked by consuming schnapps that contained gold flecks. Each cleared after several months of avoiding the gold-containing liquor.

Occupational Gold Allergy

Soluble gold salts can cause occupational dermatitis. Exposure to gold salts may take place in porcelain, gold plating, gilding glass, and photography.

Gold Dermatitis in the Gilding Industry

Nava and Briatico Vangoso (246) described six cases of allergy to gold salt. Four workers engaged in gilding presented dermatoses in acroexposed sites. An administrative employee showed urticaria, the origin of which must be attributed, besides the exposure to gold salts, to sensitivity to foods and other contact antigens. In the sixth patient, who had urticaria and past eczema at sites of gold objects (ring and watch), the dermatitis was attributed to gold, whereas the urticaria was due to food, fungi, and drugs.

Skin and Nail Lesions from Gold Potassium Cyanide

Budden and Wilkinson (247) reported a man whose work consisted of cleaning gold electrode contacts. These electrode contacts were placed in a basket containing a mixture of potassium cyanide and an oxidizing agent, metanitrobenzene sulfonic acid. The mixture resulted in the formation of gold potassium cyanide, $KAu(CN_2)$.

Four days before he was seen at the clinic, the patient developed some scattered pustules on the backs of the fingers of the right hand and erosions and crusting of the lower lip. A culture of pustules was sterile. The patient remained off work for 2 weeks, and both sets of lesions healed uneventfully. When he was seen at the end of that time, however, he had developed a purplish brown discoloration with some partial onycholysis of the free ends of most of his finger nails on the right hand. Four weeks later, his fingernails had also returned to normal.

> Gold allergy is much more common than previously thought. Most patients are female, and most have gold dental work. Dermatitis of the eyelids or other remote sites may be seen even if the fingers are unaffected. Lichen planus may sometimes be related to gold allergy.

INDIUM

Indium is found in dental restoration alloys. Marcussen et al. (248) reported allergy to indium in individuals with suspected sensitivity to dental materials. In all, nine had at least a 2+ reaction to indium sulfide 10% aq, and one reacted to indium chloride 10% aq. Several concentrations of both indium sulfide and indium chloride were tested, with indium sulfide 10% aq the most likely to give a reaction. Unfortunately, no comment was made regarding possible irritant reactions or clinical relevance.

IRIDIUM

In the same study, five patients reacted to iridium chloride 1% aq. Ammonium hexachloroiridate was also used for testing, with poor results (248). Iridium is of the platinum group of metals. In industry it is often found in association with platinum, which is a fairly common airborne allergen. There is one report of contact urticaria and respiratory hypersensitivity to iridium in an electrochemical process worker (249).

IRON

Discoloration and Dermatitis Due to Iron Salts

Hemmer et al. (250) tested 623 patients with suspected metal allergy to ferric chloride (2% aq) and ferrous sulfate (5% pet). They saw only five positive and two questionable reactions. On testing with a dilution series, only two reacted. Both were also allergic to nickel and cobalt. Relevance was doubtful.

Nater (251) reported an instance of epidermal hypersensitivity to iron, but the patch test reaction may have been the nonspecific pustular variety. Baer (252) cited a metalworker with an allergic reaction to iron who had a positive (eczematous) patch test reaction.

One patient has been reported to be allergic to yellow iron oxide in a mascara (253).

Seven of 190 Italian ceramics workers were positive to patch testing with red iron oxide (2% pet) (254). A number of other metal salts used for decorative coloring of pottery also gave positive patch tests. The only one more common, however, was nickel (15% vs 3.6%).

Allergic contact dermatitis due to iron is apparently rare.

Ferroxyl Test for Iron

The ferroxyl test may be used to show the presence of free iron in corroded metallic objects. The metallic article is immersed in a gel containing 1% sodium chloride and 0.2% ferricyanide. A positive reaction is indicated by a blue growth that resembles seaweed from the corroded metal.

Pigmentation and Tattooing from Iron

Monsel's solution (a ferric chloride solution) has long been used as a hemostyptic. The application of old or concentrated solutions, particularly to abraded skin sites, may produce a permanent red-brown pigmented iron tattoo. Monsel's solution should be fresh and well shaken before being used on cosmetically exposed areas such as the face, the breast, or the upper back (255). Aluminum chloride may be used as an alternative styptic, which is free of complicating pigmentation.

Exogenous Siderosis—Pigmentation of Skin from Iron Particles

Jirasek (256) reported a red-brown, tattoo-like eruption in welders doing spot welding, which he labeled "exogenous siderosis." Exogenous siderosis of the skin, also called "millers' disease," has occurred in the past in millers and in millstone cutters and was caused by penetration of minute fragments of steel flying from cutters during millstone shaping. Similar manifestations occurred in file makers. The same manifestations occurred in gasfitters in whom particles of soot, dust, and rust penetrated into the skin when scouring gas pipes with compressed air.

Exogenous siderosis took the form of a perifollicular, punctate, red-brown pigmentation of the forearm in a man whose work was dipping iron parts into hydrochloric acid. After an acute dermatitis had healed, permanent rusty hyperpigmentation persisted in the affected areas on the volar aspect of the wrist. Histologic examination confirmed the presence of an exogenous iron pigment in the upper layer of the corium.

Jirasek (256) stated that the occupational hyperpigmentation reported by him has undoubtedly the same features as the exogenous siderosis of the skin reported earlier in millers, file makers, gasfitters, and other workers. Such hyperpigmentation is not a disease but is an interesting occupational stigma, which, for the affected individuals, is only of cosmetic significance, although it is not negligible from the aesthetic aspect.

Allergic reactions to iron are rare; pigmentation from Monsel's solution and from industrial exposure to iron particles is more common.

Kasteler and Fowler have seen a patient with extensive iron deposition in a surgical scar (JS Kasteler, M.D., Louisville, KY, personal communication, 2000) A young woman underwent placement of stabilizing rods in the back and shortly thereafter was given an intravenous iron preparation. She developed brownish speckled dots throughout the long vertical scars. Histologic examination confirmed the presence of iron.

LEAD

The rarity of allergic reaction to lead is emphasized by Fregert (257), who, reporting a "possible" case of lead allergy, asked, "Has anyone else seen patch-test reactions to lead salts?" Fregert's case was a truck driver who had, for several years, charged the accumulators used in trucks. He developed dermatitis on the distal part of the fingers, and he himself suspected that the dermatitis was due to the lead electrodes and the hydrochloric acid. Patch testing in a standard series gave negative reactions. Two different samples of lead chloride (0.2% aq) and lead acetate (0.5% aq) gave positive reactions; lead metal gave a negative reaction. The dermatitis was possibly caused by lead dissolved in hydrochloric acid.

Dermatitis Associated with Lead Poisoning

Czarnecki and Fritsch (258) reported a case of contact sensitization to lead, which presented as an acute bullous contact dermatitis after application of an ointment containing lead oxide (unguentum diachylon Hebra). In patch testing, the patient reacted strongly to lead oxide and lead acetate. Further examination revealed chronic lead intoxication with neurologic and labyrinthine involvement. As a painter, the patient had had professional contact with lead paints up to 25 years ago for a period of 30 years. He had never noticed any contact allergies to his working materials.

Allen et al. (259) studied three patients who had blistering on exposed areas of the skin and who had biochemical evidence of lead poisoning. A causal relationship through abnormalities in porphyrin metabolism is suggested.

It should be noted that thousands of men, and now women, have used a hair preparation called Grecian Formula containing lead salts to darken hair without any reports of allergic or toxic reactions. The preparation contains an aqueous solution of lead acetate and glycerin with a small quantity of suspended sulfur.

> **Allergic dermatitis from lead or its salts is rare. Grecian Formula, used to darken hair, is not known to be an allergen. Dermatitis associated with lead poisoning may occur.**

MANGANESE

Manganese is a component of the pesticide maneb, which may cause ACD. Manganese dioxide (10% pet) gave a positive patch test reaction in 2 of 190 ceramics workers (67).

METALLIC (ELEMENTARY) MERCURY

Mercury is one of the oldest metals known. From a standpoint of exposure, allergy to mercury must be considered differently from other metals. With the other common metal allergens, exposure to the metal itself is by far the most common situation, whereas exposure to primary solutions or metal salts is unusual. Exposure to metallic mercury, however, rarely occurs except in dental materials, whereas exposure to organic mercurials such as thimerosal is fairly frequent. Allergy to organic mercurials is discussed in Chapter 17. For our purposes here, it is sufficient to note that a patch test reaction to thimerosal usually indicates mercury allergy but may also indicate allergy to the thiosalicylic acid portion of the molecule (260). An unusual cutaneous side effect caused by mercury led to the origin of patch testing. In 1895, Jadassohn (261) described a patient with acute eczematous dermatitis confined to the sites to which a gray mercurial ointment had been previously applied for treatment of pediculosis pubis. Subsequent application of the gray ointment to unaffected sites produced eczematous reactions. These observations were the first to show that contact sensitization can be induced by the simple application of a suspected substance to unaffected skin.

Reactions to Mercury from Broken Thermometers

Spilled mercury droplets from a broken thermometer can produce severe allergic reactions in sensitized individuals, such as dermatitis, stomatitis, encephalitis, and even death (262,263).

Spilled mercury droplets from a broken thermometer can be picked up with a clean, shiny piece of copper. A mixture of sulfur, calcium, and water or aerosol hair spray can also "fix" mercury droplets.

Swinyer (264) reported a patient with a 23-year history of recurrent eruptions after contact with mercury from a broken thermometer. The patient's initial sensitization occurred after a "romance" with mercury that started with several "backroom" experiments using the chemical from thermometers that he purposely broke. In one experiment, he "changed a penny to a dime" by spreading the copper-colored coin with the silver-colored mercury using his fingertips. Each subsequent exposure after sensitization produced a blistering rash, "like poison oak." Within 24 hours of mercury exposure, his eyes would swell shut. This reaction was followed by a rash that spread over his entire body. He joined a pipeline company, and his job necessitated limited exposure to a small pool of metallic mercury in a fuel flow measuring device. This exposure resulted in repeated severe cutaneous eruptions.

Vermeiden et al. (265) described a patient who developed erythema multiforme from inhalation of metallic mercury vapor. The patient reported that before his rash, he had cleaned up broken thermometers for 7 hours a day for 7 days in a 10-day period. This task had been performed in a locked room, and he had not worn a mask. On later inspection, the mercury was still found in the seams of the wooden floor.

Gerstner and Huff (266) pointed out that elementary mercury, such as that present in a thermometer or barometer, evaporates at room temperature and can enter the body by inhalation. Irreversible damage to the central nervous system can arise, depending on the concentration in the air and the time of exposure. Drowsiness and general malaise can also follow exposure to mercury vapors. These symptoms were observed in their patient. The reactions after mercury intoxications vary with individuals.

Nakayama et al. (267) studied patients with a generalized rash, mostly appearing 1 or 2 days after breaking a clinical thermometer or during dental treatment. Similar skin manifestations were revealed, suggestive at first glance of mercury exanthem (i.e., diffuse symmetrical erythema predominantly on major fluxural areas). An inverted triangular or V-shaped erythema on both upper anteromedial thighs was a common feature. Severe cases had miliary pustules or purpura on erythematous skin. Pruritus or burning sensation was relatively mild. Pyrexia or malaise was a complaint of more than half the patients. Most of the patients had a previous history of contact dermatitis to Mercurochrome, and by patch testing, these patients were found to have contact allergy to several mercurials, especially inorganic ones. Mercurochrome had been widely used as a topical disinfectant in Japan. This seems to be a possible cause of the high incidence of contact allergy to mercurials in Japan. Nakayama et al. believed that patients had developed systemic contact dermatitis due to inhalation of mercury vapor.

> Exposure to metallic mercury from broken thermometers, by contact or by inhalation, can produce severe allergic and systemic toxic effects, particularly in patients previously sensitized to topical mercurials, such as merthiolate, Mercurochrome, and ammoniated mercury.

Baboon Syndrome

A syndrome of striking, bright erythema of the buttocks combined with dermatitis in flexural areas has been termed the "baboon syndrome." Inhalation of mercury vapor causes this rare but distinctive eruption. As noted above, small pustules may appear in the red areas. Sometimes bullae may occur (268,269). Broken thermometers are the usual source of exposure, but one case occurred from playing a commercial English game containing mercury (270).

Mercury Amalgams

Mercury, without being heated, unites with many metals to form combinations known as amalgams. Dermatitis from amalgams may be caused by metallic mercury or the other metals. Amalgams composed of zinc, tin, and mercury are used as dental cements. In addition, amalgams of mercury with gold, silver, or copper are used as fillings for teeth (see Chapter 36).

Recently, mercury has been reexamined not only as an allergen but also as a cause of nonspecific symptoms, such as malaise, headache, and fatigue from exposure by dental fillings. Although the question of oral mercury toxicity is uncertain, allergic stomatitis and oral (and possibly systemic) lichen planus to mercury from dental exposure definitely occurs. This is discussed in depth in Chapter 36. To summarize, a number of studies have clearly documented that stomatitis, oral lichenoid lesions, or lichen planus, and sometimes orodynia, may be caused by allergy to dental metals. Mercury and gold have been most often implicated, but other metals may cause oral allergy as well (271–275).

Dental workers are also at risk for sensitization and ACD to mercury (276).

Unusual Sources of Mercury Exposure

Koch and Nickolaus (277) reported a 5-year-old boy with generalized dermatitis and positive patch tests to thimerosal (0.05% pet), amalgam (5% pet), mercury chloride (0.01% pet), and mercury ammonium chloride (1% pet). After common sources of mercury exposure were ruled out, chemical testing revealed the presence of mercury chloride in PVC boots. The authors stated that mercury may be used in both leather and plastic footwear and as an antimildew agent.

Patch Testing for Mercury Allergy

Thimerosal is a component of most patch test screening series and is the usual allergen for detecting mercury allergy. Goncalo et al. (260) stated that most positive patch tests to thimerosal indicate mercury allergy, but some detect allergy to the thiosalicylic acid portion of the molecule. Elemental mercury, amalgam, and various inorganic mercury salts may also be used to detect mercury sensitivity. Both Nakada et al. (278) and Handley et al. (279) suggest using both ionized (ammoniated mercury or mercury chloride) and nonionized mercury (metallic mercury or amalgam) for completeness.

When testing with amalgam, a 5% concentration in pet has been recommended (280). Testing with individual components would also be advisable when indicated.

MOLYBDENUM

In various stainless steel suture clips, molybdenum was present at about 1% concentration. Seven of 184 patients patch tested with ammonium heptamolybdate 1% had a 1+ reaction, and 4 had a 2+ or 3+ reaction. Correlation with delayed wound healing and local reactions was not well documented for molybdenum but was present in nickel allergy (281).

NICKEL—THE UBIQUITOUS CONTACT ALLERGEN

"The Romance of Nickel," a brochure distributed by the International Nickel Company (282), will no doubt intrigue nickel-sensitive persons—particularly the statement that reads, "Nickel is with you and does things for you from the time you get up in the morning until you go to sleep at night." This almost continuous exposure is reflected in the increasing number of patients who are sensitized to nickel (283). Throughout the world, nickel is reported to be one of the most common causes of allergic contact dermatitis, particularly in women (284–286). Nickel produces more cases of allergic contact dermatitis than all the other metals combined.

In men, nickel dermatitis is predominantly of occupational origin (Table 35.10). It should be noted that industrial nickel solutions can pass through rubber gloves; heavy-duty vinyl gloves should be used instead. In women, the most common cause of nickel dermatitis is direct contact, primarily from jewelry, garments, and wristwatches, and secondarily from such occupations as metal industry, hair dressing, tailoring, and hotel and restaurant work.

Once an individual acquires nickel dermatitis, allergic sensitivity to nickel persists indefinitely. Table 35.11 gives the location and source of the nickel objects that produced nickel dermatitis on 100 sensitized individuals in the general population. A study of Table 35.11 reveals that no por-

TABLE 35.10. *Industrial Exposures to Nickel*

Alkaline batteries
Blackening zinc and brass
Ceramics
Coating (electroplating)
Duplicating fluids and fluxes (brazing)
Dyes
Electrical wiring
Enamel (green: nickel oxides)
Fuel additives
Hardening of fats (acts as a catalyst)
Insecticides
Magnet cores
Mordant in dyeing and printing fabrics
Nickel alloys
Nickel plating
Paint for glass
Pigments for paint and wallpaper
Reagents and catalysts (plastics)

Note: Rubber gloves are not protective. Use heavy-duty vinyl gloves.

TABLE 35.11. *Sites and Sources of Nickel Dermatitis in the General Population*

Location	Nickel source causing dermatitis
Scalp	Hairpins, curlers, and bobby pins
Eyelids	Eyelash curler
Earlobes	Earrings (earlobe dermatitis almost pathognomonic)
Ear canals	Insertion of metallic objects
Back of ears	Spectacle frames
Sides of nose	Nickel coin (patient rubbed nose with coin)
Sides of face	Bobby pins, curlers, and dental instruments
Lips	Metal pins held in mouth and in metal lipstick holder
Neck	Clasp of necklace and zipper
Upper chest	Medallions and metal identification tags
Abdomen	Blue jean metal button
Axilla	Zipper (unilateral involvement usually)
Breast	Wire support of brassiere
Thighs	Garter clasps, metal chairs, and metal coins in pockets
Palms	Handles of doors, handbags, carriages, and umbrellas
Fingers	Thimbles, needles, scissors, coins, and pens
Wrist	Watchbands and bracelets
Arms	Bracelets
Antecubital area	Metal handle of handbag (resembles atopic eczema)
Ankles	Bracelet
Dorsum of foot	Metallic eyelets of shoes
Leg	Zipper of boots
Plantar aspect foot	Metal arch support
Pubic area and vulva	Safety pin on napkin
Bullet wounds	Nickel alloys in bullets and shrapnel[a]
Postoperative sites	Screws, bolts, and plates in orthopedic implants[a]
Acupuncture sites	Nickel-plated needles
Sites of Dermo-Jet injections	Nickel-plated Dermo-Jet

[a]May be true for alloys other than stainless steel.

tion of the skin from the scalp to the soles is invulnerable to nickel dermatitis. As an occupational disease in workers exposed to massive amounts of nickel salts, the eruption may be generalized and resemble scabies.

> **Nickel, which causes more dermatitis than all the other metals combined, is difficult to avoid in daily life. Women are more commonly sensitized by nonoccupational contacts. Men are particularly sensitized by industrial exposure. Industrial nickel solutions penetrate rubber gloves; heavy-duty vinyl gloves should be used instead.**

Epidemiology of Nickel Allergy

Table 35.9 reviews a number of studies regarding prevalence of positive patch test reactions to metals. It can be seen that women are more commonly allergic than men by a factor of 2 to 6 times. There is general agreement that this is due to jewelry usage, specifically ear piercing. Larsson-Stymne (288) and Windstrom (287) found that 13% of 960 schoolgirls age 8 to 15 with pierced ears were nickel allergic, whereas only 1% of those without pierced ears were allergic. Christophersen et al. (288), using multivariate analysis, examined various factors in nickel allergy. In addition to an increase in women, absence of atopy and presence of hand eczema independently correlated with nickel allergy (Table 35.12). Schubert et al. (289) found that of 104 patients, 68 were free of nickel dermatitis 3 years after patch testing, and 13 had chronic hand eczema. Dietary nickel modification was not tried. Forty-two had changed jobs, 36 of whom had cleared.

Nonindustrial Nickel Dermatitis in Men

Only in Kuwait are more men sensitized to nickel than women. Kanan (290) reported that the men are sensitized by the nickel-plated studs in their underwear.

Peltonen (291) stated that the most common sensitizers of men outside occupations dealing with metals seem to be wristwatches and watchstrap buckles. Like women, men are sensitized by the accessories on their clothing, particularly by buttons in jeans and belt buckles, but also by cheap jewelry. It was found that the participants of the study were not exposed to nickel in their occupations and that nickel sensitivity was found in men only in the young age group (which is more prone to wear jeans and jewelry). The inci-

TABLE 35.12. *Metal Allergy Demographics*

Nickel
    Female > male
    Incidence increasing overall
    Younger > older
    Association with hand eczema, systemic ACD
    Nonatopics > atopics
    Association with cobalt
    Association with ear piercing
    Association with palladium
Chromate
    Male > female
    Incidence decreasing or stable
    Older > younger
Cobalt
    Female > male
    Incidence increasing
    Younger > older
    Association with nickel

From Reference 1.

dence of nickel sensitization in men will increase if more men pierce their ears to wear earrings. Men, however, may tend to wear fewer different earrings of higher quality, so they may not be as readily sensitized.

Dietary Component of Nickel Dermatitis

Even today, in the new millennium, the role of dietary nickel in causing and maintaining nickel dermatitis is vastly underappreciated. The simple fact, documented by a variety of studies, is that enough nickel in the diet of a sensitive individual can provoke dermatitis. The hands are the most common location for systemic nickel dermatitis, with manifestations including pompholyx or "regular" hand dermatitis. Other body areas may be affected as well. Evidence for the role of dietary nickel includes (a) flare of eczema and/or patch test sites upon oral nickel challenge; (b) improvement of dermatitis with a reduced nickel diet; (c) improvement of dermatitis by oral disulfiram, which chelates nickel and increases its excretion; and (d) preliminary suggestions that children with orthodontic devices (braces), who are therefore exposed to low continuous levels of ingested nickel, may have less subsequent nickel ACD.

The amount of nickel absorbed from food and water has been shown to vary considerably. Nielsen et al. (292) showed that peak serum nickel concentration was 13 times greater if nickel in water was given 30 minutes before a meal of scrambled eggs as compared to giving it simultaneously with the meal.

Nickel in Food

The normal daily intake of nickel by American adults has been calculated at 0.3 to 0.6 mg (293). About 1% to 10% of nickel in food is absorbed in the gastrointestinal tract, and the remainder is excreted. The nickel content of foods is partially determined by the components of the soil in which it is grown, fungicides used on it, and the equipment used in handling the food.

Nickel in food may vary considerably from region to region. Certain foods are routinely high in nickel content. Legumes, nuts, grains, potatoes, chocolate, and fish are among the foods high in nickel (294). (See Chapter 39 for a low-nickel diet.)

Horak and Sunderman (295) stated that fecal excretion is the major route for elimination of nickel from the human body. Hence, comprehensive evaluations of environmental or occupational exposures to nickel should include analyses of nickel in feces, as well as analyses of serum, urine, and hair.

It may be noted that appreciable losses of nickel also occur in the sweat. This observation may account for the diminished concentration of serum nickel in blast-furnace workers who were chronically exposed to extreme heat. The only other known route for the excretion of appreciable amounts of nickel is in a mother's milk.

> **Most nickel in food is eliminated in the feces. Appreciable amounts appear in sweat and in a mother's milk.**

Nickel in Tap Water

Fregert (296) stated that many nickel-sensitive patients with hand dermatitis suspect that tap water contains nickel and that their dermatitis is worsened by exposure to such water. In a previous study, Fregert had found no nickel, or only traces, when various samples of tap water that had been submitted by patients were analyzed. More recently, however, a nickel-sensitive woman with hand dermatitis reported that her condition was always worse when she was living in her own apartment but improved when she was in her parents' house. The first liters of running water obtained from the patient's home contained considerable amounts of nickel, especially from the hot tap (up to 0.13 mg/L), apparently due to corrosion of the tap and the linings of the boiler and tubes. Another factor may be the previous nickel-plating of chromium-plated metal; after long use, the nickel may reach the surface on water taps. On the basis of these findings, Fregert advised, "Nickel-sensitive persons should let the first liter of water run away in the morning."

On the basis of analyses of nickel concentrations in 969 water supplies in the United States during 1969 and 1970, Kopp and Kramer (297) found that the average concentration of nickel in water samples taken at the consumer's taps was 4.8 µg/L (297). With an estimated daily intake of 2 L of water, an adult would consume approximately 10 µg of nickel in drinking water each day. These investigators found the highest concentration of nickel in tap water from the Ohio River and Lake Erie river basins.

McNeely et al. (298) found that tap water from Sudbury, Ontario, the site of the largest open-pit nickel mines in North America, contained 200 μg/L of nickel—182 times greater than the concentration in tap water from Hartford, Connecticut, which contained 1.1 μg/L. In addition, the serum and urine concentrations of nickel in persons living in Sudbury were significantly higher than in those living in Hartford. These authors emphasized that there is no evidence that environmental exposures to nickel in Sudbury, Ontario, are associated with adverse effects in humans or animals or are deleterious in any way to the health of the inhabitants.

Ingested Nickel as a Cause of Dermatitis

Fowler (299) reviewed the various studies of nickel intake in relation to flares of dermatitis. Various amounts of nickel, up to 5 or 6 mg, have been given in capsule form. Other studies have attempted dietary intervention to reduce nickel intake. With rare exceptions, ingestion of enough nickel can result in a flare of dermatitis, especially hand eczema of the "pompholyx" type. Kaaber et al. (300), for example, found that 17 patients flared after ingestion of 2.5 mg of nickel. Nine of these improved after 6 weeks on a reduced-nickel diet. In another study, weekly nickel administration worsened dermatitis in 75% of 12 subjects, whereas only 25% on placebo worsened (301).

Veien (302) was enthusiastic about the benefits of a low-nickel diet, with at least some improvement being common, although total clearing may not occur. Further evidence for the role of systemic nickel in causing dermatitis is the finding that disulfiram, a nickel chelator, may result in improvement in nickel dermatitis and definitely increases nickel excretion (303).

In a study of nine nickel-sensitive patients with various forms of hand eczema, Fowler (303) found that eight improved significantly after treatment with disulfiram 250 mg/day. None improved with placebo treatment. Side effects may include liver function abnormalities and drowsiness. Avoidance of alcohol during treatment must be absolute. An initial flare, caused by temporary mobilization of systemic nickel, may occur. Once improvement is achieved, intermittent treatment may maintain clearing.

Role of Cooking Utensils in Nickel Dermatitis

Katz and Samitz (304) found that sweat and household detergents were shown to have the capacity to release nickel from stainless steel. This finding substantiates the thesis that stainless-steel utensils can be sources of skin contact allergy with nickel.

Christensen and Möller (305) measured the release of nickel to boiling water from new and used saucepans of different materials. No nickel was released from aluminum, Teflon, and enamel. Certain amounts of nickel were released from stainless steel, but only at acid pH. When the pH was lowered, appreciable amounts of nickel were leached out into the boiling water from new as well as used saucepans. It was even shown that the amounts released were positively correlated with the acidity of the water. Patients with nickel allergy should thus avoid stainless-steel cooking utensils because some foodstuffs may provide an acid milieu during processing.

The amount of nickel released from cooking utensils in the present study was fairly small in comparison to the dose used in oral provocation.

> **Because boiling water and detergents may release nickel from stainless-steel cooking utensils, aluminum, Teflon, or enamel kitchenware can be substituted.**

In summary, then, ingested nickel from food, beverages, or cooking utensils can cause a flare of dermatitis in some individuals. Accordingly, well-motivated patients may see improvement if they can reduce their body burden of nickel through either dietary changes or disulfiram therapy.

> **Dietary nickel is a contributing factor to worsening of dermatitis in some nickel-sensitive persons. Reduction of intake yields clinical improvement in these patients.**

Possible Role of Metals in Diet in Patch Test–Negative Patients

Veien et al. (306) claimed that the dermatitis of some patients with patch test–negative vesicular hand eczema flares after oral challenge with nickel, cobalt, or chromium salts.

In a controlled study, 202 patients, 68 males and 134 females, with patch test–negative, symmetrical vesicular hand eczema, were challenged orally with 2.5 mg of nickel, 2.5 mg of chromium, and 1 mg of cobalt given as salts of the respective metals. A mixture of the three metal salts was given initially, and if this produced a flare of the eczema, the salts were administered individually at 1-week intervals.

Fifty-five patients reacted to the mixture of salts as well as to one or two of the individual salts. Three other patients were challenged openly with nickel alone. Male patients reacted primarily to chromate and cobalt, whereas female patients more commonly reacted to nickel and cobalt.

Fifty-six patients were instructed to follow diets planned to reduce the daily intake of the respective metals. The dermatitis of 36 patients cleared or improved markedly after 1 month of dieting. Responses to a questionnaire sent to these 36 patients indicated that 28 of them had followed the prescribed diet rigorously or intermittently for at least 1 year, because they experienced recurrence of the dermatitis if they stopped dieting. Six patients noted no long-term benefit, and two did not respond. The diet instructions for cobalt in this experiment are listed in Table 35.9.

Veien et al. (307) then challenged patients with various chronic dermatoses of obscure origin as follows: The 299 patients with chronic dermatitis of obscure origin were challenged orally in a controlled study, with 2.5 mg of nickel, 2.5 mg of chromium, and 1 mg of cobalt given as salts of the respective metals.

Flares of the dermatitis were seen in 12 of 61 patients with patch test–negative hyperkeratotic eczema, in 9 of 32 patients with patch test–negative perianal eczema, and in 7 of 143 patients with various other patch test–negative eczemas. In this latter group, flares were seen only among patients with nummular eczema or hand eczema. Among 34 patients with various positive patch tests not relevant to the current dermatitis, 3 patients with hand eczema experienced flares.

Patients who reacted to oral challenges with the metal salt to which they had a positive patch test included 3 of 9 with nickel allergy, 2 of 5 with cobalt allergy, and 6 of 15 with chromate allergy. These patients were tested openly.

Low metal diets were prescribed for 33 patients who had flares after oral challenge with specific metal salts. The dermatitis cleared or improved markedly for 23 of these patients after following the diet for at least 2 weeks. Responses to a questionnaire sent to the 23 patients indicated that 16 had followed the prescribed diet rigorously or intermittently for at least 1 year.

> **Some patients with chronic hand eczema and various chronic dermatoses of obscure origin, whether or not they show positive reactions to nickel, chromates, or cobalt, benefit by diets low in these metals.**

Nickel in Urine

Menné et al. (308), commenting that the importance of internal exposure to nickel in patients with recurrent hand eczema and nickel allergy has become evident, undertook a study to investigate the value of urinary nickel determinations as an index of oral nickel intake. After administering 5.6 mg of nickel orally (as the sulfate), Menné et al. found increased nickel excretion over the next 2 to 3 days.

This study showed that oral administration of 5.6 mg of nickel was followed by increased nickel excretion over 2 to 3 days. Spruit and Bongaarts (309) also produced results showing increased urinary nickel levels for more than 24 hours after the administration of 5 mg of nickel to two healthy volunteers. DeJongh and Spruit (310), however, found only limited correlation between the course of the urinary nickel concentration and the clinical activity of the

nickel dermatitis in a woman with marked nickel sensitivity. They concluded from preliminary results that it will be necessary to investigate the influence of various factors on the ion climate of the internal body fluid in more detail, because possible variables include diet, menstruation, stress, and especially the liberation of nickel ions from depot sites of complex compounds in the body. These investigators stressed that it is important to explain the factors influencing the variation of the urinary nickel concentration under "normal" circumstances during the day and night. McNeely et al. (311) found that such diverse conditions as myocardial infarction, stroke, burns, hepatic cirrhosis, and uremia could produce abnormal concentrations of nickel in serum and, presumably, urine.

Spruit (312) found that the nickel (Ni) concentration in the urine of a rheumatic nonhypersensitive person that was usually about 1 μg Ni/L urine, increased to 9 μg Ni/L urine (range: 6 to 13 μg Ni/L) by the oral ingestion of 3 $\times$ 25 mg indomethacin per day over a period of 5 days. Prolonged ingestion of a medicine with food may thus increase the internal nickel absorption and possibly cause an exacerbation of nickel eczema in patients hypersensitive to that metal.

It is comforting for the clinician to learn that the nickel concentrations of blood plasma, urine, and scalp hair do not differ between patients who are hypersensitive and those who are nonsensitive to nickel. Even persons exposed occupationally to nickel, who may have 10 times more nickel in their plasma, urine, and hair than the normal "control" population, do not necessarily become allergic to nickel (311).

> **Many factors besides diet can affect the amount of nickel in the urine. Heart, kidney, and liver disease, as well as burns and indomethacin, produce high concentrations of nickel in serum and urine.**

Nickel in Hair

Katz et al. (313) reported that the nickel content of human hair was found to be more dependent on the sex of the donor than on other parameters and that nickel sensitivity was not reflected in the nickel content of women's hair, although there is a significant difference between the nickel content of men's and women's hair.

Nickel and the Law

In response to the high rate of nickel allergy, the Danish Ministry of the Environment, on 27 June 1989, released Statutory Order No. 472 (314). The order essentially prohibits the sale of nickel-containing jewelry, eyeglass frames, or clothing accessories that give a positive dimethylglyoxime test. Penalty for violation may be a fine or imprisonment. Enforcement today seems to be uncertain.

Nickel Sensitivity as a Cause of Infusion Reactions

Stoddart (315) reported that skin reactions developed in two patients who had had intravenous infusions and that in one of these there was also an alarming anaphylactoid reaction. It was suggested that sensitivity to the nickel in the infusion cannulas was the cause. Because nickel sensitivity is relatively common, Stoddart theorized that a portion of the hitherto unexplained infusion reactions may have been due to sensitivity to nickel in infusion cannulas, which may produce manifestations of the immediate or delayed type of hypersensitivity.

Smeenk and Teunissen (316) described seven patients with a contact allergy to nickel in whom cutaneous lesions, sometimes with fever, developed after administration of an intravenous infusion. The lesions consisted of vesiculobullous eruptions on the hands, more or less generalized exanthems, and occasional flares at the sites of earlier contact eczema due to nickel. It could be demonstrated experimentally that minute amounts of nickel, sufficient to cause the symptoms described, may be eluted from metallic needles by the infusion fluid. Their experiment consisted of a closed system in which 500 mL of physiologic saline was circulated four times during a 24-hour period through a stainless steel (8% nickel, 18% chrome) needle; 7 μg/L of nickel could be found in the solution. In a similar experiment lasting 48 hours (recirculated eight times), 80 μg/L of nickel was found.

> **Nickel concentrations in urine, plasma, feces, and scalp hair do not differ between patients who are allergic or nonallergic to nickel.**

Types of Nickel Eruptions

Calnan (317) classified nickel dermatitis into two groups: (a) primary: areas in direct contact with metal (such eruptions are usually eczematous but are occasionally papular); and (b) secondary: selective symmetrical areas that are involved when the dermatitis spreads.

The secondary eruption behaves like an autosensitive hematogenous spread similar to an "id" phenomenon. It is usually symmetrical and is related to the activity of the primary site. The secondary site may be the elbow flexure, eyelids, sides of neck, and face. The eruption is sometimes said to become generalized.

The secondary or idlike eruption may be manifest occasionally as a noneczematous dermatitis, such as erythema multiforme, urticaria, or prurigo. It should be noted that, at present, this type of secondary symmetrical eruption is not often seen. Instead, a pompholyx type of eruption has been extensively described.

Both Calnan (317) and Epstein (318) remarked that nickel dermatitis is "peculiar," in that at times nickel dermatitis spreads without contact with nickel and at other times the dermatitis does not always appear at all sites of contact.

In our opinion, however, the spread of nickel dermatitis to distant areas without contact with nickel may be more apparent than real. A careful history may reveal that in reality nickel did contact all the affected areas. Nickel-plated objects in wearing apparel may have a wide range of excursion on the skin. Bracelets and various other nickel-plated trinkets may move from the wrist to the elbows. Such bracelets may also contact the chest and abdomen if they are not removed when the patient undresses or bathes. Moreover, wandering, perspiring fingers may convey nickel in solution from metallic objects to distant sites.

> **Perspiring fingers contaminated with nickel and wide excursions of nickel-plated bracelets and necklaces may produce widespread nickel dermatitis.**

The factor of perspiration has to be recognized in relationship to the production of nickel dermatitis. Because certain areas of skin may perspire more than others, it is to be expected that not all areas of the skin making contact with metallic nickel will necessarily dissolve out nickel salt in the same concentrations. Nickel-plated objects contacting relatively "dry" areas of skin may not produce dermatitis in nickel-sensitive individuals.

Many nickel-sensitive persons report that the dermatitis due to nickel is much worse in the summer. Several women stated that when they were perspiring freely, their costume jewelry would cause an itching, prickly sensation within 15 to 20 minutes and that an eruption would appear in about 45 to 60 minutes. These same persons can wear nickel-plated objects for several hours in the winter, or when they were not perspiring, without any symptoms of dermatitis. The chloride radical in sweat is apparently an important factor in dissolving the metallic nickel, permitting the soluble nickel salts to act.

The proof that the chloride in sweat can release nickel from a metallic object was demonstrated by placing a nickel-plated object in each of three jars. The first contained a solution resembling sweat (0.5% sodium chloride, 0.5% urea, and 0.17% lactic acid). The second jar contained alcohol. The third jar contained distilled water. The nickel coins were allowed to remain in the jars for 2 hours. A spot test with dimethylglyoxime was then done with the solutions remaining after the nickel objects were removed. Only the first jar gave a positive test result for nickel (319). In addition, it should be noted that considerable amounts of nickel are excreted in sweat.

Other factors to be considered are friction and pressure. Adequate pressure is undoubtedly necessary to produce nickel dermatitis. Those areas in most intimate contact with nickel are the most likely to show nickel dermatitis. When pressure is avoided, dermatitis may not occur even in patients with marked hypersensitivity to nickel.

> **The presence of sweat, friction, and pressure will determine whether a nickel-plated object will produce dermatitis in a nickel-sensitive individual.**

Talcum or other absorbent powder placed under a nickel-plated object may prevent dermatitis in nickel-sensitive persons for a short time. The powder acts both as a mechanical barrier, preventing contact of the nickel object with the skin, and as a sponge, absorbing perspiration that ordinarily would dissolve and remove soluble nickel salts from the metallic objects.

Types of Nickel Hand Dermatitis

Hand dermatitis to nickel may be due to actual contact with nickel in sensitized individuals or to internal exposure (pompholyx).

Direct Contact

In men, nickel dermatitis of the hands is usually due to industrial exposure. In women, contact with inexpensive rings, knitting needles, or prolonged contact with nickel-plated objects will localize the dermatitis.

The prognosis is good in the industrial worker if the worker changes his or her job or if industrial hygiene improves.

Very low and short contact nickel exposure can flare hand dermatitis. Nielsen et al. (320) immersed one finger of 17 nickel-allergic volunteers for 10 minutes in a nickel solution of 10 ppm. This was done daily for one week, followed by 100 ppm daily for one week. Development of vesicles at day 14 was significantly higher ($p > .05$) in subjects compared to 18 controls.

Pompholyx

The other type of hand dermatitis, which is preceded by external nickel sensitization, is pompholyx. This dermatitis is accompanied by recurring itching and vesicles in the palms and on the sides of the fingers.

Christensen (321) gave a follow-up report of 63 female patients with nickel allergy and hand eczema who were reinvestigated 6 years after the primary investigation. Christensen discovered that 30% of the patients were healed. Patients with the pompholyx eczema had the worst prognosis. The start of hand eczema was not correlated to any particular occupation. There was a strong correlation between a history of metal sensitivity and a positive patch test reaction. High frequencies of personal and family atopy were found, and atopy made the prognosis worse. Determination of serum IgE was of no use in predicting the prognosis in patients with nickel allergy and hand eczema.

> **No study of hand eczema is complete unless patch testing is performed and nickel dietary reduction attempted in allergic individuals.**

Patch Tests for Nickel Sensitivity

Patch testing with nickel is a common field of study. The following questions have been posed (322): (a) What is the best vehicle for patch testing with nickel sulfate? (b) What is the optimum patch test concentration for nickel sulfate? (c) What are the indications for intradermal patch testing with nickel? and (d) Are there patients with allergic hypersensitivity to nickel in whom patch test results to nickel are negative?

Vehicles for Testing with Nickel Sulfate

Most investigators use petrolatum as the diluent vehicle for nickel sulfate. In comparing patch test results of nickel sulfate in petrolatum with aqueous nickel sulfate, Fisher stated that 5% nickel sulfate in petrolatum gives an occasional negative reaction, whereas the aqueous solution in the same concentration gives a strongly positive patch test reaction.

In petrolatum, nickel and some other allergens may not always be evenly dispersed. Thus, there are nickel-poor or even nickel-free areas in these petrolatum patch test materials that could give rise to false-negative patch test reactions. In aqueous solutions of nickel sulfate, there is always an even distribution of the nickel salt.

Wahlberg (323) pointed out, in his experiments with humans and guinea pigs, that distilled water was slightly more reliable than petrolatum as the suitable material for patch testing with metal compounds. He also pointed out, however, the following advantages of using petrolatum: (a) It possesses sealing capacity, (b) there is less risk of decomposition of the test substances in storage, and (c) petrolatum is somewhat better than water when using nonocclusive tapes.

> **Patch tests with 2.5% nickel in petrolatum in "standard" trays are reliable. When in doubt, retest with 5% aqueous solution.**

Van Ketel (324,325) agreed that distilled water is more reliable than petrolatum as a suitable vehicle for metal compounds. He stated, however, that in certain patients with a definite nickel dermatitis, patch testing with nickel sulfate 2.5% to 5% in water did not give positive reactions. In these cases, the use of nickel sulfate 2.5% in dimethyl sulfoxide (DMSO) resulted in more positive patch test reactions than when dissolved in water. Originally, van Ketel tested with nickel sulfate 2.5% in 50% DMSO.

Van Ketel (326) concluded that in the case of clear histories of nickel allergy, the test vehicle is important.

When Wall and Calnan (327) investigated an outbreak of occupational dermatitis in an electroforming plant in which there was a heavy exposure to nickel, they found that nickel chloride was a more reliable patch test allergen than nickel sulfate in petrolatum.

Nickel chloride, in a gel vehicle, such as the T.R.U.E. test, has been suggested to be somewhat more accurate than nickel sulfate in petrolatum because of better dispersion in the gel (328,329).

Concentration of Nickel Sulfate for Patch Testing

Cronin (328) evaluated the efficacy of patch testing with 5% and 2.5% nickel sulfate in petrolatum by applying them concurrently to two series of routine patients, first in 1968 and again in 1973. In the first group, there were 75 nickel-sensitive patients, and in the second group there were 64. In both series, the weaker concentration (2.5%) failed to detect 20% of these sensitized persons. In the two groups, a few patients (8 of 139, or 6%) had positive test results to the 2.5% and negative results to the 5% concentration. This anomalous result was probably due to a fault in the technique, to greater pressure or occlusion of the weaker patch test, or to irregularities in nickel dispersion.

Cronin (328) concluded that the most suitable concentration for routine patch testing was 5% nickel sulfate in petrolatum and that because this concentration is a mild irritant in some patients, a purely poral or follicular reaction should be checked by repeating the 5% test, applying 2.5%, and checking the history.

Dooms-Goossens et al. (329) studied two women with histories of contact dermatitis to nickel-containing jewelry (dimethylglyoxime test positive) who failed to react to patch testing with 5% nickel sulfate in yellow petrolatum. Further patch testing was performed with nickel sulfate 2.5% and 5% in water and with 2.5% in DMSO 50%; no positive reactions were obtained. An intradermal test with 1:10,000 dilution in water also gave negative results.

Both patients were again patch tested with 10% nickel sulfate in yellow petrolatum, which resulted in positive reactions after 48 and 96 hours. These investigators point out that if both patients had not insisted and if the anamnesis had not been so clear, two diagnoses of nickel contact allergy would have been overlooked on the basis of the standard 5% concentration.

Occasionally, particularly in atopic individuals, pustular patch test reactions are obtained with nickel. These are nonspecific reactions of no clinical significance.

> **Pustular, patch test reactions to nickel are nonspecific and are not clinically significant; they tend to occur more often in atopic individuals.**

In Fisher's material (322), a positive patch test reaction to 5% nickel sulfate solution was invariably strongly positive in individuals with proved allergic hypersensitivity to nickel. In a series of 50 individuals with nickel dermatitis, all showed a strongly positive patch test reaction, and 49 individuals showed positive intradermal reactions. In no instance did the intradermal test with nickel show any superiority over the patch test.

In Fisher's experience, every patient with proved nickel sensitivity also showed a positive patch test reaction to nickel coins. Moreover, a follow-up study revealed that more than 90% of the patients retained such strongly positive patch test reactions over a period of 2 to 17 years.

Threshold Level of Nickel Reactivity

In a study by Emmett et al. (330), 12 nickel-sensitive patients were tested with various dilutions of nickel sulfate in pet or water. The lowest amount producing a reaction was 0.47 μg (0.01%) in pet. The lowest amount to react in a significant number of patients was 1.5 μg (0.0316%). These low levels are easily attainable by sweat leaching of jewelry, for example.

> **Intradermal nickel tests are an investigative procedure.**

Dimethylglyoxime Nickel Spot Test

The dimethylglyoxime (DMG) spot test for the detection of nickel has been modified and popularized by Fisher (331). The spot test kit contains 1% dimethylglyoxime in alcohol solution (1 fl oz) and 10% ammonium hydroxide solution (1 fl oz). The directions are as follows: Add a few drops of each solution to the metallic object, solution, or skin to be tested. There is a positive reaction when a red precipitate occurs, indicating the presence of available nickel in sufficient concentration (at least 1:10,000) to produce dermatitis in nickel-sensitive persons. Most metal alloys containing nickel give a positive reaction, except stainless steel, which is usually safe for use by those who are nickel-sensitive. The DMG spot test can detect the presence of nickel in "gold" and other jewelry when the patient and the jeweler are unaware of available nickel content.

Dr. Ronald Shore of the Hahnemann Medical College and Hospital of Philadelphia described a "modification" of the dimethylglyoxime test, as follows:

In our modification of this procedure, a few drops of dimethylglyoxime and ammonium hydroxide are successively placed on a cotton-tipped applicator, and the cotton tip is then rubbed against the test object. A positive result with this technique is the formation of a red precipitate on the applicator tip.

We have found the previously described spot test applicable for most situations. However, we believe our modification has certain advantages and can enhance what is already a very useful procedure. With our modification it is much easier to test vertical surfaces such as chair legs, convex surfaces such as doorknobs and tiny objects such as small pieces of jewelry. There is no spillage of test solutions off such objects, which could occur if they were tested by the previously described technique. Also, because one rubs the applicator tip against the object (and thereby presumably exposes more nickel to the test solution), positive reactions tend to be stronger, faster, and easier to read. This may be important with objects containing very low concentrations of soluble nickel. We have had several of our nickel-sensitive patients employ this test on a wide variety of their belongings at home and in our office to determine how they might have been exposed to nickel. Almost invariably they have discovered they were exposed to high concentrations of the metal through contact with scissors, a letter opener, keys, a telephone, a television dial, a table edge, a wheel chair frame, and other sources they had not considered previously. In several cases such testing has provided the explanation for what was, until that time, an unexplained distribution of dermatitis.

> The use of the dimethylglyoxime test for nickel is **indispensable in the management of nickel dermatitis. All nickel-sensitive patients should be taught how to perform the test to help prevent further dermatitis. A substance that gives a negative result is unlikely to cause nickel dermatitis.**

For investigative procedures involving solutions, Fleigel's text (332) gave the following procedures: A drop of the test solution and a drop of 1% alcoholic dimethylglyoxime solution are placed on filter paper and are held over ammonia, or they are mixed on a spot plate and a small drop of dilute ammonia is added. The formation of a red fleck or circle on paper or of a precipitate or color on the spot plate indicates the presence of nickel.

Limit of identification: 0.16 μg of nickel; limit of dilution: 1:300,000.

The test is considerably more sensitive when a drop of the test solution is placed on dried filter paper that has been impregnated with the reagent. The impregnation is best carried out using a warm saturated solution of the reagent in acetone. In this way, as little as 0.015 μg of nickel can be detected.

Limit of identification: 0.5 μg of nickel; limit of dilution: 1:100,000.

In the presence of 1,000 times the amounts of iron in 2 N hydrochloric acid solution.

Limit of identification: 1.25 μg nickel; limit of dilution: 1:40,000.

In the presence of 200 times the amount of cobalt.

Some caution is needed, however, because the precipitation of nickel may be prevented by the presence of large amounts of oxidizing substances (halogens, hydrogen peroxide, and nitrates), ferrous salts, and copper salts, which may also produce red or violet-colored complexes. When the test is performed in the regular manner, the presence of high concentrations of cobalt also reduces greatly the sensitivity of the test by binding the reagent. Palladium and platinum give yellow precipitates. Lucas (333) pointed out that, despite these reservations, a metal or a substance giving a negative test reaction is unlikely to provoke a nickel dermatitis.

Earrings: The "Earlobe Sign" of Nickel Sensitivity

Practically every woman with nickel sensitivity has had earlobe dermatitis from wearing "cheap" earrings, which are nickel-plated and which give a positive reaction to dimethylglyoxime. Nickel sensitivity will occur in 10% to 15% of patients if nickel-plated earrings are inserted after the ears are pierced.

> Ear piercing should be done with a stainless-steel needle, and stainless steel or more expensive earrings should be inserted for at least 3 weeks to reduce sensitization from nickel.

Ear Piercing and Nickel Sensitivity

Many individuals become sensitized to nickel when their ears are pierced. Because injury to the skin from mechanical, physical, or chemical agents followed by intimate contact with nickel-plated earrings favors the development of allergic eczematous nickel dermatitis, piercing of earlobes followed by contact with jewelry containing nickel readily induces nickel sensitivity.

Ears should be pierced with stainless-steel instruments or needles, and only stainless-steel earrings should be worn for at least 3 weeks until the pierced opening is completely epithelialized. There are many so-called hypoallergenic earrings on the market, but no earrings should be recommended for nickel-allergic persons unless one obtains a negative result from a nickel dimethylglyoxime spot test.

> **Earrings should not be labeled "hypoallergenic" unless they give a negative dimethylglyoxime test. Many "expensive" gold earrings may contain nickel.**

The idea that the piercing of earlobes is important in developing nickel allergy is strongly supported by Rystedt and Fischer's investigations (334). Among the nickel-allergic women, 95% had pierced earlobes. Piercing at an early age seems to increase the risk of incurring nickel sensitivity.

The piercing agent is probably not the main offender in nickel allergy. The nickel earrings used frequently after piercing are usually the cause of allergy. The environment of the hole in the earlobe is closed, and humid and irritant reactions often develop, especially after hair washing, when the rings are left in the earlobes. The shampoo that remains may cause an irritant contact dermatitis, which can induce nickel sensitivity.

Boss and Menné (335) agreed that the main cause of nickel sensitization in females is the piercing of ears. They stated that the manner of ear piercing today and the use of nickel-plated jewelry result in a nickel-sensitization rate of a minimum of 20% (11/53) among young females.

In a study of 700 Finnish teenagers, 31% with pierced ears were allergic to nickel, but only 2% without pierced ears were allergic (336).

Nickel-sensitive individuals must wear stainless-steel earrings or the more expensive gold earrings free of nickel. Some individuals coat "favorite" dermatitis-producing earrings with nail lacquer and can thus wear the earrings for hours without symptoms appearing.

Patented ear-piercing instruments and stainless-steel earrings are available from H & A Enterprises, New York. The Roman Research Co. sells hypoallergenic stainless-steel costume jewelry and replacement posts and hoops for other earrings under the brand name Whispers.

Jean Nickel Button Dermatitis

Brandrup and Larsen (337) examined 79 nickel-sensitive patients (65 woman and 14 men) with regard to a present or past eczema corresponding to contact with metallic buttons in jeans; 63% of the women and 64% of the men had or had had eczema of this kind. Among 40% of the women younger than 30 years of age, this was the primary site of manifestation. The seriousness of this sensitivity is illustrated by the fact that two-thirds of the nickel-sensitive patients with button dermatitis had or had had eczema of the hands. The conclusion is that jean buttons should be made of a material that does not contain nickel, such as zinc alloys, which are used for some metallic buttons, or they should be designed in such a way that the button does not

come in contact directly with the skin (338). Brandrup and Larsen stated that they had investigated the nickel release from 10 metallic buttons suspected of provoking contact dermatitis. The buttons represented identical types, although of various makes, and were used by 10 nickel-sensitive female patients whose nickel sensitivity was verified by positive patch tests.

The nickel release varied considerably. Two buttons had a particularly high release and were suspected of causing primary sensitization according to anamnestic information. Five buttons did not release more nickel than the blank synthetic sweat solution, but two of these buttons were dimethylglyoxime-positive. The dimethylglyoxime test seems to be better than the synthetic sweat/flameless atomic absorption model in predicting the risk of metallic alloys.

The jean nickel button dermatitis is usually most prominent in the navel area. The eruption may at times cover a large portion of the mid-abdomen. When the nickel-plated button is handled by someone with perspiring fingers, nickel dermatitis may occur in "ectopic" areas.

Brass or bone buttons may be substituted for the nickel-plated variety.

> **Jean nickel button, perinavel dermatitis is not uncommon in sensitized individuals. Brass or bone buttons may be substituted.**

Nickel in Eyeshadow

Goh et al. (339) reported a nickel-allergic patient who reacted when wearing certain eyeshadow cosmetics. Patch test to the cosmetic was negative, but the sensitive eyelid skin reacted. The researchers found from 13 to 70 µg/g of nickel in some eyeshadows, well above the threshold for reactivity.

Eyeshadows, and possibly other cosmetics, should be considered as occult causes of dermatitis in nickel-allergic patients.

Dermo-Jet Nickel Dermatitis

LaChapelle and Tennstedt (340) reported that 10 women allergic to nickel developed skin reactions at injection sites with a Dermo-Jet of 2% lidocaine solution and 0.9% saline solution. Ten women (age-matched), who were not allergic to nickel, were selected as controls and submitted to the same injections; they had no positive reactions. Nickel was leached out of the Dermo-Jet by tissue fluids producing the reaction.

LaChapelle et al. (341) demonstrated the release of nickel into triamcinolone acetonide suspensions stored in the reservoir of a Dermo-Jet by electrothermal atomic absorption spectrometry. Increased urinary nickel excretion was found for 3 days after intradermal injections (with the Dermo-Jet) of triamcinolone acetonide in patients suffering from alopecia areata. The dimethylglyoxime test showed that the internal rod of the reservoir as well as metallic internal parts of the nozzle leached appreciable amounts of nickel even before any clinical use.

De Corret et al. (342) reported that 20 blood donors developed a dermatitis at the site of venipuncture within a few hours of giving blood. A local anesthetic administered with a Dermo-Jet had been used before extracting blood. Sensitivity to the local anesthetic was found in only two patients. In the other patients, the reaction was caused by nickel released from the Dermo-Jet. The quantity of nickel released is greater from the anesthetic solution than from deionized water, and it increases during the time that the anesthetic remains in the Dermo-Jet. A used Dermo-Jet releases more nickel than a new Dermo-Jet.

> **Dermo-Jets containing nickel-plated parts may produce dermatitis in nickel-sensitive individuals. "All" stainless-steel Dermo-Jets are available.**

Occupational Nickel Exposure

Shah et al. (343) evaluated 386 nickel-allergic patients for workplace exposure. In 84 (22.8%), nickel was felt to be a definite or possible occupational allergen. Hand dermatitis, as expected, was more common in the occupational group, and irritant dermatitis often coexisted. Commonly affected workers included hairdressers, retail clerks, food service workers, cleaners, and metal workers.

Nickel Dermatitis in Hairdressers from Permanent-Wave Solutions

Wahlberg (344) showed that hairdressers often develop nickel hypersensitivity through contact with utensils such as scissors and clips. Dahlquist et al. (345) demonstrated that hairdressers are in contact with permanent-wave liquids, which contain ammonium and glyceryl thioglycollate. Thioglycollic acid can form complexes with nickel ions (345). Dahlquist et al. showed that commercial permanent-wave liquids readily release nickel from nickel-plated utensils used by hairdressers, but that similar objects, which are made of stainless steel, do not release any nickel.

> **Hairdressers should use stainless-steel scissors and clips because permanent-wave solutions readily release nickel from nickel-plated utensils but not from stainless steel.**

Unusual Sources of Nickel Exposure

A worker making molded bricks developed ACD from nickel (346).

In two reports, nickel in chalk apparently caused hand dermatitis in teachers (347,348).

A metal strap to dissipate static electricity caused ACD in an electronics worker (349).

Nickel allergy from a bedwetting alarm was confused with genital herpes in a 5-year-old girl (350). In another case, a swallowed coin caused generalized dermatitis in a child (351).

Reactions to Nickel-Containing Heart Valves

Lyell et al. (352) stated that life-threatening periprosthetic incompetence developed with two successive nickel-containing mitral-valve prostheses in a patient allergic to nickel. Neither prosthesis had been incorporated satisfactorily. The patient's present nickel-free prosthesis seemed to be satisfactory 22 months after insertion. Because allergy to nickel may have been involved in the failure of these prostheses, it is recommended that nickel-sensitive patients should be given nickel-free prostheses. (See Chapter 20 for further discussion of the role of nickel in the failure of metal prostheses.)

Use of Chelating Agents in Chronic Nickel Dermatitis

Chelating agents such as disulfiram (Antabuse) have proved effective in nickel carbonyl poisoning. Menné and Kaaber (353) stated that the ingestion of nickel is important for the chronicity of hand eczema in nickel-sensitive patients. They tried the effect of chelating agents, because diethyldithiocarbamate (DDC) and tetraethylthiuram disulfide (TETD, Antabuse) have proved effective in the treatment of nickel carbonyl poisoning. A 66-year-old woman suffering from severe nickel dermatitis was treated in three periods: in the first period with DDC 100 mg four times daily (QID) for 20 days and later for two periods with TETD 100 mg three times daily (TID). An improvement was observed in all three experiments.

Christensen and Kristensen (354) and Kaaber et al. (355) conducted further studies with disulfiram (DSM). Using various dosages, these authors found that more often than not, DSM was helpful for nickel-sensitive hand eczema. However, hepatitic toxicity may occasionally occur with DSM use. In one patient, a 49-year-old woman with no prior liver problems, elevated liver enzymes occurred after 8 weeks of taking DSM 200 mg/day (356). The enzymes returned to normal after stopping the drug, then went up again on drug rechallenge.

Fowler (299) published a double-blind placebo-controlled crossover study showing that while on DSM 250 mg/day, eight of nine patients improved. In contrast, on placebo four patients had no change and five worsened.

Side effects were minimal. Occasionally mild fatigue or lethargy may occur with the drug. Liver enzyme elevations have returned to normal when the drug is discontinued, but should be checked for.

Certainly, not all patients with cutaneous allergy to nickel are candidates for treatment with DSM. Some patients may not be willing to abstain from alcohol during treatment periods. Also, patients allergic to thiurams used in rubber processing may develop a systemic allergic reaction if given DSM, which is chemically related. Many patients with nickel allergy apparently react primarily to topical rather than systemic nickel. Avoidance of the allergen, topical corticosteroids and emollients, systemic antihistamines, and occasional systemic steroid usage will control many patients with nickel contact dermatitis. However, despite these measures some patients have recurrent problems.

One other chelating agent, triethylenetetramine (Trientine), also chelates nickel, but is more effective at removing copper. Burrows et al. (357) found it to be ineffective in nickel hand eczema. It did not increase urinary nickel significantly, although copper excretion went up dramatically.

Topical chelation of nickel by L-histidine or ethylenediamine tetra-acetate acid (EDTA) in skin cleansers was effective in removing more nickel from the skin than control cleansers (358). Perhaps incorporation of these agents in commercial skin cleansers would be useful in occupational nickel allergy.

Unusual Reactions Associated with Nickel Allergy

Veien et al. (302) reported that the vesicular eruptions on palms and fingers, as well as urticaria and other noneczematous reactions following internal exposure to nickel, may be due to mechanisms other than delayed hypersensitivity. Precipitating antibodies against nickel sulfate bound to human albumin have been found in some patients with widespread erythema after oral challenge.

Chronic urticaria due to nickel has been reported by Warin (358A). McConnell et al. (359) reported asthma due to nickel sulfate in a metal-plate worker; a bronchoprovocation challenge test with nickel sulfate duplicated the patient's symptoms, and circulating antibodies were found by hemagglutination tests. Block and Yeung (361) reported a second case study of asthma induced by nickel sulfate.

Espana et al. (361) carefully documented a case of chronic urticaria due to nickel in false teeth. In addition to a positive test, the patient had a positive response with severe urticaria and fever after ingesting a test dose of nickel sulfate. After removal of the dental prosthesis, she remained clear of skin lesions for 2 years. Oral lesions were not present.

In another case, localized urticaria of the upper lips was attributed to nickel in a dental implant. Removal was curative (362).

> **Nickel allergy may, on rare occasions, cause urticaria, erythema, vasculitis, asthma, and anaphylactoid reactions.**

Hjorth (363) found that nickel sensitivity could produce vasculitis. Estlander et al. of Helsinki, Finland, in a lecture entitled "Contact Allergy, Contact Urticaria, and Asthma Due to Nickel," described one patient, a 27-year-old woman, who had performed manual machine grinding of metal castings, which contain 9% nickel, for 2 years. She had used a respirator with a changeable filter at work. She had a long-standing cough and paroxysmal dyspnea followed by occasional urticaria on both arms after 2 months' employment. Both her cough and dyspnea grew worse during the second year of employment. Cheap metal objects had caused dermatitis since she was 14 years old. Epicutaneous tests showed only a 2+ allergic reaction to 2.5% nickel sulfate ($NiSO_4$) in petrolatum. Skin prick tests showed no reactions to any common inhalant allergens. A scratch chamber test elicited a pseudopodial reaction to $NiSO_4$ at a concentration of 10 mg/mL. An open test on the volar aspect of the right arm with the same $NiSO_4$ solution elicited contact urticaria in 15 minutes. Bronchial and nasal provocation tests with the same $NiSO_4$ solution also were positive. The RAST test was positive to nickel.

The patient became sensitized to nickel partly at her work. The nickel caused both urticarial and respiratory symptoms. Positive RAST testing to nickel indicates an IgE-mediated reaction.

Cook (364) reported a patient with urticaria multiforme associated with nickel and cobalt dermatitis.

"Mechanical" Prevention of Nickel Dermatitis

Some nickel-sensitive patients use adhesive or cellophane tape to cover nickel objects, and pearl clasps are sometimes substituted for metal clasps. Foam rubber covered with cotton flannel may protect an individual from nickel garter clasps. Substitution of plastic for metallic knitting needles and plastic bobby pins for the metallic variety was instrumental in clearing several cases of nickel dermatitis. Plastic sleeves and plastic covers for eyeglass frames and nickel handles protected several patients from exposure to nickel. Cellophane tape applied to pens and metal desks protected one patient.

Two patients found that talcum powder under metallic objects worn next to the skin protected them for several hours. Talcum powder as temporary prevention of nickel dermatitis may act in one of two ways: It may act as a mechanical barrier against the contact of nickel with the skin, and it may absorb perspiration, which dissolves some of the nickel from the metal object.

TABLE 35.13. *Instructions for Nickel-Sensitive Individuals*

1. You are allergic to nickel and will probably remain so indefinitely.
2. You will be especially susceptible to a rash when the weather is hot and when you are perspiring.
3. Sweat can readily dissolve nickel out of metal, even through a layer of cloth, paint, nail polish, and adhesive tape.
4. Very small quantities of nickel can produce a rash where the nickel contacts the skin, and may even be conveyed by perspiring fingers to distant areas.
5. Many metals contain some nickel, including 14K yellow and white gold. Stainless steel contains nickel, but the nickel is so firmly bound in the steel that it does not leach out with ordinary contact, and so will not cause a rash. Thus, hundreds of nickel-sensitive people have used stainless-steel earrings without difficulty.
6. Some earrings are marked "hypoallergenic" for nickel-sensitive individuals, but have proved to cause a rash because they are made of metals that release nickel.
7. You should learn how to do the chemical test for nickel called the dimethylglyoxime test. This will enable you to avoid buying jewelry that contains nickel-releasing metals and to test various metal objects to see whether they are safe for you to contact.
8. Be careful of the following wearing apparel: garter snaps, wire brassiere cup supports, zippers, hooks and snaps on undergarments, eyelets on shoes, metal arch supports, shoe and belt buckles, jewelry, medallions, ID tags, watch bands, metallic buttons on jeans. Substitute plastic snaps, buttons, and Velcro fasteners.
9. Unless you hold a nickel-releasing coin more than 3 minutes, you are unlikely to develop a rash. Coins can produce a rash if kept loose in a pocket for a prolonged period. Keep coins in a plastic bag.
10. Metal keys can cause a rash. You can substitute keys made of aluminum.
11. Be careful of household utensils, vacuum cleaners, sewing machines, needles, scissors, thimbles, drawer handles, paper clips, and telephone dials (dial with a pencil).
12. Substitute wood for metal chairs and armrests, or put seat covers on and cover armrests with thick fabric. Many chrome-plated objects contain nickel.
13. Purchase all-plastic eyeglass frames. Some nickel-sensitive people continue to use metal eyeglass frames by buffing the metal with grade 0 steel wool, then coating with polyurethane varnish, then repeating the buffing and recoating. However, this is only a temporary measure.
14. If you have a rash on your hands, you may be contacting one or more of the following: cigarette lighter, lipstick case, pens, pencils, scissors, needles, vacuum cleaners, razors, door handles, handbags, carriages, kitchen utensils, thimbles, typewriter parts, bicycle handle bars, metal sinks, or umbrellas.
15. A rash on your head and face including the eyelids may be caused by the following: hairpins, curlers, bobby pins, eyelash curler (you can get an all plastic curler), earrings, spectacle frames, metal pins held in the mouth, and applying lipstick with a metal lipstick holder.
16. On the rest of your body you may get a rash from any of the following: necklaces, medallions, metal identification tags, brassiere wire supports, zippers, watch bands, bracelets, metal arch supports, metallic eyelets of shoes, and buttons on jeans.
17. There are reports that nickel in food can produce persistent blisters on the hands without your touching nickel. If you have such blisters, try cooking your food in stainless-steel, Teflon, or aluminum pots and pans. Sometimes a diet low in nickel content is said to be helpful in clearing hand blisters. This is a difficult diet that often does not help.
18. When you go for medical or dental treatment, tell your doctors that you are allergic to nickel so that they will avoid using nickel-plated instruments, including Dermo-Jets, epilating needles, acupuncture needles, and white gold crowns. All of these are available in stainless steel.
19. Should you require orthopedic surgery with the insertion of metal parts, your orthopedic surgeon may decide that you need special metals if you are nickel sensitive. The same holds true for a nickel-sensitive patient who may need a metallic heart valve installed.
20. If you contact nickel-containing liquids at work, remember that such liquids can penetrate rubber gloves. Heavy-duty vinyl gloves are more protective.

Some patients found that the avoidance of pressure prevented nickel objects from causing nickel dermatitis; that is, wearing nickel objects so that they touched the skin lightly often prevented the dermatitis. Some patients noted that they could tolerate nickel objects after losing weight. Two patients found that nickel dermatitis of the thighs could be prevented if they did not cross their legs and thus avoided pressure on garter clasps.

Wall (365) demonstrated that nickel can penetrate rubber, but not vinyl gloves.

Substituting Alternatives to Prevent Nickel Dermatitis

1. Earrings may be made of stainless steel or gold, which give a negative dimethylglyoxime test.

2. The wearing of panty hose obviates the need for stocking garter clips. If stockings are worn, plastic garter clips should replace the metallic variety.
3. Jewelry may be coated with nail polish or resin solutions. (Caution: The patient may become allergic to these solutions.) Also, a jeweler may apply rhodium or platinum plating to the inner surface of rings or other jewelry. Do not use palladium, as cross-reactions with nickel occur.
4. Metallic buttons on jeans should be replaced with the stainless-steel variety, with plastic buttons, or with brass buttons.
5. Cooking utensils made of aluminum, Teflon, and enamel are safest for nickel-sensitive individuals.
6. In industry, nickel-sensitive workers should wear heavy-duty vinyl gloves, because nickel salts can penetrate rubber gloves.

Industrial nickel compounds can penetrate rubber gloves; thus, workers should be protected with heavy-duty vinyl gloves.

---

7. Medical devices, such as various needles, including acupuncture needles, Dermo-Jets, and heart valves, should be made of "all" stainless steel.
8. Hairdressers and barbers should use stainless-steel products.

Table 35.13 lists suggested instructions for nickel-sensitive patients in order to prevent the recurrence and prolongation of nickel dermatitis.

It should be noted that the instructions include the use of the dimethylglyoxime test (see page 648). The advantages of having the patient perform such tests are emphasized by Wilkinson and Hambly (366), who stated: "As Fisher has pointed out, it is helpful to teach nickel-sensitive persons to use a nickel spot test so that they can identify the objects containing this metal at home."

PALLADIUM SENSITIVITY

Palladium is a precious metal that may be used as a substitute for platinum. It may be found as a component of white gold and other jewelry alloys. It is becoming more commonly used in dental alloys. Exposure may also occur in the electronics and chemical industries. Some palladium salts are strong contact irritants, whereas others, such as palladium chloride, show minimum irritancy (367).

Before the 1980s, only two reports of palladium allergy were found (368,369). In 1991, however, a joint European study found 42 positive reactions in 1,521 patients (2.7%) (370). This suggests that the prevalence of allergy to palladium is either increasing or has been previously overlooked. Probably both of these conclusions are true.

Both occupational and nonoccupational cases have been reported. Stomatitis and dermatitis are seen, depending on the exposure source (371). Koch and Baum (372) reported a case of stomatitis due to combined allergy to platinum and palladium. The patient reacted to ammonium tetrachloroplatinate (0.25% pet) as well as palladium chloride (1% pet) and cleared upon removal of the dental prosthesis, which contained these metals. Jewelry and dental materials constitute the most likely route of exposure in nonoccupational cases. The majority of reported patients have been women. Not surprisingly, patients allergic to palladium may not react to the pure metal, but only to the dissolved allergen (373,374).

Almost all patients with palladium allergy are also allergic to nickel (Table 35.2). Many also react to cobalt. Because palladium and nickel are in the same group of metals (group VIII of the periodic table), it would seem that cross-reactivity might occur. Wahlberg and Boman (375) executed a precisely designed study in guinea pigs to answer this question. Nickel, as a more common allergen, might be expected to be the primary sensitizer, with palladium as a secondary cross-reactor. In fact, however, no animals sensitized to nickel reacted on challenge with palladium. In contrast, a number of animals sensitized only to palladium later reacted to nickel. This suggests that cross-reactivity works in the direction of palladium to nickel only.

Clinically, palladium allergy may explain why some nickel-sensitive patients still react to "hypoallergenic" jewelry. Just as gold allergy has been overlooked, unsuspected palladium allergy may be occurring. Palladium should be suspected in jewelry allergy or allergic stomatitis.

Palladium allergy may be much more common than previously suspected. Most patients are also allergic to nickel. Testing should be done with palladium chloride 1% pet.

Some authors have suggested that the multitude of reactions to palladium may not be clinically important because few patients reacted to discs of palladium metal (375,376). Obviously, the subject bears further study.

Aberer et al. (371) were alarmed at the frequency of positive reactions (8.3% of 1,382 consecutive patients). Only eight patients reacted to palladium alone, the rest being allergic to nickel. Six of these patients had oral complaints. These authors are concerned that increasing use of palladium in dental alloys may lead to a rise in stomatitis and other oral complaints.

PLATINUM DERMATITIS

In industry, soluble platinum salts, liquid platinum sprays, and splashes of platinum salts have been reported as causing dermatitis and asthma (376,377).

Metallic platinum, as used in jewelry, photography, dentistry, and the chemical and electrical industries, rarely causes contact dermatitis, although dermatitis due to a platinum ring has been reported (369). Rhodium is often used to plate white gold and platinum, and in this instance, the platinum dermatitis occurred when the rhodium plating wore off. Sometimes, if the ring is replated with rhodium, the platinum-sensitized individual can wear the ring again without difficulty. Most jewelry made of platinum is either pure platinum or 90% platinum and 10% iridium.

Platinosis is a disease caused, not by metallic platinum, but usually by its complex salts, primarily chloroplatinates, and affects mainly workers in platinum-refining workshops (377). The cutaneous manifestations include pruritus, erythema, eczema, and urticaria, which are usually seen on the parts of the body exposed during work.

In a review of platinum sensitivity, Levene (378) reported the following adverse reactions to platinum salts: allergic conjunctivitis and rhinitis, asthma, urticaria, and contact dermatitis.

Roberts (379) coined the term "platinosis" for the symptom complex produced by platinum and its salts. He noted that once disabling symptoms arose in any one case, that person never again became asymptomatic in a platinum-containing atmosphere. His observations concurred exactly with the other reports, and it was advised that sufferers from the effects of platinum salts should be transferred to other work. Roberts carried out scratch tests with aqueous solutions of sodium chloroplatinate on 60 platinum workers. He found that all subjects developed a 1+ reaction with a 1:10 dilution of the salt and that following the onset of symptoms, of either the cutaneous or the respiratory type, a reaction was always obtained with a 1:1,000 dilution. Roberts decided that initial scratch testing was an unreliable index of liability to develop future symptoms, and he claimed that a person with a strong personal or family history of atopic manifestations or of contact dermatitis was more likely to succumb to platinosis than others.

Baker et al. (380) reported that 15 of 107 platinum refinery workers had positive skin prick tests to platinum. Five of these had dermatitis. The researchers tested with disodium hexachloroplatinate and ammonium hexachloroplatinate at concentrations of 0.1% to 0.000001%. Thirty-nine controls were negative.

It is worth pointing out that scratch or intradermal testing can be hazardous to the point of being life-threatening in these patients. A single intradermal test using potassium hexachloroplatinate at a concentration of 1 μg/mL produced an anaphylactic reaction in the patient of Freedman and Krupey (381). It is wise for these patients to be protected by systemic antihistamine prior to skin testing.

Successful hyposensitization was achieved in an analytical chemist who exhibited typical severe symptoms of hay fever, asthma, and contact urticaria when exposed to platinum complex salts in the course of his work (382).

Patch Testing with Platinum Salts

Complex salts of platinum are not readily soluble in distilled water, but solubility is improved if physiologic saline is used. These compounds dissolve in dilute hydrochloric acid, but such solutions are not suitable for patch testing.

Levene (378) pointed out that it is likely that allergic contact sensitivity can occur, but this has not yet been convincingly proven by patch tests in appropriate cases. Allergic contact sensitivity is a delayed hypersensitivity reaction, and the situation is complicated by the well-documented ability of these salts to produce urticaria on contact. It is not even clear what is an appropriate concentration to be used for patch testing.

In a study with mice, ACD was easily induced by repeat applications of sodium hexachloroplatinate (Na_2PtCl_6) 5% in acetone. This solution, however, caused a local irritant reaction on application. Sensitization was documented 6 days later with a 2% solution (383).

This confirms the possibility of ACD to platinum, but does not help determine proper patch test materials for humans.

Although contact dermatitis to metallic platinum is rare, eczematous dermatitis and contact urticaria may occur from exposure to the platinum salts. "Platinosis"—a symptom complex of allergic rhinitis and asthma—is more common.

RHODIUM ALLERGY

Rhodium has twice been reported to cause ACD, both times in jewelers, specifically in goldsmiths (384,385). In one case, patch test with rhodium sulfate (0.05% aq) was positive, although 40 controls were negative. Both cases also reacted to cobalt but not to gold. Currently, rhodium allergy from wearing jewelry has not been reported. Rhodium may be used to plate the inside of rings to attempt to block allergy to other metals.

Rhodium, like other platinum group metals, can cause respiratory IgE-mediated reactions (249).

RUBIDIUM

Rubidium iodide (tested at 1% pet) was implicated as a cause of a facial dermatitis (386). Eyedrops were the source of the rubidium. Testing in 20 controls was negative.

REACTIONS TO SILVER AND ITS SALTS

Metallic silver in jewelry or wire rarely causes dermatitis. Gaul (387) reported a patient with allergic reactions to silver coins, pure silver, and silver nitrate.

Silver Nitrate

Silver nitrate is kept in dark bottles because on exposure to air and light it decomposes, forming small amounts of nitric acid, silver nitrite, and colloidal silver, which liberate silver ions. Testing with old solutions of silver nitrate may, therefore, give irritant reactions.

Allergic Reactions to Silver Nitrate

Marcussen (388) reported an allergic reaction to silver nitrate, as did Gaul and Underwood (389). Gaul and Underwood's patient developed a vesicular reaction to the 10% silver nitrate used for marking patch tests. He recalled having applied in the past a solution of silver nitrate to an area of eczema on his heel and having to stop it after 2 weeks because the eczema suddenly worsened and spread. On patch testing, he reacted to 5% and 10% aged silver nitrate but not to 10% fresh silver nitrate.

Topical silver nitrate may produce allergic reactions and argyria.

The ionized silver was thought to be the sensitizer in this patient and explained the discrepancy between the results of testing with old and with fresh solutions.

Argyria from Topical Silver Nitrate and Other Silver Salts

Marshall and Schneider (390) reported a case of systemic argyria secondary to the topical use of silver nitrate for bleeding gums caused by poorly fitting dentures.

Localized argyria may result from topical silver salts through either medicinal or occupational exposure. Buckley (391) reported a case of a duplicating-machine operator who developed localized argyria of her hands from daily immersion in photographic developing solutions. Handling of silver metal by silversmiths and the oral suctioning of silver nitrate solutions in the preparation of silver beads are other causes of reported occupational argyria (392). The use of colloidal silver compounds such as mild silver protein (Argyrol) and strong silver protein (Protargol) for such varied indications as bladder irrigation, urethritis, nasal drops for cold prevention, mucosal ulcerations, cervicovaginitis, and conjunctivitis has been practiced. In the early twentieth century the use of silver arsphenamine for the treatment of syphilis was associated with a significant incidence of at least localized argyria. In 1935, Gaul and Staud (393) reported 70 cases of argyria secondary to oral, intranasal, or pharyngeal use of organic and colloidal silver compounds. It appears that Marcussen's series marked the end of widespread use of the silver colloid solutions, as no subsequent reports have rivaled his in number of cases

or in frequency of detection. The current use of silver sulfadizine in the treatment of burns must be scrutinized carefully to avoid excessive systemic absorption of silver from the wounds.

"Immediate" Reaction to Argyrol

Criep (394) reported that argyrol, which is a colloidal solution of silver or silver oxide in alkaline proteins, produced immediate-type hypersensitivity after its use in the nose and as a pharyngeal spray (394). Scratch testing with 1% argyrol was positive and intradermal testing gave a severe local reaction and constitutional symptoms.

Dermatitis from Miscellaneous Silver Salts

Silver Coat

Heyl (395) stated that a patient acquired dermatitis from "silver coat." Silver coat is a powder consisting of silver cyanide with small amounts of sodium carbonate, sodium cyanide, and sodium nitrate. The patient's work involved the weighing of various precious metal salts for electroplating purposes, mainly salts of gold, silver, platinum, and palladium in powder form. Patch tests revealed a 3+ positive reaction to a 1% aq solution of "silver coat" but negative for gold potassium cyanide and silver metal.

Silver Fulminate

Although fulminates were widely used in the past as explosives, they are now little encountered. Fulminate itch is of historical interest. White and Rycroft (396) investigated a factory using silver fulminate in the manufacture of explosive snaps. Silver fulminate, known in the trade as "white salt," may produce stomatitis, particularly in women.

Ionic Silver Chloride Complexed with Thiosulfate

Marks (397) reported that a radiographer, who processed films by hand, developed a papular eczema under her watch strap. Patch tests were positive to 1% silver chloride complexed with sodium thiosulfate, to 1% silver nitrate, and to the fixing fluid. Although silver chloride is insoluble, it was suggested that it formed a soluble complex with sodium thiosulfate in the fixing tank and that this complex contaminated the patient's wristwatch strap. Ionic silver was postulated as the sensitizer.

TIN

Menné et al. (398) described the first findings of positive patch tests to tin. They found 6 of 73 patients tested to tin-coated copper discs who gave 2 or 3+ reactions. All patients were nickel sensitive. The authors stated that no nickel contaminated the tin. They did not test patients to copper or other metals. The same authors later reported five positive reactions from 2,206 consecutive patients tested with tin chloride 1% pet (399). None were nickel positive. The total of doubtful or irritant reactions was 25. No relevance was found for the five positive reactions, so it is possible the reactions were irritant. The authors stated that biopsies from four of the patients, however, were believed to be allergic, histologically.

A probable case of true ACD to tin was recently reported (400). A metalworker with heavy exposure to tin-containing metal dust developed airborne ACD on exposed surfaces. Patch testing was positive only to tin (SnCl$_2$), at 0.25%, 0.5%, and 1% in pet. Lymphocyte testing was performed but did not yield positive results.

Tributyl tin oxide, a biocide in paint, is a well-known irritant (401).

TITANIUM

Titanium is an inert metal used for some orthopedic devices and medical implants. Compared to other metals, titanium allergy is rarely reported.

There have been several reports of allergy to titanium in cardiac pacemakers. Granulomatous dermatitis in one case, with negative patch tests, was felt to be caused by titanium, because titanium was found on electron probe microanalysis in the granulomas (402). Two other cases of granuloma without positive patch tests have been reported (403,404). In three other cases, positive patch tests confirmed titanium allergy (405–407).

A frequent query to dermatologists from our patients and orthopedic colleagues involves concern over metallic orthopedic implants in metal-allergic individuals. Holgers et al. (408) studied 445 patients with titanium implants. In nine patients, a local skin reaction developed. None were allergic to titanium. In six cases, staphylococcal infection was causative, and in the others allergy to other agents occurred.

Dujardin et al. (409) reviewed the literature in 1995 and found no cases of titanium allergy among 54 cases of dermatitis related to orthopedic implants. In a Japanese report, dermatitis following a stainless-steel implant resolved when a titanium implant was substituted (410).

Based on current reports, appropriate advice to our orthopedic colleagues would be:

1. Dermatitis from stainless-steel implants is unusual but may occur in metal-sensitive persons.
2. Titanium allergy is exceedingly rare.
3. Titanium implants should be used in cases where metal allergy may present clinical or medicolegal concerns. Patch testing should be undertaken to document metal allergy where concern exists.

VANADIUM

Vanadium pentoxide (10% pet) was positive in 1 of 190 ceramics workers. No irritant reactions were seen (254).

ZINC DERMATITIS AND DISCOLORATIONS

Zinc Oxide and Zinc Pox

Although zinc oxide is completely inert allergenically, it is probably the most common cause of black dermographism produced by jewelry. Zinc oxide present in cosmetics, lotions, and dentifrices is much harder than most metals in jewelry and coins, leading to abrasion and deposition of minute metal particles. Zinc stearate is so soft that it cannot cause black dermographism. Zinc oxide ointment may be used as a "sun block," particularly for protecting the nose and lips of lifeguards at the beach.

Calnan (411) described metal fume fever as an influenza-like illness due to inhalation of fumes of zinc oxide and other metals.

Zinc pox is an eruption from zinc oxide dust, especially localized to the moist intertriginous areas such as the axillae and the groin. A secondary infection may occur (412).

Zinc Chloride

Zinc chloride is a strong primary irritant and can produce ulcerations resembling those produced by chromic acid. Allergic reactions to this caustic zinc salt are rare. Sources of exposure are dental fillings, preservation and fireproofing of timber, solder flux, and Moh's chemosurgery for skin cancer.

Zinc Chromate

This yellow pigment, made of zinc oxide and chromic acid, is widely used as an anticorrosion agent as an undercoat. Zinc chromate can cause chromate dermatitis in chromium-sensitive individuals.

Industrial exposure to zinc particles and dusts may produce "zinc pox" in the intertriginous areas and can cause "metal fever" when inhaled.

Zinc Metal Allergy

Zinc was implicated as the cause of dermatitis localized at sites of acupuncture therapy (413). Patch tests were positive only to zinc sulfate (2% pet), but no controls were tested.

Zinc Pyrithione

Zinc pyrithione has become a popular ingredient in many American antiseborrheic shampoos. Zinc pyrithione sensitivity is rare.

Yates and Finn (414) and Muston et al. (415) reported that this antidandruff agent produced allergic contact dermatitis. In addition, the patient of Yates and Finn had an actinic reticuloid syndrome.

Calnan (416) stated that scalp and facial dermatitis developed in a patient after the use of ZP11 shampoo, which contains zinc pyrithione. The patient also showed a positive patch test reaction to ethylenediamine hydrochloride. Calnan reported that zinc pyrithione also cross-reacts with piperazine hydrochloride. There is a report that a patient with occupational piperazine dermatitis was also allergic to ethylenediamine (417). A more recent case implicated zinc pyrithione in a combination of ACD and a flare of pustular psoriasis. Patch test to zinc pyrithione was positive (418).

The dermatologist treating a patient sensitive to zinc pyrithione or ethylenediamine hydrochloride must be aware of the following: (a) Zinc pyrithione cross-reacts with piperazine; (b) piperazine used for the treatment of pinworms can form hydroxyzine in the body; (c) hydroxyzine hydrochloride (Atarax, Vistaril) is an ethylenediamine derivative; therefore, (d) zinc pyrithione, piperazine, Atarax, Vistaril, and ethylenediamine hydrochloride may cross-react.

Antidandruff shampoos containing zinc pyrithione should be used with caution in ethylenediamine- and piperazine-sensitive individuals.

Zinc acexamate, an oral medication used to treat gastric ulcers, caused a generalized dermatitis in a Spanish man. Patch test and oral challenge tests were positive (419).

Zinc Insulin Allergy

Feinglos and Jegasothy (420), in an investigation of two unrelated patients who had local cutaneous hypersensitivity reactions after injection of any commercially available insulin preparation, have shown that the cause of the allergy was zinc. Zinc insulin– and zinc sulfate–induced transformation and proliferation of peripheral blood lymphocytes from these patients; they also induced the production of a specific leukocyte inhibitory factor. Intradermal skin tests for zinc were positive in both patients. Similar studies carried out in a patient whose cutaneous allergy to insulin was corrected by changing from mixed beef-pork to pure pork insulin were negative. Zinc-free insulin did not produce any allergy in the first patient. The number of patients in whom zinc (which is present in all commercially available insulin preparations) is a cause of "insulin" allergy is unknown. These patients may be identified by intradermal skin tests. This previously unrecognized allergy should be considered in all patients whose insulin allergy does not respond to conventional therapy.

ZIRCONIUM GRANULOMAS

These granulomas of the skin, originally seen following the use of zirconium sodium lactate as a deodorant, are also seen following the use of zirconium oxide for the treatment of rhus plant dermatitis (421,422).

Soluble salts were used in the deodorants that produced granulomas. In the topical preparations for rhus dermatitis, mostly insoluble salts are used.

Palmer and Welton (421) reported a case of lupus miliaris disseminatus faciei in an individual who was exposed to a zirconium oven in a metal-alloy factory.

Zirconium, like beryllium, can produce sarcoid-like granuloma (423).

Clinical Appearance

The lesions usually appear 4 to 6 weeks after initial use of the zirconium preparation and are limited to the sites of contact. They appear as persistent, firm, shiny, erythematous, flesh- or apple-jelly-colored papules, which are solitary, grouped, or coalescent. Eczematous changes are also usually present. Pruritus is minimal or absent (424,425).

Zirconium salts used in deodorants and rhus plant dermatitis may produce sarcoid granulomas in sensitized individuals.

Histologic Appearance

The epidermis is normal. In the dermis, large aggregates or tubercles of distinctive epithelioid and Langerhans cells are present. A minimal inflammatory reaction is occasionally present. Foreign body material is not detected by polarized light microscopy. Differentiation from sarcoidosis may not be possible histologically (426,427).

Mechanism of Production of Zirconium Granuloma

Zirconium granulomas may be produced by either soluble or insoluble salts, but they must first be introduced into the skin. The granulomas then develop in individuals who have acquired an allergic hypersensitivity to zirconium. Any defect in the protective layer of the skin enhances the development of hypersensitivity.

In the axillae, minute abrasions from shaving, as well as excess friction and sweating, enhance the penetration of the zirconium salts of the deodorants. The preparations containing zirconium salts used for treatment of rhus dermatitis readily penetrate through the acutely inflamed skin and through denuded areas, vesicles, and bullae.

Tests for Zirconium Hypersensitivity

Either patch or intracutaneous testing may be used to determine allergic hypersensitivity to zirconium salts.

In patch testing, the zirconium preparation may be rubbed into a test site that has been prepared by multiple scratches or denuded by a dermal curet. The site is then covered with an occlusive dressing for 2 days. In sensitized individuals, a positive reaction consists of the development of reddish brown papules in about 4 weeks. Such papules show a sarcoidal granulomatous infiltrate histologically.

In intracutaneous testing, a small wheal is made by injecting a 1:10,000 dilution of sodium zirconium lactate. A positive reaction consists of a discrete papule, which appears in 8 to 14 days. In about a month, the papule clinically and histologically has the appearance of a sarcoid lesion. It may persist for 6 to 24 months.

Prognosis

Axillary granulomas produced by soluble zirconium lactate in deodorants usually disappear within a few months. Lesions produced by insoluble zirconium oxide preparations used for rhus plant therapy usually remain unchanged for several months to years and are refractory to therapy. Temporary improvement is obtained by the use of corticosteroids either systemically or intralesionally (428).

TABLE 35.14. *Industrial Exposure to Zirconium and Its Salts*

Zirconium metals
  Alloys
  Nuclear reactors
  Superconductors
  Surgical implants
  Vacuum tube parts
Zirconium acetate
  High-temperature electrical conductors
  Refactory applications
  Water repellents
  Zinc boride
  Zinc carbide
Zirconium hydroxide
  Pigments in glass
Zirconium naphthenate
  Ceramics
  Lubricants
  Paints
  Varnishes
Zirconium nitrate (as a preservative)
  Electronics
  Ceramic glazes
  Special glasses
Zirconium oxychloride
  Cosmetics
  Greases
  Textiles
Zirconium potassium fluoride in welding fluxes
Zirconium sulfate
  Chemicals
  Lubricants
  Reagent and catalysts
  Retannage
  Tanning of white leather
Zirconium tetrafluoride
  A component of molten salts for nuclear reactors

Because zirconium compounds used for poison ivy dermatitis can produce intractable granulomas and are of questionable value, consideration should be given to discontinuing their use. Table 35.14 lists the industrial exposures to zirconium and its salts.

MISCELLANEOUS COMPOUNDS SOMETIMES CLASSIFIED WITH METALS

The following compounds are sometimes included with metals, although strictly speaking, they are not typical metals.

Phosphorus

A foundry worker with work-related hand dermatitis reacted to sodium hypophosphate (NaH_2PO_2) used in steel processing at both 1% and 5% aq. He also reacted to phosphorus sesquisulfide (P_4S_3) (429). Controls were not tested. No other explanation of the dermatitis could be found.

Phosphorus sesquisulfide has been previously reported to cause contact urticaria and dermatitis from safety matches (430). Postinflammatory hypopigmentation has also been noted.

Selenium

Stedman's Medical Dictionary defines selenium as a metallic element chemically similar to sulfur. *Webster's Dictionary* and *Random House College Dictionary* define selenium as nonmetallic.

Selenium is often found together with tellurium. It is a semiconductor and acts as a rectifier and photoconductor. It is widely used in electronics, glass, and ceramics and as a rubber accelerator (selenium diethyldithiocarbamate), catalyst, and trace element in animal feeds.

Selenium oxychloride (seleninyl chloride), a powerful solvent for metals and a chlorinating agent, is a strong vesicant that rapidly destroys the skin unless immediately removed by washing.

Some compounds of selenium are severe irritants and are readily absorbed through the lungs, gastrointestinal tract, and damaged skin. The most characteristic sign of absorption is the smell of garlic from the breath. Selenium dioxide, which is important in industry, is a light powder that dissolves in water or sweat to form noxious selenious acid. When selenium dioxide is inhaled, it causes pulmonary edema, conjunctivitis in the eyes, and burns or irritant dermatitis on the exposed skin. The nail beds become painful if it penetrates under the nails (431).

In a selenium refinery plant, 11 employees developed dermatitis, conjunctivitis, and inflammation of the upper respiratory tract. Investigation showed no evidence of sensitization, and it was concluded that all of the effects were due to irritation (432).

Senff et al. (433) report a well-documented case of selenium allergy. A laboratory technician developed hand eczema only when handling a selenite (Na_2SeO_3) containing culture medium. The only positive patch test was to selenite down to a dilution of 0.1% aq. Multiple control subjects were negative. Avoidance of the broth resulted in clearing.

Selenium sulfide is used in several topical agents, such as shampoos, for the treatment of seborrheic dermatitis and for the treatment of tinea versicolor. Allergic reactions to these preparations are rare.

Silica and Silicone Granulomas

Shelley and Hurley (434) described silica granulomas as a nonallergic foreign body epithelioid reaction to silica in the colloidal form. Silicone powder can also produce granulomas.

Mason and Apisarnthanarax (435) reported a 38-year-old woman who had a migratory silicone granuloma of the left upper portion of the chest and left upper arm secondary to a ruptured breast implant. The initial diagnosis was factitial panniculitis. With the common use of silicone in cosmetic surgery, physicians should inquire into a possible history of silicone injections or implants before ascribing a factitial cause of foreign-body granulomas.

Silicone (dimethylpolysiloxane) has been popular for use in cosmetic reconstructive surgery for many years. Numerous reports on tissue reactions to silicone have appeared in the literature. Although pure silicone is relatively inert and usually causes only minimal tissue reactions, it has also been reported to evoke a definite foreign-body or lupus-like reaction. It was thought that silastic gel implants would circumvent many of the problems encountered with injectable silicones. The silicone used in the implants varies, however, in consistency and cohesiveness, depending on the manufacturer, despite the fact that these characteristics are believed to be under strict production controls in the United States.

Silicone sprays have not been reported as producing dermatitis. They can be used for waterproofing adhesive tape so that patients can bathe or swim. Such sprays can also be used to prevent runs or tears in nylon stockings.

Silicone adhesives are used for bonding silicone elastomer (silastic medical adhesive) to itself or other implantable synthetics, such as Dacron, Teflon, and acrylic. A silicone adhesive has been implicated as a cause of dermatitis associated with an implanted cardiac pacemaker (436).

Contact urticaria to silicone rubber in a military gas mask has been reported (437).

Tellurium

Tellurium is used in the vulcanization of rubber, in alloys, as a color for glass, as a catalyst, and in a diagnostic test for diphtheria.

Blackadder and Manderson (438) reported poisoning in two research workers, both of whom had the characteristic smell of sour garlic in their breath, sweat, and urine. An unusual feature was a bluish black discoloration of the skin in streaks on the face and neck and in patches in the finger webs. This was thought to be due to the absorption of tellurium esters through the skin and the deposition of tellurium in the dermis and subcutaneous tissues. The patients recovered without treatment.

Uranium

Thiers et al. (439) reported two men preparing uranium for an atomic energy plant who developed hand eczema. They were patch tested with 2% sodium and calcium salts of uranium, to which they reacted.

REFERENCES

1. Fowler JF. Allergic contact dermatitis to metals. *Am J Cont Derm* 1990;1:212.
2. Marks J, Belsito D, DeLeo V, et al. North American Contact Dermatitis Group patch test results, 1996–1998. *Arch Dermatol* 2000; 136:534–536.
3. Wilkinson JV. Some metallurgical aspects of orthodontic stainless steel. *Am J Orthod* 1962;48:192.
4. Liden C, Menné T, Burrows D. Nickel containing alloys and platings and their ability to cause dermatitis. *Br J Dermatol* 1996;134:193–198.
5. Liden C, Rondell E, Skare L, et al. Nickel release from tools on the Swedish market. *Contact Dermatitis* 1998;39:127–131.
6. Ingber A, et al. Detergents and bleaches are sources of chromium contact dermatitis in Israel. *Contact Dermatitis* 1998;38:101–104.
7. Malten KE. Nickel sensitization and detergents. *Acta Derm Venereol* (Stockh) 1969;49:10.
8. Malten KE, Spruit D. The relative importance of various environmental exposures to nickel in causing contact hypersensitivity. *Acta Derm Venereol* (Stockh) 1969;49:14.
9. Quinones PA, Garcia Munox CM. Contact allergy due to nickel and chrome: presence of these compounds in detergents used in the household. *Ann Derm Syph* 1965;92:383.
10. Vilaplana J, et al. Cobalt content of household cleaning products. *Contact Dermatitis* 1987;16:139.
11. Zugerman C. Contact dermatitis to yellow iron oxide. *Contact Dermatitis* 1985;13:107.
12. Levy J, Sewell M, Goldstein N. II. A short history of tattooing. *J Derm Surg Oncol* 1979;5:851.
13. Sulzberger MB, Tolmach JA. Allergic flareup reactions in red tattooing: Observations on development and subsidence of mercurial sensitivity and on allergic granulomatous and sarcoid reactions. *Hautarzt* 1959;10:110.
14. Biro L, Klein WP. Unusual complications of mercurial (cinnabar) tattoo. *Arch Dermatol* 1967;96:2.
15. Lowenthal LJA. Reactions in green tattoos. *Arch Dermatol* 1960;82: 237.
16. Bjoernber A. Allergic reaction to cobalt in light blue tattoo markings. *Acta Derm Venereol* (Stockh) 1961;41:259.
17. Bjoernber A. Reactions to light in yellow tattoos from cadmium sulfide. *Arch Dermatol* 1963;88:267.
18. Goldstein N. Mercury-cadmium sensitivity in tattoos: photoallergic reaction in red pigment. *Ann Intern Med* 1967;67:948.
19. Waldmann I, Vakilzadeh F. Allergische spatty preaktion auf roten azofarbdtoff in tatowiernngen. *Hautarzt* 1997;48:666–670.
20. Scutt R, Gotch C. *The mystery of tattooing, skin deep.* London: Peter Davies, 1974.
21. Nguyen LQ, Allen HB. Reactions to manganese and cadmium in tattoos. *Cutis* 1979;23:71.

22. Rubianes EI, Sánchez JL. Granulomatous dermatitis to iron oxide after permanent pigmentation of the eyebrows. *J Derm Surg Oncol* 1993;19:14.
23. Flint GN. A metallurgical approach to metal contact dermatitis. *Contact Dermatitis* 1998;39:213–221.
24. Buckley WR, Lewis CE. The ruster in industry. *J Occup Med* 1960;2:25.
25. Burton JL, Pye RJ, Brooks DB. Metal corrosion by chloride in sweat. *Br J Dermatol* 1976;95:417.
26. Bang-Petersen N. Topical treatment of a "ruster." *Br J Dermatol* 1977;96:332.
27. Bang Pedersen N, Fregert S, Brodeilius P, Gruvberger B. Release of nickel from silver coins. *Acta Derm Venereol* (Stockh) 1974;54:231.
28. Husain SL. Nickel coin dermatitis. *Br Med J* 1977;2:998.
29. Morgan JF. Observations on persistence of skin sensitivity with references to nickel eczema. *Br J Dermatol* 1953;65:84.
30. Yeatman GW, van Dang V. Çao Gio (coin rubbing): Vietnamese attitudes toward health care. *JAMA* 1980;244:2748.
31. Ellerstein NS. The cutaneous manifestations of child abuse and neglect. *Am J Dis Child* 1979;133:906.
32. Gellis SS, Feingold M. Cao gio (pseudo-battering in Vietnamese children). *Am J Dis Child* 1976;130:857.
33. Yeatman GW, Shaw CS, Barlow MJ, et al. Pseudobattering in Vietnamese children. *Pediatrics* 1976;58:616.
34. Nong TA. "Pseudo-battered child" syndrome. *JAMA* 1976;623:2288.
35. Keller EL, Apthorp J. Folk remedies vs child battering. *Am J Dis Child* 1977;131:1173.
36. Tan A. Coin rubbing and related folk medicine. *JAMA* 1981;245:1819.
37. Seigle R. Coin rubbing and related folk medicine. *JAMA* 1981;245:1819.
38. Kranke B, Aberer W. Multiple sensitivities to metals. *Contact Dermatitis* 1996;34:225.
39. Rystedt I. Relationship between nickel and cobalt sensitization in hard metal workers. *Contact Dermatitis* 1983;9:195.
40. Lammintausta K, et al. Inter-relationship of nickel and cobalt sensitization. *Contact Dermatitis* 1985;13:148.
41. Simonetti V, Manzini BM, Seidenari S. Patch testing with nickel sulfates comparison between 2 nickel sulfate preparations and 2 different test sites on the back. *Contact Dermatitis* 1998;39:187–191.
42. Seidenari S, Manzini BM, Belletti B. Pretreatment of the test area with 1-day occlusion improves the response rate to NiSO4 5% pet. patch tests in subjects with a positive history of nickel allergy. *Contact Dermatitis* 1995;33:152–156.
43. Seidenari S, Motolese A, Belletti B. Pre-treatment of nickel test areas with sodium lauryl sulfate detects nickel sensitivity in subjects reacting negatively to routine performed patch tests. *Contact Dermatitis* 1996;34:88–92.
44. Uter W, Fuchs T, Hausser M, et al. Patch test results with serial dilutions of nickel sulfate (with and without detergent), palladium chloride, and nickel and palladium metal plates. *Contact Dermatitis* 1995;32:135–142.
45. Meneghini C, Angelini G. Intradermal test in contact allergy to metals. *Acta Derm Venereol* (Stockh) 1979;59:123.
46. Epstein S. Contact dermatitis due to nickel and chromate. *Arch Dermatol* 1956;73:236.
47. Epstein S. Dermal contact dermatitis. Sensitivity to rivanol and gentian violet. *Dermatologica* 1958;117:287.
48. Epstein S, Pinkus H. Penicillin dermatitis based on tuberculin-type sensitivity. *Ann Allergy* 1946;4:186.
49. Marcussen PV. Comparison of intradermal test and patch test using nickel sulfate and formaldehyde. *J Invest Dermatol* 1963;40:263.
50. Möller H. Intradermal testing in doubtful cases of contact allergy to metals. *Contact Dermatitis* 1989;20:120.
51. Urbach E, Pillsbury DM. Black dermagraphism. *JAMA* 1943;121:485.
52. Fisher AA. Black dermographism. A physical phenomenon. *Cutis* 1974;13:187.
53. Hurley HJ. Black dermographism (society transactions). *Arch Dermatol* 1960;81:329.
54. Fisher AA. What causes gold smudge? *Jewelers' Circular-Keystone* 1971;141:64.
55. Rapson WS. Skin contact with gold and gold alloys. *Contact Dermatitis* 1985;13:56.
56. Steinegeer S. Endemic skin lesions near an aluminum factory. *Fluoride Quart Rept* 1969;2:37.
57. Hemmer W, Wantke F, Focke M, et al. Evaluation of cutaneous hypersensitivity to aluminum by routine patch testing with AlCl3. *Contact Dermatitis* 1996;34:217–218.
58. Slater DN, et al. Aluminum hydroxide granulomas: light and electron microscopic studies and X-ray microanalysis. *Br J Dermatol* 1982;107:103.
59. Kaaber K, Nielsen AD, Veien, NK. Vaccination granulomas and aluminum allergy: course and prognostic factors. *Contact Dermatitis* 1992;26:304.
60. O'Driscoll J, et al. Contact Dermatitis to aluminum acetate eardrops. *Contact Dermatitis* 1991;24:156–157.
61. Kalveram K-J, Rapp-Frisk C, Sorck G. Misleading patch test results with aluminum Finn chambers® and mercury salts. *Contact Dermatitis* 1980;6:507.
62. Fischer T, Maibach H. Aluminum in Finn chambers® reacts with cobalt and nickel salts in patch test materials. *Contact Dermatitis* 1985;12:200.
63. Veien NK, Hattel T, Laurberg G. Systemically aggravated contact dermatitis caused by aluminum in toothpaste. *Contact Dermatitis* 1993;28:199.
64. Stevenson CJ. Antimony spots. *Trans St Johns Hosp Derm Soc* 1965;51:40.
65. White GP, Mathias CGT, Davin JS. Dermatitis in workers exposed in antimony in a melting process. *J Occupational Med* 1993;35:392.
66. Paschoud J. Occupational arsenic and antimony contact eczema. *Dermatologica* 1964;129:410.
67. Motolesa A, Truzzi M, Giannini A, et al. Contact dermatitis and contact sensitization among enamellers and decorators in the ceramics industry. *Contact Dermatitis* 1993;28:59–62.
68. Birmingham D, Key MM. An outbreak of arsenical dermatitis in a mining community. *Arch Dermatol* 1965;91:457.
69. Holinquist R. Occupational arsenical dermatitis. *Acta Derm Venereol* (Stockh) 1951;31:26.
70. Barbaud A, Mougedelle J, Schnutz J. Contact hypersensitivity to arsenic in a crystal factory worker. *Contact Dermatitis* 1995;33:272–273.
71. Curtis CH. Cutaneous hypersensitivity to beryllium. *Arch Dermatol* 1951;64:470.
72. Nichol AD, Dominiquez R. Cutaneous granuloma from accidental contamination with beryllium phosphorus. *JAMA* 1949;140:855.
73. Davis C, Cooper MM, Grimes OF. Skin granuloma following laceration by a fluorescent lamp. *CA Med* 1951;71:203.
74. Helwig EB. Chemical granuloma (beryllium) of skin. *Milit Surg* 1951;109:540.
75. Kennedy BF. Effect of adrenocorticotropic hormone (ACTH) on beryllium granulomatosis and silicosis. *Am J Med* 1951;10:134.
76. Dobson RL. General discussion on the treatment of chronic beryllium poisoning with ACTH and cortisone. *AMA Arch Indus Hyg* 1951;3:543.
77. Fisher AA. Nonsurgical treatment of cutaneous beryllium granuloma. *Arch Dermatol* 1953;68:214.
78. Folesky H. Some aspects of beryllium granuloma. *Berufsdermatosen* 1967;15:93.
79. Jones Williams W. Granulomatous diseases. *Proc Roy Soc Med* 1971;64:946.
80. Haberman AL, Pratt M, Storrs FJ. Contact dermatitis from beryllium in dental alloys. *Contact Dermatitis* 1993;28:157.
81. Vilaplana J, Romaguera C, Grimalt F. Occupational and nonoccupational allergic contact dermatitis from beryllium. *Contact Dermatitis* 1992;26:295–298.
82. Balkisson R, Newman L. Beryllium copper alloy (2%) causes chronic beryllium disease. *J Occup Med* 1999;41:304–308.
83. Vilaplana J, Romaguera C, Grimalt F. Occupational and non-occupational allergic contact dermatitis from 2 nickel containing dental prostheses in a nickel-allergic patient. *Contact Dermatitis* 1989;21:204.
84. Rudner E, et al. Epidemiology of contact dermatitis in North America. *Arch Derm* 1973;108:537.
85. Raith L, Schubert H, Goring H-D. Contact dermatitis from cadmium chloride? *Contact Dermatitis* 1982;8:267.
86. Wahlberg JE. Routine patch testing with cadmium chloride. *Contact Dermatitis* 1977;3:293.

87. Kaaber S, Cramers M, Jepsen FL. The role of cadmium as a skin sensitizing agent in denture and non-denture wearers. *Contact Dermatitis* 1982;8:308.

88. Gebhardt M, Geier J. Evaluation of patch test results with denture materials series. *Contact Dermatitis* 1996;34:191–195.

89. Geier J, Vieluf D, Fuchs T. Patch testing with cadmium chloride. *Contact Dermatitis* 1996;34:73–74.

90. Friedman AA. Dermatitis of the breast from "lead" pencils. *Arch Dermatol* 1956;73:384.

91. Capusan I, Mauksch J. Occupational dermatoses of workers of a carbon black producing factory. *Berufsdermatosen* 1969;17:28.

92. Nater JP. Possible causes of chromate eczema. *Dermatologica* 1963;126:160.

93. Fregert S. Occupational dermatitis in a 10 year material. *Contact Dermatitis* 1975;1:96.

94. Burry JN, Kirk J. Environmental dermatitis: chrome cripples. *Med J Aust* 1975;2:720.

95. Burrows D. Prognosis in industrial dermatitis. *Br J Dermatol* 1972;87:145.

96. Breit R, Turk RBM. The medical and social fate of the dichromate allergic patient. *Br J Dermatol* 1976;94:349.

97. Cronin D. Chromate dermatitis in men. *Br J Dermatol* 1971;85:95.

98. Fregert S. Occupational dermatitis in a 10 year old material. *Contact Dermatitis* 1975;1:96.

99. Avnstorp C. Follow-up of workers from the prefabricated concrete industry after the addition of ferrous sulphate to Danish cement. *Contact Dermatitis* 1989;20:365.

100. Fregert S, et al. Reduction of chromate in cement by iron sulfate. *Contact Dermatitis* 1979;5:39.

101. Avnstorp C. Risk factors for cement eczema. *Contact Dermatitis* 1991;25:81.

102. Halbert AR, Gebauer KA, Wall LM. Prognosis of occupational chromate dermatitis. *Contact Dermatitis* 1992;27:214.

103. Zachariae CO, Agner T, Menne T. Chromium allergy in consecutive patients in a country where ferrous sulfate has been added to cement since 1981. *Contact Dermatitis* 1996;35:83–85.

104. Olsavsky R, et al. Contact sensitivity to chromate: comparison at a London contact dermatitis clinic over a 10-year period. *Contact Dermatitis* 1998;38:329–331.

105. Freeman S. Shoe dermatitis. *Contact Dermatitis* 1997;36:247–251.

106. Bajaj A, Gupta S, Chatterjee A, Singh K. Shoe dermatitis in India. *Contact Dermatitis* 1991;24:149–151.

107. Nater JP. Possible causes of chromate eczema. *Dermatologica* 1963;126:160.

108. Hostynek J, Maibach H. Chromium in US household bleach. *Contact Dermatitis* 1988;18:206.

109. Feuerman EJ. Housewives' eczema and the role of chromates. *Acta Derm Venereol* (Stockh) 1969;39:288.

110. Tritsch H, Orfanos C, Luckerath I. Experiments on the allergic skin reaction to chromated catgut. *Hautarzt* 1967;18:355.

111. Nethercott JR, Holness DL. Dermatologic problems of musicians. *J Am Acad Dermatol* 1991;25:870.

112. Fregert S. Otitis externa due to chromate of matches. *Acta Derm Venereol* (Stockh) 1962;42:473.

113. Fregert S. Book matches as a source of chromate. *Arch Dermatol* 1963;88:546.

114. Fregert S. Chromate eczema and matches. *Acta Derm Venereol* (Stockh) 1962;42:473.

115. Morris GE. Chromate dermatitis from chrome glue and other aspects of the chrome problem. *AMA Arch Industr Health* 1955;11:368.

116. Lück H, Jentsch G. Chromium dermatitis caused by epoxy resin. *Contact Dermatitis* 1988;19:154.

117. Fregert S, Hjorth N, Gruyberger B. Chromate in bridge table felt. *Contact Dermatitis Newsletter* 1970;8:173.

118. Fisher AA. Blackjack disease and other chromate puzzles. *Cutis* 1976;18:21.

119. Burrows D. Chromium and the skin. *Br J Dermatol* 1978;99:587.

120. Donaldson RM, Barreras RF. Intestinal absorption of trace elements of chromium. *J Lab Clin Med* 1966;68:484.

121. Kaaber K, Veien NK. The significance of chromate ingestions in patients allergic to chromate. *Acta Derm Venereol* (Stockh) 1977;57:321.

122. Veien NK, Kaaber K. Nickel, cobalt and chromium sensitivity in patients with pompholyx (dyshidrotic eczema). *Contact Dermatitis* 1979;5:371.

123. Van Ulsen J, Stolz E, Van Joost TH. Chromate dermatitis from a homeopathic drug. *Contact Dermatitis* 1987;16:53.

124. Fowler J. Systemic contact dermatitis caused by chromium picolinate. *Cutis* 2000;65:116–117.

125. Fisher AA. Chromates: prime causes of industrial allergic contact dermatitis. *Cutis* 1983;32:24.

126. Ros AM, Bang-Pedersen NB. Chromate in a defatting solvent. *Contact Dermatitis* 1977;3:105.

127. Bang-Pedersen NB. Chromate in the food laboratory. *Contact Dermatitis* 1977;3:105.

128. Fregert S, Gruyberger B. Factors decreasing the content of water-soluble chromate in cement. *Acta Derm Venereol* (Stockh) 1973;53:267.

129. Fregert S, Gruyberger B, Mitchell JC. Chromate in postage stamps. *Contact Dermatitis* 1975;1:328.

130. Einarsson O, Kylin B, Lindstedt G, Wahlberg JE. Chromium, cobalt and nickel in used cutting fluids. *Contact Dermatitis* 1975;1:182.

131. Malten KE. Cobalt and chromium in offset printing. *Contact Dermatitis* 1975;1:120.

132. Rudsky E, Czerwinska-Dihnz I. Sensitivity to dichromate milk testers: 6 cases of chromate allergy in milk testers. *Contact Dermatitis* 1977;3:107.

133. Huriez CL, Martin P, Lefebvre M. Sensitivity to dichromate in a milk analysis laboratory. *Contact Dermatitis* 1975;1:247.

134. Rogers S, Burrows D. Contact dermatitis to chromate in milk testers. *Contact Dermatitis* 1975;1:387.

135. Stevenson CJ. Fluorescence as a clue to contamination in TV workers. *Contact Dermatitis* 1975;1:242.

136. Varelzides A, Katsambas A, Georgala S, et al. Shoe dermatitis in Greece. *Dermatologica* 1974;149:236.

137. Weiler K-J, Von Russel HA. Das Chromekzem durch Branntkalk. *Berufsdermatosen* 1974;22:116.

138. Krook G, Fregert S, Gruyberger B. Chromate and cobalt eczema due to magnetic tapes. *Contact Dermatitis* 1977;3:60.

139. Garcia-Perez A, Martin-Pascual A, Sanchez-Misiego A. Chrome content in bleaches and detergents: its relationship to hand dermatitis in women. *Acta Derm Venereol* (Stockh) 1973;53:353.

140. Rycroft RJR, Calnan CD. Chromate dermatitis from a boiler lining. *Contact Dermatitis* 1977;3:198.

141. Engel HO, Calnan CD. Chromate dermatitis from paint. *Br J Ind Med* 1963;20:192.

142. Newhouse NL. A cause of chromate dermatitis among assemblers in an automobile factory. *Br J Ind Med* 1963;20:199.

143. Fregert S, Gruyberger B, Heijer A. Sensitization to chromium and cobalt in processing of sulphate pulp. *Acta Derm Venereol* (Stockh) 1972;52:221.

144. Samitz MH, Shrager J, Katz S. Studies on the prevention of injurious effects of chromates in industry. *Industr Med Surg* 1962;31:427.

145. Richter G, Heidelbach U. Chromate eczema after glass polishing with corundum. *Berufsdermatosen* 1969;17:8.

146. Lee HS, Goh CL. Occupational dermatoses among chrome platers. *Contact Dermatitis* 1988;18:89.

147. Fregert S. Chromate in welding fumes with special reference to contact dermatitis. *Acta Derm Venereol* (Stockh) 1963;43:119.

148. Shelley WG. Chromium in welding fumes as a cause of eczematous hand eruption. *JAMA* 1964;189:772.

149. Zugerman C. Chromium in welding fumes. *Contact Dermatitis* 1982;8:69.

150. Burrows D, Andersen RE, Camarasa JS. Trial of 0.5% versus 0.375% potassium dichromate. *Contact Dermatitis* 1989;21:351.

151. Nethercott J, et al. A study of chromium-induced allergic contact dermatitis with 54 volunteers: implications for environmental risk assessment. *Occup Environ Med* 1994;51:371.

152. Kosann M, Brancaccio R, Shupack J, et al. Six-hour versus 48 hour patch testing with varying concentrations of potassium dichromate. *Am J Contact Dermatitis* 1998;9:92–95.

153. Siegenthaler U. Studies on contact sensitivity to chromium in the guinea pig. *J Invest Derm* 1983;80:44.

154. Samitz MH, Epstein E. Experimental cutaneous chromate ulcers in guinea pigs. *Arch Environ Health* 1962;5:463.

155. Samitz MH. Some dermatologic aspects of the chromate problem. *Arch Industr Health* 1955;11:361.

156. Anderson FE. Cement and oil dermatitis: the part played by chrome sensitivity. *Br J Dermatol* 1960;72:108.

157. Goh CL, Gan SL. Change in cement manufacturing process, a cause

for decline in chromate allergy? *Contact Dermatitis* 1996;34:51–54.

158. Conde-Salazar L, Guimaraens D, Villegas C, et al. Occupational allergic contact dermatitis in construction workers. *Contact Dermatitis* 1995;33:226–230.

159. Fisher AA. Cement burns resulting in necrotic ulcers due to kneeling in wet cement. *Cutis* 1979;23:272.

160. Rowe RJ, Williams GH. Severe reaction to cement. *Arch Environ Health* 1963;7:709.

161. Hannuksela M, Suhonen R, Karvonen J. Caustic ulcers caused by cement. *Br J Dermatol* 1976;95:547.

162. Tosti A, Peluso AM, Varotti C. Skin burns due to transit-mixed Portland cement. *Contact Dermatitis* 1989;21:58.

163. Junger H, Witzani R. Cement ulcers. *Dermatosen Beruf Umwelt* 1978;26:121.

164. Ackroyd TNW. *Cement: properties and manufacture.* Oxford: Pergamon Press, 1962.

165. Stoermer D, Wolz G. Cement burns. *Contact Dermatitis* 1983;9:421.

166. Fowler J, Kauffman L, Marks J, et al. An environmental hazard assessment of low level dermal exposure to hexavalent chromium in solution among chromium sensitized volunteers. *J Occup of Environ Med* 1999;41:150–160

167. Wall LM. Chromate dermatitis and sodium dithionite. *Contact Dermatitis* 1982;8:291.

168. Romaguera C, et al. Formulation of a barrier cream against chromate. *Contact Dermatitis* 1985;13:49.

169. Miyachi Y, et al. Auto-oxidative damage in cement dermatitis. *Arch Dermatol Res* 1985;277:288.

170. Gollhausen R, et al. Trends in allergic contact sensitizations. *Contact Dermatitis* 1988;18:147.

171. Young E, Van Weelden H, Van Osch L. Age and sex distribution of contact sensitivity to standard allergens. *Contact Dermatitis* 1988; 19:307.

172. Christophersen J, et al. Clinical patch test data evaluated by multivariate analysis. *Contact Dermatitis* 1989;21:291.

173. Edman B. Sites of contact dermatitis in relationship to particular allergens. *Contact Dermatitis* 1985;13:129.

174. Marcussen PV. Cobalt dermatitis. Clinical picture. *Acta Derm Venereol* (Stockh) 1963;43:231.

175. Price ML, MacDonald DM. Cheilitis and cobalt allergy related to ingestion of vitamin B12. *Contact Dermatitis* 1981;7:352.

176. Rostenberg Jr A, Perkins AJ. Nickel and cobalt dermatitis. *J Allergy* 1951;22:467.

177. Fisher AA. Contact dermatitis at home and abroad. *Cutis* 1972;10:719.

178. Young WC, Ulrich CW, Fouts PJ. Sensitivity to vitamin B12 concentrate. *JAMA* 1950;143:893.

179. Kalensky J, Schwank R. Hypersensitivity to cobalt caused by an antihydrotic cream. *Cesk Derm* 1962;43:423.

180. Skog E. Skin affections caused by hard metal dust. *Industr Med Surg* 1963;32:266.

181. Fischer T, Rystedt I. Cobalt allergy in hard metal workers. *Contact Dermatitis* 1983;9:115.

182. McDermott FT. Dust in the cemented carbide industry. *J Am Ind Hyg Assoc* 1971;32:188.

183. Bourne LB, Milner FJM. Polyester resin hazards. *Br J Industr Med* 1963;200:100.

184. Pirila V. On occupational diseases of skin among paint factory workers, painters, polishers and varnishers in Finland: clinical and experimental study. *Acta Derm Venereol* (Stockh) 1947;27[Suppl 16]:1.

185. Nater JP. Cement eczema. *Nederl T Geneesk* 1958;102:250.

186. García J, Armisen A. Cement dermatitis with isolated cobalt sensitivity. *Contact Dermatitis* 1985;12:52.

187. Camarasa GJM. Cobalt contact dermatitis. *Acta Derm Venereol* (Stockh) 1967;47:287.

188. DeFonseca A. Joint sensitization with chromium, cobalt and nickel in cement eczema. *Acta Derm Sifilgiogr* 1970;61:151.

189. Mueller R, Breucker G. Cobalt as work-dependent eczematogen and as co-allergen with chromium and nickel. *Derm Wochenschr* 1968; 154:276.

190. Bhushan M, Craven NM, Beck MH. Contact allergy to methyl ethyl ketone peroxide and cobalt in the manufacture of fibreglass-reinforced plastics. *Contact Dermatitis* 1998;39:203.

191. Jolanki R, Tarvainen K, Tatar T, et al. Occupational dermatoses from exposure to epoxy resin compounds in a ski factory. *Contact Dermatitis* 1996;34:390–396.

192. Schena D, Rosina P, Chieregato C, et al. Lymphomatoid-like contact dermatitis from cobalt naphthenate. *Contact Dermatitis* 1995;33: 197–198.

193. Pirila V. Sensitization to cobalt in pottery workers. *Acta Derm Venereol* (Stockh) 1953;33:193.

194. Tuomi ML, Rasanen L. Contact allergy to tylosin and cobalt in a pig farmer. *Contact Dermatitis* 1995;33:285.

195. Ratcliffe J, English JS. Allergic contact dermatitis from cobalt in animal feed. *Contact Dermatitis* 1998;39:201–202.

196. Kanerva L, Jolanki R, Estlander T. Offset printer's occupational allergic contact dermatitis caused by cobalt-2-ethylhexoate. *Contact Dermatitis* 1996;34:67–68.

197. Zelger J. Cobalt allergy. *Derm Wochenshr* 1962;146:425.

198. Nurnberger F, Arnold W. Quincke's edema as a manifestation of a cobalt allergy due to a sensitization of cobaltous shell splinters. *Berufsdermatosen* 1969;17:21.

199. Camarasa JG, Alomar A. Photosensitization to cobalt in a bricklayer. *Contact Dermatitis* 1981;7:154.

200. Romaguera C, Lech M, Grimalt F, et al. Photocontact dermatitis to cobalt salts. *Contact Dermatitis* 1982;8:383.

201. Allenby CF, Basketter DA. Minimum eliciting patch test concentrations of cobalt. *Contact Dermatitis* 1989;20:185.

202. Marcussen PV. Intradermal test using cobalt chloride. *Acta Derm Venereol* (Stockh) 1963;43:472.

203. Saltzer EI. Allergic contact dermatitis due to copper. *Arch Dermatol* 1968;98:37.

204. Foussereau J, et al. Allergy to copper gas. *Med France* 1969;76: 4489.

205. Santosh V, et al. Results of patch testing with dental materials. *Contact Dermatitis* 1999;40:50–51.

206. Cohen SR. A review of the health hazards from copper exposure. *J Occup Med* 1974;16:621.

207. Oster G, Salgo MP. The copper intrauterine device and its mode of action. *N Engl J Med* 1975;239:432.

208. Barranco VP. Eczematous dermatitis caused by internal exposure to copper. *Arch Dermatol* 1972;106:386.

209. Forck G, Kastner H, Wagner H. One case of allergic reaction due to copper-T. Second International Symposium of Contact Dermatitis, Elsinore, Denmark, March 1977.

210. Barkoff JR. Urticaria secondary to a copper intrauterine device. *Int J Dermatol* 1976;15:594.

211. Dry J, Leynadier F, Bennani A, et al. Intrauterine copper contraceptive devices and allergy to copper and nickel. *Ann Allergy* 1978;41: 194.

212. Romaguera C, Grimalt F. Contact dermatitis from a copper-containing intrauterine contraceptive device. *Contact Dermatitis* 1981;7: 163.

213. Karlberg A-T, Boman A, Wahlberg JE. Copper—a rare sensitizer. *Contact Dermatitis* 1983;9:134.

214. Dhir G, et al. Contact dermatitis caused by copper sulfate used as coloring material in commercial alcohol. *Ann Allergy* 1977;39:204.

215. Van Joost T, Habets JMW, Stolz I. The meaning of positive patch test to copper sulphate in nickel allergy. *Contact Dermatitis* 1988;8: 101.

216. Pande RS, Gupta YN. Thrombocytopenic purpura following copper sulfate therapy. *J Indian Med Assoc* 1969;52:227.

217. Reid DJ. Allergic reaction to copper cement. *Br Dent J* 1968;124:92.

218. Fregert S, Hjorth N. In: Rook AJ, et al., eds. *Textbook of dermatology.* Oxford: Blackwell Scientific Publications, 1968.

219. Fox JM, Kennedy R, Rostenberg Jr A. Eczematous contact-sensitivity to gold. *Arch Dermatol* 1061;83:956.

220. Malten KE, Mali J. Contact eczema due to gold. *Allergic Asthma* 1966;12:31.

221. Elgart ML, Higdon RS. Allergic contact dermatitis to gold. *Arch Dermatol* 1971;103:649.

222. Bruze M, Edman B, Bjorkner B, et al. Clinical relevance of contact allergy to gold sodium thiosulfate. *J Am Acad Dermatol* 1994;31: 579–583.

223. Fowler J. Allergic contact dermatitis to gold. *Arch Dermatol* 1988;124:181–182.

224. Koch P, Bahmer F. Oral lesions and symptoms relating to metals in dental restorations. *J Am Acad Dermatol* 1999;41:422–430.

225. Bjorkner B, Bruze M, Moller H. High frequency of contact allergy to gold sodium thiosulfate. *Contact Dermatitis* 1994;30:144–151.

226. Fowler JF. Selection of patch test materials for gold allergy. *Contact Dermatitis* 1987;3:280.

227. Koch P, Kiehn M, Frosch P. Epikutane Testung mit Goldsalzen. Zwei Multicenterstudien der Deutschen Kontaktallergiegruppe. *Hautarzt* 1997;48:812–816.

228. Kligman A. The identification of contact allergies by human assay. *J Invest Dermatol* 1966;47:393.

229. Bruze M, Andersen K. Gold—a controversial sensitizer. *Contact Dermatitis* 1999;40:295–299.

230. Fisher AA. Metallic gold: the cause of persistent allergic "dermal" contact dermatitis. *Cutis* 1974;14:177.

231. Shelley WB, Epstein E. Contact-sensitivity to gold as a chronic papular-eruption. *Arch Dermatol* 1963;87:388.

232. Bowyer A. Epidermal reactions and prolonged dermal reactions to patch testing with gold salts. *Acta Derm Venereol* (Stockh) 1967;47:9.

233. Petros H, Macmillan AJ. Allergic contact sensitivity to gold with unusual features. *Br J Dermatol* 1973;88:505.

234. Suzuki H. Nickel and gold in skin lesions of pierced earlobes with contact dermatitis. *Arch Dermatol Res* 1998;290:523–527.

235. Kalimo K, Rasanen L, Aho H, et al. Persistent cutaneous pseudo lymphoma after intradermal gold injection. *J Cutan Pathol* 1996;23:328–334.

236. Fisher AA. Ear piercing hazard of nickel-gold sensitization. [Letter]. *JAMA* 1974;228:1226.

237. Malten KE, Mali J. Contact eczema due to gold. *Allergy Asthma* 1966;12:31.

238. Comaish S. A case of contact hypersensitivity to metallic gold. *Arch Dermatol* 1969;99:720.

239. Rytter M, Schubert H. Allergy due to a golden ring by primary epicutaneous sensitization. *Dermatologica* 1971;142:209.

240. Choy E, Gambling L, Best S, et al. Nickel contamination of gold salts: link with gold induced skin rash. *Br J Rheumatol* 1997;36:1054.

241. Möller H, Svensson A, Bjorkner B, et al. Contact allergy to gold and gold therapy in patients with rheumatoid arthritis. *Acta Derm Venereol* 1997;77:370–373.

242. Möller H, Bjorkner B, Bruze M. Clinical reactions to systemic provocation with gold sodium thiomalate in patients with contact allergy to gold. *Br J Dermatol* 1996;135:423–427.

243. Jeffrey D, Biggs D, Percy J, et al. Quantitation of gold in skin in chrysiasis. *J Rheumatol* 1975;2:28.

244. Miller M, Harford R, Yeager J, et al. A case of chrysiasis. *Cutis* 1997;59:256–258.

245. Russell M, Langley M, Truett A, et al. Lichenoid dermatitis after consumption of gold containing liquor. *J Am Acad Dermatol* 1997;36:841–844.

246. Nava C, Briatico Vangosa G. Allergy to gold salts. *Med Lavoro* (Milano) 1971;62:572.

247. Budden MG, Wilkinson DS. Skin and nail lesions from gold potassium cyanide. *Contact Dermatitis* 1978;4:172.

248. Marcussen J, Cederbrant K, Heilborn J. Indium and iridium allergy in patients exposed to dental alloys. *Contact Dermatitis* 1998;38:297–298.

249. Bergman A, Suedberg U, Nilsson E. Contact urticaria with anaphylactic reactions caused by occupational exposure to iridium salt. *Contact Dermatitis* 1995;32:14–17.

250. Hemmer W, Focke M, Wanke F, et al. Contact hypersensitivity to iron. *Contact Dermatitis* 1996;34:219–220.

251. Nater JP. Epidermal hypersensitivity to iron. *Hautarzt* 1960;11:223.

252. Baer R. Allergic contact sensitization to iron. *J Allergy Clin Immunol* 1973;51:35.

253. Zugerman C. Contact dermatitis to yellow iron oxide. *Contact Dermatitis* 1985;13:107–109.

254. Motolese A, et al. Contact dermatitis and contact sensitization among enamellers and decorators in the ceramics industry. *Contact Dermatitis* 1993;28:59.

255. Brehm G. Pigmentierung nach lokaler Anwendung von Eisenchloridlosung. *Akt Dermatol* 1976;3:117.

256. Jirasek L. Occupational exogenous siderosis of the skin. *Contact Dermatitis* 1979;5:334.

257. Fregert S. Allergic contact dermatitis from lead? *Contact Dermatitis Newsletter* 1973;13:352.

258. Czarnecki N, Fritsch P. Contact allergy to lead. *Hautarzt* 1978;29:445.

259. Allen BR, Hunter JAA, Beatties AD, Moore MR. Lead poisoning and blistering of the skin. *Scot Med* 1974;19:3.

260. Goncalo M, Figueiredo A, Goncalo S. Hypersensitivity to thimerosal: the sensitizing moiety. *Contact Dermatitis* 1996;34:201–203.

261. Sulzberger MB. *Dermatologic allergy*. Springfield, IL: Charles C Thomas Publisher, 1940.

262. Frykholm KO, Wahlgren F. A fatal case of mercurial dermatitis with complication. *Acta Derm Syph* 1964;44:362.

263. Miedler LH, Forbes JD. Allergic contact dermatitis due to metallic mercury. *Arch Environ Health* 1964;17:960.

264. Swinyer LJ. Allergic contact dermatitis from metallic mercury. *Contact Dermatitis* 1980;6:226.

265. Vermeiden I, Oranje AP, Vuzevski VD, Stolz E. Mercury exanthem as occupational dermatitis. *Contact Dermatitis* 1980;6:88.

266. Gerstner HB, Huff JE. Selected case histories and epidemiologic examples of human mercury poisoning. *Clin Toxicol* 1977;11:131.

267. Nakayama H, Niki F, Shono M, Hada S. Mercury exanthem. *Contact Dermatitis* 1983;9:411.

268. Zimmer J, Grange F, Straub P, et al. Mercury erythema after accidental exposure to mercury vapor. *Ann Med Interne Paris* 1997;148:317–320.

269. Andersen K, Hjorth N, Menné T. The baboon syndrome: systemically induced allergic contact dermatitis. *Contact Dermatitis* 1984;10:97–100.

270. Le-Coz CJ, Boos V, Cribier BJ, et al. An unusual case of mercurial baboon syndrome. *Contact Dermatitis* 1996;35:112.

271. Veron C, Hildebrand HF, Martin P. Amalgames dentaires et allergie. *J Biol Buccale* 1986;14:83.

272. Laine J, et al. Resolution of oral lichenoid lesions after replacement of amalgam restorations in patients allergic to mercury compounds. *Br J Dermatol* 1992;126:10.

273. Laine J, Kalimo K, Happonen RP. Contact allergy to dental restorative materials in patients with oral lichenoid lesions. *Contact Dermatitis* 1997;36:141–146.

274. Camisa C, Taylor JS, Bernat Jr, et al. Contact hypersensitivity to mercury in amalgam restorations may mimic oral lichen planus. *Cutis* 1999;63:189–192.

275. Koch P, Bahmer FA. Oral lichenoid lesions, mercury hypersensitivity and combined hypersensitivity to mercury and other metals: histologically proven reproduction of the reaction by patch testing with metal salts. *Contact Dermatitis* 1995;33:323–328.

276. Kanerva L, Lahtinen A, Toikkanen J, et al. Increase in occupational skin diseases of dental personnel. *Contact Dermatitis* 1999;40:104–108.

277. Koch P, Nickolaus G. Allergic contact dermatitis and mercury exanthem due to mercury chloride in plastic boots. *Contact Dermatitis* 1996;34:405–409.

278. Nakada T, Higo N, Iijima M, et al. Patch test materials for mercury allergic contact dermatitis. *Contact Dermatitis* 1997;36:237–239.

279. Handley J, et al. Mercury allergy in a contact dermatitis clinic in Northern Ireland. *Contact Dermatitis* 1993;29:258–261.

280. von Mayenburg J, Rakoski J, Szliska C. Patch testing with amalgam at various concentrations. *Contact Dermatitis* 1991;24:266.

281. Lhotka C, Szekeres T, Fritzer-Szekeres M, et al. Are allergic reactions to skin clips associated with delayed wound healing? *Am J of Surg* 1998;176:320–323.

282. *The romance of nickel.* New York: International Nickel Co, 1960.

283. Fisher AA. Nickel—the ubiquitous contact allergen—possible significance of its presence in food, water, urine, hair and infusion fluids. *Cutis* 1978;22:544.

284. Hogan D, et al. Results of routine patch testing of 542 patients in Saskatoon, Canada. *Contact Dermatitis* 1988;19:120.

285. Marks J, Belsito D, DeLeo V, et al. North American Contact Dermatitis Group patch test results for the detection of delayed-type hypersensitivity to topical allergens. *J Am Acad Dermatol* 1998;38: 911–918.

286. Lee T, Lam T. Patch testing of 490 patients in Hong Kong. *Contact Dermatitis* 1996;35:23–26.

287. Larsson-Stymne B, Windstrom L. Ear piercing—a cause of nickel allergy in school-girls. *Contact Dermatitis* 1985;13:289.

288. Christophersen J, et al. Clinical patch test data evaluated by multivariate analysis. *Contact Dermatitis* 1989;21:291.

289. Schubert H, et al. Epidemiology of nickel allergy: results of a follow-up analysis of patients with positive patch tests to nickel. *Contact Dermatitis* 1988;18:237.

290. Kanan MW. Contact dermatitis in Kuwait. *J Kwt Med Assoc* 1969;3:129.

291. Peltonen L. Nickel sensitivity in the general population. *Contact Dermatitis* 1979;5:27.

292. Nielsen GD, Soderberg U, Jorgensen PJ, et al. Absorption and retention of nickel from drinking water in relation to food intake and nickel sensitivity. *Toxicol Appl Pharmacol* 1999;154:67–75.

293. Murphy G, Rhea K, Peeler JT. Levels of copper, nickel, rubidium and strontium in institutional total diets. *Environ Sci Tech* 1973;7:1.

294. Flyvholm M-A, Nielson GD, Andersen A. Nickel content of food and estimation of dietary intake. *Z Lebensm Unters Forsch* 1984;179:427.

295. Horak E, Sunderman Jr EW. Fecal nickel excretion by healthy adults. *Clin Chem* 1973;19:429.

296. Fregert S. Nickel in tap water. *Contact Dermatitis Newsletter* 1971;9:202.

297. Kopp JF, Kramer RC. *Trace metals in waters in the United States.* Cincinnati: US Department of the Interior, Division of Pollution Surveillance, 1967.

298. McNeely MD, Neckay MW, Sunderman Jr EW. Measurements of nickel in serum and urine as indices of environmental exposure to nickel. *Clin Chem* 1972;18:992.

299. Fowler JF. Allergic contact dermatitis to metals. *Am J Contact Dermatitis* 1990;1:212.

300. Kaaber K, Veien NK, Tjell JC. Low nickel diet in the treatment of patients with chronic nickel dermatitis. *Br J Dermatol* 1978;98:197.

301. Sjovall P, Christensen OP, Möller H. Oral hyposensitization in nickel allergy. *J Am Acad Dermatol* 1987;17:774.

302. Veien NK. Systemically induced eczema in adults. *Acta Derm Venereol* (Suppl) 1989;69:147.

303. Fowler JF. Disulfiram is effective for nickel allergic hand eczema. *Am J Contact Dermatitis* 1992;3:175.

304. Katz SA, Samitz MH. Leaching of nickel from stainless steel consumer commodities. *Acta Derm Venereol* (Stockh) 1975;55:113.

305. Christensen, OB, Möller, H. Release of nickel from cooking utensils. *Contact Dermatitis* 1978;4:343.

306. Veien NK, Hattel T, Justesen O, Norholm A. Oral challenge with metal salts: 1. Vesicular patch-test-negative hand eczema. *Contact Dermatitis* 1983;9:402.

307. Veien NK, Hattel T, Justesen O, Norholm A. Oral challenge with metal salts: 2. Various types of eczema. *Contact Dermatitis* 1983;9:407.

308. Menné T, Mikkelsen HI, Solgaard P. Nickel excretion in urine after oral administration. *Contact Dermatitis* 1978;4:106.

309. Spruit JC, Bongaarts PFM. Nickel content of plasma, urine and hair in contact dermatitis. *Dermatologica* 1977;154:291.

310. DeJongh GH, Spruit D. Factors influencing nickel dermatitis: II. *Contact Dermatitis* 1978;4:149.

311. McNeely MD, Sunderman Jr EW, Nechay MW, et al. Abnormal concentrations of nickel in serum in cases of myocardial infarction, stroke, burns, hepatic cirrhosis, and uremia. *Clin Chem* 1971;17:1123.

312. Spruit D. Increased nickel absorption following Indomethacin therapy. *Contact Dermatitis* 1979;5:62.

313. Katz SA, Bowen HJM, Comaish JS, et al. Tissue nickel levels and nickel dermatitis. *Br J Dermatol* 1975;92:187.

314. Menné T, Rasmussen K. Regulation of nickel exposure in Denmark. *Contact Dermatitis* 1990;23:57.

315. Stoddart JC. Nickel sensitivity as a cause of infusion reactions. *Lancet* 1960;2:741.

316. Smeenk G, Teunissen PC. Allergic reactions to nickel from infusion equipment. *Ned Tijdschr Geneeskd* 1977;121:4.

317. Calnan CD. Nickel sensitivity in women. *Arch Allerg Appl Immunol* 1957;11:73.

318. Epstein S. Epidermal and dermal reactions in a case of sensitivity to nickel. *J Invest Dermatol* 1962;38:37, 1962.

319. Fisher AA. Nickel dermatitis. *Cutis* 1967;1:298.

320. Nielsen N, Menné T, Kristiansen J, et al. Effects of repeated skin exposure to low nickel concentrations: a model for allergic contact dermatitis to nickel in the hands. *Br J of Derm* 1999;141:676–682.

321. Christensen OB. Prognosis in nickel allergy and hand eczema. *Contact Dermatitis* 1982;8:7.

322. Fisher AA. Problems attending patch testing for nickel sensitivity. *Cutis* 1982;29:148.

323. Wahlberg JE. Petrolatum—a reliable vehicle for metal allergens? *Contact Dermatitis* 1980;6:134.

324. Van Ketel WG. Petrolatum. *Contact Dermatitis* 1981;7:60

325. Van Ketel WG. Patch testing with nickel sulphate in DMSO. *Contact Dermatitis* 1978;4:167.

326. Van Ketel WG. Petrolatum again: an adequate vehicle in cases of metal allergy? *Contact Dermatitis* 1979;5:192.

327. Wall LM, Calnan CD. Occupational nickel dermatitis in the electroforming industry. *Contact Dermatitis* 1980;6:414.

328. Cronin E. Patch testing with nickel. *Contact Dermatitis* 1975;1:56.

329. Dooms-Goossens A, Naert C, Chrispeels MI, et al. Is a 5 percent nickel sulphate patch test concentration adequate? *Contact Dermatitis* 1980;6:232.

330. Emmett EA, et al. Allergic contact dermatitis to nickel: bioavailability from consumer products and provocation threshold. *J Am Acad Dermatol* 1988;19:314.

331. Fisher AA. The dimethylglyoxime test in the prevention and management of nickel dermatitis. *Cutis* 1990;46:467.

332. Fleigel F. *Qualitative analysis by spot test,* 3rd ed. New York: Elsevier, 1946.

333. Lucas JB. Common industrial dermatoses. *Cutis* 1974;13:533.

334. Rystedt I, Fischer T. Relationship between nickel and cobalt sensitization in hard metal workers. *Contact Dermatitis* 1983;9:195.

335. Boss A, Menné T. Nickel sensitization from ear piercing. *Contact Dermatitis* 1982;8:211.

336. Kerosuo H, Kullaa A, Kerosuo E, et al. Nickel allergy in adolescents in relation to orthodontic treatment and piercing of ears. *Am J Orthod Dentofacial Orthop* 1996;109:148–154.

337. Brandrup F, Larsen FS. Nickel dermatitis provoked by buttons in blue jeans. *Contact Dermatitis* 1979;5:148.

338. Larsen ES, Brandrup F. Nickel release from metallic buttons in blue jeans. *Contact Dermatitis* 1980;6:298.

339. Goh CL, Ng SK, Kwok SF. Allergic contact dermatitis from nickel in eyeshadow. *Contact Dermatitis* 1989;20:380.

340. LaChapelle JM, Tennstedt D. An anatomo-clinical study of delayed skin allergic reactions to nickel following intradermal injections of lidocaine with a Dermo-Jet. *Contact Dermatitis* 1982;8:193.

341. LaChapelle JM, Tennstedt D, Lauwerys R, et al. Release of nickel into fluids stored in the reservoir of Dermo-Jets. *Contact Dermatitis* 1982;8:122.

342. de Correst LF, Garrastazu MT, Soloeta R, Escayol P. Nickel contact dermatitis in a blood bank. *Contact Dermatitis* 1982;8:32.

343. Shah M, Lewis FM, Gawkrodger DJ. Nickel as an occupational allergen: a survey of 368 nickel sensitive subjects. *Arch Dermatol* 1998;134:1231–1236.

344. Wahlberg JE. Nickel allergy and atopy in hairdressers. *Contact Dermatitis* 1975;1:161.

345. Dahlquist I, Fregert S, Gruvberger B. Release of nickel from plated utensils in permanent wave liquids. *Contact Dermatitis* 1979;5:52.

346. Hegyi E, Gaspařík J. The nickel content of moulded bricks as building material. *Contact Dermatitis* 1989;21:63.

347. Raith L, Jaeger K. The nickel content of chalk-cause of dermatitis? *Contact Dermatitis* 1986;14:61.

348. Zanca A, et al. The release of nickel from blackboard chalk may cause contact dermatitis. *Contact Dermatitis* 1988;19:143.

349. Widstrîm L, Bergstrôm B, Wennerholm C. Nickel allergy and wrist strap to dissipate static electricity. *Contact Dermatitis* 1986;15:299.

350. Hanks JW, Venters WJ. Nickel allergy from a bed-wetting alarm confused with herpes genitalis and child abuse. *Pediatrics* 1992;90:458.

351. Lacroix J, Morin CL, Collin P-P. Nickel dermatitis from a foreign body in the stomach. *J Pediatr* 1979;95:428.

352. Lyell A, Bain WH, Thomson RM. Repeated failure of nickel-containing prosthetic heart valves in a patient allergic to nickel. *Lancet* 1978;2:658.

353. Menné T, Kaaber K. Treatment of pompholyx due to nickel allergy with chelating agents. *Contact Dermatitis* 1978;4:289.

354. Christensen OB, Kristensen M. Treatment with disulfiram in chronic hand nickel dermatitis. *Contact Dermatitis* 1979;4:221.

355. Kaaber K, Menné T, Hougaard P. Treatment of nickel dermatitis with Antabuse: double blind study. *Contact Dermatitis* 1983;9:297.

356. Kristensen ME. Toxic hepatitis induced by disulfiram in a non-alcoholic. *Acta Med Scand* 1981;209:335.

357. Burrows D, et al. Treatment of nickel dermatitis with Trientene. *Contact Dermatitis* 1986;15:55.

358. Healy J, Johnson S, Little MC, et al. An in vitro study of the use of chelating agents in cleaning nickel contaminated skin: an alternative approach to preventing nickel allergic contact dermatitis. *Contact Dermatitis* 1998;39:171–181.

358A.Warin RP. Chronic urticaria. *Contact Dermatitis* 1982;8:117.

359. McConnell LH, Fink JN, Schlueter DP, et al. Asthma caused by nickel sensitivity. *Ann Intern Med* 1973;78:888.

360. Block GT, Yeung M. Asthma induced by nickel. *JAMA* 1982;247:1600.

361. Espana A, et al. Chronic urticaria after implantation of 2 nickel-containing dental prostheses in a nickel-allergic patient. *Contact Dermatitis* 1989;21:204.

362. Fernandez-Redondo V, Gomez-Centeno P, Toribio J. Chronic urticaria from a dental bridge. *Contact Dermatitis* 1998;38:178–179.

363. Hjorth N. Nickel vasculitis. *Contact Dermatitis* 1976;2:356.

364. Cook LJ. Associated nickel and cobalt contact dermatitis presenting as erythema multiforme. *Contact Dermatitis* 1982;8:280.

365. Wall LM. Nickel penetration through rubber gloves. *Contact Dermatitis* 1980;6:461.

366. Wilkinson DS, Hambly EM. Nickel spot testing at home. *Contact Dermatitis* 1978;4:114.

367. Campbell KI, et al. Dermal irritancy of metal compounds. *Arch Environ Health* 1975;30:168.

368. Munro-Ashman D, Munro DD, Hughes TH. Contact dermatitis from palladium. *Trans St John Hosp Derm Soc* 1969;55:196.

369. Sheard Jr C. Contact dermatitis from platinum and related metals: report of case. *Arch Dermatol* 1955;71:357.

370. Camarasa JG, et al. Palladium contact sensitivity. *Contact Dermatitis* 1991;24:370.

371. Aberer W, et al. Palladium in dental alloys—the dermatologists' responsibility to warn? *Contact Dermatitis* 1993;28:163.

372. Koch P, Baum H. Contact stomatitis due to palladium and platinum in dental alloys. *Contact Dermatitis* 1996;34:253–257.

373. Dodd DJ, Burrows D. Patch testing with pure palladium metal in patients with sensitivity to palladium chloride. *Contact Dermatitis* 1992;26:327.

374. DeFine Olivarius F, Menné T. Contact dermatitis from metallic palladium in patients reacting to palladium chloride. *Contact Dermatitis* 1992;27:71.

375. Wahlberg JE, Boman A. Palladium chloride—a potent sensitizer in the guinea pig. *Am J Contact Dermatitis* 1990;1:112.

376. Marshall J. Toxicity of platinum. *S Afr Med J* 1952;26:8.

377. Roberts AE. Platinosis. *Arch Industr Hyg* 1951;4:549.

378. Levene GM. Platinum sensitivity. *Br J Dermatol* 1971;85:590.

379. Roberts AE. Platinosis. A five-year study of the effects of soluble platinum salts on employees in a platinum laboratory and refinery. *AMA Arch Industr Hyg Occup Med* 1951;4:549.

380. Baker DB, et al. Cross-sectional study of platinum salts sensitization among precious metals refinery workers. *Am J Indus Med* 1990;18:653.

381. Freedman SO, Krupey J. Respiratory allergy caused by platinum salts. *J Allergy* 1968;42:233.

382. Levene GM, Calnan CD. Platinum hypersensitivity: treatment by specific hyposensitization. *Clin Allergy* 1971;1:75.

383. Schuppe H, Kir G, Lerchenmuller C, et al. Contact hypersensitivity to disodium hexachloroplatinate in mice. *Toxicol Lett* 1997;93:125–133.

384. de la Cuadra J. Occupational contact dermatitis from rhodium and cobalt. *Contact Dermatitis* 1991;25:182.

385. Bodello P. Contact dermatitis to rhodium. *Contact Dermatitis* 1987;17:111.

386. Cameli N, et al. Contact dermatitis from rubidium iodide in eyedrops. *Contact Dermatitis* 1990;23:377.

387. Gaul LE. Incidence of sensitivity to chromium, nickel, gold, silver and copper compared to reactions to their aqueous salts including cobalt sulphate. *Ann Allergy* 1954;12:429.

388. Marcussen PV. Eczematous allergy to metals. *Acta Allergolog* 1962;17:311.

389. Gaul LE, Underwood GB. The effects of aging a solution of silver nitrate on its cutaneous reaction. *J Invest Dermatol* 1948;11:7.

390. Marshall JP, Schneider RP. Systemic argyria secondary to topical silver nitrate. *Arch Dermatol* 1977;113:1077.

391. Buckley WR. Localized argyria. *Arch Dermatol* 1963;88:531.

392. Gettler AO, Rhoads CP, Weiss S. A contribution to the pathology of generalized argyria with a discussion of the fate of silver in the human body. *Am J Pathol* 1927;3:631.

393. Gaul LE, Staud AH. Clinical spectroscopy. *JAMA* 1935;104:1387.

394. Criep LH. Allergy to argyrol. *JAMA* 1943;121:421.

395. Heyl T. Contact dermatitis from silver coat. *Contact Dermatitis* 1979;5:197.

396. White IR, Rycroft RJG. Contact dermatitis from silver fulminate itch. *Contact Dermatitis* 1982;8:159.

397. Marks R. Contact dermatitis due to silver. Case report. *Br J Dermatol* 1966;78:606.

398. Menné T, Andersen K, Kaaber K, et al. Tin: an overlooked sensitizer. *Contact Dermatitis* 1987;16:9.

399. De Fine-Olivarius F, et al. Skin reactivity to tin chloride and metallic tin. *Contact Dermatitis* 1993;29:110.

400. Nielsen N, Skov L. Occupational allergic contact dermatitis in a patient with a positive patch test to tin. *Contact Dermatitis* 1998;39:97–100.

401. Goh C. Irritant dermatitis from tri-n-butyl tin oxide in paint. *Contact Dermatitis* 1985;12:161.

402. Viraben R, Boulinguez S, Alba C. Granulomatous dermatitis after implantation of a titanium containing pacemaker. *Contact Dermatitis* 1995;33:437.

403. Verbov J. Pacemaker contact sensitivity. *Contact Dermatitis* 1985;12:173.

404. Brun R, Hunziker N. Pacemaker dermatitis. *Contact Dermatitis* 1980;6:212–213.

405. Abdallah HI, Balsara RK, O'Riordan AC. Pacemaker contact sensitivity: clinical recognition and management. *Ann Thorac Surg* 1994;57:1017–1018.

406. Peters MS, Schroeter AL, van Hale HM, et al. Pacemaker contact sensitivity. *Contact Dermatitis* 1984;11:214–218.

407. Rueda M, Pons-Guirard AQ. Allergie au pacemaker. *Nouv Dermatol* 1994;13:183–187.

408. Holgers K, et al. Clinical, immunological, and bacteriological evaluation of adverse reactions to skin-penetrating titanium implants in the head and neck region. *Contact Dermatitis* 1992;27:1.

409. Dujardin F, Fevrier V, Lecorvaisier C, et al. Allergic dermatitis caused by metallic implants in orthopedic surgery. *Rev Chir Orthop Reparatrice Appar Mot* 1995;81:473–474.

410. Tan M, Suzuki H. Usefulness of titanium implants for systemic contact dermatitis due to orthopaedic prostheses. *Contact Dermatitis* 1995;33:202.

411. Calnan CD. Metal fume fever. *Contact Dermatitis* 1979;5:124.

412. Schwartz L, Tullipan L, Birmingham DS. *Occupational diseases of the skin,* 3rd ed. Philadelphia: Lea & Febiger, 1957.

413. Koizumi H, et al. Acupuncture needle dermatitis. *Contact Dermatitis* 1989;21:352.

414. Yates YM, Finn OA. Contact allergic sensitivity dermatitis and actinic reticuloid syndrome. *Contact Dermatitis* 1980;6:349.

415. Muston HL, Messenger AG, Byrne JPH. Contact dermatitis from zinc pyrithione, an antidandruff agent. *Contact Dermatitis* 1979;5:276.

416. Calnan CD. In: Fisher AA, ed. Highlights of the first international symposium on contact dermatitis. *Cutis* 1976;18:645.

417. Calnan CD. Occupational piperazine dermatitis. *Contact Dermatitis* 1975;1:126.

418. Nielsen N, Menné T. Allergic contact dermatitis caused by zinc pyrithione associated with pustular psoriasis. *Amer J of Contact Derm* 1997;8:170–171.

419. Galindo P, Garrido J, Gomez E, et al. Zinc acexamate allergy. *Contact Dermatitis* 1998;38:301–302.

420. Feinglos MN, Jegasothy BV. Insulin allergy due to zinc. *Lancet* 1979;1:122.

421. Palmer L, Welton W. Lupus miliaris disseminatus faciei: zirconium hypersensitivity as possible cause. *Cutis* 1967;7:74.

422. Rublin L. Granulomas of axillae caused by deodorants. *JAMA* 1956;162:953.

423. Shelley WB, et al. Intradermal tests with metals and other inorganic elements in sarcoidosis and anthraco-silicosis. *J Invest Dermatol* 1958;31:301.

424. Williams RM, Skipworth GB. Zirconium granulomas of glabrous skin following treatment of rhus dermatitis. *AMA Arch Dermatol* 1959;80:273.

425. Epstein WL, Allen JR. Granulomatous hypersensitivity after use of zirconium-containing poison oak lotions. *JAMA* 1964;190:162.

426. Baler GR. Granulomas from topical zirconium in poison ivy dermatitis. *Arch Dermatol* 1965;91:145.

427. Shelley WB, Hurley HJ. Allergic origin of zirconium deodorant granulomas. *Br J Dermatol* 1958;70:75.

428. LoPresti PJ, Hambril GW. Zirconium granuloma following treatment of rhus dermatitis. *Arch Dermatol* 1965;92:188.

429. Costa C, Hunziker, N. Occupational dermatitis due to sodium hypophosphite. *Contact Dermatitis* 1988;19:313.

430. Payero M, et al. Contact urticaria and dermatitis from phosphorus sesquisulphide. *Contact Dermatitis* 1985;13:126.

431. Glover JR. Some medical problems concerning selenium in industry. *Trans Assoc Industr Med Officers* 1954;4:94.

432. Jirasek L, Kalensky J. Hypersensitivity to platinum, rhodium, gold, copper, antimony and other precious metals and occupational dermatitis caused by selenium. *Cesk Dermatol* 1975;50:361.

433. Senff H, et al. Allergic Contact dermatitis from selenite. *Contact Dermatitis* 1988;19:73.

434. Shelley WB, Hurley HJ. The pathogenesis of silica granulomas in man: a non-allergic colloidal phenomenon. *J Invest Dermatol* 1960;34:107.

435. Mason J, Apisarnthanarax P. Migratory silicone granuloma. *Arch Dermatol* 1981;117:366.

436. Raque C, Goldschmidt H. Dermatitis associated with an implanted cardiac pacemaker. *Arch Dermatol* 1970;102:647.

437. Elmer K, George R. Contact urticaria to the MCV-2A/P gas mask. *Mil-Med* 1996;164:377–378.

438. Blackadder ES, Manderson WG. Occupational absorption of tellurium: a report of two cases. *Br J Industr Med* 1975;32:59.

439. Thiers MM, Chanial G, Rivoire J, Muller F. Dermites professionnelles par sensibilisation aux urantes de sodium et de calcium. *Arch Des Malades Professionelles Méd Travail Soc* 1961;22:168.

CHAPTER 36

Contact Stomatitis and Cheilitis

The oral mucosa, like the skin, is subject to two types of local reactions—primary irritation and allergic sensitization. In general, the mucosa is more resistant to primary irritants and is not as readily sensitized as is the skin, possibly because the keratin layer of the skin may contain proteins that more readily combine with simple chemicals to form allergens (1).

The oral mucosa is constantly bathed in saliva, which washes food particles, debris, irritants, and sensitizers from the mucosal surface. Saliva also plays a considerable role in digestion through the action of enzymes, such as amylase and maltase. Saliva may solubilize allergens. In addition, saliva may contain yeasts, which can modify the clinical picture of the stomatitis.

> **Mucosal reactions to contractants are modified by the presence of saliva, which cleanses, buffers, and contains yeasts, and by the abundant vascularity of the oral mucosa as compared to the skin.**

CLINICAL PICTURE OF CONTACT STOMATITIS AND CHEILITIS

Often the subjective symptoms of contact stomatitis are more prominent than the physical signs. Patients may complain of loss of taste, numbness, a burning sensation, and pain in the involved area. Itching is not a usual symptom.

The appearance of the mucous membrane varies from a barely visible, mild erythema to a fiery red color with or without edema. Lingual papillae may disappear. In the presence of considerable edema, the mucosa takes on a smooth, waxy, glazed appearance. Vesiculation of the oral mucosa is rarely seen, because vesicles rupture quickly to form erosions. Erosions may be seen with allergy but also with primary immunobullous disease such as pemphigus, pemphigoid, or lupus erythematosus. Vitamin deficiency and various infections are included in the differential diagnosis of stomatitis. Oral lichen planus may be idiopathic or allergic in nature.

In allergic reactions to denture base material, there is often a sharp line between the red, inflamed mucosa covered by the denture and the adjacent uninvolved area. The irritation of an ill-fitting plate may, however, give an appearance identical to that of allergic denture stomatitis. Similarly, allergic stomatitis from metal or acrylics used in dental implants or crowns often shows a sharp border just around the treated teeth. However, occasional cases of allergic stomatitis may not have localized lesions. Some cases of diffuse stomatitis or burning mouth syndrome without lesions may be due to allergy.

> **Allergic contact stomatitis may mimic the oral changes of a vitamin deficiency. Loss of taste, numbness, and burning sensations rather than itching are prominent symptoms.**

Allergic stomatitis is often accompanied by cheilitis. The usual picture of allergic cheilitis, whether secondary to stomatitis or caused by contactants applied directly to the lips, is one of dryness, scaliness, fissuring, and angular cheilitis. Edema and vesiculation of the lips are rarely present. Itching may be prominent. A riboflavin deficiency syndrome may be simulated.

In contrast to the distinct disease "perioral dermatitis," allergic cheilitis usually does not have a "grenz zone" of normal skin immediately adjacent to the vermilion border. Perioral dermatitis is more akin to acne than dermatitis, although it may have features of both.

Primary Irritation of the Oral Mucosa by Heat and Chemicals

Irritation Due to Heat

The oral mucosa can usually withstand excessively hot liquids and spicy foods with little or no evidence of irritation. The ingestion of hot liquids or hot foods, such as melted cheese in grilled cheese sandwiches and pizzas, however, may sometimes inflict severe, painful thermal burns with

TABLE 36.1. *Causes of Irritant Stomatitis*

Heat	Nicotine
Chemicals	Uremia
Aspirin	
Denture cleaners	
Solvents	
Acids, alkalis	

the formation of vesicles or bullae, particularly on the palate, tongue, and lips. The patient may treat such burns by sucking on ice chips or by applying ice-cold glycerin to the affected areas. If pain persists, a topical anesthetic such as lidocaine (Xylocaine, Viscous) may then be applied to painful sites. Table 36.1 lists some causes of irritant stomatitis.

Stomatitis Due to Chemical Injury

A common cause of chemical injury is repeated placement of aspirin tablets against a painful tooth. Prolonged contact of acetyl-salicyclic acid with the oral mucosa often results in superficial ulceration. Chewing gum containing aspirin may also produce oral ulceration (2,3). Jolly (4) stated that the majority of chemical burns of the oral mucosa are produced by aspirin intentionally held in the mouth. The patient treats a toothache (unwisely) by packing an aspirin-based analgesic around the tooth and holding it in the mouth as long as possible. Although aspirin has no local anesthetic properties, it does have a strong caustic action on oral mucosa and can rapidly cause complete separation and sloughing of the epithelium.

The prolonged use of undiluted perborate or hydrogen peroxide may also produce painful, superficial erosions of the oral mucosa.

The most severe injury from chemicals occurs in individuals who swallow lye for suicidal purposes and in young children who accidentally ingest household caustics and acids. Such strong chemicals may cause severe necrosis and sloughing of the mucosa. In addition, caustic chemicals such as phenol, silver nitrate, and nitric acid may be accidentally placed against the mucosa during dental procedures.

If the patient can be treated immediately after exposure to a strong chemical, the affected mucosa should be rinsed liberally with cold water and the chemical should be neutralized. Alkalis are neutralized by weak acetic acid or vinegar, acids by a solution of bicarbonate of soda, and phenol by alcohol.

Caustic Burns of Mouth and Throat Caused by Denture Cleaners

Denture cleaners come in powder, pill, and cream form. Abramson (5) wrote that after having been soaked in a warm solution of a denture cleaner, "store teeth" should be rinsed thoroughly before being put back into the wearer's mouth. Cleaner and mouth were never intended to meet.

Several children who chewed or swallowed denture cleaners have suffered severe mouth and throat burns. Most active ingredients in the cleaners are acid, alkali, or oxygenating compounds, or a combination. Abramson (5) pointed out that studies indicate that alkalis are particularly destructive to esophageal tissue because they penetrate deep into tissue layers by liquefaction necrosis; acid burns are less destructive because they produce coagulation necrosis that blocks deeper penetration.

Denture wearers and those who soak "bite plates" overnight in these cleaners may acquire irritant stomatitis if the cleaners are not rinsed off thoroughly before dentures and bite plates are inserted into the mouth.

Stomatitis Due to Shohl's Solution

Necrotic and ulcerative lesions of the oral mucous membranes may be produced in patients receiving a solution of 9.8% sodium citrate and 14% citric acid (Shohl's solution) orally to alleviate metabolic acidosis. The lesions are due to a direct primary irritant effect of the solution. Shohl's solution should be diluted when used by patients who have difficulty swallowing or poor oral hygiene. Water, fruit juices, or a carbonated beverage may be used as a diluent. Effective treatment consists of discontinuing the use of Shohl's solution and employing hydrogen peroxide and antibiotic suspension as mouthwashes.

Stomatitis Nicotina

Prolonged smoking may produce distinct umbilicated papules on the palate (6). The lesions arise from the ducts of the salivary glands and not from the glands themselves.

Reddy et al. (7) reported that 550 people with nicotine stomatitis (a precancerous lesion) and a control group of 2,850 were surveyed with respect to their smoking and other habits. The most important factor in the development of this type of stomatitis is reverse smoking of homemade *chuttas*. Other methods of smoking produce lesions less frequently and in a milder form. Women have more chance of developing stomatitis than men because many form a habit of smoking only the reverse way, whereas most men smoke either the ordinary way or the reverse way and so have less chance of developing lesions.

> **Aspirin tablets, chewing gum, hot foods, caustics, perborate, peroxides, and antienzymes in dentifrices may produce irritation and erosions of the oral mucosa.**

Trauma

Prolonged, low-grade irritation and trauma of the oral mucosa from jagged teeth or ill-fitting dentures may lead to erosions, keratinization, leukoplakia, and malignant degeneration. Traumatic ulcers can be caused by tooth brushing or by chronic irritation from jagged teeth, rough dental restorations, and ill-fitting dentures. These ulcers are usually shallow, surrounded by an erythematous margin, and variable in shape; an ulcer in the buccal sulcus resulting from denture pressure tends to be linear. Removal of the cause of trauma should result in healing of the ulcer.

Any traumatic ulcer that persists for longer than 2 weeks should be biopsied to exclude malignant change.

Cotton Roll Stomatitis

"Cotton roll stomatitis" is a complication of oral surgery. The saliva-absorbing cotton roll strips off tissue when it is removed, causing a superficial ulceration.

> **Superficial ulcerations of the mouth can occur from hot pizza (pizza palate) and the use of cotton roll strips in oral surgery.**

"White" Lesions of the Mouth Caused by Chemicals

A variety of chemicals may accidentally burn the mouth, such as gasoline siphoned from a car, pipetted caustic agents, or chemicals inadvertently applied during dental treatment. A mild irritant may simply produce local inflammation, but a strong caustic will cause tissue necrosis that appears clinically as white lesions (4).

Uremic Stomatitis

Uremia may cause stomatitis (8). Six of 10 patients reported died within 10 months of the onset of stomatitis. It was postulated that in these patients the stomatitis was a chemical burn caused by the action of bacterial urease on the salivary urea with subsequent liberation of ammonia.

> **The breakdown of salivary urea into ammonia is said to be the cause of uremic stomatitis.**

Ulcerative Stomatitis in Infants

Oral ulcerations in newborns and infants are commonly due to infectious diseases such as herpes simplex. Coxsackie virus (hand-foot-mouth disease), and moniliasis. Physical or thermal trauma may also produce oral lesions. Mennie et al. (9) reported a case of oral ulcers in a 17-day-old baby apparently due to direct irritation from contact with a solution of 18% sodium chloride with hypochlorous acid that the mother used to "disinfect" her breasts.

Hyperkeratrophic or Hyperplastic Stomatitis

In sensitized individuals, nickel, chrome, cobalt, and other metals in dental appliances may produce hypertrophic and leukoplakia-like lesions at the sites of contact. Individuals who use snuff or chew tobacco may develop diffuse hyperplasia of the oral mucosa, which at times may mimic papillomas or verrucae. A viral cause has been attributed to focal epithelial hyperplasia, which is characterized by multiple painless, soft papules and nodules of the oral mucosa having the same color as the adjacent normal mucosa. These lesions are of variable size and shape and usually cause no discomfort.

ALLERGIC CONTACT STOMATITIS

Allergic contact stomatitis occurs less frequently than allergic contact dermatitis, probably because of the following factors.

1. With the exception of dental appliances, the period of contact of sensitizers with the buccal mucous membranes is brief.
2. Saliva dilutes and removes potential allergens and may buffer and neutralize chemicals.
3. The anatomical structure of the buccal mucosa, with its extensive vascularization, aids in rapid dispersion and absorption of the allergen, thereby preventing prolonged contact of the allergen with the mucosa.

When the skin is the original surface sensitized, the mucous membrane may or may not be involved on a clinical level. However, when the mucous membrane is first sensitized, the skin is usually involved. For example, sensitization to an ingredient in a dentifrice may produce allergic stomatitis, cheilitis, and circumoral dermatitis upon exposure to the allergen (Table 36.2).

Lowney (10) showed that a series of applications of dinitrochlorobenzene to the buccal mucosa induces a mild contact sensitivity in some subjects and not in others. Virtually all subjects then were refractory to subsequent attempts to induce sensitivity or raise the level of sensitivity previously induced. This finding, that partial tolerance to dinitrochlorobenzene can be induced by buccal administration of the compound, may become of importance if this technique works with other chemicals.

TABLE 36.2. *Causes of Allergic Stomatitis*

Foods and flavors: balsam of Peru, cinnamon and derivatives, menthol, peppermint, etc.
Preservatives and components of dentifrices: parabens, prolylene glycol, formo-cresol, etc.
Dental materials: metals, acrylics, other plastics and resins, eugenol, etc.

Although allergic contact sensitivity is usually generalized, affecting the skin and oral mucosa simultaneously, experiments with dinitrochlorobenzene indicate that sensitization by way of the buccal mucosa may increase skin tolerance.

Flavorings, a Common Cause of Allergic Stomatitis and Cheilitis

Cinnamon flavorings, particularly cinnamic aldehyde, are probably the most frequent cause of allergic stomatitis from dentrifices and foods. On patch testing, a positive result to balsam of Peru, used as a screening allergen, suggests that these flavorings should be avoided in the appropriate clinical setting.

Three patients developed an allergic cheilitis and stomatitis from the use of toothpaste containing cinnamic aldehyde. One patient experienced a flare-up of the condition after she added cinnamon to her coffee as a flavoring agent. Patch tests with 1% cinnamic aldehyde gave strongly positive reactions in the three patients.

Drake and Maibach (11) described a patient who had acute stomatitis and dermatitis from a popular toothpaste containing cinnamon oil flavor. Magnusson and Wilkinson (12) studied 16 patients for whom patch tests gave positive results who developed "oral" symptoms from a newly formulated "spicy" toothpaste containing cinnamic aldehyde. Kirton and Wilkinson (13) reported five additional cases of toothpaste cheilitis and stomatitis caused by cinnamic aldehyde. Table 36.3 lists some toothpastes that do not contain cinnamic aldehyde (13).

Another report linked cinnamon-containing or cinnamon-flavored oral preparations with red or white oral mucosal plaques and lichenoid oral lesions (14). Histology revealed hyperkeratosis and a lichenoid infiltrate with many plasma cells.

Cinnamic aldehyde in dentrifices may produce irritant, stinging sensations and allergic cheilitis, stomatitis, and lichenoid lesions.

TABLE 36.3. *Toothpastes Not Containing Cinnamic Aldehyde*

Aim
Arm and Hammer Dental Care Tartar Control
Crest Tartar Protection Smooth Mint Gel
Crest Cavity Protection Icy Mint Stripe
Crest Gum Care
Crest Multi Care
Mentadent
Pepsodent
Ultrabrite Whitening

A report from Korea indicates that a product called Eundan used as a breath freshener and smoking deterrent may cause allergic and/or irritant stomatitis. One herb, *Tinula helenium,* was shown to be a direct irritant. Another component, *Glycyrrhiza uralensis,* apparently acted as an allergen (15).

Essential Oils

In dentistry, essential oils are chiefly used as pharmaceutical aids, as mild antiseptics and anodynes, and as flavoring for dentrifices and mouthwashes. Several of these oils can produce allergic stomatitis and cheilitis.

The essential oils, particularly clove oil and cinnamon oil, may cross-react with balsam of Peru, which is used in dental cement liquids. In addition, these oils may cross-react with benzoin, rosin, vanilla, and the essential oils of orange peel (16,17).

An orange peel may be used externally for the removal of zinc oxide-eugenol cements. Orange peel may cross-react with balsam of Peru, celery, bergamot, caraway, dill, and lemon turpentine.

Anise oil is used as a flavoring agent, especially to disguise substances of disagreeable taste.

Cinnamon oil (cassia oil) is a very weak antiseptic. In dentistry, it is used primarily as a flavoring agent. Oil of cinnamon has further been identified as the cause of allergic cheilitis and stomatitis from toothpaste (18), bubble gum, and lipstick. Ingestion of oil of cinnamon in dry vermouth may provoke a flare-up of preexisting allergic contact dermatitis in sensitized individuals (19). Cross-sensitization to balsam of Peru may result from primary sensitivity to oil of cinnamon.

Many irritants and allergens in medicaments, dentrifices, cosmetics, foods, and metallic objects may produce cheilitis, which may mimic vitamin B deficiency syndrome or candidiasis.

Menthol, USP

Menthol is used as a flavoring agent, as a component of zinc oxide-eugenol cements, and as a mint flavoring and cooling agent in toothpastes and mouthwashes, cough drops, candy, chewing gum, food, cigarettes, liqueurs, and mixed drinks (20). Papa and Shelley (21) described dermatitis, cheilitis, and stomatitis from methol.

Morton et al. (22) presented data on 12 patients with oral symptoms and allergy to methanol and/or peppermint. Five patients had burning mouth syndrome, four had oral ulcers, and three had oral lichen planus. Patch tests were positive to menthol (5% pet), peppermint oil (1% pet), or both. In six of nine that could be contacted later complete or significant clearing occurred with allergen avoidance. One other patient cleared with removal of a mercury filling.

Eugenol

This is the main constituent of clove oil, oil of carnation, pimento oil, and oil of bay. In dentistry, eugenol is used in periodontal dressings, zinc oxide cement, and impression pastes.

Goransson et al. (23) observed three cases of eugenol hypersensitivity. In one, a eugenol impression paste produced allergic cheilitis and stomatitis. In the other two, an allergic eczematous reaction was produced from handling eugenol. Koch et al. (24) showed that eugenol is a potent sensitizer.

A case of a 10-year-old girl allergic to eugenol in chewing gum has been reported (25). She had no oral lesions but only a circumoral dermatitis. Her chewing gum was shown to contain eugenol. In addition to eugenol, she was positive to isoeugenol, balsam of Peru, and fragrance mix.

Eugenol may cross-react with balsam of Peru, diethylstilbestrol, and benzoin.

> **Eugenol, the main ingredient in clove oil, is used in periodontal dressings, zinc oxide cement, and impression pastes, and may readily sensitize the mucous membrane and skin.**

Allergic Stomatitis and Lichen Planus Caused by Metals

A wide variety of metals have been used by dentists and oral surgeons for fillings and prostheses, including aluminum, antimony, beryllium, chromium, cobalt, copper, gold, indium iridium, mercury, nickel, osmium, palladium, platinum, rhodium, ruthenium, silicon, silver, tin, and tungsten. Of these metals used in dentistry, mercury and gold have most commonly been implicated as a producer of allergic reactions (26), including lichen planus (LP). All dental amalgams contain mercury and in addition may contain copper, silver, tin, and other metals. According to the number of metals they contain, amalgams are classified as binary, tertiary, quaternary, and so forth (27). Metal dentures containing chromium, nickel, and other metals may produce dermatitis, stomatitis, and LP, or lichenoid oral lesions (28).

Mercury

Probably the most common contact with mercury in the general population occurs from mercury amalgam dental fillings. The possibility of toxicity from dental mercury is currently a popular topic for debate. Essentially there are questions relating to putative mercury sensitivity: (a) Can dental mercury cause oral lesions, including lichenoid lesions? (b) Can dental mercury cause cutaneous urticaria, dermatitis, or LP in sensitive individuals? and (c) Can den-

tal mercury cause nonspecific systemic complaints such as fatigue, malaise, and headache?

Generally, older reports suggested that mercury is unlikely to cause oral lesions, whereas virtually all recent literature implicates mercury (and other metals) as possible causes of stomatitis and LP.

Gaul (29) reported on three patients with mercury dermatitis in whom epidermal sensitivity to mercury was demonstrated. In all three patients, however, silver amalgam dental fillings, containing approximately 50% metallic mercury, produced no irritation within the mouth. Epstein (30) stated that the contact antigen formed with mercury is given specificity for the epidermis by protein conjugates characteristic of, or present only in, the epidermis, and that mercury sensitivity does not extend to the oral mucosa.

> **Silver amalgam fillings contain metallic mercury, which can produce generalized dermatitis or localized erosions in mercury-sensitive individuals.**

However, Fernstreom et al. (31) stated that patients who had previously been sensitized to mercury and had acquired a mercury dermatitis subsequently developed a stomatitis and a flare-up of the dermatitis when mercury amalgam fillings were used. These patients had a prompt remission when their mercury amalgam fillings were removed. Such flare-ups were attributed to mercury vapor, which is liberated by the amalgam fillings, both when the amalgam is being prepared and during insertion into the cavity. The authors consider the amount liberated from the filling after treatment to be negligible in comparison to the amount liberated while the filling is being inserted.

Juhlin and Ohman (32) found that erosions of the oral mucosa occurred adjacent to amalgam fillings in mercury-sensitive individuals.

Nordlind and Liden (33) found that 5 of 12 patients with oral lesions adjacent to amalgam reacted to mercury in the form of mercuric chloride 0.1% aq. Several reacted to other metals, including copper, gold, and palladium. In contrast, only 1 of 11 patients with oral lesions not related to amalgam reacted to mercuric chloride. The authors believed that the reactions were significant and that $HgCl_2$ (0.1% pet) should be tested in all patients with oral lesions.

Oral lichen planus may also be induced by metal allergy. In one study, 11 of 67 patients with oral LP reacted to mercury and/or a mercury salt (34). Seven reacted to nickel. Because the metal was not removed from the patients, no definite clinical correlation could be made.

Koch and Bahmer (35) presented what is probably the largest and most definitive study to date with extensive patch testing of 19 patients with oral LP adjacent to fillings, 42 with oral LP not anatomically related to fillings, 28 with other oral diseases, 46 with burning mouth syndrome, and 59 controls with no oral symptoms or pathology. Fifteen of the 19 in the first group were positive to inorganic mercury, sometimes with positive reactions only developing after 10 to 17 days. Thirteen of these 15 had total or significant clearing after removal of the dental mercury. Mercury was positive in only 7 of the other 116 patients, suggesting that other oral lesions or symptoms are less likely to be related to dental metals. Gold allergy was found in 17 patients, and in 2 the gold was removed with lesional resolution. Palladium was positive in 19 patients and 8 controls with uncertain relevance. Biopsies from patch test reactions frequently showed lichenoid histology.

Cutaneous Reactions to Dental Mercury

Johnson et al. (36) found that the removal of mercury amalgam fillings cleared recalcitrant eczemas in mercury-sensitive individuals. Sidi and Casalis (37) described mercury-sensitive patients with chronic eczema that persisted until amalgam fillings were removed. Vickers (38) reported on a mercury-sensitive individual who developed a widespread, eczematous eruption, starting 24 to 48 hours after a mercury amalgam filling had been inserted. No oral lesions were described. Vickers speculated that the generalized dermatitis was due to mercury dropped on the mucosal surface of the mouth during the dental operation.

Spilled mercury may be picked up with a clean, shiny piece of copper. Hair sprays may be used to "immobilize" and then remove mercury in other inaccessible regions.

Spector (39) described a patient in whom there was a sudden appearance of extensive edema and urticaria involving the neck, face, and upper part of the back following installation of an amalgam filling. This reaction recurred on two occasions when the patient underwent dental treatment with silver amalgam. The eruption persisted for 7 to 10 days, then disappeared spontaneously without removal of the filling.

Spector performed patch tests with minute portions of the silver alloy alone, the mercury alone, and a combination of both. The patient had a negative patch test reaction to the silver alloy alone. When the mercury alone was used, the patient developed severe local erythema at the test site, with vesiculation, edema, and urticarial reactions on the elbows and neck. A similar reaction was noted when the combination of both was used. Spector concluded that this was a rare instance of mercury sensitivity manifested by urticaria, edema, and a vesiculation.

Thomson and Russel (40) described a patient who, on several occasions after mercury amalgam dental restorations, developed first an urticarial and then an eczematous eruption on her face, trunk, and extremities. Her history revealed that she had previously developed an eczematous eruption on the lower part of the abdomen and thighs and a vaginitis from the use of a contraceptive jelly containing a phenylmercuric salt. Patch tests were positive to 0.1% mercuric-chloride and silver amalgam. The dermatitis on each occasion lasted 10 to 14 days, then subsided, although the mercury amalgam fillings were not removed.

It may be justifiable to replace silver amalgam filling in mercury-sensitive individuals with non-metallic or gold fillings if they suffer from persistent urticaria or a generalized eczematous dermatitis.

Frykholm (41) tried to determine whether exposure to mercury in amalgam restorations can be deleterious to health. First, he tried to measure the amount of mercury that escaped from the amalgam and the amount that was absorbed. Second, he endeavored to measure the quantity of mercury excreted in the urine and feces.

Frykholm found that the average amount of mercury per millimeter of respired air in 30 minutes of treatment was 0.02 mg to 0.4 mg but that the upper values occurred only if copper amalgam was used. If the fillings were coated with saliva, the amount of vapor evolved was instantly reduced. His experiments on the solubility of mercury amalgam fillings in saliva and gastric juice showed that the freshly triturated amalgam was only slightly soluble. The amount of mercury reaching the circulation appeared to be insignificant. He concluded that amalgam restoration treatment exposes the patients to a small quantity of mercury mainly during insertion and that reports of reactions after amalgam restorations, even in mercury-sensitive persons, are uncommon, and the few cases reported usually involved a history of allergic contact to mercury.

In the cases discussed above, the usual time of onset of eczema or urticaria in mercury-sensitive patients is a few hours after an amalgam filling has been inserted. The eruption usually persists for 10 to 14 days, which fits well into Frykholm's work on mercury liberation after amalgam insertion.

The answers to the questions posed above would, at this time with current information, seem to be as follows. Mercury and other metal may produce oral lesions, including lichen planus–like lesions, at sites of mucosal contact. Generalized skin reactions and lesions elsewhere in the mouth are uncommonly related to dental metals but may occur.

Patch testing with mercury and its salts is somewhat tricky because irritant reactions may occur. Von Mayenburg et al. (42) found that 13 of 27 patients with reactions to mercury salts also reacted to 20% amalgam in pet. The amalgam contained 51% mercury, 34% silver, with the remainder being tin, zinc, and copper. Ten of the 13 reacted down to 5% amalgam in pet. The authors suggested using a 5% or 10% concentration for testing. It should be remembered that mercury may react with aluminum in Finn chambers. Whether this is of clinical significance is unknown. If desired, plastic chambers may be used instead.

Mercury toxicity with noncutaneous constitutional symptoms has not been documented scientifically. Patch testing with mercury of a patient with nonspecific symptoms without oral or cutaneous findings may be unreliable and lead to invalid conclusion due to the frequency of irritant and allergic reactions. However, patch testing in patients with unexplained oral LP is definitely indicated.

Nickel

Foussereau and Laugier (43) cited a case of generalized eczema that occurred after a chromium-nickel denture had been fitted. Skin tests were strongly positive to nickel and chromium, and the dermatitis subsided after the denture was removed. No mention is made of oral reactions. In most instances in which an allergic reaction is attributed to a metallic chrome object, the nickel content is the actual sensitizer. Nickel readily penetrates the micropores in chrome-plated objects.

Van Loon et al. (44) showed that nickel in the mouth can produce allergic stomatitis in patients who exhibit positive nickel patch tests. Five such patients had a small nickel plate glued to a tooth for 7 days. All five patients developed stomatitis at the site, which showed histologic features of an allergic reaction on biopsy.

Allergic contact stomatitis and cheilitis can occur from nickel-plated instruments used in dental procedures (45). Many nickel-sensitive individuals have acquired allergic stomatitis and cheilitis by holding between the lips nickel-plated objects, such as needles, pins, bobby pins, and metal lipstick holders (46). Perlèche may be clearly simulated in nickel-sensitive individuals who hold nickel-plated coins, keys, and other objects at the corners of their mouths. One patient developed erosions of the gums resembling aphthous ulcers from holding metal bobby pins between the teeth (47).

Copper

Allergic sensitivity to this metal is rare. Saltzer and Wilson (48) reported on a case of allergic contact dermatitis caused by copper. Frykholm et al. (28) reported that allergy to copper derived from dental alloys may produce oral lesions of lichen planus.

Another report showed 2 of 12 patients with lichenoid stomatitis reacted to copper sulfate 5% aq, as did 1 of 36 controls (33). Testing with 1% concentration of copper sulfate would be less likely to give a false-positive result.

Gold

Elgart and Higdon (49) described a case of allergic sensitivity to gold in which the gingival mucosa sloughed from contact with a gold crown and sites of previous gold contact dermatitis to jewelry flared. The cutaneous lesions subsided when the crown was removed.

Gold is becoming recognized as a more common allergen than was previously appreciated.

Marcusson (50) tested 397 patients presenting to a patch test clinic with oral symptoms that were not specified in his report. The complaints, however, seemed to be temporally related to dental work. Twenty-three percent were positive to gold, a much higher rate than the 4% to 9% seen in most patch testing centers. Twenty-two percent were allergic to nickel, which is somewhat more than expected. Cobalt and chromate allergies were also slightly overrepresented.

Schaffran et al. (51) pointed out that individuals with gold dental work and no oral symptoms at all are often patch test positive to gold. Of those with gold in the mouth, 34% were positive, whereas only 11% without dental gold were positive.

The mere fact of having gold dental work, therefore, seems to predispose to gold allergy even in the absence of clinical symptoms.

Chrome-Cobalt Combination

Brendlinger and Tarsitano (52) described a woman with severe dermatitis and allergic reactions to several metals who recovered only after removal of a cast chrome-cobalt partial denture. Replacement with an all-acrylic resin partial denture was satisfactory.

Chrome-cobalt pins used to fasten porcelain teeth to acrylic dentures may produce stomatitis in individuals sensitized to cobalt. In a case observed by Fisher, such pins produced an extensive stomatitis and cheilitis in a cobalt-nickel-sensitized individual. The reaction occurred after the acrylic portion of the denture had worn away, exposing the pins. When the pins were covered with self-curing acrylic resin, the stomatitis cleared.

Ovrutsky and Ulyanov (53) and Moffa et al. (54) reported generalized and eczematous reactions from such chromium-containing dental casting alloys.

Platinum and Palladium

Sheard (55) stated that both metallic platinum and its salts are potent allergens and that the reactions to dentists' platinum wiring may be allergic.

Palladium is becoming well recognized as an allergen usually in combination with nickel sensitivity (56). It is used in dental alloys and therefore may be expected to cause stomatitis occasionally. However, three patients with a positive patch test to palladium chloride (2.5% aq) did not show any reactions to a palladium metal plate placed in the mouth for 7 days (44). Perhaps a longer duration of exposure is needed for the palladium ions to be released, or perhaps the patch tests were irritant false-positives.

A case of linear facial LP with a "peculiar sensation" in the mouth was caused by allergy to palladium. Patch tests were positive to both palladium and platinum. Removal of the palladium-containing dental work resulted in total resolution of symptoms (57). A case of combined palladium and platinum allergy causing lichenoid stomatitis was reported from Germany (58).

Beryllium

Beryllium has also been reported to cause two cases of allergic stomatitis (59). The alloy rexillium was used in making dental prostheses.

Because of the rising cost of gold, a number of base metal alloys are being substituted. Two major types of base metal alloys are available: a high nickel type (70% to 84% Ni) and a nickel-free type based in cobalt and chromium. Some of these alloys contain beryllium.

> **Because of high cost of gold alloys, nickel, cobalt, chromium, and beryllium are being substituted.**

Allergic and Irritant Stomatitis from Other Dental Materials

Corticosteroids

Allergy to topical corticosteroids is becoming recognized. Tixocortal pivalate is a good patch test marker for steroid hypersensitivity. In a report from Switzerland, three women were allergic to tixocortal in a nasal spray, and one also had stomatitis from an oral lozenge containing the drug (60).

Dental Impression Compounds

These preparations may contain stearin, stearic acid, paraffin wax, beeswax, and gutta-percha with synthetic or natural resins, such as shellac copak (kauri), coumarone-indene resins, and fillers. Of these ingredients, the resin is most likely to cause sensitization stomatitis.

Some of the fluxes contain borax, boric acid, silica, and potassium fluoride. Most fluxes are strong irritants. Waxes such as paraffin, beeswax, carnauba, candelilla, and petrolatum are used by dentists.

Several types of plaster containing mineral gypsum, potassium sulfate, potash alum, and alizarin S are used.

Van Groeningen and Nater (61) reported that of approximately 2,000 persons treated with Scutan, an epimine plastic for temporary crowns and bridges, and Impregum, a polyether impression material, a total of 10 patients complained of untoward reactions. Patch tests with the basic materials were performed on 4 of the 10 patients. Positive allergic reactions were obtained to patch tests with the catalyst methyl-*p*-toluene sulfonate 0.1% in dibenzyltoluol

present in Scutan, and the catalyst methyldichlorobenzene sulfonate 0.1% in dibenzyltoluol present in Impregum. Four control subjects did not react to these concentrations.

Scutan, the temporary dental splint material, contains no monomers and is not an acrylic derivative. Impregum is an impression rubber material used for the construction of inlays, crowns, and bridges. It is usually in contact with the oral mucosa for only a short period.

Resinous Substances Used in Dentistry

Allergic contact dermatitis and urticaria from dental resin-based products are considered rare (62). However, it is difficult to assess which materials are present in a patient's mouth. Very little is known about how components released from dental restorations act as sensitizers or cause dermatologic sequelae in presensitized individuals.

Balsam of Peru

Balsamic resin of plant origin, composed principally of resin and cinnamic and benzoic acid esters, is a component of some cement liquids.

Copal

This substance consists of mixed resins of plant origin and is a constituent of some cavity varnishes. This resin should not be confused with Copalite, which is a synthetic resin.

Mastic

This substance is composed principally of masticinic acid and used in some cavity varnishes.

> **Rosin (colophony) and other resinous substances used in dental cement, liquids, and cavity varnishes may cross-react with perfume and other odoriferous substances.**

Rosin

Also called colophony, rosin is an ingredient of many mixtures used for sealing pulp canals. Rosin in chloroform solution has been used as a varnish for pulp protection in deep cavities. It has been added to zinc oxide or to eugenol as an ingredient of pulp capping preparations, surgical packs, impression pastes, and other preparations (63).

Resins, Epoxy, and Acrylate

Hensten-Pettersen (64) reported that, over the last 15 years, more than 100 similar new brands of resin-based cold-curing materials have been introduced. Resin-based unfilled and composite materials, pit and fissure sealants, orthodontic adhesives, glazes, veneers and repair kits for porcelain-fused-to-metal restorations, root canal sealers, and temporary crowns are today used in a large segment of the population and occasionally cause allergy.

Depending on the composition, the polymerization is induced by chemical agents or ultraviolet or visible light sources. The materials are based on monomers of different types: methacrylate monomers and urethane-based-dimethacrylates, epoxybispheno resins, and ethylene-amino derivatives.

> **Modern bonding adhesive materials may contain acrylic monomers and epoxy resins and hardeners that may cause allergic reactions.**

In addition, the chemicals involved in the polymerization processes are present: benzoyl peroxide, hydroquinone, camphoroquinone, phthalates, tertiary aromatic and aliphatic amines, benzoin ethers, ultraviolet stabilizers, and antioxidants and their derivatives (65). Even though the materials set to a hard state in the oral environment, the amount of residual unreacted endgroups of dimethyl acrylates may vary from 15% to 50%, leading to a slow release of degradation products such as formaldehyde (66).

One case of oral lichen planus documented by biopsy was thought to be caused by resin that was exposed to the mucosa from a broken denture (63). Removal of the material cleared the eruption.

In the United States, bis-GMA (2,2 bis(4(2-hydroxy-3 methacryloxypyloxy)phenyl-)-propane is the chemical generally used for most bonding. "Bis" stands for the epoxy resin bisphenol A, which reacts with glycidyl methacrylate. The plastic is generally combined with quartz, lithium aluminum silicate, glass, or silicon dioxide to modify the physical properties of the resin. The size of these particles is generally 0.04 μ to 40.0 μ (BF Bollack, D.D.S., Director, Dental Materials Research, Mt. Sinai Medical Center, New York, NY, personal communication).

Davidson et al. (67) reported on the basis of animal testing that tissue reactions may occur from dental bonding adhesives and that reactions may occur in the patient, the operator, and office personnel.

For orthodontists and patients who are allergic to the usual bonding material, General Orthodontic Lab, 659 Eagle Rock Avenue, West Orange, NJ 07052, manufactures Contacto, in which the hydroxy group replaces epoxy and acrylic acid replaces acrylic monomer.

Thompson et al. (68) studied the unpolymerized material extracted from cured orthodontic bonding resin, which was analyzed by ultraviolet spectrophotometry. Under certain conditions, substantial amounts of the material (approximately 14%) were leached from bracketed teeth (68). Significant amounts of unpolymerized material remaining in cured orthodontic bonding resins can be readily leached out by various aqueous solutions, such as saliva, water, soda water, and ethanol solutions. Resin monomers are not leached from cured specimens by aqueous solutions containing citrate. The ultraviolet spectra of the material extracted by various test solutions demonstrated that ethenol and dimethyl sulfoxide preferentially extracted material that absorbed light in the range of 265 nm to 280 nm.

> **Saliva, water, soda water, and alcohol can leach out any unpolymerized material remaining in "cured" orthodontic bonding resins.**

Acrylic Denture Materials

Most dentures today are processed from acrylic resins that are heat cured. Self-curing acrylics that harden without heat are available for repairing and relining. Heat-cured acrylic dentures rarely cause allergic reactions (69).

The acrylic monomer usually contains an inhibitor or stabilizer, such as hydroquinone, and the polymer, an initiator, such as benzoyl peroxide or dimethyl-*p*-toluidine (or a tertiary amine). When the monomer and polymer are mixed in the cold, the benzoyl peroxide initiates the reaction and a hard, solid, high-molecular-weight polymer is produced. The mixture can also be heat cured, when no initiator is required. In the heat process the reaction is essentially complete, but after cold cure it is likely that very small amounts of the monomer will be left unpolymerized. This residual monomer is capable of inducing stomatitis and angular cheilitis in sensitized individuals.

Certain additives in acrylic denture material may also be sensitizers. Thus, hydroquinone, the inhibitor in the monomer, may be the sensitizer rather than the acrylic monomer itself. Benzoxyl peroxide may account for some instances of methacrylate sensitivity.

Crissey (70) cited four instances in which hypersensitivity stomatitis venenata resulted from heat-cured acrylic dentures. The onset of symptoms followed fitting of the acrylic dentures by periods varying from 1 week to 4 years. These cases had the following features in common: (a) the clinical picture of stomatitis venenata, including angular stomatitis; (b) relief of symptoms when the dentures were removed, and subsequent flare-up on reinsertion; (c) positive patch test reactions (cheek) to filings from the heat-cured acrylic prostheses and the acrylic monomer; and (d) negative patch test reactions to polystyrene denture material.

In a report from India, two patients with oral lesions reacted to triethyleneglycol dimethacrylate (71).

Acrylic dentures may also contain plasticizers (dibutyl or dimethyl phthalate), pigments (mercuric sulfate, ferric oxide, carbon black, and selenium compounds), and cross-linking agents (glycol dimethyl acrylate and divinyl benzene) to prevent crazing, and an inhibitor, such as hydroquinone.

Tosti et al. (72) reported one case of contact stomatitis in a 62-year-old woman traced to N,N'-dimethyl-para-toluidine used as an accelerator for the acrylic reaction.

Hydroquinone, used to stabilize acrylic monomer, caused cheilitis and stomatitis in one patient who was also allergic to several metals (73). Van Joost et al. (74) reported four denture reactors. One person reacted to methyl methacrylate, one to bisphenol A, and two to a product called Lurene, in which the allergen was not identified.

Patients often complain of a burning sensation for several hours after first use of an acrylic denture that has been relined or repaired. Such complaints may be related to the presence of solvents such as ethyl or amyl acetate, diethyl carbonate, and glycerol triacetate.

Nonallergic Causes of Denture Stomatitis

Inflammation of the mucous membrane beneath artificial dentures is often referred to as "denture-sore mouth." The oral mucosa of the palate and the maxillary edentulous alveolar ridges are the most common sites of involvement. The tissue beneath the denture may appear bright red and edematous, and the patient may complain of soreness, rawness, dryness, and burning sensations in the area in contact with the denture. Occasionally perlèche may be the only sign of denture stomatitis. Usually these reactions are irritant in nature due to poor-fitting dentures or trapped food particles (75).

Wakkers-Garritsen et al. (76) stated that it is remarkable that the denture-sore mouth (DSM) syndrome appears to occur mainly in women patients. In their group of 24 persons, 19 were women. The DSM complaints generally started between ages 40 and 60 years; the mean age was 49 years. In most cases, complaints commenced with the first prosthesis. Using other prostheses from different materials made no appreciable difference; in one case, seven successive dentures were made of different compounds without any real improvement.

These data, combined with the fact that in 12 of 24 cases complaints started within 1 hour of mucosal contact, indicate the nonallergic cause of the complaints. This is supported by the negative results of the patch test reactions. Mechanical factors are difficult to assess. In many cases, however, patients stated that the fitting of their dentures was correct, a fact that was confirmed by functional analysis. Evidence of heat accumulation beneath the dental plates in patients complaining of DSM could not be detected. Finally, the investigators could not confirm the suggested causal role of *Candida albicans* or related yeasts.

These investigators had an impression that all patients included in this investigation were very tense and nervous. Further studies to elicit these psychologic factors are necessary.

> The "denture-sore-mouth" syndrome occurs principally in women; no cause has as yet been discovered. Many patients have tried half a dozen dentures of different materials without relief of symptoms.

The Dry Mouth Syndrome

Klein (77) stated that "dry mouth syndrome" is one of the most prevalent complaints after age 65. This is one of the factors contributing to the increase in dental caries, inability to wear dentures, burning sensation in the mouth, and decreased sensitivity of the taste buds of many individuals in this age group. The source of this problem is diminution of salivary flow caused by acinar destruction and hyalinization, adhesions and obstructions with atrophy of salivary ducts, and infection or disease within the stoma of the glands themselves. Not every individual develops this condition, and many aged patients have adequate salivary flow well into the 80s or even beyond. Sjogren's syndrome, tumors of the salivary glands, and diabetes may also cause dry mouth syndrome.

Traumatic Suction Effect of Ill-Fitting Dentures

Nonallergic denture-sore mouth caused by trauma is quite common. Traumatic denture-sore mouth produces an erythematous, "cluster of grapes" appearance owing to a suction effect produced by the rocking back and forth of ill-fitting dentures. When a denture is constructed, a depression is created in this area to prevent "denture rock." This depression causes a suction effect that may produce papillary hyperplasia, which may be a precancerous lesion. To prevent this condition, it is strongly recommended that all denture patients leave their dentures out overnight.

The Role of Candidiasis in Denture Stomatitis

Jolly (4) stated that denture stomatitis may be caused by oral candidiasis and, like acute atrophic candidiasis, is a red rather than a white lesion. It occurs as a uniform or patchy atrophic erythematous lesion, almost exclusively limited to the palate of denture wearers. It is usually, but not always, seen under dirty dentures that are worn 24 hours a day. It is generally described as sore or burning rather than painful and occurs more commonly in women than men.

Two predisposing factors stand out:

1. The space between denture and palate can be regarded as an ideal culture chamber.
2. The denture acts in the manner of an occlusive dressing, keeping any organisms on its surface in close contact with the mucosa.

Taaffe and Rigott (78) found that *Candida* occurred more commonly in the oral mucosa of denture-wearing patients than in the control subjects. There was no evidence of increased prevalence of *Candida* at other mucocutaneous sites, and the amount of *Candida* recovered from the stools did not suggest involvement at other sites in the alimentary system. Countercurrent immunoelectrophoresis did not produce indirect serologic evidence of a heavy *Candida* antigen load. Lymphocyte transformation with phytohemagglutinin and migration inhibition on challenge with tubercle and *Candida* antigen was normal in all cases. Apart from mechanical or hygienic factors, it seems unlikely that these patients have a predisposition to become targets for *Candida* infection. The demonstration of increased debris (measured gravimetrically) on the dentures of the patient group suggests that *Candida* may be more important as an opportunist infection than as the primary initiating factor.

A large proportion of patients with this condition also have angular cheilitis (perlèche), similarly infected with *C. albicans*. The dentures are often implicated in that their shape and dimensions allow deep creasing or folding at the angles of the mouth. These creases are continually wet because they form a capillary channel between the inside of the mouth and the facial skin.

Treatment involves soaking the dentures in antifungal solution at night, and perhaps construction of new dentures. Oral Nystatin suspensions or troches containing clotrimazole are also helpful. Systemic agents such as fluconazole may be quite useful as well.

> **Oral candidiasis is a frequent complication of ill-fitting dentures, which promote accumulation of food debris under the denture. These patients usually do not have monilia infections elsewhere in the body.**

Antiseptics and Preservatives in Oral Medications and Foods

Certain antiseptics that are added to dentifrices, mouthwashes, and topical oral medications and anesthetics to retard or prevent microbial growth have been shown to be sensitizers. Such chemicals include parahydroxybenzoic acid (parabens), dichlorophene (G-4), hexachlorophene (G-11), phenylmercuric nitrate, Merthiolate, ethylenediamine hydrochloride, the quaternary ammonium compounds, benzoic gum, and benzyl benzoate.

Parabens

Parabens (parahydroxybenzoate) are bacteriostatic, fungistatic, and antioxidant in their action and are widely employed as preservatives (see Chapter 17).

The US Food and Drug Administration requires that the labels on foods and topical prescription drugs indicate the presence of parabens. This requirement does not apply to oral preparations and dentifrices. Sensitive patients may therefore find it difficult to avoid contact with these agents. Elimination of paraben-containing dentifrices or cosmetics is a difficult problem, because there is no law to impel a manufacturer of toothpastes, for example, to indicate the presence of preservatives in his product.

Parabens in dentifrices may produce cheilitis and circumoral dermatitis. Fortunately, even paraben-sensitive individuals usually tolerate paraben-containing oral medications, provided the mucosa is intact.

Dichlorophene (G-4) and Hexachlorophene (G-11)

Dichlorophene in dentifrices has caused many instances of allergic cheilitis. Patients have become sensitized to this preservative and have developed stomatitis with a cherry-red tongue and loss of taste and numbness. The lips become dry and scaly, and fissuring at the corners of the mouth suggests vitamin B deficiency. Hexachlorophene, in contrast, has almost never produced allergic sensitivity.

Formaldehyde

This chemical, present in Thermodent dentifrice and in desensitizing agents and used in root canal therapy as Formo-Cresol, may produce allergic stomatitis. Fowler has seen a case of hand eczema in a dental office worker due to Formo-Cresol (J. Fowler, Louisville, KY, 1998).

Sodium Perborate

This oxidizing agent is an occasional sensitizer. In the United States, sodium perborate sensitivity is rare. Sodium perborate is present in Kleenite, a denture cleansing preparation.

Quaternary Ammonium Compounds

The members of this chemical family, which includes benzalkonium chloride (Zephiran) and benzethonium chloride (Phemerol), are rare sensitizers, but may produce irritant reactions.

Merthiolate and Phenylmercuric Nitrate

Merthiolate contains not only a mercurial component but also thiosalicylic acid. Allergic stomatitis and cheilitis may occur in sensitized individuals. Mercury in dental fillings is more often a cause of stomatitis.

Gallates

The gallates (octyl, propyl, and lauryl or dodecyl) are used as preservatives in foods and cosmetics, especially ones containing fats or oils. Cheilitis and stomatitis occasionally have been reported to these agents (79). In one case, a 6-year-old boy had recurrent lip swelling for 1 year due to lauryl gallate in margarine (80).

BHA

Butylated hydroxyanisole (BHA) caused lip swelling in a woman (81). Food challenge test was positive.

Ethylenediamine Hydrochloride

This stabilizer, present in Mycolog Cream, has produced many instances of allergic cheilitis and circumoral dermatitis. Flare-ups of the cheilitis may be produced by the administration of aminophyllin, which contains ethylene diamine hydrochloride as one of its ingredients. In addition, flare-ups may be produced by the administration of such antihistamines as Pyribenzamine and Antistine, which are ethylenediamine derivatives (see Chapter 17).

Antiseptics Used in Dental Surgery

Maurice et al. (81) reported severe allergic contact stomatitis and dermatitis around the mouth from iodoform in a ribbon gauze known as BIPP used in packing a dental socket. Systemic iodine toxicity has occurred using this gauze in large cavities, but apparently no other allergic reactions to it have been noted.

The sensitizing and irritant phenolic compounds used in root canal work and periapical infections include creosote and the parachlorophenols. Thymol and hexylresorcinol may produce cross-reactions with resorcin.

Merk et al. (82) reported allergic contact stomatitis from hexetidine in a gargle.

Penicillin

The topical use of penicillin is now being avoided. Contact sensitivity has been widely reported after use of topical oral penicillin preparations, such as troches. Penicillin may still occasionally be used with streptomycin and other antibiotics in the local treatment of infected pulp canals. Severe anaphylactoid reactions have occurred in penicillin-sensitive individuals after the endodontic use of a paste containing penicillin, bacitracin, dihydrostreptomycin, and sodium caprylate (83).

Tetracyclines

Undesirable oral mucosal reactions have been noted from the use of lozenges containing tetracycline, and patients being treated systemically and topically with this antibiotic may develop a transitory yellowish brown discoloration of the tongue, which is not allergic in nature.

Allergic mucosal reaction to antibiotic-containing lozenges may be due to the antibiotic or coloring or flavoring agents. In one case of stomatitis caused by Aureomycin troches, the allergic reaction was due to sensitization to a certified yellow dye in the preparation.

Eczematous eruptions of the fixed type do occasionally result from systemic administration of tetracyclines (84). Furthermore, cross-fixed drug reactions from systemic use of Aureomycin, Achromycin, and Terramycin have been described (85). Such reactions may produce erosions of the mouth and lips.

> "Fixed" drug eruptions caused by tetracycline may appear on the lips and buccal mucosa, simulating aphthous ulcers or herpes.

Reactions to Lozenges and Troches

These preparations may contain antibiotics, quaternary ammonium compounds, local anesthetics (particularly benzocaine), hexylresorcinol, iodine compounds, or tyrothricin. Allergic reactions to antibiotic-containing lozenges may be due to the antibiotic or to the coloring or flavoring agents.

When an oral topical medication is suspected of producing allergic contact stomatitis, testing must be performed with all the individual ingredients in the preparation, regardless of whether they are active or inert. Inert flavoring and coloring agents and preservatives are just as important causes of allergic contact stomatitis and cheilitis as are the active antiseptic or anesthetic chemicals present in the lozenges and troches.

> Antiseptics, antibiotics, anesthetics, flavoring agents (essential oils), certified dyes in dentifrices, and topical dental medication may produce stomatitis and cheilitis.

Surface or Topical Anesthetics as Mucosal Sensitizers with Special Reference to Benzocaine

Benzocaine, a common sensitizer, continues to be used in many topical anesthetic compounds.

Table 36.4 lists some topical oral preparations that contain benzocaine. Such preparations are often used as mouthwash or gargle in the treatment of aphthous stomatitis, "teething pains," herpes simplex, denture irritation, trench mouth, cheilosis, avitaminosis, thrush, gingivitis, and throat irritations.

TABLE 36.4. *Some Oral Topical Medications Containing Benzocaine*

Benzocaine ointment with oil of cloves
Benzodent
Noval-Benzocaine-Tetracaine solution
Topical anesthetic liquid, ointment, and spray
Cepacol anesthetic troches
Orabase with benzocaine analgesic oral protective paste
Dalidyne
Anbesol
Dental Poultice (Dent)
Dent's Toothache Gum
Gum-20R
Kank-A-Viscous Liquid
Numzit
OraJel
Rid-A-Pain Gel
Tamac Liquid, Solid, Roll-On
Toothache Drops (Dewitt)

Inhalation of topical benzocaine aerosol sprays in benzocaine-sensitive individuals may produce marked edema of the mouth and larynx with resulting respiratory distress and syncope.

The topical administration of anesthetic aerosol sprays can produce in benzocaine-sensitive individuals a shocklike syndrome. Lidocaine (Xylocaine), mepivacaine (Carbocaine), or dyclonine hydrochloride (Dyclone) usually can be safely substituted in benzocaine-sensitive patients when surface anesthesia is required.

Benzocaine-sensitive patients may show cross-reactions with the following injectable local anesthetics that are derived from para-aminobenzoic acid: procaine (Novocain), butethamine (Monocaine), tetracaine (Pontocaine), and propoxycaine (Ravocaine). Metabutethamine (Unacaine), which is based on meta-aminobenzoic acid, meprylcaine (Oracaine), and isobucaine (Kincaine), which is based on benzoic acid, may also cause cross-reactions with benzocaine.

The injection of these local anesthetics into benzocaine-sensitive individuals may lead to localized swelling of the oral mucosa at the site of injection. On rare occasions, generalized urticaria or anaphylaxis will result from the injection of procaine into benzocaine-sensitive patients.

The following injectable local anesthetics rarely cross-react with benzocaine and, because they are based on an "amide" structure, should be used in benzocaine-sensitive patients or in those who are sensitive to local anesthetics derived from esters of para-aminobenzoic acid, meta-aminobenzoic acid, or benzoic acid: lidocaine (Xylocaine), mepivacaine (Carbocaine), prilocaine (Citanest), and pyrrocaine (Dynacaine). Patch testing with the individual allergens should be performed, however, even though cross-reactivity is rare.

It should be emphasized that patch tests with local anesthetics do not reveal the immediate, urticarial, or anaphylactic type of reaction. Scratch, intradermal, or nasal testing may be helpful in this regard.

Avoid use of procaine- (Novocaine-) type anesthesia in benzocaine-sensitive individuals. "Amide" injectables such as Xylocaine (lidocaine) usually can be used safely.

Ingredients of Dentifrices and Mouthwashes

In 1995, Sainio and Kanerva (86) published a list of 48 toothpastes then on the Finnish market, many of which are also available in the United States. About 50% contained one or more allergens, such as peppermint oil, parabens, other flavors, and other preservatives.

Most powder and paste dentifrices contain flavoring, coloring agents (certified dyes), abrasives, and soaps or synthetic detergents, particularly "foaming" alkyl sulfates or sarcosinates. In addition, toothpastes may contain glycerine, propylene glycol, sorbital solution, alcohol, and thickeners, such as tragacanth, alginate, carrageen (Irish moss), and cellulose derivatives. Some dentifrices include antiseptics, preservatives, fluorides, and ammonium compounds. Saccharin and the cyclamates may be added (87,88) (Table 36.5).

Mouthwashes are medicated liquids used for cleansing the mouth for therapeutic or cosmetic purposes and, like dentifrices, may contain alcohol, flavorings, antiseptics, and preservatives (Table 36.6).

The alkyl sulfates, sarcosinates, and sulfonates are synthetic "foaming" detergents. So-called antienzyme dentifrices may contain these surfactants, which are claimed to prevent transformation of sugar to acid in the oral cavity. These surface-active agents very rarely produce allergic reactions.

TABLE 36.5. *Some Popular Dentifrices and Their Active Ingredients*

Gleem—calcium pyrophosphate
Colgate (with MFP)—sodium monofluorophosphate, sodium-N-alkyl sarcosinate
Crest—sodium fluoride, sodium alkyl sulfate, sodium monoglyceride sulfonate
MacLeans—sodium alkyl sulfate, magnesium, aluminum silicate, calcium carbonate
Pepsodent—sodium alkyl sulfate, titanium dioxide
Pycopay Tooth Powder—sodium chloride and sodium bicarbonate as abrasives
Sensodyne—strontium chloride
Ultrabrite—sodium alkyl sulfate, sodium-N-alkyl-sarcosinate, titanium dioxide

TABLE 36.6. *Some Widely Used Mouthwashes and Their "Active" Ingredients*

Act—sodium fluoride, cetylpyridinium chloride (propylene glycol)
Astringosol—zinc chloride, fluid extract of myrrh
Cepacol—cetylpyridinium chloride
Cepastat—phenol, eugenol, menthol
Chloraseptic—menthol, phenol
Fluorigard—sodium fluoride
Forma-Zincol—formaldehyde, zinc chloride
Gly-Oxide—carbamide peroxide
Colgate 100—benzothonium chloride, alcohol
Isodine—povidone-iodine
Kasdenol—oxychlorosene (calcium hypochlorite)
Lavoris—zinc chloride, cinnamaldehyde, clove oil
Listerine—thymol, eucalyptol, methyl salicylate, menthol, benzoic acid, alcohol
Micrin—cetylpyridinium chloride, dequalinium (quaternary ammonium compounds), oil of peppermint, menthol, alcohol
Oral B—cetylpyridinium chloride, alcohol (parabens)
Oral Pentacresol—amyltricresols
Plax—tetrasodium pyrophosphate, alcohol, benzoic acid
Polident—alcohol, sodium lauryl sulfate
Reef—cetylpyridinium chloride, menthol, methyl salicylate, alcohol
Rembrandt—methylparaben, sodium lauryl sulfate
Scope—cetylpyridinium chloride, domiphen bromide (both quaternary compounds)
Sterisol—hexetidine
S.T. 37—hexylresorcinol
Targon—alcohol
Tyrolaris—Tyrothricin, alcohol-uinaria extract
Viadent—SD alcohol, zinc chloride
Vinee—sodium perborate, calcium carbonate, sodium aluminum sulfate, flavors

Sims (89) claimed that antienzyme dentifrices may produce ulcerative lesions of the oral mucosa and sore tongue in patients with allergic sensitivity to the antienzyme. Sodium lauryl sarcosinate, a foaming, surface-active agent in some dentifrices, has been claimed to act as an antienzyme. Allergic reactions to this agent have not been proved. Sensitivity to so-called antienzymes is probably not due to an allergic mechanism.

The abrasives in dentifrices (e.g., chalk, calcium carbonate, bentonite, pumice, hydrated aluminum, calcium phosphate, zinc oxide, sodium chloride, sodium bicarbonate, and the magnesium salts) are very rare sensitizers. The quaternary ammonium compounds are very rare sensitizers. The preservatives, essential oils, formalin, flavorings, antiseptics, antibiotic agents, and alcohol are more common sensitizers.

The coloring agents (certified dyes) in modern dentifrices and mouthwashes are mostly of the aniline or azo variety. Certification of a dye relates only to its toxicity and not to its allergic potential. Allergic sensitization to these dyes is rare, and when it occurs, cross-reaction with paraphenylenediamine is present in about 25% of cases. Natural colors, such as cudbear and cochineal, are rarely used at present.

If not properly diluted, many mouthwashes may produce an irritant stomatitis from the presence of such antiseptics and astringents as sodium perborate, zinc chloride, borax, menthol, thymol, phenol, iodine, methyl salicylate, alcohol, boric acid, creosols, surfactants, and flavors.

> **The following ingredients of dentifrices and mouthwashes have produced allergic stomatitis: formaldehyde, antiseptics (mercurial antiseptics), benzalkonium chloride, dichlorophene (G-4), antibiotic agents, essential oils used as flavors, alcohol, and coloring agents (certified dyes).**

The fluorides are very rare sensitizers (90,91) but frequently produce nonspecific nonallergenic pustular patch test reactions (92). Virtually all mass-marketed toothpastes produced in the United States now contain fluoride.

Saunders (93) claimed that fluoride toothpastes can produce circumoral dermatitis.

There is one report of a possible urticarial reaction to a fluoride dental treatment solution in an atopic child (94).

Ammoniated dentifrices, such as Dr. Lyons Powder, Colgate Ammoniated Powder, and Ammident, contain di-ammonium compounds and carbamides (urea). These ammonium compounds are not sensitizers.

Ulcers Caused by Contact Allergens

On rare occasions, contact of the sensitized patient's oral mucosa with the specific allergen may produce erosions or ulcers rather than a diffuse stomatitis. Such lesions may be indistinguishable from aphthous ulcers (95).

Sugarman (96) cited a case of hypersensitivity to a mint chewing gum in which the lesions were characterized by an aphthous ulcer. Kutcher et al. (97) could not confirm the finding of Tuft and Girsh (98) that aphthous ulcers were due to sensitivity to citric or acetic acid.

Cancellieri (99) listed contact sensitivity to dentifrices, teeth whiteners, mouth purifiers, chewing gum, drugs, food, acrylic resin liquid, and monomers in dentures as capable of producing chronic aphthous ulcers. Fisher (26) observed nickel-sensitive women with ulcers of the lips and oral mucosa caused by the holding of nickel-plated objects, such as bobby pins or hair clips, in their mouths. Fregert et al. (100) studied a patient with allergic hypersensitivity to alcohol, as shown by positive patch test reactions, who developed a burning sensation, erythema, and aphthae of the oral mucosa whenever she ingested alcoholic beverages.

> **The term "aphthous ulcer" should be reserved for idiopathic oral lesions and should not be used in connection with known allergic lesions.**

CHEILITIS AND PERLÈCHE

The vermilion border of the lips has a modified epithelium, which is much more likely to develop allergic contact sensitivity reactions than is the oral mucosa. Allergens in contact with both the oral mucosa and the lips often produce only cheilitis.

An angular cheilitis may be the only manifestation of allergic hypersensitivity to denture materials and dental fillings, and it may closely mimic a vitamin B deficiency. Allergic cheilitis may first manifest itself merely with dryness and fissuring. Edema and crusting may supervene from contact with strong allergens over a prolonged period.

Freeman and Stevens (101) retrospectively analyzed 75 cases of cheilitis seen in a contact dermatitis clinic. Irritant cheilitis was diagnosed in 36%, mostly attributed to chronic lip licking. Allergy was found in 25%. Common allergens included fragrances and flavorings, preservatives, lanolin, oxybenzone, and colophony. Sunscreens, lipsticks, toothpastes, medicaments, and cosmetics were causative, along with one case of nickel allergy in a flutist. Atopic dermatitis was found in 9%. Women accounted for two-thirds of the cases, and the ages ranged from 9 to 79 years.

Allergic contact cheilitis may result from contact with allergens in dental preparations and oral care products; topical agents directly applied to the lips, such as antichap agents, lipsticks, and sunscreens; foods and flavorings; and allergens transported by touching the lips, such as nail polish, metals in jewelry, or other contactants. Because the hands are relatively resistant, cheilitis or facial dermatitis may occur in the absence of hand dermatitis. Patients with nickel sensitivity may develop cheilitis from holding hairpins, bobby pins, or metal pens in their mouths. Individuals who chew poison ivy leaves, either inadvertently or to produce a hyposensitization effect, often develop a severe cheilitis, sometimes accompanied by a mucositis of the tongue and mouth. Rubber-sensitive individuals who chew on the rubber erasers of pencils may develop allergic cheilitis.

> **The lips are more readily sensitized than is the oral mucosa.**

Selected Causes of Allergic Cheilitis and Perlèche

Cheilitis from Dentifrices

Bactericidal agents, essential oils, and preservatives in toothpastes and mouthwashes may produce allergic cheilitis (102). Examples of these allergens are listed above.

Lipstick Cheilitis

A number of additives in lipsticks may produce allergic cheilitis. The most common are flavoring agents and preservatives. Dyes and other components are rare allergens (see Chapter 17).

Lip Salve Cheilitis

Lip salves have a softer base than do ordinary lipsticks and may be uncolored or colored with carmine, the aluminum lake of the pigment from cochineal obtained by precipitation with inorganic salts and aluminum. This dye, which is also present in lip rouge, has been shown by Sarkany and Everall (103) to be capable of producing allergic cheilitis.

Cheilitis Caused by Nail Polish and Nail Hardeners

Patients allergic to nail polish who bite their nails may develop cheilitis and perlèche. The usual sensitizer in nail polish is tosylamide-formaldehyde resin. So-called hypoallergenic nail polish contains an alkyd resin. Acrylates in artificial nails may cause cheilitis and facial dermatitis.

Huldin (104) observed three cases of hemorrhage of the lips in nail-biting patients who used nail hardeners, which contain formaldehyde. This phenomenon disappeared with discontinuation of the nail hardener and recurred when it was reused. Examination of the lips revealed many small (1 mm to 3 mm) hemorrhages in the midportion of the lips, which blended out toward the angle of the mouth. Most of these changes were noted on the vermilion border of the lower lip. There were no other petechial-type lesions of the conjunctivae or the extremities.

> **Nail biters may develop cheilitis, perlèche, and hemorrhages of the lip from nail polish and nail hardeners.**

Cheilitis Caused by Foods

Klauder (115) described a patient with sensitivity to carrots who developed a cheilitis and perioral dermatitis when she ate this vegetable raw or cooked.

Patients who are sensitized to poison ivy may acquire an allergic cheilitis from eating mango, which contains a catechol related to poison ivy oleoresin.

Individuals who remove orange peels with their teeth may develop an allergic cheilitis from orange peel. The specific sensitizer is limonene, an essential oil. Mitchell and Rook (106) reported a case of cheilitis caused by the volatile oil of oranges. The volatile orange oils may produce not only cheilitis but also circumoral dermatitis and hyperpigmentation.

Lupton (107) described a persistent cheilitis caused by coffee. In this instance, the coffee also produced a positive patch test reaction on the skin.

> **Carrots, orange peel, coffee, and menthol may produce allergic cheilitis. Nickel, rubber, and nail polish have produced "allergic" perlèche in sensitized individuals.**

Perlèche Caused by Nickel

Nickel-sensitive individuals who habitually place between the lips nickel-plated objects such as hairpins, bobby pins, pens, pencils, and metal lipstick holders, readily develop "allergic" nickel perlèche. In several instances of "nickel" perlèche, there was sufficient nickel present in the labial commissures to give a positive reaction to dimethylglyoxime (108).

Perlèche Caused by Rubber

Rubber-sensitive individuals who chew on rubber pencil erasers, rubber bands, and the rubber tips of toothbrushes have acquired this type of perlèche. In one instance, a rubber dam used in a dental procedure produced "allergic" perlèche. In five of six instances of "rubber" perlèche, the actual sensitizer proved to be mercaptobenzothiazole, a rubber accelerator.

Other Causes of Cheilitis or Perlèche

Allergic cheilitis has resulted from application of triamcinolone acetonide (Mycolog Cream) for angular cheilitis presumably caused by monilia. In these instances, the actual sensitizer was the ethylenediamine stabilizer in the cream (109).

The erythrosin in disclosing tablets (Xpose and Red Cote), which are used to identify dental plaque, is a photosensitizer. If the disclosing solution made with this dye contaminates the lips and is not removed, exposure to sunlight may produce a photosensitizing cheilitis. Other disclosing solutions and tablets may contain iodine or Mercurochrome.

Irritant Perlèche and Cheilitis

The Role of Saliva in Production of "Irritant" Perlèche

"Perlèche" (from the French word, *perlècher*, meaning "to lick thoroughly") is used to describe inflammatory processes occurring at the angles of the mouth.

Perlèche caused by contact irritants or sensitizers may exactly mimic the angular cheilitis resulting from monilia, riboflavin deficiency, and the split papules of secondary syphilis. Saliva plays a major role in the production of perlèche, particularly the irritant variety (108).

The salivary enzymes such as amylase and maltase, which play a role in the digestion of food, probably are irritating when they are in contact with the skin. Other enzymes present in saliva, such as acid and alkaline phosphatase, cholinesterase, lipase, sulfatase, galactosidase, lysozyme, hyaluronidase, catalase, glycogenase, hexokinase, carbonic anhydrase, and mucinase, are no doubt also irritants when in intimate, prolonged contact with the skin.

Any process that increases the flow of saliva, which, in turn, becomes trapped at the angles of the mouth, will produce perlèche. Chewing tobacco and gum, which increases the flow of saliva, can produce an angular cheilitis. Probably the most exotic variety of "chewer's perlèche" is observed in eastern India, where betel chewing is a common practice among both men and women. The betel leaf is coated with a paste of lime and various astringents, placed in the mouth, and chewed. The constant chewing keeps the mouth full of saliva, which trickles to the labial commissures. The continuous friction and rubbing of the moist opposing surfaces at the angles of the mouth produces perlèche with maceration, erosion, and fissures (110).

Excess salivation with drooling and moisture at the corners of the lips favors irritation and secondary infection. Those "lickers" who habitually place the tongue moistened with saliva at the corners of their mouth soon acquire perlèche.

"Pickers" who excoriate the labial fissures with their nails or other objects develop a "mechanical" form of perlèche. Irritant metabolic products formed in saliva are capable of producing irritation at the corners of the mouth. Thus, the first sign of uremic stomatitis may be an angular cheilitis that gradually extends to the entire buccal mucosa. This type of stomatitis is due to ammonia produced by the action of bacterial urease on the increased salivary urea (111).

> **Any condition, process, or product that increases the flow of saliva may be a factor in the production of perlèche, which may also be an early sign of uremia.**

Saliva also plays an important role in the formation of angular cheilitis in which faulty dentition is a factor. In edentulous individuals, in those wearing ill-fitting dentures, or in elderly individuals with marked attrition of the teeth, there is a closing of the vertical dimension so that the jaws approximate one another more closely, resulting in a folding of the skin and mucosa at the angles of the lips. These folds trap saliva and moisture. The saliva accumulating in the retaining folds irritates and macerates the labial fissures, producing perlèche.

Male patients with chronic angular cheilosis often keep the lips firmly approximated when shaving because of the discomfort after cutting over the inflamed tissues. They thus maintain abrasive areas of "stubble" in the contiguous portions of skin of the upper and lower lips. Consequently, an intact epidermis cannot develop. Such patients should be instructed to shave over the infected areas with the mouth stretched wide open.

Differential Diagnosis

A careful history and proper patch tests may help clinch a diagnosis of allergic contact angular cheilitis and aid in the differential diagnosis of the following types of perlèche:

1. Riboflavin deficiency—angular stomatitis (angular cheilitis, cheilosis) is the most common and characteristic oral manifestation of riboflavin deficiency. The lesion may be unilateral or bilateral. The first visible alteration is a whitening or pallor of the mucosa of the labial commissures. This is followed by maceration of the area, with pain or irritation upon opening the mouth. As the lesions progress, there is fissuring or cracking with ulceration. Often the lesions are complicated by secondary bacterial infection.

2. Moniliasis—This variety of perlèche is most common in diabetics, debilitated individuals, those taking antibiotics for long periods, and HIV patients. Occasionally moniliasis will complicate perlèche caused by contact allergy or some dental problems.

3. *Streptococcus* or *Staphylococcus* infections—Such infections occur particularly in sick or ill-nourished children and may occur in epidemic form.

4. Atopic and seborrheic dermatitis involving the face—Such dermatoses may be associated with angular cheilitis.

5. Angular fistulae—Congenital fistulae at the angles of the mouth, sometimes associated with oral sinuses, rarely produce a recurrent or refractory angular cheilitis (112).

6. Isotretinoin users—Patients taking isotretinoin (Accutane) for acne often develop dry skin of the face with inflammation of the angles of the mouth and scaling of the lips.

7. Thomas et al. (113) warned that factitious cheilitis must be distinguished from contact and actinic cheilitis on the basis of history and laboratory examination. Actinic cheilitis usually occurs with a background of obvious facial actinic damage in fair-skinned individuals.

Goldman (114) cited trauma from the use of dental floss as a factor in the development of perlèche on the right side of the mouth. The patients called attention to this problem. Unwaxed dental floss applied to the bicuspids and molars rubbed against the commissure area of the lips, especially when the mouth was wide open. Recurrences of the perlèche were prevented by stopping the use of dental floss. If dental floss is needed for dental hygiene, especially for teeth at the back of the mouth, such as the molars, waxed floss should be used and the mouth should not be opened too widely. With the extensive use of dental floss, such irritation of the commissures must not be uncommon.

The differential diagnosis of contact angular cheilitis includes riboflavin deficiency, moniliasis, bacterial infections, congenital fistulae, uremic stomatitis, and dental floss trauma.

The Management of Perlèche

Schoenfeld and Schoenfeld (115) emphasized the following factors in the management of perlèche.

The dermatologist should take a close look at the palate. If inflammation is present, either a new denture or a relining of the old denture is probably indicated.

Drooling, nocturnal or otherwise, contributes a great deal to angular cheilitis. Indeed, without the macerating action of saliva (along with its function as a vehicle for *Candida albicans*), many cases would not occur. Anything that promotes drooling, such as sucking on a pipe, pencil, or thumb in the corner of the mouth, predisposes the patient to this condition.

Orthodontic appliances cause a temporary change in lip contour and promote salivation that together can cause drooling and subsequent cheilitis. A teenager wearing braces and taking antibiotics for acne is obviously a good candidate for the condition. Luckily, both treatments are relatively temporary, and the eventual prognosis is excellent.

Persistent mouth breathing caused by any one or combination of factors, such as class 2 malocclusion, persistent rhinitis, or enlarged adenoids, allows saliva to collect in the angles of the mouth with subsequent cheilitis.

Therapy for angular cheilitis consists of two parts. The main approach should be first, to correct the underlying causes, then to treat with antibiotic preparations locally, which will accomplish permanent clearing of the lesions. Topical nystatin or other antifungal agents. Frequent application is required, because the area is constantly bathed by saliva. Sometimes simple elimination of the focus of irritation will clear the condition. Intralesional injection of diluted triamcinolone may reduce inflammation. Combining a low-strength topical corticosteroid with the antifungal agent may be helpful. Lip balms should be used cautiously because they often contain sensitizers. Petrolatum may be used safely if desired.

Although palliative treatment of angular cheilitis is simple and effective, recurrences will continue to plague the patient unless all the etiologic factors are treated.

PATCH TESTING IN STOMATITIS, CHEILITIS, AND PERLÈCHE

Screening patch test trays contain a number of allergens that may cause stomatitis, cheilitis, and perlèche. These include some metals, rubber allergens, preservatives, flavorings (balsam of Peru and the fragrance mix), and topical medications. Supplemental allergens, such as acrylates, other metals, dental resins, cosmetic ingredients, sunscreens, and other items listed in this chapter, may be useful for complete diagnostic accuracy. Cosmetic products such as lipsticks and salves can usually be tested as is. However, testing with dental materials and dentifrices themselves requires caution (Table 36.7).

Precautions for Patch Testing with Dentifrices and Mouthwashes

Soaps or synthetic detergents in a dentifrice may produce primary irritant reactions under a closed patch test. Positive

TABLE 36.7. *Ingredients of Dentifrices and Mouthwashes—Concentrations and Vehicles for Patch Testing*

Contactant	Concentration and vehicle	Comment
Abietic acid	2% pet	In denture adhesive powders
Acacia (gum arabic)	As is	Binder in denture adhesive powders
Acetic acid	3% aq	Astringent in mouthwash
Acetone (dimethyl ketone)	As is (open)	Solvent for celluloid-like material in dentifrices
Alcohol, USP 70%	As is (open)	Solvent and astringent in mouthwashes
Alum	10% aq	Aluminum and potassium sulfates, astringent in mouthwashes
Aluminum acetate	10% aq	Astringent
Aluminum chlorhydroxide	10% aq	Astringent
Aluminum chloride	2% aq	Astringent
Aluminum sulfate	2% aq	Astringent
Aluminum sulfocarbolate	2% aq	Astringent
Ammonium fluoride	2% aq	May produce nonspecific pustular patch test reaction
Ammonium persulfate	2% aq	Ammoniated dentifrices
Ammonium phosphate	2% aq	Ammoniated dentifrices
Amyltricresols	1% aq	Phenol-mercury compound in oral Pentacresol mouthwash
Anise oil	25% co	Flavoring agent
Bacitracin	As is	Present in Wybiotic troches
Balsam of Peru	10% pet	Present in denture cement liquids, may cross-react with cinnamates, essential oil flavors, and eugenol
Benzalkonium chloride, USP	0.1% aq	Present in mouthwashes; commercial names: Zephiran, benzalkonium
Benzocaine	5% pet	Present in Orafix Medicated, Benzodent, Parcain, topical anesthetic
Benzoic acid	5% pet	Antibacterial agent in mouthwashes
Benzothonium chloride (Phemerol)	0.1% aq	Present in Colgate 100 mouthwash
Benzoyl peroxide	10% pet	Used in acrylic resins, may cross-react with benzoic acid and cinnamon derivatives
Benzyl alcohol	5% pet	Present in flavoring agents
Betadine solution (povidone-iodine)	As is	Mouthwash and gargle
Betanaphthol	10% oo	Antibacterial agent in mouthwash
Borax (sodium borate)	Sat aq	Chloraseptic, Dobell's solution
Boric acid	Powder as is	Antiseptic in mouthwash
Camphor oil	10% pet	Some camphors contain oil of laurel, a flavoring agent; may be used in dentistry as camphorated parachlorophenol
Caraway seed oil	25% co	Flavoring agent
Carbamide (urea)	2% aq	Dr. Lyons, Colgate Powder, and Ammident toothpaste
Carnation oil	10% aq	Flavoring agent; present in some eugenol preparations
Cassia flavor	5% oo	Chinese cinnamon flavoring agent
Cetylpyridinium chloride	0.1% aq	Quaternary ammonium compounds present in Cepacol, Micrin, Reef, and Scope
Chloroform	40% oo	Solvent for gutta-percha, gum copal, and acrylic denture material
Chlorophyllin, sodium copper	5% aq	Present in Green Mint mouthwash
Chlorothymol	2% aq	Antiseptic in mouthwash
Cinnamic acid	5% pet	Flavoring agent
Cinnamic aldehyde	2% pet	Flavoring agent (Lavoris)
Cinnamon oil	5% oo	Flavoring agent
Citric acid	1% aq	Astringent in mouthwash
Clove oil	25% co	Eugenol is chief constituent, flavoring agent (Lavoris)
Coriander oil	10% co	Flavoring agent
Coumarin	5% pet	A cinnamic acid flavor
Dequalinium	0.1% aq	Quaternary ammonium compound in Micrin mouthwash
Dichlorophene (G-4, Baxin)	2% aq	Preservative in toothpaste
Domiphen bromide	0.1% aq	Quaternary ammonium compound in Scope mouthwash
Essential oils	1% alc	Flavoring, antiseptic, and anodyne agents
Ethylenediamine	10% pet	Stabilizing agent
Ethylenediamine tetra-acetic acid (versene)	10% aq	Stabilizing agent
Eucalyptus oil	1% alc	Flavoring agent
Eugenol	5% pet	Flavoring agent (derived from clove oil)
Formaldehyde	1% aq	Present in Thermodent toothpaste
Geraniol	10% pet	Flavoring agent
Ginger oil	25% co	Flavoring agent

continued

TABLE 36.7. *(Continued)*

Contactant	Concentration and vehicle	Comment
Glycerine	As is	Humectant and sweetener
Glycol	10% aq	Humectant
Glyoxide	As is (open)	Contains urea peroxide, mouthwash providing hydrogen peroxide
Gramacidin	As is	Antibacterial in mouthwash
Gum arabic (acacia)	As is	Binder in denture adhesive powders
Hexachlorophene (G-11) (gamophen)	2% aq	Antibacterial in some detergent mouthwash preparations
Hexetidine (ethylhexyl, hexahydro, methyl, imidiaso, imidazolol)	1% aq	Antibacterial agent present in Sterisol mouthwash
Hexylresorcinol	As is	Antiseptic in mouthwash
Hypochlorite, calcium	10% aq	Present in oxychlorosene in Kasdenol mouthwash
Irish moss (carrageen)	As is	Trade names: Sea Kem, Viscarin, and Chondrus Extract; binder in many toothpastes
Isodine	As is	Mouthwash with povidone-iodine
Javelle water (potassium hypochlorite)	10% aq	Antiseptic mouthwash
Karaya gum (sterculia gum)	As is	Denture adhesive powders
Krameria, tincture (tinctura rhatanhiae)	5% alc	Astringent in mouthwash
Lactic acid	3% aq	Astringent in mouthwash
Laurel oil	25% co	Flavoring agent
Lavender oil	1% alc	Flavoring agent
Limonene, oil of	1% alc	Flavoring agent
Linalool	10% pet	Flavoring agent
Mace, oil of (nutmeg)	10% alc	Flavoring agent
Magnesium peroxide	As is	Oxidizing agent in MacLeans toothpaste
Menthol	1% pet	Flavoring agent in Listerine, Reef, Chloraseptic
Methylbenzathonium chloride	0.1% aq	Quaternary ammonium disinfectant
Methyl cellulose	As is	Binder in dentifrices
Methyl salicylate	2% oo	Flavor in Listerine and Reef
Myrrh, tincture	10% alc	Disinfectant—Astringosol
Neomycin	20% pet	Present in Wybiotic troches
Nitrobenzene (oil of mirbane)	10% oo	Flavoring agent; artificial oil of bitter almonds
Nitrofurazone	1% pet	Antibacterial agent in mouthwash
Nutmeg oil (mace)	10% alc	Flavoring agent
Oleyl alcohol	20% pet	Solvent for essential oils
Orange oil	1% alc	Flavoring agent
Orris root	Powder pure	Flavoring agent present in adhesive dentifrices
Oxychlorosene	1% aq	Hypochlorite in Kasdenol mouthwash
Pancreatin	As is	Mixture of enzymes in Pycopay toothpowder
Peppermint oil	25% co	Flavoring agent
Phemerol	0.1% aq	See benzothonium chloride
Phenol	1% aq	Present in Chloraseptic mouthwash
Phenolic compounds	1% aq	Amyl, heptyl, and octyl phenols used in mouthwashes
Pimiento	10% co	Flavoring agent
Polyethylene glycol	10% aq	Humectant and solvent
Polysorbate 80, USP	10% pet	Emulsifier and dispersing agent in dentifrices
Potassium chlorate	10% aq	Antiseptic oxidizing agent in mouthwash
Propylene glycol	10% aq	Humectant and binder
Quaternary ammonium compounds	0.1% aq	Antibacterial agent in detergents
Sassafras	2% oo	Flavoring agent
Sodium alginate (Algin)	As is	Emulsifier in dentifrices
Sodium alkyl sulfate	2% aq	"Foaming" surfactant in Ultrabrite, Gleem, Stripe, MacLeans, Pepsodent
Sodium fluoride	0.5% aq	May give nonspecific pustular patch test reaction
Sodium hypochlorite	10% aq	Antiseptic in Zonite
Sodium monofluorophosphate	0.5% aq	Present in Colgate toothpaste with MFP
Sodium monoglyceride sulfonate	2% aq	"Foaming" surfactant in Gleem
Sodium laurel sulfate	2% aq	"Foaming" agent in dentifrice
Sodium-N-alkyl sarcosinate	2% aq	"Foaming" agent in Ultrabrite and Colgate with MFP
Sodium perborate	Powder as is	Oxidizing agent in Vince and Amosan
Sorbisol	10% aq	Humectant in dentifrices
Spearmint, oil of	1% alc	Flavoring agent
Stannus fluoride	0.5% aq	Present in Crest, Cue, Fat, and Superstripe

continued

TABLE 36.7. *(Continued)*

Contactant	Concentration and vehicle	Comment
Sterculia gum (karaya)	As is	Denture adhesive powders
Strontium chloride	2% aq	Present in Sensodyne dentifrice
Tannic acid	1% aq	Astringent mouthwash
Thyme, oil of	25% co	Flavoring agent
Thymol (isopropyl metacresol)	1% pet	Antibacterial agent present in Listerine, Chloraseptic
Tragacanth	1% aq	Emulsifier and binder in dentifrices
Tween	5% aq	Polyethylene sorbitan monooleate; emulsifying agent in mouthwashes
Tyrothricin	As is	Present in Tyrolaris mouthwash
Urea (carbamide)	10% aq	Ammoniated toothpastes
Wintergreen, oil of (gaultheria oil)	1% alc	Flavoring agent
Zinc chloride	2% aq	Astringent in Lavoris, Astringosol
Zinc oxide	As is	Used in combination with eugenol in many dental preparations
Zinc peroxide	As is	Astringent, antiseptic
Zinc sulfate	5% aq	Astringent
Zinc sulfocarbolate	5% aq	Astringent

alc, alcohol; aq, aqueous; as is, full strength; co, castor oil; oo, olive oil; open, uncovered; pet, petrolatum; sat, saturated

reactions to tests with a dentifrice or mouthwash should always be checked by testing at least five controls. If they also show positive reactions, the product is a primary irritant as tested (116). Those containing soaps or detergents should first be tested uncovered on the back or forearm, and only tested with a closed patch under dilution.

Mouthwashes often contain alcohol and other ingredients that may partially evaporate and cause irritation under a closed patch test.

A repeated open application test (ROAT) may be helpful in testing these agents. Apply the product to the antecubital space twice daily for 5 days. A positive test implies allergy, if controls are negative. A negative test, however, may be falsely negative due to inadequate concentration of an allergen in the product.

In the event that an allergic patch test reaction is obtained with a dentifrice or mouthwash, an effort should be made to ascertain the specific sensitizing ingredient. Furthermore, aimed testing may be possible with the cooperation of the product manufacturer. Such knowledge will enable the patient to avoid the sensitizer and prevent recurrent stomatitis and dermatitis.

Direct Testing of Oral Mucosa

If a dentifrice or mouthwash is suspected of causing an allergic stomatitis or cheilitis, and skin patch tests with the suspected preparation or its ingredients are negative, direct testing of the buccal mucosa may occasionally be indicated.

The suspected ingredient is incorporated into Orabase, which is an adhering paste composed of pectin, gelatin, sodium carboxymethylcellulose, and plasticized hydrocarbon gel. The mixture is applied to the inner side of the dried lip

and left in place for 24 hours. Positive reactions marked by erythema of the mucosa may occur the next day, with the reaction reaching its peak at 48 hours after the allergen has been applied.

Another method of direct testing of the mucosa is to place the allergen inside a rubber or plastic cup that is then tied to the surface of the teeth in such a fashion that the allergen, held in the cup with collodion, is in contact with the buccal fold.

Dentures may be used to keep suspected allergens against the mucosa in those who use such appliances.

Using any of these nonstandard testing methods can produce false-positive irritant reactions as well as false-negative reactions, so clinical correlation is essential.

Testing for Allergic Sensitivity to Acrylic Dentures

Patch testing by strapping the denture to the forearm may lead to diagnostic errors, because redness, papulation, vesiculation, and even bullae may result from nonspecific pressure effects. This practice is not recommended. Patch testing with heat-cured dentures or with denture grindings also may give false reactions. Testing with the monomer and other separate ingredients avoids false-positive reaction from the hardness of the denture or the sharpness of filings (Table 36.8).

The identification of specific allergens in denture materials can be difficult, because many combinations of chemicals and additives may be used. Even if a positive patch test reaction is obtained with a single chemical, the patient can sometimes use dentures containing the chemical provided the denture is cured by heat. For example, dental mechanics with allergic hypersensitivity to the acrylic monomer or the

TABLE 36.8. *Suggested Screening Tray for Patch Testing for Stomatitis, Cheilitis, and Perlèche*

Metals
  Nickel sulfate
  Cobalt chloride
  Gold sodium thiosulfate
  Potassium dichromate
  Metallic mercury
  Ammoniated mercury
  Palladium chloride
  Platinum
  Copper sulfate
  Beryllium sulfate
  Indium sulfate
  Iridium chloride
Acrylates and plastics
  Methyl methacrylate
  Rosin
  Epoxy resin
  Bis-GMA
Flavorings
  Balsam of Peru
  Eugenol
  Fragrance mix
  Benzyl alcohol
  Clove oil
  Menthol
  Cinnamic aldehyde
Disinfectants and preservatives
  Benzalkonium chloride
  Domiphen
  Cetylpyridinium chloride
  Sodium benzoate
  Benzethonium chloride
  Dichlorophene (G-4)
  Hexylresorcinol
  Paraben mix
  Propylene glycol

hydroquinone may develop severe contact dermatitis of the hands. These individuals nevertheless can wear heat-cured dentures without difficulty (117).

Kaaber et al. (118) studied the significance of sensitizing compounds in the denture base for the etiology of the burning mouth syndrome (BMS) in 53 denture-wearing persons, 7 males and 46 females. Patch tests were performed with standard concentrations of benzoyl peroxide, dibutylphthalate, dimethyl-*p*-toluidine, formaldehyde, hydroquinone, methylmethyl acrylate, and *p*-phenylenediamine, as well as cadmium sulfate, potassium dichromate, cobalt chloride, and nickel sulfate. Furthermore, patch testing was performed with filings from the denture mixed with the patients' own saliva. Positive skin reactions to dimethyl-*p*-toluidine, hydroquinone, formaldehyde, methylmethyl acrylate, *p*-phenylenediamine, potassium dichromate, cobalt chloride, and nickel sulfate were observed in 15 persons, including 3 patients with reactions to filings from their dentures.

In 12 cases a causal connection could be traced between the oral symptoms and the denture base, indicating that contact sensitivity to base materials of the denture plate plays a greater role in the pathogenesis of BMS in edentulous persons than was previously suggested.

In our experience, patch testing with dentures or with filings of dentures often produces false-positive reactions from nonspecific pressure of hard particulate matter. Patch tests should be performed with commercially available allergens if at all possible. The liquid monomer or the other basic denture materials in solution or in petrolatum may be tested, but must be highly diluted to avoid irritant reactions and active sensitization.

Fowler (119) has seen a case of a dental worker allergic to acrylates wherein positive reactions were seen 4 weeks after testing, performed on two separate occasions.

THERAPY OF ALLERGIC CHEILITIS AND STOMATITIS

In mild cases, prompt removal of the specific contact allergen is all that is necessary to effect a cure.

For swelling of the lips with an intact epithelium, the application of petrolatum on which is superimposed ice-cold water compresses is helpful. When the swelling of the lips is accompanied by fissuring and crusting, a nonsensitizing topical antibiotic ointment such as mupirocin may be used, along with a topical steroid such as desonide ointment. Ointments are preferable because they generally contain less sensitizers. Bland emollients such as petrolatum may be used as well.

When there is edema of the oral mucosa, sucking on ice chips is indicated. Painful erosions or ulcers may be covered with triamcinolone acetonide (Kenalog in Orabase) or other topical steroids. An effective way to apply the topical steroid is to place the gel or ointment on a gauze pad, then place the pad against the affected area for 15 to 30 minutes. It may be held in place by the teeth or tongue. For painful lesions, lidocaine (Xylocaine Viscous) or other local anesthetics may be applied. Ulcer-Ease Mouth Rinse (Med-Derm Co., Kingsport, TN) is an over-the-counter mouth rinse with antiseptic and analgesic properties.

According to Dr. J. Litt (personal communication), patients obtain marked relief by gargling with diphenhydramine hydrochloride (Benadryl Elixer) and by dissolving a 250-mg capsule of tetracycline in 2 oz of warm water and swirling it around in the mouth for 5 minutes every 3 to 4 hours.

REFERENCES

1. Fisher A A. Contact stomatitis, glossitis, and cheilitis. *Otolaryngol Clin North Am* 1974;7:827.
2. Claman H N. Mouth ulcers associated with prolonged chewing of gum containing aspirin. *JAMA* 1967;202:651.

3. Cohen L. Ulcerative lesions of the oral cavity. *Int J Dermatol* 1980; 19:62.

4. Jolly M. White lesions of the mouth. *Int J Dermatol* 1977;5:719.

5. Abramson A. Causes of stomatitis. *Medical World News,* 28 June 1974, p. 19.

6. Forsey R R, Sullivan T J. Stomatitis nicotina. *Arch Dermatol* 1961; 83:112.

7. Reddy C R R M, Ramulu C, Raju M V S, Reddy P G. Relation of reverse smoking and other habits to the development of stomatitis nicotina. *Indian J Cancer* 1972;91:223.

8. Gruskin S E, Tolman D E, Wagoner R D. Oral manifestations of uremia. *Minn Med* 1970;53:495.

9. Mennie S, Piccinno R, Pistritto M G. Ulcerative stomatitis in a neonate due to a chlorine antiseptic. *Contact Dermatitis* 1988;18:320.

10. Lowney E D. Unresponsiveness to a contact sensitizer in man. *J Invest Dermatol* 1968;51:411.

11. Drake T E, Maibach H I. Allergic contact dermatitis and stomatitis caused by a cinnamic-aldehyde flavored toothpaste. *Arch Dermatol* 1976;112:202.

12. Magnusson B, Wilkinson D S. Cinnamic aldehyde in toothpaste: 1. clinical aspects and patch tests. *Contact Dermatitis* 1975;1:70.

13. Kirton V, Wilkinson W. Sensitivity to cinnamic aldehyde in a toothpaste: 2. further studies. *Contact Dermatitis* 1975;1:77.

14. Miller R L, Gould A R, Bernstein M L. Cinnamon-induced stomatitis venata. *Oral Surg Oral Med Oral Pathol* 1992;73:708.

15. Kim S C, Hong K T, Kim D H. Contact stomatitis from a breath refresher (Eundan). *Contact Dermatitis* 1988;19:309.

16. Hjorth N. *Eczematous allergy to balsams.* Copenhagen: Munksgaard, 1961.

17. Calap Calatayud J. Allergy to balsam of Peru. *Med Esp* 1969;61:119.

18. Fisher A A. Allergic contact stomatitis. *Cutis* 1975;15:149.

19. Kern A N. Contact dermatitis from cinnamon. *Arch Dermatol* 1960;81:599.

20. Camarasa G, Alomar A. Menthol dermatitis from cigarettes. *Contact Dermatitis* 1978;4:169.

21. Papa C M, Shelley W B. Menthol hypersensitivity. *JAMA* 1964;189: 546.

22. Morton C A, Garioch J, Todd P, et al. Contact sensitivity to menthol and peppermint in patients with intra-oral symptoms. *Contact Dermatitis* 1995;32:281–284.

23. Goransson J, et al. Some cases of eugenol sensitivity. *Svensk Tandlak T* 1967;60:545.

24. Koch G, Magnusson B, Nyquist G. Contact allergy to medicaments and materials used in dentistry: II. Sensitivity to eugenol and colophony. *Odont Rev* 1971;22:275.

25. Beswick S J, Ramsay H M, Tan B B. Contact dermatitis from flavourings in chewing gum. *Contact Dermatitis* 1999;40:49–50.

26. Fisher A A. Allergic reactions due to metals used in dentistry. *Cutis* 1974;14:797.

27. Foussereau J, Laugier P. Allergic eczema from metallic foreign bodies (tooth fillings and denture alloys). *Clin Dermatol* 1966;52: 221.

28. Frykholm K O, Frithiof A, Fernstrom A I, et al. Allergy to copper derived from dental alloys as a possible cause of oral lesions of lichen planus. *Acta Derm Venereol* 1969;49:268.

29. Gaul L E. Immunity of the oral mucosa in epidermal sensitization to mercury. *Arch Dermatol* 1966;93:45.

30. Epstein S. The antigen-antibody reaction in contact dermatitis. *Ann Allergy* 1952;10:633.

31. Fernstreom A E B, et al. Mercury allergy with eczematous dermatitis due to silver amalgam fillings. *Br Dent J* 1962;113:206.

32. Juhlin L, Ohman S. Allergic reaction to mercury in red tattoos and in mercury adjacent to amalgam fillings. *Acta Derm Venereol* 1968;48: 103.

33. Nordlind K, Liden S. Patch test reactions to metal salts in patients with oral mucosal lesions associated with amalgam restorations. *Contact Dermatitis* 1992;27:157.

34. Mobacken H, et al. Oral lichen planus: hypersensitivity to dental restoration material. *Contact Dermatitis* 1991;24:277.

35. Koch P, Bahmer F. Oral lesions and symptoms related to metals used in dental restoration: a clinical, allergological, and histologic study. *J Am Acad Dermatol* 1999;41:422–430.

36. Johnson H H, Schonberg I L, Bach N F. Chronic atopic dermatitis, with pronounced mercury sensitivity: partial clearing after extraction of teeth containing mercury amalgam fillings. *Arch Derm Syph* 1951;63:279.

37. Sidi E, Casalis J. Les intolerances de la muqueuse buccale. *Presse Med* 1951;59:730.

38. Vickers C F. Mercury sensitivity. *Contact Dermatol Newsletter* 1961;2:000.

39. Spector L S. Allergic manifestations to mercury. *JAMA* 1951;42:320.

40. Thomson J, Russell J A. Dermatitis due to mercury following amalgam dental restoration. *Br J Dermatol* 1970;82:292.

41. Frykholm K O. On mercury from dental amalgam: its toxic and allergic effects and some comments on occupational hygiene. *Acta Odontol Scand* 1957;22[Suppl 15]:230.

42. von Mayenburg J, Rakoski J, Szliska C. Patch testing with amalgam at various concentrations. *Contact Dermatitis* 1991;24:266.

43. Foussereau J, Laugier P. Allergic eczema from metallic foreign bodies (tooth fillings and denture alloys). *Clin Dermatol* 1966;52: 221.

44. van Loon L A J, et al. Contact stomatitis and dermatitis to nickel and palladium. *Contact Dermatitis* 1984;11:294.

45. Fisher A A, Shapiro A. Allergic eczematous contact dermatitis due to metallic nickel. *JAMA* 1956;161:717.

46. Wilson H T. Nickel dermatitis. *Br J Dermatol* 1955;67:291.

47. Calnan C D. Nickel sensitivity in women. *Int Arch Allergy* 1957;1: 73.

48. Saltzer E J, Wilson J W. Allergic contact dermatitis due to copper. *Arch Dermatol* 1968;98:375.

49. Elgart M L, Higdon R S. Allergic contact dermatitis to gold. *Arch Dermatol* 1971;103:649.

50. Marcusson J A. Contact allergies to nickel sulfate, gold sodium thiosulfate and palladium chloride in patients claiming side-effects from dental alloy components. *Contact Dermatitis* 1996;34:320–323.

51. Schaffran R, Storrs F, Schalock P. Prevalence of gold sensitivity in asymptomatic individuals with gold dental restorations. *Am J Contact Dermatitis* 1999;10:201–206.

52. Brendlinger D L, Tarsitano J J. Generalized dermatitis due to sensitivity to a chromebalt removable partial denture. *J Am Dent Assoc* 1970;81:395.

53. Ovrutsky G D, Ulyanov A D. Allergy to chromium using steel dental prosthesis. *Stomatologia* 1976;55:660.

54. Moffa J P, Beck W D, Hoke A W. Allergic response to nickel-containing dental alloys. *J Dent Res* 1977;56[Special Issue B]:107.

55. Sheard Jr C. Contact dermatitis from platinum and related metals. *Arch Dermatol* 1955;71:357.

56. Fowler J F. Allergic contact dermatitis to metals. *Am J Contact Dermatitis* 1990;1:212.

57. Mizoguchi S, Setoyama M, Kanzaki T. Linear lichen planus in the region of the mandibular nerve caused by an allergy to palladium in dental metals. *Dermatology* 1998;196:268–270.

58. Koch P, Baum H P. Contact stomatitis due to palladium and platinum in dental alloys. *Contact Dermatitis* 1996;34:253–257.

59. Haberman A L, Pratt M, Storrs F J. Contact dermatitis from beryllium in dental alloys. *Contact Dermatitis* 1993;28:157.

60. Bircher A J, Pelloni F, Langauer-Messmer S, Muller D. Delayed hypersensitivity reactions to corticosteroids applied to mucous membranes. *Br J Dermatol* 1996;135:310–313.

61. Van Groeningen G, Nater J P. Reactions to dental impression materials. *Contact Dermatitis* 1975;1:373.

62. Tinkelman D G, Tinkelman C L. An unusual etiology of urticaria. *Pediatrics* 1979;63:339.

63. Garcia-Bravo B, Pons A, Rodriguez-Richardo A. Oral lichen planus from colophony. *Contact Dermatitis* 1992;26:279.

64. Hensten-Pettersen C. Dermatitis and dental materials. *Contact Dermatitis* 1981;7:174.

65. Bowen R L. Compatibility of various materials with oral tissues: 1. the components in composite restorations. *J Dent Res* 1979;58:1493.

66. Ruyter I F, Svendsen S A. Remaining methacrylate groups in composite restorative materials. *Acta Odontol Scand* 1978;36:75.

67. Davidson W M, Sheinis E M, Shepherd S R. Tissue reaction to orthodontic adhesives. *Am J Orthod* 1982;82:502.

68. Thompson L R, Miller E G, Bowles W H. Leaching of unpolymerized materials from orthodontic bonding resin. *J Dent Res* 1982;61: 989.

69. Fisher A A. Allergic sensitization of the skin and oral mucosa to acrylic denture materials. *JAMA* 1954;156:238.

70. Crissey J T. Stomatitis, dermatitis and denture materials. *Arch Dermatol* 1965;92:45.
71. Santosh, et al. Results of patch testing with dental materials. *Contact Dermatitis* 1999;40:50–51.
72. Tosti A, et al. Contact stomatitis due to N_1N-dimethyl-para-toluidine. *Contact Dermatitis* 1990;22:113.
73. Torres V, et al. Allergic contact cheilitis and stomatitis from hydroquinone in an acrylic dental prosthesis. *Contact Dermatitis* 1993;19:102.
74. van Joost T H, van Ulsen J, Van Loon J. Contact allergy to denture materials in the burning mouth syndrome. *Contact Dermatitis* 1988;18:97.
75. Fisher A. Allergic sensitization of the skin and oral mucosa to acrylic resin denture materials. *J Prosthet Dent* 1956;6:600.
76. Wakkers-Garritsen B G, Timmer L H, Nater J P. Etiological factors in the denture sore mouth syndrome: an investigation of 24 patients. *Contact Dermatitis* 1975;1:337.
77. Klein D R. Oral soft tissue changes in geriatric patients. *Bull NY Acad Med* 1980;56:721.
78. Taaffe A, Riggott J M. Aetiological factors in denture stomatitis. *Br J Dermatol* 1982;107:38.
79. Pemberton M, et al. Allergy to octyl gallate causing stomatitis. *Br Dent J* 1993;175:106–108.
80. Lewis F M, Shah M, Gawkrodger D J. Contact sensitivity to food additives can cause oral and perioral symptoms. *Contact Dermatitis* 1995;33:429–430.
81. Maurice P D L, et al. Allergic contact stomatitis and cheilitis from iodoform used in a dental dressing. *Contact Dermatitis* 1988;18:114.
82. Merk H, Ebert L, Goerz G. Allergic contact dermatitis due to the fungicide hexetidine. *Contact Dermatitis* 1982;8:216.
83. Epstein S. Dermal contact dermatitis from neomycin. *Ann Allergy* 1958;16:268.
84. Welsh L. The fixed drug eruption. *Arch Dermatol* 1961;84:1012.
85. Welsh L. Cross-fixed drug eruption from three antibiotics. *Arch Dermatol* 1955;71:521.
86. Sainio E L, Kanerva L. Contact allergens in toothpastes and a review of their hypersensitivity. *Contact Dermatitis* 1995;33:100–105.
87. Kierland R. What's new. *Int J Dermatol* 1971;10:208.
88. *Accepted dental therapeutics,* 33rd ed. Chicago: American Dental Association, 1968.
89. Sims W B. Oral lesions caused by antienzyme dentifrices. *US Armed Forces J* 1955;6:995.
90. Shea J J, Gillespie S M, Waldbott G. Allergy to fluoride. *Ann Allergy* 1967;25:388.
91. Douglas T E. Fluoride dentifrice and stomatitis. *Northwest Med* 1957;56:1037.
92. Fisher A A, et al. Pustular patch test reactions. *Arch Dermatol* 1959;80:742.
93. Saunders M J. Fluoride toothpastes: a cause of acne-like eruptions. *Arch Dermatol* 1975;111:793.
94. Camarasa J G, et al. Contact urticaria from sodium fluoride. *Contact Dermatitis* 1993;28:294.
95. Pay D K, Shelley W B. Necrotic ulcerations secondary to oral neomycin troches. *Arch Dermatol* 1965;91:136.
96. Sugarman M M. Contact allergy due to mint chewing gum. *Oral Surg* 1950;3:1145.
97. Kutcher A H, et al. Citric acid sensitivity in recurrent ulcerative (aphthous stomatitis). *J Allergy* 1958;29:438.
98. Tuft L, Girsh L S. Buccal mucosal tests in patients with canker sores (aphthous stomatitis). *J Allergy* 1958;29:503.
99. Cancellieri C P. Chronic aphthous ulcers (canker sores) due to inhalant allergen sensitivity. *J Allergy* 1958;29:503.
100. Fregert S, et al. Alcohol dermatitis. *Acta Derm Venereol* 1969;49:493.
101. Freeman S, Stephens R. Cheilitis: analysis of 75 cases referred to a contact dermatitis clinic. *Am J Contact Dermatitis* 1999;10:198–200.
102. Dooms-Goossens A, Degreef H, Verhoeve L. Hidden contact allergens in ORL—pharmaceutical preparations. *Acta Otorhinolaryngol Belg* 1979;33:474.
103. Sarkany R H, Everall J. Cheilitis due to carmine in lip salve. *Trans St John Hosp Derm Soc* 1961;46:39.
104. Huldin D H. Hemorrhages of the lips secondary to nail hardeners. *Cutis* 1968;4:709.
105. Klauder J V. Sensitization to carrots. *Arch Dermatol* 1956;74:149.
106. Mitchell J, Rook JC. *Botanical dermatology—plants and plants injurious to the skin.* Philadelphia: Lea & Febiger, 1979.
107. Lupton E S. Cheilitis due to coffee. *Arch Dermatol* 1961;84:798.
108. Fisher A A. Perleche (angular cheilitis) due to contactants. *Cutis* 1974;14:499.
109. Epstein E, Maibach H I. Ethylenediamine allergic contact dermatitis. *Arch Dermatol* 1968;98:476.
110. Singh G. Betel chewers perleche. *Br J Dermatol* 1973;89:98.
111. Gruskin S E, Tolman D E, Wagoner R D. Oral manifestations of uremia. *Minn Med* 1970;53:495.
112. McCarthy P L, Shklar G. *Diseases of the oral mucosa.* New York: McGraw-Hill, 1964.
113. Thomas III J R, Greene S L, Dicken C H. Factitious cheilitis. *J Am Acad Dermatol* 1983;8:368.
114. Goldman L. Dental floss as a factor in the development of perleche. *Arch Dermatol* 1979;115:108.
115. Schoenfeld R J, Schoenfeld F I. Angular cheilitis. *Cutis* 1977;19:213.
116. Fisher A A. Patch tests for allergic reactions to dentifrices and mouthwashes. *Cutis* 1970;6:554.
117. Nyquist G. Sensitivity to methyl methacrylate. *Trans Roy School Dent* 1958;35.
118. Kaaber S, Thulin H, Nielsen E. Skin sensitivity to denture base materials in the burning mouth syndrome. *Contact Dermatitis* 1979;5:90.
119. Fowler J. Late patch test reactions to acrylates in a dental worker. *Am J Contact Dermatitis* 1999;10:224–225.

CHAPTER 37

Aquatic Dermatoses

It is paradoxical that, in this age of modern technological advances and myriad amusements, humans' primitive urge for sea and surf seems to be accelerating.

There are many recreational, commercial, military, and scientific divers in the United States. Add to this the untold numbers of swimmers, surfers, snorklers, water skiers, and fishing and boating enthusiasts, and one can begin to appreciate the lure that salt water holds for millions of Americans. The same draw holds true for many other nations around the world for both economic and recreational reasons.

Little wonder, then, that water-related injuries and diseases have become commonplace and that aquatic medicine has developed as a specialty in its own right. However, the important field of aquatic dermatology has been comparatively neglected—despite the empiric observations of both coastal and inland dermatologists that they are seeing more and more patients with water-related dermatoses.

Oceans, lakes, swamps, swimming pools—even fish tanks—contain numerous creatures and plants, large and small, as well as a multitude of microscopic organisms. Many of these water organisms have evolved self-protective stinging, biting, and envenomating mechanisms capable of producing unique and various skin eruptions, along with occasional systemic reactions.

In addition to the considerable variety of water-related skin manifestations, mobility further complicates management of aquatic dermatoses. Patients jet to distant locales on vacation or business, immerse themselves in strange oceans, lakes, and rivers—and frequently return with "imported" water-related skin lesions. Because some of the skin manifestations do not appear for weeks or even months, the dermatologist in Connecticut or Tennessee may well be required to manage an unfamiliar condition originating in Bermuda or Anguilla. By the same token, the patient presenting to a California or Idaho dermatologist with an apparent water-related dermatosis may have recently returned from the Great Lakes region—a frequent source of cercarial dermatitis produced by freshwater schistosomes.

Although many of these conditions are self-limiting, they nevertheless require attention. Appropriate first-aid treatment is certainly indicated for such symptoms as pruritus,

painful lesions, bullae, or wounds. More importantly, related systemic disorders can lead to disastrous consequences if left untreated. A high index of suspicion is essential. In many instances, prompt and accurate diagnosis is vital and even lifesaving (1).

M. B. Strauss, M.D., assistant director of the Baromedical Department, Memorial Hospital Medical Center, Long Beach, California, suggests that divers carry with them the summary of treatment for marine animals shown in Table 37.1. Ricardo Mandojana, M.D., a frequent lecturer at the annual meetings of the American Academy of Dermatology, recommends a diver's first-aid kit for treatment of bites and stings (Table 37.2).

DERMATITIS CAUSED BY PORTUGUESE MAN-OF-WAR, JELLYFISH, AND RELATED COELENTERATES

An individual emerging from the sea with complaints of itching or burning is generally unaware that he or she may have struck a marine creature equipped with nematocysts, or "stinging capsules." However, careful history taking should immediately alert the clinician to such a possibility. History is particularly essential because nematocysts can often remain harmlessly deposited on the skin for a time, only to "fire" later when activated by a specific stimulus.

Nematocysts are found only within the phylum Coelenterata. Coelenterates are radially symmetrical animals of simple structure. The mouth opens into a single cavity, and the body wall is formed by two layers of cells with structureless jelly between them. Almost all coelenterates possess nematocysts. Thousands of these "stinging capsules" or "nettle cells" are concentrated on the tentacles.

This large and variegated phylum is particularly abundant in all tropical and subtropical waters. Of the 9,000 or so species that have been identified, approximately 100—including jellyfish, sea anemones, fire corals, and the Portuguese man-of-war—are capable of producing injuries to humans. The classes within this phylum and several clinically significant species are shown in Table 37.3. Table 37.4 lists the geographic areas in which the venomous coelenterates are found.

TABLE 37.1. *Recommended Summary of Treatment*

Summary: Marine animal injuries/treatments

Class	Mechanism	Examples	Emergency Rx
1	Bites (trauma)	Shark Barracuda	Control bleeding and shock
2	Nematocyst (stings)	Jellyfish Anemones Coral Hydras	1. Inactive (vinegar, etc.) 2. Coalesce and remove tentacles 3. Neutralize (soda, ammonia)
3	Spines (puncture)	Urchins Cones Stingrays Sculpins	Inactivate with hot water
4	Fangs (px bites)	Octupus Sea snake	Control shock
5	Poisonings, shocks, indolent wounds, rashes	Scombroids Corals, barnacles Parasites	Usually not an emergency at time of dive Treatments per symptoms

---

> **The coelenterates include sessile forms such as hydroids (corals and sea anemones) and free-floating forms (jellyfish and Portuguese man-of-war) moving on the surface of the sea. All of these organisms contain nematocysts.**

The Nature of Nematocysts

The nematocyst is contained within an outer capsule called the cnidoblast. Projecting from one surface of the cnidoblast is a sensitive trigger-like apparatus called a cnidocil. The nematocyst is fluid filled and contains a hollow, coiled, threadlike tube. The fluid within the nematocyst is the venom.

The envenomation process begins when a swimmer or diver brushes against the cnidocil. This stimulates the cnidoblast to open a trap-door mechanism, the operculum. The thread tube containing the venom is ejected forcefully and rapidly, causing its sharp tip to penetrate the human skin. This inoculates the venom into the skin. Thousands of nematocysts can sting the victim at the same time, causing a severe local irritation and a generalized reaction.

The stimulation necessary to discharge a nematocyst apparently involves both chemical and mechanical factors. It has been shown that freshwater stimulates the "firing" of nematocysts. Friction may also cause nematocysts to fire, and patients suspected of being contaminated with nematocysts should be advised to avoid rubbing or scratching the affected areas.

TABLE 37.2. *Recommended Supplies for Divers**

Tourniquet, compresses, gauze, waterproof Band-AIDS
Vinegar (some jellys)
Drying (talc, flour, soda, etc.) powder
Bicarbonate of soda or ammonia solution (coral and some jellyfish)
Water heating device
CPR equipment
Pointed tweezers (sea urchins)
Hydrogen peroxide or polysporin ointment
Meat tenderizer (stings)
Olive oil (sea urchins)
Iodine (coral)
Lemon juice (itching from corals, hydroids, etc.)
Oral diphenhydramine, topical corticosteroids, Elamax or EMLA cream

*Modified from Ricardo Mandojana, M.D., lecture to annual meeting of the American Academy of Dermatology, 1998.

TABLE 37.3. *The Phylum Coelenterata*

Class: Hydrozoa
  Order: Siphonophora
    Species: *Physalia physalis* (Portuguese man-of-war)
  Physalia utriculus (bluebottle)
  Vella vella (purple sail)
  Order: Calcyophora (glassy nectophore)
Difficult to see because of same index of refraction as seawater
  Order: Leptomedusae (feather hydroids)
  Order: Milleporina
  Millepora sp. (stinging coral [not a true coral])
Class: Scyphozoa (true jellyfish)
  Order: Cubomedusae
    Species: *Chironex fleckeri* (sea wasp)
  Cyanea (sea nettles)
  Chiropsalmus quadrigatus
Class: Anthozoa
  Subclass: Zoantharia
    Order: Actiniaria (sea anemones)
    Scleractinia (true coral)

TABLE 37.4 *Important Venomous Coelenterates*

Species	Where found	Comments
Physalia physalis Portuguese man-of-war Bluebottle	Tropical and subtropical waters	Pelagic; conspicuous gas-filled float; tentacles up to 12 m long
Millepora sp. Fire coral	Tropical waters	Typical reef inhabitants
Stephanoscyphus racemosus *Halecium* sp. *Lytocarpus* sp. Stinging hydroids	Tropical and subtropical waters; more common in Indo-Pacific	Characteristic of reefs but may attach to pilings, rafts, and other structures
Chironex fleckeri Australian sea wasp	Waters off northern Australia	Most dangerous of coelenterates
Chiropsalmus sp. *Sarbdea* sp. Sea wasps; box jellies	Widespread in tropical and subtropical waters, especially Indo-Pacific	Cause severe stings but less dangerous than *Chironex*
Cyanea capillata Lion's mane or giant jellyfish	Most of Pacific; north Atlantic	Largest of jellyfish; bell diameter up to 3 m, tentacles up to 36 m long
Chrysaora quinquecirrha Sea nettle	Tropical and north temperate waters	Common off Atlantic coast of United States; severe stinger; tentacles up to 1.2 m long
Anemonia sulcata European stinging anemone	Eastern Atlantic and Mediterranean	Common shallow-water species; can inflict a severe sting
Rhodactis howesi Matamutu anemone	Tropical Pacific and Indian oceans	Often eaten in Polynesia; toxic on ingestion if uncooked; also reported to cause stings

---

> **Nematocysts unique to the phylum Coelenterata can discharge their venom by freshwater (not saltwater) stimulation or by mechanical means such as friction from scratching or rubbing the affected area.**

The Nature of Nematocyst Venom

High molecular weight toxins isolated from nematocysts have been shown to be heat labile, nondialyzable, and degradable by proteolytic agents. In many species, these toxins appear to inhibit nerve activity by altering ionic permeability. The toxins may also induce cardiac dysfunction (2).

Experimental studies have shown that animals contacting or receiving the venom parenterally experience severe pain and paralysis in the central nervous system soon after envenomization. Other sequelae may include urticaria, pruritus, edema, paralysis, cardiac arrest, and death.

A toxic, protein-tetramine, polypeptide complex seems to be operative in coelenterate extracts. Paralysis and central nervous system effects appear to be related primarily to toxic proteins and peptides and secondarily to the presence of tetramine. Burning pain and urticaria can probably be explained by the presence of serotonin, histamine, or histamine-releasing agents in the venom.

Dermatitis and Systemic Reactions to Nematocysts

Dermatitis resulting from contact with nematocyst-containing tentacles varies with the concentration of stings and the toxicity of the venom. Pain, which usually is the first symptom, ranges from mild stinging to a marked burning sensation. There is usually a linear, red, elevated eruption accompanied by erythema and edema from jellyfish and Portuguese man-of-war stings. Anemone and fire coral stings are usually blotchy or punctate rather than linear.

The lesion may require 24 hours or so for full development and may persist up to a few weeks. Vesiculation and local necrosis have been reported but are rare. Systemic symptoms accompanying severe stings include muscular cramps, cough, dyspnea, and vomiting.

Urticarial eruptions can occur, sometimes accompanied by anaphylactic reactions with marked weakness and a cough caused by edema of the throat and larynx. Shock and death may ensue in children and in those with exceptional hypersensitivity. Vesiculation and local necrosis may also occur. In the United States, most severe stings are caused by the *Physalia physalis* (Portuguese man-of-war).

> **Long, linear, papular, or urticarial eruptions that are characteristic of jellyfish or Portuguese man-of-war envenomization may be accompanied by syncope.**

Variations of Reactions from the Different Members of the Coelenterata Phylum

Contact with the sessile forms, such as hydroids, corals, and sea anemones, usually occurs in scuba divers who touch these animals. Stings from these sessile forms are not as severe as stings from the free-floating forms, such as the jellyfish and Portuguese man-of-war.

Stings may also be inflicted by marine animals stranded on the beach or by detached tentacles that adhere to fish nets or mooring lines. The severity of the sting depends chiefly on the number of nematocysts that discharge into the skin, but species differences in venoms are also important (3). Minton (4) stated that in most severe coelenterate stings, tentacles remain attached to the skin. The undischarged nematocysts in these tentacles must be inactivated promptly. This can be best accomplished by immediately applying vinegar, although alcohol or sodium bicarbonate may be used if vinegar is unavailable (T Millington, M.D., personal communication, Camarillo, CA, 1999). On the research vessel *Alpha Helix* during diving operations in Australian and Philippine waters, a 1-liter plastic bottle of methyl alcohol was kept in all dive boats. Salt, sugar, or dry sand may be substituted, but they are less effective. After about 15 minutes, the inactivated tentacles may be scraped off. Vinegar has been reported to be able to inactivate nematocysts in some species in Australia (5).

> The nematocysts of detached tentacles adhering to fish nets or mooring lines are still "active" on the skin.

Portuguese Man-of-War Dermatitis

The Portuguese man-of-war (*Physalia physalis*) may travel in a fleet. Its red, blue, or green air-filled iridescent bag (measuring as much as 14 inches across) floats on the waves and acts as a kind of sail to catch the wind. This marine animal, incapable of rhythmic contractions, is entirely subject to wind and wave action, and therefore has no control over its destination (6–11).

Although the sac is quite harmless, the trailing mass of tentacles, which may be more than 100 feet long below the surface of the water, is dangerous. Each tentacle is studded with thousands of nematocysts, which can sting any surface they contact. Nematocysts detached from the tentacles of the Portuguese man-of-war remain capable of firing for at least several months. In addition, the tentacles may still be venomous for weeks after the Portuguese man-of-war has been washed ashore and died. Upon discharge, the stinging capsules penetrate the skin and inject a fluid containing a neurotoxin. This toxin is believed to be a multicomponent

system apparently made up of phospholipases A and B, several neutral lipids, enzymes with high proteolytic activity, and biologically active peptides.

After contact with the tentacles of the Portuguese man-of-war, the patient may experience a sharp stinging sensation, burning, numbness, and severe paresthesia. Skin inflammation may vary from linear urticarial lesions to ulceration to a "string of beads." A vesicular dermatitis is a fairly common sequela after erythema, edema, itching, and burning. Acute conjunctivitis may develop in children who grasp the tentacles of the Portuguese man-of-war, then rub their eyes.

Systemic manifestations that often occur soon after contact may include lacrimation, coryza, muscular pains, dyspnea, and a feeling of constriction in the chest.

Despite the intense pain and discomfort experienced by the patient, collapse and death are relatively rare. Death may occur if the areas stung are extensive in relation to the size of the patient. Collapse is generally presaged by nausea and backache experienced 10 or 15 minutes after initial dermatologic symptoms become apparent. More commonly, recovery occurs within several hours, although the skin lesions may pass through a stage of hemorrhagic necrosis before healing. Healed lesions may leave pigmented striae for weeks or months. Permanent scarring occasionally results.

> The tentacles of dead Portuguese man-of-war and nematocysts detached from such tentacles are venomous for long periods.

Bluebottle Stings

Physalia utriculus, the Pacific species of Portuguese man-of-war, is much smaller than its Atlantic cousin. According to Arnold (12), the Hawaiian species of bluebottle rarely grows as long as 3 or 4 inches, with tentacles rarely exceeding 10 or 15 feet.

Reactions to the bluebottle sting are rarely serious, and dermatologic reactions are similar to the larger forms of Portuguese man-of-war.

Velella Velella Dermatitis (By-the-Wind Sailor or Purple Sail Dermatitis)

Velella velella, a siphonophore, is a purple-edged, thin triangular sail on an oval float. It drifts on the water, much as the Portuguese man-of-war, and has trailing tentacles with nematocysts, which it uses to capture prey.

The dermatitis produced by it is a mild papulourticarial eruption.

Calycophora Dermatitis (Stinging Water Dermatitis)

This order of the phylum Coelenterata is extremely elusive because the animal, almost the same index of refraction as seawater, can be seen only when sunlight strikes it directly. Contact with this small glassy nectophore may result in a markedly pruritic eruption that may persist from several hours to several days. The nectophore is found particularly in deep seawater.

Feather Hydroid Dermatitis

Feather hydroids are fairly abundant in tropical and subtropical water. Swimmers climbing onto offshore rafts or swimming around pilings are most commonly afflicted by this hydrozoan.

The feather hydroid venom affects the skin more slowly than does jellyfish venom. The venom may cause two types of skin eruptions: urticaria, developing within a few minutes after contact, and delayed papular, hemorrhagic, or zosteriform reaction, occurring 4 to 12 hours after contact.

Characteristic bands of dermatitis 20 cm wide may be produced, accompanied by erythema multiforme and morbilliform eruptions. The patient may experience marked anxiety and apprehension. Systemic reactions may include severe abdominal pain and muscle spasms, diarrhea, and fever.

The patient should be warned against repeated exposure to feather hydroids. Such exposure may lead to allergic sensitization, possibly resulting in anaphylactic shock.

Sea Bathers' Eruption and Swimmers' Itch

Sea bathers' eruption has been identified as a dermatitis resulting from contact with the larvae of the jellyfish *Linuche unguiculata*. Tomchik et al. (13) reported that this eruption has become increasingly common since the late 1980s along the South Florida coast and in the Caribbean.

The acute dermatitis begins a short time after bathing in the sea. Erythematous macules, papules, or wheals are observed within a few hours after exposure (14). These lesions are localized on covered parts, such as the abdomen, buttocks, and thighs, and on the breasts of female patients. Accompanying symptoms may include chills, a low-grade 24-hour temperature, a burning sensation, and pruritus.

Some patients suffer repeatedly after seawater bathing, whereas other swimmers in the same area remain unaffected—suggesting that individual susceptibility or sensitization may be operative. Other than avoiding swimming in infested waters, the only practical method of prophylaxis consists of wiping the skin dry on emerging from the water.

The disorder is usually self-limiting, rarely persisting for more than 7 days. Therapy is palliative, consisting of calamine lotion with 1% menthol. Parenteral antihistamines usually control the eruption and itching. Rarely, systemic corticosteroids may be required.

Sea Nettle Dermatitis

Jellyfish, native to both saltwater and freshwater, are among the most ubiquitous of sea creatures. Certain species, such as *Chironex fleckeri* (sea wasp), and *Cyanea* and *Chrysaora* (sea nettles), are extremely troublesome to humans and may even be deadly. They are often found congregated, brought close to land or washed ashore by storms. The small freshwater jellyfish *Craspedacusta* is similar in structure to its frequently larger saltwater relatives.

Symptoms vary according to the venom of a particular species, as well as to the number of nematocysts that have penetrated the victim's skin. Shock and death may ensue if the victim is young, particularly sensitive, or stung by the deadly sea wasp.

It is often possible to identify the species of offending jellyfish by microscopic study of the nematocysts on the patient's skin. In certain cases, identification may also be made by noting the type of eruption and the linear patterns of the lesions, each pattern being specific for a particular species of jellyfish. The initial lesions caused by *Chironex fleckeri*, for example, are multiple linear wheals with transverse bars. The purple or brown marks from the tentacles form a whiplash skin lesion.

Gloves should be worn when removing tentacles that have become attached to the patient's skin. Rinsing with seawater may also aid in the removal of tentacles and nematocysts, if alcohol or other agents are unavailable.

Adriatic Sea Jellyfish

Kokelj et al. (15) reported that of 10 species of jellyfish found in the Adriatic, 5 are known to be toxic to humans. These include *Corybdea marsupialis*, *Aurelia aurita*, *Chrysaora hysoscella*, *Peligin noctilucs*, and *Rhizostoma pulmo*.

> The severity of reaction from contact with jellyfish nematocysts varies with the species, age of the patient, number of stinging capsules contacted, and degree of allergic sensitivity.

Chironex Fleckeri (Sea Wasp)

The most dangerous jellyfish, *Chironexfleckeri*, is found off northern Australia. Over 70 deaths, mostly children, have been reported (5). The bell may be up to 20 cm in diameter, and there may be 40 to 60 tentacles up to 3 m long. Three toxins have been identified . The most important is a cardiotoxin that may lead to arrhythmia and cardiac arrest.

Neuromuscular and respiratory paralysis may also occur. There are also hemolytic and dermonecrotic toxins.

At the site of a sting, a distinctive ladder-like pattern occurs with red, brown, and purple lesions. Shock and death may ensue within minutes. Holmes stated that vinegar should be applied but never alcohol or freshwater (5). Antivenom, which may be lifesaving, is available in Australia.

Carukia Barnesia

This small (1–2 cm) jellyfish causes a distinctive "syndrome." There is initial stinging of variable severity with or without subsequent local pain. A patch of erythema is followed by small papules and excessive local sweating. After 30 to 40 minutes systemic symptoms develop, including widespread pain and severe headache. A sympathomimetic response occurs, and cardiogenic shock may develop. Use of vinegar is unhelpful. Antivenom and supportive care are helpful.

Toxic Versus Allergic Reactions to Jellyfish

Burnett and Calton (16) and Hartman et al. (17) stated that the principal clinical reaction to envenomation from the jellyfish appears to result from toxicity rather than allergy because (a) no cases of immune resistance have been reported, (b) victims can be repeatedly stung without differences in symptoms, and (c) venom injection into different mammals induces similar clinical results. Other reports, however, have demonstrated the presence of venom-specific human immunoglobulins in envenomated patients (18,19). This fact suggests that both toxic and allergic mechanisms may be important in the pathogenesis of the stings.

Burnett et al. (16) reported the case histories of three patients with unusual reactions to jellyfish envenomations or increased amounts of antijellyfish serum antibodies. These cases demonstrated the following facts: (a) Allergic reactions may play a significant pathophysiologic role in jellyfish envenomation of humans; (b) elevated specific antijellyfish immunoglobulins may persist for several years; (c) recurrence of the clinical cutaneous reaction to jellyfish stings may occur within a few weeks without additional contact with the tentacles; and (d) it is apparent that serologic cross-reactivity between the sea nettle and the Portuguese man-of-war occur, as do false-positive enzyme-linked immunosorbent assay (ELISA) serologic tests to either jellyfish venom.

> Most reactions to jellyfish are caused by toxicity and a few by allergy, which accounts for recurrent skin reactions to jellyfish without additional contact.

A report by Tamanaha and Izumi (20) indicates that a persistent reaction, rather than simple immediate toxicity, can occur after a sting by the Hawaian box jellyfish (*Carybdea alata*). A patient developed persistent pruritic papular lesions that lasted 7 months. Histology revealed a spongiotic dermatitis with dense lymphocytic infiltrate and scattered eosinophils.

More definitive evidence of allergy to jellyfish venom is presented by Kokelj et al. (15). Using antigen prepared from nematocysts of *Olindras sambaquensis*, a small transparent jellyfish found near South America, a patient who had a history of multiple stings reacted on patch and "scratch-patch" tests. Ten controls were negative. Prick tests were negative in all, suggesting absence of an IgE-mediated response.

Apparently, IgE antibodies to some jellyfish venoms can develop, causing subsequent attacks to become more severe. However, IgG-blocking antibodies may develop in some individuals, rendering subsequent attack less severe.

Burnett and Calton (18) emphasized that elevated levels of serum anti–sea nettle venom IgE persisted for several years in two patients who had exaggerated reactions to jellyfish (sea nettle, *Chrysaora quinquecirrha*) stings. These antibodies also cross-reacted with Portuguese man-of-war venom. The determination of increased antigen-specific IgE concentrations may be of value in identifying patients at risk or in diagnosing stings by "unseen" animals.

> The IgE radioallergosorbent test (RAST) may be of value in identifying patients at risk or in diagnosing stings by "unseen" animals.

Ohtaki et al. (21) determined that allergic contact reactions play an important role in addition to immediate toxic reactions after exposure to the jellyfish *Corybdea rastonii*. Twenty-five volunteers had tentacles from the jellyfish applied to the forearm. Immediate pain and urticaria developed that resolved over 1 to 3 days. One to 2 weeks later, lesions of dermatitis erupted in the exposed areas in 15 of the 25 volunteers. Histology suggested allergic contact dermatitis and lymphocyte stimulation tests to jellyfish venom were elevated over controls in most of the subjects.

Sea Anemone Dermatitis (Sponge Fisherman's or Sponge Diver's Disease)

Animal sea anemones belong to the phylum Coelenterata, class Anthozoa. All species have nematocysts. Because of their variety of colors, animal sea anemones frequently have a flower-like appearance similar to plant anemones. Unfortunately, they are not as harmless as their botanical namesakes.

The characteristic contact dermatitis produced by a sea anemone is related to the specific toxicity of the venom of the offending species. *Actinia* induces painful urticarial reactions, whereas *Anemonia* causes an itching, burning sensation at the sting site, accompanied by swelling and erythema.

The most common skin condition caused by animal sea anemones is *Sagartia* dermatitis—"sponge fisherman's disease," as it is termed in some Mediterranean areas. *Sagartia* has the shape of a flower. It is approximately 4 cm long and has a hollow polypoid cylinder with two rows of graceful tentacles radially arranged.

This small sea anemone attaches itself symbiotically to the base of sponges. Sponge divers locate the sponges by feeling along the ocean floor with their hands. After uprooting the sponges and cleaning them by removing stones and other encrusted debris, they place the sponges in nets suspended from their necks. During such activity, sponge divers have ample opportunity to come in contact with the stinging tentacles of *Sagartia*.

Within a few minutes after contact, the patient experiences an itching, burning sensation, accompanied by erythema and vesicles. The lesion is initially swollen and red, changing later to a deep purple. Headache, nausea, vomiting, fever, chills, and muscle spasms are frequent complaints.

Immediate treatment is similar to that instituted for jellyfish stings: Remove tentacles while wearing gloves, and rinse affected area with seawater or alcohol. The healing process may be relatively slow. In addition, multiple abscesses with sloughing ulcers may develop, necessitating antibiotic treatment.

Sea anemone dermatitis (sponge fisherman's or sponge diver's disease) is produced by a flower-like coelenterate attached symbiotically to sponges.

Coral Dermatitis and Coral Cuts

The skin lesions produced by the Coelenterate corals, Milleporina, are caused by a combination of factors—effects of the nematocyst venom, laceration by the razor-sharp exoskeleton of the coral, foreign-body reaction, and secondary infection. True corals are structures of various sizes and shapes, formed by the cementing of tiny limestone exoskeletons or polyps, of the order Scleractinia.

Coral cuts occur among divers, fishermen, and others whose activities bring them into contact with living coral. These injuries are not particularly painful, but they heal slowly and often result in ulcers. The pathogenesis is not well understood. A foreign-body reaction and bacterial infection may be chiefly responsible, although the possibility of sensitization to antigens on the surface of live coral cannot be discounted. Envenomation from the nematocysts is probably not significant. In sports divers and tourists, the ulcers usually remain shallow and heal promptly, especially if the victim returns to a temperate climate. In residents of tropical seacoasts, however, large, deep, indolent ulcers are not uncommon. This may result from repeated trauma and infection with underlying malnutrition.

True coral, such as the elk-horn coral of the West Indies, causes severe stings. Toxic coral abrasions often result in a nonpruritic morbilliform rash within 8 hours that resolves in several days.

Nematocysts of true coral are usually fairly innocuous, and the resulting dermatitis—a pruritic erythema—can be effectively treated with a simple cooling lotion such as calamine lotion or alcohol.

Coral cuts should be treated vigorously to prevent secondary infection and ulceration. The following procedures are suggested.

1. Using soap and water, scrub the lesions with a soft brush or rough towel. Such vigorous cleansing is necessary to remove any calcareous pieces of coral that may become embedded in the lesion and produce an indolent wound.
2. Apply hydrogen peroxide and allow to "boil" for several minutes. Dry the wound.
3. Apply isopropyl alcohol and place an antibiotic ointment or the contents of a capsule of tetracycline over the still-wet wound. Pat into a paste with an applicator and allow the paste to dry.

The crust that is formed serves as a covering on the wound, remaining intact after bathing and allowing the lesion to heal from its outer edges. No bandage is necessary.

4. If the wound does not heal promptly, surgical debridement under a local anesthetic may become necessary.

Stinging or Fire Coral Dermatitis

The species *Millepora alcincornis* is not a coral at all. However, it looks like coral and acts like coral at least in one respect—it has nematocysts that cause skin eruptions. The nematocysts are located in the organism's wet mucus.

Fire coral is found living among true coral in the tropical Pacific Ocean, Indian Ocean, Red Sea, and Caribbean Sea. It can be recognized by its yellowish brown color, somewhat like mustard.

Tropical fire coral, a stinging coral, has earned its appellation by virtue of the tender, erythematous, burning lesion it produces upon contact, resulting from the high concentration of formic acid near the outer edge of the shell. The lesion usually resolves spontaneously, although application of ammonia may neutralize the formic acid.

Coral cuts should be vigorously cleansed to remove calcareous coral particles and the wound treated with antibiotic powder or ointment.

Dogger Bank Itch

English and other European fishermen, operating trawlers in the North Sea, may suffer from Dogger Bank itch. Contact with the causative agent *Alcyonidrium* sp., bryozoan coral, occurs when handling nets that have scraped along the seabed. Ashworth et al. have identified several other corals as causing a similar eruption. Exposed areas, such as the hands and the arms, are affected. In winter, the responsible organisms are reduced in number, so the disease shows a seasonal pattern of occurrence (22,23,23A).

"Indirect" Coelenterate Dermatitis

It may be possible for coelenterate dermatitis to develop without actual direct contact with any species in the phylum. This can occur in three ways:

1. Two species of nudibranch, *Glaucus atlanticus* and *Glaucus glaucilla*, eat the nematocysts and tentacles of the Portuguese man-of-war. The nematocysts pass through these sea slugs undigested and are deposited in the dorsal papillae. Bathers coming into contact with these armed nudibranchs can be stung by the nematocysts, resulting in the condition known as nudibranch dermatitis, which in reality is a nematocyst dermatitis.

2. Coelenterates may release antigenic and allergenic venomous substances into their aquatic environment. Allergens in the venom may sensitize individuals without immediate contact with nematocysts. Subsequently, severe allergic dermatitis may result if the sensitized individual comes into contact with a ruptured stinging capsule.

3. During severe storms, nematocysts detached from tentacles, particularly from jellyfish, may become free-floating and capable of discharging venom for several months. Thus, one may acquire nematocyst dermatitis without actual contact with a coelenterate. Lifeguards are aware of "epidemics" of a mild itching, papular eruption that may occur after such storms. Because characteristic linear lesions are not formed, nematocyst dermatitis may not be suspected.

> **During severe storms, nematocysts may become detached from coelenterates, particularly jellyfish. Such detached nematocysts may become free-floating and cause an "epidemic" of nematocyst dermatitis.**

Delayed, Persistent, Cutaneous Reactions to Coelenterates

Reed et al. (24) reported three patients who developed firm, persistent papules and plaques at sites of previous contact with two species of coelenterates. Histologically, a predom-

inantly mononuclear inflammatory cell infiltrate located primarily in the reticular dermis was observed with destruction of hair follicle epithelium and arrectores pilorum. Epidermal changes included focal spongiosis and exocytosis of lymphocytes. The eruptions subsided no sooner than 7 weeks from time of onset. It is hypothesized that this cutaneous reaction represents a persistent delayed hypersensitivity response to an antigenic component of the coelenterate nematocyst.

Principles of Treatment of Nematocyst Envenomization

In the past, various recommendations for the alleviation of coelenterate stings included the application of vinegar, alcohol, ammonia, urine, ice water, hot water, potassium permanganate crystals, formalin, barnacle juice, and meat tenderizer.

Current responsible opinion would seem to indicate the following measures.

1. Avoid the use of freshwater, as it activates nematocysts. Never allow the victim to enter a fresh shower after exposure to a coelenterate until the nematocyst toxin has been neutralized. The result could be extreme intensification of symptoms, even shock. The patient's skin may, however, be gently rinsed with seawater without adverse effect.

2. Apply vinegar to inactivate the toxin introduced by the nematocyst. If unavailable, use sodium bicarbonate or alcohol. Virtually any type of alcohol available is adequate, including rubbing alcohol, liquor, toilet water, cologne, or perfume. Be sure the liquid is applied over the entire affected area.

3. Alternatively, apply proteolytic meat tenderizer. This acts in a fashion similar to alcohol.

4. Avoid formalin, which is too toxic for routine use.

5. If nothing else is available, saltwater heated to the limit of tolerance may help neutralize the venom.

6. To help remove clinging tentacles, a paste of seawater and baking soda may be applied 5 minutes after the alcohol. Application of flour or talcum will serve the same purpose, coalescing the tentacles, which may then be readily scraped off with a knife or sharp instrument. Dry sand may be used if powders are not available. (Tentacles should not be removed with the ungloved hand.)

7. Wash the areas again with saltwater.

8. In severe cases—especially if the victim is a child—tourniquets on the exposed limbs may be lifesaving. The purpose of the tourniquet is not to stop arterial flow, but to reduce venous return. Always use a rubber tourniquet, and apply it so that a finger can be slipped underneath. Release the tourniquet for 3 or 4 minutes every hour.

9. Use local anesthetic ointments, creams, lotions, or aerosols to alleviate burning or pruritus. (Avoid doxepin preparations. Instead, use lidocaine derivatives.)

10. Clean ulcerating lesions three times a day. Apply an antibiotic ointment, preferably one not containing neomycin, which is commonly sensitizing.

Prevention of Nematocyst Envenomization

It is important to bear in mind that the tentacles of some species of jellyfish may trail a great distance from the body of the animal—as much as 50 feet or more, in some instances. Consequently, jellyfish should be given wide berth. Tight-fitting nylon or woolen underwear or rubber skin diving suits are useful in affording protection from attacks from these creatures. Divers working in tropical waters should be completely clothed. Even though appearing dead, jellyfish washed up on the beach may be quite capable of inflicting a serious sting. The tentacles of some jellyfish may cling to the skin. Swimming soon after a storm in tropical water in which large numbers of jellyfish were previously present may result in multiple severe stings from remnants of damaged tentacles floating in the water.

DERMATITIS CAUSED BY ECHINODERMS (SPINY CREATURES)

The phylum Echinodermata includes sea urchins, starfish, and sea cucumbers.

The literature on coral reef echinoderms goes back to the earliest phases of sea exploration. Aristotle wrote several notable passages on species of starfish and sea urchins.

Echinoderms are shy, nonaggressive, slow-moving animals who are continually at the mercy of their environment. Unfortunately for humans who come into contact with these creatures, one of the echinoderm's principal means of defense is an array of sharp or toxic spines. There are approximately 6,000 species of echinoderms, of which at least 80 are known to be venomous or poisonous.

Injuries from sea urchin spines are a familiar occupational hazard of fishermen in the Mediterranean and many tropical areas. In addition, the growing popularity of underwater activities among vacationers in these regions is presenting many dermatologists with a new diagnostic problem. Awareness of the hazard is the key to proper management.

Sea Urchin Dermatitis

Sea urchins are spherical organisms generally found on the rocky bottoms of bodies of saltwater, although some species prefer to burrow in the sand. They are covered with numerous movable spines, the length of which varies with the species. Formed by the calcification of a cylindrical projection of subepidermal connective tissue (25), these spines are extremely brittle and may break off easily in the victim's skin. The spines of some species are venomous and may contain a neurotoxin.

Intermingled among the spines are pedicellariae, pincerlike organs or fangs. These organs are attached to stalks that may be shorter or longer than the spines. Venom from the pedicellariae may be injected into the victim's skin via hooklike jaws or valves.

Diagnosis of sea urchin dermatitis is relatively simple if the patient recalls and mentions the original injury. In many cases, however, the immediate reaction may have been so slight that the patient failed to even notice initial contact with the organism. The diagnostician should be aware that some sea urchin spines contain a dye that may discolor the patient's skin and subcutaneous tissues, thereby giving the false impression that the spine is embedded in the skin. X-ray examination can diagnose the presence of spines.

Two types of sea urchin reactions have been noted:

1. *Immediate reactions.* A severe burning pain that may persist for several hours, with or without edema, is the chief immediate symptom of sea urchin dermatitis. Some patients bleed profusely.

Secondary infection may introduce further complications and may be severe when multiple lesions are present. Infected discharging wounds may be a means by which the tissues get rid of infecting spines.

Treat painful edematous lesions with water as hot as can be tolerated until the symptoms disappear. Application of an antibiotic is indicated when secondary infection is present. In the absence of secondary infection, lesions usually heal within 1 or 2 weeks, providing no portion of the spine remains within the wound.

Certain sea urchin spines are readily phagocytosed in the tissues and dissolve without difficulty. If the spine does not dissolve, surgical removal should be considered. In the acute stage, such removal may be rendered difficult by the fragility of undissolved spines and the presence of dyes, which interfere with proper visualization. Removal of spines should not be attempted unless they are easily seen. Visualization via X-ray examination is essential prior to surgical removal.

Strauss and McDonald (26) stressed that complications may arise, particularly when spines are embedded over bony prominences within joints or are in contact with nerves. These authors described a previously unreported case of neuropathy associated with sea urchin injuries. They emphasized that when sea urchin injuries necessitate exploration, aseptic surgical technique is required.

2. *Delayed reactions.* After an interval of 2 or 3 months after the initial injury, delayed reactions may develop. These reactions may be nodular or diffuse. Lesions of both types are very persistent, and although spontaneous resolution may ultimately occur, it cannot be relied upon as a consistent eventuality.

The nodular form of a granulomatous lesion consists of small, firm nodules. Some nodules are flesh colored, although others take on the color of the dye in the spines.

Asada et al. (27) reported a woman who developed a granulomatous dermatitis 10 days after a sea urchin sting. X-rays revealed no spines in the tissue. Several weeks later, ground sea urchin spines extract showed a 2+ patch test reaction with negative controls. This apparently confirmed the possibility of allergic contact dermatitis to residual allergen as a cause of late reactions to aquatic stings.

> The spines of sea urchins are very brittle and easily break off in the skin. They are difficult to remove. The spines have a dye that comes off on the tissue and makes it difficult to tell if anything is left. Secondary infection is common.

Intralesional injections of a corticosteroid are sometimes effective in treating such lesions. If the presence of spines is revealed upon X-ray examination, surgical removal is indicated.

Meneghini (28) reported on a clinical experiment in which he used water-alcohol extracts from the spines of sea urchins. These extracts produced a positive allergic delayed intradermal reaction in two fishermen with sea urchin granulomas. Control subjects did not develop such reaction.

Histologic changes associated with sea urchin lesions show a wide range of variation. There may be microabscesses or a chronic granulomatous inflammatory reaction of foreign-body type (29), and double refractable particles may sometimes be detected (30). However, the histology of the skeletal granulomas may give no clue as to their origin (31).

Halstead (19) emphasized that some sea urchins are of concern to skin divers because of their abundance and the ability of their sharp spines to penetrate sandals, shoes, and flippers. The long-spined tropical sea urchin (*Diadema* and its relatives) is especially hazardous. People diving in the West Indies should take special care because of the great abundance of these urchins in shallow water areas in many of the Caribbean islands. Sea urchins are most commonly encountered under rocks, in crevices, or in other sheltered areas among corals. Sometimes they are found in open sandy flats. The spines inflict mechanical injury and may contain a venom that is not as toxic as that produced by the pedicellariae.

The Pedicellariae

One of the primary functions of pedicellariae is defense. When the sea urchin is at rest in calm water, the valves are generally extended, moving slowly about, awaiting prey. When a foreign body comes in contact with the sea urchin, it is immediately seized. The pedicellariae do not release their hold as long as the object moves, and if it is too strong to be held, the pedicellariae are torn from the test, or shell, but continue to bite the object. Detached pedicellariae may remain alive for several hours after being removed from the sea urchin and may continue to secrete venom into the victim.

> The spines of the sea urchin are less venomous but can produce severe injury. The pedicellariae are more venomous and can continue to secrete venom even after being detached from the sea urchin.

Neurotropic Toxic Effects

Manowitz and Rosenthal (32) stated that urchins of the *Tripneustes* genus, found exclusively in the Pacific Ocean, are capable of liberating histamine and bradykinin-like products. Injury by this organism is followed by severe pain, dyspnea, and giddiness. The toxin appears to be neurotropic for cranial, in particular, facial, nerves. Multiple cranial nerve palsies follow massive envenomation. The local pain remits within 1 hour, but facial nerve paralysis may persist for up to 6 hours.

> Pacific Ocean sea urchins produce a neurotropic toxin that can produce cranial nerve paralysis for several hours.

Treatment

The treatment of sea urchin wounds caused by their spines varies with the type of spine and the area of the body involved. Most sea urchin spines are friable and break off quite easily when grasped with a pair of forceps. Generally, it is difficult to remove sea urchin spines without surgical intervention. If the spine is situated in soft tissue away from bone, it sometimes can be crushed by pummeling the area with the fist. (Local anesthesia may be required for pain.) This tends to fragment the spine, and usually the pieces will be absorbed and disappear in a few days. In other cases, the spines may become encrusted and remain for many months, sometimes migrating to another site, where they may have to be surgically removed. Sea urchin spines penetrating a bone joint should be x-rayed and surgically removed. Failure to remove them may result in a severe chronic inflammatory reaction. Because sea urchin wounds frequently become infected, hot soaks and antibiotic therapy may be required. Pedicellariae envenomations may produce severe reactions because they are more potent than the venom found in the spines of sea urchins. Any pedicellariae clinging to the skin should be promptly removed. Bathing the wound with alcohol or some other antiseptic solution is usually helpful. The affected part should be immersed in hot water (120°F, or 50°C), with care taken not to scald the patient. Artificial respiration may be required. Any allergic reactions can usually be controlled with the use of Adrenalin and antihistamines. Antibiotics may be required.

Preventive Measures

No sea urchin having elongated, needle-like spines should be handled. Moreover, leather and canvas gloves, shoes, and flippers do not afford protection. Care should be taken in handling any tropical species of short-spined sea urchin without gloves because of the pedicellariae. Because of the danger of coming in contact with sea urchins, a diver working at night in coral areas must exercise extreme care.

Starfish Dermatitis

Starfish have simple thorny spines of calcium carbonate crystal (calcite) intermingled with organic substances. The spines arc held erect by a number of muscles. Specialized glandular tissue embedded in the calcite is capable of secreting a toxin that can be discharged into the water or perhaps directly into the skin.

The toxic substance exuded by starfish is apparently diffusible in water and alcohol. Consequently, when large numbers of starfish are present, contact with the surrounding water may produce a pruritic, papulourticarial eruption. Calamine lotion with 0.5% menthol is a soothing preparation for such dermatitis.

The starfish *Acanthaster planci* (crown of thorns) can inflict a painful sting when its venomous aboral spines pierce the skin. Such injury may produce granulomatous lesions requiring surgical excision.

Contact with the spines of the venomous starfish may cause extremely painful wounds accompanied by redness, swelling, numbness, and possible paralysis. Nausea and vomiting may be present, and the wound may become infected. Some persons are sensitive to the slime of this starfish, and contact with the slime may cause a dermatitis.

Sea Cucumber Dermatitis

The visceral liquid ejected by the animal sea cucumbers *Cucumaria* and *Stichopus* can cause irritation of the skin and the eyes (33). The skin manifestation is a papular eruption caused by the toxic material holothurin, which is produced in the body wall of the sea cucumber. Holothurin consists of cardiac glycosides or steroid saponins (34), such as have been previously identified in plants.

In a personal communication to W. L. Orris, M.D., formerly director of Medical Services, Scripps Institution of Oceanography, University of California, San Diego, A. H. Banner, professor of zoology at the University of Hawaii, reported that "when my children were small they took delight in throwing apodous holothurian, *Opheodesoma spectabilis*, at each other. I had finally to forbid it because it caused a skin rash; whether it was from the anchor-shaped spicules or from toxic compounds, I do not know."

Some sea cucumbers feed on the nematocysts of coelenterates and retain the stinging nematocyst apparatus in an intact state for use in their own defense. The clinician should be aware of this possibility in managing skin reactions resulting from contact with sea cucumbers. The application of alcohol to skin that has come in contact with such sea cucumbers will detoxify any nematocysts present.

When the venom of the sea cucumber is expelled into the water and comes in contact with the skin, it produces an inflammatory reaction; if it comes into contact with the eyes, it can cause blindness.

ERUPTIONS AND REACTIONS CAUSED BY MOLLUSKS

The phylum Mollusca consists of unsegmented, soft-bodied invertebrates, most of which secrete calcareous shells. Mollusks respire by means of gills or a modified primitive pulmonary sac; some species are equipped with jaws.

It has been estimated that 45,000 species of mollusks inhabit the waters of the globe, probably constituting the largest single group of biotoxic marine invertebrates of direct importance to humans. Within the phylum Mollusca, the pelecypods (scallops, oysters, clams, etc.) appear to cause the greatest number of human intoxications annually. The next most important group in terms of biotoxicity are the gastropods (snails, slugs), with the cephalopods (squid, octopus, cuttlefish, etc.) ranking third (25).

Only two classes—Gastropoda and Cephalopoda—have been definitely implicated in the precipitation of dermatologic reactions.

Cone Shells

The most dangerous members of the class Gastropoda are of the genus Conus, family Conidae. Many tropical and subtropical species—notably *Conus aulicus, C. geographus, C. gloria-maris, C. marmoreus, C. omaria, C. striatus, C. textile,* and *C. tulipa*—have a venom apparatus well developed enough to inflict human fatalities. A 15% to 20% mortality rate has been reported for some of the more deadly of these gastropods found in Australia and California (35). Off the Florida coast, species such as the Chinese alphabet cone (*C. spurius Auct*) and the queen cone (*C. regius Chemnitz*), have been suspected of being dangerous (36).

Because of the attractiveness of the shells, Conidae varieties are avidly sought after for private and public collections. Hence, victims tend to be careless collectors who have not taken proper precautions.

These potentially deadly creatures are usually only about 4 inches in length. For the most part, they are shallow-water inhabitants. Some species are found in the attached algae of coral reefs; others crawl in the vicinity of coral heads; still others feel most at home in a sandy or coral rubble substrate. Species most hazardous to humans are those that inhabit the sand or rubble. Cone shells are nocturnal creatures; they burrow in the sand or coral in the daytime and emerge to feed at night on a varied fare that includes other gastropods, as well as octopuses, pelecypods, and small fish.

Stinging or venomous mollusks of concern to the skin diver fall largely into two categories: (a) gastropods or univalve mollusks and (b) cephalopods—octopuses and squids.

Envenomization Mechanism

Cone shells inflict their stings by means of venomous radular (rasping) teeth, which lie dormant in a sheath when not in use. When needed, a single tooth passes from the sheath through the pharynx, where it is charged with venom produced in the venom duct. The tooth then passes from the pharynx into the anterior opening of the proboscis and is held there, ready to pierce the victim. The chemistry and pharmacology of cone shell venom have yet to be clearly elucidated; there is some evidence that cone shell venoms vary from one species to the next (37).

Dermatologic Symptoms

Cone shell stings are of the puncture-wound variety. Initial symptoms generally include a sharp stinging or burning sensation, or localized ischemia, cyanosis, and numbness in the area of the wound. Pain is variable. One patient will complain that the pain is excruciating, whereas another will report that it is no greater than an insect sting. Generalized pruritus may be a problem in some patients.

Systemic Symptoms

Numbness, swelling, and paresthesia beginning at the wound site may spread rapidly and involve the entire body, particularly the lips and mouth. In severe cases, early paralysis of the voluntary muscles may be followed by a complete generalized muscular paralysis. Aphonia and dysphagia, if present, may be marked and cause the victim great distress. Blurred vision and diplopia are common symptoms. Gastrointestinal symptoms, with the exception of nausea, are usually absent. Coma and cardiac failure may ensue.

Halstead (37) stated that cone shell stings should be treated like snakebite, with ligature, incision, and removal of the venom by suction. Incision and suction are of little value if more than 1 hour has lapsed since the wound was inflicted. The patient should rest and be moved to a hospital as soon as possible.

When the patient arrives at the hospital, cardiac massage, defibrillation, vasopressor drugs, and so on, may be required. Respiratory depressants should be avoided, and respiratory stimulants are probably useless because of the neuromuscular blocking action of the cone shell venom. Unfortunately, there are no specific antivenins available for cone shell envenomations.

Cone shell stings should be treated like snakebite.

Local Treatment

Treatment of cone shell stings is entirely empiric and symptomatic. Although local measures are usually of little value, syringing the wound with a strong soap solution should be attempted. Heat treatments have been reported to be useful. Local injection of epinephrine has been recommended, but its value remains unproven (38).

Preventive Measures

Collectors who fancy cone shells should always wear gloves. The cone shell should be picked up by the large posterior end of the shell and should be dropped immediately if the proboscis is extended from the pointed anterior end. Cone shells should never be held in the hand any longer than necessary. Most stings have occurred while the collector was attempting to scrape encrusted organic debris from the shell. Possibly, the scraping process stimulates the cone to strike.

Venomous cone shells are capable of releasing a serotonin-like toxin virulent enough to kill young children. Mild cases of cone shell envenomation resemble bee or wasp stings. Severe reactions may lead to paresthesia, paresis, dysphagia, chest tightness, blurred vision, and eventually cardiovascular collapse. Paralysis of the respiratory center is believed to be the usual cause of death.

Sea Butterflies

Pteropods, or sea butterflies, are small gastropods rarely exceeding 1 inch in length. Although they are found in abundance in open seas throughout the world, biologic data about sea butterflies are scarce. Briefly, it is known that they are hermaphroditic and that they feed essentially on protozoans and microscopic algae. There is a total of some 60 species.

Pteropod stings evoke a maculopapular rash resembling that produced by certain coelenterates. However, unlike the dermatologic sequelae associated with coelenterates, sea butterfly stings do not appear to elicit serious dermatologic manifestations following the initial sting.

An outbreak of stingings, presumably caused by the straight-needle pteropod *Creseis acicula*, was reported off St. Petersburg, Florida. The stings were believed to have occurred when these needle-like gastropods penetrated swimmers' bathing suits. Whether the lesions resulted from the mechanical effects of contact or from a toxic substance has never been established. Treatment, when necessary, depends entirely on symptoms.

Octopuses and Other Cephalopods

Few marine creatures have received as much popular attention as the octopus, a member of the Cephalopoda class of mollusks, which also includes squids and cuttlefish. Despite the fabled reputation of "giant octopuses" that threaten ships and attack divers, octopuses and squids are generally harmless and retiring; few are believed to be venomous. The chief exception, ironically, appears to be the tiny *Hapalochlaena maculosa*, or blue-ringed octopus—only 3 to 4 inches long and found mainly in Australian coastal waters. It has been called the world's most deadly octopus—even more deadly, according to Dr. J. Trinka, deputy director of the Commonwealth Serum Laboratories of Australia, than Australian snakes, which are considered the world's most lethal (39). Some experts have reported a 25% mortality rate after bites by the blue-ringed octopus. Normally *H. maculosa* is a rather inconspicuous creature, but when threatened or angered the bluish patterns on its predominantly yellowish brown body and arms become an iridescent peacock blue. These bright colors often attract bathers and divers.

Human fatalities and near fatalities seem to follow a fairly identical pattern (40). The octopus, found stranded in a rock pool, is placed on the back of the hand or arm and displayed to interested parties, or carried to the beach. Frequently the victim is unaware of any actual bite, but symptoms occur within 5 or 10 minutes.

The bite usually manifests as two small puncture wounds produced by the sharp, parrot-like jaws of the cephalopod. Pain, when immediately present, is a burning and stinging sensation; some patients describe it as similar to that of a bee sting. Initially localized, the pain may radiate to include the entire appendage. Within a few minutes, a tingling or pulsating sensation develops in the area of the wound. The profuse and prolonged bleeding characteristic of these stings suggests that coagulation time is retarded. Swelling, redness, and heat generally develop around the wound, and some victims complain of an intense pruritus. Allergic urticarial reaction has also been reported (41).

In severe cases, systemic symptoms may include numbness of the mouth and tongue, blurring of vision, difficulty in speech and swallowing, loss of tactile sensation and equilibrium, and muscular paralysis. Death, when it occurs, appears to be associated with respiratory failure.

DERMATITIS CAUSED BY SPONGES, ALGAE, AND MOSSES

Sponges are stationary animals living attached to the sea bottom. Our familiar bath sponges are in fact the skeletons of certain Porifera that inhabit warm waters. These skeletons are composed of spongin, a fibrous material that retains its elastic properties long after the sponge is dead. Sponges were recorded as plants for many centuries but received animal status from zoologists in 1835. Mitchell reports that in a textbook on dermatology, a paper on a skin reaction from the sponge, *Tedania ignis*, is erroneously listed under dermatitis from plants. Both freshwater animal sponges and marine animal sponges can cause contact dermatitis.

Fire Sponge Dermatitis

Tedania ignis, also known as fire sponge, is abundant in the Miami area and near the shore along the Florida Keys. The nickname is appropriate when one considers both the fire sponge's color and its stinging apparatus. The color is normally a brilliant vermilion or reddish orange, although orange or yellowish orange fire sponges are occasionally seen. The sponge grows as a bunch of branches or "fingers" extending upward from a main base. Despite its stinging powers, it usually harbors a host of marine worms, shrimps, and other small crustacea that live unharmed in the central cavity.

The fire sponge has no commercial value but is nonetheless a beautiful creature.

If detached, or particularly if one of the "fingers" is broken, the fire sponge is capable of producing a dermatitis resembling that of poison ivy. The patient initially experiences an itching or prickling sensation, followed in a few hours by swelling, stiffness, and considerable discomfort. If the fingers are stung, they become immovable within 1 day; any attempt to flex them is accompanied by pain. Symptoms usually subside within 2 days, when there is a gradual reduction of swelling and return of normal movement in the affected area. Treatment of fire sponge dermatitis is the same as for severe poison ivy dermatitis.

In addition to the skin reaction, fire sponge can produce an erythema multiforme–type of eruption. This reaction has been attributed to a pharmacologically active substance that may also be a sensitizer.

Poison Bun Sponge Dermatitis

Less common than *Tedania,* the poison bun sponge *(Fibula nolitangere)* ranges into somewhat deeper water. The appellation *nolitangere* ("do not touch") is appropriate: *Fibula's* sting is reported to produce an even more violent reaction than that of the fire sponge.

The poison bun sponge is relatively difficult to recognize, because it closely resembles a number of other common sponges in size, shape, and color. It generally grows in small masses, occasionally in small lumps, and the oscula (holes) are usually large enough to admit a finger. Fibula is brownish on the outside and drab on the inside with a soft "bready" texture. The skin is exposed to the toxic substance when one contacts the surface of this sponge or breaks it.

Red Sponge Dermatitis

The red sponge *(Microciona prolifera)* may produce erythema and edema of the hands and stiffness of the joints in oyster fishermen and others who handle it. Subsequently, bullae develop and may become purulent. If not properly treated, the eruption may persist for several months.

A patch test with a small piece of sponge confirms the diagnosis. The treatment is the same as for severe poison ivy dermatitis.

Sponge Spicule Dermatitis

In addition to the stinging sponges, which produce dermatitis via chemical action, some sponges can cause traumatic injuries. Certain sponges are equipped with a skeletal matrix containing silicon dioxide spicules or calcium carbonate spicules. Both types may produce an irritation when broken off in the skin, and both are difficult to remove once they have penetrated.

The application of adhesive tape to the affected area is sometimes efficacious, because the spicules may adhere to the tape. Isopropyl alcohol should be applied after the adhesive tape is removed. Patients should be advised to wear canvas gloves when handling living sponges that can cause injuries.

Commercial sponges have no spicules.

Sponge and Anemone

Because the coelenterate, the sea anemone, may live symbiotically with sponges, exposure may produce a nematocyst dermatitis.

Seaweed Dermatitis Due to Algae

Approximately 30,000 species of algae have been identified. Although they are included among the lowest divisions of the vegetable kingdom and most contain chlorophyll, many algae are equipped with flagella and propel themselves through the water very much like animals (42). Algae grow in a variety of sizes, shapes, and colors. The smallest are microscopic, such as the snowflake-like diatoms, which are barely a micron in diameter. The giant kelp, which may attain a length of 300 feet, is among the largest algae.

One of the plant kingdom's most ubiquitous members, algae may be found in almost every type of environment. Primitive blue-green algae thrive in the water of hot springs that attain a temperature of 160°F; others may be found in freshwater and saltwater and in the snow, ice, and waters of the Arctic regions (43). Some are saprophytic or symbiotic—growing in or on other plants and animals. Viable, growing algae have been found at ocean depths of 12,000 feet, despite the fact that sunlight can only penetrate ocean waters to a depth of 900 feet. The algae of medical importance to the dermatologist are those found in running waters, ponds, lakes, and oceans. These consist mainly of the blue-green alga *(Lyngbya majuscul). Lyngbya* looks somewhat like hair. Not all strains are toxic. One area may have a toxic strain, although the algae just a few miles away may be nontoxic. *Lyngbya* occurs in abundance from the intertidal zone to a depth of 100 feet—representing a hazard to sensitized swimmers.

Grauer and Arnold (44) reported 125 cases of seaweed dermatitis treated in Hawaii after contact with *Lyngbya.* Hundreds of other mild, unreported cases were suspected. The cases occurred at beaches from Laie and Kaawa to Lanikai—and possibly Waimanalo—with no instances of occurrence in Kaneohe Bay. (Later, Hawaiian dermatologists saw similar cases where the alga was encountered on the windward beaches.) The following pattern emerged during this epidemic of *Lyngbya* dermatitis (44).

1. The patient had been swimming, often in water made turbid by suspended fragments of seaweed.
2. He or she continued to wear the wet bathing suit after leaving the ocean and before showering.
3. A gradual onset of itching and burning occurred within a few minutes to a few hours after emerging from the ocean.
4. Visible dermatitis beginning with redness appeared after 3 to 8 hours.

The initial symptoms are followed by blisters and deep desquamation, leaving a moist, bright red, tender, and painful area on the scrotum, perineum, or perianal region. The eruption appears on the area of the body covered by the bathing suit; male patients are especially affected on the most dependent part of the scrotum, producing "great balls of fire." Women patients, especially those wearing close-fitting brassieres, are occasionally affected on the breasts.

A few instances of skin reactions to freshwater blue-green algae have also been reported (45,46).

A number of similarities between seaweed dermatitis and sea bathers' eruption have been noted. Both eruptions occur in the same body region after the patients swim in salt water at a time when an unusually large amount of seaweed is found on the beaches or in the water. The disorders have a seasonal incidence, occurring in the spring and summer (March to September in Florida and June to September in Hawaii). Finally, both are characterized by a pruritic eruption ensuing within a few hours after swimming, persisting for a few days, and subsiding spontaneously. Obviously, therefore, differential diagnosis between the two conditions may be necessary.

An eruption confined to areas of the skin covered by a bathing suit or a scuba wet or dry suit suggests dermatitis caused by blue-green alga (Lyngbya majuscula), which is common from near the water surface to a depth of about 30 meters (100 ft).

The most effective measures are prophylactic. Advise patients who swim or dive in a seaweed-rich area to bathe with soap and water immediately after emerging from the water to prevent L. majuscula dermatitis. They should also wash bathing suits to remove bits of clinging seaweed. Cleaning the beach of accumulated seaweed is also helpful. Specific treatment is not usually necessary, but severe dermatitis may require systemic corticosteroids.

Solomon and Stoughton (47) demonstrated that cutaneous inflammation was induced by debromoaplysiatoxin, a purified toxin extracted from L. majuscula Gomont. This alga causes a seaweed dermatitis that occurs in persons who have swum off the coast of Oahu in Hawaii. By topical application, the toxin was found to produce an irritant pustular folliculitis in humans and to cause a severe cutaneous inflammatory reaction in rabbits and in hairless mice.

> **Hawaiian seaweed dermatitis is an irritant dermatitis caused by a toxin in a blue-green alga. In males the scrotum may be severely affected.**

Cardellina et al. (48) also reported that a highly inflammatory and vesicatory substance, lyngbyatoxin A, has been isolated from the lipid extract of L. majuscula Gomont; its gross structure was determined from chemical and spectral data. Lyngbyatoxin A is closely related to teleocidin B, a poisonous substance associated with several strains of Streptomyces.

The condition should be treated in the same manner as a mild poison ivy dermatitis. Proper protective clothing usually prevents occurrence of the eruption.

Iodide Eruption Caused by Ingestion of Kelp (a Giant Alga)

Pustular eruptions or exacerbation of acne may be related to eating kelp, a giant brown alga, or taking kelp tablets, a practice common among health food enthusiasts. Kelp contains a great deal of iodide; the eruption is, in fact, iododerma.

Protothecosis

Protothecosis is a cutaneous or disseminated infection caused by Prototheca, an achloric mutant of the green alga, Chlorella.

In general, the principal importance of algae to medicine and sanitation has been related to toxicoses and the production of an offensive odor or taste in contaminated water supplies. The blue-green algae often are indicators of sewage contamination of streams or lakes (49).

Prototheca has been found in fresh and marine water and in sewage treatment systems. Although several species have been described, only two—P. segbwema and P. wickerhamii—have been demonstrated as pathogens in humans. There is some evidence indicating that achloric mutants of other genera of algae also exist and that some may have medical significance (50).

Protothecosis has diverse clinical manifestations. It is probable that infection is initiated via entry of the organism through preexisting openings in the skin. Immunosuppressed individuals are at special risk of infection with these algae.

Florida Seaweed Dermatitis

Sargassum natans has been reported to cause an acute, mildly pruritic urticarial eruption upon contact (51). This alga occurs commonly in waters off southeastern Florida in the winter months. The eruption occurred in two children playing with the seaweed, and reproduction of the eruption was demonstrated in a volunteer. The reaction occurred within seconds to minutes and was self-limited, requiring no treatment. No nematodes were seen upon inspection of the seaweed.

Japanese Sargassum Allergy

Two eel fishermen were shown to have positive patch test to Japanese sargassum (Sargassum muticum), which is a brown algae of the order Fucales (52). Further study revealed positive patch tests to potassium iodide as well. Brown algae contain high amounts of iodine, up to 2.5 mg/kg of dried material (48).

> **Kelp, which is a giant alga, contains iodine, which may produce an iodide eruption in health food enthusiasts taking kelp tablets.**

Red Moss Dermatitis

Although the animal named red moss (Microciona) has been reported to cause a contact reaction on the hands of fishermen, anemones living on the moss actually may be responsible (53).

Skin reactions attributed to plant moss (*Iosthecium*) are probably caused by contamination of the moss by allergenic chemical compounds of the liverwort plant *(Frullania)*, which grows among the moss (54).

DERMATITIS CAUSED BY AQUATIC WORMS OR THEIR LARVAE

Aquatic worms that may affect the skin of man include the cercarial stage of tropical schistosomes, the adult bristle-worms, and leeches.

Schistosome Cercarial Dermatitis

Cercarial dermatitis is an infestation resulting from penetration of the skin by the cercariae of schistosomes, the larval forms of digenetic (requiring at least two separate hosts for completion of their life cycle) trematodes. These schistosomes are parasitic flatworms having one or more external suckers. Their cercariae—immature larval forms—are usually microscopic and are provided with tails.

The flukes are members of the phylum Platyhelminthes, which includes the class Turbellaria (the planarians), the class Cestoda (the tapeworms), and the class Trematoda (the flukes). Under normal circumstances, the definitive hosts of many fluke species are parasites of a wide variety of vertebrates, including human beings in some instances. In the case of marine schistosomal dermatitis, the definitive host is a marine bird or some other marine vertebrate (55).

Schistosome cercarial dermatitis is sometimes referred to as a "disease of the place," exemplifying the widespread geographic distribution of the condition. Reports of schistosome cercarial dermatitis have come from virtually every area of the globe—Occident, Orient, Arctic, temperate and tropical zones, in fresh, brackish, or salt water.

According to health officials, schistosomal infestation—including the dermatitis-producing type—may rival malaria as the world's number one health problem. In western Africa, the Orient, and the West Indies, many agricultural workers are endangered by this infestation while in irrigation waters. Swimming and diving activities have become a serious hazard in infested streams or lakes.

Although serious schistosomal infestation is not common in North America, cercarial dermatitis has become a vexing problem on certain freshwater and even saltwater beaches. Snails and birds inhabiting the lake areas of Wisconsin, Michigan, and neighboring north central states are the intermediate hosts for the infestation.

Terminology

The discussion of schistosome cercarial dermatitis is cluttered by various synonyms that are sometimes used interchangeably: clam-diggers' itch, swimmers' itch, and sea bathers' eruption. Some observers have insisted on a distinction between swimmers' itch and sea bathers' eruption, limiting swimmers' itch to the eruption on exposed areas and sea bathers' eruption to a dermatitis resulting from ocean bathing.

These distinctions are artificial and confusing. It is more appropriate to speak of schistosome cercarial dermatitis when such organisms have been identified, while continuing to use sea bathers' eruption for cases in which no specified organism has been implicated.

Ecologic Cycle

Cercarial dermatitis results when a person becomes an unwitting interloper in a rather complex ecologic cycle. The adults of the dermatitis-producing schistosomes are blood parasites of birds or mammals. The typical cycle begins with the hatching of the schistosome eggs, which are present in the droppings of infested animals (56). Appropriate species of snails become infested upon contact with the miracidia hatched from the eggs, and the snails then serve as an intermediate host.

Environmental factors, including water temperature and light, trigger the release of cercariae from the snail into the surrounding water, at which point they swim about in search of a definitive vertebrate host, usually a water fowl but on occasion a terrestrial mammal such as a mouse, vole, muskrat, or deer (32). The cercariae attempt to penetrate the skin of any organism with which they come in contact, including human being. Cercariae in humans do not usually complete their life cycle, which includes systemic invasion, since humans are not their natural hosts. This ecologic chain is completed when the adult worms produce eggs. Although penetration of cercariae may take place in the water, it usually occurs as the film of water evaporates on the skin (57).

Thus, the diver or swimmer who contracts schistosome cercarial dermatitis has accidentally intruded into the normal life cycle of these parasites.

Clinical Features

Schistosome cercarial dermatitis is a skin infestation characterized by an intensely pruritic maculopapular rash caused by an immune response in a person, an unnatural host. Further infestations tend to become more severe as sensitization takes place. The response induces local destruction of cercariae, producing an allergic reaction to dead cercariae. The cercariae are actually walled off and destroyed in the epithelial layers of the skin. Wood et al. (55) described the histopathology as follows: The cercariae are apparently unable to penetrate beyond the papillary dermis; histologic examination of infested tissue shows intraepithelial burrows and abscesses surrounded by and filled with eosinophils, polymorphonuclear leukocytes, and lymphocytes. Cercariae themselves are not seen in serial sections.

The patient initially experiences a prickling sensation, followed by rapid development of urticarial wheals. These wheals subside in about a half hour, leaving minute macules. Severe itching and edema occur after some hours. Transformation of macules into papules—and occasionally pustules—reaches maximum intensity in 2 to 3 days. The papular and sometimes hemorrhagic rash heals in 1 to 2 weeks but may be complicated by excoriated lesions. Secondary infection with the formation of purulent lesions is common.

Barnes (57) described cercarial dermatitis as essentially a sensitization phenomenon. He noted that local skin lesions produced by the schistosomes are slight, but with continuous reinfestation, sensitized persons may show a definite dermatitis. Repeated infestations tend to become increasingly severe.

There has been some discussion whether the dermatitis-producing schistosome cercariae of North America can also induce systemic infestation. Most commentators have dismissed this possibility.

Walther (58) reported that a 17-year-old boy with chronic papules of the scrotum showed no improvement after topical therapy. A skin biopsy specimen showed *Schistosoma mansoni* eggs. No evidence of bladder or bowel involvement was found. No treatment is necessary for schistosomal infections without severe symptoms or excessive egg production.

The clinical findings in a group of persons exposed to cercariae in a Delaware state park have been reviewed. Thirty of 37 persons who waded in a coastal shellfishing area developed dermatitis. Twenty-four started itching within 2 hours after exposure. All developed itching and papules after 12 hours. Vesicles occurred in 25 (83%) and secondary bacterial infection in 4. The eruptions were self-limited, with only two of the patients requiring systemic corticosteroids (59).

Microbilharzia variglandis was the offending schistosome.

Bastert et al. (60) described a case of cercarial dermatitis in an aquarium hobbyist. The eruption was localized to hands and arms and occurred after cleaning an aquarium containing local cold-water snails. The causative organism was of the genus *trichobilharzia*.

Differential Diagnosis

Differential diagnosis would include insect bites, scabies, drug eruption, and contact dermatitis. A distribution that excludes the bathing suit area would make scabies less likely, and knowledge of multiple cases and association with swimming should suggest the correct diagnosis.

Zaki and Nuzzi (61) of the Department of Health Services, County of Suffolk, Long Island, New York, reported that there are many instances of sea bathers' eruption on Long Island. Particularly during the bathing season (although not confined to that period), the department receives complaints concerning the development of rashes on exposed areas of the skin after direct contact with coastal waters. The complainant is generally apprehensive, fearing that he or she may have been in contact with polluted waters, and the complaint is often accompanied by a request to sample the waters in question for bacteriologic quality.

Leeches

Leeches have played a Jekyll and Hyde role in the existence of humans. In its Jekyll guise, the medicinal leech was used routinely for bloodletting from ancient times until the nineteenth century. In many areas of the world, it is still a time-honored therapy.

In its Hyde aspect, the leech has been implicated in a number of disastrous historic events. Tennent (62) described how land leeches routed an entire battalion of English soldiers from their wooded encampment in Ceylon. Harmer and Shipley (63) reported on a genus of freshwater leeches that harassed Napoleon's soldiers in the Nile region.

Leeches are classified in the phylum Annelida (segmented worms), in which they constitute the class Hirudinea. They can be further categorized under marine, freshwater, and terrestrial types. Marine leeches have a salt-water habitat and feed on fishes. Freshwater leeches—still used as therapeutic agents in certain regions—are present in lakes, ponds, and creeks. Terrestrial leeches are especially common in tropical rain forests.

Leeches attach themselves to the skin, feed until engorged, then fall off. At the site of attachment, the leech introduces an anticoagulant, hirudin, as well as antigenic substances that have not been specifically identified. The leech draws out blood in considerable excess of its maximum needs.

The wound bleeds freely and heals slowly in unsensitized individuals, even when not infected by pyogenic organisms. If sensitization has developed, reaction to the bite may be urticarial, bullous, or necrotic. Heldt (64) reported that the bite of the leech can cause serious allergic reactions, including anaphylaxis.

Individuals walking through streams or marshes are the usual victims of leech bites; in areas where leeches are still used medicinally, allergic reactions may complicate treatment.

Removal of leeches may be facilitated by application of a few drops of brine, alcohol, or strong vinegar, or a match flame applied near the site of attachment. These measures force the leech to release its hold. Leeches should never be pulled off the skin, lest the jaws remain in the wounds and induce phagedenic ulcers.

Reactions to bites of leeches include freely bleeding wound; necrotic, urticarial, or bullous reactions; and anaphylaxis.

In removing a leech, do not pull it from the skin, because the jaws may remain in the wound and produce a phagedenic ulcer. Apply salt water, alcohol, vinegar, or a match flame near the site of attachment.

Bristle Worm Dermatitis

Certain sea worms belonging to the family Amphinomidae are equipped with tufts of silky chitinous bristles arranged in rows around their bodies. When a worm is touched or stimulated in some other fashion, the bristles are raised in defense, and the body of the worm contracts simultaneously. Thus, an almost continuous defensive armor of bristles is presented to those who disturb the worm.

These bristles detach easily, penetrating the skin in much the same way as the spines of the prickly pear cactus. The spines are as difficult to remove as cactus spines; each spine has to be removed individually.

The common bristle worm of the lower east coast of Florida and the Florida Keys is *Hermodice carunculata* Kinberg. Commonly attaining a length of a foot or more and a width of nearly an inch, this species is generally found on coral, rock slabs, and sponges, as well as in porous rock. The worm itself is green with reddish markings along the sides, and the white bristles are tipped with dull red. Although the bristle tufts appear small when the worm is not in a fighting mood, these white tufts "blossom" impressively when *H. carunculata* is disturbed.

Amphinema brasiliensis resembles *H. carunculata* except that the gills are red; their bristle stings are similar.

In contrast to *Hermodice*—which is a sea bottom worm—*Chloeia euglochis* Ehlers is a freely swimming bristle worm often found near the water surface, swimming by means of short, wavelike undulations. There are instances of *Chloeia* being caught on a hook as they attempt to settle on the bait (65).

In various parts of the world, the following worms produce a bristle-worm dermatitis:

Chloeia flava (Pallas), Malayan coast
C. viridis (Schmarda), West Indies, Gulf of California, Mexico south to Panama
Euythoe complanata (Pallas), Australia and the tropical seas
Hermodice carunculata (Pallas), tropical eastern America and eastern Gulf of Mexico

Bristle worm dermatitis is caused by penetration of bristles into the skin. Each bristle must be removed individually.

Contact with a bristle worm produces a burning sensation accompanied by moderate edema, a papular eruption, and occasionally necrotic lesions. Itching, pain, and paresthesia are frequent symptoms.

In treating worm "stings," the bristles must be removed carefully with forceps. Scraping is usually ineffective, as the bristles tend to break off and remain embedded in the skin. However, an effective method of removing bristles is to cover them with adhesive tape. When the tape is pulled off, the attached bristles are usually removed with it. After removal, application of diluted ammonia water or alcohol can be soothing. In an emergency situation, rubbing the affected area may have an immediate palliative effect.

Worm Bites

Certain segmented worms bite with chitinous jaws, producing a stinging pain. Edema and itching may follow. The application of cold compresses or alcohol is soothing. Handling of any sea worms should be avoided unless gloves are worn.

Blood Worm (Glycera)

The chitinous jaws of *Glycera* are able to penetrate the skin and produce a painful sensation similar to that of a bee sting. The marks from the jaws are oval-shaped and are about as large as the inner circle of the following letter *O,* in the center of which is a small reddish spot usually indicating where the jaws have pierced the skin, and are bordered by a surrounding area of blanching. The wounded area may become hot and swollen and may remain so for a day or two. The swelling may be followed by numbness and itching.

Biting Reef Worm (Eunice Aphroditois)

Eunice aphroditois may attain a length of 5 feet (1.5 m) and is equipped with large chitinous jaws that are capable of inflicting a nasty bite. The wounds may be a few millimeters in diameter, soon becoming swollen, hot, and inflamed. These wounds can become infected.

Some aquatic worms can inflict a painful bite; they should be handled with gloves.

DERMATITIS CAUSED BY OTHER MACROSCOPIC ORGANISMS

Crab Larvae Irritation

Burnett and Cargo (66) reported that a cutaneous irritation on exposed skin surfaces can be induced by crab larvae.

The larvae, which are small, gray, translucent bodies, feel like "floating sand particles" or "small gray seeds." A large flotilla of them touching bathers is described as "pine needles sticking skin." Neither urticaria nor any other type of eruption occurs following contact. The unusual sensations appear rapidly and disappear when the larval forms are removed from the body.

> **Crab larvae may produce a "prickling" sensation without dermatitis, particularly when embedded under a bathing suit.**

These larvae have calcified spines that can induce injury in humans. The lack of resultant eruption in the area of irritation supports the hypothesis that the sensation is traumatically induced rather than mediated by a venom. Additionally, no glandlike structure has been reported at the base of these spines.

A more recent report indicated that the larvae form of a xanthid crab (Rhithropanopeus harisii) which is found along the East Coast of the United States, can cause this type of eruption. The blue crab (Callinectes sapidus) which occurs in the Atlantic Ocean off Maryland, can cause a similar eruption (67).

Sea Louse Dermatitis

Although water skiers, skin divers, and swimmers who frequent the waters of the Southern California coast have long been acquainted with the sharp bite of sea lice, sea louse dermatitis (cymothoidism) has only recently found its way into the medical literature (68).

Sea lice are actually small marine crustaceans of the order Isopoda, suborder Cymothoidea of the crab family. These active and free-swimming crustaceans generally inhabit the shoal waters of tropical and temperate estuarial shorelines (69). Frequently burying themselves in the sandy bottom below the water level, cymothoids will readily prey on any organism that intrudes on their immediate domain (70). Although they usually feed on higher marine animals, sea lice will also, as suggested, attack humans.

Cymothoids are equipped with a powerful biting apparatus that can quickly attach itself to fish or human extremities. The bite is rapid and sharp, causing punctate hemorrhagic wounds at the site.

The injured area should be cleansed with hydrogen peroxide, and an antibiotic ointment should be applied to the hemorrhagic crusts that usually form.

> **The bite of the sea louse typically produces hemorrhagic puncture wounds.**

Soapfish Dermatitis

Fishermen in the Virgin Islands and Puerto Rico are aware that keeping a soapfish in a restricted volume of seawater with other fish often results in the death of the other fish. Fortunately, human contact with a soapfish (Rypticus saponaceus), family Grammistidae, produces nothing worse than dermatitis.

The soapfish receives its name from the soapy mucus it releases when handled or otherwise disturbed. The skin irritant in this mucus is called grammistin.

Similar irritant substances have been isolated from certain species of boxfish and sea bass (71,72).

As with any acute irritant dermatitis, cold compresses of Burrow's solution allay the burning and itching sensation produced by contact with the mucus of these fish.

Randall et al. (73) reported the following experience with a soapfish:

> While diving in the Florida Keys, [I] became aware, in an unusual way, that something exuded from the soapfish . . . is very noxious. About a 9-inch (228.6-mm) adult was speared. . . . Rather than carry the fish all the way to the boat at the surface, it was temporarily stored inside [my] bathing trunks. Very soon it became apparent that a secretion from this fish was a powerful urethral irritant, and it was promptly removed from the bathing suit.

Soapfish dermatitis is caused by the irritant effect of a toxin (grammistin) in the soapy mucus released by irritated soapfish, boxfish, and sea bass.

INJURIES AND ERUPTIONS CAUSED BY VENOMOUS FISH SPINES AND FISH SKIN

Dermatitis Caused by Poison Spines

Many species of fish are capable of inflicting painful and dangerous lacerations by means of dorsal or caudal spines provided with complex venom glands.

In warmer waters, the species of stingray, scorpion fish, catfish, rabbit fish, stargazers, and toadfish are the most common fish that produce poison spine dermatitis.

In colder waters, the weaver, the spiny dogfish, the Norwegian haddock, and several species of stingray found on the Atlantic coast can inflict serious wounds.

The puncture wounds and lacerations of fish spines may produce intense pain for several hours. Edema and erythema around penetrated skin may stimulate a bacterial cellulitis. The wound may, indeed, become infected and may be very slow in healing. Certain poison spines quickly produce systemic symptoms. Shock, vomiting, abdominal pain, profuse sweating, and tachycardia may be followed by muscular paralysis and death.

Little is known of the chemical and pharmacologic nature of fish spine venom, except that it is heat labile. Therefore, wounds from "poison" fish spines should be treated with heat.

> **The venom introduced by certain fish spines is heat labile.**

There is a division of opinion regarding the advisability and efficacy of using a ligature in the treatment of fish stings. If more than 10 minutes has lapsed since the sting was made, it is doubtful that a ligature is of any value. If used, the ligature should be placed at once between the site of the sting and the body, but as near the wound as possible. The ligature should be released every few minutes to maintain adequate circulation. Most doctors recommend soaking the injured member in hot water for 30 minutes to 1 hour. The water should be maintained at as high a temperature (120°F, or 50°C) as the patient can tolerate without injury, and the treatment should be instituted as soon as possible. If the wound is on the face or body, hot moist compresses should be used. The heat may have an attenuating effect on the venom because heating readily destroys stingray venom *in vitro*. Intravenous calcium gluconate injections are sometimes helpful. The addition of magnesium sulfate or Epsom salts to the water is believed to be useful. Infiltration of the wound area with 0.5% to 2% procaine has been used with good results. If local measures fail to prove satisfactory, intramuscular or intravenous Demerol will generally be efficacious. Following the soaking procedure, debridement and further cleansing of the wound may be desirable. Lacerated wounds should be closed with dermal sutures. If the wound is large, a small drain should be left in it for 1 or 2 days. The injured area should be covered with an antiseptic and sterile dressing.

Stingray Envenomization

Depicted as "demons of the sea," "denizens of the deep," or "devil fish," stingrays are elasmobranchs that have been recognized as venomous since ancient times. They were known to Aristotle and Pliny; Dioscorides (c. 100 B.C.) gave the first detailed description of convulsions and death due to stingray envenomation. Eleven species of stingrays have been identified on the coasts of the United States: seven in the Atlantic Ocean and four in the Pacific Ocean.

These flat, smooth sea creatures have a characteristic round, kite, or diamond shape and a long whiplike tail. They range in size from a diameter of several inches to a breadth of 4 to 5 feet. *Dasyatis sabina*, especially abundant in Tampa Bay, reaches a maximum breadth of about 1 foot. Other species may attain a length of more than 14 feet. Most people afflicted with stingray wounds acquire them via contact with the smaller species that frequent shallow waters around rocky areas and burrow themselves in the sand.

Stingrays are mainly scavengers, feeding on small crustaceans and fish scraps. They glide slowly about with alternate winglike motions of their pectoral fins. When they come to rest with a sudden quick movement of the fins, they stir up a cloud of sand that covers their entire body except for their eyes. Stingrays are not aggressive. When startled, the ray will usually hasten away at great speed, leaving behind a muddy wake. But their habit of lying motionless in shallow water makes them easily stepped on by the unwary bather or wader.

Venom Apparatus

The "sting" of the stingray is a bilaterally serrated, dentinal caudal spine located on the dorsum of the animal's tail. Within this dentinal structure are venomous canals containing loose, reticular tissues and small, thin-walled blood vessels. A thin layer of compact matrix is seen at the surface of the spine. The spine is encased in an integumentary sheath, and the venom is contained within the ventrolateral grooves.

When the stingray is accidentally stepped on, pressure of the foot on the dorsum of the fish provokes it to thrust its tail upward and forward, driving its sting into the victim's foot or leg. When the sting enters the flesh, the integumentary sheath is ruptured, releasing the venom into the victim's tissues. As the spine is withdrawn, the integumentary sheath may be torn free and remain embedded in the wound.

> **The venomous spines of the stingray are located in the animal's tail, which lashes forcefully in response to danger.**

Symptoms

Stingray wounds may be large and severely lacerated. Russell (74) reported that a sting no wider than 5 mm may produce a wound approximately 3 cm long, and larger stings may produce wounds as long as 7 inches.

Patients stung by stingrays (usually in the foot or leg) describe the experience as similar to having received a sharp, painful stab. The stinging is followed by the immediate onset of intense pain. The pain can be quite excruciating, increasing in severity during the first 90 minutes after contact. The pain appears to be out of proportion to that which might be produced by nonvenomous fish or by stepping on a broken bottle or bivalve.

Examination generally reveals a freely bleeding puncture or laceration, often contaminated with parts of the stingray's integumentary sheath. Discoloration is generally not pronounced immediately after the injury, but within 2 hours discoloration around the edges may extend several centimeters from the wound. If left untreated, necrosis of this area is fairly common. Edema is a frequent finding and may persist for several weeks in untreated patients.

Although symptoms and signs of envenomization are usually localized to the injured area, a number of systemic symptoms can occur. These range from syncope, weakness, nausea, and anxiety, to generalized cramps, fasciculations in the muscles of the affected extremity, inguinal or axillary pain, and respiratory distress. Arrhythmias, paresthesia, and convulsions may also occur.

Treatment

The wound should be debrided of all pieces of spine and sheath, and heat should be applied immediately—preferably by immersion in hot water or by means of hot, wet compresses. High temperatures may be attained if the extremity is first immersed in comfortably hot water; hotter water can be added as acclimatization takes place (75).

Relief from pain is usually immediate. Continue hot soaking for at least 30 minutes, and repeat if the pain returns. Occasionally, several heat treatments may prove necessary to neutralize all the venom present.

In severe envenomization, a tourniquet induces slow venous return and may be lifesaving. Use elastic material applied just tight enough to allow insertion of the index finger under the tourniquet. Treatment for shock may be necessary. Tetanus prophylaxis should be given after any penetrating marine injury (76).

Prevention

Stings may also be inflicted by rays speared or caught in nets or on lines. There is no reliable report of a ray stinging while swimming free. Patients should be advised to exercise considerable care when wading in shallow waters known to be inhabited by stingrays.

Freshwater Rays

Freshwater stingrays are found in the Atlantic rivers of tropical and temperate South America and Africa and in the Mekong River of Laos. In all of these regions, the sting of the freshwater rays is greatly feared. Stingrays are widely distributed in streams of the Amazon River and Rio de la Plata, and numerous stories and superstitions attest to the fear inspired by this creature in pioneers and natives. The subject of freshwater stingray envenomization has been intensively studied only in recent years. General clinical features and treatment measures appear to be similar to those associated with envenomization caused by the saltwater species (77).

Scorpion Fish and Stonefish Envenomization

Scorpion fish are the most venomous of all fish. The spine venom found in several species that inhabit tropical seas—especially the venom of the notorious stonefish (Synanceja)—has been compared to cobra venom in its neurotoxicity. The stonefish has been justifiably described as the most dangerous of all stinging fishes.

Members of the family Scorpaenidae, scorpion fishes have been classified into 350 separate species, including the lionfish, zebra fish, bullrout, and waspfish. Widely distributed throughout all tropical and most temperate seas, the greatest number of species are found in the tropical Indo-Pacific. Some scorpion fish closely resemble sea bass, although others are exquisitely modified to mimic patches of seaweed in shape and color. The most dangerous are remarkably camouflaged to resemble algae-covered rocks or to blend in with the small coral masses among which they live (78).

Although the spine venom of local species of scorpion fish is less toxic than that of Indo-Pacific species, it should be remembered that they are nonetheless highly venomous and have the potential to cause severe dermatologic and systemic effects. Scorpion fish are common about the Florida Keys, the Caribbean, the Gulf of Mexico, and Southern California; the California species is often called sculpin.

Most scorpion fish stings result when an individual removes the fish from a hook or net and is jabbed by the venomous spines. Stonefish are especially dangerous because of the difficulty of detecting them from their surroundings. One should use caution when placing one's hand in the crevices or in holes inhabited by these fish. Knowledge of the habits and appearance of these fish is important.

The venom of scorpion fish is contained within the tissues that envelop certain of the dorsal, pelvic, and anal fin spines. The number of venomous spines varies with the species, as does the structure of the venom gland or venom-containing tissues. Envenomization occurs from mechanical pressure on the spine, which tears the integumentary sheath and allows the venom to escape into the wound.

Stonefish venom is heat labile with neurotoxic and myotoxic effects primarily. Hemolytic effects are not clinically significant (79).

Because of their protective coloring and their habit of lying motionless on the rocky bottoms or burying themselves in the sand, scorpion fish are easily stepped on. When this occurs, the spine sheaths are depressed and the poison glands are stimulated into releasing their contents; the stinging action is virtually automatic.

Intense pain, localized swelling, discoloration, and paresthesia around the wound are common reactions. Systemic symptoms and signs may include lymphadenitis, nausea, vomiting, weakness, pallor, and syncope. Untreated patients may suffer respiratory distress, shock, and coma.

The poison spines of scorpion fish produce a wound that should be treated like snakebite and for which an antivenin is available.

First-aid treatment for scorpion fish stings is similar to that used in cases of snakebite. The wound should be opened with a knife or lancet and the surrounding area squeezed or sucked to remove as much poison as possible. Sucking with the lips will not have harmful effects, since any poison that may be swallowed is quickly neutralized by stomach acids. If bleeding is not too profuse, it can be allowed to continue for 1 or 2 minutes. However, prolonged bleeding should be stopped by placing a tourniquet at the nearest joint adjacent to the wound.

Immersion of the limb in hot water may bring symptomatic relief and is recommended to deactivate the toxins.

The Commonwealth Laboratories of Melbourne, Australia, have made available an antivenom for the treatment of stonefish spine poisoning, but it is uncertain if this is available in the United States.

Zebra Fish (Lionfish)

Zebra fish are among the most beautiful and ornate of coral reef fish. They are generally found in shallow water, hovering about in a crevice or at times swimming unconcernedly in the open. They are also called turkey fish because of their interesting habit of swimming around slowly and spreading their fanlike pectorals and lacy dorsal fins like a turkey gobbler displaying its plumes. These fish are frequently observed swimming in pairs and are apparently fearless in their movements. Acceptance of an invitation to reach out and grab one of these fish results in an extremely painful experience, because hidden under the "lace" are needle-sharp fin stings. The fearlessness of the zebra fish makes it a particular menace to anyone working in its habitat, the shallow water coral reef areas.

Lionfish respond aggressively to perceived threats by erecting spines with which they pierce the invader's skin, releasing venom into the wound. The toxicity of *Pterois* venom is attributable to a nondialyzable protein that produces profound hypotension, probably vasodilation, muscular weakness, and death by respiratory arrest in experimental animals.

The Centers for Disease Control (CDC), Atlanta, stated that in humans, such stings usually cause local cyanosis, inflammation, swelling, severe pain, and occasionally necrosis of surrounding tissue with sloughing but no fatalities.

Thousands of zebra fish are imported annually to the United States from the Philippines and end up in private fish collections, with some risk to those unfamiliar with them. CDC officials recommend immediate irrigation of the wound and encouragement of bleeding. The affected area then should be immersed for 30 to 90 minutes in water as hot as can be tolerated without tissue injury. Magnesium sulfate added to the water will act as an analgesic.

Catfish Envenomization

The ability of catfish to inflict extremely painful wounds with their pectoral and dorsal spines has been well established. Although most of the documented stings have resulted from contact with saltwater species, freshwater catfish—abundant in the rivers and streams of North America—can also administer a painful and very distressing sting to humans.

The common sea catfish (*Galeichthys felis*) has four barbels on its chin. Its body is smooth and scaleless, dark silvery gray above and white beneath, and it spans a length of about 1 foot. A shore fish, it prefers the muddy areas around docks and boat slips. The ability of catfish to eat and digest virtually any food they can swallow is almost legendary (80).

Although the North American marine species are rarely eaten, freshwater catfish are commonly included in the diets of many Americans. Freshwater catfish of North America include the brown bullhead, the Carolina mudtom, the channel catfish, the blue catfish, and the white catfish. All are primarily bottom feeders, with the same lack of discrimination in diet as their saltwater cousins.

The venom apparatus of the saltwater catfish includes dorsal and pectoral stings and the axillary venom glands. Dorsal and pectoral stings are comprised of modified or coalescent soft rays that have become ossified. In most catfish, these spines are so constructed that they can be locked in the extended position at the will of the fish. Thus, the creature is equipped with a formidable and efficient defensive weapon (81).

The victim of catfish envenomization experiences an instantaneous stinging, throbbing, or scalding sensation that may be localized or that may radiate up the affected limb. Severity of symptoms varies with the species of catfish and the amount of venom received. Discomfort produced by the less toxic species generally subsides within 30 minutes or less, whereas the more potent tropical species may produce a violent pain lasting 48 hours or more.

Immediately after the patient is stung, the area surrounding the wound becomes ischemic. The pallor is followed by cyanosis, then by redness and swelling. Patients with extreme wounds may develop a massive edema involving an entire limb, accompanied by lymphadenopathy, numbness, and localized gangrene.

The sting of North American catfish is generally mild in nature, with symptoms subsiding within several hours. Although sequelae are rare, necrosis of the involved tissues has been observed with severe envenomization. Improper wound care may result in secondary bacterial infection (82).

Therapy depends on symptoms. The treatment of choice is immersion in hot water, although potent analgesia may be necessary in severe cases. Infections are treated with appropriate antibiotics.

Patten (83) reported that most catfishermen in the Gulf of Mexico region carry a thermos of hot water in their boats as the specific remedy to apply if they are stung.

> **Catfish envenomization is characterized by severe local injury often accompanied by protracted pain. In extreme cases, potent analgesia may be required.**

MISCELLANEOUS AQUATIC DERMATOSES

Frictional Irritation

Elasmobrach (sharks, skater, and rays) have smooth skin studded with tiny scales called dermal denticles, which are constructed similar to fish teeth. Frictional injury and skin tearing can occur if one of these animals brushes against a person. Manta ray dermatitis is a name for this irritation, which occurs after "riding" manta rays.

Stingray Hickey

A bite mark or "hickey" can occur when recreational divers attempt to feed stingrays. These bites, which usually occur on the arm or hand, are surrounded by a bruise and are self-limited (84).

Scombroid Dermatitis

Scombroid dermatitis is caused by a primary irritant found in the skin and flesh of scombroid fish, which include tuna, skipjack, and bonito. This dermatitis appears in workers handling scombroid fish without wearing gloves. The irritant appears to be more concentrated in spoiled than in fresh fish.

The irritant dermatitis of the hands is treated with the application of corticosteroid cream. In the presence of fissures and denuded, excoriated, or infected skin, an erythromycin ointment should also be applied.

> **Scombroid dermatitis and red feed dermatitis are irritant occupational hazards of fishermen who handle, without gloves, scombroid fish or certain mackerel.**

Scombroid Poisoning

Ingestion of scombroid fish that have been improperly preserved may result in upper body and facial flushing, urticaria, and anaphylactoid symptoms. It is caused by toxins that include histamine and saurine formed by bacterial activity.

Red Feed Dermatitis

Red feed is a reddish orange crustacean (*Calanus* sp.) eaten by mackerel from June to September. Ingested red feed accelerates the proteolytic breakdown of the gastric wall of the fish, releasing the gastric juices. Handling of fish that have eaten red feed results in edema, erythema, and superficial ulcerations of the skin of the hands.

Dr. Paul J. Cheung (pathologist, Osborne Laboratory of Marine Sciences, New York Zoological Society, personal communication) stated, "The red feed dermatitis is a form of edema and dermatitis that occurs in fishermen who, with bare hands, handle the red-colored contents (possibly the red-tide organism) of the gut of herrings and mackerel, which (between June and September) feed on red-pigmented copepods of the genus *Calanus.*"

"Red Tide" Dermatitis

Certain unicellular organisms known as dinoflagellates, which have been designated as "plant-animals," may "bloom" in vast numbers and may cause a phenomenon known as "red tide."

Swarming of these organisms known as "red tide" can lead to poisoning and skin reactions from eating mollusks that contain the dinoflagellates.

Marine Animals that Shock Electrically

Individuals who emerge from the sea in a dazed condition with no visible eruption may be suffering from electric shock produced by certain marine animals, including catfish, stargazers, electric eels, and electric rays.

These marine animals possess electricity-generating organs that can discharge 8 to 200 volts of current. The amperage is very low, and if the victim is in good health, injury is insignificant. Contact with a large marine "shocker" may result in an electric shock strong enough to knock over or temporarily disable the victim.

The electric eel found in the freshwater streams of South America is the most powerful of electric fish.

Recovery is usually uneventful. In severe cases the treatment is the same as for any form of electric shock.

> **Several marine animals can produce electric shocks, which are usually not severe.**

DERMATITIS AND INFECTIONS CAUSED BY MARINE BACTERIA

A number of cutaneous and systemic infections may occur in relationship to water exposure or exposure to aquatic creatures. These may include bacterial, fungal, and mycobacterial diseases. Previous editions of this text have discussed some of these infections in more detail. However, consideration here will be limited to several conditions that may be confused with contact dermatitis.

Erysipelothrix Dermatitis

This dermatitis is sometimes known as erysipeloid of Rosenbach. It also has several more colorful appellations, including "speck finger" and "blubber finger." The condition is most common in fish handlers but can occur in anyone working with marine food products or aquariums. On the Atlantic Coast, erysipeloid infection frequently occurs among workers who handle crabs and live fish, and it is believed to be one of the main causes of temporary disability in such occupations (85).

Erysipelothrix Rausopathlae, the causative organism, is a gram-positive coccoid that later becomes a gram-positive bacillus. This organism is a slender rod that may be either curved or straight and that usually shows elongated filaments. It is nonmotile and does not form spores or capsules (86). Closely related bacteriologically to *Listeria,* the organism may be easily confused with streptococci or diphtheroids.

Erysipelothrix enters the skin through an opening, usually a small puncture wound on the finger. After a 1- to 5-day incubation period, a spreading erythema is observed, accompanied by pain and itching (87).

Three forms of the disease have been reported: (a) a mild localized cutaneous form; (b) a severe generalized cutaneous form; and (c) a systemic form, sometimes complicated by endocarditis.

The localized form involves the fingers and hands. It begins as a sharply defined violent red area around the site of infection. Prickling, itching, and pain are frequent accompanying symptoms. Occasionally the lesion becomes purulent. Aching or burning digits may interfere with the patient's sleep.

The lesion characteristically progresses up the edge of the finger into the web, then descends the adjoining finger. It commonly spreads to the dorsum of the hand but seldom affects the palm.

Inasmuch as erysipeloid is a self-limiting condition—usually running its course within 1 to 3 weeks—conservative treatment is indicated. Administration of appropriate antibiotics follows culture identification and sensitivity tests. Penicillin or cephalosporin therapy is generally helpful. Reporting on 10 patients with the condition, Lamphier (85) found that duration of the disease was doubled in 5 patients who underwent surgery.

Erysipelothrix dermatitis is an occupational hazard in fishermen and those working with marine food products and in aquariums.

Pseudomonas: Hot Tub Folliculitis

Pseudomonas folliculitis is a cutaneous infection that develops 8 to 72 hours after contact with a whirlpool, hot tub, or swimming pool contaminated with *Pseudomonas.* The striking clinical finding is multiple groups of dark red urticarial papules and pustules occurring mostly under areas of the bathing suit, with open skin generally spared. Although there may be some pruritus, the more common complaint is pain and tenderness on pressure. In addition to the highly characteristic skin lesions, patients often develop fever, malaise, headache, and prostration (88–90).

Usually groups of people are affected in a "mini-epidemic" pattern. Although home whirlpools may serve as the source of exposure, public hot tubs and swimming pools are more often responsible. Heavy bather loads may overwhelm the pool's disinfectant level.

The differential diagnosis clinically includes scabies, insect bites, contact dermatitis, viral eruption, bacterial folliculitis, perforating folliculitis, iododerma, and bromoderma.

Histologically, the lesions demonstrate minimal epidermal change, but the follicular epithelium is perforated, with an inflammatory infiltrate adjacent to the areas of the disrupted follicular epithelium. Although normal skin is resistant to invasion by *Pseudomonas,* it is known that superhydration of the stratum corneum leads to high surface levels of *Pseudomonas* (91). The organism does not invade living tissue and therefore does not survive long on the human skin.

Treatment

Therapy may not be necessary, as most cases are self-limited and resolve within several days. Usually only debilitated or immunologically deficient persons are at risk for serious disease. Ciprofloxacin orally is effective against *Pseudomonas* and is useful if treatment is deemed necessary.

Pseudomonas Cepacia *Dermatitis*

Foot lesions associated with *Pseudomonas cepacia* are variously known as jungle rot, foot rot, swamp rot, or trench foot.

The organism has been isolated from lesions of the feet, hands, and groin. Invasion takes place through intact, sodden skin. Soldiers exposed to swampy, wet terrain are most frequently affected. The lesions are characterized by maceration, hyperkeratosis, and fissuring (92). The toe webs are often involved.

Prophylaxis consists of cleanliness and dryness.

Green Nail Syndrome

Pseudomonal infection of the nail bed is readily diagnosed clinically by the characteristic dark-green discoloration.

Systemic symptoms are absent in this chronic infection. Trapping of moisture under a damaged nail is probably responsible. Treatment with topical antibiotics such as colistin sulfate (Colymycin Otic) for several weeks is usually curative.

DERMATITIS RELATED TO SWIMMING AND SWIMMING POOLS

Dermatitis from Swimming Pool Disinfectants

Chlorine

Chlorine is the most widely used swimming pool disinfectant. Irritant dermatitis is uncommon, and allergic reactions are extremely rare (93). For chlorine-sensitive individuals with their own swimming pools, Betadine Solution (Purdue Frederick Co.) may be used (94).

Bromine

Bromine is much less widely used than chlorine, and, like chlorine, irritant and allergic reactions are rare.

In the United States, bromine-based disinfectants are used more often in spas or hot tubs, whereas chlorine is used most commonly in swimming pools. Rycroft and Penny (95) reported 48 patients with eczema presumed to be associated with use of brominated pools or spas. However, only one was patch tested with negative results. Most patients tolerated chlorinated pools. A more recent report implicates a compound called Halobrome (1-bromo-3-chloro-5,5-dimethylhydantoin) (96). All patients were patch test positive to the chemical at both 1.0% aq and 0.1% aq. Controls were negative, and patients were negative to all screening allergens.

UNDERWATER EQUIPMENT–RELATED DERMATOSES

Diving Suit Dermatitis

A 27-year-old diver had a severe contact dermatitis of the neck, trunk, and extremities whenever he wore his rubber diving suit. Results of patch tests to a piece of the diving suit were strongly positive. It was finally determined that the patient was allergic to a thiourea compound similar to the one that had produced sneaker dermatitis. N,N'-diethylurea is used to cement the nylon lining to the rubber diving suit. Persons allergic to thiourea must obtain rubber suits without nylon linings (97).

A maker of diving suit material, the Rubatex Corp. (Bedford, VA), writes as follows: "to your inquiry concerning information on thiourea-free wet diving suits. Rubatex Corporation manufactures two grades of closed-cell neoprene for use in the manufacture of wet suits. Rubatex does not manufacture wet suits. We supply the closed-cell neoprene with or without nylon stretch fabric bonded to one or two sides of the sheet. In order to be absolutely free of thiourea, one must obtain a suit of G-231-N with no nylon on the inside."

> **Wet diving suit dermatitis may be caused by thiourea adhesive, which binds nylon linings to the rubber.**

Skin Reactions to Underwater Masks and Mouthpieces

The facial condition known as "mask burn," frequently noted by both physicians and patients, is usually dismissed as a necessary annoyance of snorkeling and scuba diving. However, more severe reactions have been described (98). Although some patients experience only a reddish imprint of the mask on the face, others suffer a severe, painful, and at times disabling eruption characterized by vesiculation, weeping, and crusting.

Mouthpieces may result in only minor oral insults without disabling symptoms that last for long periods of time. However, severe intraoral irritation and inflammation accompanied by vesiculation of the oral mucosa, gingiva, and tongue may eventually develop in patients who become sensitized to the mouthpiece. Chemical constituents in the equipment may be the causative allergens of these reactions. Rubber masks and mouthpieces contain antioxidants similar to those that are known to cause contact dermatitis in some surgeons after the use of rubber gloves. In particular, mercaptobenzothiazole has caused such instances of rubber dermatitis.

Maibach (99) studied a series of patients who each had a characteristic facial dermatitis caused by contact with a scuba diver face mask. The dermatitis occurred on those parts of the face that were in direct contact with the mask. The dermatitis that appeared 8 to 48 hours after wearing the mask spared the central portion of the face, including the eyes and nose.

Patch testing on the back with very thinly shaven 2-cm square patches of the rubber from the mask applied with an occlusive adhesive tape produced a spreading dermatitis present at 48 and 96 hours. The manufacturer provided samples of the main rubber additives used in the mask. The offending agent proved to be N-isopropyl-N-phenylparaphenylenediamine (IPPDA), a rubber antioxidant. Patch testing with 0.05% IPPDA in petrolatum produced a strong positive reaction at 48 and 96 hours. No response was produced in five controls. These patients were able to use masks in which the IPPDA derivative was not used.

For patients who experience severe and frequent reactions, the use of "hypoallergenic" masks and mouthpieces is mandatory. Masks and mouthpieces made of silicone rubber or PVC plastics are hypoallergenic.

> Underwater masks and mouthpieces may cause irritant and allergic reactions. The allergic reactions are due to rubber accelerators or antioxidants in the rubber, which are not present in silicone rubber.

Skin "Bends" Dermatitis

A skin "bends" condition is due to increased water pressure and may produce pruritus, erythematous papules, marbling, cyanotic discoloration, and purpura. The dermatologic condition may require treatment in a pressurized chamber.

The so-called nitrogen rash may be related to skin "bends." Physiologic nitrogen rash occurs in scuba divers when they surpass the maximal time underwater at any given depth. The condition is said to be caused by the dissolution of nitrogen in the subcutaneous adipose tissue at more than one atmosphere of pressure. The eruption, which consists of tender, pruritic, erythematous lesions that appear primarily on the elbows and flanks, usually resolves within several hours. It is advisable that diving not be resumed until the lesions are completely healed.

REFERENCES

1. Fisher AA. *Atlas of aquatic dermatology*. New York: Grune & Stratton, 1978.
2. Baslow MH. Marine toxins. *Annu Rev Pharmacol* 1971;11:447.
3. Mitchell JC. Biochemical basis of geographic ecology. *Int J Dermatol* 1975;14:239.
4. Minton SS. Spines and stings and sea snakes. *Consultant* 1977;5:45.
5. Holmes JL. Marine stingers in Far North Queensland Australia. *J of Derma Toc* 1996;37:523–526.
6. Halstead BW. *Poisonous and venomous marine animals of the world*, vol 1, *Invertebrates*. Washington, DC: US Government Printing Office, 1965.
7. Marr II. Portuguese man-of-war envenomization. *JAMA* 1967;199: 337.
8. Ioannides G, Davis JH. Portuguese man-of-war stinging. *Arch Dermatol* 1965;91:448.
9. Russell FE. Physalia stings: a report of two cases. *Toxicon* 1966;4:65.
10. Stillway CW, Lane CE. Phospholipase in the nematocyst toxin of *Physalia physalis*. *Toxicon* 1971;9:193.
11. Russell FE, Carlson RW. Jellyfish stings. In: Conn HF, ed. *Current therapy*. Philadelphia: WB Saunders, 1975.
12. Arnold HL. Portuguese man-of-war ("blue-bottle") stings: treatment with papain. *Straub Clin Proc* 1971;37:30.
13. Tomchik R, Russell M, Szmani A, Black N. Clinical perspectives on seabathers eruption also known as sea lice. *JAMA* 1993;269:1669.
14. Osment L. Update: seabather's eruption and swimmer's itch. *Cutis* 1976;18:545.
15. Kokelj F, Stinco G, Avian M et al. Cell mediated sensitization to jellyfish antigens confirmed by positive patch test to *Olindas sambaquiensis* preparations. *J Am Acad Dermatol* 1995;33:307–309.
16. Burnett JW, Calton GJ. The chemistry and toxicology of some venomous pelagic coelenterates. *Toxicon* 1977;15:117.
17. Hartman KR, Calton GJ, Burnett JW. Use of the radioallergosorbent test for the study of coelenterate toxin-specific immunoglobulin E. *Int Arch Allergy Appl Immunol* 1980;61:389.
18. Burnett JW, Calton GJ. Use of IgE antibody determinations in cutaneous coelenterate envenomations. *Cutis* 1981;27:50.
19. Halstead BW. Phylum coelenterate. In: *Poisonous and venomous marine animals of the world*, vol 1, *Invertebrates*. Washington, DC: US Government Printing Office, 1965.
20. Tamanaha R, Izumi A. Persistent cutaneous hypersensitivity reaction after a Hawaiian box jellyfish sting *(Carybdea alata)*. *JAAD* 1996;35: 991–993.
21. Ohtaki N, et al. Cutaneous reactions caused by experimental exposure to jellyfish, *Carybdea Rastoonii*. *J Dermatol* 1990;17:108.
22. Newhouse ML. Dogger Bank itch: survey of trawlermen. *Rehabilitation* 1967;60:941.
23. Carle JS, Thybo H, Christophersen C. Dogger Bank itch (3). Isolation structure determination and synthesis of a hapten. *Contact Dermatitis* 1982;8:43.
23A. Ashworth J, et al: Occupational contact dermatitis in East Coast of England Fishermen. *Contact Dermatitis* 1990;22:185–186.
24. Reed KM, Bronstein BR, Baden HP. Delayed and persistent cutaneous reactions to coelenterates. *J Am Acad Dermatol* 1984;10:462.
25. Nicholas D. *Echinoderms*. London: Hutchinson, 1962.
26. Strauss MB, McDonald RI. Hand injuries from sea urchins. *Clin Orthop* 1976;114:216.
27. Asada M, et al. A case of delayed hypersensitivity reaction following a sea urchin sting. *Dermatologica* 1990;180:99.
28. Meneghini CL. Cases of sea urchin granuloma with positive intradermal test to spine extracts. *Contact Dermatitis Newsletter* 1972;12:316.
29. O'Neal RL, et al. Injury to human tissues from sea urchin stings. *Calif Med* 1964;101:199.
30. Rocha G, Fraga S. Sea urchin granuloma of the skin. *Arch Dermatol* 1962;85:406.
31. Mortensen T. *A monograph of the Echinoidea: Index to Vols I–V*. Copenhagen: Carlsberg-Fund, CA Reitzel 1951.
32. Manowitz NR, Rosenthal RR. Cutaneous-systemic reactions to toxins and venoms of common marine organisms. *Cutis* 1979;23:450.
33. Halstead BW. *Poisonous and venomous marine animals of the world*, vol 2, *Invertebrates*. Washington, DC: US Government Printing Office, 1965.
34. Rothberg I, et al. Terpenoids. LXVIII. 23-epsilon-acetoxy-17—deoxy-7, 8-dihydroholothurinogen, a new triteripenoid sapogenin from a sea cucumber. *J Org Chem* 1973;38:209.
35. Rosco D. Treatment of venomous and poisonous marine animal injuries. *Int Soc Aquat Med Newsletter* 1976;2:6.
36. Phillips C, Brady WH. *Sea pests—poisonous or harmful sea life of Florida and the West Indies*. Miami: University of Miami Press, 1953.
37. Halstead BW. Marine biotoxicology. In: Coulston F, ed. *EQS environmental quality and safety*, vol 3. New York: Academic Press, 1960.
38. Russell F. Animal venoms. In: *Practice of medicine*, vol 9. Hagerstown, MD: Harper & Row, 1975.
39. Deas W. Venomous octopus. *Sea Frontiers* 1970;16:357.
40. Sutherland SK, Lane WR. Toxins and mode of envenomation of the common ringed or blue-banded octopus. *Med J Aust* 1969;1:893.
41. Edmonds C. A non-fatal case of blue-ringed octopus bite. *Med J Aust* 1969;2:601.
42. Tiffany HL. *Algae, the grass of many waters*. Springfield, IL: Charles C Thomas Publisher, 1968.
43. Kavaler L. *The wonders of algae*. New York: The John Day Co, 1961.
44. Grauer FH, Arnold HL. Seaweed dermatitis. *Arch Dermatol* 1961; 84:720.
45. Cohen SG, Reif CB. Cutaneous sensitization to blue-green algae. *J Allergy* 1953;24:452.
46. Heise II HA. Microcystis: another form of algae producing allergenic reactions. *Ann Allergy* 1951;9:100.
47. Solomon AE, Stoughton RB. Dermatitis from purified sea algae toxin *(Debromoaplysiatoxin)*. *Arch Dermatol* 1978;114:1333.
48. Cardellina II JH, Marner F-J, Moore RE. Seaweed dermatitis: structure of lyngbyatoxin A. *Science* 1979;204:193.
49. Davies RR, Spencer H, Wakelin PO. A case of human protothecosis. *Trans R Soc Trop Med Hyg* 1964;58:448.
50. Klintworth GK, Fetter BF, Nielsen Jr HS. Protothecosis, an algal infection: report of a case in man. *J Med Microbiol* 1968;1:211.
51. Burnett J, Burnett H, Burnett M. Sargassum dermatitis. *Cutis* 1997; 59:303–304.
52. van der Willigen A, et al. Contact allergy to iodine in Japanese sargassum. *Contact Dermatitis* 1988;18:251.
53. Corson EF, Pratt AG. "Red moss" dermatitis. *Arch Derm Syph* 1943;47:574.

54. Mitchell JC. Biochemical basis of geographic ecology. *Int Dermatol* 1975;14:239.

55. Wood MG, Srolovitz H, Schetman D. Schistosomiasis: paraplegia and ectopic skin lesions as admission symptoms. *Arch Dermatol* 1976;112:690.

56. Chu GWT. Pacific area distribution of freshwater and marine cercarial dermatitis. *Pacific Sci* 1958;12:299.

57. Barnes RD. Invertebrate zoology. *Clinical parasitology.* Philadelphia: Appleton-Century-Crofts, 1958.

58. Walther RR. Chronic papular dermatitis of the scrotum due to *Schistosoma mansoni*. *Arch Derm* 1979;115:869.

59. Wiley R. Cercarial dermatitis outbreak at a state park—Delaware, 1991. *J Am Med Assoc* 1992;267:2581.

60. Bastert J, Sing A, Wollenberg A, Korting H. Aquarium dermatitis; cercarial dermatitis in an aquarist. *Dermatology* 1998;197:84–86.

61. Zaki MH, Nuzzi R. Unusual health effects associated with surface waters. *NY State J Med* 1982.

62. Tennent JE. *Ceylon, an account of the island, physical, historical, and topographical, with notes on its natural history, antiquities, and productions,* vol 1. London: Longman, Green, Longman & Roberts, 1859.

63. Harmer SF, Shipley AE. *Cambridge natural history,* vol 2. London: Macmillan, 1896.

64. Heldt TJ. Allergy to leeches. *Henry Ford Hosp Med Bull* 1961;9:498.

65. Phillips C, Brady WH. *Sea pests, poisonous or harmful sea life of Florida and the West Indies.* Miami: University of Miami Press, 1953.

66. Burnett JW, Cargo DG. Cutaneous irritation induced by crab larvae. *J Am Acad Dermatol* 1979;1:42.

67. Burnett H, Burnett P, Burnett J. Cutaneous irritation produced by oceanic crab larvae. *Cutis,* 1999;61:208.

68. Best WC, Sablan RG. Cymothoidism (sea louse dermatis). *Arch Dermatol* 1964;90:177.

69. Bassler RS. Shelled invertebrates of past and present. *Smithson Sci Ser* 1934;10:157.

70. Noble ER, Noble GA. *Parasitology,* 1st ed. Philadelphia: Lea & Febiger, 1961.

71. Boylan, DB, Scheuer PJ. Pahutoxin: a fish poison. *Science* 1967;155:52.

72. Hashimoto Y, Kamiya H. Occurrence of a toxic substance in the skin of a sea bass *Pogonoperca punctala*. *Toxicon* 1980;7:65–70.

73. Randall JE, Aida K, Hibiya T, et al. Grammistin, the skin toxin of soapfishes, and its significance in the classification of Grammistidae. *Publ Seto Marine Biol Lab* 1971;19:157.

74. Russell FE. The stingray: national history, venom apparatus, chemistry and toxicology, and clinical problem. In: *Poisonous marine animals.* Neptune, NJ: TFH Publications, 1971.

75. Mullanney PJ. Treatment of stingray wounds. *Clin Toxicol* 1970;3:613.

76. Castex MN. Freshwater venomous rays. In: Russell FE, Saunders PR, eds. *Animal toxins: international symposium on animal toxins.* New York: Pergamon Press, 1967.

77. Rodrigues RJ. Pharmacology of South American freshwater stingray venom (*Potamotrygon motoro*). *Trans NY Acad Sci* 1972;34:677.

78. Schaeffer Jr RC, Carlson RW, Russell FE. Some chemical properties of the venom of the scorpionfish *Scorpaena guttata*. *Toxicon* 1971;9:69.

79. Burnett J. Aquatic adversaries: stonefish. *Cutis* 1998;62:269–270.

80. Scoggin CH. Catfish stings. *JAMA* 1975;231:176.

81. Halstead BW, Kuninobu LS, Hebard HG. Catfish stings and the venom apparatus of the Mexican catfish. *Galeichthys felis* (Linnaeus). *Trans Am Microscopical Soc* 1953;72:297.

82. Wintrobe MM, Thorne GW, Adams RD, et al. *Harrison's principles of internal medicine,* 7th ed. New York: McGraw-Hill, 1974.

83. Patten BM. More on catfish stings. *JAMA* 1975;232:248.

84. Evans L, Evans C. Stingray hickey. *Cutis* 1996;58:208–210.

85. Lamphier TA. Erysipeloid infection of digits. *J Fla Med Assoc* 1971;58:39.

86. Barnett J, Estes S, Wirmon J, et al. Erysipeloid. *J Am Acad Dermatol* 1983;9:116–123.

87. Burnett JW. Uncommon bacterial infections of the skin. *Arch Dermatol* 1962;85:597.

88. Fowler J, Stege G. Pseudomonas "hot tub" folliculitis. *J Ky Med Assoc* 1990;39:66.

89. Washburn J, Jacobson JA, Marston E, et al. Pseudomonas aeruginosa rash with a whirlpool. *JAMA* 1976;235:2205.

90. McCausland WJ, Cox PJ. Pseudomonas infection traced to motel whirlpool. *J Environ Sci Health* 1975;37:455.

91. Hojo-Tomoka MT, Marples PP, Kligman AM. *Pseudomonas* infection in superhydrated skin. *Arch Dermatol* 1973;107:723.

92. Taplin D, Bassett DCJ. Foot lesions associated with *Pseudomonas cepacia*. *Lancet* 1971;2:568.

93. Fisher AA. Dermatitis from chlorine and certain chlorinated products. *Cutis* 1984;33:20.

94. Black AP, Keirn MA, Smith JJ, et al. The disinfection of swimming pool waters. (1) comparison of iodine and chlorine as swimming pool disinfectants. *Am J Public Health* 1970;60:535.

95. Rycroft R, Penny P. Dermatoses associated with brominated swimming pools. *Br Med J* 1983;287:462.

96. Fitzgerald D, Wilkinson S, Bhaggoe R, et al. Spa pool dermatitis. *Contact Dermatitis* 1995;33:53.

97. Fisher AA. Water related dermatoses. *Cutis* 1980;25:132.

98. Alexander JE. Allergic reactions to mask skirts, regulator mouthpieces. *Pressure* 1976;5:10.

99. Maibach H. Scuba diver facial dermatitis: allergic contact dermatitis to *N*-isopropyl-*N*-phenylparaphenylenediamine. *Contact Dermatitis* 1975;1:330.

SUGGESTED READINGS

Halstead BW. *Poisonous and venomous marine animals,* vols 1, 2, and 3. Washington, DC: US Government Printing Office, 1965.

Mitchell JC. Biochemical basis of geographic ecology. *Int Dermatol* 1975;14:239.

Strauss MB. Beneath the waters, exotic wounds for the unwary. *Phys Sports Med* 1974;2:22.

CHAPTER 38

Treatment of Contact Dermatitis

ACUTE CONTACT DERMATITIS

Acute poison ivy dermatitis is the most common example of an acute allergic contact dermatitis. Systemic corticosteroid therapy is of great benefit and should be considered in all but mild cases of acute allergic contact dermatitis. For adults, 40 to 60 mg of prednisone per day, in two or three divided doses, is the treatment of choice. Generally, this dosage should be tapered gradually, resulting in a total treatment time of 10 to 14 days. An easily remembered dosage schedule for prednisone is 10 mg four times daily for 3 days, three times daily for 3 days, two times daily for 3 days, then once daily for 3 days. Further tapering is not necessary, and steroid side effects, although possible, are very rare with this length of treatment. Tapering the treatment too soon often results in a rebound of the initial dermatitis.

In cases of localized acute contact dermatitis, or in patients in whom even a short course of systemic steroids is contraindicated, a potent topical corticosteroid cream can be used. Fluorinated steroids such as these, however, should not be used on the face or intertriginous areas except for periods of less than 1 to 2 weeks. Cream bases, which may provide some drying effect, are preferable to ointments, which may trap moisture.

To further enhance the drying of acute, weepy lesions, moist compresses that have a soothing effect and remove crust and debris are helpful. Moisten a clean, absorbent cloth with an astringent, such as aluminum sulfate and calcium acetate (Domeboro), or even plain tap water, and apply for 20 to 30 minutes several times a day. Alternatively, bathing in oatmeal baths (Aveeno) is useful when large body areas are involved.

Itching is often severe in acute contact dermatitis and is usually best treated by steroids rather than antihistamines. However, antihistamines initially may have an added effect and also may induce drowsiness, which may be beneficial to the patient. Hydroxyzine, 10 to 25 mg, or diphenhydramine, 25 to 50 mg two to four times daily as needed and tolerated, may be useful. Other sedating antihistamines may be used, but sometimes nonsedating antihistamines such as cetirizine may be helpful.

CHRONIC CONTACT DERMATITIS

In contrast to their use in the treatment of acute contact dermatitis, systemic steroids should be used cautiously in the treatment of chronic contact dermatitis because the condition may require months or even years of therapy. The first line of treatment beyond prevention and avoidance is the use of emollients to decrease itching and reduce dryness and scaling. Lotions containing alpha-hydroxy acids, such as glycolic acid or lactic acid, are available over the counter and are especially useful for thick, scaly plaques. Low- to medium-strength topical steroids, such as hydrocortisone valerate, alclometasone, or desonide, are useful. Some ointments, however, are greasy; the patient's acceptance of them must be considered when prescribing these products.

Intralesional injection of triamcinolone acetonide (Kenalog), 4 to 10 mg per ml, is useful in occasional thick plaques, but caution must be exercised because of the potential for atrophy. Antihistamines are of some benefit in minimizing itching, but intolerance may develop, thus limiting their effectiveness. In selected cases, Kenalog 40 mg to 60 mg intramuscularly, which has a beneficial effect of 3 to 6 weeks' duration, may be used without serious risk of adverse effects.

TREATMENT OF DERMATITIS IN SPECIAL CIRCUMSTANCES

Nickel Dermatitis

Systemic nickel dermatitis may sometimes occur in the form of dyshidrosiform hand eczema or may occur in other areas of the body. A low-nickel diet, as discussed elsewhere in this text, may be helpful. If both external and internal allergen avoidance is not successful, disulfiram 250 mg four times daily may be tried. This agent binds nickel and allows it to be excreted in the urine and stool. Absolute avoidance of alcohol is essential in taking this drug because alcohol intake will result in nausea and vomiting. In addition, liver function test results should be monitored before and during treatment. Readers should check the references and review the studies on this agent before prescribing it.

Skin-Protective Products

Generally, skin protectants or "barrier creams" have proven unsatisfactory in the care of patients with contact dermatitis. However, a number of new products that may prove to be of some use have been introduced to the marketplace as of this writing. Also, in occasional cases some of the older barrier creams used in industry may have some benefit. It must be kept in mind, however, that barrier creams may trap allergens, actually worsening dermatitis. Furthermore, individuals may be allergic to some components of barrier creams.

The one barrier product that has been proven of definite use is IvyBlock Lotion for the prevention of dermatitis from poison ivy, oak, and sumac. The protective nature of this product has been well documented. It should be applied to all exposed areas before possible contact with the offending plants. Protection is expected for at least 4 hours but may last as long as 8 hours. The mechanism of action is uncertain, but perhaps the active ingredient in IvyBlock (quaternium-18 bentonite) may bind the urushiol allergen and prevent its penetration. Accordingly, after exposure any exposed areas should be washed with soap and water. It is uncertain at this time whether IvyBlock Lotion provides protection from other allergens. Fowler (personal observation) has noted some success in using this product in individuals with airborne Compositae dermatitis.

NONCORTICOSTEROID MANAGEMENT OPTIONS FOR CONTACT DERMATITIS

Grenz Ray Treatment

Grenz rays are useful in the management of chronic dermatitis, including chronic contact dermatitis. The equipment to perform this treatment is not as commonly available as it once was due to concerns about the hazards of ionizing radiation. Grenz rays are softer than superficial X rays. In a study of chronic symmetrical hand eczema, significant benefit was demonstrated using 3 Gy (300 rad) weekly for 6 weeks (1). In a study of six patients who were nickel sensitive, a dilution series of nickel patch tests were placed on both sides of the back, and one side was treated with 3 Gy weekly for 3 weeks. Almost nothing was seen at the sites treated with grenz rays, and monoclonal antibody staining of skin biopsy specimens showed severe depletion of Langerhans cells at the treated sites (2). A similar study of irritant reactions found a slight but not significant difference between sodium lauryl sulfate patch tests applied to skin pretreated with grenz rays (3).

Phototherapy

A comparison of ultraviolet B (UVB) light versus bath PUVA (psoralen plus ultraviolet A) phototherapy for the management of hand dermatitis in 13 patients treated for 6 weeks found no significant difference (4).

PUVA has been successfully used to manage photosensitive Compositae-sensitive patients, however. The dose of methoxsalen used was 0.3 mg/kg. The patients were started on 60 mg of prednisone at the same time that they started PUVA at 1 joule less than the minimal phototoxic dose (MPD). Treatments were administered on a Monday-Wednesday-Friday schedule, 1.5 hours after ingestion of methoxsalen. Treatments were increased 1 J if the MPD was greater than 6 J, or increased by 0.5 J if the MPD was 6 J or less. The prednisone dose was decreased to 40 mg at week 2, further tapered to 20 mg at week 3, and then discontinued. The maximum UVA exposure was 10 J per treatment. The frequency of phototherapy was tapered after 6 weeks to twice a week and then once a week. This schedule was successful (5).

Azathioprine

For patients with chronic parthenium dermatitis, an alternative to the phototherapy approach outlined in the previous section is the use of azathioprine. In a study of 15 Parthenium-sensitive patients with extensive contact dermatitis who had contraindications to corticosteroids, oral azathioprine (100–150 mg per day) was used. This produced a slow improvement. No significant side effects occurred in this study, but it took between 6 and 12 months to obtain substantial benefit. By the end of the year of treatment, near total clearing had occurred (6).

Cyclosporine

Oral cyclosporine at a dose of 3 mg/kg per day for 6 weeks was used to treat 27 patients with hand dermatitis. The mean decrease in disease activity was 54% (7), which is somewhat disappointing. Topical use of cyclosporine has also been disappointing (8). A comparison between cyclosporine and betamethasone-17,21-diproprionate in 41 patients found that 50% improved with cyclosporine and 30% improved with betamethasone (9).

Topical Tacrolimus

Topical tacrolimus (FK 506) has been shown to inhibit both irritant and allergic contact dermatitis in the guinea pig (10). In rats, its inhibitory action was stronger than alclometasone dipropionate, and it is thought to inhibit the activation of sensitized T lymphocytes (11). The benefits of tacrolimus ointment in atopic dermatitis make it a potentially useful drug for the management of some cases of contact dermatitis (12).

SDZ ASM 981

The novel anti-inflammatory drug SDZ ASM 981 is still in development. It has been shown to be effective in the treatment of atopic dermatitis (13). It down-regulates the production of cytokines associated with antigen-specific activation of T cells (14). At the Twelfth International Contact Dermatitis Symposium in 1999, Cherill and colleagues from Novartis and the Oregon Health Sciences University reported that 1% SDZ ASM 981 was safe, well tolerated, and more effective than placebo in the treatment of irritant contact dermatitis of the hands (15).

TREATMENT OF IRRITANT CONTACT DERMATITIS

In the acute phase of irritant contact dermatitis of the feet, the use of foot baths with cool Burow's solution (1 part to 20 parts water for 20 minutes twice daily) reduces inflammation and edema. In the presence of secondary infection, appropriate antibiotics should be prescribed. After the foot baths, zinc oxide ointment or plain Lassar's paste may be applied. If the dermatitis is oozing, an absorbent paste composed of the following substances can be applied:

- Burow's solution 10 mL
- Anhydrous lanolin 20 g
- Plain Lassar's paste up to 60 g

In the presence of fissuring, the following ointment may be used:

- Mastisol (Ferndale Laboratories) 2 mL
- Zinc oxide ointment up to 20 g

The dermatitis produced by saliva and food juices often does not respond to creams and ointments. Adherent, protective pastes, such as plain Lassar's paste, give better results. When an infant's skin is bathed constantly by saliva or irritating fluids, the application of an absorbent and protective paste composed of the following substances is useful:

- Burow's solution 5 mL
- Anhydrous lanolin 10 g
- Talc USP 10 g
- Zinc oxide ointment up to 6 g

MANAGEMENT OF CHRONIC OTITIS

Patients who have chronic or infectious eczematoid dermatitis of the ear should have patch tests performed.

VoSol HC is an otic solution containing 1% hydrocortisone in an acid-nonaqueous propylene glycol solution that, although free of antibiotics, is antibacterial, antifungal, and anti-inflammatory. This is an effective solution except for individuals who are sensitive to propylene glycol.

> VoSol HC solution, free of antibiotics, is effective except for propylene glycol–sensitive persons, in whom a modified carbol-fuchsin paint free of phenol may be used.

TABLE 38.1 *Otic Preparations Free of Propylene Glycol*

Americaine Otic[a]
Auralgan Otic Solution[a]
Coly-Mycin S Otic with Neomycin and Hydrocortisone[b]
Debrox Drops
Decadron Phosphate Sterile Ophthalmic Solution[c]
Metreton Ophthalmic Solution Sterile[c]
Otic Domeboro Solution
Otobiotic Otic Suspension
Otocort Ear Drops[b]

[a]Not recommended because of benzocaine content.
[b]Not recommended because of neomycin content.
[c]Advocated for both ophthalmic and otic use.

When everything else fails in the treatment of dermatitis and itching of the external ear canal, carbol-fuchsin paint is effective. The deep red color of the solution, however, is a disadvantage.

Cerumenex Eardrops to soften wax may produce an acute otitis externa with spreading dermatitis to the face, neck, and back. The actual sensitizer in Cerumenex was a polypeptide in several reported cases (16–18). Propylene glycol in Cerumenex may also be a sensitizer. Table 38.1 lists propylene glycol–free otic preparations.

INSTRUCTIONS FOR THE PREVENTION OF IRRITANT DERMATITIS IN INDIVIDUALS WHO HAVE ATOPIC DERMATITIS

- *Clothing:* Clothes worn close to the skin should be smooth and loose. Rough and starched cuffs and collars are irritating. Avoid contact with wool. Linen, cotton, poplin, gabardine, suede, chamois, and synthetic fibers, such as orlon and nylon, are usually well tolerated. Wash all new clothing before use, and be sure that all soaps and detergents are removed after each washing. Wear sandals or perforated shoes whenever possible. Avoid prolonged use of tennis shoes.
- *Furniture and room furnishings:* Keep rooms, especially the bedroom, as uncluttered as possible. Avoid dust-gathering draperies and carpets. Small cotton scatter rugs are permitted. Avoid use of upholstered furniture. Plain wooden furniture is preferable.
- *Toys:* Avoid fuzzy or woolen toys, such as teddy bears. Toys made of wood, rubber, paper, or plastics are permitted.
- *Pets:* It is best not to allow dogs, cats, or birds in the house. If the presence of such pets is necessary, they must be excluded from the bedroom. Turtles and fish are permitted anywhere in the house.
- *Dust and molds:* Exposure to all kinds of dust must be avoided as much as possible. Dust on the skin is irritating, and the inhalation of dust may also cause increased itching. Moldy objects should also be avoided for the same reasons.

- *Overheating and excessive perspiration:* Patients should indulge in activities that involve minimal sweating. Swimming, particularly in salt water, seems to agree with most patients who have atopic dermatitis.
- *Tension:* Nervous excitement and tension may cause itching and scratching. If trying situations, such as school examinations or difficult business or social situations, are anticipated, taking prescribed medication beforehand may be helpful.
- *Scratching:* Scratched skin quickly becomes inflamed and damaged, with resultant retardation in healing. Patting or rubbing may be less harmful than scratching. Keep fingernails short. The application of ice or ice-cold water on cotton cloths to localized areas may stop the itching.
- *Soaps and cleaning agents:* Strong detergents, cleansers, and solvents, such as turpentine and benzene, are particularly harmful to atopic skin. Mild soaps may be tolerated. Because one cannot predict the soap substitute that will work for a particular individual, several, such as Soydome, Lowila, Dermolate, or Aveeno Bar, may have to be tried.

Adults who have atopic dermatitis of the hands present special problems. Frequently, atopic dermatitis clears with the exception of the hands, where the eruption may remain for prolonged periods. The use of rubber or cotton-lined gloves is unsuccessful because atopic skin does not tolerate the occlusion and the resulting sweat retention and maceration. People who have atopic dermatitis of the hands should use long-handled brushes for dishwashing, cleaning, and doing most other household chores.

TREATMENT OF CONTACT DERMATITIS SUPERIMPOSED ON ATOPIC DERMATITIS

In general, treatment of contact dermatitis complicating an atopic eczema is the same as that of contact dermatitis on nonatopic skin, with the exceptions noted in this section.

Wet Dressings

Potassium permanganate or silver nitrate dressings should be avoided because they are often irritating to atopic skin. Burow's solution (1 part to 20 parts water) or wet dressings of a 1% boric acid solution are better tolerated. Occasionally, even these dressings are too drying. If the inflamed skin is dry, hot, and edematous, the application of a thin layer of plain petrolatum and a superimposed ice bag or ice-cold water compresses may be more soothing.

Tub Baths

In generalized acute cases, tub baths may be indicated. An ointment-based moisturizer or corticosteroid should be used after bathing to prevent overdrying.

Topical Corticosteroid Therapy

In uncomplicated atopic dermatitis, topical corticosteroid creams and ointments are often efficacious. Occlusive dressings with Saran Wrap generally are tolerated in air-conditioned circumstances or cool climates but not in ambient surroundings that lead to sweating. Even in a cool setting, occlusion will be tolerated only for 1 to 2 hours. If intense pruritus occurs, treatment will be counterproductive and should be abandoned.

Systemic Corticosteroid Therapy

In general, the use of systemic corticosteroid therapy is avoided in atopic dermatitis because of the chronicity of the disease and because the patient may become dependent on this mode of therapy. In the presence of severe or generalized contact dermatitis in the atopic individual, however, systemic corticosteroid therapy should be used in the absence of contraindications. Such systemic therapy is indicated particularly when the contact dermatitis is of an allergic nature and the contactant has been discovered. In such instances, systemic therapy does not need to be prolonged for more than 2 or 3 weeks.

An efficient, economical method of systemic corticosteroid therapy in such cases is the administration of 60 g of prednisone daily for 2 days, 40 mg daily for 3 days, 30 mg daily for 2 days, 20 mg daily during the second week, and finally 10 mg daily during the third week. A gradual tapering of the steroid over 2 to 3 weeks tends to prevent a severe rebound dermatitis. Children may receive 20 mg of prednisone for 3 days and then a gradually decreasing dose for 3 weeks.

MANAGEMENT OF EPOXY-RESIN DERMATITIS

Most problems encountered with handling epoxy-resin or curing-agent systems can be prevented by following good personal hygiene and safety practices that include protection for the skin and eyes; good ventilation, including exhaust hood facilities; avoidance of inhalation of vapors; and use of fire prevention safeguards.

Pegum (19) has shown that epoxy resins penetrate rubber gloves. Better protection is obtained with heavy-duty vinyl gloves.

Epoxy resin can be removed by acetone, alcohol, or methyl ethyl ketone followed by acid-type cleansers and a conditioning cream; however, overuse of these solvents can provoke an irritant dermatitis.

Epoxy resin can penetrate nitrile gloves. Use heavy-duty vinyl gloves instead.

INSTRUCTIONS FOR PATIENTS WHO HAVE HOUSEHOLD ECZEMA ("DISHPAN HANDS")

1. Use long-handled brushes for dishwashing and for cleaning and scouring pots, stoves, and dishwashing machines (20).

2. Heating and sweating inside a rubber glove may be as bad for the hands as the irritation from soaps and cleansers. White cotton gloves must be worn inside the rubber gloves. Loose-fitting gloves may be more comfortable and less irritating than gloves that fit snugly. Try not to wear rubber gloves for more than 30 minutes at a time. Do not put hands into very hot water when wearing rubber gloves, because the heat may penetrate the gloves and irritate the hands. Many patients have found that rubber gloves sometimes make their hands worse because they have become allergic to the rubber. If this occurs, switch to light-weight or heavy-duty vinyl gloves. Soak dishes in hot, soapy water for 30 minutes and let the water cool before washing so that the hands are not overheated by the hot water.

3. Bathe babies with one's bare hands, because soaps used for this purpose are mild and do not usually irritate the skin. If the hand dermatitis is acute and rubber gloves are worn, however, put a pair of cotton gloves over the rubber gloves so that the baby can be handled without danger of slipping through the wet rubber gloves.

4. Handling diapers, which contain much ammonia, may irritate the hands. Pick up such diapers with forceps or tongs, place them into a basin containing 1 teaspoon of boric acid powder to 1 quart of water, and allow them to remain in this solution for about 1 hour to neutralize the ammonia.

5. Wear cotton gloves to prevent the hands from getting excessively soiled while doing dry, dusty, and dirty housework. This makes the need for excessive cleaning of the hands unnecessary. If the fingertips are free of dermatitis, cut off the tips of the gloves to allow air to circulate about the hands and thereby prevent excessive sweating.

6. Contact of the hands with fruit juices, fruits, vegetables, and raw meats may irritate the skin. Use canned or frozen products until the hands are better. Avoid direct contact of the inflamed skin with the irritating juices of onions and garlic.

7. Wool causes itching and irritation in many individuals; contact with it should be minimized.

8. Avoid exposure of the hands to hair tonics and lotions. Use a brush or cotton-tipped swab to apply such preparations to the scalp.

9. When pouring or measuring detergents or bleaches, be careful that they do not splash onto the hands and forearms. Patients who have hand eczema should use bleaches in powder form or those that are premeasured and packaged in plastic containers.

10. Cleansing of the skin in hand dermatitis:

    A. Do not use household cleansers on the hands. These products are made to remove dirt from dishes, clothes, walls, and floors and are too harsh for use on the skin. Also avoid the use of solvents such as turpentine or benzene. These chemicals are harsh because they defat the skin and cause marked dryness and cracking. Do not use deodorant soaps or antibacterial soaps, because they have chemicals that can irritate or cause allergic reactions. Use plain, unscented soaps. If the hands are dry, use a superfatted soap.

    B. Avoid prolonged or too frequent washing of the skin. Gently pat the skin dry with a soft cloth or tissues. Avoid vigorous rubbing. Remember that some people seem to tolerate unlimited washings of the hands with soap and water, whereas others get dry and irritated skin even with minimal washing. Do not use soaps that sting and are excessively drying.

    C. Even the mildest soap must be rinsed off the hands gently and thoroughly.

    D. In the acute stage, when the hands are swollen and red, avoid cleansing the skin with soap. Bathe the hands in Burow's solution (1 part to 20 parts water). If the skin feels dry after this procedure, gently swab it with olive oil and apply the prescribed medication. Remove rings from fingers when washing the hands.

Principles of Treatment of Hand Dermatitis

The following directions are general guidelines only; they may need to be modified to suit individual cases.

1. Use an unscented soap or hand cleanser free of color, antiseptics, deodorants, vitamins, and tar.

2. Wash hands with lukewarm water and use the soap sparingly. Rinse hands thoroughly. Dry gently with a clean towel and do not forget to dry between the fingers. Wash the hands as infrequently as possible, preferably no more than two or three times daily.

3. Take off rings when washing hands. Soap caught under a ring may produce a flare-up of hand dermatitis.

4. Avoid hobbies or household chores that involve direct contact with solvents, turpentine, waxes, adhesives, and epoxy resins unless protective gloves can be worn.

5. Do not use strong corticosteroid topical medications over prolonged periods. These may produce skin atrophy.

6. If the skin is dry, a corticosteroid ointment gives better results than a cream. If an ointment is considered too messy, use a cream in the daytime and an ointment at night.

7. Wear thin polyethylene gloves at night for several hours to enhance the effect of the ointment and to prevent spread of the ointment to the bedclothes.

8. Avoid use of creams that contain anything you are shown to be allergic to on patch testing. Use a fragrance-free moisturizing cream liberally, as recommended by your physician.

9. Guidelines regarding gloves:

   A. Plastic (vinyl) gloves are better protection against some chemicals than latex rubber gloves, to which some people become allergic. Try to limit the wearing of gloves to approximately 30 minutes or less at a time. Wear thin cotton gloves underneath vinyl gloves to absorb perspiration.

   B. While doing dry, dusty, and dirty work, wear cotton gloves to prevent the hands from getting excessively soiled. Wash your gloves, not your hands.

   C. Woolen gloves cause irritation of many people's hands.

   D. Neither vinyl nor rubber gloves stop penetration of some chemicals, such as hair perming chemicals and many solvents. A plastic polymer glove, such as the 4-H Glove, is usually more protective against these chemicals.

10. Avoid handling the following items with bare hands:

   A. Fruit juices and the inside of the skin of fruits; raw meats, fish, and vegetables, especially raw onions and garlic

   B. Detergents, turpentine, and kerosene

   C. Hair tonics (Use a cotton-tipped swab or a brush.)

   D. Shampoos (Use vinyl gloves.)

General Measures in the Management of Hand Dermatitis

In addition to the special measures and instructions already suggested in this chapter, most patients who have contact dermatitis of the hands require antieczematous and antibacterial therapy and may benefit from the following suggestions.

- *Wet dressings:* In the acute phase, when itching, edema, and oozing are features, compresses with cold water to which crushed ice has been added are valuable, except in the presence of vascular disease of the hands, particularly Raynaud's syndrome. In the presence of infection, the addition of Burow's solution (1 tablespoon to a pint of cold water) is indicated. In most instances, it is inadvisable to use wet potassium permanganate dressings on the hands because it produces uncomfortable drying and crusting and discoloration of the nails, which may be embarrassing to the ambulatory patient. Another water additive used to make a wet dressing is Prophyllin Powder (Dystan), a copper-chlorophyll product that produces a soothing compress solution.

- *Proper cleansing:* Avoid excessive hand washing. The skin of the hands does not have to be cleansed completely before each application of a topical remedy. Only those scales, crusts, and debris that come away easily with gentle cleansing should be removed.

- *Topical medication:* Following the use of the wet dressings, topical corticosteroid medications may be applied to the hands. For ambulatory patients, creams may be used in the daytime, whereas ointments are applied overnight. Often, ointments are more effective than creams on the palms. Such ointments may be kept in place and their effect enhanced with plastic gloves, which are used for several hours at a time.

  Dermatitis of the hands readily becomes secondarily infected. Practically all fissured, crusted hand eczemas are infected and can benefit from antibiotic treatment. Fisher recommends a corticosteroid cream for daytime use and erythromycin ointment (Ilotycin) for nighttime use. Oral erythromycin or another antibiotics active against staphylococcal and streptococcal infections may be helpful.

- *Systemic treatment:* Systemic corticosteroid therapy may be indicated when the dermatitis of the hands is severe and spreading and does not respond quickly to topical remedies. In the absence of the usual contraindications to such therapy, 40 to 60 mg of prednisone or its equivalent may be given for several days. The dosage should be decreased by 10 to 15 mg every few days over a 10- to 14-day period. Such gradual tapering of steroid therapy prevents the rebound of the contact dermatitis that may take place when corticosteroid therapy is stopped too abruptly. Alternatively, 40 to 60 mg intramuscularly of triamcinolone acetonide (Kenalog and others) may be useful for its prolonged duration of action. The offending contactant should be searched for and eliminated in order to prevent recurrences.

- *Treatment of fissures:* Fissures can be carefully coated with a cyanoacrylate glue such as Krazy Glue or Super Glue. Care must be taken that the fingers are not glued together.

- *Occlusive dressings:* In the chronic phase of a hand dermatitis, the use of corticosteroid ointments covered with an occlusive dressing such as Saran Wrap may expedite healing. This form of therapy should be avoided in individuals who have atopic backgrounds and who have hyperhidrosis.

- *Protective bandages:* The patient should avoid the use of Band-Aids and other adhesives directly on the skin. Light, white cotton gloves are useful to protect the hands and to keep topical remedies in place. Even an ordinary gauze bandage may irritate the skin of the hands. Soft, closely woven cotton or linen dressings are preferred.

- *Sedation:* For the tense, pruritic, sleepless patient, cyproheptadine hydrochloride (Periactin) 4 mg twice a day or hydroxyzine hydrochloride (Atarax) 10 mg three times daily may be prescribed for their antipruritic and sedative effects. Other antihistamines may be similarly used.

- *Scale reduction:* In thick, keratotic hand eczema, the following mixture may be useful: salicylic acid (2%), liquor carbonis detergens (LCD) (2%), hydrocortisone (2.5% cream) or triamcinolone (0.1% cream 60 g), and Velvachol (as much as suffices, up to 240 g).

- *Other treatments:* Hand PUVA or grenz ray therapy may be useful in stubborn chronic cases of hand eczema. Care must be taken with topical psoralen products because burning is more likely than with systemic psoralen administration.

REFERENCES

1. Lindelof B, Wrangsjo K, Liden S. A double-blind study of grenz ray therapy in chronic eczema of the hands. Br J Dermatol 1987;117:77.
2. Lindelof B, Liden S, Lagerholm B. The effect of grenz rays on the expression of allergic contact dermatitis in man. Scand J Immunol 1985;21:463.
3. Lindelof B, Lindberg M. The effect of grenz rays on irritant skin reactions in man. Acta Derm Venereol 1987;67:128.
4. Simons JR, Bohnen IJ, van der Valk PG. A left-right comparison of UVB phototherapy and topical photochemotherapy in bilateral chronic hand dermatitis after 6 weeks' treatment. Clin Exp Derm 1997;22:7.
5. Burke DA, Corey G, Storrs FJ. Psoralen plus UVA protocol for Compositae photosensitivity. Am J Contact Dermat 1996;7:171.
6. Sharma VK, Chakrabarti A, Mahajan V. Azathioprine in the treatment of Parthenium dermatitis. Int J Dermatol 1998;37:299.
7. Granlund H, Erkko P, Reitamo S. Long-term follow-up of eczema patients treated with cyclosporine. Acta Derm Venereol 1998;78:40.
8. De Rie MA, Meinardi MM, Bos JD. Lack of efficacy of topical cyclosporin A in atopic dermatitis and allergic contact dermatitis. Acta Derm Venereol 1991;71:452.
9. Granlund H, Erkko P, Eriksson E, Reitamo S. Comparison of cyclosporine and topical betamethasone-17,21-dipropionate in the treatment of severe chronic hand eczema. Acta Derm Venereol 1996; 76:371.
10. Lauerma AI, Stein BD, Homey B, et al. Topical FK 506: suppression of allergic and irritant contact dermatitis in the guinea pig. Arch Dermatol Res 1994;286: 337.
11. Sengoku T, Moritak, Sakuma S, et al. Possible inhibitory mechanism of FK 506 (tacrolimus hydrate) ointment for atopic dermatitis based on animal models. Eur J Pharmacol 1999;379:183.
12. Fleischer AB Jr. Treatment of atopic dermatitis: role of tacrolimus ointment as a topical noncorticosteroidal therapy. J Allergy Clin Immunol 1999;104(3 pt 2):S126.
13. Van Leent EJ, Graber M, Thurston M, et al. Effectiveness of the ascomycin macrolactam SDZ ASM 981 in the topical treatment of atopic dermatitis. Arch Dermatol 1998;134:805.
14. Grassberger M, Baumruker T, Enz A, et al. A novel anti-inflammatory drug, SDZ ASM 981, for the treatment of skin diseases: in vitro pharmacology. Br J Dermatol 1999;141:264.
15. Cherill Tofte S, MacNaul R, et al. One-percent SDZ ASM 981 cream effective in the treatment of chronic irritant hand dermatitis: A 6-week, randomized, double-blind, vehiclec-vehicled, single-center study. Presented at the Twelfth International Contact Dermatitis Symposium, October 1999, San Francisco, CA.
16. Kroon S. Contact dermatitis from oleyl polypeptide in Xeruminex ear drops. Contact Dermatitis 1981;7:271.
17. Boxley JD, Dawber RP. Contact dermatitis to one ingredient of Xeruminex ear drops. Contact Dermatitis 1976;2:233.
18. Grice K, Johnstone CI. Contact dermatitis from Xerumenex. Br Med J 1972;1·508.
19. Pegum JS. Penetration of protective gloves by epoxy resin. Contact Dermatitis 1979;5:281.
20. Grimalt F, Romaguera C. Dry and fissured skin limited to the index finger of the right hand as a unique manifestation of housewife's dermatitis. Contact Dermatitis 1977;3:54.

CHAPTER 39

Specific Instructions for Patients with Common Contact Allergens

GENERAL INSTRUCTIONS FOR A POSITIVE PATCH TEST

1. A positive test indicates an adverse reaction may occur if your skin comes in contact with the identified substance. Usually this will be a rash that itches and persists for several days or even several weeks.
2. It is important to avoid direct skin contact with your allergen as no method like "allergy shots" to desensitize to this type of allergen is presently available.
3. When an allergen is avoided, improvement in skin rashes starts slowly, and in most cases the full benefit of the avoidance will occur within 3 weeks, but with severe or prolonged skin problems the benefit may continue to increase for up to 3 months.
4. Being in the same room with an allergen that has been identified by patch testing is generally not a problem unless the substance can be blown into the air or is extremely volatile.
5. The parts of the skin that come in greatest contact with the allergen will usually have the greatest amount of rash. Areas protected from direct exposure to the allergen will usually show little or no rash.
6. If the instructions you are given as to what should be avoided do not make sense or skin contact with materials thought to contain your allergen fails to result in a rash within a few days, something is wrong. There may be an additional allergen to worry about, or allergy may not be your only problem. Some people do not clear as quickly as others because they have "sensitive skin" that is more easily irritated by everyday, normally harmless exposures. Discuss this with your doctor.

NEOMYCIN

The substance to which you are allergic is one that will normally be found on labels. If you are purchasing anything for use on your skin, first inspect the package for the ingredient list. If you have products at home that do not have a label or the container does not list the ingredients, it would be best to go to the store where the product was purchased and inspect the original package. In the United States, products that are sold for consumer use on the skin as a cosmetic or toiletry item must be labeled with the ingredients listed in decreasing order of concentration. The first item listed is present in the greatest concentration, and the last listed is at the lowest concentration. Many of the allergenic materials are present in very low concentrations and are listed near the end of the ingredient list. Products sold as medical devices at present only have to reveal the "active" ingredients.

Sometimes a product will contain so little of a material that you are allergic to that skin contact may be harmless. However, you cannot count on this and should try to avoid all the products that have the potential to cause trouble.

You are allergic to neomycin. This antibiotic is a common ingredient in over-the-counter triple antibiotic ointments. Examples would be Neosporin, Neopolycin, and Mycitracin. It will be listed on the ingredient label. It is common to also be allergic to bacitracin if you are allergic to neomycin, and it would be wise to avoid both. Betadine ointment is a chemically unrelated antibiotic that you could substitute for neomycin. Also, a prescription ointment called mupirocin is safe for you. Let your doctors know that you are allergic to neomycin and related antibiotics.These include gentamycin and tobramycin and are called aminoglycosides. You should avoid these.

BENZOCAINE

The substance to which you are allergic is one that will normally be found on labels. If you are purchasing anything for use on your skin, first inspect the package for the ingredient list. If you have products at home that do not have a label or the container does not list the ingredients, it would be best to go to the store where the product was purchased and inspect the original package. In the United States, products that are sold for consumer use on the skin as a cosmetic or toiletry item must be labeled with the ingredients listed in decreasing order of concentration. The first item listed is present in the greatest concentration, and the last listed is at the lowest concentration. Many of the allergenic materials are present in very low concentrations and are listed near the end of the ingredient list. Products sold as medical devices at present only have to reveal the "active" ingredients.

Sometimes a product will contain so little of a material that you are allergic to that skin contact may be harmless. However, you cannot count on this and should try to avoid all the products that have the potential to cause trouble.

You are allergic to benzocaine. This is an anesthetic and is used to numb the skin or make the nerve endings in the skin less sensitive. It is commonly found in skin care products for burns, cuts, sores, and rashes. Benzocaine is a common ingredient found in medication for teething babies, hemorrhoidal preparations, and some cough and sore throat medications. Many other anesthetics that end in "caine" may also cause your skin to break out, but one that is safe for use is lidocaine (Xylocaine). You should let your doctor know you are allergic to benzocaine so that no such materials are used on your skin, mouth, or gums at the dentist's or doctor's office or in any of your prescriptions. Always check labels for this, as it will be noted if it is present.

THIMEROSAL

The substance to which you are allergic is one that will normally be found on labels. If you are purchasing anything for use on your skin, first inspect the package for the ingredient list. If you have products at home that do not have a label or the container does not list the ingredients, it would be best to go to the store where the product was purchased and inspect the original package. In the United States, products that are sold for consumer use on the skin as a cosmetic or

toiletry item must be labeled with the ingredients listed in decreasing order of concentration. The first item listed is present in the greatest concentration, and the last listed is at the lowest concentration. Many of the allergenic materials are present in very low concentrations and are listed near the end of the ingredient list. Products sold as medical devices at present only have to reveal the "active" ingredients.

Sometimes a product will contain so little of a material that you are allergic to that skin contact may be harmless. However, you cannot count on this and should try to avoid all the products that have the potential to cause trouble.

You are allergic to thimerosal. This is also known as Merthiolate. Some immunizations contain thimerosal that can lead to strong local reactions, but systemic reactions almost never occur. Most products with thimerosal are used on moist areas of the body, such as around the eyes, ears, nose, and genital areas. Contact lens solutions may be sources of thimerosal.

IMIDAZOLIDINYL UREA

The substance to which you are allergic is one that will normally be found on labels. If you are purchasing anything for use on your skin, first inspect the package for the ingredient list. If you have products at home that do not have a label or the container does not list the ingredients, it would be best to go to the store where the product was purchased and inspect the original package. In the United States, products that are sold for consumer use on the skin as a cosmetic or toiletry item must be labeled with the ingredients listed in decreasing order of concentration. The first item listed is present in the greatest concentration, and the last listed is at the lowest concentration. Many of the allergenic materials are present in very low concentrations and are listed near the end of the ingredient list. Products sold as medical devices at present only have to reveal the "active" ingredients.

Sometimes a product will contain so little of a material that you are allergic to that skin contact may be harmless. However, you cannot count on this and should try to avoid all the products that have the potential to cause trouble.

You are allergic to imidazolidinyl urea. This is a preservative commonly used in skin care products. By reading labels, you should be very successful at avoiding this allergen. A similar preservative called diazolidinyl urea should probably also be avoided, because many, but not all, people who are allergic to one may react to both.

QUATERNIUM-15

The substance to which you are allergic is one that will normally be found on labels. If you are purchasing anything for use on your skin, first inspect the package for the ingredient list. If you have products at home that do not have a label or the container does not list the ingredients, it would be best to go to the store where the product was purchased and inspect the original package. In the United States, products that are sold for consumer use on the skin as a cosmetic or toiletry item must be labeled with the ingredients listed in decreasing order of concentration. The first item listed is present in the greatest concentration, and the last listed is at the lowest concentration. Many of the allergenic materials are present in very low concentrations and are listed near the end of the ingredient list. Products sold as medical devices at present only have to reveal the "active" ingredients.

Sometimes a product will contain so little of a material that you are allergic to that skin contact may be harmless. However, you cannot count on this and should try to avoid all the products that have the potential to cause trouble.

You are allergic to quaternium-15, which is a preservative. It is also used to purify some water-soluble coolants in industrial settings. In industry, it is known as Dowicil 200. Quaternium compounds with other numbers are usually totally different and generally not of concern. It may be present in products frequently recommended by dermatologists, but you should avoid these if quaternium-15 is on the label.

LANOLIN

The substance to which you are allergic is one that will normally be found on labels. If you are purchasing anything for use on your skin, first inspect the package for the ingredient list. If you have products at home that do not have a label or the container does not list the ingredients, it would be best to go to the store where the product was purchased and inspect the original package. In the United States, products that are sold for consumer use on the skin as a cosmetic or toiletry item must be labeled with the ingredients listed in decreasing order of concentration. The first item listed is present in the greatest concentration, and the last listed is at the lowest concentration. Many of the allergenic materials are present in very low concentrations and are listed near the end of the ingredient list. Products sold as medical devices at present only have to reveal the "active" ingredients.

Sometimes a product will contain so little of a material of which you are allergic that skin contact may be harmless. However, you cannot count on this and should try to avoid all the products that have the potential to cause trouble.

You are allergic to lanolin, which is also known as wool alcohol or wool wax alcohol. Another very similar chemical that you should avoid is called Amerchol. Lanolin is derived from sheep's wool. Because it is a biologic product, the amount of allergen may vary from batch to batch. You may find an occasional lanolin-containing product that you can use, but this is not to be considered as an invalidation of the test results. Prudence would dictate avoidance of all lanolin products.

RUBBER ALLERGENS

You have been found to be allergic to a rubber chemical. Although some forms of rubber are familiar, others are not. Elastic materials are generally rubber based and may contain your allergen. Rubber cements are used to hold together many items where flexibility is required, such as shoes. Adhesives and tapes may contain these materials, as may hoses and belts.

Some rubber allergens are found in agricultural products, such as fungicides, although others may be found in pet care products. Some polyurethane foam rubber products have been found to contain these allergens. Cloth-covered foam materials and clothing that contains spandex are other possible sources.

Specific rubber allergen groups are listed below.

Mercaptobenzothiazole and Mercapto Mix

In addition to the above, pay attention to pesticides, animal repellents, and veterinarian products.

Thiuram Mix

May be found in Playtex rubber gloves. Cotton liners do not protect against this allergen. May also be found in fungicides and the prescription drug Antabuse.

Carba Mix

Also found in the same items noted for thiuram mix. Both have been found in polyurethane foam rubber. Might cross-react with iodopropynyl butylcarbamate, a preservative in skin care products.

Black Rubber Mix

This is more common in industrial black rubber and automobile tires. Sometimes other colors of rubber contain these chemicals. These allergens have been found in some undergarment elastic. Some persons allergic to this mix have problems from dyes used on synthetic fabrics, such as rayon, polyester, and acrylics.

If you are having a problem with gloves, vinyl gloves do not contain rubber chemicals and should be safe for you.

CINNAMIC ALCOHOL AND ALDEHYDE

You are allergic to a form of cinnamon (either cinnamic alcohol or cinnamic aldehyde). This is both a flavor and a fragrance. Use of unscented or fragrance-free products is necessary to minimize skin contact with cinnamon. Sometimes cinnamon is part of a mixture of flavor chemicals and not readily apparent by taste or smell.

Ingestion of cinnamon-flavored items may cause some, but not all, cinnamon-sensitive people to have a rash or itching. If you feel this is a possible cause for your symptoms, you should avoid obvious cinnamon-flavored food and beverage items, as well as colas, sweet vermouth, bitters, and chocolate.

Cassia oil is another name for these allergens.

EPOXY RESIN

You are allergic to epoxy resin. This is generally found in two-part glue and paints or other coatings that have to be mixed shortly before use. Dentists use epoxies; therefore, you should inform your dentist of your allergy. Sometimes epoxy resin may remain in some plastics. If you are concerned about a plastic item, it must come in contact with your skin and the rash should occur at this site. Heated epoxy resins may become fumes that lead to rashes on sensitive exposed skin, such as the eyelids.

PARATERTIARY BUTYLPHENOL FORMALDEHYDE RESIN

You are allergic to paratertiary butylphenol formaldehyde resin. This is found in glues, such as those used in shoes and other adhesives. Rubber items may contain this substance. It has also been found in duplicating paper, printing inks, and some plastics. Some handles on cookware are made of plastic containing this allergen. Some plywood is glued together with it. Commercial deodorants and commercial germicidal detergents may contain it. It is also often found in adhesives used for leather goods, such as wallets, wristwatch straps, and handbags.

COLOPHONY

You are allergic to colophony or rosin. This is obtained from the sap of pine trees. It is frequently used to make things sticky, such as glues and adhesives. Adhesive tape is one example. Polish for furniture, floors, and cars may contain colophony. Solder used in electronics contains rosin, as does some welding flux. Paper products contain colophony, as does printer's ink. Some putty and wood doughs are sources of this allergen. The rosin bag on the pitcher's mound and rosin for violin bows are familiar sources of this allergen. Occasionally, cosmetics may contain colophony, especially eye cosmetics.

PARAPHENYLENEDIAMINE

You are allergic to paraphenylenediamine. This is a black dye. In general, once the dye has "set," it is nonallergenic. The most common problem with this allergen is in dying hair. It can similarly cause problems if it gets on your skin while you are dying other objects, such as furs or cloth. Photographic chemicals may contain paraphenylenediamine. Some clothing dyes may cause reactions, but for this to explain your rash, the skin that has the rash would have to be the skin contacted by the suspect clothing. Similarly, some rubber goods may have chemical contents that will cause your skin to develop a rash. Some industrial chemicals that are found in rubber may be chemical cousins to this allergen and cause rashes when in contact with skin.

The labels on hair dyes may have names that are somewhat different from paraphenylenediamine, but cause just as much of a problem. Avoid the following:

p-toluenediamine
1,4-benzenediamine
p-aminodiphenylamine
1,4-phenylenediamine
2,4-diaminoanisole
p-aminoaniline
o-aminophenol

Some people with this allergy also have trouble with sulfa drugs and sunscreens based on PABA (para-aminobenzoic acid). Others may have trouble with anesthetics such as benzocaine. Your doctor should tell you if these are concerns in your case.

Henna is a safe hair coloring. Also, most people allergic to this chemical can tolerate semipermanent hair coloring rinses.

FORMALDEHYDE

You are allergic to formaldehyde. Skin contact with formaldehyde is required for this to cause a rash. Avoid contact with items that list formaldehyde as an ingredient on the label. If the product is a shampoo or similar product that is applied to skin and washed off, you may be able to tolerate this brief contact, but prudence would dictate that you avoid such contact if at all possible. Some formaldehyde-sensitive persons cannot tolerate even the tiniest amount of skin contact with formaldehyde, but most are not this severely sensitive. There are five commonly used topical preservatives that are in the formaldehyde family: quaternium-15, imidazolidinyl urea, diazolidinyl urea, bronopol, and DMDM hydantoin. Most formaldehyde-allergic people need to avoid all of these, but occasionally you may tolerate a product with a low level of one of these.

If your occupation brings you in contact with some of the following circumstances, you may be getting formaldehyde on your skin and causing rashes: embalming fluid; photographic chemicals; industrial disinfectants and fumigations; automotive fluids; medical dialysis fluids and the medications Mandelamine and Urised; paints; leather processing; some printing processes such as etching. The manufacturing process of plastics and plywood is often a source of formaldehyde exposure to workers.

Fumes of formaldehyde will not usually cause difficulty because the concentration is so low. If your rash is in skin exposed to air and the most sensitive areas of that exposed skin are a prominent part of your problem, then fumes of formaldehyde may be of concern. Smoke from fires or cigarettes will contain formaldehyde.

Clothing that is permanent press is treated with formaldehyde-related materials. At one time the dominant chemical used was formaldehyde, and multiple washings of the clothing reduced the formaldehyde concentration. Now a group of more complex chemicals is used, and although these are related to formaldehyde, the likelihood of this causing your rash can best be tested with the specific fabric finishes. You should not be concerned about clothing as part of your problem unless the areas of rash correspond to places that clothing comes in contact with the skin bearing the rash.

ETHYLENEDIAMINE

You are allergic to ethylenediamine. This chemical is an ingredient in the original formula of Mycolog Cream. The company that makes Mycolog no longer makes a formula that contains your allergen. Mycolog II is safe for use from an allergen standpoint. However, the generic forms of Mycolog are made with the original formula, which should be avoided.

If you have asthma, your doctor may wish to give you an intravenous medication that is known as aminophylline. It breaks down into your allergen and should be avoided. You should let your doctor know about your allergy.

Some medicines used for itching may cause you to have a rash. They are chemically almost identical with ethylenediamine and may be mistaken as the same chemical by your body. It may be wise to avoid these closely related materials, which are in the antihistamine category:

hydroxyzine (Atarax, Visteril)
tripelennamine (Pyribenzamine)
meclizine (Bonine, Antivert)
chlorcyclizine (Mantadil)
cyclizine (Marezine)
buclizine (Bucladin-S)

Tincture of Merthiolate contains ethylenediamine and should be avoided. There are industrial exposures that may apply to your case if you work with electroplating, film developing chemicals, some dying processes, and some other solvents. Epoxy hardeners often contain chemicals related to ethylenediamine.

BALSAM OF PERU

You are allergic to balsam of Peru. This is a sweet-smelling natural substance from pine or fir trees. Allergy to balsam of Peru most frequently means that you are allergic to a fragrance chemical or perfume. However, because this is a natural product and contains many different substances, it is difficult to be exact as to which fragrance chemical is at fault. The prudent person would avoid scented products and favor fragrance-free or unscented ones instead.

Some medical products will contain balsam of Peru, and it may be listed on the ingredient label in some cases. Check products that may be used in the diaper area and for hemorrhoid treatment. There are closely related chemicals that enjoy a medical use, such as benzoin and benzyl alcohol, and if these appear on the label of a skin care product, it would be best to avoid them.

Naturally occurring ingredients in foods may contain substances so closely related or identical to substances present in balsam of Peru that when ingested they may cause your rash. If avoiding external sources of balsam of Peru has not resulted in clearing of your problem, then a period of dietary avoidance of the substances listed below may be worthwhile. (Dietary restrictions may take 3 to 4 weeks to show benefit. If you improve, you should add back one food per week to see if avoidance really makes any difference. Frequently, only one or two foods are truly found to be at fault, but it is still necessary to eliminate all the other possible causes for the diet restrictions to be properly evaluated.)

Avoid citrus peel and related flavors in any food, such as candy, gum, baked goods, spiced teas, tobaccos, ice cream, cola, and citrus soft drinks. Avoid spices, such as cinnamon, cloves, vanilla, curry, tomato ketchup, chili sauce, chutney, pickled herring, pickled vegetables, paté, vermouth, and bitters.

POTASSIUM DICHROMATE

You are allergic to chromates. This allergen is found in a variety of substances. The powdered form of cement and some wet cement contain chromates that cause problems mainly for members of the construction trades. If the powdered form of cement is blown by wind onto your skin, a rash may develop on the exposed areas; otherwise, direct skin contact with the material is required for a rash to develop. Other construction materials including brick, mortar, and drywall may contain chromates. Leather goods are treated with chromates and may cause you to have a rash. This is usually a problem when the leather becomes wet by sweat or moisture from other sources. Some chromate-allergic people have no trouble with leather shoes as long as they wear socks and their shoes do not get wet.

Coatings used to prevent rust generally are chromates and must be kept off your skin. These are used in industry to galvanize sheet metal and protect metals in general, and they are also found in home-use rust preventatives. Yellow and green paints are also a potential source of chromates. Other items may be of concern, such as some textiles, cosmetics, and the green felt on pool tables, and nongreen items such as blueprints, lithography fluids, match heads, and wood preservatives.

KATHON (METHYLCHLOROISOTHIAZOLINONE/METHYLISOTHIAZOLINONE)

This preservative is starting to come into common use in the United States, after having been in use in Europe for some time. It is now present in many shampoos sold in the United States, especially in cosmetic and skin care products. Usually the name Kathon is not listed on the label, but the longer name noted above (methylchloroisothiazolinone/methylisothiazolinone) is what you will see on the label. You need to read very carefully to be sure you do not use any products that contain this chemical. This chemical is used in industry in water-cooling plants and metalworking fluids.

NICKEL

You are allergic to nickel. This metal allergen accounts for most, but not all, costume jewelry reactions. Nickel objects often are shiny and appear chrome plated. Not all metal will contain nickel. Direct skin contact with the metal object containing nickel will cause a rash at that specific site. For example, metal eyelash curlers may cause eyelid rashes. Cleaning your ears with a metal bobby pin may cause ear canal rashes. Metal pins and snaps in clothing may cause spots of itchy, reddened skin at such sites, such as around the belly button.

Stainless steel contains nickel, but it is so tightly bound to the metal that it will not get into your skin and cause problems. In general, it takes about 3 minutes of skin con-

tact with a metal object to start to move the nickel from the metal into your skin. Wet contact with metal will shorten the length of time for the transfer to occur and start a rash.

A test kit is available from Allerderm Laboratories, P.O. Box 2070, Petaluma, CA 94953. This kit will allow you to test metal items for the presence of nickel at home or work. Keep in mind that nickel will go through rubber gloves with or without cotton liners. Avoidance of skin contact is the key to getting better.

Diet Instructions for Nickel-Sensitive People

Sometimes after avoiding all skin contact with an allergen, such as nickel or chromate, the rash may persist. In some cases, the same amounts of these allergens that occur naturally in foods will be responsible for the rash continuing. When this is the case, it is necessary to avoid the foods listed below for 3 to 4 weeks to rid the body of a continued stimulation that could be causing the rash. If your skin improves with the diet, you may add back one food per week to see if your rash returns or flares. This will confirm the importance of continuing to avoid the food in question. It will also ensure that you are not needlessly giving up a food you enjoy. Frequently, only one or two food items will be critical to your getting better. It is necessary to begin with strict avoidance of all the possibilities in order to determine the role of diet in your care.

Various food items and drinks can aggravate nickel eczema even though the nickel content of these foods may be low. Such food items include beer, wine (in particular, red wine), herring, mackerel, tuna, tomato, onion, carrot, and certain fruits, in particular, apples and citrus fruits (juice). The vegetables mentioned can usually be tolerated when cooked.

The first liter (quart) of water taken from the tap in the morning should not be used in food preparation, as nickel may be released from the tap during the night. Nickel-plated kitchen utensils, such as eggbeaters and tea balls, should be replaced.

Acid foods, such as stewed fruits and rhubarb, cooked in stainless-steel utensils should be avoided. The acids in the foods can cause nickel to be released from the utensils. Tinned foods should be eaten only in moderation.

Provided by: Niels K. Veien, M.D., Ph.D., The Dermatology Clinic, Vesterbro 99, DK-9000 Alborg, Denmark.

These foods are OK	Avoid these foods
Meat, fish, etc.	
Eggs	Shellfish, such as shrimp,
Fish	mussels, and crawfish
Meat (all kinds)	
Poultry	
Dairy products	
Butter	Chocolate milk
Cheese	
Milk in all forms	
Yogurt (unflavored)	

Vegetables

These foods are OK	Avoid these foods
Asparagus	Beans (green, brown,
Beets, red	white)
Broccoli	Kale
Brussels sprouts	Leeks
Cabbage, white	Lentils
Cauliflower	Lettuce
Chinese cabbage	Peas (green and split)
Corn	Soy protein powder (used
Cucumber	in sausages, sandwich
Dill	meat, products made
Eggplant	from minced meat,
Garlic (in moderation)	bread, soup
Mushrooms	concentrates,
Onions (in moderation)	bouillon, etc.)
Parsley	Spinach
Peppers, green, red	Sprouts made from beans
Potatoes	and alfalfa

Grains and grains products

Breakfast foods made of rice	Bran
Cakes and biscuits *not*	Buckwheat
containing almonds or	Millet
other nuts, cocoa, or	Muesli and other similar
chocolate	breakfast cereal
Cornflakes	products
Cornmeal	Multigrain breads
Cornstarch	Oatmeal
Macaroni	Rice (unpolished)
Popcorn	Rye bran
Rice (polished, white rice	Sesame seeds
in moderation)	Sunflower seeds
Spaghetti	Wheat bran and other bran
Wheat flour	and fiber products,
Whole grain rye and wheat	including cereals, bran
bread (in moderation)	biscuits, and fiber tablets
	Whole grain breads and
	biscuits

Fruit, berries, etc.

Bananas (in moderation)	Dates
Berries (all *except*	Figs
raspberries)	Pineapple
Peaches	Prunes
Pears	Raspberries
Raisins	
Rhubarb	

Drinks

Alcoholic beverages	Chocolate and cocoa
(distilled products	drinks
and drinks made from	Tea from drink dispensers
these)	
Carbonated beverages	
Coffee and tea (not too strong	
and in moderation)	

Miscellaneous

Margarine	Almonds
Yeast	Baking powder (in large
	amounts)
	Hazel nuts and other nuts
	Linseed, linseed oil
	Peanuts
	Sweets containing
	chocolate, marzipan,
	nuts, and strong licorice
	Vitamins containing nickel

COBALT

This is a metal found in some costume jewelry and other everyday inexpensive metal objects. In addition, it may be found in construction materials such as concrete, drywall, brick, and mortar. Occasionally, it is found in cosmetics as a coloring agent and may be found in wet, uncured pottery.

Many individuals allergic to cobalt are also allergic to nickel and chromate. These metals also are often found in jewelry and construction materials, as noted above. Cobalt is occasionally used in industry in the manufacture of plastic and rubber materials, but this should only be a problem for workers in these industries, not for consumers handling plastic or rubber.

COCAMIDOPROPYL BETAINE

This is a substance found in many skin care products, especially soaps, shampoos, and hair conditioners, but also other products, including skin lotions, makeup removers, and even contact lens cleaners. This chemical is called a surfactant, which means it is used to help dissolve oils and to let other substances mix together. It should be fairly easy to avoid this substance because it should be listed on labeling by this name.

It may also be found in some household cleaning products.

FRAGRANCES

Fragrance allergy may be difficult to deal with because there are literally several hundred individual chemicals, both natural and synthetic, that are used in fragrances. A person who is allergic to fragrances on patch testing may have problems with perfumes and colognes but also with the fragrances in other skin and hair care products, laundry products, and so on. Therefore, individuals with a fragrance allergy should use fragrance-free products as much as possible. If an individual wishes to use a fragrance-containing product, the product should be site tested by applying a small amount of the product to the inside of one elbow twice a day in the same spot for 7 days. If no redness or itching develops at that site, then that particular fragrance-containing product is probably safe for use.

It is generally not advised that individuals with a fragrance allergy apply fragrance materials to their clothing. Some individuals with a fragrance allergy may develop dermatitis when eating certain foods and spices in the family of balsams. Your doctor can discuss this more fully with you if this is suspected.

GLUTARALDEHYDE

This chemical is also called glutaral. This is a sterilizing solution and preservative that is commonly found in medical and dental offices. It is occasionally used in dental products and shampoos. It is commonly found in industrial hand cleaners as a disinfectant. It is also present in embalming fluid and is used as a tanning agent for some leather products. Many people have problems from exposure to medical and dental instruments that have been cleaned with this chemical. It is also used as an agent in some photographic processes.

GLYCERYL THIOGLYCOLATE

This is a chemical that is the main ingredient in most currently used hair permanent solutions that are known as acid perms or heat perms. There is an older permanent solution that contains another chemical called ammonium thioglycolate. Most people who are allergic to the glyceryl thioglycolate can tolerate ammonium thioglycolate. Unfortunately, glyceryl thioglycolate is a chemical that penetrates normal rubber gloves; therefore, these do not protect individuals from this chemical. 4-H gloves provide a good barrier and will not allow the chemical to penetrate. These can be obtained from commercial glove suppliers.

GOLD

Gold allergy is much more common than previously believed. Obviously, some people will react at sites where their skin comes in contact with gold jewelry, such as the ears, fingers, and neck. However, some people do not react on the hands because the skin there is relatively strong and does not break out as easily. Some individuals will develop dermatitis on the face, eyelids, or other sensitive areas of the body just by touching and wearing gold jewelry. Because these areas are more sensitive, occasional contact of jewelry on the skin can cause problems. It is recommended that people who are allergic to gold should avoid wearing gold jewelry as much as possible. Use on special occasions for short times is probably acceptable. Platinum or sterling silver can be worn safely, but white gold should be avoided as well. For special jewelry items an individual may wish to wear, a jeweler can usually plate the back of the jewelry with rhodium or platinum, which helps to block the contact of gold with the skin. Many individuals with gold allergy have gold dental work. It is unlikely that gold dental work will cause problems on the skin. However, if an individual has mouth sores in areas of contact with gold dental work, then this problem may be helped by changing to a dental filling to which the patient is not allergic. In addition, there are some cases of lichen planus that have been shown to be related to gold allergy in dental work.

PARABENS

These are chemicals that are commonly used as preservatives to kill microorganisms in skin and hair care products. You will often see a prefix before the word "paraben" on label ingredients, such as "butyl" or "propyl." Any of the parabens must be avoided. Occasionally, these chemicals may be used as preservatives in medications taken internally. If there is any question about this, your pharmacist should be consulted, and he or she should be able to determine if parabens are present in a medication you are taking. Sometimes individuals can tolerate using a preparation that contains these chemicals on normal skin, but if the same preparation is used on skin that is already irritated, then an allergic reaction may develop. Also, sensitive areas such as the face are more likely to react than other skin surfaces.

PROPYLENE GLYCOL

This is a thick, liquid substance that is used in many skin care products and cosmetics as a thickener and to give an antibacterial effect. It should be in the ingredient list on products. It is also found in many prescription and over-the-counter cortisone-type creams. In addition, propylene glycol may be used as a swimming pool or mobile home antifreeze. It is also used in some food products, especially condiments, salad dressings, and prepared baked goods. However, it is sometimes found in other unexpected food products, such as some cake mixes. It should be included in food ingredient labeling. In most cases, individuals allergic to propylene glycol do not need to avoid other glycols, including butylene glycol, hexylene glycol, and polyethylene glycol.

DIAZOLIDINYL UREA

The substance to which you are allergic is one that will normally be found on labels. If you are purchasing anything for use on your skin, first inspect the package for the ingredient list. If you have products at home that do not have a label or the container does not list the ingredients, it would be best to go to the store where the product was purchased and inspect the original package. In the United States, products that are sold for consumer use on the skin as a cosmetic or toiletry must be labeled with the ingredients listed in decreasing order of concentration. The first item listed is present in the greatest concentration, and the last listed is at the lowest concentration. Many of the allergenic materials are present in very low concentrations and are listed near the end of the ingredient list. Products sold as medical devices at present only have to reveal the "active" ingredients.

Sometimes a product will contain so little of a material to which you are allergic that skin contact may be harmless. However, you cannot count on this and should try to avoid all the products that have the potential to cause trouble.

You are allergic to diazolidinyl urea. This is a preservative commonly used in skin care products. By reading labels, you should be very successful at avoiding this allergen.

BACITRACIN

The substance to which you are allergic is one that will normally be found on labels. If you are purchasing anything for use on your skin, first inspect the package for the ingredient list. If you have products at home that do not have a label or the container does not list the ingredients, it would be best to go to the store where the product was purchased and inspect the original package. In the United States, products that are sold for consumer use on the skin as a cosmetic or toiletry must be labeled with the ingredients listed in decreasing order of concentration. The first item listed is present in the greatest concentration, and the last listed is at the lowest concentration. Many of the allergenic materials are present in very low concentrations and are listed near the end of the ingredient list. Products sold as medical devices at present only have to reveal the "active" ingredients.

Sometimes a product will contain so little of a material to which you are allergic that skin contact may be harmless. However, you cannot count on this and should try to avoid all the products that have the potential to cause trouble.

You are allergic to bacitracin. This antibiotic is a common ingredient in over-the-counter triple antibiotic ointments. Examples are be Neosporin, Neo-Polycin, and Mycitracin. Bacitracin is also available by itself and is found in Betadine healing ointment. It will be listed on the ingredient label. Povodone-iodine ointment is a chemically unrelated antibiotic that you could substitute for bacitracin; this is also known as Betadine ointment, which should not be confused with Betadine healing ointment.

BUDESONIDE

You are allergic to budesonide, a type of corticosteroid or cortisone that is a marker for allergy to a wide range of cortisone products. It would be best to avoid the following corticosteroids, even though some of them may be safe for use on your skin surface. Avoid triamcinolone, amcinonide, fluocinolone acetonide, halcinonide, flucinonide, desonide, hydrocortisone-17-butyrate, hydrocortisone butyrate and valerate, clobetasol propionate and butyrate, betamethasone valerate and dipropionate, prednicarbate, fluocortolone hexanoate and pivalate, and alclometasone dipropionate. There may be corticosteroids that you can safely take. Cortisone allergy is not as rare as once believed, and many doctors are unfamiliar with cortisone allergy. Internal cortisones that you may be able to safely take include dexamethasone and betamethasone (oral or injectable forms only).

TIXOCORTOL-21-PIVALATE

You are allergic to a corticosteroid known as tixocortol-21-pivalate. The cortisone is representative of a class of cortisone that you should avoid. The more common members of this class are hydrocortisone, prednisone, prednisolone, and methylprednisolone. There may be other cortisones that you can safely take, but these are best avoided. Cortisone allergy is something with which many doctors are unfamiliar. It is not as rare as once believed. High doses of cortisones like prednisone may appear to give benefit because of their pharmacological properties, but as the dose is reduced, the immunologic reaction (allergy) becomes apparent. Potentially safer internal corticosteroids include dexamethasone and betamethasone.

MIXED DIALKYL THIOUREAS

Diethyl thiourea and dibutyl thiourea are included in the allergen referred to as mixed dialkyl thioureas. These are chemicals added to neoprene rubber products. Common sources of exposure to these chemicals are rubber weather stripping, wet suits for diving, some polyvinyl chloride adhesives, neoprene rubber gloves, orthopedic knee and elbow sleeves, and the insoles of athletic shoes. Industrial anticorrosive compounds may contain these thioureas, as may some industrial detergents. Diazo copy paper, which is used for industrial textile patterns and architectural plans, also contains these agents.

TOSYLAMIDE FORMALDEHYDE RESIN

You are allergic to a chemical found in nail polish. This material imparts durability to the polish and is not associated with any specific color. It is even found in clear nail polish. You should choose a nail polish that does not contain this material, such as Clinique and Almay nail polishes. You may also check the labels of nail polish of other companies to determine if they will be safe for your use. Older bottles of nail polish may list this ingredient under the name toluene-sulfonamide formaldehyde resin. The new name is tosylamide formaldehyde resin, but the ingredient is the same.

ETHYLENEUREA MELAMINE FORMALDEHYDE RESIN

You are allergic to a chemical used to make fabric wrinkle resistant or permanent press. This allergen will not appear on the label of the garments you buy. Several very closely related chemicals are also used to make fabrics wrinkle resistant, and because they are all very similar chemically, you should avoid all permanent press clothing. These chemicals are related to formaldehyde, to which you may also be sensitive.

Some types of fabric are more likely to be treated with your allergen. These include cotton-polyester blends, 100% cotton wrinkle-resistant fabrics, wrinkle-resistant linen, shrink-proof woolens, rayon, corduroy, and any blends of cotton, rayon, wool, or other synthetic or natural fibers. It is important to remember that 100% cotton is not a guarantee of safety, as cotton can be treated with these chemicals. If a garment wrinkles and requires ironing, it is likely to be safe.

Fabrics that are unlikely to be treated with these chemicals include 100% cotton denim, 100% linen, 100% silk, 100% polyester, 100% nylon, and 100% ultrasuede.

CHLOROXYLENOL

The substance to which you are allergic is one that will normally be found on labels. If you are purchasing anything for use on your skin, first inspect the package for the ingredient list. If you have products at home that do not have a label or the container does not list the ingredients, it would be best to go to the store where the product was purchased and inspect the original package. In the United States, products that are sold for consumer use on the skin as a cosmetic or toiletry must be labeled with the ingredients listed in decreasing order of concentration. The first item listed is present in the greatest concentration, and the last listed is at the lowest concentration. Many of the allergenic materials are present in very low concentrations and are listed near the end of the ingredient list. Products sold as medical devices at present only have to reveal the "active" ingredients.

Sometimes a product will contain so little of a material to which you are allergic that skin contact may be harmless. However, you cannot count on this and should try to avoid all the products that have the potential to cause trouble.

You are allergic to chloroxylenol. This is a preservative commonly used in skin care products. By reading labels, you should be very successful at avoiding this allergen. It may be found in products such as burn remedies, hair dressings, Absorbine Jr., carbolated Vaseline, feminine hygiene products, and in some prescription topical corticosteroids. It is found in powders such as ZeaSORB, Desitin, and Aveeno. It is also known as PCMX, p-chloro-meta-xylenol, and 4-chloro-3,4-xylenol.

IODOPROPYNYL BUTYLCARBAMATE

The substance to which you are allergic is one that will normally be found on labels. If you are purchasing anything for use on your skin, first inspect the package for the ingredient list. If you have products at home that do not have a label or the container does not list the ingredients, it would be best to go to the store where the product was purchased and inspect the original package. In the United States, products that are sold for consumer use on the skin as a cosmetic or toiletry must be labeled with the ingredients listed in decreasing order of concentration. The first item listed is present in the greatest concentration, and the last listed is at the lowest connection. Many of the allergenic materials are present in very low concentrations and are listed near the end of the ingredient list. Products sold as medical devices at present only have to reveal the "active" ingredients.

Sometimes a product will contain so little of a material to which you are allergic that skin contact may be harmless. However, you cannot count on this and should try to avoid all the products that have the potential to cause trouble.

You are allergic to iodopropynyl butylcarbamate. This is a preservative commonly used in skin care products. By reading labels, you should be very successful at avoiding this allergen.

2-BROMO-2-NITROPROPANE-1,3-DIOL

The substance to which you are allergic is one that will normally be found on labels. If you are purchasing anything for use on your skin, first inspect the package for the ingredient list. If you have products at home that do not have a label or the container does not list the ingredients, it would be best to go to the store where the product was purchased and inspect the original package. In the United States, products that are sold for consumer use on the skin as a cosmetic or toiletry must be labeled with the ingredients listed in decreasing order of concentration. The first item listed is present in the greatest concentration, and the last listed is at the lowest concentration. Many of the allergenic materials are present in very low concentrations and are listed near the end of the ingredient list. Products sold as medical devices at present only have to reveal the "active" ingredients.

Sometimes a product will contain so little of a material to which you are allergic that skin contact may be harmless. However, you cannot count on this and should try to avoid all the products that have the potential to cause trouble.

You are allergic to 2-bromo-2-nitropropane-1,3-diol. This is a biocide and preservative. It can be found in skin care products and is used in industry to prevent the growth of microorganisms in water-based fluids such as coolants used by machinists. By reading labels, you should be very successful at avoiding this allergen in consumer products. The material safety data sheet on water-soluble coolants should be consulted for the presence of this material in industry. Industrially, it may be referred to as Bronopol.

METHYLDIBROMOGLUTARONITRILE

The substance to which you are allergic is one that will normally be found on labels. If you are purchasing anything for use on your skin, first inspect the package for the ingredient list. If you have products at home that do not have a label or the container does not list the ingredients, it would be best to go to the store where the product was purchased and inspect the original package. In the United States, products that are sold for consumer use on the skin as a cosmetic or toiletry must be labeled with the ingredients listed in decreasing order of concentration. The first item listed is present in the greatest concentration, and the last listed is at the lowest concentration. Many of the allergenic materials are present in very low concentrations and are listed near the end of the ingredient list. Products sold as medical devices at present only have to reveal the "active" ingredients.

Sometimes a product will contain so little of a material to which you are allergic that skin contact may be harmless. However, you cannot count on this and should try to avoid all the products that have the potential to cause trouble.

You are allergic to methyldibromoglutaronitrile. This is a preservative commonly used in skin care products. By reading labels, you should be very successful at avoiding this allergen. You may find this listed on labels as methyldibromoglutaronitrile/phenoxyethanol. This is another form of your allergen, and you should avoid this too. Some Lubriderm products contain this material, as may other skin care products. In some countries this compound is called dibromodicyanobutane+phenoxyethanol. Another name for this chemical is Euxyl K 400.

DMDM HYDANTOIN

The substance to which you are allergic is one that will normally be found on labels. If you are purchasing anything for use on your skin, first inspect the package for the ingredient list. If you have products at home that do not have a label or the container does not list the ingredients, it would be best to go to the store where the product was purchased and inspect the original package. In the United States, products that are sold for consumer use on the skin as a cosmetic or toiletry must be labeled with the ingredients listed in decreasing order of concentration. The first item listed is present in the greatest concentration, and the last listed is at the lowest concentration. Many of the allergenic materials are present in very low concentrations and are listed near the end of the ingredient list. Products sold as medical devices at present only have to reveal the "active" ingredients.

Sometimes a product will contain so little of a material to which you are allergic that skin contact may be harmless. However, you cannot count on this and should try to avoid all the products that have the potential to cause trouble.

You are allergic to DMDM hydantoin. This is a preservative commonly used in skin care products. By reading labels, you should be very successful at avoiding this allergen.

Appendix

EXPLANATION OF TERMS USED IN THE APPENDIX

1. *Primary sensitizer.* Testing with this substance may sensitize the patient. The patch test reaction usually is delayed for at least 5 days.
2. *Photosensitizer.* This substance should be tested both covered and with exposure to sunlight or ultraviolet radiation.
3. *Controls.* The substance may be a primary irritant. The patch test reaction should be checked with at least three normal controls.
4. *Para-amino.* This refers to chemicals that have an amino group in the para position, including paraphenylenediamine, paraaminobenzoic acid, and aminosalicylic acid. Cross-reactions occur with certain local anesthetics, sulfonamides, sunscreens and azo, and aniline dyes.
5. *Sensitizes to alcohol.* Exposure to this chemical combined with the ingestion of alcohol produces an aldehyde syndrome consisting of flushing of the skin, nausea, and vomiting.

KEY TO ABBREVIATIONS USED IN THE APPENDIX

acet.:	acetone
alc.:	alcohol 70%
aq.:	aqueous
as is:	undiluted
chlor.:	chloroform
c.o.:	castor oil
con.:	concentration
mek.:	methylethylketone
o.o.:	olive oil
pdr.:	powder
pet.:	petrolatum
sat.:	saturated
sol.:	solution
veh.:	vehicle

Contactant	Concentration and Vehicle	Exposure	Cross-Reactions	Comment
Abietic acid	2% pet.	Rosins, colophony, adhesives, balsams, typewriting paper, denture adhesive powder, pine resin	Hydroabietalcohols	Forms about 80% of American rosin
Abieto-formo-phenolic resin	2% pet.	Printing ink	Rosin	
Abitol (dihydroabietyl alcohol)	1% pet.	Cosmetics, plastics, adhesives	Rosin	
Acacia (gum arabic)	50% aq.	Ink, matches, lithography, mucilage, pharmaceutical vehicle, offset sprays in printing, adhesives, stiffeners for rayon, pastry, denture adhesive powder		May contain alcohol
Acetanilide	5% pet.	Analgesics, antipyretics, dye manufacture, cellulose ester varnishes		
Acetarsol	1% pet.	Vaginal suppositories, amoebic dysentery, toothpaste, mouthwash		
2-Acetexycyclonhexahone oxime	1% pet.	In the synthesis of lysine		
Acetic acid	3% aq. sol.	Vinegar, flavoring agent, wart remedy, astringent mouthwash		Causes aphthous ulcer?
Acetone	10% o.o.	Industrial solvent, nail polish remover, diabetic urine, solvent for celluloid material in dentifrices		Anti-irritant
1-Acetyl-2-phenylhydrazine	1% pet.	Anaerobic sealant		A dimethacrylate
Achromycin Ointment (Lederle)	As is	Topical medication	Tetracyclines	
Acid fuchsin	1% pet.	Azo dyes	Para-amino compounds	
Acridine	1% pet.	Yellow dyes, acriflavine, tar		Photosensitizer
Acriflavine	1% pet.			An acridine dye photosensitizer
Acrylic monomer (methyl methacrylate)	10% o.o.	Synthetic resins, dentures, artificial nails, adhesives, paints, plastic, glass, sealer of screws in automobile industry, orthopedic prostheses		Can penetrate rubber gloves. May contain hydroquinone benzoyl peroxide, tertiary amines, can cause contact urticaria

Contactant	Concentration and Vehicle	Exposure	Cross-Reactions	Comment
Acrylonitrile	0.1% pet.	Used in Plexidur plastic splints		
Acyclovir	1% pet.	Topical and systemic		
Adhesive tape (acrylate)	As is	Dermicel (J & J), Steri-strip Brand Skin Closures, Micropore Brand Surgical Tape (3M)		Some brands colophony
Adhesive tape (rubber)	As is			May contain rubber additives, rosin, turpentine, and lanolin
Aerosol OT (dioctylester of sodium sulfosuccinic acid)	1% aq. sol.	Surfactant, anionic synthetic detergents, bubble baths		Controls
Akrinol Cream (acrisorcin; Schering)	As is		Hexylresorcinol	
Alantolactone	0.1% pet.	Sensitizer in Compositae plants		Known as Helenin in Denmark
Alcohol (industrial denatured)	As is			Contains methyl alcohol and acetone
Alcohol (ethyl)	70–95%		Amyl, butyl, methyl, isopropyl alcohol	Test reaction may occur very rapidly; may cause contact urticaria
Alcohol (isopropyl, "rubbing")	As is	Cosmetics, medicinal preparations		Denaturing agents include tartar emetic, quinine, salicylic acid, colchicine, alkaloids and azo dyes
Alcohol (methyl, methanol, wood)	As is	Chemical synthesis, antifreeze, solvent in shellac, varnish, paint remover, denaturant in denatured alcohol		*Synonyms*: methyl hydrate, methyl hydroxide, acetone, alcohol, wood spirits, wood naphtha, Columbian spirits, carrinol

Contactant	Concentration and Vehicle	Exposure	Cross-Reactions	Comment
Alizarin dyes:				
Alizarin red	As is	Synthetic dyes, red paints, hair dyes, chemical indicators		
Alizarin 778	1% alc.			
Alizarin sulfate	10% aq. sol.			
Alkyl ethoxy sulfate	1% pet.	Liquid dishwashing products		
Alkyl phenoxyl polyethoxy ethanols	2% aq.	Wetting agent and emulsifier		
Allantoin	0.5% aq. sol.	Topical medications, "healing agent," cosmetics, vaginal creams, shampoos		Uric acid derivative
Allyl glycidyl ether	0.25% MEK[a]	Reactive epoxy diluent		
Allyl phenoxyacetate	1% pet.	Carpet shampoo		
Almond oil	As is	Brilliantines, hair dressings, spices, flavoring agents		
Aloe arborescens	As is	Plant and laxative		
Aloe vera	10% pet.	Anthraquinone compound	Benzoin and Balsam of Peru (topical medicinal)	
Alpha-chlorobenzaldehyde phenylhydrazone	0.1% aq. sol.	To prepare optical fluorescing compound as an optical whitener		
Alpha-phenyl-indol in PVC	2% pet.	Stabilizer in polyvinyl chloride		
Alpha-terthienyl	1% pet.	Thiophene compound present in Chrysanthemum family of plants		
Alprenolol	2% aq. sol.	Beta-adrenergic blocking agent		
Alrosol C (fatty acid amide condensate)	1% aq. sol.	Surfactant, nonionic synthetic detergents		Controls irritant
Alstroemeria	As is	South American plant		
Alum (aluminum and potassium sulfate)	10% aq. sol.	Styptic agents, purification of water, baking powders, mouthwashes, astringents		

[a]MEK, methyl ethyl ketone.

Contactant	Concentration and Vehicle	Exposure	Cross-Reactions	Comment
Aluminum acetate	10% aq. sol.	Mordants, siccatives, astringents, deodorants, fur dyeing, fabric finishing, waterproofing, dye compounds, disinfectants		Rare sensitizer. May produce nonspecific follicular reaction
Aluminum chlorhydroxide	10% aq. sol.	Deodorants, antiperspirants, astringents		
Aluminum chloride	2% aq. sol.	Astringents, antiseptics, antiperspirants		Rare sensitizer. Irritation from pore closure
Aluminum metal	As is	Finn-Chambers		
Aluminum powder	As is in pet.	Astringents, instruments		Rare sensitizer
Aluminum sulfate	2% aq. sol.	Astringents, antiseptics, antiperspirants		Rare sensitizer. Irritation from pore closure
Aluminum sulfocarbolate	2% aq. sol.	Astringents, antiseptics, antiperspirants		Rare sensitizer. Irritation from pore closure
Amaranth pink	5% pet.	Color elixir phenobarbital, foods, alcohol		
Amerchol L-101	1% pet.	Lanolin alcohol	Lanolin	
Amino-azobenzene	0.25% pet.	Leather dyes, textiles	Para-amino compounds	
Amino-azotoluene hydrochloride	1% pet.	Leather dyes	Para-amino compounds	
Amino-azotoluene	1% pet.	Scarlet red topical medications	Para-amino compounds	
3-Amino-1,2,4-triazole	5% pet.	Herbicide		
Aminoethylethanolamine	1% aq. sol.	Aluminum cables		Used to solder aluminum electric wires
Aminoguanidine hydrochloride	5% pet.	Herbicide		
o-Aminophenol	10% pet.	Fur and hair dye		Paraphenylenediamine
Aminophylline	1% aq. sol.	Pharmaceutical industry, rectal suppositories (Rectalad, Aminet, Heogen)	Phenergan, pyribenzamine	Composed of ethylenediamine and theophylline

Contactant	Concentration and Vehicle	Exposure	Cross-Reactions	Comment
Ammoniated mercury	2% pet.	Topical medications	Organic and inorganic mercurials, mercury amalgam	Incompatible with sulfur and iodine pigment changes
Ammonium fluoride	2% aq. sol.	Glass industry, insecticides, rust removers, dentistry, Aluminum Brite (Copper Brite Co.)		Patch tests may produce large nonspecific pustules. Keep in dark wax-coated bottle
Ammonium persulfate	2% aq. sol.	Flour and hair bleaches, disinfectants, deodorants, ammoniated dentifrices	Potassium-sodium persulfate	May produce urticaria, shock by contact
Ammonium phosphate	2% aq. sol.	Ammoniated dentifrices		
Ammonium rhodanate	1% pet.	Photography		
Ammonium thioglycolate	5% aq. test open			
Ammonyx Io	5% aq. sol.	Surfactant and antiseptic for surgical scrubs Present in chlorhexidine		
Ampholyt G	1% aq.	Disinfectant, present in Tego		
Ampicillin sodium	5% aq. sol.	Use fresh preparation		Occupational hazard in nursing personnel
Amyl acetate (banana oil) Amyl cinnamic alcohol Amyl cinnamic aldehyde	10% o.o. 5% terpene 5% terpene	Solvents, nail polish removers, waterproofing, sheet metal, enamelware, woodworking		
Amyl dimethylaminobenzoate	1% pet.	Ultraviolet cured ink		
Amyltricresol	1% aq. sol.	A phenol mercury compound in Pentacresol Mouthwash		
Anethole	5% pet.	Toothpaste flavoring		Found in oils of anise, star anise, and fennel
Anileridine	As is	Injectable narcotic		Occurs in pharmacists and those who inject narcotics

Contactant	Concentration and Vehicle	Exposure	Cross-Reactions	Comment
Aniline	10% o.o.	Dyes, drugs, cloth marking inks, paints, paint removers	Para-amino compounds	A colorless aminobenzene. May contain naphthylamine
Aniline black	10% o.o.	Fur dyes	Para-amino compounds	
Aniline blue	2% pet.	Cosmetics, carbons, fur dyeing, hair dyes, nail polish, rubber, photographics, inks, colored pencils, crayons	Para-amino compounds	
Aniline dyes	5% pet.	Crayons, diaper markings, shoe polishes	Para-amino compounds	Toxic to infants when used for diaper markings
Anise oil	25% c.o.	Flavoring agents in dentistry, liqueurs (anisette), confectioneries, perfumes, soaps		Derived from seeds of carrot family
Anisyl alcohol	5% pet.			
Anthracene	Pure	Tar		Photosensitizer
Anthralin ointment (Cignolin)	0.05% pet.	Anthra-Derm Ointment (Dermik), Anthryl (Reed & Carnrick)		Irritant when covered. Controls
Anthraquinone	2% pet.	Yellow vat dyes, makes seeds distasteful to birds, laxatives		From anthracine, a coal tar derivative
Antimony chloride Antimony oxide	2% aq. sol. Pure	Alloys, type metals, batteries, foils, ceramics, safety matches, ant pastes, textiles, tartar emetic, Fuadin, base for paints, vitreous enamels, fireproofing plastics		Irritant and toxic
Antimony sulfide	2% aq. sol.	Matches, putty		
Antipyrine (phenazone)	5% pet.	Auralgan Ear Drops (Ayerst), Tympagesic Ear Drops (Warren-Teed)		Auralgan also contains benzocaine and hydroquinoline. May cause erythema multiforme
Antisapstain	1% pet.	Antifungal agent for timber		Can cause irritant and allergic reactions

Contactant	Concentration and Vehicle	Exposure	Cross-Reactions	Comment
Antistine (antazoline)	0.5% aq. sol or 1% pet.	Eye and nose drops	Pyribenzamine, Neoantergan, Diatrin, Neohetramine, Trimeton, Benadryl, aminophylline	Derivative of ethylenediamine
Antivy (CIBA)	As is (patch-scratch)			Contains zirconium oxide. Allergic granuloma
Apomorphine	1% aq. scratch test	For the treatment of alcoholism. Exposure nurses, pharmacists who dispense the drug.		
Aquaphor (Duke Lab.)	As is		Lanolin	Cholesterolated Vaseline and lanolin alcohol. Cholesterolated absorbent ointment base
Aracel C (Sorbitan sesquioleate)	5% o.o.	Pharmaceuticals		In Polysorb Hydrate
Araldite 502	0.1% acet.	Low molecular weight epoxy resins		
Araldite 6060	10% acet.	High molecular weight epoxy resins		
Arctic Syntex M (sodium monoglyceride sulfide)	5% aq. sol.	Surfactant, synthetic detergents		Controls
Argyrol	10% aq. sol. (open)	Antiseptics		
Arlacel	10% aq. sol.	Emulsifier in soaks and detergents		
Arlacel A (mannide monooleate)	5% aq. sol.	Surfactant, nonionic synthetic detergents; pharmaceuticals		Controls
Arnica, tincture of	20% alc.	Rubefacients	Chrysanthemum	Arnica and chrysanthemum, belonging to the aster family or Compositae
Arning's Tincture	As is (open)		Balsam of Peru	Contains anthrarobin, tumenol ammonium, ether, tincture of benzoin

Contactant	Concentration and Vehicle	Exposure	Cross-Reactions	Comment
Arsenate (potassium)	1% aq. sol.	Fowler's solution		
Arsenate (sodium)	1% aq. sol.	Insecticides, ant poisons, weed killers, wallpaper paints, glass, ceramics	Other arsenicals	Frequent pustular patch test reaction
Arsenic trioxide (white arsenic)	5% in starch pdr.	Insecticides, soaps, hair tonics, depilatories, caustics, weed killers, poison baits, fungicides, glasses, enamels, alloys	Sodium arsenate	Frequent pustular patch test reaction
Artemesia	As is	Compositae plant-test		Ingested as folk remedy; may cause systemic contact dermatitis.
Artichoke	Patch test with stem as is or alcohol extract of stem	Food handlers and gardeners	Cross-reacts with Compositae	
Arylalcanoic acids	1% pet.	Rubifacient used in Europe		Present in Motrin
Asterol (diamthazole)	5% pet.	Antifungal agents		
Atranorin	0.1% pet.	Lichen substance present in oak moss		
Atronin	1% pet.	May be photosensitizer. Present in lichens and perfumes		
Aureomycin Ointment, Powder (Lederle)	As is		Tetracyclines	
Azidamphenicol	5% pet.	Antibiotic closely related to chloramphenicol		
Azo dyes	2% pet.	Foods, drugs, cosmetics, clothes, ballpoint pens, ink	Para-amino compounds	
Azodicarbonamide	1% pet.	Used in the manufacture of polyvinyl chloride Polyolefin plastics		

Contactant	Concentration and Vehicle	Exposure	Cross-Reactions	Comment
Bacitracin	20% pet.	Wybiotic Troches, Tyrotrace, Baciguent, Baci-Wax, Mycitracin, Epimycin A, Bacimycin, Cortisporin, Polysporin, Neo-polycin, Neosporin, Tetrazets	Polymyxin B colistine	May coreact with neomycin. Can cause contact urticaria
Balsam of Peru	25% pet.	Topical medications, cements, liquids in dentistry, Anusol Suppositories (Warner-Chilcott), Rectocaine Suppositories (Moore Kirk), Endacaine Compound Suppositories, Granulex, Rectal Medicone Suppositories and Ointment, Wyanoids HC, Calmol 4, Melynor Ointment (Davies Rose Hoyt), cosmetics, hair tonics, perfumes, flavoring industry, china painting, oil painting	Benzoin, rosin, benzoic acid, benzyl alcohol, cinnamic acid, essential oils, orange peel, eugenol, cinnamon, clove, Tolu balsam, storax, benzyl benzoate, wood tars	An important sensitizer A perfume allergy indicator May cause contact urticaria
Balsam of tolu	1% alc.	Cough mixtures, throat lozenges, benzoin tincture, tolu varnish, coating for pills, perfumes	Benzoin tincture, balsam of Peru	
Barium sulfide	2% aq. sol.	Depilatories	Freshly prepared	
Bay rum	As is	Hair tonics	Eugenol, clove oil, cinnamon oil	Combination of Jamaica rum and oil of bay
Bee glue (propolis)	As is			May contain raw beeswax
Beeswax (cera alba [bleached], cera flava [unbleached])	30% pet.	Adhesives, plasters, textile waterproofing agent, ointments, cosmetics, polishes, cosmetic stiffeners	Balsam of Peru	May be contaminated with bee glue
Beeswax-turpentine mixture	5% pet.	Eyeglass frames		To produce smooth gloss on plastics
Benadryl (diphenhydramine hydrochloride; Parke, Davis)	2% pet.	Caladryl Ointment (Parke, Davis)	Dramamine	
Benomyl (benlate)	1% pet.	Insecticide		
Benoquin (monobenzone; Elder)	As is	Depigmenting agent	Hydroquinone	Contains monobenzylether of hydroquinone

Contactant	Concentration and Vehicle	Exposure	Cross-Reactions	Comment
Benzaldehyde	5% pet.	Oil of bitter almond, preservatives, biologicals	Vanilla, balsam of Peru	Contact urticaria
Benzalkonium chloride	1:1000 aq. sol. = 0.1%	Antiseptic detergents, mouthwashes, preservative in ophthalmic solutions, Zephiran solution, medicated paper tissues (Zephiran towelettes)		May be irritant
Benzene (benzol)	5% o.o.	Coal tar distillates, motor fuels, commercial solvents		Synonyms: phenyl hydride, coal tar naphtha
Benzene hexachloride	5% pet.	Insecticide Kwell (Reed & Carnrick)		May cause chloracne, porphyria
Benzethonium chloride (Phemerol)	1:1000 aq. sol. = 0.1%	Antiseptic detergents		Present in Colgate mouthwash, feminine hygiene sprays
Benzidine (para-diaminodiphenyl)	3% alc.	Tests for blood, derivatives are optical bleaches		
Benzine	50% o.o.	Petroleum solvents		Synonyms: petroleum benzine, petroleum ether
Benzisothiazoline	1% pet.	Preservative in gum arabic Industrial preservative Biocide in pottery industry		
Benzocaine	5% pet.	Numerous topical anesthetic compounds (see text)	Para-amino compounds	Synonyms: anethesin, ethyl aminobenzoate, Anesthone, parathesin. May cause contact urticaria. Rare photosensitizer
Benzoic acid	5% pet.	Balsam of Peru, Whitfield's ointment, essential oils, mouthwashes, preservatives for fruit, pharmaceuticals		Extremely rare sensitizer

Contactant	Concentration and Vehicle	Exposure	Cross-Reactions	Comment
Benzoin	10% alc.	Tincture of benzoin, compound tincture of benzoin, Arning's tincture, benzo-inated lard (adeps benzoatus), antioxidant in creams, perfumes, expectorants, throat lozenges, raw beeswax, bee glue, preservative in adhesives, gums of myrrh, locust, golbam	Balsam of Peru, benzyl cinnamate, benzyl alcohol, eugenol, vanilla, alpha-pinene Storax	
Benzophenone	5% pet.	Sunscreens (Solbar, Sunguard, Uval), textiles, plastics, rubber products, paints, varnishes, cosmetics		May produce urticarial and contact sensitivity. Synonyms: Spectra Sorb UV 284
Benzoquinone	1% pet.	Present in plants and wood		
Benzotriazole	0.5% pet.			
Benzoyl peroxide	1% pet.	Polyester and acrylic resins, Quinolor Ointment (Squibb), burn dusting powder, flour improver, benzoyl peroxide ointment. Acne medications: Persadox, Benoxyl, Loroxide, Vanoxide, Oxy 5, Oxy 5 HC, etc.	Benzoic acid derivatives, cinnamon, cocaine, Surfacaine, Metacaine	Not stable Irritant Discolors Textiles
Benzyl alcohol	5% pet.	Essential oils, balsam of Peru, food flavorings, perfumes, antiseptic and local anesthetics	Balsam of Peru Perfumes	Preservative in allergy extracts and injectables
Benzyl benzoate	2% pet.	Balsam of Peru, balsam of tolu, perfumes, nail polish plasticizer, Topocide (Lilly)	Diethylstilbestrol	
Benzyl salicylate	2% pet.	Perfumes, detergents, sunscreens (methoxsalen), psoralens	Essential oil	May enhance photosensitization
Bergamot, oil of	2% pet.	Eau de Cologne Shalimar, hair tonics, toilet water, china painting, ceramics		A photosensitizer. Test open and closed
Beryllium nitrate	1% aq. sol. 0.5% aq. sol.	Cathode tube and fluorescent lights, alloys, electrical equipment, ceramics, fluorophors		May produce granulomas as can beryllium SO$_4$ and beryllium chloride

Contactant	Concentration and Vehicle	Exposure	Cross-Reactions	Comment
Betadine (povidone-iodine; Purdue Frederick)	As is (open)			Iodine in polyvinyl pyrrolidine; irritant
Betanal	2% aq.	Herbicide (phenmedipham)		
Betanaphthol	10% o.o.	Glues, adhesive solvent, book binding, mouthwashes, hair tonics		
Bioban P-1487	0.5% pet.	Cutting oils		Formaldehyde releaser?
Biocide (Tektamer 38)	1% pet.	In paste glue		
Bis-(4-chlorophenoyl) methyl chloride	1% chlor.	Insecticide-related DDT		
Bis(diethyl and dibutyldithio-carbamato) zinc	1% pet.	Rubber	Thiuram Comp.	
Bismark brown	5% pet.	Dyeing silks, wools, leathers	Para-amino compounds	
Bisphenol A	1% acet.	Epoxy resin converter, antioxidant, component of oil-soluble phenolic resins	Diethylstilbestrol, organic silicone compounds, monobenzylether of hy-droquinone	
Bithionol	1% pet.	Antiseptic no longer used in US	Chlorinated salicylanilides	Photosensitizer
Bitrex	2% pet.	Disinfectant		
Bitter almond, oil of	10% o.o.		Benzoin, balsam of Peru	A benzaldehyde poison
Borax (sodium borate)	Sat. aq. sol.	Refrigerant, antiseptics, soaps, deter-gents, abrasives, bath salts, cosmet-ics, flux		
Boric acid	3% aq.	Antiseptics, detergents, cosmetics		
Boron trifluoride-ethylamine	1% pet.	Epoxy resin hardener (formaldehyde-releasing agent)		
Brilliant green	2% aq. sol.	Dyes		
British antilewisite (BAL; 2-3, dithiopropanol; dimer-caprol)	5% pet.	Chelating agents		
9-Bromofluorene	Do not test	Chemistry laboratory		Erythema multiform re-action

Contactant	Concentration and Vehicle	Exposure	Cross-Reactions	Comment
Bronopol	0.25% pet.	Preservative in cosmetics		
Brucine	1% pet.	Denatured alcohol		A strychnine compound
Brut	2% pet.	Perfume containing musk ambrette, sensitizer and photosensitizer		
BTC (lauryl dimethyl benzyl-ammonium chloride)	0.1% aq.	Surfactant, cationic synthetic deter-gents, bubble baths		Irritants
Budesonide	0.1% pet.	Topical corticosteroids	Grp. B corticosteroids	
Bufexamac	1% pet.	Topical analgesic in Italy and Belgium		
Burow's solution (liquor alu-minum acetatis)	10% aq. sol.	Astringents, antiseptics		Very rarely sensitizes
Butacaine	5% pet.	Topical anesthetic	Para-amino-compound	Based on para-aminobenzoic acid
Butethamine (Monocaine)	5% pet.	Local anesthetic	Para-amino compound	Based on para-aminobenzoic acid
Butyl acetate	25% o.o.	Solvents, nail polish removers		
Butyl acrylate	0.1% pet.	Plastics, spectacle frames		
Butyl aminobenzoate	As is	Local anesthetic	Procaine, benzocaine	Butesin picrate Proprietary name
Butyl glycidyl ether	1% o.o.	Reactive epoxy resin diluent		
p-tert-Butylcatechol	0.1% acet.	Oil antioxidant		May cause depigmenta-tion
Butylhydroxyanisol	1% pet.	Antioxidant		
Butylhydroxytoluene	1% pet.	Antioxidant		
p-tert-Butylphenol formalde-hyde resin	10% pet.	Adhesive—contains little or no formaldehyde		
Butyrolactone (Antara)	As is	Organic solvent		Useful solvent for patch testing of resins
Cadmium sulfide (Capsebon)	1% aq. sol.	Tattoos, photo-conducting material, forms pink pigment in acrylic den-tures with cadmium selenide		Photoallergic

Contactant	Concentration and Vehicle	Exposure	Cross-Reactions	Comment
Calcium chloride	2% aq. sol.	EEG Electrode Paste, dehydrating agents, antimildew		A primary irritant
Calcium cyanamide	1% aq.	Fertilizer and pesticide anthelmintic		Found in Carbodiimide—irritant—does not produce cyanide effects
Calcium lignosulfonate	10% aq. sol.	Animal food	Paper pulp	Paper and wood
Calcium oxide (quicklime)	Do not patch test	Unslaked lime, caustic lime, burnt lime		Not a sensitizer. Burns skin when moistened. See also lime, slaked
Calcium thioglycollate	5% aq. sol.	Depilatories		
Camomile, oil of	25% o.o.	Cosmetics, mirror manufacturing, vegetable hair dyes		Compositae
Camphor oil Camphor powder Camphor crystals	10% pet.	Used in dentistry as camphorated chlorophenol, preservatives, plasticizer, nail polish, lacquers, varnishes, moth repellents, embalming fluids, explosives, pharmaceuticals		Some camphors contain oil of laurel
Canada balsam	25% pet.	Cement for lenses, fine lacquers, mounting slides	Turpentine, balsam of Peru	
Cantharidin	1% alc.	Skin vesicant, rubefacient in hair tonics, Cantharone (Ingram), wart remedy Verrusol (C & M)		
Capsicum, tincture of	1% alc.	Hair tonics, rubefacient, tear gas (On Guard)		
Captan	0.25% pet.	Pesticide, antifungal	Phaltan	A dicarboximide
Captopril	10% aq.		Other ACE inhibitors usually negative	
Caraway seed oil	25% c.o.	Spices in baking, liqueurs, soaps, flavor in dentifrices		May cause contact urticaria
Carbamide (urea)	10% aq. sol.	Therapeutic agent, Ammident, Colgate and Dr. Lyons toothpaste		
Carbitol (diethylene glycol)	10% aq. sol.	Solvents, stabilizer of emulsions		

Contactant	Concentration and Vehicle	Exposure	Cross-Reactions	Comment
Carbocaine Hydrochloride (mepivacaine; Winthrop)	2% aq. sol.	Local anesthetics	Lidocaine	Not based on para-amino-benzoic acid
Carbolfuchsin paint (Castellani's paint)	As is (open)			Contains resorcin. Keep in dark bottle
Carbon disulfide	10% o.o.	Industrial solvents, laboratories, rayon industry		
Carbon paper	As is	Typing, lithography, blue printing, photocopying		*Reported sensitizers:* Triphenyl phosphate, oleyl alcohol, nigrosine
Carbon tetrachloride	10% o.o.	Solvents, floor waxes, cleansers, fire extinguisher fluids, insecticide sprays, antiseborrheic lotion		Synonyms: carbon tet, tetrachloromethane and perchloromethane
Carbowax	As is	Cosmetics, pharmaceutical vehicles		Solid polyethylene glycols
Carboxylase (co-carboxylase, coenzyme B)	10% aq. sol.	Manufacture of thiamine	Thiamine chloride	
Carboxyphenyl	As is	Manufacturer of photo processing		
Carbromal (bromodiethyl-acetylurea)	1% in propylene glycol	Carbrital (Parke, Davis), Taborea (Table Rock)	Barbiturates	Purpuric patch test
Carbyne	1% aq. sol.	Herbicide		
Cardamom	50% aq. sol.	Confectionary spice		
Carmine dye	5% pet.	Rouge, lip pomade, ink, stains, food	Terpenes	Contains cochineal, a dried insect
Carnation oil	5% pet.	Eugenol, "Flubber" putty, flavoring agent, perfume		
Carnauba wax	50% mineral oil	Orange skin protective, old phonograph records, furniture, shoe and floor waxes, candles, electrical insulation, cosmetics, lipsticks, cologne sticks		Obtained from South American palm trees. A solid that becomes fluid when rubbed with a circular motion

Contactant	Concentration and Vehicle	Exposure	Cross-Reactions	Comment
Casalic green	2% aq. sol.	Chromium oxide powder, green tattoos, Guinget Cream		
Cashew nut oil	3% alc.	Voodoo dolls, swizzle sticks, mucilage, printer's ink, varnishes	Rhus and other Anacardiaceae	
Cassia flavor	5% o.o.	Chinese cinnamon		
Castor oil	As is	Cosmetic emollient		
Catechol	3% o.o.	Plastic industry, rubber	Resorcin, hydroquinone	
Cauliflower	As is	Cruciferae plant	Cabbage, brussels sprout, grape seed	
CD-2 (amino diethylamino monohydrochloride; diethyl paraphenylenediamine)	1% aq. sol.	Color film developers		Lichen planus type of eruption
CD-3 (color developer) (amino-4-N-ethyl-N-(methane-sulfon-aminoethyl)-m-toluidine)	1% pet.			
Cedarwood oil	10% o.o.	Essential perfume oil		A photosensitizer
Cellulose	As is	Sodium carbomethyl cellulose used in Japanese cake mix Surgical is oxidized regenerated cellulose		
Cement (clay and limestone)	As is (open)	Construction industry irritant		May contain cobalt, nickel and chromates
Cephalosporin	As is or scratch test 0.5% aq. sol.	Handling or taking drug	Penicillin	Positive patch test in adverse drug reaction
Ceramol	30% pet.			Blend of cetyl and stearyl alcohol with sodium lauryl sulfate
Ceresin (ozokerite)	30% pet.	Cosmetic stiffeners		
Cerium oxide	As is	Polishing eyeglass lenses		May cause depigmentation

Contactant	Concentration and Vehicle	Exposure	Cross-Reactions	Comment
Cetyl alcohol	30% pet.	Fatty alcohol present in lanolin, Chloromycetin Cream, Vioform HC Lotion, Neo-Cord-Dome Lotion, Pragmatar	Stearyl alcohol	Synonyms: hexadecyl or palmityl alcohol Can cause contact urticaria
Cetyl pyridinium bromide	1:1000 aq. sol.			Used in Hungarian contraceptives
Cetyl pyridinium chloride (Ceepryn)	1:1000 aq. sol.	Cepacol, Micrin, Reef, Scope		A quaternary ammonium compound
Chalk dyes	1% pet.	Colored chalk dyes Pigment red, pigment yellow		
Chamomile tea	5% aq. sol.	Artemesia and mugwart		May cause severe bullous eruption
Chicory	Leaf or juice as is	Handling of plants		Used as coffee substitute
Chloracetopenone (CN)	0.1% alc.	Tear gas		Test open. A severe irritant and primary sensitizer
Chloral hydrate	10% aq. sol.	Hair tonics, suppositories, Calmitol Ointment, veterinary anesthetics	Chlorobutanol	
Chloramine	2% aq. sol.	Water disinfectants	Sod. hypochlorite	
Chloramphenicol	2% pet.	Antibiotic		
Chloramphenicol (Chloromycetin [Parke, Davis])	5% pet.	Antibiotic cream, Genetris Pessaries	DNCB	
Chlordane	5% acet.	Insecticides		
Chlordantoin	1% pet.	Antifungal agent found in Clocandil vaginal cream		
Chlorhexidene	1% aq. sol.	Antiseptic		May be irritant
Chlorhexidine digluconate	0.5% aq.	Antiseptic		
Chlorinated alkalies	0.5% aq. sol.	Javelle water, Labarraque's solution, Carrel-Dakin's solution, Clorox, chlorinated lime, chloramine	Sodium hypochlorite	

Contactant	Concentration and Vehicle	Exposure	Cross-Reactions	Comment
Chlorinated naphthalene	As is	Electric wires, motors, electrical equipment, transformers		Produces acneiform eruptions
Chloroacetamide	0.2% aq. sol.	Preservative in cosmetics, pharmaceuticals, coolant oils, pesticides		
Chlorobenzene	5% o.o.	Insecticides		Produces acneiform eruptions
Chlorobenzylidene malonitrile (CS)	1% alc. (open)	Tear gas		Test open. A severe irritant and primary sensitizer
Chlorobutanol crystals	5% o.o.	Dentalone (Parke, Davis), sedative dressing (Krutchen), local anesthetics, preservative for parenteral solutions and pharmaceuticals, biological fluids	Chloral hydrate	
Chlorocresol	2% pet.	Valisone Cream, topical medications, pesticides	Chloroxylenol	
Chloroform	40% o.o.	Solvent for gutta percha, gum copal, acrylic dentures, Ultra Brite and McLean's Toothpaste, anesthetics, liniments		
Chloro-meta-cresol	1% pet.	Preservative		p-Chloro-meta-cresol
Chloromethylisothiazolinone	0.5% pet.	Antibacterial preservative in cosmetics and shampoos		Present in Kathon
p-Chloro-o-cresol	0.1% alc.	Preservative		Phenolic compound
Chloro-2-phenylphenol (Dowicide 32)	1% pet. (open and closed)	Liquid soap, disinfectants, fungicides		Photosensitizer
Chlorphenesin	1% pet.	Plant growth inhibitor found in fungicides		
Chlorophyll	1% pet.	Deodorizers		
Chlorophyllins	5% aq. sol.	Deodorizers, cosmetics, suntan preparations, Green Mint Mouthwash		

Contactant	Concentration and Vehicle	Exposure	Cross-Reactions	Comment
Chloroquin	5% pet.	Pharmaceuticals	Atabrine	
Chlorosalicylamide	1% white pet.	Antimycotic agent (Jadit)		Photosensitizer
Chlorothalonil	0.0001% aq.	Paint, wood preservative, floriculture		Vapors at 0.4 ppm cause airborne dermatitis
Chlorothion	1% alc. (open)	Insecticides		
Chlorothymol	2% alc. or 0.1% aq.	N.F. Antiseptic Solution. *Antiseptic solutions:* Gray Cross, C.S.I. *Foot powders:* Upjohn Medicated, Dr. Solvey, Ward's Foot Balm, K4. *Douches:* Lanteen, Verazeptol. *Liniments:* Neurabalm, Balsam of Myrrh, Rex Rub. Key Nose Drops. Formula DC Vaginal Jelly. *With benzocaine:* Idol, Lanocaine		
Chloroxylenol	1% pet.	Chloroxylenol Solution B.P., Absorbine, Jr., Redux EGG Paste, Nullo Foot Cream, Rezamid Cream Lotion, Acne Aid, Cenathesin, First aid petroleum jelly. *Sprays:* Feminine hygiene "My Own" (Emko), Unburn, Unguentine, Top Brass, Stopette Deodorant. *Powders:* ZeaSORB, Desitin, Aveeno	Chlorocresol	Synonyms: p-chloro-meta-xylenol; 4-chloro-3,5-xylenol; Ottasept; PCMX; Bezytol
Chlorpromazine chloride (Thorazine)	1% pet.	Medical, nursing and chemistry personnel	Phenothiazines	Photoallergic and phototoxic
Chromium sulfate	2% aq. sol.	Textile inks, paints, varnishes, leather processing, lithographing, fur dyeing, electroplating, blueprinting		Trivalent chromium
Chromium trichloride	0.5% aq. sol.	See Chromium sulfate		Use 1/100 for intradermal testing
Chrysarobin	0.03% pet.	Topical medications		Obtained from goa powder (Indian tree)

Contactant	Concentration and Vehicle	Exposure	Cross-Reactions	Comment
Chrysoidine brown	5% pet.	Leather dyes	Para-amino compounds	
Cidex	1% aq. sol.	Cold sterilizing solution	To be freshly prepared	Is 2% buffered glutaraldehyde
Cinchona, tincture of	1% alc.	Hair tonics, rubefacients		
Cinnabar (red mercuric sulfide)	1% pet.	Red tattoos, topical medications		Only mercurial compatible with sulfur. May cause lichenoid and granulomatous allergic reactions.
Cinnamates (2-ethoxyethyl-p-methoxy)	1% pet.	Sunscreens		Photosensitizer
Cinnamic acid	5% pet.	Styrax, balsam of Peru, menthyl and benzyl cinnamates in sunscreens: RVPaque (Elder), SunDare Lotion (Texas Pharmacal), Sun Bath (Revlon), Sun Tan Gelee (Rexall)		Contact urticaria
Cinnamic aldehyde	1% pet.	Cinnamon oil, cassia oil, cinnamon powder, patchouli oil, flavoring agents, toilet soaps, perfumes	Balsam of Peru, benzoin	Depigmentation Contact urticaria
Cinnamon oil	2% pet.	Cassia bark, flavoring agents, vermouths, gum, toothpastes, confections, cola beverages, tobacco, bubble gum, lipsticks	Balsam of Peru, cinnamic aldehyde, bay leaf, marjoram	Contact urticaria
Citric acid (citron oil)	1% aq. sol.	Transfusions, nicotine stain remover, astringent mouthwash		Cause of aphthous ulcers?
Citronella oil (lemon grass oil)	1% pet.	Perfumes, insect repellents		
Citrus Red 2	2% acet.	Dye for Florida orange peel		An azo dye
Clindamycin	1% aq. sol.	Antibiotic		
Clorox	1% aq. sol.	Detergents, chlorinated alkalines		
Clove oil	1% pet.	Eugenol, antiseptics, local anesthetics, mucilage, perfumes, condiments, chewing gum	Balsam of Peru, diethylstilbestrol, benzoin	

Contactant	Concentration and Vehicle	Exposure	Cross-Reactions	Comment
Coal tar	5% pet.	Adhesives, creosotes, insecticides, phenols, wood working, preservation of wood		Photosensitizing
Cobalt chloride	2% aq. sol. or 1% pet.	Tattoos, pottery, clays, cements, hematinics, alloys, anodes, glass enamels, adhesives, fly paper, hair dyes, carbides, pigments	Vitamin B_{12}	Vitamin B_{12} (Cobione) is a cobalt compound
Cobalt naphthenate	2% pet.	Polyester resins, rubber industry	Other cobalt salts	
Cobalt sulfate	2% aq. sol.	Alloys, dyeing, lacquers, glass, paints, oilcloth colors, enamels, permanent ink for porcelain		
Cobaltous aluminate (azure or cobalt blue)	2% aq. sol.	Blue tattoo pigment		
Cocaine hydrochloride	1% aq. sol.			Based on benzoic acid
Cocaine liquid	1% aq. sol.	Topical anesthetics, mydriatic		Based on benzoic acid
Cocamidopropyl betaine	1% aq.	Hair and bath products		Non-ionic surfactant
Cocoanut oil	Pure	Soaps, oleomargarine, cooking fat, baking ingredients, confections		
Cocoanut soap (sodium salt)	2% aq. sol.	Surfactant, synthetic detergents, bubble baths		Control
Cocobolo wood	As is	Musical instruments, kitchen utensil handles, wood-working industry		
Coins, U.S.A.	As is	Penny Nickel Dime Quarter Half dollar	95% copper, 5% zinc 75% copper, 25% nickel 90% copper, 8% nickel 90% copper, 8% nickel 60% copper, 40% nickel (All U.S. coins except the penny give a positive dimethylglyoxime test reaction)	

Contactant	Concentration and Vehicle	Exposure	Cross-Reactions	Comment
Collodion	As is			Contains ether, absolute ethyl alcohol and pyroxylin
Collodion, flexible	As is			Contains colophony (rosin) and castor oil
Colocynth extract	1% alc.	Denaturing agent in alcohol		
Colophony	See Rosin			
Congo red	2% pet.	Azo dye		Diagnostic aid in amyloidosis, indicator of free HCl in gastric contents
Coniferyl benzoate	1% pet.	Benzoin	Benzyl cinnamate, benzyl alcohol, eugenol, benzoin, vanilla	
Copper sulfate	5% aq. sol.	Insecticides, fungicides, food processing, fertilizers, mordant in fur dyeing, coin alloys, D'Alibour solution		A rare sensitizer
Coriander, oil of	10% c.o.	Flavoring agents		
Costus root oil	0.1% pet	Plants		
Cottonseed oil	As is	Cosmetics, margarine, vegetable shortening		
Coumarin	10% o.o.	Flavorings (including vanilla), perfumes, cosmetics, optical bleaches		A cinnamic acid derivative; Photosensitizer
Creosote (creosote oil)	10% o.o.	Expectorants, preserving wood, waterproofing, lumber industry		A photosensitizer
Cresol	1% aq. sol.	Antiseptics		
Crotamiton	5% pet.	Scabies treatment		
Crystal violet	1% aq. sol.	Gentian violet		
Cutting oil	As is (open) or 50% o.o.			Controls. May contain additives

Contactant	Concentration and Vehicle	Exposure	Cross-Reactions	Comment
Cyclaine (hexylcaine hydrochloride; Merck Sharp & Dohme)	1% aq. sol.	Local anesthetics	Procaine p-Amino-compounds	
Cyclohexamide (actidione)	1% pet.	Culture media, garden spray	Neomycin	
Cyclohexanol peroxide	0.5% pet.	Polyester resin hardener		
n-Cyclohexyl benzothiazyl sulfenamide	1% pet.	Rubber	Mercapto derivatives	
Dammar resin	20% pet.	Plasters, varnishes, lacquers		Resin from East Indies plant
Dangard	0.25% pet.	Q.E.D. Shampoo sold by barbers		
DDT (dichlorodiphenyltrichloroethane)	1% pet.	Insecticides, chlorobenzene derivatives		May produce chloracne and possibly porphyria
Decyl alcohol	5% pet.	Lanolin		An aliphatic alcohol
Depilatories	As is (open)			Controls
Dequalinium chloride	0.1% aq. sol.	Micrin Mouthwash, antiseptics		A quaternary ammonium compound
Desenex (WTS-Pharmacraft)	As is	Antifungal agents		Rare sensitizer
Detergent 1011 (secondary amide of lauric acid)	1% aq. sol.	Surfactant, nonionic synthetic detergents		Controls
Detergent, enzyme	0.25% aq. sol.			Test the pure subtilisms 0.1% aq.
Diallyl phthalate	0.1% acet.	Polyester resin industry		A strong irritant
Diaminodiphenylmethane	0.5% pet.	Rubber antioxidant, epoxy resin curing agent, intermediate in germicides, surface active agents, pharmaceuticals, corrosion inhibitors, phosphate insecticides	Amino compounds Polyurethane resins	Photosensitizer
Diazolidinyl Urea (Germall II)	1% aq. sol.	Preservative in cosmetics		

Contactant	Concentration and Vehicle	Exposure	Cross-Reactions	Comment
Diazonium	1% alc. (open)	Phosphate insecticides		
Diazonium compounds	10% aq. sol.	Ozalid photocopy paper		Contains 4-nn'-diethyl-amino benzene diazonium chloride
Dibenzothiazyl disulfide	1% pet.	Rubber	Mercapto derivatives	
Di-beta-naphthyl para-phenylenediamine	1% pet.	Rubber	Paraphenylene derivatives	
Dibromsalan (dibromosalicylanilide)	1% pet.	Deodorant soaps, White Lifebuoy		Photoallergic
Dibutyl phthalate	5% pet.	Plasticizer for synthetic resins, nail lacquer		
Dibutyl tin maleate	1% pet.	Plasticizer in plastic (Elastiglass)		
Dichlorobenzene	5% chloroform	Mothballs		A primary sensitizer
Dichlorodiphenyl (methyl carbinol)	5% acet. (open)	Organic insecticides		
1,2,4-Dichloronitrobenzene (dinitrochlorobenzine) (DNCB)	0.1% acet.	Algicide in air conditioner NALCO-205		A primary sensitizer
Dichlorophene (G4)	1% aq. sol.	Fungicides, antimildew agents, preservative in creams, dentifrices	Hexachlorophene	
Dichloropropane	1% pet.	Used in production of plastic products		
Diethylenetriamine	0.1% aq. sol.	Epoxy resin amine	Ethylenediamine HCL	
Diethylethanolamine	0.1% aq. sol.	Amine polyurethane catalyst		
Diethyl-meta-toluamide (DEET)	5% alc. (open)	Black Flag, Off, 7—11, RVPellent (Elder)		May produce bullous eruption
Diethylparaphenylenediamine (CD$_2$)	1% pet.	Color film developers	Para-amino compound	Lichen planus reaction

Contactant	Concentration and Vehicle	Exposure	Cross-Reactions	Comment
Diethylstilbestrol	0.1% in ethyl alc.	Aquarant "E" (Webster), Furestrol Suppositories (Eaton), diethylstilbestrol suppositories (Lilly)	Dienestrol, hexestrol, bisphenol A, monobenzyl-ether of hydroquinone, eugenol, stilbene benzophenone benzylbenzoate	Contact urticaria
Diethylthiourea	1% pet.			Sensitizer in diver's wet suit
Difluorodiphenyl-trichloroethane	5% acet.	Insecticides		
Difolantan	1:1000 aq.	Fungicide for farm crops		Derivative of dicarbox-imide
Digalloyltrioleate	3% pet.	A-Fil, Neo-A-Fil (Texas Pharmacal), Sunprotectol (Lamond)		Sunscreens may be photosensitive
Dihydrostreptomycin sulfate	20% pet.	Pharmaceutical and nursing personnel	Neomycin, kanamycin, streptomycin	
Dihydroxyacetone	10% aq. sol.	Man Tan, Magictan, Positan, Tan-O-Rama, Tansation, Tanfastic		Rare sensitizer
Dihydroxyphenyl	0.1% pet.	Rubber		
Diisocyanatohexane	1% aq.	Textile finish		Usually occupational
Diisopropyl fluorophosphate	1% alc. (open)	Insecticides		
Dilan	5% acet. (open)	Insecticides		
Dimethoxane	1% pet.	Preservative in water systems and emulsions		
Dimethylaminopropylamine	1% pet.	Epoxy resin hardener		Irritant
Dimethylaniline	1% pet.	Polyester resin accelerator		
Dimethylglyoxime	10% in Carbowax	Chemical test for nickel		
Dimethyl paratoluidine	2% pet.	Accelerators, acrylic resins		

Contactant	Concentration and Vehicle	Exposure	Cross-Reactions	Comment
Dimethyl phthalate	20% pet.	Plasticizer for synthetic resins, insect repellents		
Dimethyl sulfate	*Do not test*			Forms sulfuric acid
Dimethyl sulfoxide (DMSO)	90% aq. sol.	Industrial solvents, topical medicaments		Primary urticariogenic agent
Dimethylol dihydroxy ethylene urea (Fixapret CPN)	4.5% aq.	Permanent press clothing	Other textile resins	
Dimethylol urea formaldehyde	10% pet.	Crease resistant, drip dry clothing		Releases formaldehyde
Dimite dichlorodiphenylethanol	5% acet. (open)	Insecticides		
Di-β-naphthyl-p-phenylenediamine	1% pet.	Rubber antioxidant	IPPD	
Dinitrochlorobenzene (DNCB)	0.1% acet.	Investigative sensitizer, algicide in water cooling systems	Chloromycetin (chloramphenicol)?	A primary sensitizer
Dinobuton	1% pet.	Insecticide in Acrex		
Dioctyl phthalate	1% pet.	Plastics and rubber		
Dioctyl sodium sulfosuccinate	1% aq. sol.	Wetting compounds, anionic surfactant		
Diodoquin (diiodohydroxyquin; Searle)	5% pet.	Amebicides	Vioform, Quinolor, Sterosan	
Dioxane	1% aq.	Degreasing solvent		
Dipentamethylene thiuram disulfide	1% pet.	Rubber	Other thiuram compounds	
Diphenyl	2% pet.	Dielectrics	Fungicide for oranges	
Diphenylcyclopropenone	0.1% acet.	Chemistry experiments		
Diphenylguanidine	1% pet.	Rubber accelerator		
Diphenylparaphenylenediamine	1% pet.	Rubber accelerator (black rubber)	PPDA derivative	
Dipropylenetriamine	1% pet.	Epoxy resin hardener		
Dithiomorpholine	1% pet.	Rubber vulcanizer		

Contactant	Concentration and Vehicle	Exposure	Cross-Reactions	Comment
Dithionone	1% pet.	Pesticide		Merck product
Divinyl benzene (styrene)	1% o.o.	See Styrene		
DMDM Hydantoin	1% aq. sol.	Preservative		Other names: Bis-(hydroxymethyl) dimethylimidazolidinedione, Dimethylol-Dimethyl Hydantoin Glydant, Imidazolidinedione-Bis(hydroxymethyl) Dimethyl
Domiphen bromide	0.1% aq. sol.	Quaternary compound in Scope Mouthwash		A "Quat" compound
Dowicide(s)	1% pet.	Germicides, fungicides, antiseptics, disinfectants		A series of phenolic substances
Dowicide A (sodium-o-phenyl phenate)	1% pet.	Dowicide A, B, and G used in paper money		Not absorbed through skin. An oil solution (5%) is well-tolerated on human skin, but aqueous solutions of the sodium salt are irritating in concentrations exceeding 0.5%
Dowicide B (sodium 2,3,5-trichlorophenate)	1% pet.	Water-soluble fungicide		
Dowicide C (sodium chloro-o-phenyl phenate)	1% pet.	Water-soluble antiseptic		
Dowicide D (2-chloro-4-phenyl-phenol sodium)	1% pet.	Germicide		
Dowicide E (2-bromo-4-phenyl-phenol sodium)	1% pet.	Fungicide		
Dowicide F (sodium tetra-chlorophenate)	1% pet.	Used as germicide, antiseptic, fungicide		

Contactant	Concentration and Vehicle	Exposure	Cross-Reactions	Comment
Dowicide G (sodium pentachlorophenate)	1% pet.	Industrial antiseptic		
Dowicide H (sodium tetrachlorophenoxide)	1% pet.	Industrial antiseptic		
Dowicide 1 (o-phenyl phenol)	1% pet.	Germicide, antiseptic, fungicide		
Dowicide 3 (chloro-phenyl phenol)	1% pet.	Germicide, antiseptic, fungicide		
Dowicide 4 (2-chloro-4-phenyl phenol)	1% pet.	High-efficiency germicide		
Dowicide 6 (tetrachlorophenol)	1% pet.	Germicide, antiseptic, fungicide		
Dowicide 7 (pentachlorophenol)	1% pet.	Oil-soluble antiseptic, germicide, fungicide		
Dowicil 200	1% pet.	Bactericide		Release formaldehyde
Duponol WA (sodium lauryl sulfate)	1% aq. sol.	Surfactant, anionic synthetic detergents		Controls
Duraspan (International Latex)	As is	Polyurethane elastomer (spandex)		
Dyclone (dyclonine hydrochloride; Dow Chemical)	1% aq. sol.	Local anesthetics		Not based on para-aminobenzoic acid
Dyes Certified Disperse Orange 3 Blue Disperse Yellow 3 Red	2% pet. 1% pet.	Foods, drugs, cosmetics Nylon dyes	Para-amino compounds	
Ecogaine	2% aq. sol.	Local anesthetics	Procaine, benzocaine P-amino compound	Based on para-aminobenzoic acid
Edathamil (calcium EDTA versenate)	1% aq. sol.	Chelating agent		
Eldoquin (Elder)	See Hydroquinone			
Emulsifying wax	30% pet.			Contains alkyl stearyl alcohol
Eosin	50% pet.	Fluorescent dyes, pharmaceuticals		A photosensitizer

Contactant	Concentration and Vehicle	Exposure	Cross-Reactions	Comment
Ephedrine	1% pet.	Nose drops		
Epichlorhydrin	0.1% alc.	Epoxy resin	Propene oxide	
Epon 828	1% acet.	Epoxy resins		
Epon 1001	1% acet.	Epoxy resins		
Epoxy acrylate	0.5% pet.	UV inks and varnishes	Other acrylates	
Epoxy glue hardener	0.5% pet.	One part of 2 tube preparation, household glue, collages, sculptures		May contain triethylenetetramine or diaminodiphenylmethane
Epoxy glue resin	1% acet.			Has caused contact urticaria
Epoxy glycidyl ether	0.1% acet.			Epoxy resin diluent
Erythromycin stearate	1% pet.	Antibiotic		
Erythrosin	2% pet.	Fluorescent dyes		A photosensitizer
Esoterica (Mitchum)	As is	Skin-lightening cream		Contains ammoniated mercury
Essential oils	1% alc. or 2% pet.	Flavor in dentifrices, mouthwashes, medicinal elixirs, perfumes		May be photosensitizer
Ether	60% o.o.	Anesthetics, solvents		May be irritant
Ethoxyethyl-p-methoxycinnamate	5% pet.	Sunscreen		Photosensitivity
Ethoxyquin	1% o.o.	Apple packing, animal feed additive		A quinoline
Ethyl acetate	5% mek.	Solvent for varnishes, lacquers and nitrocellulose plastics, component of nail polish removers		Trace amounts in foods and alcoholic beverages
Ethyl acrylate	0.1% pet.	Cross-link agent in rubber		
Ethyl butyl thiourea	1% pet.	Neoprene adhesive		
Ethyl cetab (cetylethyldimethyl-ammonium bromide)	0.1% aq. sol.	Surfactant, cationic synthetic detergents		Controls "Quat" compound

Contactant	Concentration and Vehicle	Exposure	Cross-Reactions	Comment
Ethyl hexyl acrylate	0.5% pet.			
Ethyl parahydroxybenzoate	5% pet.	Preservative in pharmaceuticals, cosmetics, foods, cleansers	Other parabens	May cause systemic contact dermatitis
Ethylene dichloride	50% o.o.	Solvents, plastics, rubber, insecticides, hobby crafts		
Ethylene glycol	5% alc.	Antifreeze solvent	Propylene glycol	
Ethylene glycol monomethyl ether acetate (Egmea)	1% mek.	Used to cement nose pads to eyeglass frames		May contain traces of ethyl acetate
Ethylene oxide	0.01% aq.	Sterilizing gas for surgical instruments, towels, sheets, gloves, anesthesia masks, chemical reactor		Powerful vesicant
Ethylene urea, melamine formaldehyde resin (Fixapret AC)	5% pet.	Permanent press clothing	Other textile resins	
Ethylenediamine hydrochloride	1% pet.	Mycolog Cream, parent substance of certain antihistamines and aminophylline; dyes, rubber, fungicides, waxes, resins, insecticides, asphalt; present in Tincture Merthiolate (Lilly)	Aminophylline, Pyribenzamine, Antistine, Diethyltetramine Piperaine citrate Piperazine	Can cause systemic contact dermatitis
Ethylenediamine tetraacetate (Versene)	1% aq. sol.	Stabilizing agent in many ophthalmic solutions, chelating agent		
1,3-Ethylhexanediol	5% o.o.	Insect repellent		Irritant
Eucalyptus oil	1% alc.	Gutta percha for root canal fillings	Balsam of Peru, benzoin, vanilla, oil of orange peel	
Eugenol	25% pet.	Oil of carnation (hyacinth), oil of bay, pimento oil (allspice), clove oil, flower oils, cinnamon oil, food spices, perfumes, zinc oxide dental cement, flavoring agent, dental impression agent	Iso-Eugenol Balsam Peru Benzoin Propanoid	Derived from clove oil Has caused contact urticaria

Contactant	Concentration and Vehicle	Exposure	Cross-Reactions	Comment
Eurax Cream and Lotion (10% n-ethyl-o-crotonotoluide; Geigy)	As is	Scabicide		
Euxyl K400	0.5% pet.	Cosmetics, skin care products	Mix of phenoxyethanol and methyldibromoglutaronitrile	
Evafanol AS-1	1% aq.	Fabric finish		Anti-"pilling" agent
Evans Blue Dye	1% aq. sol.	Azo dye		Used in lymphangiography
Eyeglass frames, plastic	Shavings (controls)			*Possible allergens:* cellulose acetate, cellulose propionate, resorcinol monobenzoate, anthraquinone p-tertiarybutyl phenol, azo dyes, beeswax-turpentine mixture, ethylene glycol, ethylene oxide and ethyl acetate
Eyeglass nose pad				Ethylene glycol monomethyl ether acetate (welds nose pad to eyeglass frames)
Fentichlor	1% pet. (open and closed)	Antiseptic and fungicide, cosmetics, pharmaceuticals		A photosensitizer
Ferric chloride	2% aq. sol.	Monsel's solution, styptic		Very rare sensitizer
Flit	25% o.o.	Insecticide		
Fluorescein	10% pet.	Dyes, eyeglass cleaner		Photosensitizer
Fluorouracil	5% pet.	Cytotoxic drug		Phototoxic?
Formaldehyde resins		Plastics, textile finishes		
Urea formaldehyde	10% pet.			
Melamine formaldehyde	10% pet.			

Contactant	Concentration and Vehicle	Exposure	Cross-Reactions	Comment
Others	1% pet. or 1% isopropyl alcohol	Glues, plastics, textile finishes		
Formalin (40% sol. of formaldehyde gas)	1 or 2% aq. sol.	*Cosmetics:* shampoos, antiperspirants, Sub-Rosa Cream Deodorant, nail hardener, nail polish, resins, Thermodent Toothpaste, soaps, permanent wave lotions. *Medical:* root canal preparation (Formo-Cresol) disinfectant, wart remedies, fungicides, insecticides, tissue fixative, embalming fluid, denatured alcohol, orthopedic casts, renal dialysis unit, vaccines. *Industrial:* tanning white leather, textile finish (antiwrinkle), synthetic gums and adhesives, synthetic resins and rubber, paper, photography, antimildew in leather, glues, wet strength paper	Glutaraldehyde?	Hexamethylenetetramine (methenamine) liberates formaldehyde in the presence of acids. Formaldehyde-releasing agents. May cause contact urticaria
Formic acid spirits	1% aq. sol.	Hair tonics		
Fowler's solution (potassium arsenite solution)	As is			Equivalent to 1% arsenic trioxide
Fuchsin	1% pet.	Basic fuchsin, rosaniline, therapeutic dye, fuchsin-silver nitrate. Marking patch test sites—irritant		
Fumaronitrile	Do not test	Plasticizer for vinyl resin herbicide, soil fumigant		A potent irritant and vesicant. May also be allergen.
Furacin (nitrofurazone; Eaton)	As is	Topical bacterial agent	Contains Carbowax	Water-soluble Furacin preparations have a base of polyethylene glycols
Garamycin (Gentamycin)	20% pet.	Antiseptic topical medication	Neomycin, kanamycin	Contact urticaria

Contactant	Concentration and Vehicle	Exposure	Cross-Reactions	Comment
Garlic	5% aq. extract		Balsam of Peru, tars, onion	Controls
Gasoline	50% o.o.			
Gentian violet (methylrosaniline chloride)	1% aq. sol.	Stain, indicator, antiseptics, vaginal creams, tablets, aerosols	Rivanol	Intradermal test with 0.05 ml. of a 1:5000 dilution
Geraniol	5% pet.	Flavoring agent, perfume, geranium oil		
Ginger oil	25% c.o.	Condiments, candy gastric medications, rubefacient		
Ginkgo fruit pulp	1:10 acet.		Rhus, cashew	Ginkgo tree is a member of Anacardium genus
Glospan (Globe Manufacturing Co.)	As is	Polyurethane elastomer (spandex)		Lycra spandex is free of mercaptobenzothiazole
Glue	As is open or 10% acet.	Furniture, shoes, books, toys, waterproofing		Rubber, epoxies, chromates, formaldehyde, polyvinyl acetate resins
Glutaraldehyde	1% aq. sol. freshly prepared	Tissue fixative, antiperspirants, antiseptics, tanning agent for soft leather, embalming fluids, shampoo preservative, dentifrices	Formaldehyde?	Tans and dries skin May discolor skin
Glycerin	10% aq.	Emollient, pharmaceutical vehicle, mounting medium in microscopy		Very rare sensitizer
Glyceryl monooleate	30% pet.	Emulsifier, soaps, cosmetics		
Glyceryl monostearate	30% pet.	Emulsifier, cosmetics, food products, medicinals		
Glyceryl monothioglycolate	2.5% pet.	Permanent waves		
Glycol dimethyl acrylate	5% o.o.	Synthetic resins		Prevents crazing, cracking of resins
Gly-Oxide	As is	Mouthwash providing hydrogen peroxide		Contains urea peroxide

Contactant	Concentration and Vehicle	Exposure	Cross-Reactions	Comment
Gold chloride	1% aq. sol.	Photographers		Pustular patch test reaction
Gold cohesive	As is	Dentistry		
Gold leaf	As is	Gilding, topical ulcer medication		
Gold sodium thiosulfate	0.5% pet.	Jewelry, dental		Persistent positive
Gold trichloride	1% aq. sol.	Jewelry		
Gramicidin	5% pet.	Antibacterial topical agent, mouthwashes		
Graphite (black lead)	As is	Lead pencils, crucibles, rubber surfaces, lubricants		
Grotan BK	2% pet.			
Grotan HD-2	0.15% pet.			
Grotan K	1% pet.			
Guaiacol	5% pet			
Guaiazulene	1% pet.	Used in Italian lipsticks, dentifrices; antiinflammatory agent		
Guanine (2-amino-6-hydroxy purine)	5% pet.	Pearly nail lacquer		Obtained from fish scales
Guignet's green (chromium oxide)	2% aq. sol.	Green tattoo pigment		
Gum(s)	50% aq. sol.	Resinous plant exudates		Contains carbohydrates forming mucilaginous substances with water
Gum arabic (acacia)	50% aq. sol.	See Acacia		
Gutta percha	As is aqueous suspension brittle when exposed to air	Resins, rosins, root canal mixtures		Latex of Malaysian trees contains more resin than does rubber

Contactant	Concentration and Vehicle	Exposure	Cross-Reactions	Comment
Hair lotions, tonics, and sprays	As is (open)			May contain: *rubefacient*—chloral hydrate, formic acid spirits, quinine salts, tincture capsicum or cinchona, cantharidin; *phenolic compounds*—chlorthymol, resorcinol, betanaphthol; *other antiseptics*—salicylic acid, formaldehyde, mercury bichloride; *tars*—coal tar derivatives, oil of cade; *vehicle*—alcohol and volatile solvents, perfumes
Haloprogin	1% pet.	Antifungal, antibacterial		
Henna	10 mg powder in 100 ml water or ether	Vegetable dye, synthetic henna (Lawsonia, hydroxynaphthoquinone—the coloring matter of henna leaves)		Rarely sensitizes. May cause contact urticaria
Hexachlorophene (G-11)	1% pet.	Soaps, detergents, creams, oils, pharmaceuticals	Bithionol, chlorinated salicylanilides Dichlorophene	Now restricted by FDA primarily to prescription items, photosensitizer
Hexahydrophthalic anhydride	1% pet.			
Hexamethylenetetramine (methenamine)	1% pet.	Many proprietary urinary antiseptics often combined with mandelic acid. Also a rubber accelerator	Formaldehyde	Liberates formaldehyde in the presence of acids
Hexanedioldiacrylate	0.1% pet.	Ultraviolet cured inks		Photosensitizer
Hexetidine	alc.	Antibacterial agent in Sterisol mouthwash, douches		Synonyms: ethylhexyl, hexahydro, methylimidaso, imidasolel

Contactant	Concentration and Vehicle	Exposure	Cross-Reactions	Comment
Hexylresorcinol	1% pet.	Contraceptives, Sucrettes, Tetrazets, ST 37, Crystoids, Caprikol (Merck), Akrinol Cream, Listerine, Lanteen Jelly (Esta), Nymore	Resorcin	
Holocaine (phenacaine) Hcl.	1% aq. sol.	Local anesthetics	Benzocaine, procaine, p-amino compounds	
Homatropine	1% aq. sol.	Eye drops		
Hyamine 1622 (p-diisobutyl phenoxyethoxy ethyldimethyl benzyl-ammonium chloride)	0.1% aq. sol.	Surfactant, cationic synthetic detergents, bubble baths, Clesk Lotion (Dara), Quinette Inserts (Arnar-Stone)		"Quat"
Hydralizine hydrochloride, bromide or sulfate	1% aq. sol. or 1% pet.	Wide industrial exposure, metal, plastics, rubber products, rocket fuel, photography, insecticides, fungicides, preservatives. Parent substance for drugs listed in adjacent column	Apresoline, isonicotinic acid, hydrazide, phenyl-hydrazine, Nardil (derived from hydrazine hydrobromide)	
Hydroabietyl alcohol (abitol)	10% pet.	Film former in mascara and adhesive		Abietic acid
Hydrochloric acid	1% aq. sol.	Chemical industry, Acidulin (Lilly), Convertin (Ascher), Muripsin (Norgine), Normacid (Stuart)		Rarely sensitizes Irritant
Hydrocortisone	2.5% alc.			
Hydrocortisone acetate or free alcohol	2.5% alc.			
Hydrofluoric acid	0.2% aq. sol.	Corrosive agents, glass etching, electric lamp manufacturing, dry cleaning		Pustular patch test reaction Irritant
Hydrogen peroxide solution	3% aq. sol.	Bleaches, oxidizing agents, antiseptics		
Hydrogen sulfide	2% aq. sol.	Petroleum refineries, tunnels, mines, rayon plants		Irritant

Contactant	Concentration and Vehicle	Exposure	Cross-Reactions	Comment
Hydrophilic ointment U.S.P.	As is			Contains sodium lauryl sulfate, propylene glycol, stearyl alcohol, methyl paraben, propyl paraben, white petrolatum, distilled water
Modified				Modified hydrophilic ointment contains glycerin instead of propylene glycol
Hydrophilic petrolatum (U.S.P.)	As is			Contains stearyl alcohol, cholesterol, white wax, white petrolatum
Hydroquinone	1% pet.	Rubber inhilbitor polyester, acrylic, photography, Eldoquin and Eldopaque (Elder), Artra (White), Derma-blanch (Brayten)	Resorcin, pyrocatechol, monobenzylether of hydroquinone	Depigmenting agent May be irritant
Hydroquinone, monobenzylether of	See Monobenzylether of hydroquinone			
Hydroxycitronell	1% pet.	Perfume		Causes hyperpigmentation
Hydroxyethyl methacrylate	5% pet.	Anaerobic metal sealant		
8-Hydroxyquinoline	5% pet.	Antibacterial		Bioform, Diodoquin
Hypochloride	2% aq. sol.	Kasenol Mouthwash, Oxychlorosene		
Ibuprofen	10% pet.			
Ichthyol (ichthammol; sulfonated bitumen)	10% pet.	Topical medications, Derma Medicone (Medicone), Ichthymall (Mallinckrodt)		Rarely sensitizes
Idoxuridine	1% pet.	Antiviral agent	Other pyrimidine drugs	

Contactant	Concentration and Vehicle	Exposure	Cross-Reactions	Comment
Igepal (nonylphenoxy polyethylene oxyethanol)	1% aq. sol.	Surfactant, synthetic detergents, bubble baths		Controls
Igepon T.H.C. (sodium oleyl laurate)	1% aq. sol.	Surfactant, synthetic detergents, bubble baths		Controls
Imidazolidinyl urea (Germall 115)	2% pet.	Antibacterial, antifungal		
Indalone	As is (open)	Insect repellents		
Indane	5% acet. (open)	Insecticides: chlordane, heptachlor, aldrin, dieldrin, endrin, diendrin		
Indigo	5% pet.	Tattoos, stains, blue dye		
Ink(s)	As is (open)			Acid and basic dyes, iron salts, tannic acid, gallates, phenol, silver nitrate, alkalies, castor oil
Ink eradicator	As is (open)			Active agents are tin chloride, sodium bisulfite, sodium hypochlorite, sodium chloride
Iodine crystals	0.5% alc.	Betadine	Iodoform, radiopaque iodine, iodized medications, thymol iodide	Old iodine solutions exposed to light are irritants. Incompatible with sulfur and mercury.
Iodine, tincture of	As is (open)		Same as Iodine crystals.	Is an irritant when covered
Iodochlorhydroxyquin	3% pet.	Vioform, Sterosan, Chinoform, Clioquinol	Chloroquinadol Hydroxyquinoline	Topical agents may produce irritant & allergic reaction
Iodoform (formyl triiodide)	5% pet.	Local anesthetics, antiseptics	Iodine, formaldehyde	
Ioprep	As is (open)			Irritant when occluded

Contactant	Concentration and Vehicle	Exposure	Cross-Reactions	Comment
Irgasan GF3 (Cloflucarban [Geigy])	0.5% pet.	Safeguard soap; used abroad as bacteriostat in vinyl gloves; shampoos		A carbanilide
Irgasan DP 300 (Triclosan [Geigy]; 2,4,4-trichloro-2-hydroxydiphenyl ether)	0.5% aq.	Surgical scrub soaps; Dial, Colgate P300, Palmolive and Calgan antiseptic soaps; Right Guard, Calm and Dial underarm deodorants and antiperspirants; commercial laundry products, disposable paper products, paper lining for rodent cages, industrial fabric softener, fabric bacteriostat		Widely used bacteriostat
Irish moss (carrageen)	As is	Cosmetics, wave sets, dentifrices, mucilage		Trade names: Sea Kem, Viscarin, Chondrus extract
Isobutyl-p-aminobenzoate	5% pet.	Sunscreen	p-amino compounds	
Isocyanate monomer	1.1% acet.	Polyurethane resins	Diaminodiphenyl methane	
Isodine	As is	Mouthwash		Like Betadine, is iodine in PVP
Iso-eugenol	5% pet.	Balsam of Peru—Eugenol		
Isophorone diamine	0.1% o.o.	Epoxy resin hardener		
Isopropyl alcohol	10% aq.	Antiseptic, solvent		
Isopropyl myristate	10% alc. or 2% pet.	Cosmetics, pharmaceuticals, Decaspray, aerosol sprays		Alcohol ester of fatty acid
Isopropyl-n-phenyl paraphenylene-diamine (IPPD)	0.1% pet.	Rubber antioxidant (black rubber)	Hair dye, paraphenylene-diamine derivatives	May cause lichenoid or purpuric eruptions. Trade names: Cysone, Eastone, Fleezwax, Flexaone, Santoflex, Nonox-2A
Isothane (laurylisoquinolinium bromide)	0.1% aq. sol.	Surfactant, cationic synthetic detergents, bubble baths		Controls "Quat" compounds
Isothiouronium (PBA-1)	0.1% aq.	Persulfate bleach accelerator		
Jaborandi leaves, tincture of	As is (open)	Hair tonics		

Contactant	Concentration and Vehicle	Exposure	Cross-Reactions	Comment
Jasmin absolute	10% pet.	Perfume		
Jasmin, oil	10% pet.	Fragrance		Causes pigmented cosmetic dermatitis
Jasmine synthetic	10% pet.	Perfume		
Javelle water (potassium hypochlorite)	10% aq. sol.	Disinfecting and bleaching agents	Chloramine	European preparations may contain dichromates
Jojoba oil	20% o.o.	Cosmetics		Replacement for spermacetic OTC treatment—wrinkles, dry skin
Juniper tar (oil of cade)	25% c.o.	Alma-Tar (Schieffelin)		
Kanamycin	20% pet.	Antibiotic		Neomycin
Karaya gum (Sterculia gum)	As is 10% aq.	Hair-waving lotions, denture adhesive powders, cement for ileostomy appliances, furniture polishes		Obtained from sterculia ureus
Kathon	0.5% pet.	Antibacterial preservative in cosmetics, shampoos	Contains methylchloro-isothiazolinone and methylisothiazolinone	
Kerosene	60% o.o.	Solvents, curing tobacco, heating, cooking, lighting, waterless hand cleansers		Irritant
Ketone	10% o.o.	Organic solvents, acetone		
Ketoprofen	2.5% pet. or commercial vehicle	Topical NSAID	Ibuproxam	Photoallergy (UVA)
Krameria, tincture of (tinctura rhatanhiae)	5% alc.	Poultices for hemorrhoids, oral and mucosal astringents, combined with tincture of myrrh		Primary sensitizer
Kwell (Reed & Carnrick)	As is	Pediculosis remedy		Contains benzene hexachloride
Lactic acid	3% aq. sol.	Astringent mouthwash, pharmaceutical creams		

Contactant	Concentration and Vehicle	Exposure	Cross-Reactions	Comment
Lanolin	As is	Wool fat, wool wax, adhesives, cosmetics, pharmaceuticals	Eucerin Wool alcohols	Wool alcohols may be the specific sensitizers
Lantrol (dewaxed lanolin)	As is			
Latex	As is	Rubber, gutta percha, chicle, balata, fig		Fig tree latex is a sensitizer and photosensitizer
Laurel oil	2% pet.	Flavoring agent, felt hats, camphor laurel, plastics, perfumes, pharmaceuticals		
Lauryl alcohol	20% pet.	Lanolin		An aliphatic alcohol
Lauryl gallate	0.1% pet.	Antioxidant in margarine and cosmetics		
Lavender oil	1% alc. or pet.	Colognes, cosmetics, soaps, china, ceramics and paintings	Balsam of Peru, rosin, wood tar, essential oils	A photosensitizer, pigmentation, essential oil
Lead acetate	1% aq. sol.	Dyeing and printing cottons, weighing silks, laboratory determinations		
Lead arsenate	20% pet.	Fungicides, insecticides		
Lead chloride	2% pet.	Fur processing, felt processing, mordants, printing, solder, and flux		
Lead oxide (red lead)	2% alc.	Matches, glazes for ceramics, paints		
Lemon grass oil	2% pet.	Perfume		
Lemon oil	2% pet.	Perfume		
Lidocaine (Xylocaine)	1% pet.	Anesthetic		Amide
Lime, slaked (calcium hydroxide)	As is	Hydrated lime		Controls. See also Calcium oxide (quicklime)
Limonene, oil of (Pipentene)	2% pet.	Orange, lemon peel, perfumes, lemon wood	Turpentine, celery, bergamot, dill	Main sensitizer of orange and lemon peel
Linalool, oil of	10% pet.	Flavoring in dentifrices		

Contactant	Concentration and Vehicle	Exposure	Cross-Reactions	Comment
Lindane	1% pet.	Pesticide		Hexachlorocyclohexane, gamma-hexane Has caused urticaria
Linseed oil	As is	Paints, varnishes, sculpturing, furniture polishes, refinishing waxes, carron oil, putty, folk medicine		
Lipstick	As is			Indelible variety may photosensitize
Lycra (Du Pont)	As is	Polyurethane elastomer (spandex)		
Lysol (compound cresol solution)	1% aq. sol.	Disinfectant		
Mace, oil of (nutmeg)	1% alc.	Flavoring agent		
Mafenide acetate	8% pet.	Burn remedy (Sulfamylon Cream)		
Magnesium peroxide	10% pet.	Oxidizing agent—McLean's Toothpaste		
Malachite green	2% aq. sol.	Dye		
Malathion	1% alc. (open) 0.5% pet.	Insecticides		A primary sensitizer
Maleic anhydride	1% aq. sol.	Epoxy resin		
Maneb	1% pet.	Present in fungicides, pesticides, known as manganese ethylene bis-dithiocarbamate		
Manganese oxide	10% pet.	Pigment in rubber goods, alloy in iron and steel, dry batteries, brick, pottery, dyeing industry, drying paints and varnishes, glass making, printing, dyeing textiles		
Mastic	As is (open)	Varnishes, styptic, astringent, cements, microscopy, dentistry		Resin of European mastic tree

Contactant	Concentration and Vehicle	Exposure	Cross-Reactions	Comment
Matches and match boxes (striking surfaces)	As is			Principal ingredients are potassium chlorate, red phosphorus, phosphorus sesquisulfide (phosphorus trisulfide), antimony sulfide, chromates, red lead, glue, cornstarch, coloring agents, rosin, paraffin May cause airborne dermatitis and contact urticaria.
Melamine formaldehyde	10% pet.	Clothing finishes, epoxy resins, synthetic resins		
Menthol	1% pet.	Flavoring agents, rubefacients, dusting powders, douches, foods, cigarettes, liqueurs, mixed drinks, Listerine, Reef, Chloraseptic, face cream, toothpaste, mint candies, cough drops, aerosol room spray		Contact urticaria
Mercaptans	10% aq.	Depilatories, glue	Thioglycolic acid, BAL (dimercaprol)	
Mercaptobenimidazole	1% pet.			
Mercaptobenzothiazole	1% pet.	Rubber accelerator	Mercapto derivatives	
Mercolized cream (Dearborn)	As lis	Skin lightener cream		Contains ammoniated mercury Irritant
Mercresin Tincture (Upjohn)	As is (open)		Organic and inorganic mercurials	Irritant when covered. Contains organic mercury and cresol
Mercurochrome Solution (merbromin; Hynson, Westcott & Dunning)	As is	Organic mercurial antiseptic	Organic and inorganic mercurials Metallic mercury	

Contactant	Concentration and Vehicle	Exposure	Cross-Reactions	Comment
Mercurous chloride (calomel)	0.5% pet.	Topical and systemic medicaments	Organic and inorganic mercurials Metallic mercury	May produce eczematous "contact-type" dermatitis medicamentosa
Mercury (metallic)	0.5% pet.	Dentistry, thermometer		
Mercury bichloride	0.05% aq. sol.	Disinfectants, processing artificial silk, bronzing, dental laboratories, electric wiring, electroplating, electric equipment, paints, electric storage batteries, reagents, embalming fluid, fur processing, felt curing, engraving, printing, thermometers, metal work, mirror finishing, lamp bulbs, photography, photogravure, insecticides, skin lighteners	Organic and inorganic mercurials Metallic mercury	May cause nonspecific pustular patch test reactions Irritant
Mercury-salicylic ointment	As is (open)	Topical medications		May irritate glabrous skin
Merthiolate (thimerosal)	0.1% pet.	Preservative in cosmetics, topical medications, dentifrices, germicides Contact lens solutions		Contains an organic mercurial and thiosalicylic acid. Tincture of Merthiolate contains ethylenediamine
Metacide	1% alc. (open)	Insecticides		
Metaphen (nitromersol; Abbott)	0.5% pet.	Germicides	Inorganic mercurials	
Metaphenylenediamine	0.1% aq. sol.	Epoxy hardeners		
Methoxychlor	5% acet.	Insecticides		
8-Methoxypsoralen	0.001% alc.	Plants of Umbelliferae family, perfume oils (oil of bergamot), Trisoralen (Elder)		A photosensitizer
Methyl acetate	10% o.o.	Organic solvents		
Methyl acrylate	0.1% pet.	Textiles, leather		Susceptible to cold and water

Contactant	Concentration and Vehicle	Exposure	Cross-Reactions	Comment
Methyl alcohol (methanol)	Pure as is	Solvents, thinners, artificial leather manufacture, dry cleaning, antifreeze, rubber cement, celluloid, gums, resins, chemical processing		Synonyms: methyl hydrate, methyl hydroxide, acetone, alcohol, wood spirits, wood naphtha, carbinol, Columbian spirits, colonial spirits
Methyl bromide	Do not test	Fire extinguisher fluid, refrigerants, fumigants		Severe irritant
Methyl cellulose	2% aq.	Binder in dentifrices		
6-Methyl coumarin	10% alc.	Perfume		Photosensitizer
Methyl dichlorobenzene sulfonate	0.1% acet.	Dental impression material		
Methyl diisocyanate (MDI)	1% pet.			
Methyl ethyl ketone	As is (open)	Solvents		
Methyl ethyl ketone peroxide	0.5% acet.	Polyester resin catalyst		
MEK peroxide (methyl ethyl ketone peroxide)	1% pet.			
Methyl heptene carbonate	0.1% alc.	Perfumes, blend fixatives in lipsticks, soaps		
Methyl methacrylate	2% pet.	Resin used in dentistry, bone cement, adhesive artificial nails		
Methyl morpholine	0.1% aq. sol.	Polyurethane catalyst		
Methyl orange	2% pet.	Indicator		
Methyl parahydroxybenzoate	5% pet.	Preservatives, pharmaceuticals, cosmetics, food, cleansers	"Parabens"	May cause systemic contact dermatitis
Methyl salicylate	2% o.o.	Flavoring in dentifrices, Listerine, Reef, oil of wintergreen, rubefacients	Sodium salicylate aspirin	A primary sensitizer; May cause systemic contact dermatitis
Methylbenzethonium chloride	0.1% aq. sol.	Germicides, disinfectants, Diaparene (Breon)		Quaternary ammonium disinfectant

Contactant	Concentration and Vehicle	Exposure	Cross-Reactions	Comment
Methylchloroisothiazolinone/methylisothiazolone (MCI/MI or Kathon CG)	100 ppm	Cosmetics, skin and hair care products Industrial water systems, cutting oils		
Methylene blue	2% pet.	Dyes, platinum bleach	Phenothiazines	A photosensitizer
Methylisothiazolinone	0.5% pet.	Antibacterial preservative in cosmetics, shampoos		Present in Kathon
n-Methylol-chloracetamide	5% pet.	Preservative, coolant oils, and cosmetics found in Danish Product Parmetol		
n-Methylolacrylamide	0.1% pet.	Combined with vinyl acetate coatings, adhesives, varnishes		
Metol	1% pet.	Photography	p-amino compound	p-Methylaminophenol sulfate
Metycaine (piperocaine; Lilly) HCL	1% aq. sol.	Local anesthetics, suppositories, ophthalmic ointment		Based on benzoic acid, not on para-amino-benzoic acid
Miconazole nitrate	2% pet.	Antifungal agents		
Miconazole nitrate	2% pet.	Antimycotic agent		
Miranol HM (Lauroyl imidazoline)	2% aq. sol.	Surfactant, synthetic detergents, bubble baths		Controls
Miranol SM (capryl imidazoline derivative)	1% aq. sol.	Surfactant, synthetic detergents, bubble baths		Controls
Mirbane oil	10% o.o.			
Mirbane oil (nitrobenzene)	25% c.o.	Substitute for oil of bitter almonds, manufacturing aniline dyes		
Mitomycin C	0.1% pet.	Bladder instillation		Acral eruption
Monobenzylether of hydroquinone (agerite alba; monobenzone)	1% pet.	Rubber antioxidant, depigmenting agent, Benoquin (Elder)	Hydroquinone	Sensitizer and producer of leukoderma
Monoglycerol para-aminobenzoate	5% pet.	Sunscreening agents	Para-amino compounds	A photosensitizer
Monosulph (sulfated castor oil)	2% aq. sol.	Surfactant, synthetic detergents, bubble baths		Controls

Contactant	Concentration and Vehicle	Exposure	Cross-Reactions	Comment
Monsel's solution	As is (open)	Styptic		Contains approximately 20% iron
Morphine	1% aq. sol.		Apomorphine	Primarily urticariogenic on scratch or intracutaneous testing
Morpholine	1% pet.	Present in Sulfasan—vulcanizing agent		
Morpholinylmercaptobenzo-thiazole	1% pet.	Rubber accelerator	Other mercapto derivatives	
Mucilage	As is			Plant substances forming adhesive liquids with water
Musk ambrette	5% alc.	After shave lotion, perfume		Photosensitizer
Musk ambrette	5% pet.	Perfume		Photosensitizer
Mustard oil	0.1% pet.	Flavoring in food products, soaps, drugs, folk medicine		Contains allyl thiocyanate
Myristyl alcohol	5% pet.	Lanolin Pharmaceuticals		
Myrrh, tincture	10% alc.	Astringosol and Odora Lorvic Disinfectants		
Nacconol NRSF (alkylaryl sulfonate)	1% aq. sol.	Surfactant, anionic synthetic detergents, bubble baths		Controls
Nail polish	As is			Sulfonamide resin most common sensitizer. Dye may be photosensitizer
Naphtha	50% o.o.	Solvents, dry cleaning agents, varnishes, fuel		
Naphthalene	2% alc.	Mothballs, moth flakes, deodorant cakes, synthetic intermediate		
Naphthol A-S	1% pet.	Textiles		Dye coupler
Neomycin	20% pet.	Topical medications, cosmetics, soaps, deodorants	Other aminoglycosides, antibiotics	If reaction to patch test is negative, check with 1/100 intradermal testing

Contactant	Concentration and Vehicle	Exposure	Cross-Reactions	Comment
Neoprene	20% in equal parts of toluene and ethyl acetate	Rubber industry		A photosensitizer
Neroli, oil of	2% pet.	Essential perfume oil, liqueurs		
Nesacaine (chloroprocaine hydrochloride; Strasenburgh)	2% aq. sol.	Local anesthetics	Para-amino compounds	
Neutral red	0.1% aq.	Dye added to quaternary ammonium salts to control pH		Neutral red is red at pH 6.8 and yellow at 8.0 Photosensitizer
Neutronyx 600 (aromatic polyglycol ether condensate)	1% aq. sol.	Surfactant, nonionic synthetic detergents, bubble baths		Controls
Nickel sulfate	5% aq. sol. or 5% pet.	Hairpins, curlers, bobby pins, eyelash curlers, earrings, eyeglass frames, nickel coins, dental instruments, metal lipstick holders, clasps of necklaces, zippers, medallions, metal identification tags, wire support of brassiere cups, garter clasps, metal chairs, handles of doors, handbags, carriages, umbrellas, thimbles, needles, scissors, pens, watchbands, metallic eyelets of shoes, metal arch supports, safety pins on sanitary napkins, hair dyes and bleaches, electric wiring, telephone wiring, silver work, mordant in dyes, insecticides, fungicides, nickel plating, nickel-containing alloys		Pustular patch test reactions
Nicotine (base)	10% aq.	Transdermal patches		
Nicotine sulfate	5% aq. sol.	Agricultural sprays, insecticides, "black leaf"		Do not test with nicotine base

Contactant	Concentration and Vehicle	Exposure	Cross-Reactions	Comment
Nigrosine	2% pet.	Dye, varnish leather, platinum blond hair bleach		
Nigrosine base (Solvent black 7)	1% pet. or 1% mek.	Carbon paper, shoe polish, crayons, typewriter ribbon, inks, leather finish		
Ninol 2012 (fatty acid alkanolamine condensate)	1% aq. sol.	Surfactant, nonionic synthetic detergents, bubble baths		Controls
Nitric acid	Do not test	Explosives, dyes, celluloid manufacture, artificial pearls, precious stones		Powerful irritant
Nitrobenzene (oil of mirbane; artificial oil of bitter almonds	10% o.o.	Shoe dyes, flavoring in foods, soaps, perfumes		Odor like that of oil of bitter almonds
Nitrofurazone	1% pet.	Antibacterial agent, mouthwashes, Furacin (Eaton)		
Nitrogen mustard	As is	Topical agent for mycosis fungoides		May produce urticaria and anaphylaxis
Nitroglycerin	0.2 mg/ml in water	Angina treatment		Ointment, disc
Nitrose dimethyl aniline	1% alc.	Dye		Primary sensitizer
Nomic 218	2% aq. sol.	Surfactant, nonionic synthetic detergents, bubble baths		Control
Nonoxynol-6	0.5% aq. sol.	Industrial waterless hand cleanser		
Nonoxynol-9	0.5% aq. sol.	Spermicidal in emulsifying agent; birth control sponges		
Nordihydroguaiaretic acid	2% pet.	Fat antioxidant		
Novocain (procaine; Winthrop)	5% pet.		Para-aminobenzoic acid esters	Does not cross-react with Xylocaine. Based on para-aminobenzoic acid
Nupercaine (Cinchocaine hydrochloride)	1% pet.	Anesthetic		

Contactant	Concentration and Vehicle	Exposure	Cross-Reactions	Comment
Nutmeg oil (mace)	1% alc.	Condiments, flavoring agent		
Nylon dyes	1% pet.			Disperse Orange 3 and Yellow 3
Nystatin	3% alc.	Mycolog Cream, Nystaform-HC, Mycostatin, Nilstat, Nysta-Dome, Achrostatin, Declostatin, Florotic, Myconef, O-V Statin, Tetrex-F		Rare sensitizer
Oak moss, absolute	2.0% pet.	Perfume	Atranorin	
Oak moss, synthetic	5% pet.	Perfume		
Octyl alcohol	20% pet.	Lanolin		
2-Octyl dodecanol	30% pet.	Lanolin		
Oleyl alcohol	30% pet.	Lanolin, hair lotions, brilliantines, cosmetics, superfatting agent, solvent for essential oils	Stearyl alcohol	
Omite	1% pet.	Plant Parasiticide (Japanese)		Irritant
Optical bleaches	1% aq. sol.	"Whiter-than-white" detergent, blancophores, stilbene derivative, Solium methyl umbelliferones		Photosensitizers
Orange peel	As is	May be covered with carnauba wax, colored with azo dye (Citrus Red 2), sprayed with arsenic	o-Phenyl phenol	Controls. Orange peel may be irritant under patch
Orange peel, oil of	1% alc.	Colognes, perfumes, baking, candies, beverages	Turpentine, celery, bergamot, caraway, dill, balsam of Peru	Contains terpenes, oil of limonene, carotene
Orcinol (dihydroxytoluene)	2% alc.	Antiseptic	Resorcinol	5-Methyl resorcinol
Orris root	Pdr. pure	Dentifrices, perfumes, teething rings, adhesives, back plasters		
Orthodichlorbenzene	5% alc.	Leather dyes		
Orthoform	25% pet.	Topical anesthetics	Para-amino compounds	Based on para-aminobenzoic acid, primary sensitizer

Contactant	Concentration and Vehicle	Exposure	Cross-Reactions	Comment
Ortho-phenyl phenol	1% pet.	Cosmetic preservative Preservative in paper linings of lids of cosmetic jars. Same as Dowicide 1		May cause depigmentation
Orvus WA (sodium lauryl sulfate)	1% aq. sol.	Surfactant, anionic synthetic detergents, bubble baths		Controls
Ovotran	5% acet.	Insecticides		
Oxaine (oxethazine; Wyeth) HCl.	2% aq. sol.	Gastrointestinal topical anesthetics		
Oxalic acid	0.1% aq.	Bleaches, stain removers, rust removers, metal cleansers		Irritant
Oxybenzone (Benzophenone-3) (Eusolex 4360)	2.0% pet.	Sunscreens, cosmetics		Regular and photo ACD
Oxychlorosene	1% aq. sol.	Hypochlorite in Kasdenol Mouthwash		Prepare fresh for testing
Oxyquinoline sulfate	1% pet.	Contraceptive, antiseptic		
Ozokerite (ceresin)	30% pet.	Cosmetics, candles, waxes		
Paints	As is (open) or 10% pet.			
Palladium chloride	1% pet.	Jewelry, dental	Nickel	
Palladium sodium dichloride	0.1% aq.	Jewelry, dental alloy		
Pancreatin	5% pet.	Enzyme mixture, Pycopay Toothpaste	Trypsine, chemotrypsine	
Panthenol (pantothenol)	30% pet.	Vitamin B_5, Aquasol A, Panthoderm		Alcohol of pantothenic acid
d-Panthenyl Ethyl Ether	1% pet.	Present in hair lotion and cosmetics, part vitamin B complex		
Paper money	As is		U.S. paper bills may contain formaldehyde and Dowicides (chlorinated phenols) to prevent mildew	
Para-aminobenzene	1% pet.	Organic dye		Para-amino compounds

Contactant	Concentration and Vehicle	Exposure	Cross-Reactions	Comment
Para-aminobenzoic acid (aminobenzoic acid)	10% pet.	Pabafilm sunscreening agent, Solar Cream (Doak), synthesis of local anesthetics, vitamin B complex, brewer's yeast	Paraphenylenediamine, procaine, sulfonamides, azo dyes, benzocaine P-amino compounds	The acid is less soluble and less sensitizing than are its salts Photosensitizer
Para-aminophenol	2% pet.	Analgesics, fur dyes	Paraphenylenediamine	
Paraben mixture	15% pet.	Preservative in topical agents, cosmetics, foods, cleansers		3% each of ethyl, methyl, propyl, butyl and propyl parahydroxy-benzoic acid
Para-chloro-meta-xylenol	1% pet.	Cosmetic and topical medication	May cross-react with chloro-meta-cresol	
Parachlorophenol	1% aq. sol.			
Paradichlorobenzene	1% alc.	Mothproofing, toilet bowls, deodorants		May produce purpura
Paraffin	Equal parts soft paraffin	Petrolatum (soft yellow paraffin)		
Parahydroxybenzoic acid (methyl and ethyl propyl parabens)	5% pet.	Parabens as preservatives in pharmaceuticals, cosmetics, foods		Sensitizer in topical creams
Para-oxon	1% alc. (open)	Insecticides		
Paraphenylenediamine (PPDA)	2% pet. in a dark bottle	Hair dyes, fur dyes, leather processing, rubber vulcanizing, printer's ink, photographic work, x-ray fluids, lithographing	Azo and aniline dyes, procaine, benzocaine, para-aminobenzoic acid, HydroDIURIL, carbutamide sulfonamides, para-aminosalicylic acid	Many weakly positive patch test reactions are *not* significant Has caused "tightness" of the chest
o-nitro-Paraphenylenediamine	1% pet.			
Pararosaniline	Sat. sol.	Dye		
Para-tertiary butyl phenol	1% pet.	Adhesive, resins, duplicating paper, rubber industry, leather industry		May cause leukoderma Antioxidant
Para-tertiary butyl phenol formaldehyde resin (PTBFR)	1% pet.	Adhesives shoes/leather	PTBP	

Contactant	Concentration and Vehicle	Exposure	Cross-Reactions	Comment
Parathion	1% alc. (open)	Insecticides		
Paratoluenediamine sulfate	1% pet.	Chemistry laboratories		
Paris green (Schweinfurt or emerald green)	2% acet.	Paint pigment, wood preservative, insecticide sprays	P-amino compound	Copper acetoarsenite compound
Parsnip, parsley (wild)	As is (moist)			Photosensitizer
Parsol 1789 (4-tert-butyl-4'-methoxydibenzoyl-methane)	2% pet.	Sunscreen		Photo ACD UVA absorber
Patchouli, oil of	1% pet.	Cosmetics, perfume	Essential oils	
Pearl essence Natural	As is	Frosted nail polish		A suspension of guanine crystals (from fish scales) in amyl acetate or acetone
Synthetic	As is	Lacquers, plastics		Metal stearates, lead, barium hypophosphites, bismuth oxychloride, metallic silver, zinc ammonium phosphate and hydrolysis of products of titanium chloride on protein films
Pencil colors				Lead (graphite) is not a sensitizer. Indelible pencils—methyl or crystal violet—are not sensitizers. Green and yellow colored pencils may contain lead chromate
d-Penicillamine	1% aq.	Ophthalmic or systemic	Penicillin	
Penicillin (powder or ointment)	10,000 IU/gram pet.	Topical use, pharmaceuticals, nursing and medical professions, cheese processers, fruit handlers		Contact allergy may be accompanied by anaphylactic variety
Pentachloronitrobenzene (PCNB)	0.5% pet.	Agricultural fungicide		

Contactant	Concentration and Vehicle	Exposure	Cross-Reactions	Comment
Pentachlorophenol	1% alc.	Weed killers, insecticides, wood preservatives, adhesives		
3-Pentadecylcatechol	0.1% pet.	Anacardiaceae: rhus, mango, cashew, India nut marking tree		A primary sensitizer
Pentaerythritol triacrylate (PETA)	0.1% pet.	UVR cured ink		Phototoxic
Pentoxol	As is	Organic solvents		
Peppermint oil	1% pet.	Flavoring agent, perfumes	Balsam of Peru, rosin, wood	An essential oil
Perchlorethylene (tetra-chloroethylene)	25% o.o.	Dry cleaning		Sensitizes to alcohol
Perfumes	As is (open and closed)		Balsam of Peru, benzyl salicylate, phenylac-etaldehyde	May produce berloque dermatitis
Permanent wave solutions	2% aq. sol.			Rare sensitizers
Permanganate, potassium	1% aq. sol.	Oxidizing agents, neutralizer of alka-loids, disinfectants		
Peroxide catalysts Acetyl Benzoyl peroxide Cumene hydroperoxide Cyclohexanone Lauroyl Methyl ethyl ketone	0.5% acet. or 1% pet.	Polyester resins Acrylate resins		
Petitgrain Oil	5% pet.	Perfume oil		A photosensitizer
Petrolatum	As is	Vaseline, soft yellow paraffin or white		Best vehicle for most patch test substances, rarely sensitizing
Petroleum	20% o.o.	Insecticides, rodenticides, gasoline, solvents		
Phenanthrene	1% pet.	Tar		A photosensitizer

Contactant	Concentration and Vehicle	Exposure	Cross-Reactions	Comment
Phenergan Cream (Wyeth)	As is		Promethazine, phenothiazine (Thorazine, Thephorin)	A photosensitizer
Phenol (carbolic acid)	1% aq. sol.	Dermal Chemabrasive (Budkon), Carbolated Vaseline, carbolfuchsin, Chloraseptic Lozenges and Mouthwash (Eaton), P&S Liquid and Ointment, Panscol Ointment (Baker)	Resorcin, cresols, hydroquinone	Irritant
Phenolformaldehyde	5% pet. or 1% alc.	Clothing, finishes, epoxy resins		
Phenolic compounds	1% aq. sol.	Mouthwashes		Amyl, heptyl and actyl phenols in mouthwashes
Phenolphthalein	0.5% alc.	Indicator, laxative		Test at site of fixed drug eruption
Phenothiazine	1% aq. sol. (photosensitizer—1% pet. test open and closed)	Veterinarian anthelmintic, fly control, methylene blue Chloropromazine Phenothiazine HCl. Tripenelamine	Phenergan	Present in Sparine, Thorazine, Compazine, Stelazine, Temaril, Largon, Tindal, Dartal, Mellaril, Vesprin, Prolixin, Repoise, Dermitil
Phenyl indole	2% pet.	Found in polyvinyl chloride fabrics		
Phenoxybenzamine	0.1% pet.	Chemical laboratory		Irritant
Phenoxyethenol	1% pet.	Preservative in cosmetics Antimicrobial		Rare sensitizer
Phenylacetaldehyde	2% pet. or 0.5% alc.	Perfumes, flavoring agents		
Phenylbetanaphthylamine	1% pet.	Rubber antioxidant		
Phenylcycloparaphenylenediamine	1% pet.	Rubber, Black Rubber		
Phenylephrine	1% pet.	Eye drops—Mydriatic eye drops		
Phenylglycidyl ether	1% o.o.	Epoxy resin		
Phenylglycidyl ether	0.25% acet.	Epoxy resin		

Contactant	Concentration and Vehicle	Exposure	Cross-Reactions	Comment
Phenylisopropyl para-phenylenediamine (IPPD)	0.1% pet.	Rubber (black)		Can cause lichenoid or purpuric eruptions
Phenylmercuric acetate and borate	0.1% pet.	Fungicides, germicides, preservatives in cosmetics, contraceptives, Nylmerate (Holland-Rantos)	Organic and inorganic mercurials	May be a primary irritant in 0.1% aq. sol.
Phenylmercuric nitrate	0.05% pet.	Preservatives, vaginal cream, contraceptives, Pher-Mer-Nite, Merpectogel		
Phenyl salicylate (salol)	1% pet.	Plastics, lacquers, adhesives, waxes, polishes, suntan oils, plasticizers		
Phosphorus trisulfide (phosphorus sesquisulfide)	As is	Safety matchboxes, matches, ignition paper, diesel motors, high-pressure lubricants, asphalt		Airborne allergen May cause contact urticaria
Phthalic anhydride	1% alc.	Epoxy resins		A primary sensitizer
Phytomenadione	10% pet.	Vitamin K₁ parenteral		
Picric acid (trinitrophenol)	5% aq. sol.	Dye industry, explosives, artificial flowers, antiseptics		
Picryl chloride	1% acet.			A primary sensitizer
Pimaric acid	10% pet.			
Pimento	10% c.o.	Flavoring agent, all spice		
Pine oil	5% pet.	Disinfectants, deodorants, liquid scrub soaps		Controls Irritant
Pine tar	25% pet.			
Pinene	15% o.o.			
Piperazine	1% aq. sol.	Vermifuges, Antepar, Pipizan, Multifuge, Perin, Ascarey	Ethylenediamine HCl.	May flare from ingestion of Atarax (hydroxyzine hydrochloride)
Pitch	As is (open)	Various tars		A photosensitizer
Plants	As is—leaf, flower, pollen bulb			Risk of false positive reaction

Contactant	Concentration and Vehicle	Exposure	Cross-Reactions	Comment
Plaster of Paris (gypsum; calcium sulfate)	As is	Cast, moldings		Some reinforced with formaldehyde resin
Plastibase (Squibb)	As is	Quinolor Ointment		Contains 5% polyethylene plastic resin
Plastic(s)				
Monomer	0.1–1% acet. or pet.			
Polymer	As is			
Plastic cement	As is (open)	Industrial, toys, models, glue sniffers		Contains volatile hydrocarbons and solvents, formaldehyde, formaldehyde resins, nitrocellulose
Platinum bleaches for hair	As is	Methyl violet, methylene blue, nigrosine		Applied after peroxide bleach
Platinum chloride	1% aq. sol.			May cause a pustular reaction
Plexoderm (Crookes-Barnes)	As is		Balsam of Peru	Contains salicylic acid, allantoin and styrax
Poison ivy extract or oleoresin	0.1% acet.	Identical to poison sumac and poison oak	Oleoresin of Japanese lacquer tree, cashew nut, mango fruit, India ink tree, ginkgo tree	A primary sensitizer
Polyester (unsaturated)	1% acet.			
Polyester monomer	10% acet.	Polyester resin		
Polyethylene glycol	4% pet.	Polyethylene glycol ointment (U.S.P.), Furacin (Eaton), Plastibase (Squibb), Carbowax, hair dressings		Nos. 200 to 700 are liquids. Nos. 1000 to 6000 are solids (Carbowax) Rare sensitizer
Polymethyl methacrylate (acrylic polymer powder)	As is	Dentistry, synthetic resins		Acrylic *monomer* may sensitize; the *polymer* very rarely does so

Contactant	Concentration and Vehicle	Exposure	Cross-Reactions	Comment
Polymyxin B sulfate	3% pet	Numerous topical medications		Rare sensitizer
Polysorb-80 U.S.P. Polysorbate-80	5% aq.	Emulsifier and dispersing agent, surfactant		Tween 80
Polysorb Hydrate (Fougera)	5% o.o.			Sorbitan sesquioleate in wax-petrolatum
Polysulfide liquid polymer	1% acet.	Epoxy resin plasticizer		
Polyvinyl pyrrolidone	As is	Hair lacquers, cosmetics, pharmaceuticals, Betadine, Isodine		Not a sensitizer
Pontamine black powder	2% pet.	Fur dyes		
Pontocaine (tetracaine hydrochloride; Winthrop)	2% aq. sol.	Local anesthetics	P-amino compounds	
Potassium aurocyanide	0.01% aq.			
Potassium carbonate	1% aq. sol.	Soaps, cleaning agents, lye, Drano, Pronto		
Potassium chlorate	1% aq. sol.	Matches, oxidizer in mouthwashes		
Potassium dichromate	0.5% pet.	*General:* leather, bleaches, matches, yellow paints, spackle compounds, detergents. *Industrial:* fur industry, photography, photoengraving lithography, electroplating, tanning agents, mordants in dyeing, yellow and orange paints, ink manufacture, stainless steel, chrome plating, match making, polishing steel, diesel engine radiator fluid, welding, acetylene workers, cement, rubber, glass, linoleum, wood impregnated with chromated zinc chloride, alloys, containing chrome, antirust compounds	Trivalent chromium compounds	Sensitizer, also irritant and producer of chrome ulcers. False positive reactions common in patients with acute dermatitis or irritable skin and in atopics
Potassium hydroxide	Do not test	Soaps, cleaning agents, cuticle remover		Irritant

Contactant	Concentration and Vehicle	Exposure	Cross-Reactions	Comment
Potassium iodide	30% pet.	Photographic emulsions, animal and poultry feed, table salt, medications		Halogens often produce pustular patch test reactions. Control test in Duhring's disease with potassium bromide
Potassium persulfate	2.5% aq. sol.	Bleaches, germicides	Ammonium persulfate	
Potassium and sodium di-cyanoaurate	0.001% ethanol			
Potosan	1% alc. (open)	Insecticides		
Pramoxine hydrochloride (4-n-butoxyphenyl gamma-mor-pholino-propyl ether hy-drochloride)	1% aq. sol.	Topical anesthetics: Anugesic Ointment and Suppositories (Warner-Chilcott), Aural Acute (Saron), Drotic Ear Drops (Ascher), Phorm Ointment (Ascher), Tronothane Hy-drochloride (Abbott), Vio-Hydro-cortisone Cream (North American Pharmacal), Pramasone Lotion (Ferndale), Prax Cream (Ferndale)		Does not cross-react with benzocaine or xylocaine
Primin (6-methoxy-2n-pentyl-p-benzoquinone)	0.0025% ethyl ether	Allergen in primula plant		
Primrose (Primula obconica) Expressed Leaf	25% aq. sol. As is	Main English plant sensitizer Main English plant sensitizer	Daisy family Daisy family	Primary sensitizer Primary sensitizer
Procaine hydrochloride (Novocain)	2% aq. sol.	Other local anesthetics based on p-amino compound (benzocaine)	Benzocaine, para-aminobenzoic acid, para-aminosalicylic acid, paraphenylenedi-amine	Does *not* cross react with Xylocaine
Proflavine dihydrochloride	1% pet.	Topical fluorescent dye		Advocated for herpes simplex. Caution: a sensitizer

Contactant	Concentration and Vehicle	Exposure	Cross-Reactions	Comment
Promethazine HCl	2% pet.		Phenothiazines	Photosensitizer; has caused contact urticaria
Propantheline bromide	1% aq. sol.	Pro-Banthine (Searle) when incorporated in topical agents as an antiperspirant		Treatment of axillary hyperhidrosis
Propolis	As is	Cosmetics, medicaments		"Bee glue"
Propylene glycol	5% aq. sol.	Vehicle for 5-fluorouracil, humectant, cosmetics, Synalar Solution, Lidosporin		
Propylene oxide	1% alc.	Chemical intermediate in preparing polyurethanes; also used in solvent, fumigant; present in Danish product Medi-Swab		
Propyl gallate	1% pet.	Cosmetics, lipsticks	Other gallates?	Antioxidant
Propyl parahydroxybenzoate (propyl paraben)	5% pet.	Preservative in topical agents, cosmetics, foods, cleansers	Other parabens	
Psoriasis Lotion (Rexall)	As is			Mercuric oleate
Pyrethrum powder	2% pet.	Insecticides, mothproofing	Chrysanthemum, turpentine, ragweed	Contains pyrethrins and cinerins
Pyribenzamine hydrochloride (tripelennamine)	2% pet.	Antihistamine	Sulfapyradine, Antistine	An ethylenediamine derivative
Pyridine	30% o.o.	Tar		A photosensitizer
Pyrocatechol	2% in 95% alc.		Hydroquinone, resorcin	
Pyrogallol	1% pet. or 3% aq. sol.	Hair dyes, tars	Resorcin	
Pyrrolinitrin	1% pet.	European antimycotic medication		
Quassin (extract of Jamaica bitter wood)	2% acet.	Lacquers, paper, waterproofing, denatured alcohol		Contains sucrose octaacetate
Quaternary ammonium compounds	0.1% aq.	Cetrimide, antiseptic detergents such as Phemerol, Zephiran, Ceepryn, Diaprene		Rare sensitizers, may cause ulceration of genitalia in concentrated solutions

Contactant	Concentration and Vehicle	Exposure	Cross-Reactions	Comment
Quaternium-15 (Dowicil 200)	2% pet.	Preservative		Formaldehyde-releasing agent
Quicklime (unslaked lime; calcium oxide)	Caustic; do not test	Mortar, cement, fertilizers, soap, glass, metals, depilatories, manufacture of calcium cyanide, calcium carbide		See Lime, slaked and Calcium oxide
Quillaja	1% alc.	Emulsifying agent, solution of coal tar, cosmetics		Derived from South American rosaceous tree bark
Quince seed	As is	Hair straighteners, mucilage, gums, cosmetics		
Quinidine sulfate	1% aq. sol.	Pharmaceutical industry, contraceptives		Eczematous or purpuric patch test reaction
Quinine sulfate or hydrochloride	1% aq. sol.	Contraceptives, sunscreens, hair tonics, quinine tablets, vermouth, gin, vodka, denatured alcohol		Photosensitizer
Quinolor Compound Ointment (Squibb)	Half strength with pet.		Vioform, Sterosan, Diodoquin	Contains chlorhydroxyquinoline, benzoyl peroxide, methyl salicylate, menthol and eugenol in Plastibase vehicle. Some preparations contain eucalyptol, white thyme oil
Quinoxaline dioxide	5% pet.	Growth promoter animal foodstuffs		
Quotane Ointment and Lotion (dimethisoquin hydrochloride; Smith, Kline & French)	As is	Topical anesthetic		Not related to para-aminobenzoic acid
Ragweed	1:1000 acet.		Chrysanthemum, pyrethrum, turpentine	Plant leaves and pollen may also be used for testing
Ranitidine (Zantac)	5% pet.	H₂ antagonist		

Contactant	Concentration and Vehicle	Exposure	Cross-Reactions	Comment
Rapeseed oil (Factice)	As is	Adhesives, lubricant		
Red mercuric oxide	3% pet.	Antiseptics, bleaching agents	Organic and inorganic mercurials	
Resorcin	5% pet.	Acne remedies, hair tonics, suppositories, eye drops, tanning, explosives, resins, dyes, cosmetics, freckle cream, dyeing and printing	Euresol, phenol, hexylresorcinol, orcinol, hydroquinone, pyrocatechol, pyrogallol, hydroxyquinone	Deteriorates when exposed to light. Dispense in dark bottle. May be irritant
Resorcin green	2% pet.	Azo dye	Para-amino compounds	
Resorcinol monoacetate (Euresol [knoll])	5% aq. sol.	Clantis (Dara), Resulin Resorcitate (Schieffelin), Sulforcin (Texas Pharmacal), RMS Lotion (Ar-Ex), Acne-Dome (Dome)	Resorcin	
Resorcinol monobenzoate	1% pet.	Colored eyeglass frames	Balsam of Peru	Ultraviolet inhibitor
Retinoid acid	0.1% pet.	Acne therapy		
Rezifilm (Squibb)	As is			Contains tetramethylthiuram disulfide
Rhodamine	5% pet.	Red lipstick dye		A photosensitizer
Rhulicream, Rhulispray, Rhulitol (Lederle)	As is (patch scratch)	Topical agent for plant dermatitis		Allergic granuloma from zirconium
Riasol (Shield)	As is	Proprietary preparation for psoriasis		Mercury as cocoanut oil soap
Rigithane 112	1% alc.	Polyurethane resins		
Rigithane catalyst	10% aq. sol.	Polyurethane resins		
Roccal (alkyldimethyl-benzyl-ammonium chloride)	0.1% aq. sol.	Surfactants, cationic synthetic detergents, bubble baths, benzalkonium chloride		Controls "Quat"
Rodannitrobenzene	1% pet.	Pesticides	Paraphenylenediamine	
Rosaniline (basic fuchsin)	2% aq. sol.	Therapeutic dye		
Rose bengal	2.5% pet.	Dyes		Photosensitizing

Contactant	Concentration and Vehicle	Exposure	Cross-Reactions	Comment
Rose, oil of	1% alc./1% pet.	Perfume, unguentum aquae rosae		
Rosin (colophony): gum rosin (from turpentine), wood rosin (from pine stump)	10% pet.	Yellow bar soap, adhesive tape, insulating tape, Scotch Tape, glossy paper, flypaper, polish, paints, inks, epilating wax, rosin bags for ball players, rosin for violin bows	Balsam of Peru, turpentine (gum rosin) Wood tars Methyl abieate	Contains abietic acid and 1-pinearic acid
Rotenone powder (Derris root)	5% in talcum	Insecticide		From roots of rotenone-bearing plants (Derris and Lonchocarpus)
Rubber accelerators	1% pet.	Mercaptobenzothiazole, tetramethyl-thiuram monosulfide, diphenyl-guanidine		Of the rubber accelerators, these are the most common sensitizers
Rubber antioxidants	1% pet.	Monobenzylether of hydroquinone, phenyl-beta-naphthylamine, iso-propyl paraphenylenediamine		Of the rubber antioxidants, these are the most common sensitizers
Rubber, finished products	As is	Rubber box toes of shoes, rubber cements, dress shields, elastic in hair-nets, panties, dental plates, edge of eyelash curler, kneeling pads, rubber support pessary and diaphragms, dental sheeting, head rests, condoms, rubberbands, finger guards, art gum erasers, stethoscopes, rubber hand grip of vibrators, aprons, mammary prostheses, goggles, adhesive tape, "Flubber' (a putty-like toy), tire treads, tubes, wire insulation, drug sundries, calendered stocks		Rubber accelerators and antioxidants are the most common cause of rubber dermatitis
Rubber peptizer	1% pet.	Thio-beta-naphthol		Keeps rubber soft

Contactant	Concentration and Vehicle	Exposure	Cross-Reactions	Comment
Rust removers	Do not test (see comment)			Contains irritants such as naphtha, ammonium sulfide, oxalic acid, hydrofluoric acid, concentrated solution of phosphoric acid, inorganic heavy metal salts. For testing, see individual chemicals or begin with 1% solutions and use controls
Salicylates	2% o.o.		Aminosalicylic acid	Amyl, benzyl, glyceryl, menthyl, ethylhexyl phenyl and propylene salicylates may be used as sunscreens
Salicylic acid	1% pet.	Many topical agents, including Whitfield's ointment		Rare sensitizer. Salicylic acid and mercury combinations may be irritants when covered
Saligenin (salicyl alcohol)	2% aq. sol.	Topical local anesthetics		Rarely sensitizes
Sandalwood oil	1% pet.			Photosensitizer
Sassafras oil	1% pet.	Flavoring agents		
Sawdust	As is			Test dry and moist
Scarlet red (aminoazotoluene)	As is 2.5% pet.	Dye, therapeutic agent for burns and ulcers	Para-amino compounds	
Sedormid	Sat. sol. in propylene glycol	This drug is not being made at present		Purpuric patch test reaction
Selenium sulfide	3% pet.	Selsun (Abbott), glass, photoelectric cells, coloring of acrylic dentures		May be irritant
Selsun (Abbott)	As is (open)	Therapeutic shampoo		Contains selenium sulfide

Contactant	Concentration and Vehicle	Exposure	Cross-Reactions	Comment
Sesame oil	50% o.o.	Vehicle for intramuscular medications, synergist for pyrethrins, cosmetics, pharmaceuticals		
Shampoos	5% aq. sol (open) 2% aq. sol. (closed)			Controls
Shellac	As is	Paint, varnish, hair dressings, waxes		May have methyl alcohol and arsenic trisulfide. Controls
Shoe polish	5% pet.			
Silicone fluids (dimethyl polysiloxanes)	As is	Cosmetics, greases, antifog agent, eyeglasses, glass		May cause blepharitis, lacrimation
Silver bromide	2% aq. sol.	Photography, mirror finishing		
Silver nitrate	2% aq. sol. (open)	Caustic pencils and hair dyes		Pustular patch test reaction
Simazine	1% pet.			
Siroil (Siroil)	As is	Proprietary psoriasis remedy		Contains mercury, irritant
Soaps	1% aq. sol.			Controls
Sodium alginate (algin)	As is	Emulsifiers, mucilage, ice cream, wave sets		
Sodium alkyl sulfate	0.5% aq. sol.	Foaming surfactant in detergents, Ultrabrite, Gleem, McLeans, Pepsodent, pharmaceuticals, cosmetic creams		May contain formaldehyde
Sodium amidotrizoate	10% aq.	A radiopaque substance in angiography and renography		
Sodium arsenate	10% aq. sol.	Arsenical soaps, insecticides, hair tonics		
Sodium bisulfite	10% aq. sol.	Antioxidant in food		May cause anaphylaxis in asthmatic patients
Sodium carbonate	10% aq. sol.	Soap additives		Irritant

Contactant	Concentration and Vehicle	Exposure	Cross-Reactions	Comment
Sodium diethyldithiocarbamate	10% in Carbowax	Treatment of nickel carbonyl poisoning		
Sodium fluoride	0.5% aq. sol.	Glass etchings, dentifrices		Pustular patch test reaction common
Sodium fusidate	2% pet.	Fucidin Ointment		
Sodium hydroxide	Do not test	Soaps, cleaning agents, lye—Drano, Pronto		Powerful irritant
Sodium hypochlorite	0.5% aq. sol.	Bleaching solutions, cleansing agents Antiseptic	Chloramine	Controls, irritant
Sodium hyposulfite	0.5% aq.	Antiseptic		
Sodium lauryl sulfate (Duponal C)	1% aq. sol.	Emulsifying agent in cosmetics, pharmaceuticals, "foaming" dentifrices		Fatty alcohol sulfate. Primary irritant. Controls
Sodium metabisulfite	2% pet.	Antioxidant in pharmaceuticals, printing, and photography		
Sodium monofluorophosphate	0.5% aq. sol.	Surfactant (Colgate Toothpaste)		Pustular patch test reactions
Sodium monoglyceride sulfonate	1% aq. sol.	Surfactant (Gleem Toothpaste)		Controls
Sodium n-lauroyl sarcosinate	1% aq. sol.	Antienzyme, dentifrices, emulsifiers, surfactant in cosmetics, pharmaceuticals		Controls
Sodium perborate	10% pet.	Dentures, household cleansers, cold hair-waving neutralizers, mouthwashes, Vince, Amosan		
Sodium pyrithione	0.3% aq.	Metal-working fluids, water-based printer's ink, antidandruff shampoo		Also known as sodium omadine
Sodium stearate	1% aq. sol.	Cosmetics		Controls
Sodium sulfide	2% aq. sol.	Bleaching agent for cotton, paper, stain remover for tetryl and potassium permanganate, preservative for dyes and foods, Wandex (Research Supplies)		Controls Has caused contact urticaria Unstable in solution

Contactant	Concentration and Vehicle	Exposure	Cross-Reactions	Comment
Sodium sulfide	2% aq. sol.	Sulfur dyes, hides, insecticides, depilatories		
Sodium thiosulfate	5% aq. sol.	Fungicides, stain removers, hair dye developers, Tinver, Komed Lotion, Microsyn		
Solithane 113	1% alc.	Polyurethane prepolymer		
Solithane catalysts C-113-300 C-113-328	1% alc. 2% aq. sol.	Polyurethane catalyst Polyurethane catalyst		
Sorbic acid	2% pet.	Preservative, Hytone Cream (Dermik), Aristocort Cream (Lederle), Fluorone Cr. (Upjohn), Maxiflor (Herbert), Kenalog Cr. (Squibb), Pramasone Cr. (Ferndale)		Present in many fruits, especially strawberries. Urticariogenic agent
Sorbitol	10% aq. sol.	Humectants, cosmetics, pharmaceuticals		
Sorsis Cream (Ar-Ex)	As is	Topical agent for psoriasis		Contains ammoniated mercury
Span 20 (sorbitan monolaurate)	5% o.o.	Surfactant, nonionic synthetic detergents, bubble baths	Other Spans	Controls
Span 80 (sorbitan monooleate)	5% o.o.	Surfactant, nonionic synthetic detergents, bubble baths	Other Spans	Controls
Spandelle (Firestone)	As is	Polyurethane elastomer (spandex)		Not a sensitizer
Sparklers				*Green sparklers* contain barium nitrate, potassium perchlorate and aluminum powder; *red sparklers* contain strontium carbonate, nitrate, potassium perchlorate and aluminum powder

Contactant	Concentration and Vehicle	Exposure	Cross-Reactions	Comment
Spearmint oil	2% pet.	Flavoring agents		
Spermaceti	As is	Cosmetics, pharmaceuticals, candles		
Spice, oil of	5% pet.			
Spiramycin	1% pet.	Veterinary antibiotic		
Stannous fluoride	0.5% aq. sol.	Dentifrices, including Crest, Cue, Fact, Superstripe, Dr. Lyons Fluoride, McKesson Fluoride		Pustular patch test reaction
Stearamidoethyl Diethylamine Phosphate	0.5% pet.	Cosmetic emulsifier		
Stearic acid	5% pet.	Cosmetics, soaps		Pustular patch test reaction common
Stearyl alcohol	30% pet.	Lanolin, aliphatic alcohol in lanolin, cosmetics, textile finishes, antifoam agent, lubricant	Oleyl alcohol Cetyl alcohol	May cause contact urticaria
Sterosan Cream (Geigy) (chlorquinaldol)	As is	Bacteriostatic and fungistatic cream and ointment	Vioform, Diodoquin, Quinolor	Free of iodine
Stilbene triazine	0.5% aq. sol.	Optical bleaches, brightening agents, soaps, detergents, cosmetics, textiles		Photosensitizer
Stoddard Solvent (high flash point petroleum distillate)	25% o.o.	Dry cleaning, paint thinner		
Streptomycin	2.5% aq. sol. 1% pet.	Medical, nursing and pharmaceutical personnel	Dihydrostreptomycin, kanamycin, neomycin	Has caused systemic contact dermatitis
Strontium chloride	2% aq. sol.	Sensodyne dentifrice		
Strontium sulfide	2% aq. sol.	Depilatories		
Styrax USO (storax)	2% pet.	Plexoderm, perfumes, contains topical medication	Benzoin styrene, balsam of Peru	A balsam with cinnamic acid
Styrene (vinyl benzene)	1% o.o.	Synthetic rubber, alkyd, acrylic and polyester resins, extractive of storax balsam, compound tincture of benzoin, soaps, wines, berries	Benzoin compounds	

Contactant	Concentration and Vehicle	Exposure	Cross-Reactions	Comment
Styrene oxide	1% o.o.	Reactive epoxy diluent		
Subtilins	0.1% aq. sol.	Detergent enzymes		
Sulfacetamide, topical	5% pet.	Sultrin (Ortho), many ophthalmic and acne topical medications		Rarely sensitizes
Sulfanilamide, topical	5% pet.	AVC, Otomide, Vagitrol, Sufamil	Para-amino compounds	A photosensitizer
Sulfobromophthalein	5% aq. sol.	Diagnostic dyes		Anaphylactic or immediate rather than delayed allergens
Sulfonamide	5% pet.	Blexcon (Madland), Gantrisin (Roche), Vagitrol (Syntex)	Para-amino compounds	Sulfonamide diuretics may be photosensitizers
Sulfonamide-formaldehyde resin	10% pet.	Main sensitizer in nail lacquer		
Sulfonated imidazole	0.5% aq. sol.	Optical bleaches, brightening agents, soaps, detergents, cosmetics, textiles		Photosensitizer
Sulfur	5% pet.	Topical medications, gunpowder, matches, bleaches, insecticides, fungicides		*Precipitated sulfur* contains calcium sulfide; *sublimed* sulfur is a pure yellow sulfur powder. Incompatible with iodine and mercury
Sulfuric acid	Do not test			Strong irritant
Sulisobenzone (2-hydroxy-4-methoxy-benzophenone-5-sulfonic acid)	10% pet.	Sungard, Uval, Spectra Sorb UV 284, Uvinulms-40		Sunscreen
Surfacaine (cyclomethycaine; Lilly)	1% pet.	Topical anesthetic, Surfacaine Compound, Surfadil		Not based on para-aminobenzoic acid
Synthetic detergents	2% aq. sol.			
Tagamet (Cimetidine)	1% pet.	Pharmacist		Controls
Talc (talcum) U.S.P.	As is	Cosmetics, pharmaceuticals		May produce granulomas in wounds

Contactant	Concentration and Vehicle	Exposure	Cross-Reactions	Comment
Tannic acid	0.25% aq. sol.	Mordant in dyes, sizing paper and silk, polished fabrics, tortoise shell frames, rubber manufacture, tanning leather, photography, sunscreens and medicines for burns, Dalidyne (Dalin), Astringent lotion, Onycho-Phytex (Unimed), artificial nail preparation, tannic jelly		Rare sensitizer
Tar				
Coal	5% pet.	Alphosyl, Balnetar, Carbo-Cort, Dax-alan, Ionil T, Polytar, Pragmatar, Sebical Tar Shampoo, Sebutone, Supertah, Tarbonis, Tar Distillate, Tarpaste, Topigel, Tropsor Lotion, Unguentum Bossi, Ze-Tar-Quin, Zetar Shampoo and Emulsion		Photosensitizer
Coal tar solution	As is	Liquor carbonis detergens, Epidol, Tri-dentar (Spirt), Hydro-Tar (Schiefflin), Pentarcort (Dalin), Methatar (Borden), Ulcortar (Ulmer), Cor-Tar-Quin Cream and Lotion (Dome)		Photosensitizers. Contains coal tar, Quillaja bark, alcohol
Wood	12% (3% each of pine, beech, juniper and birch)	Almay-Tar (Schieffelin), oil of cade (juniper tar)		Not photosensitizers
Tartar emetic	3% aq. sol.	Dye mordant, counterirritant, denaturing agent in rubbing alcohol		
Tashan Cream (Hoffman-La Roche)	As is			The vitamin E in this preparation reported to be a sensitizer. See Vitamin E

Contactant	Concentration and Vehicle	Exposure	Cross-Reactions	Comment
Tattoo pigments		Blue—Cobalt Blue—Cobalt Chloride 2% pet. Green—Chromium—Potassium Dichromate 0.5% pet. Red—Mercury sulfide—Mercury 0.5% pet. Yellow—Cadmium Sulfide—1% aq. sol. Purple—Manganese—Manganese oxide Pure		*Black:* carbon, iron oxide, logwood (may contain potassium dichromate). *Blue:* cobaltous aluminate. *Brown:* ferric sulfate. *Flesh:* iron oxide. *Green:* Chromium oxide, chromium sesquioxide (casalis green), hydrous chromium oxide (Guignet's green), copper salts mixed with azo dyes. *Red:* cadmium selenide, cinnabar, sienna. *Violet:* manganese violet. *White:* Zinc oxide. *Yellow:* cadmium sulfide
TEA-Coco a/k/a Potassium pyrosulfite	5% aq.	Pharmaceutical antioxidant. Printing, photography. Shampoos, cosmetics		
TEGON	0.1% aq. sol.	European antiseptic detergent		Dodecylic aminoethyl glycine hydrochloride
Terpineol	5% pet.	Thyme, pharmaceutical		
Terraclor	0.5% pet.			
Tertiary butyl catechol	1% acet.	Polyester resin inhibitor, antioxidant, lubricating oils, paint, rubber, plastics		May produce leukoderma
Tertiary butyl phenol	1% acet.	Detergents, synthetic oils, disinfectants		May produce leukoderma
p-Tertiary butyl phenol formaldehyde, resin	1% pet.	Resins, glues		
Tetrabromofluorescein + eosin	50% pet.	Dye in lipsticks, pharmaceuticals		Photosensitizer

Contactant	Concentration and Vehicle	Exposure	Cross-Reactions	Comment
Tetracaine (Pontocaine [Winthrop])	2% aq. sol.	Local anesthetics, PNS suppositories (Winthrop), Vertussin Loz- tablets (Warren-Teed), Rectodyne Ointment (Semed)	Procaine, benzocaine	Based on para-amino-benzoic acid
Amethocaine	1% pet.		P-amino compounds	
Tetrachlorodiphenylethane (TDE)	5% acet.	Insecticides		
Tetrachloroisophthalonitrile (TCPN)	0.01% acet.	Agricultural fungicide		
Tetrachlorosalicylanilide (TCSA, Impregon)	0.5% pet.	Antiseptic used in soaps	Tribromosalicylanilide, bithionol, hex-achlorophene	A photosensitizer
Tetraethylthiuram disulfide (disulfiram, Antabuse)	1% pet.	Rubber industry, medications	Thiram compound Carbamates	Sensitizes to alcohol
Tetrahydroxy benzophenone	1% pet.			
Tetralin (tetrahydronaphtha-lene)	25% o.o.	Plumbing, steam fitting	Thiram compounds	
Tetramethylthiuram disulfide (thiram, febram, fermate)	1% pet.	Rubber industry, insecticides, fungicides, germicides, Rezifilm (Squibb)	Disulfiram, Antabuse, Carbamates, Thiram	Sensitizes to alcohol
Tetramethylthiuram monosul-fide	1% pet.	Rubber accelerator	Tetrathiuram disulfides, carbamates	Sensitizes to alcohol
Tetryl	Sat. sol. in ether	Munitions		Produces yellow stain; often causes folliculitis
Thallium sulfate	1% aq. sol.	Rodenticides, insecticides, depilatories		Toxic hair loss
Thephorin (phenindamine tar-trate; Hoffman-La Roche)	2.5% pet.			Potential topical sensi-tizer
Thermometer fluids (Metallic mercury)	0.5% pet.			*Clinical:* mercury. *Indoor and outdoor:* triethyl phosphate, toluene, xylene, alcohol
Thiamine chloride (vitamin B₁)	50% aq. sol.	Pharmaceuticals	Cocarboxylase (coenzyme B)	

Contactant	Concentration and Vehicle	Exposure	Cross-Reactions	Comment
Thimerosal	See Merthiolate			
Thio-beta-naphthol	1% pet.	Rubber peptizer		
Thioglycolic acid	5% aq. sol.	Depilatories		
Thiokol polysulfide polymers	1% acet.	Epoxy resin systems		
Thiophene compound	1% pet.	Phototoxic Compositae plants		
Thiophenol	0.1% alc.	Merthiolate (Lilly)		Sensitizer in thiosalicylic acid
Thiosalicylic acid	0.1% alc.	Merthiolate (Lilly)		
Thiourea, dialkyl esters	0.1% pet.	Rubber Diazo paper	Thiuram?	
Thorazine (Smith Kline & French)	1% pet.	Medical, nursing, pharmaceutical personnel handling and injecting the drug. Excreted in urine (contaminated linen)	Phenothiazine drugs, Phenergan, Theruhistin, Pyrrolazote	Photosensitizer
Thyme, oil of	1% alc.	Waterproofing, flavoring agent, Quinolor Compound (Squibb)	Niaouli Oil	
Thymol (isopropyl metacresol)	1% pet.	Dentifrices, mouthwashes, antiseptics, antimildew, Listerine, Chloraseptic, douches		
Thymol iodide	25% pet.	Antiseptics		
Tiger Balm	As is	Chinese proprietary ointment	Balsam of Peru	Contains balsams
Tin (stannic chloride)	10% aq. sol.	Metal, plating		
Tinactin (Schering)	As is	Fungicide		Contains tolnaftate 1%, butylated hydroxy-toluene polyethylene glycol
Tinuvin-P (hydroxy-5-methyl-phenyl benzotriazole)	1% pet.	UV absorber, plastics, dyes, dental, cosmetics, spandex, ostomy bags, plastic watch straps		
Titanium tetrachloride	Do not test			Vesicant

Contactant	Concentration and Vehicle	Exposure	Cross-Reactions	Comment
Tixocortol pivalate	1% pet.	Corticosteroid allergy marker	Hydrocortisone	
Tobacco	As is			
dl-alpha-Tocopherol	10% pet.	Vitamin E		
Toilet water	As is			Photosensitizer
Tolnaftate	1% pet.	Tinactin Solution Antifungal medication		Iso-z-naphthyl-m-n-di-methylthiocarbanilate
Toluene	50% o.o.	Solvents, rubber, adhesives, dyes, perfumes, thermometer fluids, nonclinical thermometer fluids		
Toluene diisocyanate (TDI)	1% pet.	Isocyanate compounds—pulmonary toxin		
Toluene sulfonamide resin	2% pet.			
p-Toluenesulfonyl chloride	0.5% alc.	Furan plastics, dye manufacture, synthetic tanning		
Toluidine Red	10% o.o.	Aniline dye		Photosensitizer
Toothpastes and powders Soapless With soap or detergent	As is (open) 2% aq. sol.			Controls
Topocide (Lilly)	As is	Miticide, insecticide		Benzyl benzoate, benzocaine, and DDT
Trafuril Ointment (European)	5% pet.	Primary urticariogenic agent		
Tragacanth	1% aq. sol.	Powders, cosmetics, candy manufacture, calico printing, drying agent, drug filler, sizing paper, printing, wave-setting fluids		Vegetable gum
Trenimon (2,3,5-triethylene-imino-1,4-benzoquinone)	0.05% pet.	Chemotherapeutic agent		
Tretinoin	0.005% alc.			Retin A, retinoic acid
Triacetin (glyceryl triacetate)	As is	Cigarette filters, Enzactin (Ayerst), antifungal agent		
Triazine	0.5% aq. sol.	Film hardener		

Contactant	Concentration and Vehicle	Exposure	Cross-Reactions	Comment
Tribromosalicylanilide (TBS)	1% pet.	Antiseptic in soaps—Green Lifebuoy, Praise, Safeguard	Tetrachlorosalicylanilide, bithionol, hexachlorophene	A photosensitizer
Trichloroacetic acid	Do not test			Primary irritant
Trichloroethylene (ethylene trichloride, acetylene trichloride)	5% o.o.	Metal degreasing, solvent for oils, greases, paints, varnishes, dye; leather manufacturing, dry cleaning, refrigerant, anesthetics, insecticides, perfumes		Sensitizes to alcohol
Triclosan (Irgasan DP 300)	2% pet.	Antiseptic		
Tricresyl ethyl phthalate	5% pet.	Plasticizer in nail adhesive		
Tricresylphosphate (tritolyl phosphate)	5% pet.	*Plasticizer:* vinyl films, resins, polyester, cellulose, nail lacquer. *Lead scavenger:* in gasoline, fire retardant. *Carbon paper*	Triphenylphosphate	
Triethanolamine	5% pet.	Cosmetics, pharmaceuticals, epoxy hardener		
Triethanolamine	1% pet.	Cosmetic surfactant		
Triethylenediamine	0.1% aq. sol. 0.5% pet.	Polyurethane resin catalyst, epoxy hardener		
Triethylenetetramine	0.1% aq. sol. 0.5% pet.	Epoxy resin		
Trimethylolpropane triacrylate (TMPTA)	0.1% pet.	UVR Cured ink		
Trimeton Ointment (prophenpyridamine; Schering)	As is	Tripoton, Inhiston	Antistine	
Trinitrobenzene	1% acet.			Primary sensitizer
Trinitrotoluene	20% pet.	Explosives		Causes yellow discoloration
Tri-ortho-cresyl-phosphate	Do not test (very toxic)	Plastic coatings, fireproofers, lubricants, gasoline		In Morocco, vegetable oil adulterated with this compound produced paralysis in thousands

Contactant	Concentration and Vehicle	Exposure	Cross-Reactions	Comment
Triphenylmethane	1% pet.	Dyes		
Triphenyl phosphate	5% pet.	Cellulose acetate carbon paper		
Trisodium phosphate	2% aq. sol.	A "builder" added to detergents and soaps		
Triton 25 (para-octyl phenol ethylene oxide)	0.1% aq. sol.	Wetting agent in cosmetic and pharmaceutical preparations, textiles, metal cleaning, dry cleaning solvent, solvent in ballpoint inks		
Triton X-100 (alkylated aryl polyether alcohol)	1% aq. sol.	Surfactant, nonionic synthetic detergents, bubble baths		Controls
Triton X-200 (sodium salt of alkylated aryl polyether sulfonate)	1% aq. sol.	Surfactant, anionic synthetic detergents, bubble baths		Controls
Triton X-400 (stearyldimethyl-benzylammonium chloride)	0.1% aq. sol.	Surfactant, cationic synthetic detergents, bubble baths		Controls "Quat"
Tromantadine	0.5% pet.	Antiviral drug		
Turkey Red Oil	1% o.o.	Surfactant, agricultural textile industry		
Turpentine	10% o.o. or (turpentine peroxides) 0.3% pet.	Synthetic resins, pine oleoresins, furniture and stove polish, varnish, wax solvent, cleaning fluid, paint thinner, adhesives, insecticides. *Liniments:* Sloans, Minards, Johnson's Anodyne, Mentholatum, Penetromide	Chrysanthemum, ragweed, pyrethrum, colophony (rosin), balsams (pine and spruce)	Sensitizer is alpha-carene or alpha-pinene Irritant
Turpentine peroxide	0.3% pet.	Present in Sloan's Liniment and Secaderm Cream		
Tween 20 (sorbitan monolaurate polyoxyethylene derivative)	5% aq. sol.	Surfactant, nonionic synthetic detergents, bubble baths		Controls
Tween 80 (sorbitan monooleate polyoxyethylene derivative)	5% aq. sol.	Surfactant, nonionic synthetic detergents, bubble baths		Controls
Tylosin (Tylan)	5% pet.	Animal feed	Spiramycin?	Antibiotic
Tyrothricin	20% pet.	Tyrolaris Mouthwash, Creams and Ointments, Isodettes, Otalgine Drops (Purdue Frederick)		

Contactant	Concentration and Vehicle	Exposure	Cross-Reactions	Comment
Ultrawet K (sodium aralkyl sulfonate)	1% aq. sol.	Surfactant, synthetic detergents, bubble baths		Controls
Umbelliferone (7-hydroxy-coumarin)	2% pet.	Sunscreening agents, optical bleaches	Furocoumarin	A cinnamic acid derivative. Photosensitizer
Undecylenic acid	2.5% pet.	Sweat, topical antifungal medications		Rare sensitizer
Unguentum Bossi (Doak)	As is	Psoriasis remedy		Contains ammoniated mercury, tar and sulfosalicylic acid
Urea (carbamide)	10% aq. sol.	Amino Cerv (Milex), Carbamine (Key Pharmaceuticals), Carmol Cream (Ingram), Debrox (International Pharmaceutical), Gly-Oxide (International Pharmaceutical), Kerid Drops (Blair), Otomide (Schering), Panafil Ointment (Rystan), Panafil-White Ointment (Rystan), Ureaphil (Abbott), Stilbamidine, deodorants, dentifrices, hand creams (Aquacare), formaldehyde resins		Rare sensitizer. Urea frost (urea particles of face in uremia). Cause of ammoniacal dermatitis and stomatitis. Tsyrkunol, L: Occupational Skin Diseases in Workers Engaged in Production of Nitrogen-Mineral Fertilizers, P. Westnder-Vener., 6, 31, 1963. Synthetic urea is an irritant
Urea formaldehyde	10% pet.	Plastics, finishes		
Urea peroxide (Gly-Oxide)	As is			
Uric acid	1% aq. sol.	Allantoin (a derivative of uric acid)		
Usnic acid	1% pet.	Lichens, lichen mosses, clothing dyes, litmus paper	Furocoumarins	Rarely sensitizes
Vanilla (alcoholic extract)	10% acet.	Flavoring agent in foods, tobacco, beverages, perfumes	Balsam of Peru, benzoin, oil of cloves Coumarin	Vanilla lichen—a dermatitis due to mites infesting vanilla pods
Vanillin	10% pet.	Aromatic crystalline principle of vanilla	Balsam of Peru, benzoin, oil of cloves, eugenol Coumarin	Vanillism—allergic dermatitis, rhinitis and asthma from vanilla

Contactant	Concentration and Vehicle	Exposure	Cross-Reactions	Comment
Vegetable gums	1% pet.			Karaya, gum arabic (acacia) and tragacanth are the most sensitizing gums
Vermouth	As is (open)	Handlers and imbibers		Some vermouths contain oil of cinnamon and quinine
Vinegar	As is	Condiments, preservative, fermenting beer, cider, malt, wine, lead subacetate		Acetic acid content causes aphthous ulcers?
Vinyl benzene (styrene)	1% o.o.	See Styrene		
Vinyl films	As is			Sensitizers in vinyl films may be *plasticizers,* such as tricresylphosphate, dioctyl-phthalate, ester of adipic acid, and epoxy resins, or *stabilizers,* such as dibutyl tin maleate
Vioform Ointment, Cream, Lotion (iodochlorohydroxyquin; CIBA)	As is	*Related compounds:* Entero-Vioform (CIBA), HEB-Cort V Cream and Lotion (Barnes-Hind), Hysone (Mallard), Lidaform-HC Creme and Lotion (Dome), Nystaform Ointment (Dome), Nystaform-HC Ointment and Lotion (Dome), Pentarcort (Dalin), Racetico Cream (Lemmon), Vioform Inserts (CIBA), Vioform-Hydrocortisone (CIBA), Vio-Hydrosone Cream (North American Pharmacal), Quinoform, 1-Quinn Dermaform, Domeform, Torofor (Torch), HEB-Cort, Hyquin Cream, Topigel	Diodoquin, Sterosan, Quinolor Ointment Broxyquinolene	Iodine containing hydroxyquinoline
Virginamycin	2.5% pet.		Pristinamycin	Antibiotic
Vitamin A	0.1% pet.	Hand and cosmetic creams, vitamin A and D ointment		May be tested as Retinol acid "pure"

Contactant	Concentration and Vehicle	Exposure	Cross-Reactions	Comment
Vitamin A acid (Tretinoin)	0.1% pet.	Topical acne medications		An irritant. Rare sensitizer
Vitamin B₁ (thiamine chloride, Betabion Hydrochloride, Aneurin Hydrochloride)	10% pet.	Pharmaceutical industry	Cocarboxylase, coenzyme B (diphosphothiamin)	Sensitized workers flare and acquire "systemic" contact dermatitis after ingestion or injection of thiamine chloride
Vitamin B₆ (pyridoxine; 2-methyl-3-nitro-4-methoxyly-methyl-5-cyano-6-chlopyridine)	10% pet.	Pharmaceutical industry	Pyridine derivatives in production of castor oil	Berufdermatosen, 13, 28, 1965. Allergic contact dermatitis in production of B₆ and of castor oil, another pyridine derivative
Vitamin B₁₂ (cyanocobalamine, Betalin 12, Berubigen, Cobione)	10% pet.	Pharmaceuticals Animal feed additive	Cobalt	0.4% of B₁₂ molecule is cobalt. See text for cobalt patient whose dermatitis flared from injection of B₁₂. Positive patch test reactions obtained with injectable B₁₂ preparations
Vitamin E (alpha-tocopherol)	As is in pet.	Tashan Cream, Vitamin E Deodorant Spray (Mennen), Vitamin LE Soap (Altabra from Italy)		Brodkin, R.H., et al.: Sensitivity to Topically Applied Vitamin E (in Tashan Cream). Arch Derm., 90, 76, 1965
Vitamin E Deodorant Spray (Mennen)	As is			Contains propellent, Alcohol SD-40, vitamin E, silicone fluid and perfume. (The sensitizer in many cases proved to be vitamin E in this spray)

Contactant	Concentration and Vehicle	Exposure	Cross-Reactions	Comment
Vitamin K (Menadiol sodium diphosphate [Kappadione, Synkayvite]; menadione sodium bisulfite [Hykinonel])	0.1% aq. sol.	Production of vitamin K		Jirasek, L.: Hypersensitivity to Vitamin K. Cesk. Derm., *40*, 17, 1965
White henna (magnesium carbonate)	As is in pet.	Hair bleaches		
White spirits	25% o.o.	Solvent, thinner, turpentine substitute		
Wintergreen, oil of (gaultheria oil)	1% alc.	Flavoring agent, rubefacient, antiseptic, Banalg Liniment (Cole) Ger-O-Foam (Geriatric), Panalgesic (Poythress)	Salicylates	Rich in methyl salicylate
Witch hazel (Hamamelis)	As is	Topical medications, rubefacient, Tucks Pads, Cream, Ointment (Fuller); Hazel-Balm (Arnar-Stone)		Contains tannins and 70–80% alcohol
Wood (sawdust)	As is			Risk of false positive reaction. Controls
Wood tars		See Tar, wood		
Wool alcohols	30% pet.	Lanolin, eucerin, lanolin derivatives		Main sensitizer in lanolin
Xylene (Sylol)	50% o.o.	Solvents, paint removers, lacquers, degreasing cleansers, insecticides, pesticides		
Xylocaine (lidocaine; diethylaminoacet-2,6-xylidide hydrochloride)	2% aq. sol	Local anesthetic, solution, ointment, jelly, suppositories		Does not cross-react with benzocaine
Ylang-ylang oil	5% pet.	Cosmetics		Cause pigmentation
Zephiran chloride (benzalkonium; Winthrop)	1:1000 aq. sol.	Cationic antiseptic detergent, antirust powder and tablets		
Zinc bis-diethyldithiocarbamate	1% pet.	Rubber antioxidant		
Zinc chloride	2% aq. sol.	Astringents, plumbing, welding, wood preservative		

Contactant	Concentration and Vehicle	Exposure	Cross-Reactions	Comment
Zinc ethylenebisdithiocarbamate	1% pet.	Rubber antioxidant		
Zinc oxide	10% pet.	Adhesives, paints, galvanizing, zinc plating, drying agents, dental cements, automobile tires, white ointments and powders, cosmetics		Rare sensitizer. May cause black dermographism
Zinc peroxide	10% pet.	Oxidizing medications, bleaches, healing agents, deodorants, astringents		
Zinc phenosulfonate	1% alc.	Astringents, cosmetics, deodorants (Secret, Top Brass, Arrid, Hi & Dry, Manpower)		
Zinc pyrithione	1% alc.	Dandruff therapy		Photosensitivity
Zinc stearate	10% pet.			May cause irritant granulomas
Zinc sulfate	5% aq. sol.	Astringent, styptic pencil		
Zineb	1% pet.	Pesticide	Carbamates	Ethylene-bis(dithiocarbamate) zinc
Ziradyl (Parke, Davis)	As is (patch-scratch)	Topical agent for plant dermatitis		Zirconium oxide, Benadryl. Allergic granuloma
Ziram	1% pet.	Pesticide		
Zircobarb Lotion (Vogel)	As is (patch-scratch)	Topical agent for plant dermatitis		Hydrous zirconium. Allergic granuloma
Zirconium lactate, sodium	0.1% aq. sol. (1:10,000 intracutaneous)	Antiperspirants		Allergic granuloma
Zirconium oxide	Pdr. as is (patch-scratch)	Ziradyl, Zirium, Zirnox, Rhulihist, Rhulicream, Rhulitol, Ivarest, Allergesic, Zotox		Allergic granuloma

Contactant	Concentration and Vehicle	Exposure	Cross-Reactions	Comment
Zirconium silicate	As is (patch-scratch)	Pepsodent Toothpaste		
Zirconyl hydrochloride	10% pet.	Secret Roll-on Deodorant		"Safe" zirconium?
Zirium (Ulmer)	As is (patch-scratch)	Topical agent for poison ivy dermatitis		Zirconium oxide and thenylpyramine. Allergic granuloma
Zirnox (Bristol)	As is (patch-scratch)	Topical agent for plant dermatitis		Allergic granuloma

Subject Index

Page references followed by *f* and *t* indicate figures and tables, respectively.

A

Abietic acid, 338, 366, 736
  in dentrifices and mouthwashes, 680*t*
  in oils and cooling fluids, 470*t*
  sensitization to, 366
  in typewriting paper, 438
Abieto-formo-phenolic resin, 736
Abitol, 736, 771
Abrasive agents, 273
Absorbers
  paste, 717
  for rubber, 535, 540*t*
Acacia (gum arabic), 145, 562*t*, 736, 769
  allergy to, 561
  in dentrifices and mouthwashes, 680*t*, 681*t*
  in food, 267–268, 268*t*
  pharmaceutical products that contain, 562–564, 565*t*
Acaricides, 433, 433*t*
Accessories, clothing, 304
Accroides (yacca), 563*t*
ACD. *See* Allergic contact dermatitis
Acetaminophen (Propacetamol), 199
Acetanilide, 736
Acetarsol, 736
Acetarsone, 178
2-Acetexycyclonhexahone oxime, 736
Acetic acid, 680*t*, 736
Acetic ether. *See* Ethyl acetate
Acetone, 477, 736
  in dentrifices and mouthwashes, 680*t*
  paresthesia due to, 414*t*
1-Acetyl-2-phenylhydrazine, 736
Acetyl ethyltetramethyltetralin. *See* Versalide (AETT)
Acetylene tetrachloride. *See* Tetrachloroethane
Acetylene trichloride, 810
N'-Acetylsulfanilamide, 177, 177*t*
Achromycin Ointment (Lederle), 736
Acid dyes, 296
  Acid Black 48, 298*t*
  Acid Blue 40, 298*t*
  Acid Red 118, 298*t*
  Acid Red 151, 298*t*
  Acid Red 359, 298*t*
  Acid Violet 17, 298*t*
  Acid Yellow 23, 298*t*
  Acid Yellow 61, 298*t*
  Acid Yellow 159, 298*t*
  Acid Yellow 198, 298*t*

Acid fuchsin, 736
Acne
  chloracne, 78, 79, 472
    differential diagnosis of, 471, 472*t*
    features of, 473
    systemic complications of, 473, 473*t*
    therapy for, 473
  occupational, 78–79, 471–473
    causes of, 77, 78*t*
  oil, 471–473
  from petrolatum, 115
  pomade acne, 47, 48, 77–79
Acne preparations
  that contain benzoyl peroxide, 160
  that contain mercury compounds, 153, 154*t*
  that contain resorcinol, 113, 113*t*
Acne venenata, 47–48
Acneform eruptions, 77, 78*t*, 245
Acral dermatitis, chronic, 272
Acrex. *See* Dinobuton
Acridine, 736
Acriflavine, 736
Acriflavine (acridine) dyes, 162
Acrisorcin, 737
Acrolein, 503–504, 506*t*
Acrylamides, 460*t*, 461, 503–504, 505*t*–506*t*
Acrylate
  in dentistry, 456*t*
  ethylhexyl, 337
  initiators, 501
  light-sensitive or UV-cured
    components of, 501, 501*t*
    in printing industry, 501–502
  open vs closed systems, 500–501
  in orthopedic surgery, 323
  in paint, 429*t*
  patch testing with, 507
  in pressure-sensitive acrylic adhesives, 503–504, 505*t*
  in printing plates, 502
  stomatitis from, 670–671, 683*t*
Acrylate compounds
  epoxy, 500
  in printing, 430
Acrylate-resin-based adhesive tape, 337, 737
Acrylic
  in dentistry, 456*t*
  dermatitis from, 283–284
  in paints, 428, 428*t*
  in printing, 430*t*
Acrylic acid allergy, 593–594
Acrylic bone cement, 453
  benzoyl peroxide activator of, 160

  hand dermatitis from, 453
  hand protection for orthopedic surgeons
    against, 275
  orthopedic, 507–508
    in artifical joint rejection, 508
    components of, 507, 508*t*
Acrylic compounds
  exposures to, 499, 499*t*
  patch testing with, 507
  sensitizers in, 500, 500*t*
Acrylic dentures
  allergic and irritant stomatitis from, 671–672
  testing for allergic sensitivity to, 682–683
Acrylic hand alterers and lattices, 290
Acrylic inks, ultraviolet-cured, 502
Acrylic monomer, 736
  in dentistry, 456
  patch tests with, 456
Acrylic nails, 65, 500
Acrylic plastics, 499–509
  open vs closed systems, 500–501
Acrylic pressure-sensitive adhesives, 504–507
  backing (facing) of, 507
  monomers used for, 503–504, 505*t*–506*t*
  solvent-based formulation of, 503–504, 504*t*
Acrylic resins
  general uses of, 499–500
  system components, 501, 501*t*, 508–509
Acrylimides, 503–504, 506*t*
Acrylonitrile, 737
  paresthesia due to, 414*t*
  in pressure-sensitive acrylic adhesives, 503–504, 506*t*
Actamar. *See* Bithionol
Actidione, 758
Actinic dermatitis, chronic, 407
Actinic reticuloid syndrome, 76
Acupuncture needles, 332–333
Acyclovir, 181, 737
Addiction, 81
Additives
  animal feed, 458–459, 460*t*
  chewing gum, 39, 39*t*
  in clothing, 285–287
  color, 607
  cooling fluid, 470*t*, 471
  food, 267, 267*t*, 519, 520*t*
    antioxidant, 268, 268*t*
    contact dermatitis from, 519–526
    hand dermatitis due to, 267–269
  oil, 470*t*, 471
  patch testing with vinyl resins and, 491, 491*t*
  rubber, 535–540

irritation of oral mucosa by, 663–664
laboratory, 90t
leukoderma from, 571, 572t
occupational
  desensitization procedures with, 422
  patch testing with, 421
  skin color changes due to, 572, 572t
for patch testing with rubber, 545, 545t
photoallergenic, 400, 400t
phototoxic, 398, 398t
plant, 372–374
in plasticizers, 538–539, 539t
in plastics, 312–314
in rubber, 312–314
  depigmentation from, 554
  nonrubber sources of, 554–556
  positive patch test reactions to, 542, 542t
in softeners, 538–539, 539t
stomatitis from, 664
test for chromates, 626
"white" lesions of mouth caused by, 665
Chemotechnique Diagnostics AB, 24
Chenopodiaceae (spinach family), 382–383
Chest dermatitis, 59
Chewing gum additives, 39, 39t
Chicory, 752
Childhood
  allergic dermatitis due to specific sensitizers in, 37–38
  atopic dermatitis in
    from contact with proteins, 36
    from cow's milk, 107
    from grains, 107
  caustic burns in, 33
  contact cheilitis in, 36
  contact dermatitis in, 33–37
  dermatitis of feet in, 35–36
  diaper dermatitis in, 34–35
  exposure to balsam of Peru in, 137
  patch testing in, 37
  perianal dermatitis in, 35
  perioral dermatitis in, 36
  plant dermatitis in, 36
  rosacea-like eruptions of, 81
  rubber sensitivity in, 543
  sensitizers in, 37, 38t
  strong topical corticosteroid effects in, 38
"Childproof" caps, 459, 460
Chinese rice paper plant, 376
Chironex fleckeri (sea wasp), 691–692
Chironomid, 597
Chloracetamide, 223
  in paint, 429t
  in shoes, 306t
Chloracetopenone, 752
Chloracetophene, 481
Chloracne, 78, 79, 472
  connubial, 44
  differential diagnosis of, 471, 472t
  features of, 473
  systemic complications of, 473, 473t
  therapy for, 473
Chloracnegens, 471, 472t
Chloral hydrate, 95, 752
Chloramine-T (Chloramine), 156–157, 590, 752
Chloramphenicol, 90t, 175, 175t, 752
  allergic contact urticaria from, 589

ophthalmologic, 129t
  reactions to, 175
  systemic contact dermatitis due to, 92
Chlordane, 752
Chlordantoin, 752
Chlorhexidine, 157, 228, 752
  allergic contact urticaria from, 591
  in feminine hygiene sprays, 487
Chlorhexidine diacetate, 408t
Chlorhexidine digluconate, 752
Chlorhexidine gluconate, 129t
Chlorinated alkalies, 752
Chlorinated hydrocarbons, 476–477
Chlorinated naphthalene, 753
Chlorinated products, 156–158
Chlorinated water, 156
Chlorine
  in antiseptics and disinfectants, 156–158
  dermatitis from, 711
5-Chloro-2-methyl-4-isothiazolon-3-one (Kathon CG). See Methylchloroisothiazolinone/methylisothiazolinone
Chloro-2-phenylphenol (Dowicide 32), 753
4-Chloro-3-cresol, 470t
Chloro-3-methyl. See 4-Chloro-m-cresol
4-Chloro-3-methylphenol. See 4-Chloro-m-cresol
4-Chloro-3,5-xylenol. See Chloroxylenol
2-Chloro-4-phenyl phenol, 763
2-Chloro-4-phenyl-phenol sodium, 762
4-Chloro-m-cresol, 158
p-Chloro-m-xylenol. See Chloroxylenol
Chloro-meta-cresol, 753
p-Chloro-o-cresol, 431t, 753
Chloro-phenyl phenol, 763
Chloroacetamide (Hibitane), 470t, 753
alpha-Chlorobenzaldehyde phenylhydrazone, 738
Chlorobenzene, 753
ortho-Chlorobenzylidene malnotrile (CS), 481
Chlorobenzylidene malonitrile, 753
Chlorobutanol crystals, 753
Chlorocresol, 591, 753
Chloroethanol. See Ethylene chlorohydrin
Chloroform, 476, 680t, 753
para-Chloromercuriphenol, 153
Chloromethylisothiazolinone, 753
Chloromycetin (Parke, Davis), 752
Chloronitrobenzenes, 431t
Chloroparanitraniline red
  in paint, 429t
  in printing, 430t
Chlorophene, 431t
bis-(4-Chlorophenoyl) methyl chloride, 747
Chlorophorin, 378t
Chlorophyll, 753
Chlorophyllins, 753
  sodium copper, 680t
Chloroprocaine hydrochloride, 783
Chloroquin, 754
Chlorosalicylamide, 401, 754
Chlorothalonil, 594, 754
Chlorothion, 754
Chlorothymol, 680t, 754
Chloroxine, 157
Chloroxylenol, 25, 158, 754

instructions for patients, 732
in oils and cooling fluids, 470t
products that contain, 158, 158t
Chlorpenhiramine maleate, 129t
Chlorphenesin, 753
Chlorproethazine, 201
Chlorpromazine (Thorazine), 401, 454–455, 754, 808
  allergic contact urticaria from, 590–591
  in dairy work, 434t
Chlorquinaldol, 803
Cholesterol-lowering agents, 130
Chrism, 364
Chromated catgut, 619
Chromates, 619
  allergic reactions to
    clinical features of, 618
    demographics of, 636, 638t
  blackjack disease due to, 620
  in bleaching agents, 619
  in cement dermatitis, 624
  chemical test for, 626
  dermatitis from, 619
    treatment of, 625
  in detergents, 619
  in flour, 440
  in foods, 620
  hand dermatitis due to, 264
  in industrial dermatitis, 621–622
  in matches, 620
  occupational exposures to, 621, 621t
  pompholyx from ingestion of, 263–264
  reactions to, 618–623
  in shoes, 306t, 619
  sources of exposure to, 619
  substances and industries to be avoided by individuals sensitive to, 622, 622t
Chrome
  alloys, 620
  environmental contamination by, 625
  in epoxy resin adhesive, 620
  in hide glues, 620
  patch test concentrations for, 612t
  plating, 619–620, 622
  in tanning, 308, 619
  ulcers from, 623
Chrome-cobalt combination, 669
Chrome cripples, 618
Chromium
  chronicity of dermatitis from, 618
  in food and dietary supplements, 620–621
  granulomatous reactions to, 614
  hardness of, 614, 615t
  in tattoos, 608
  valences, 623
Chromium oxide, 769
Chromium sulfate, 754
Chromium trichloride, 754
Chromonychia
  contact, 66–67
  exogenous vs endogenous, 67
  from thermal injury, 66
Chromotropic acid test, 289
Chrysanthemum, 375, 435t
Chrysarobin, 754
Chrysiasis, 633
Chrysoidine brown, 755

photoallergenic, 400, 400*t*
phototoxic, 398, 398*t*
sulfonamide, 93
topical drug addiction, 81
Dry-cleaned clothes, 304
Dry-cleaning preparations, 294
Dry contact dermatitis, 83–84
Dry mouth syndrome, 672
DUO brand surgical adhesive (Thayer Co.), 337
Duponal C. *See* Sodium lauryl sulfate
Duponol WA, 763
Durable-press allergic contact dermatitis
consequences of, 287–288
patch testing for, 288
Durable-press finishing, 280, 281*t*
cross-linking agents, 280–281, 282*t*
Duraspan (International Latex), 763
Dust
dermatitis due to, 83–84
instructions for prevention of irritant
dermatitis, 717
Dust mites, 104–105
Dyclone, 763
Dyclonine hydrochloride (Dow Chemical), 763
Dyeline paper copying, 437–438
Dyes. *See also specific colors, dyes*
acid, 296
acriflavine (acridine), 162
allergic contact dermatitis due to, 302–303
allergic contact urticaria due to, 594
allergy to
historical data on, 298
modern data, 299
screening for, 300
aniline, 300
anionic, 296
antiseptic triphenylmethane, 161–163
azo, 75, 743
cross-reactions, 295
FD&C, 527, 528
pigmented contact dermatitis due to, 75
azobenzene, 510
basic (cationic), 296
in carbon paper, 436, 436*t*
certified, 763
chemical classification of, 295–296
in clothing, 295–297, 298, 298*t*
direct, 296
disperse (plastosoluble), 297
allergic contact dermatitis from, 297
textiles for allergic patients, 302, 302*t*
in drugs
dermatitis due to, 527–529
testing for reactions to, 528
in fiber, 297
food, 267–268, 268*t*, 526–527, 527*t*
hair, 248
cobalt in, 626
metal salts in, 607
in leather shoes, 310
mordant, 296
natural, 530
nylon stocking, 298, 298*t*
oxidation base, 297
patch test concentrations for, 162, 162*t*
phototoxic, 529–530, 529*t*
pseudophytodermatitis due to, 375

reactive, 297
screening for allergy to, 299–300
shoe dye dermatitis, 310
sulfur, 296
synthetic, 530
textile
allergic contact dermatitis from, 297–299
classification of, 296–297
prevalence of allergy to, 299, 299*t*
screening for allergy to, 299–300
types of, 297
vat, 297
Dysesthesia
definition of, 413
vulvar, 61–62
Dyshidrosiform contact dermatitis, 79–80
Dyshidrotic hand eczema, 89

E

Ear
dermatitis of, 57–59
otitis of, 58–59
Ear piercing, 644–645
Ear preparations, 153, 154*t*
Earlobe dermatitis, 57
Earlobe otitis, 58
Earlobe sign of nickel sensitivity, 644–645
Earrings
hypoallergenic, 645
nickel sensitivity with, 644–645
Ears, "surgarcane," 58
East India resin, 563*t*
Ecdysis, 119–120
ECG. *See* Electrocardiography
Echinoderms, 695–697
Echothiophate iodine, 129*t*
Ecogaine, 763
Econazole, 90*t*
Ectopic flare, 15
Eczema
of amputee skin, 326–327
atopic, from flour, 439
dyshidrotic, 80
in bakers, 439
of hand, 89
hand
barrier creams for prevention of, 274
dyshidrotic, 89
epidemiology of, 262
patch test reactivity with, 261–262
patterns, 270
skin test correlations, 261, 262*t*
household, 261, 719
housewife's, 261, 263, 269–270
Eczematous dermatitis
allergic, from foods, 265–266
delayed
patch testing for, 10
from spices, 266, 266*t*
from vegetables, 266, 266*t*
from platinum salts, 650
systemic, in elderly, 40–41
Eczematous drug eruptions, 42
Eczematous fiberglass dermatoses, 514
Eczematous urticarial reactions, 599–600
Edathamil, 763
Edema, eyelid, 550

Edge effect, 16
EDTA. *See* Ethylenediamine tetra-acetate
Effector cells, 3–4
EG. *See* Ethylene glycol
Eggs, 585–586
Egmea, 765
El litre tree *(Lithraea caustica),* 353, 353*t*
Elasmobrachs, 709
Elastic hair nets, 552
Elastic leg support bandages, 339
Elastomers, 284–285
Elderly
contact dermatitis in, 39–41
allergic, 40–41
features of, 41
hair-dye dermatitis in, 40
industrial dermatitis in, 40
photodermatitis in, 40
ragweed dermatitis in, 40
systemic eczematous contact dermatitis in,
40–41
wearing-apparel dermatitis in, 40
Eldoquin (Elder), 763
Elecampane, 145, 376–377
Electric shocks, 709
Electrical burns, 331
Electrocardiography
allergic contact dermatitis associated with,
328, 329*t*
dermatologic hazards of, 328–329
electrode jelly, 328, 329
gels and pastes, 234, 328–329
nickel-plated electrodes, 329
rubber straps to fasten electrodes, 329
Electrodes
ECG, 329
TENS, 331
Electronics, 442
Electrostatic or xerographic paper copying, 438
Elemi, gum, 563*t*
Emerald green, 788
Emollients, 487*t*, 488
Empyreumatic (oleum rusci), 141
Emulgade F, 591
Emulsifiers
allergy to, 236–239
in foods, 523, 523*t*
patch test results, 236, 237*t*
in skin care preparations, 252
Emulsifying wax, 763
Emulsions, pressure-sensitive adhesive,
503–504, 504*t*
"Endogenic" contact dermatitis, systemic, 188
Endogenous steroids, 206
Endotoxins, 549–550
English ivy, 375
Enoxolone, 201
Envenomization
catfish, 708–709
cone shell, 698
nematocyst
prevention of, 695
treatment of, 694–695
scorpion fish, 707–708
stingray, 706–707
stonefish, 707–708
Environmental contamination, 625

Panties, rubber, 552
Pantothenol, 786
Pants paresthesia syndrome, 288, 414–415, 414t
Pants pressure purpura, 74
Papaine, 129t
Paper
  carbon, 436
  carbonless, 436–437
  copy, 437–438
  dermatitis from, 435–438
  dermatologist's table paper, 216–217
  diazo, 438
  eyelid dermatitis due to, 54
  formaldehyde in, 217
  perfume in, 438
  typewriter correction, 438
  typewriting, 438
Paper copying
  diazo or dyeline process, 437–438
  electrostatic or xerographic method, 438
  methods of, 437, 437t
Paper money, 786
Papular gold eruptions, 631–632
Para-aminoazobenzene, 306t
Para-aminobenzene, 786
Para-aminobenzoic acid, 403, 404, 408t, 787
Para-aminobenzoic acid esters, 403, 404, 430
Para-aminophenol, 787
Para-chloro-meta-xylenol, 787
Para-diaminodiphenyl. See Benzidine
Para-dioxane. See Dioxane
Para-octyl phenol ethylene oxide, 811
Para-oxon, 787
Para-phenylenediamine, 575
Para red
  in paint, 429t
  in printing, 430t
Para-tertiary butyl phenol formaldehyde resin,
    787
Paraben-free over-the-counter corticosteroid
    lotions and creams, 203, 204t
Paraben mix, 22, 25, 787
Paraben paradox, 52, 218–219
Parabens
  allergic stomatitis from, 673
  allergy to, 218, 219
  contact urticaria due to, 592
  in ECG monitoring jelly, 328
  in foods, 267t, 519
  immediate urticarial reactions to, 220
  instructions for patients, 730
  in medicated bandages, 339
  over-the-counter topical corticosteroids that
    contain, 203, 204t
  systemic contact dermatitis due to, 96,
    219–220
Parachlorometacresol, 158, 222–223. See also
    4-Chloro-3-cresol; 4-Chloro-m-cresol
Parachlorometaxylenol. See also Chloroxylenol
  allergy to, 222–223
  in Redux ECG paste, 329
Parachlorophenol, 787
Paradichlorobenzene, 787
Paraffin, 787. See also Kerosene
  soft. See Petrolatum
Parafinnomas, 115
Paraformaldehyde medicaments, 214, 214t

Parahydroxybenzoic acid, 787
Paraphenylenediamine, 787
  allergic contact urticaria from, 594
  in developers, 427
  hand dermatitis due to, 265
  industrial uses, 554–555, 556t
  instructions for patients, 726
  in laboratory workers, 460t
  products that contain, 554–555, 556t
  in shoes, 306t
o-nitro-Paraphenylenediamine, 787
Paraphenylenediamine mix, 547
Pararosaniline, 787
Parasites, 303–304
Paratertiary amylphenol, 573, 573t
Paratertiary butylcatechol, 573
Paratertiary butylphenol
  exposure to, 571, 572t
  germicidal phenolic detergents that contain,
    573, 573t
  leukoderma from, 571
  in shoes, 306t
Paratertiary butylphenol formaldehyde resin,
    90t, 313
  instructions for patients, 726
  management of allergy to, 315
  in shoes, 306t, 312–313
Parathion, 432t, 788
Paratoluenediamine sulfate, 788
Paratoluenesulfonamide, 429t
Paresthesia
  from contactants, 413–417, 414t
  from mohair, 415
  pants paresthesia syndrome, 414–415
  pressure, 414t, 415
  from solvents, 415
  from synthetic pyrethroid insecticides,
    413–414
  from wool, 415
Paris green, 788
Paronychia
  in bakers, 439
  from cosmetics, 245
Parsley, 381, 788
Parsnips, 788
  wild, 381
Parsol 1789. See
    Butylmethoxydibenzoylmethane
Parthenium dermatitis
  clinical features of, 369–370
  export to India, 369–370
Pastes
  Camcreme ECG, 328–329
  in electrocardiography, 328–329
Patch test clinic, 27–28
Patch testing
  acaricides, 433, 433t
  with acrylic compounds, 507
  with acrylic monomer, 456
  active sensitization due to, 14–15
  adverse reactions, 13–14, 14t
  with aluminum Finn chambers, 615–616
  anaphylactoid reactions, 16
  animal repellents, 433, 433t
  antibiotic series, 180, 180t
  in atopic individuals, 102, 103
  in atopic infants, 37

for baking industry, 440, 440t, 525t
basic assumptions of, 9–10
battery, 12
for beekeepers, 143, 143t
with bulbs, 386–387
cardinal rules for, 11
for cattle breeders, 434, 435t
for cellulose ester plastic sensitivity, 510, 510t
in cheilitis, 679–683
in childhood, 37
closed-patch testing for leukoderma, 576
in clothing dermatitis, 303
with cobalt, 629
communication with patients about results,
    13
complications due to, 14
for conjunctivitis and eyelid dermatitis, 53,
    53t
for contraceptive dermatitis, 325, 325t
cosmetics, 240, 241t–242t, 245–253
with cutting fluids, 468, 469
for dairy workers, 434, 434t
for delayed eczematous dermatitis, 10
with dentrifices, 679–682, 680t–682t
determination of relevance, 425–426
to determine hardening in industry, 422
in drug eruptions, 41–42
for durable-press allergy, 288
for dyes, 162, 162t
edge effect, 16
with emulsifiers, 236, 237t
for epoxy resins, 492, 493t, 494–495, 494t
for ethylene oxide reactions, 486
excited skin syndrome ("angry back") in,
    16–21
  strategy for dealing with, 18–19, 18t
false-negative reactions, 13, 613
false-positive reactions, 18, 613
for farmers and agricultural workers, 434,
    434t
flare-ups of earlier reactions, 89
for food dyes, 527, 527t
for forest workers, 434, 435t
with formaldehyde, 218
with formaldehyde resins, 499
fragrance mixture, 343–344, 344t
frequently used substances, 25
fungicides, 431, 431t
for gold allergy, 631
for hairdressers, 441, 441t
for hand dermatitis, 262–265
for hand eczema, 261–262
herbicides, 432, 433t
with hydroquinone, 575
hyperpigmentation due to, 15
for immediate urticarial reactions, 10
with industrial oils, 471
insecticides, 432, 432t
interpretation of, 12–13, 23–24
  distinguishing between irritant reactions
    and allergic reactions, 24
  key for, 24, 24t
  reading test results, 23–24
  in screening series, 21–22
with irritant plants, 385
irritant reactions, 15
  avoiding, 11–12

causes of, 10–12
distinguishing between allergic reactions and, 24
for lanolin sensitivity, 126–127, 238–239
for lichenoid contact dermatitis, 77
for local anesthetic reactions, 198
for mercury allergy, 636
with metals and metal salts, 611–614
with mouthwashes, 679, 680*t*–682*t*
precautions for, 679–682
naturally occurring mixes, 22
negative reactions, 13
in metal dermatitis, 611–613
with new industrial compounds, 420, 421
for nickel sensitivity, 642–644
coins for, 610
dietary metals in patch test-negative patients, 639–640
threshold level of reactions, 643
with nickel sulfate, 643
with nitrites, 46
nonspecific reactions to protein substances, 103
with occupational chemicals, 421
with occupational cutaneous impairment and disability, 425–426
for occupational sawdust allergy, 378, 378*t*
for painters, 428, 429*t*
paraben mix, 22
penicillin, 170–171
in perlèche, 679–683
petrolatum as vehicle for, 115–116
photopatch testing, 407–408
with plants, 387
with plants, 385–386
age of plants and, 386
positive reactions, 386
timing and site of, 386–387
with platinum salts, 650
for poison ivy sensitivity, 354–355
for polyester resins, 510, 510*t*
with polyethylene glycol, 235
polyrethane compound, 512
positive reactions
to fragrances, 344, 345*t*
general instructions for, 723
persistence of, 15
principles of dealing with patients with more than one, 18–21
to rubber chemicals, 542, 542*t*
to rubber mixes, 542, 543*t*
with potassium dichromate, 622–623
practical aspects of, 9–26
preemployment, 421–422
preoperative, 323
pressure effects, 16
principles of, 10, 10*t*
for printers, 430, 430*t*
for protein substance reactions in atopic individuals, 103
purpuric reactions, 74
pustular reactions, 16, 79
in atopic individuals, 103
to nickel, 643
relevance of, 12–13
with rubber, 545, 545*t*
for rubber condom sensitivity, 62

with rubber mixes, 545–547
with rubber pieces, 547
safety of, 13–16
screening, 12, 19*t*–21*t*, 23
screening kit, 22–23
sensitization by, 15
for shoe dermatitis, 306, 306*t*, 314
with soaps and detergents, 273
for stomatitis, 679–683, 683*t*
for stump dermatitis, 328
suppliers of adhesive tapes, 24–25
suppliers of devices, 24
suppliers of materials, 24–25
with synthetic resins, 490
in systemic contact dermatitis, 90–91
for TDDS allergy, 338, 338*t*
with tear gases, 483
for textile clothing, 303, 303*t*
in textile industry, 427–428, 428*t*
for textile resin allergy, 288, 288*t*
with thimerosal (merthiolate), 151
toiletries, 245–253
for veterinarians, 457–458, 458*t*
with vinyl resins and additives, 491, 491*t*
for zirconium hypersensitivity, 82
Patches
band-aid, 337
transdermal drug delivery system, 338
Patchouli, oil of, 788
Patient instructions. *See* Instructions
PBA-1. *See* Isothiouronium
PCMC. *See* Parachlorometacresol
PCMX. *See* Parachlorometaxylenol
PCNB. *See* Pentachloronitrobenzene
PE. *See* Phenoxyethanol
Pear oil. *See* Amyl acetate
Pearl essence, 788
Pectin, 562*t*
Pediamycin. *See* Erythromycin
Pedicellariae, 696
PEG. *See* Polyethylene glycol
Pencil colors, 788
Penethamate hydroiodide, 458
d-Penicillamine, 788
Penicillin, 454, 788
allergic contact urticaria from, 588, 589
allergic stomatitis from, 674
in animal feed, 460*t*
cattle breeder exposure, 434, 435*t*
positive patch test reactions, 170–171
reactions to, 169–170
systemic contact dermatitis due to, 91
Penile tourniquet syndrome, 63
Penis
irritant dermatitis of, 487
traumatic sclerosing lymphangitis of, 46
traumatic ulcers of, 46
Pens, 132
Pentachloronitrobenzene, 431*t*, 788
Pentachlorophenol, 763, 789
in fungicides, 431*t*
in herbicides, 433*t*
3-Pentadecylcatechol, 789
Pentaerythritol, 430*t*
Pentaerythritol triacrylate, 430*t*, 789
Pentane, 475
Pentanedial. *See* Glutaraldehyde

1,5-Pentanedial. *See* Glutaraldehyde
Pentoxol, 789
Pentyl acetate. *See* Amyl acetate
Pepeo tree (*Mauria puberula*), 353, 353*t*
Peppermint oil, 522, 681*t*, 789
Peptizers, rubber, 538–539, 539*t*
Perchloroethylene, 476, 789
Perchloromethane. *See* Carbon tetrachloride
Performing artists, 445
Perfumes, 789
concentrations in products, 343, 344*t*
in feminine hygiene sprays, 487, 487*t*
formulations of, 349, 349*t*
natural resins in, 562, 564*t*
in paper, 438
photoallergic contact dermatitis from, 404
reactions to, 208
in soaps and detergents, 274
use tests, 349
Periactin. *See* Heptadine hydrochloride
Perianal dermatitis, 35
Periaxillary dermatitis, 59
Perinaval dermatitis, 645
Perioral dermatitis, 36
Perioral leukoderma, 576
Periorbital depigmentation, raccoon-like, 551
Peristomal allergic and irritant contact dermatitis, 323–324
Perlèche
causes of, 677–678, 678
from foods, 677
irritant, 678–679
management of, 679
from nickel, 678
patch testing in, 679–683
from rubber, 678
Permanent-press finish clothing dermatitis
from formaldehyde resins, 286
management of, 289
Permanent-wave solutions, 789
nickel dermatitis from, in hairdressers, 646
reactions and patch testing, 247
Permanganate, potassium, 789
Peroxide catalysts, 789
Peroxides
curing agents for rubber, 535, 538*t*
in printing, 430*t*
Persistent light reactivity, 76, 405–408
classic generalized immunologic, 407
classification of, 405–407
localized specific immunologic, 405–407
localized specific nonimmunologic, 405
to topical agents, 405, 406*t*
Persistent papular gold eruptions, noneczematous, 631–632
Persistent photosensitivity, 407
Personal cleanliness products, 251
Perspiration, 718
Pessaries, rubber
dermatitis from, 550
vulvitis due to, 61
Pesticides
carbamate, 555–556
classification of, 430, 431*t*
occupational dermatitis from, 430–435
occupational exposure to, 430, 430*t*
thiuram, 555–556